D1244434

INTRODUCTION TO Anatomy & Physiology

SECOND EDITION

By

Susan J. Hall, PhD
Deputy Dean of the College of Health Sciences
University of Delaware
Newark, Delaware

Michelle A. Provost-Craig, PhD
Associate Professor of Kinesiology and Applied Physiology
University of Delaware
Newark, Delaware

William C. Rose, PhD
Associate Professor of Kinesiology and Applied Physiology
University of Delaware
Newark, Delaware

Publisher
The Goodheart-Willcox Company, Inc.
Tinley Park, IL
www.g-w.com

Manufactured in the United States of America.

ISBN 978-1-64564-020-2

1 2 3 4 5 6 7 8 9 – 21 – 24 23 22 21 20 19

Cover Image: Jane_Mori/Shutterstock.com

To the Student

Have you ever wondered why you have curly, wavy, or straight hair? Or why you may have to wear corrective lenses for your eyes? Or why diseases strike some people but not others?

Do you ever wonder if certain dietary and health habits might reduce your risk of having diabetes and coronary heart disease in later life? Did you know that it is important to maximize your bone density during early and teenage years to prevent developing osteoporosis? How can your lifestyle choices at 16 affect your body at 60? These are all considerations related to your anatomical and physiological makeup, and they are topics discussed in this book.

People have been curious about the human body for centuries. It is quite natural, since it is the body you live in. The more you know and understand about your body, the more you can choose to make intelligent choices about your own health and longevity. Knowledge about these topics can also help you to help your family and friends understand their health issues.

This textbook is your road map to understanding all of the fascinating intricacies of the human body. In addition to providing the basics of how your body works, the text highlights some of the latest research on topics of interest. Since many of you are probably curious about career opportunities in human health and healthcare, this text also features descriptions of job opportunities encompassing the ladder of jobs in healthcare.

This textbook will answer questions you have had and raise other questions you may never have thought about. As you discover the answers on these pages, we believe you will agree with us that the human body is the most interesting topic in all of science. We wish you happy reading!

Susan J. Hall

Michelle A. Provost-Craig

William C. Rose

Contributors

Goodheart-Willcox Publisher would like to thank the following classroom instructors who provided assessment questions and lab activities.

Andrea Beverly, RN, EdD
Supervisor of Career, Technical, and Adult Education
Tampa, Florida

Karen Cluck, MT(ASCP), RDA
Health Science Instructor
Holland Medical High School
Abilene, Texas

Debbie Curtin
NAF Academy Coordinator
Cal-HOSA Past Board Chair
Covina, California

Reviewers

Goodheart-Willcox Publisher would like to thank the following instructors who reviewed selected chapters and provided valuable input into the development of this textbook program.

Jean Almeida
Anatomy & Physiology Teacher
Bayside High School
Palm Bay, Florida

Holly Brooks
Science Teacher
Muscle Shoals High School
Muscle Shoals, Alabama

Heather Carter
Science Teacher
Cullman High School
Cullman, Alabama

Karen Cluck, MT(ASCP), RDA
Health Science Instructor
Holland Medical High School
Abilene, Texas

Melissa Culpepper, RN
Healthcare Science Instructor
Colquitt County High School
Norman Park, Georgia

Diane Farthing
Anatomy & Physiology Teacher
Amador Valley High School
Pleasanton, California

Jennifer Filippi
Science Teacher/Science Department Chair
Folsom High School
Folsom, California

Jamie Ford
Teacher
Carnegie Vanguard High School
Houston, Texas

Robin Gosdin, RN
Health Science Instructor, CNA Program Director
Cleburne High School
Cleburne, Texas

Dr. Joseph Scott Hardin
Teacher
Franklin High School
Franklin, Tennessee

Mary Pat Hepp
Science Instructor
Justin-Siena High School
Napa, California

Rachel Kannady
Teacher
White Station High School
Memphis, Tennessee

Julian A. Kiler
Adjunct Faculty/HSMT Instructor
Los Angeles Pierce College and Career Technical Education/Riverside County Office of Education
Los Angeles, California

Ashley Kozora
Teacher
Abilene Cooper High School
Abilene, Texas

Zakary LaFaver
Science Teacher
Spring Hill High School
Chapin, South Carolina

Joelle Lilavois
Science Teacher
James Clemens High School
Madison City, Alabama

Magdalena Molledo
Science Teacher
West Shore Jr./Sr. High School
Melbourne, Florida

Renee Ogle
Teacher
Amador Valley High School
Pleasanton, California

Lindsey Olson
Science Educator
Torrey Pines High School
San Diego, California

Kelsey Parent
Life Science Teacher
and Science Department Chair
South Forsyth High School
Cumming, Georgia

Dr. June Walker
Teacher
Orange Park High School
Orange Park, Florida

Leila Warren
Science Teacher
Chamblee Charter High School
Chamblee, Georgia

Mary Werner, RN, BSN
Health Science Teacher
Lake Norman High School
Mooresville, North Carolina

Heather Wesson, RN, BSN
Nurse Aide Instructor
Lincoln County School of Technology
Lincolnton, North Carolina

Joanne Wilson
Science Teacher
Lake Norman Charter High School
Huntersville, North Carolina

Precision Exams Certification

Goodheart-Willcox is pleased to partner with Precision Exams by correlating *Introduction to Anatomy and Physiology* to their Medical Anatomy & Physiology. Precision Exams Standards and Career Skill Exams were created in concert with industry and subject matter experts to match real-world job skills and marketplace demands. Students that pass the exam and performance portion of the exam can earn a Career Skills Certification™. Precision Exams provides:

- Access to over 150 Career Skills Exams™ with pre- and post-exams for all 16 Career Clusters.
- Instant reporting suite access to measure student academic growth.
- Easy-to-use, 100% online exam delivery system.

To see how *Introduction to Anatomy and Physiology* correlates to the Precision Exams Standards, please visit https://www.g-w.com/introduction-anatomy-physiology-2021 and click on the Correlations tab. For more information on Precision Exams, including a complete listing of their 150+ Career Skills Exams and Certificates, please visit https://www.precisionexams.com.

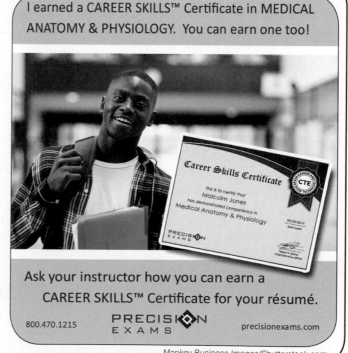

Monkey Business Images/Shutterstock.com

About the Authors

Susan J. Hall is a professor in the Department of Kinesiology and Applied Physiology at the University of Delaware. She is a fellow of the American College of Sports Medicine and the AAHPERD Research Consortium, and she has served as President of the Biomechanics Academy of AAHPERD, President of the AAHPERD Research Consortium, and Vice President of the American College of Sports Medicine. She is also the author of several successful textbooks and has served on several journal editorial boards. After graduating from Duke University, she began her career as a high school biology teacher. She earned a master's degree from Texas Woman's University and a PhD from Washington State University. She has been teaching at the college level for more than 30 years and served for many years as a department chair and deputy dean.

Michelle A. Provost-Craig is an Associate Professor in the Department of Kinesiology and Applied Physiology at the University of Delaware, where she has taught graduate and undergraduate courses in physiology, clinical exercise physiology, and electrocardiogram interpretation for more than 20 years. She is the recipient of the University's most prestigious awards for Excellence in Teaching and Excellence in Advising and Mentoring. She also received a University grant from the Center for Teaching Effectiveness to develop innovative approaches to teaching anatomy and physiology to college students. At the University of Delaware, she served as the graduate coordinator of the Masters in Exercise Science program and was the founder of their Cardiopulmonary Rehabilitation Program. Dr. Provost-Craig has served in numerous leadership roles for the United States Figure Skating Association (USFSA) and has performed physiological assessments of national and international elite ice figure skaters. She was the Vice President of the Mid-Atlantic Chapter of the Regional American College of Sports Medicine (ACSM) and has participated in several ACSM committees. Dr. Provost-Craig earned a master's degree from the University of Delaware and a PhD in Exercise Physiology from the University of Maryland.

William C. Rose is an Associate Professor in the Department of Kinesiology and Applied Physiology at the University of Delaware, where he has taught anatomy and physiology for 20 years. He is a member of the American Physiological Society and the American College of Sports Medicine. He is the author of textbook chapters and research articles in the fields of cardiovascular physiology and biomechanics. He has served as a grant proposal reviewer for the National Science Foundation and as a manuscript reviewer for scientific journals such as *Circulation* and the *American Journal of Physiology*. After graduating from Harvard University with a degree in physics, Rose earned a PhD in biomedical engineering from Johns Hopkins University. He completed a postdoctoral fellowship in cardiology at Johns Hopkins Hospital, and he worked in research and development for the DuPont Company before joining the University of Delaware.

Brief Contents

Contents

CLINICAL CASE STUDY

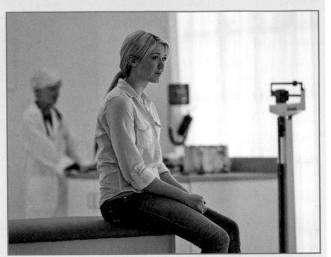

Erickson Stock/Shutterstock.com

What Research Tells Us

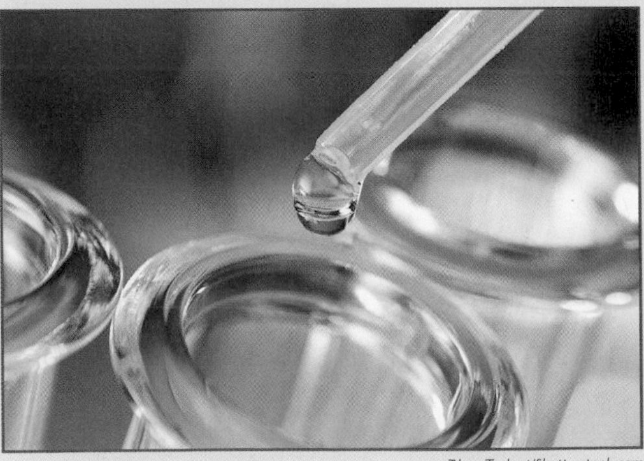

Alex_Trakset/Shutterstock.com

CAREER CORNER

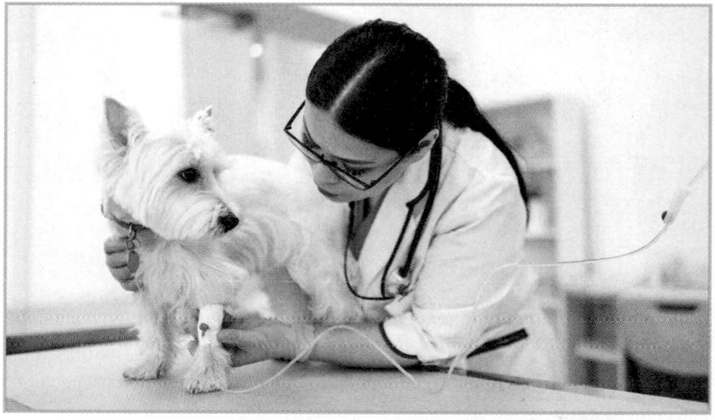

YAKOBCHUK VIACHESLAV/Shutterstock.com

LIFE SPAN DEVELOPMENT

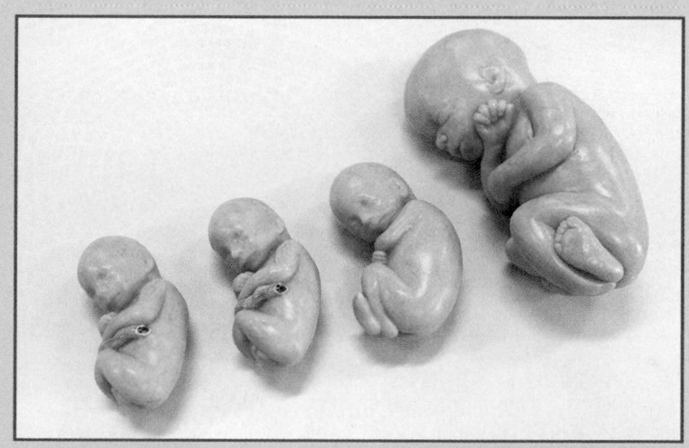

Rattiya Thongdumhyu/Shutterstock.com

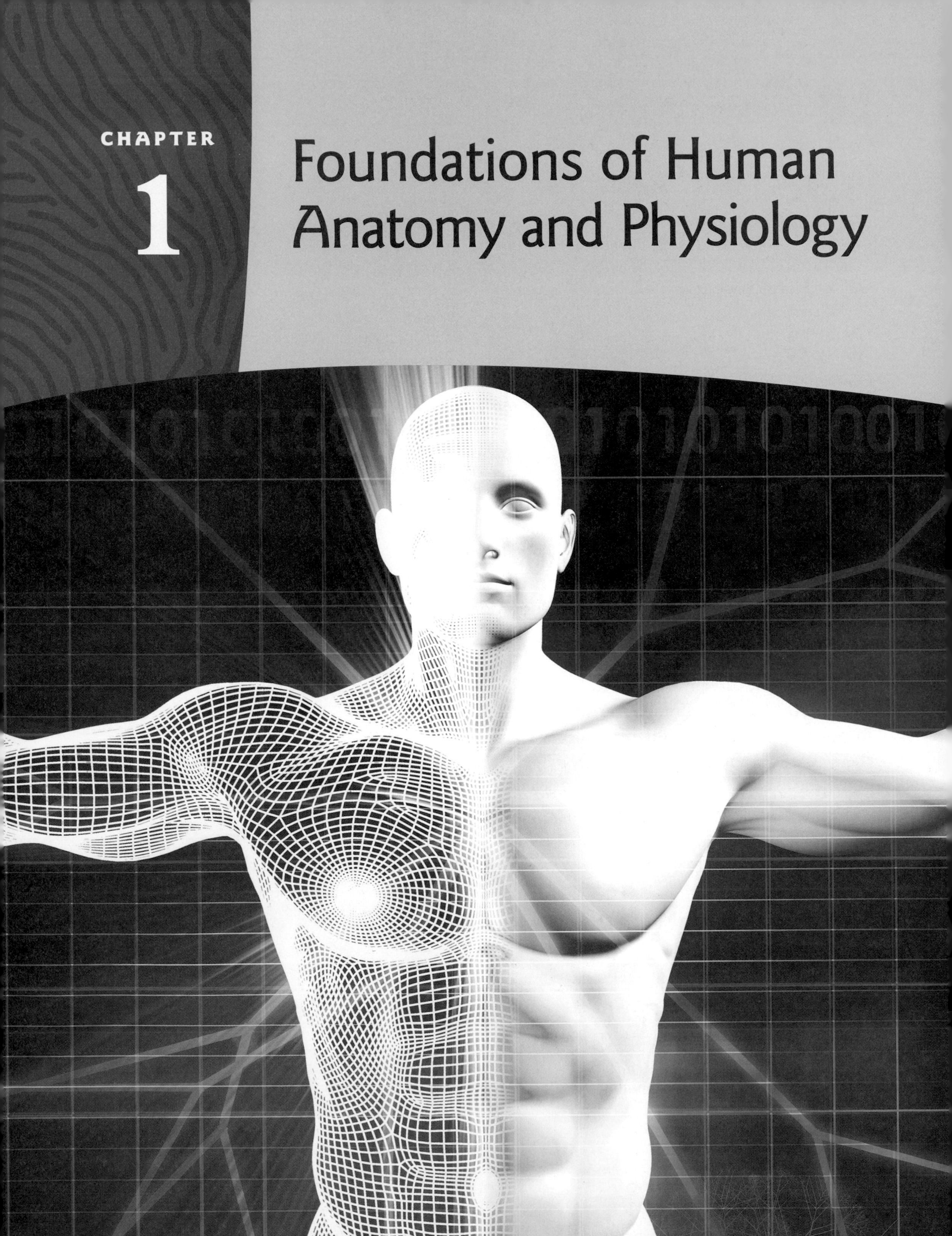

CHAPTER 1 Foundations of Human Anatomy and Physiology

How is the human body like a machine?

Humans have been interested in their own anatomy and physiology for many centuries. The human body has astonishing capabilities, including the abilities to think, speak, move, see, hear, smell, taste, remember, and feel emotions.

Human anatomy and physiology involve the study of the form and function of the human body. These ancient fields of scientific study continue today and are now sufficiently advanced such that scientists have developed precise terminology to describe them. The related, modern-day fields of biology and biomechanics also contribute new knowledge about how the human body works and interacts with the environment.

In this chapter you will learn some of the important, specialized terminology essential for the study of anatomy and physiology. You will also learn the basic, underlying physiological processes essential for life and the different ways in which forces in the environment can cause injury. In addition, the chapter looks back at the historical roots of anatomy and physiology and explores exciting advances in the fields of science and healthcare.

Chapter 1 Outline

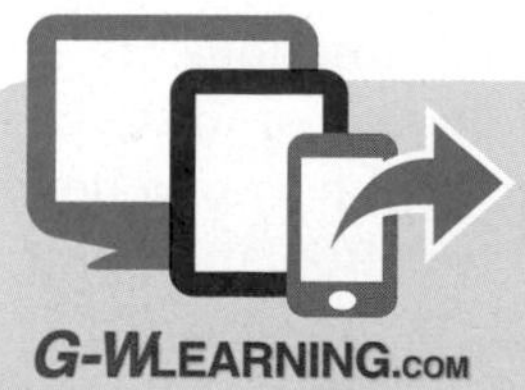

Click on the activity icon or visit www.g-wlearning.com/healthsciences/0202 to access online vocabulary activities using key terms from the chapter.

◂ kentoh/Shutterstock.com

LESSON 1.1 The Language of Anatomy and Physiology

Before You Read

Try to answer the following questions before you read this lesson.

- What body position is considered the "starting point" for describing body positions?
- Why is the metric system used in all fields of science and medicine?

Lesson Objectives

- Define *anatomy* and *physiology* and explain the relationship between them.
- Identify the anatomical position, the planes and cavities of the body, and the terms used to describe body movements.
- Discuss the choice of the metric system as the international system of measurement for all fields of science.

Key Terms

abdominal cavity	oral cavity
abdominopelvic cavity	orbital cavities
anatomical position	pelvic cavity
anatomy	physiology
anterior (ventral) body cavity	posterior (dorsal) body cavity
conversion factor	quadrant
cranial cavity	sagittal plane
frontal plane	spinal cavity
metric system	thoracic cavity
middle ear cavities	transverse plane
nasal cavity	

This lesson introduces the study of anatomy and physiology and explains how and why the two are related. Like all fields of science, anatomy and physiology rely on a specialized set of terminology for accurate descriptions of body structures and functions. This chapter introduces and explains some of the basic terminology that will be used throughout the book.

Introducing Anatomy and Physiology

When a living organism is being described, the term *anatomy* is often closely followed by the term *physiology*. Although these concepts are closely related in some respects, they are very different in others.

Anatomy is the study of the form or structure of all living things, including plants and animals. This textbook focuses on the human body, so you will be studying human anatomy. The word *anatomy* is taken from Greek words meaning "to cut apart." The study of the body structures you can see with your eyes, without looking through a microscope, is called *gross anatomy*. The study of tiny parts seen only with a microscope is termed *microscopic anatomy*.

Physiology (fiz-ee-AHL-oh-jee) is the study of how living things function or work. This textbook discusses human physiology. Looking through the table of contents, you will see that most of the chapters are about one of the systems of the human body. The muscular system, skeletal system, and cardiovascular system are familiar examples.

Branches of human physiology exist for all the different systems of the human body, including muscle physiology, skeletal physiology, and cardiovascular physiology. Each system contributes a unique capability to the human body, and some systems also exert influences on other systems.

Why is the study of anatomy and physiology combined in one book? The answer is that there is a close relationship between how the human body is structured and how it functions.

In a healthy human body, all functions are normal and painless. When a disease or injury causes a breakdown of even a small part of a body structure, however, abnormal function and pain can result. An obvious example is the case of a broken femur (upper leg bone), preventing normal leg movement. Another example is a tumor in the digestive tract that prevents normal passage of materials through the digestive system and rapidly becomes painful and life-threatening. Similarly, inhalation of harmful substances such as tobacco smoke can cause structural changes in the lungs that make breathing difficult. Understanding the normal anatomy and physiology of the human body is the first step in understanding the structures and processes that become dysfunctional with injury and disease.

Check Your Understanding

1. What is the relationship between anatomy and physiology?
2. Why are anatomy and physiology generally studied together?
3. What is gross anatomy?

Describing the Human Body

Throughout this text you will read detailed descriptions of the structures that make up the human body. Learning some specialized terminology first will help you picture and understand these structures and their functions.

The body position that serves as a "starting point" for describing positions and directions for the human body is called the **anatomical position** (**Figure 1.1**). The anatomical position is a normal standing position, with the feet slightly apart, the face and shoulders facing forward, and the palms of the hands facing forward.

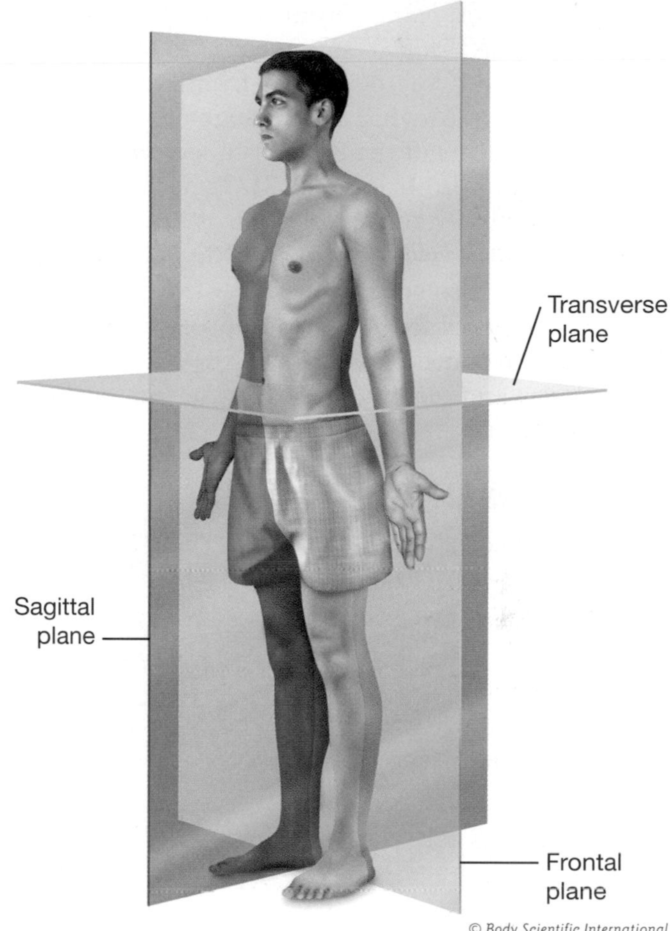

Figure 1.1 The anatomical reference position. Three imaginary planes divide the body into halves in three directions. *Along which plane is your body moving during rotational movements?*

Planes

To describe the human body and its movements, imagine that there are three planes, or flat surfaces, passing through the center of the body (**Figure 1.1**). These planes help describe motions of the body and the body segments when they are aligned with the direction of one of these planes.

MEMORY TIP

Understanding the word parts that make up anatomical terms can help you figure out the meanings of words you have not encountered before. Throughout this textbook, Memory Tips will help you understand the word roots, prefixes, and suffixes that make up medical words. You may also refer to the appendices, medical dictionaries, and the internet for more information about word parts.

- The **sagittal plane** divides the body into right and left portions—so forward and backward motions of the body or body parts are said to be *sagittal plane movements*. The three sagittal plane movements are flexion, extension, and hyperextension (**Figure 1.2A**). From the anatomical position, forward movements of the head, trunk, arm segments, and thighs are called *flexion*. Backward motion of the lower leg is also termed *flexion*. When a body segment is in a position of flexion, returning it to the anatomical position is called *extension*. Continued extension of a body segment beyond the anatomical position is called *hyperextension*.
- The **frontal plane** divides the body into front and back portions, and sideways movements are considered to be *frontal plane movements* (**Figure 1.2B**). There are two major movements

in the frontal plane. From the anatomical position, *abduction* (*abduct* means "to take away") moves a body segment away from the midline of the body. Moving a body segment closer to the midline of the body is called *adduction* (*add* means "to bring back"). In performing a jumping jack the arms and legs are simultaneously abducted and then adducted.

- There are also special terms for frontal plane movements of the foot. Rotation of the sole of the foot toward the midline of the body is called *inversion* and turning the sole of the foot outward is termed *eversion*. Running shoes with motion control are designed to keep the foot from over-rotating upon impact with the ground.
- Finally, the **transverse plane** divides the body into top and bottom portions, and rotational movements are called *transverse plane movements* (**Figure 1.2C**). From the anatomical position, rotational movements of the head, neck, and trunk are called *left rotation* and *right rotation*. Rotation of an arm or leg toward the midline of the body is termed *internal rotation*, and rotation in the opposite direction is *external rotation*.

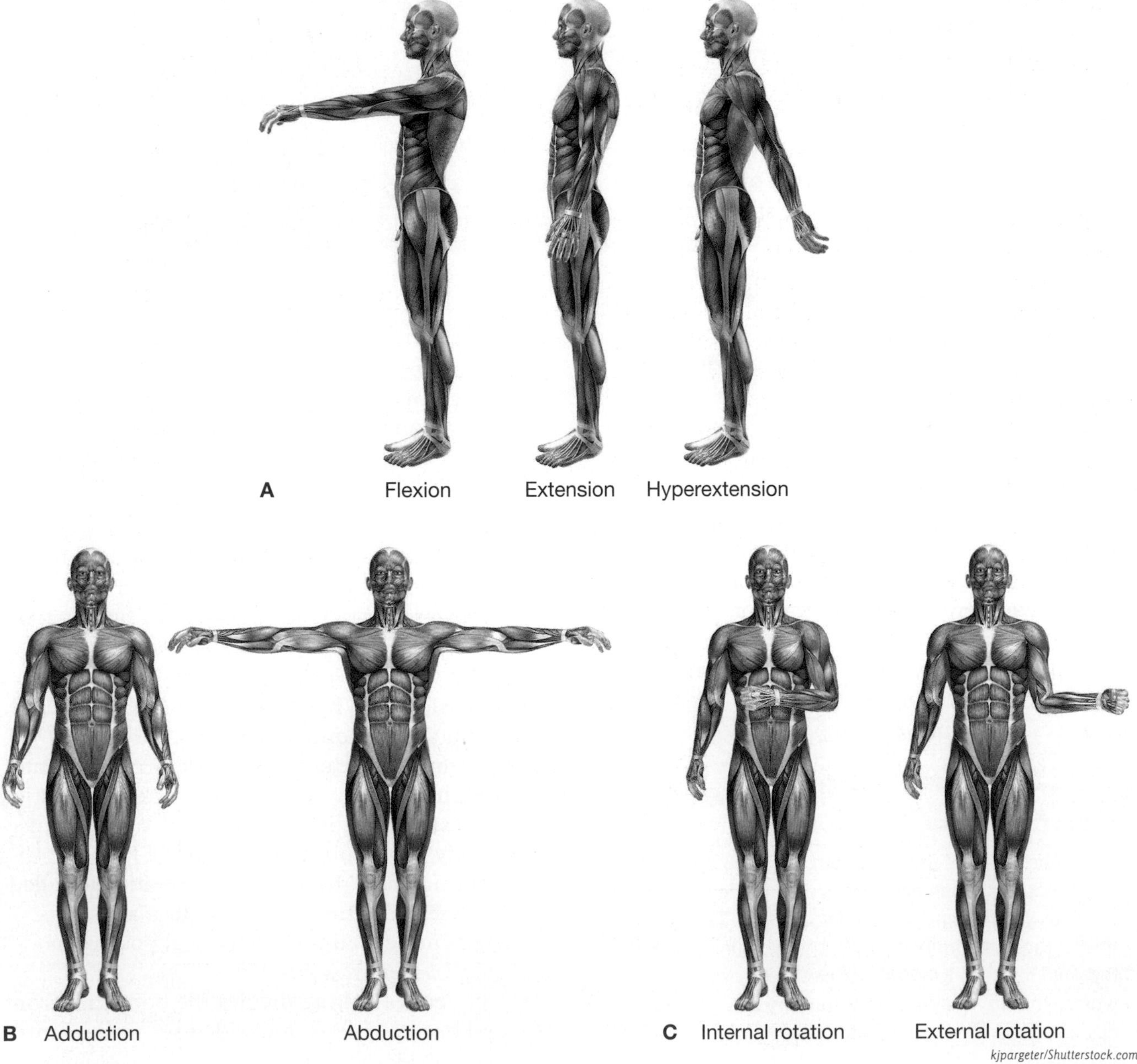

Figure 1.2 Movement terminology. A—Sagittal plane movements. B—Frontal plane movements. C—Transverse plane movements.

Of course, many body movements follow a curved path and are not lined up with any one of these three planes. Movements that do not occur in direction with one of the three planes are described as *nonplanar*.

Directions

Directional terms describe relationships between different body parts. The most commonly used directional terms are paired, describing opposite relationships. For example, the term *superior* means "above" or "over," whereas *inferior* means "below" or "under." It is therefore correct to state that the chin is superior to the knees. Alternatively, you could say that the knees are inferior to the chin (**Figure 1.3**). Other commonly used paired terms are *medial* (toward the middle) and *lateral* (away from the middle), and *anterior* (toward the front) and *posterior* (toward the back).

Quadrants and Regions

Regions of the body are often named after the anatomical structures they contain. For example, the thigh can also be referred to as the *femoral region* because it contains the femur, the major bone of the thigh. The nose is known as the nasal region because it contains the nasal cavity, and so on. Other common regional terms are listed in **Figure 1.4**.

The human abdomen is commonly divided into either four or nine regions. When four divisions are used, they are called **quadrants**. The standard terminology for these quadrants is right upper quadrant (RUQ), left upper quadrant (LUQ), right lower quadrant (RLQ), and left lower quadrant

Common Directional Terms for Anatomy

Term	Description
superior (cranial)	closer to the head
inferior (caudal)	away from the head
anterior (ventral)	toward the front of the body
posterior (dorsal)	toward the back of the body
medial	toward the midline of the body
lateral	away from the midline of the body
proximal	closer to the trunk
distal	away from the trunk
superficial	toward the surface of the body
deep	away from the surface of the body

Figure 1.3 *Goodheart-Willcox Publisher*

Regions of the Body

Anterior Term	Pronunciation	Location
abdominal	ab-DAHM-i-nal	anterior trunk, inferior to the ribs
acromial	uh-KROH-mee-al	superior, distal shoulder
antebrachial	an-tih-BRAY-kee-al	forearm
antecubital	an-tih-KYOO-bi-tal	anterior to the elbow
axillary	AK-sil-ar-ee	armpit
brachial	BRAY-kee-al	upper arm
buccal	BUCK-al	cheek of the face
carpal	KAR-pal	wrist
cervical	SER-vi-kal	neck
coxal	KAHK-sal	hip
crural	KRU-ral	lower leg
deltoid	DEL-toyd	upper arm
digital	DIJ-i-tal	fingers and toes
femoral	FEHM-oh-ral	thigh
fibular	FIB-yoo-lar	lateral, lower leg
frontal	FRUHN-tal	forehead
inguinal	ING-gwi-nal	groin
mental	MEHN-tal	chin
nasal	NAY-zal	nose
oral	OHR-al	mouth
orbital	OHR-bi-tal	eye
patellar	pa-TEHL-ar	anterior knee
pelvic	PEHL-vik	anterior pelvis
pubic	PYOO-bik	genital area
sternal	STER-nal	breastbone
tarsal	TAR-sal	ankle
thoracic	thoh-RAS-ik	chest
umbilical	uhm-BIL-i-kal	navel
Posterior Term	**Pronunciation**	**Location**
calcaneal	kal-KAY-nee-al	heel of the foot
cephalic	seh-FAL-ik	head
femoral	FEHM-oh-ral	thigh
gluteal	GLOO-tee-al	buttock
lumbar	LUHM-bar	lower back
occipital	ahk-SIP-i-tal	posterior head
olecranal	oh-LEK-ra-nal	posterior elbow
popliteal	pahp-LIH-tee-al	posterior knee

(continued)

Figure 1.4 *Goodheart-Willcox Publisher*

Regions of the Body (continued)

Posterior Term	Pronunciation	Location
plantar	PLAN-tar	sole of the foot
sacral	SAY-kral	between the hips
scapular	SKAP-yoo-lar	shoulder blades
sural	SOO-ral	calf of the leg
vertebral	VER-teh-bral	spinal column

Figure 1.4 *(continued)* *Goodheart-Willcox Publisher*

(LLQ). **Figure 1.5A** shows the quadrants. Notice that "left" and "right" refer to the patient's body as it appears in the anatomical position, not left and right from another person's viewpoint. **Figure 1.5B** shows the nine regions that are used when an abdominal area needs to be defined more specifically.

Cavities

Inside the human body are a number of open chambers called *cavities* (**Figure 1.6**). These cavities hold the internal organs of the body.

The **posterior (dorsal) body cavity**, located toward the posterior side of the body, includes two named cavities—the cranial cavity and the spinal cavity. The **cranial cavity** holds the brain, and the **spinal cavity** surrounds the spinal cord. The delicate brain and spinal cord are protected, respectively, by the bony skull and the bones of the vertebral column.

The **anterior (ventral) body cavity**, located toward the anterior side of the body, also includes subdivisions. A large, dome-shaped muscle called the *diaphragm* separates the **thoracic cavity** and **abdominopelvic** (ab-dahm-i-noh-PEHL-vik) **cavity**. The thoracic cavity houses the heart and lungs, among other organs. The abdominopelvic cavity includes the **abdominal cavity** and **pelvic cavity**. No structure separates these cavities. The abdominal cavity contains the stomach and other parts of the digestive tract and the liver, as well as other organs. The pelvic cavity holds the reproductive and excretory organs.

The body also includes several small cavities, including:

- **oral cavity**—located within the mouth
- **nasal cavity**—situated inside the nose
- **orbital cavities**—hold the eyes
- **middle ear cavities**—found in the skull; serve as chambers for transmitting and amplifying sound

Each of these small cavities is discussed in further detail in Chapter 7.

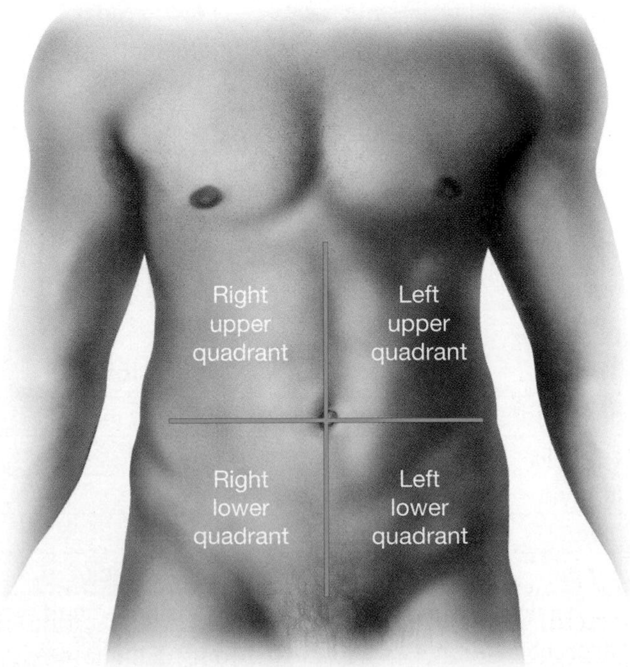

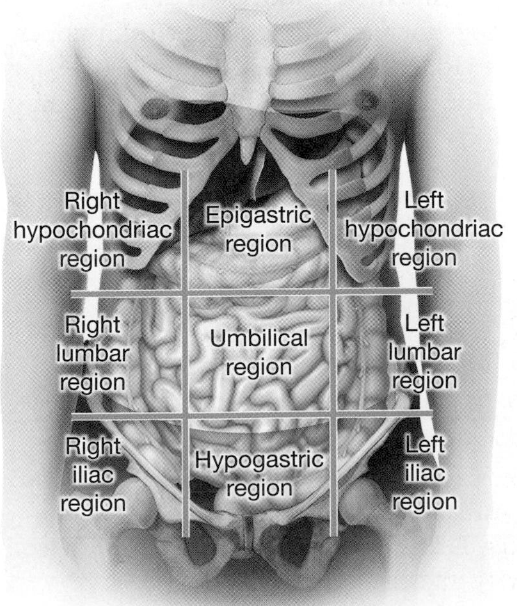

© Body Scientific International

Figure 1.5 A—Abdominal quadrants. B—Abdominal regions.

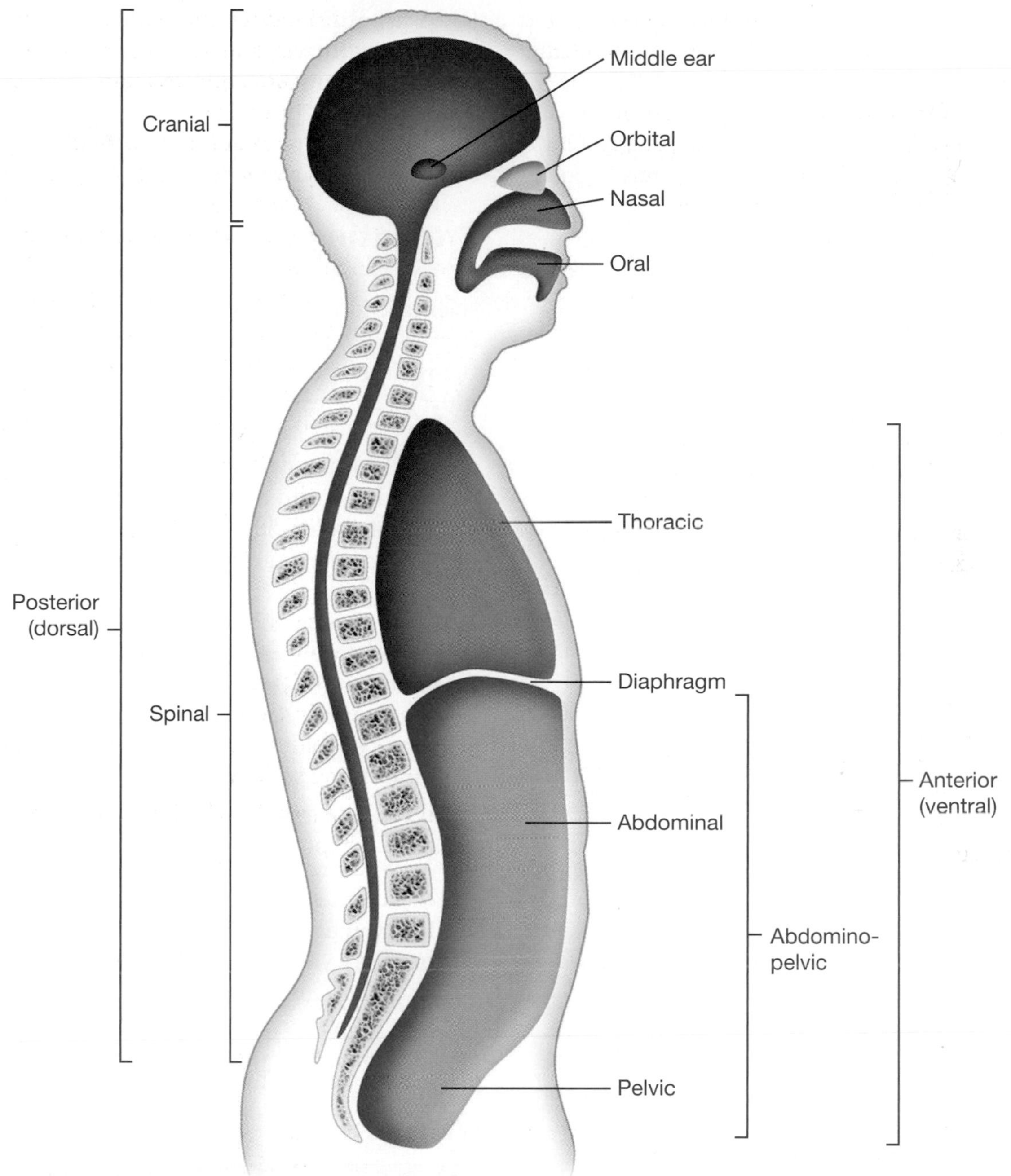

© Body Scientific International

Figure 1.6 The body cavities. *All but one of the labels in this drawing name body cavities. What is the one exception?*

Check Your Understanding

1. What three planes are commonly used to describe movements of the human body?
2. What are the two major body movements that are made in the frontal plane?
3. What larger body cavity holds both the spinal cavity and the cranial cavity?

Mathematics in Science and Medicine

Just as there are specific anatomical terms used to describe directions and regions within the human body, there is a system for numerical quantities. This system, known as the **metric system**, is used in all fields of science and medicine throughout the world, including the United States. The metric system is also used for everyday measurements by every major country in the world, except the United States.

The metric system originated as the result of a request by King Louis XVI to the French Academy of Sciences during the early 1790s. In 1875, the Treaty of the Meter was signed by 17 countries that agreed to adopt the use of the metric system.

Since that time, the metric system has become popular worldwide for several reasons:

- It involves only four base units—the meter (of length); the kilogram (of mass); the second (of time); and the degree Kelvin (of temperature).
- The base units are precisely defined, reproducible quantities that are independent of factors such as gravitational force.
- All units (except those for time) are related by factors of 10, making conversions between units easy, since you only need to move the decimal point.
- The system is used internationally.

In the United States, the system of measurement used for nonscientific purposes is called the *English system*. The English system of weights and measures arose over the course of several centuries, mainly for purposes of buying and selling goods and dividing parcels of land. Specific units came largely from royal decrees. For example, a yard was originally defined as the distance from the end of the nose of King Henry I to the thumb of his extended arm. The English system of measurement is not regular, or even logical. There are 12 inches to the foot, 3 feet to the yard, 5,280 feet to the mile, 16 ounces to the pound, and 2,000 pounds to the ton.

Converting Units of Measurement

Because in the United States people are most familiar with the English system of measurement, it is useful to understand how to convert English measurements to metric units for scientific applications. A **conversion factor** is a number that can be used to multiply the units of one measurement system into units in another measurement system. In this case, English units are being converted into metric units. The number 2.54 is the conversion factor for changing measurements in inches (in.) to centimeters (cm). For example:

$$12 \text{ in.} \times 2.54 = 30.48 \text{ cm}$$
$$1.5 \text{ in.} \times 2.54 = 3.81 \text{ cm}$$

Another commonly used conversion factor is 0.45, which converts pounds (lb) into kilograms (kg). For example:

$$10 \text{ lb} \times 0.45 = 4.5 \text{ kg}$$
$$180 \text{ lb} \times 0.45 = 81.00 \text{ kg}$$

A list of English-metric conversion factors for units of length, weight, volume, area, and temperature are presented in Appendix A. Appendix B contains a review of useful basic mathematical operations. Refer to these appendices as needed to convert units throughout this textbook.

Presenting Mathematical Data

When scientists publish research studies in scientific journals, all quantitative information is expressed in metric units. To effectively explain the results of scientific inquiry, the researchers must also determine how to best present their results. One decision that must be made is whether to present information in the text of the paper or to organize it into a table or graph.

Usually, data displaying a trend are best shown in a graph. Large amounts of quantitative data are typically best presented in a table. However, small amounts of quantitative information, such as average heights and weights of study participants, are best presented in the text. **Figure 1.7** summarizes the rules for appropriately constructing tables and graphs to display quantitative information.

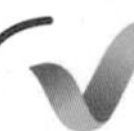

Check Your Understanding

1. How many centimeters are in 132.5 inches?
2. A patient at a medical center is weighed, and her weight is recorded as 115 lb. What is this patient's weight in kilograms?
3. In general, what is the best way to present data that display a trend?

Rules for Constructing Tables and Graphs

1. Each table or graph should "stand alone" (be fully self-explanatory without the reader having to refer to the text).
2. All units of measurement should be clearly identified in column headings for a table and on the horizontal and vertical axes for a graph.
3. The number of research participants upon which table or graph values are based should be identified either in the table/graph title or in a footnote.
4. All like table entries should read vertically and be presented to the same number of decimal places.
5. For graphs, the dependent variable is placed on the vertical axis and the independent variable on the horizontal axis.

Figure 1.7 *Goodheart-Willcox Publisher*

LESSON 1.1 Review and Assessment

Mini Glossary

Make sure that you know the meaning of each key term.

abdominal cavity space bounded by the abdominal walls, the diaphragm, and the pelvis

abdominopelvic cavity continuous internal opening that includes the abdominal and pelvic cavities

anatomical position erect standing position with arms at the sides and palms facing forward

anatomy the study of the form or structure of living things, including plants, animals, and humans

anterior (ventral) body cavity continuous internal opening that includes the thoracic and abdominopelvic cavities

conversion factor a number that can be used to multiply the units of one measurement system into units in another measurement system

cranial cavity opening inside the skull that holds the brain

frontal plane an invisible, vertical flat surface that divides the body into front and back halves

metric system international system of measurement that is used in all fields of science

middle ear cavities openings in the skull that serve as chambers for transmitting and amplifying sound

nasal cavity opening within the nose

oral cavity opening within the mouth

orbital cavities openings that hold the eyes

pelvic cavity internal opening that holds the reproductive and excretory organs

physiology the study of how living things function or work

posterior (dorsal) body cavity continuous internal opening located near the back of the body that includes the cranial and spinal cavities

quadrant four divisions of a whole; for example, the human abdomen is often divided into four quadrants for descriptive purposes

sagittal plane an invisible, vertical flat surface that divides the body into right and left halves

spinal cavity the internal opening that houses the spinal cord

thoracic cavity the internal opening that houses the heart and lungs

transverse plane an invisible, horizontal flat surface that divides the body into top and bottom halves

Know and Understand

1. What is the difference between gross anatomy and microscopic anatomy?
2. Name the three anatomical planes and the motions they are correlated with.
3. What two body cavities are named for directional terms?
4. Which small cavity is used as a passageway for air and food?
5. What are the four base units used in the metric system?
6. Why is the English system of measurement not considered practical to use as a universal system?

Analyze and Apply

7. Based on your knowledge of medical terminology, what is the meaning of the term *midsagittal plane*?
8. Compare and contrast the metric and English systems of measurement.
9. About 60% of the weight of the average human body is due to water. If Walter weighs 180 lb and Sonya weighs 150 lb, what is the difference in their water weight?
10. In the anatomical position, what is the correct anatomical term for the position of the palms of the hands?
11. Using anatomical terms, explain the position of a pain near the breastbone.

IN THE LAB

12. With a Twinkie (or similar product) positioned lengthwise (in "anatomical position") on the table in front of you, identify the following locations on the Twinkie: most superior part, anterior, posterior, lateral, most medial aspect. Next, make incisions along the sagittal plane, frontal plane, and transverse plane. How many pieces of Twinkie do you have? Which "structure" would be considered deep to the superficial surface of the Twinkie?
13. Find the most distal aspect of the hand in anatomical position. Is this structure superior or inferior to the elbow? Now, abduct your arm 180 degrees from anatomical position. Is this structure still distal? Is it now superior or inferior?
14. Measure your arm from the tip of your nose to the thumb of your extended arm using the English system. Is your measurement the same as that of King Henry I? Convert your measurement to a metric measurement.

LESSON 1.2

Basic Physiological Processes

Before You Read

Try to answer the following questions before you read this lesson.

- What are the major organ systems of the human body?
- Why is homeostasis important?

Lesson Objectives

- Explain how building blocks, beginning with atoms, combine to eventually comprise organ systems.
- Define *homeostasis* and explain how homeostatic mechanisms help maintain health.
- Explain how the body's metabolism works and what factors can influence metabolic rate.

Key Terms

atoms	metabolism
cells	molecules
control center	negative feedback
effector	organ
homeostasis	organ system
homeostatic imbalance	positive feedback
homeostatic mechanisms	receptor
metabolic rate	tissues

The human body is an elegant biological machine. This lesson provides an overview of how this machine works.

Structural and Functional Organization of the Body

The human body is organized into specialized systems that carry out precise functions. Many of these systems also influence the activities of the other systems. To appreciate these specialized systems, start by considering how they are constructed.

At the most basic level, tiny particles called **atoms** combine in different ways to form larger particles known as **molecules**. As you will learn in Chapter 2, the human body depends on many different kinds of molecules, such as water, proteins, and carbohydrates.

The smallest building blocks of all living beings are **cells**, which are composed of organized groups of various types of molecules. Groups of similar cells with a common function form **tissues**. The four basic types of tissues are *epithelial, connective, muscular*, and *neural*.

The next level of organization is the **organ**. An organ is a body part organized to perform a specific function and is composed of at least two different types of tissue. The heart, lungs, brain, and liver are all critically important organs.

An **organ system** includes two or more organs that work together. The nervous system, for example, includes the brain, spinal cord, and all the nerves located throughout the body. The cardiovascular system includes the heart and all of the blood vessels. Each of the human body's organ systems is discussed in a chapter in this book. **Figure 1.8** and **Figure 1.9** provide an overview of these organ systems.

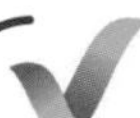

Check Your Understanding

1. List the hierarchy of structure from the smallest living thing to the largest.
2. What are the four basic types of tissue found in the human body?

Homeostasis

To maintain a healthy environment inside the body, the organ systems work together to control factors such as body temperature, blood pressure, blood sugar, water balance, and sodium levels within normal boundaries. This state of regulated physiological balance is called **homeostasis** (hoh-mee-oh-STAY-sis). The word *homeostasis* comes from Greek words that mean "staying the same."

How does homeostasis work? Organ systems work together to maintain homeostasis through processes called **homeostatic mechanisms**. The body systems that initiate most homeostatic responses are the nervous and endocrine systems.

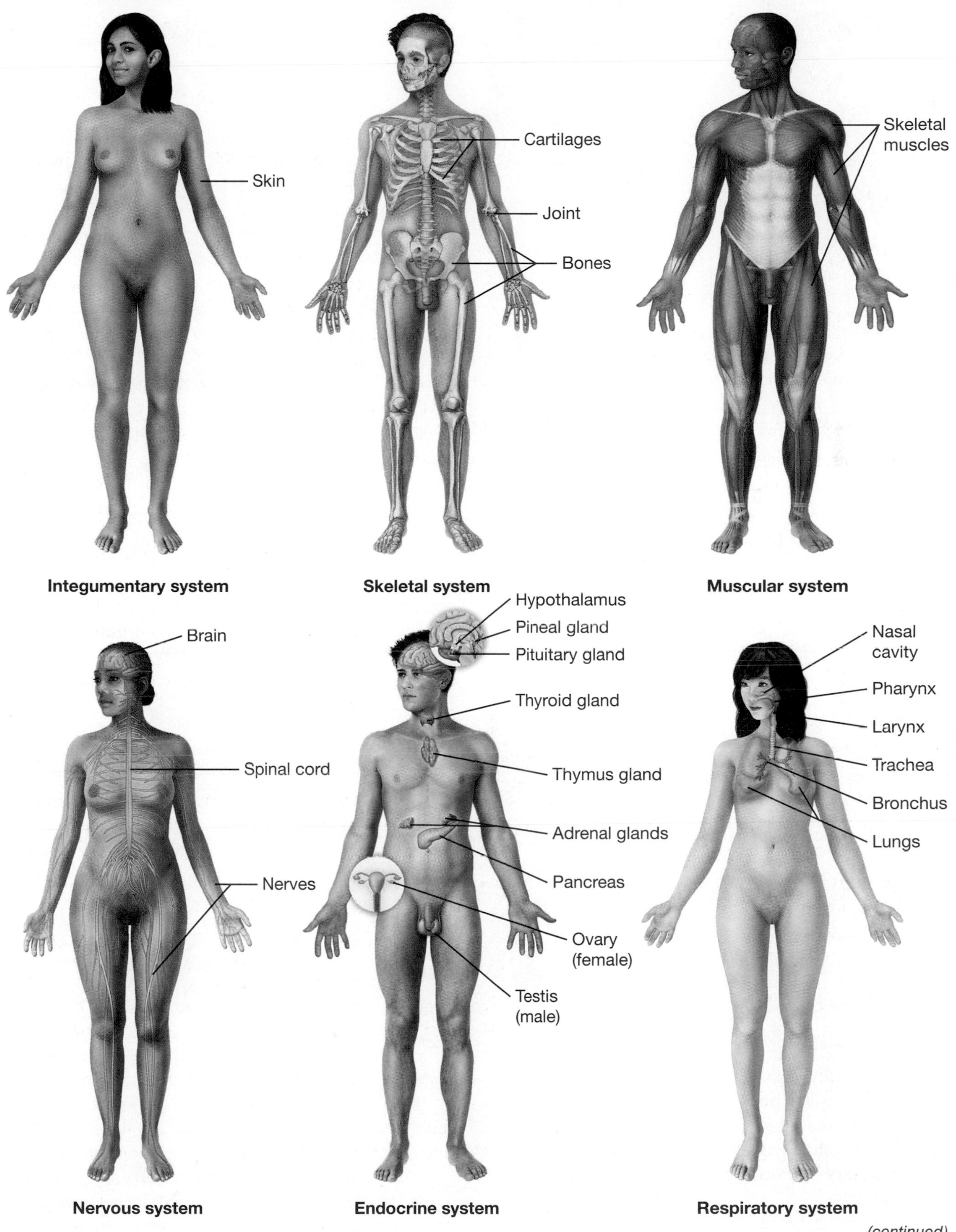

Figure 1.8 The organ systems of the body. *What are some of the ways in which organ systems work together?*

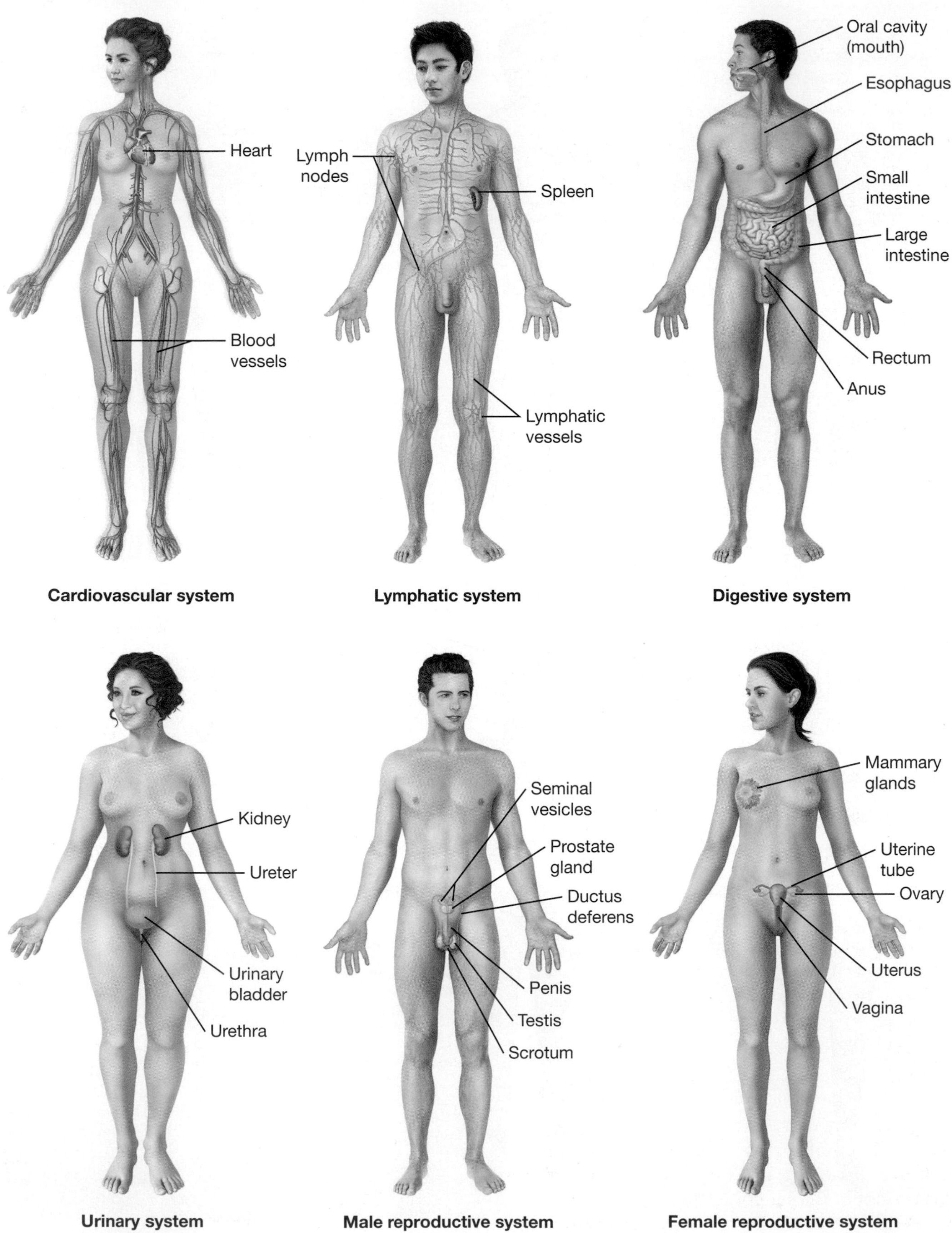

Heart
Blood vessels
Cardiovascular system
Lymph nodes
Spleen
Lymphatic vessels
Lymphatic system
Oral cavity (mouth)
Esophagus
Stomach
Small intestine
Large intestine
Rectum
Anus
Digestive system
Kidney
Ureter
Urinary bladder
Urethra
Urinary system
Seminal vesicles
Prostate gland
Ductus deferens
Penis
Testis
Scrotum
Male reproductive system
Mammary glands
Uterine tube
Ovary
Uterus
Vagina
Female reproductive system
© Body Scientific International

Figure 1.8 *(continued)*

The Human Organ Systems		
System	**Major Organs**	**Primary Functions**
Integumentary	layers of skin	protects, eliminates waste, helps regulate body temperature
Skeletal	bones, cartilage, ligaments	supports body, protects organs, produces blood cells
Muscular	cardiac, smooth, and skeletal muscle	pumps the heart, helps move materials through the digestive tract, moves the body
Nervous	brain, spinal cord, nerves, sensory receptors	receives and interprets sensory input, directs body movements, includes memory, emotions, cognition
Special sensory	eyes, ears, organs of smell and taste	enables vision, hearing, smell, and taste
Endocrine	endocrine glands	secretes hormones
Respiratory	lungs, nasal passages, pharynx, larynx, trachea	delivers oxygen and removes carbon dioxide from blood
Cardiovascular	heart, blood vessels	transports oxygen and nutrients to the body's cells and removes waste products
Lymphatic	lymphatic vessels and nodes	returns body fluids to the bloodstream
Digestive	esophagus, stomach, intestines	breaks down foods for absorption of nutrients by the body
Urinary	kidneys, bladder	removes nitrogen-containing wastes from blood
Reproductive	male: testes, scrotum, penis female: ovaries, uterus, vagina	enables production of offspring

Figure 1.9 Goodheart-Willcox Publisher

As you will learn in the chapters devoted to these systems, the systems function through a complex combination of chemical and physical processes. To maintain homeostasis, all the systems must work together and make adjustments when the body's external and internal environments change.

All homeostatic control mechanisms have three elements in common. Changes in the environment stimulate a sensory **receptor** nerve, which relays an informational message to a **control center** along an *afferent pathway*. The control center analyzes the information, and when an action is required to maintain homeostasis, the control center sends a command stimulus to an **effector** along an *efferent pathway*. The effector causes an action that helps maintain homeostasis.

Negative Feedback

Most homeostatic mechanisms work on the principle of **negative feedback**. In a negative feedback loop, conditions exceeding a set limit in one direction trigger a negative reaction in the opposite direction. This negative reaction restores the system to the set point.

A familiar example of a mechanical system that functions on negative feedback is the thermostat on a home heating or cooling system. If the temperature surrounding the thermostat rises or falls outside the set limits, the thermostat triggers either the heater or air conditioner to turn on. The heater or air conditioner stays on until the temperature is restored to the original setting.

In the human body, if the temperature begins to rise above the normal 98.6°F (37°C), the hypothalamus of the brain triggers a series of signals to different organs to cause sweating. The evaporation of sweat on the skin cools the body (**Figure 1.10**). Simultaneously, the blood vessels close to the skin dilate to help release heat.

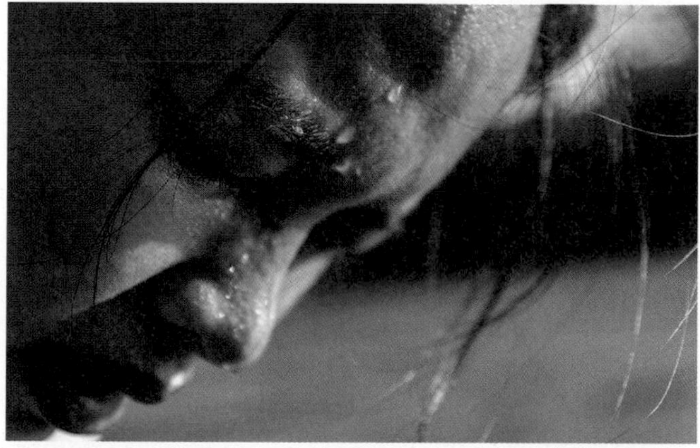

Werayuth Tes/Shutterstock.com

Figure 1.10 Sweating during vigorous exercise helps to cool the body. *Is this homeostatic mechanism an example of negative or positive feedback?*

Alternatively, when the body becomes chilled, the hypothalamus signals the muscles to cause shivering. This increased activity of the muscles produces heat, which helps warm the body. At the same time, the blood vessels close to the skin constrict to reduce heat loss through the skin.

Positive Feedback

Although most homeostatic mechanisms in the human body operate by negative feedback, positive feedback loops also occur. In contrast to negative feedback loops that reduce a disruptive influence, **positive feedback** mechanisms *increase* disruptive influences. Positive feedback is involved in accelerating blood clotting, transmitting nerve signals, and stimulating contractions during childbirth.

In the case of body temperature, however, a fever that exceeds 104°F (40°C) can provoke a dangerous positive feedback loop. Body temperature this high increases the body's metabolic rate, which increases body heat still further. This condition can be fatal if nothing is done to cool the body. Anyone experiencing symptoms of heat exhaustion, including nausea, confusion, dizziness, or fainting, should immediately be removed from the heat and cooled by the quickest means available.

Maintaining Homeostasis

Homeostasis within the human body does not mean that conditions are maintained in a perfectly constant state at all times. Rather, there are routine fluctuations of variables such as blood pressure and body temperature. These normal fluctuations occur in response to a variety of conditions in the external and internal environments. Vigorous exercise, for example, produces a normal elevation in both blood pressure and body temperature. Homeostatic mechanisms work to keep these fluctuations within a normal, healthy range.

Homeostatic Imbalances

A **homeostatic imbalance** occurs when the organ systems have a diminished ability to keep the body's internal environment within normal ranges. For example, the aging process is accompanied by many homeostatic imbalances. These imbalances can lead to changes such as the wrinkling and thinning of skin, reduced muscle mass and strength, and decreased mental acuity.

Homeostatic imbalances can also be caused by disease. For example, when you digest food, the concentration of glucose, a simple sugar in your blood, increases. The pancreas, an organ in the endocrine system, produces a hormone called *insulin* that normally controls blood sugar, keeping it within a healthy range. The insulin does this by moving glucose in the blood into the body's cells, where it can be used for fuel or stored for future use.

People with certain types of diabetes, however, are unable to move glucose out of the bloodstream because their pancreas does not make enough insulin or their cells do not respond normally to insulin. The resulting homeostatic imbalance, if not corrected, can lead to serious problems. Among those problems are kidney failure, lower limb amputations, and blindness. You will learn more about diabetes in Chapter 8.

Check Your Understanding

1. Explain the difference between positive and negative feedback in maintaining homeostasis. Give an example of each.
2. What is homeostatic imbalance? Include at least one example in your explanation.
3. Is the body always in a homeostatic state? Explain.
4. What are possible consequences of the body's failure to maintain homeostasis?

Metabolism

Metabolism is a term used to describe the multitude of chemical reactions constantly going on within the body's cells. *Metabolism* typically refers to two general types of activity: *anabolism* and *catabolism*.

Anabolism and Catabolism

Anabolism is the process through which complex molecules such as proteins are constructed from simpler ones. Catabolism is just the opposite, with complex molecules such as carbohydrates being broken down into simpler molecules.

Through catabolic processes, the complex molecules in the food and drink people consume supply the body with energy in the form of *adenosine triphosphate (ATP)*. ATP, which you will learn more about in Chapter 2, powers activities within the cells. Even while sleeping, the body needs

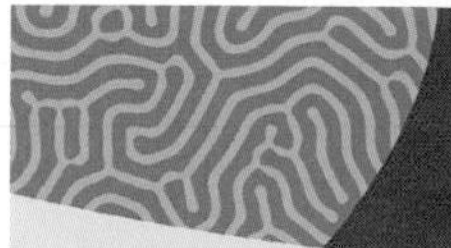

What Research Tells Us

...about Homeostatic Mechanisms during Distance Running

The number one danger associated with marathons, triathlons, and other long-distance running events is overheating. Overheating is a condition in which the body's homeostatic mechanisms for temperature control are overwhelmed. Overheating begins with heat cramps, which can progress to heat exhaustion, eventually leading to heat stroke and death. How does overheating happen, and what steps can runners take to avoid it?

Researchers have recognized that long-distance running poses a severe challenge to the body's homeostatic processes. One reason for this is that some runners do not drink sufficient fluids during long-distance events. Inadequate water intake reduces the body's ability to sweat—a process that has a cooling effect on the body. An inability to sweat leads to hyperthermia, or dangerously high body temperature. Hyperthermia encompasses both elevated core temperature and elevated skin temperature.

Inadequate water intake can also cause dehydration, which reduces total body blood volume. This limits blood supply to the working muscles, skin, and brain. As a result, the muscles fatigue, the skin is less able to release heat, and the person's judgment may be impaired. Research has shown that dehydration exceeding 3% of the total volume of body water causes increased strain on the cardiovascular system and a marked decline in aerobic performance. This makes it more difficult to sustain exercise at the same pace and increases the perception of effort. Hyperthermia may also directly affect the central nervous system, contributing to total body fatigue.

Overheating under any circumstances can lead to heat exhaustion. The symptoms of heat exhaustion can include profuse sweating, weakness, nausea, vomiting, headache, lightheadedness, and muscle cramps. Individuals experiencing any of these symptoms due to overheating should immediately be placed in a cool environment and adequately hydrated. If nausea or vomiting prevents the affected individual from drinking enough water, intravenous fluids may be required.

In cases in which the body's homeostatic mechanisms for temperature correction fail, heat exhaustion can progress to heat stroke. Body temperature of 41°C (106°F) and the absence of sweating are signs that the normal homeostatic processes have been overwhelmed. Individuals under these conditions become confused and lethargic and may have a seizure. These symptoms represent a life-threatening emergency, and immediate medical attention is needed.

Ironically, a related danger during long-distance running can be drinking too much water. Runners in the Boston, Chicago, and Big Sur marathons have died from consuming too much water during the race. The problem is that an excessive amount of water dilutes the blood. This causes the sodium concentration in the blood to fall too low, causing swelling of the brain, which can be fatal.

Under normal conditions, the body expels extra water in the form of urine. However, research has shown that during a long-distance endurance event, there is an inflammatory response that can alter hormone levels, reducing the body's ability to produce urine.

Running experts suggest weighing yourself before and after a long training run. If you've gained weight, you've consumed too much water, but if you've lost weight, you need to drink more. The recommended amount of liquid to consume is 3 to 6 ounces for every 20 minutes of vigorous exercise. You must take into account, however, that your sweating rate and the environment may necessitate drinking more or less.

Taking It Further

1. What challenges does long-distance running present to your homeostatic mechanisms?
2. Why is it so important to maintain homeostasis?

energy for activities such as breathing, circulating blood, adjusting hormone levels, and growing and repairing cells.

Metabolic Rate

A person's **metabolic rate** is the speed with which the body consumes energy, which is also the rate of ATP production. Approximately 60%–75% of the calories that an average person burns is accounted for by the basal metabolic rate, the energy needed for maintaining basic life functions. About another 10% of the calories burned is used in digesting and processing the food and drink that people consume. (For this reason, diets that are overly restrictive tend to be counterproductive for losing weight—you do not burn as many calories because there is not as much to digest.)

The remainder of the calories burned depends on the amount of physical activity a person engages in. Because muscle requires more energy for maintenance than other tissues, even at rest, muscular individuals burn more calories and are said to have "higher metabolic rates" than others.

Check Your Understanding

1. Which two processes make up metabolism? Define them.
2. What percentage of a person's total calorie consumption is burned performing basic life functions?
3. What powers all activities in a cell?

LESSON 1.2 Review and Assessment

Mini Glossary

Make sure that you know the meaning of each key term.

atoms tiny particles of matter

cells the smallest living building blocks of all organisms

control center system that receives and analyzes information from sensory receptors, then sends a command stimulus to an effector to maintain homeostasis

effector unit that receives a command stimulus from the control center and causes an action to help maintain homeostasis

homeostasis a state of regulated physiological balance

homeostatic imbalance a state in which there is a diminished ability for the organ systems to keep the body's internal environment within normal ranges

homeostatic mechanisms the processes that maintain homeostasis

metabolic rate the speed at which the body consumes energy

metabolism all chemical reactions that occur within an organism to maintain life

molecules combinations of two or more atoms

negative feedback mechanism that reverses a condition that has exceeded the normal homeostatic range to restore homeostasis

organ body part organized to perform a specific function

organ system two or more organs working together to perform specific functions

positive feedback mechanism that further increases a condition that has exceeded the normal homeostatic range

receptor transmitter that senses environmental changes

tissues organized groups of similar cells

Know and Understand

1. Which two factors define whether or not something is an organ?
2. Which two principles form the basics of homeostatic mechanisms?
3. What happens to homeostasis as a person ages?
4. Why might people who are in good shape physically have higher metabolic rates than those who are not?

Analyze and Apply

5. How might the transmission of nerve signals be an example of a positive feedback system?
6. Compare and contrast the signs and symptoms of dehydration with hyponatremia, a condition in which the amount of water in cells exceeds the amount of sodium.
7. Using a hot stove as an example, describe how afferent and efferent nerves protect us from being burned.
8. An average adult male should consume about 2,500 calories daily. One pound is equal to 3,500 calories. Noah is a 36-year-old male who is currently consuming 2,500 calories per day, but he wants to lose 6 lb in 2 weeks. How many calories must Noah restrict from his diet each day to achieve this goal? Is this a healthy way to diet? Explain your answer.
9. During a marathon, a runner fails to hydrate on the first leg of the 5K race, and she begins to experience nausea and dizziness. What explanation do you have for the runner's symptoms, and how should they be treated?

IN THE LAB

10. Create a collage that helps you remember the function of each organ system. Show your collage to your classmates. Can they determine the systems and functions in your collage?
11. Over the course of one day, keep track of the number of times you notice your body using negative feedback. Record the stimulus and the body's response (for example, you walk into a cold room and get goose bumps).
12. Run up and down some stairs 10 times. What do you notice about how your body responds to this activity? Is this an example of positive or negative feedback? Explain.

LESSON 1.3

How Forces Affect the Body

Before You Read

Try to answer the following questions before you read this lesson.

- Why does the size of the area over which a force is distributed make a difference?
- Why does the direction of stress distribution within a tissue make a difference?

Lesson Objectives

- Explain the kinetic concepts of force, mass, weight, pressure, and torque and explain their effects on the human body.
- Identify the external forces that can act on the body and explain their effects.

Key Terms

acceleration	net force
bending	plastic
combined loading	pressure
compression	shear
deformation	stress
elastic	tension
force	torque
kinetics	torsion
mass	weight

The human body both generates and resists forces during daily activities. The internal forces produced by muscles enable body movements, whereas forces such as air resistance and friction may slow the body down. Sports may involve applying forces to balls, bats, racquets, or clubs. Sports may also involve absorbing forces from impacts with balls, the ground or floor, and opponents (in contact sports). This lesson introduces key concepts to help you understand the effects that these types of activities have on the human body.

Basic Kinetic Concepts

Kinetics is the analysis of the actions of forces. The field of human biomechanics is based on analysis of the forces, both internal and external, acting on the human body. A basic knowledge of kinetic concepts is useful for understanding both the movements of the body and the effects of forces that can potentially cause injury.

Force

Force can be thought of as a push or pull acting on a structure. Force is described in terms of its size or magnitude, direction, or the point at which it acts on a structure. Body weight, friction, and air or water resistance are all forces that commonly act on the human body.

Because a force rarely acts alone, it is important to recognize that what you see and feel are the effects of **net force**. Net force is the single force resulting from the summation of all forces acting on a structure at a given time (**Figure 1.11**). Thus, net force represents the size and direction of all acting forces.

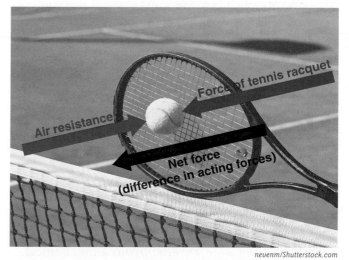

nevenm/Shutterstock.com

Figure 1.11 The net force acting on a tennis ball at the moment of impact with a racquet is the difference between the force exerted by the racquet and the opposing force of air resistance. *How does the net force determine the direction of the resulting motion?*

The size and direction of net force determines the overall effect of the forces acting on a structure. When the forces acting on a structure are balanced, or cancel each other out, there is no net force and no resulting motion. For example, if two people apply equal and opposite forces on the two sides of a swinging door simultaneously, the door won't move. However, if a net force is present, the door will move in the direction of the net force.

Mass and Weight

Mass is the quantity of matter an object contains. The action of a force causes an object's mass to accelerate, either increasing or decreasing in speed. **Weight** is a force equal to the gravitational acceleration exerted on an object's mass. As the mass of an object increases, its weight increases proportionally. If you were to travel to the moon or another planet with a different gravitational force than on Earth, your weight would be different, but your mass would remain the same.

Pressure

Pressure is defined as the amount of force distributed over a given area. You might wonder how much pressure is exerted on the floor beneath you if you shift your weight to one foot. To find out, divide your body weight by the surface area of the sole of your shoe. Thinking about this, would you prefer to have your foot stepped on by a woman wearing athletic shoes or a woman wearing stilettos (high-heel shoes)? The woman's weight would be distributed over a much smaller area in the stilettos, resulting in a much larger pressure against your unfortunate foot.

Torque

When a force causes a structure to rotate, the rotary effect of the force is called **torque**. If you pull or push a suspended bicycle wheel, the wheel begins to spin. The harder you pull or push the wheel, the faster it spins. From a mechanical perspective, you are creating torque on the bicycle wheel.

Torque can be quantified as the size of the force multiplied by the perpendicular distance from the line of force application to the center of rotation. In the case of a spinning bicycle wheel, perpendicular distance is the distance from the outside of the tire to the axis of the wheel. The greater the amount of torque acting at the center of rotation, the greater the tendency for rotation to occur.

When a muscle in the human body contracts, it applies a pulling force on a bone. A sufficiently large force causes movement of the bone, with the bone rotating at the nearby joint center. The amount of torque generated at the joint center is the size of the muscle force multiplied by the distance between the muscle attachment and the joint center. You will learn more about how to measure and calculate forces in Chapter 5, *The Muscular System*.

Check Your Understanding

1. What term describes the process of analyzing actions of forces?
2. Name and describe two forces that commonly act on the body.
3. What causes an object to rotate?

Forces and Injury to the Human Body

What factors determine whether forces acting on the human body result in injury? The effect of a given force depends not only on its size, direction, and application point but also on the duration of force application.

Directional Force Distribution within the Body

Compressive force, or **compression**, can be thought of as a squeezing force (**Figure 1.12**). An effective way to press wildflowers is to place them inside the pages of a book and to stack other books on top of that book. The weight of the books creates a compressive force on the flowers. Similarly, when you land from a jump, the weight of your body plus the force of landing set up a compressive force on the bones of your skeleton.

The opposite of compressive force is tensile force, or **tension** (**Figure 1.12**). Tension is a pulling force that creates a stretching or tightness in the object to which it is applied. When a person hangs from a pull-up bar, tension

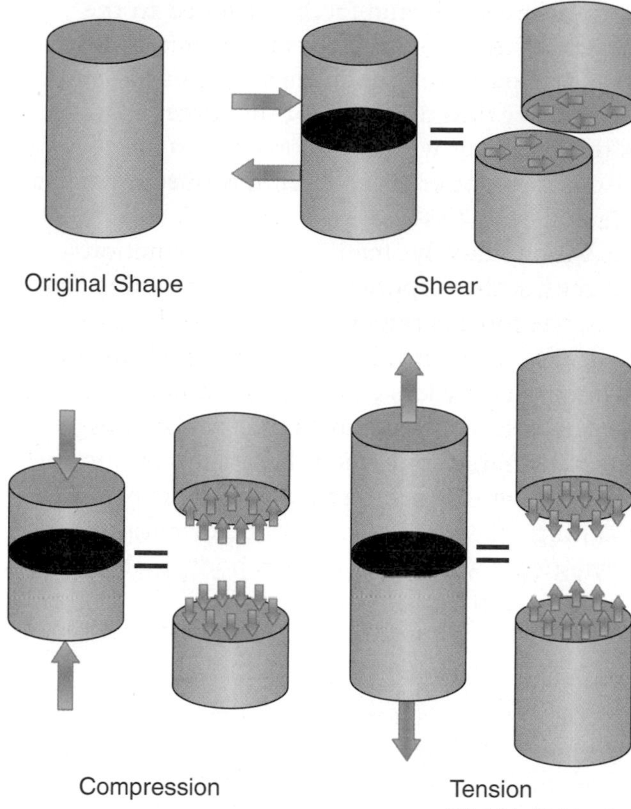

Figure 1.12 Compression, tension, and shear represent three directions of stress distribution within a body. The large arrows on the left represent the application of external force to the object. The small arrows on the right represent the resulting distribution of stress within the object. *Which directional force would be present during a shoulder dislocation injury?*

is created in the arms as they support the weight of the body. A heavier person in this position creates more tension in the arms than a lighter person. Muscles also produce tensile force that pulls on the attached bones.

A third direction of force is called **shear**. While compressive and tensile forces act along the length of a bone or other object to which they are applied, shear force acts perpendicular to the length of the object (**Figure 1.12**). Shear force tends to cause a portion of the object to slide, or shear, with respect to another portion of the object. Abrasions are caused by shear force acting on the skin. When a baseball player slides into a base, for example, the shear force created by the ground against any exposed skin can cause an abrasion.

The direction of stress distribution within a biological tissue has direct implications for injury potential. Bone, for example, is strongest in resisting compression and the weakest in resisting shear.

Mechanical Stress

Another factor that affects the outcome of forces acting on the human body is the way in which a force is distributed. While pressure represents the distribution of force outside a body, **stress** represents the resulting force distribution inside a body. Stress is quantified in the same way as pressure—the size of the force divided by the area over which the force acts. As **Figure 1.13** shows, force acting on a small surface produces greater stress than the same force acting over a larger surface.

When a blow is sustained by the human body, the likelihood of injury to body tissue is related to the magnitude and direction of the stress created by the blow. *Compressive stress*, *tensile stress*, and *shear stress* are terms that indicate the direction of the acting stress. The protective pads and helmets worn in many sports are designed to distribute forces over a large area, minimizing the stress sustained by the underlying body parts.

Combined Loads

When multiple forces act at once, more complicated force distribution patterns are set up within the body. A combination of off-center forces can create a loading pattern known as **bending** (**Figure 1.14**).

Torsion (TOR-shun) occurs when a structure is caused to twist about its length, typically when one end of the structure is fixed (**Figure 1.14**). Torsional fractures of the tibia can occur in

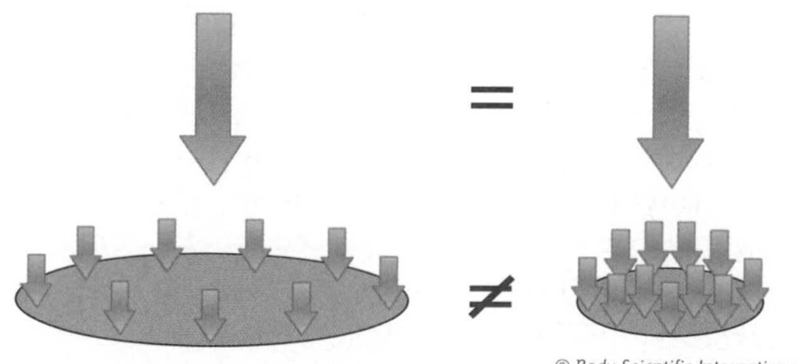

Figure 1.13 When a force of a given size is distributed over an area, the larger the area, the smaller the stress generated. *Which would generate greater amounts of stress—having your hand stepped on by the heel of a stiletto or the heel of a flip-flop sandal?*

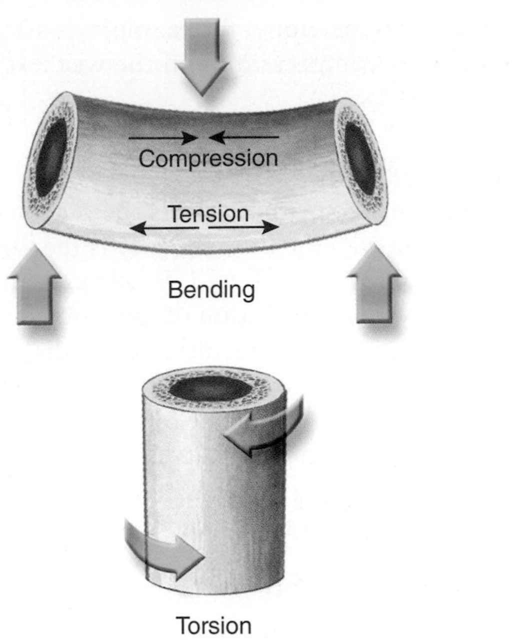

Figure 1.14 Bending and torsion are forms of combined loading.

football and skiing accidents in which the foot is held in a fixed position while the rest of the body undergoes a twist.

The simultaneous action of two or more types of forces is known as **combined loading**. Because of the variety of forces people encounter during daily activities, combined loading patterns are relatively common. Fortunately, they do not usually result in injury.

The Effects of Force Application

When a force acts on an object, there are two potential effects: acceleration and deformation. **Acceleration** is the change in velocity of the object to which the force is applied. The more massive or heavy the object, the smaller the acceleration will be.

The second effect is **deformation**, or change in shape. When a racquetball is struck with a racquet, the ball is both accelerated (put in motion in the direction of the racquet swing) and deformed (flattened on the side that is struck). The amount of deformation that occurs in response to a given force depends on the stiffness of the object acted on.

When an external force is applied to the human body, several factors influence whether an injury occurs. Among these, as discussed, are the size and direction of the force, as well as the area over which the force is distributed. Also important are the material properties of the affected body tissues.

With relatively small forces, deformation occurs but the response is **elastic**, meaning that when the force is removed, the tissue returns to its original size and shape. Stiffer materials, such as bone, display less deformation in response to a given force. Sometimes the force causes the deformation to exceed the tissue's elastic limit. When this occurs the response is **plastic**, meaning that some amount of deformation is permanent. Within the human body, a plastic response translates to injury.

Repetitive versus Acute Loads

Yet another factor that influences the likelihood of injury is whether the forces sustained by the body are repetitive or acute. When a single force causes an injury, the injury is said to be *acute*. For example, the force produced by a single check in ice hockey or the force resulting from an automobile accident may be sufficient to fracture a bone. These types of forces are acute forces.

Injury can also result from relatively small forces sustained on a repeated basis. For example, each time your foot hits the ground while you are running, a force of approximately two to three times your body weight is sustained. Although a single force of this magnitude is not likely to result in a fracture to healthy bone, many repetitions of such a force may cause a fracture in an otherwise healthy bone of the foot or lower leg. Such injuries are called *chronic injuries* or *stress injuries*.

Check Your Understanding

1. What is the difference between compression and tension?
2. Which force is acting between a baseball player and the ground when he slides into home plate?
3. What is the difference between plastic and elastic responses?

LESSON 1.3 Review and Assessment

Mini Glossary

Make sure that you know the meaning of each key term.

acceleration the change in velocity of an object to which the force is applied

bending a loading pattern created by a combination of off-center forces

combined loading the simultaneous action of two or more types of forces

compression a squeezing force that creates compression in the structure to which it is applied

deformation change in shape

elastic a response that occurs when force is removed and the structure returns to its original size and shape

force push or pull acting on a structure

kinetics the analysis of the actions of forces

mass the quantity of matter contained in an object

net force the single force resulting from the summation of all forces acting on a structure at a given time

plastic permanent deformation of an object that occurs when a force causes a deformation that exceeds the object's elastic limit

pressure force distributed over a given area

shear a force that acts along a surface and perpendicular to the length of a structure

stress force distribution inside a structure

tension a pulling force that creates tension in the structure to which it is applied

torque the rotary effect of a force

torsion a loading pattern that can cause a structure to twist about its length

weight force equal to the gravitational acceleration exerted on the mass of an object

Know and Understand

1. List at least three ways in which force can be described.
2. What is net force?
3. Compare mass and weight.
4. Which two forces act along the length of an object such as a bone?
5. What type of force causes rotation?

Analyze and Apply

6. A player gets hit by a lacrosse ball. What is the predominant type of force generated by the ball on the player?
7. Explain how a torn ligament is an example of a plastic response.
8. A linebacker and running back are running toward each other. The linebacker is hit and knocked over by the running back. Using net force as the basis for your answer, explain why the linebacker was knocked over.
9. Is a stress fracture an acute or chronic injury? Explain your answer.
10. Muscles in the human body exert force and transform it into a variety of movements. During exercise, if a person holds a weighted dumbbell and curls it toward his shoulder, what type of force is exerted on the elbow joint?

IN THE LAB

11. Grasp a tongue depressor by both ends and gently bend it as far as it will go without breaking it; hold that position for 30 seconds. What force is occurring on the top? What force is occurring on the bottom? Now release the tongue depressor. Is the tongue depressor experiencing elasticity or plasticity? Explain.
12. Using a piece of Laffy Taffy®, an Oreo® Cookie, and a soda can, develop a demonstration for the class that depicts tension, compression, and shearing forces. Determine both the causes and effects of the variances in the forces produced. Communicate your findings to the class.
13. Conduct an internet search for optical illusions. Collect at least five examples. Show each example to a partner and record your partner's first and second impressions of the image content. Then decide on a format to display your data (see Lesson 1.1). Include your own first and second impressions and those of your partner. Write an analysis of your findings. Were your perceptions the same or different?

LESSON 1.4

Understanding Science

Before You Read

Try to answer the following questions before you read this lesson.

- What is the scientific method?
- How do research hypotheses relate to theories?
- Which recent scientific advances are improving human health and the environment?

Lesson Objectives

- Describe the scientific method and explain why it is important.
- Explain what a scientific theory is and how it is derived.
- Identify the important early anatomists and physiologists and discuss the impact of their work.

Key Terms

data set
hypothesis
research question
science
scientific method
scientific theory
statistical inference
statistical significance

To many, the word *science* creates a mental image of a person wearing safety glasses and a white lab coat, swirling solutions in test tubes and scribbling down equations. But only some scientists wear lab coats and work in laboratories. Others work in a variety of settings as they study plants, animals, birds, insects, volcanos, ocean currents, weather patterns, Earth's solar system, distant galaxies, food safety, human behavior...and human anatomy and physiology.

How can the study of such markedly different topics all constitute science? The word *science* comes from the Latin word *scientia*, which means "knowledge." Thus, **science** is a systematic process that creates new knowledge and organizes that knowledge in the form of testable explanations and predictions about some aspect of the universe. Of course, *testable* is a key word in that definition. Some questions are outside the realm of science because they deal with phenomena that are not currently scientifically testable.

The Scientific Method

The **scientific method** is a systematic process that can be used to answer questions or find solutions to problems in many fields. There are seven steps involved in the scientific method.

Step 1: Identifying a Research Question

All research begins with the identification of a specific **research question** for which someone seeks an answer, or a problem that someone would like to have solved. The research question or problem is the reason for conducting the research.

Goals for Research Questions

This means, of course, that the research question or problem must be important. Investigating the research question should be worth an investment of the scientist's time and effort. And keep in mind that almost all scientists today work in teams. Because this type of team research is expensive, investing time and money in an investigation is a substantial commitment.

As mentioned earlier, a sound research question must be sufficiently specific. It should also be possible to investigate the question through the process of using various tools. These tools are used to collect, organize, analyze, and interpret data.

Data Sets

A **data set** is a group of systematically collected and recorded observations of some sort. It may consist of observations about any topic imaginable. Sometimes the data set is quantitative, consisting of numbers. In other cases, it is qualitative, consisting of recorded comments. Sometimes it is a combination of the two (**Figure 1.15**).

Step 2: Formulating One or More Hypotheses

In scientific research, a **hypothesis** is an educated guess as to what the outcome of a research study will be. It is not merely a hunch or a feeling, but an intelligent expectation based on a thorough

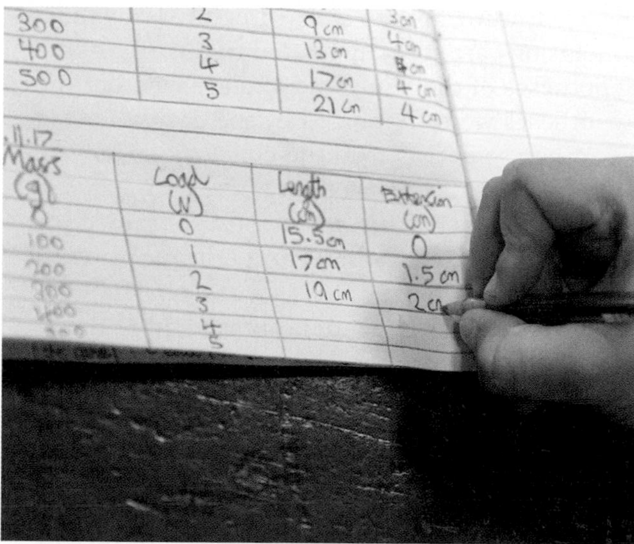

Craig Walton/Shutterstock.com

Figure 1.15 A student records data during a scientific experiment. *What are some examples of different kinds of data that they might be collecting?*

understanding of the research topic. Researchers usually base their hypotheses on related information discovered by scientists in the same field and published in research journals. Scientists are constantly communicating their findings and the information they have extracted from various sources to other scientists. They apply all of this information to refining the question they want to study.

An example of a research hypothesis might be, "We hypothesize that reaction time will be significantly longer following 24 hours of sleep deprivation." Notice that this hypothesis can be confirmed (accepted) or not confirmed (rejected) based on the results of the study. This must be the case for all legitimate scientific research hypotheses. Thus, all hypotheses are tentative, testable statements.

Step 3: Planning the Organization of the Study

The organizational aspects of a study involve determining how, where, when, and by whom the data will be collected. In studies involving human participants, organizing the study includes determining

- the criteria to be used for selection of participants;
- the number of participants needed;
- what each participant will be expected to do;
- the equipment or surveys to be used in data collection; and
- the statistical tests that will be used to analyze the data.

Step 4: Collecting the Data

Empirical research involves the recording of observations, or data. Scientists collect data in many different ways. For example, they can use various tools to take precise, accurate measurements. They can use computer-linked laboratory apparatus to record data values. They can distribute questionnaires or conduct interviews. They use tools as varied as incubators, meter sticks, calculators, and computers (**Figure 1.16**).

No matter what the data type or medium for collection, it is essential that all data be collected objectively, using the same procedures. One of the hallmarks of good research is that if other competent researchers were to repeat the study using the same procedures, they would get the same results. For this to be the case, the data collection procedures must be well controlled, and they must be accurately and fully described in the research report.

Step 5: Analyzing and Evaluating the Data with Statistical Tools

The analysis and evaluation of data using statistical tools is a vitally important step in the research process. The statistical tests used in analyzing the data determine whether the findings of a study have **statistical significance**.

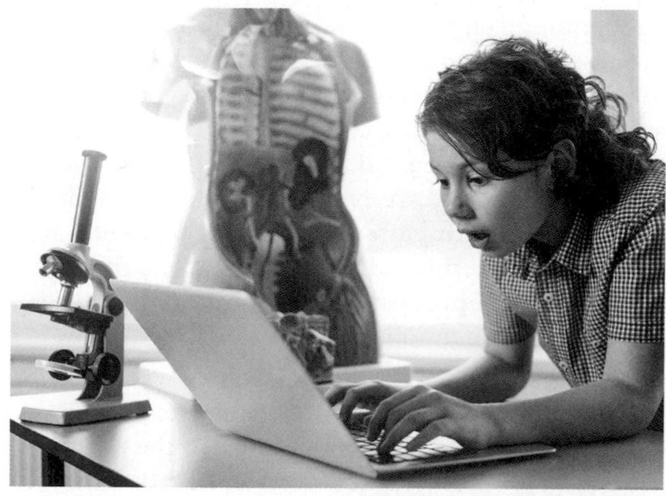

YAKOBCHUK VIACHESLAV/Shutterstock.com

Figure 1.16 Microscopes are commonly used lab equipment, and computers are often used to record observations and data.

When the results of a research study are statistically significant, it suggests that what has been observed from the data collected in the study is also true in general. When a data set is collected on human participants, statistically significant findings suggest that what is true of the participants sampled is also true of the larger population represented by the participants. This practice of translating the findings of a research study to a large population is known as **statistical inference**.

The ability to accurately predict the characteristics of a very large group based on measurements from a small subset of the large group is a powerful tool. Suppose you would like to know what percentage of US high school students take a course in human anatomy and physiology. You could survey every high school in the country and compile the information, but this would be quite tedious and time consuming. A more efficient method would be to take data from a few representative high schools and then generalize your findings to the entire United States. By looking at such data over a period of years, you could even predict trends in anatomy and physiology enrollment. How would you know that you could legitimately generalize conclusions from your findings? You could do this by making sure that your sample of representative high schools is truly "representative."

Step 6: Interpreting and Discussing the Results

Interpreting and discussing the results of a study are usually the most interesting and challenging components of the scientific research process. Unfortunately, there is no formula for discussing the results of a study. Typically, researchers discuss whether the results do or do not support the original hypotheses and compare the findings of the study to the findings of similar studies. Depending on the nature of the study, it may also be useful to discuss the reasons that the findings are important and to point out practical or clinical applications that may logically follow from the results.

Step 7: Deriving Conclusions from the Results

The conclusions of a study are composed of one or more concise statements that communicate the key findings of the study. Legitimate, valid conclusions are directly related to the original hypotheses of the study and explain whether the hypotheses were supported by the data collected.

When scientists read the conclusions of a study, they may or may not agree with or accept the conclusions. Scientists are trained to carefully analyze, evaluate, and critique scientific explanations. They do this by considering the empirical evidence (data) presented as the result of the experimental or observational testing. They also consider the logical reasoning behind the interpretation of the study results. A knowledgeable scientist also examines all sides of the scientific evidence presented in the study by considering whether the results presented are in agreement or conflict with the published results of other similar studies.

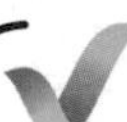

Check Your Understanding

1. What drives all research?
2. What is an educated guess, as opposed to a hunch or feeling?
3. How do you determine whether a research project is valid?
4. How are statistical significance and statistical inference related?
5. The conclusion of a research project needs to be related back to which part of the study?

Developing Scientific Theories

People often use the word *theory* when they really mean a guess or hunch. For example, "My theory is that the teacher will give the class a pop quiz tomorrow if his football team loses this evening." Sometimes the word *theory* is also used when the speaker really means an educated guess, or a hypothesis.

A **scientific theory** is an explanation of some aspect of the natural world that is based on rigorously tested, repeatedly confirmed research. When a hypothesis has been thoroughly tested through a variety of conditions and is found to accurately explain a natural or physical phenomenon, it becomes a theory.

The strength of a scientific theory is based on the extent to which it explains a diverse set of circumstances. Theories can be improved

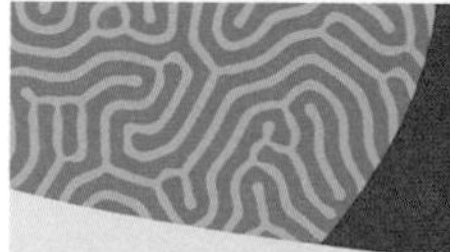

What Research Tells Us

...about Research

If you were to pursue a career in the health professions, you might become involved in research projects, even if you do not work in a setting in which research is usually done. Scientific investigations happen in laboratories, but research also happens in barns full of cows, community health clinics, pediatricians' offices, and other unconventional places. For example, a pharmaceutical company may work with community healthcare providers to monitor effectiveness and side effects of a new drug. A company that makes dentistry tools may want to get feedback from dental hygienists who have used the tools.

Safety and Resources

Whether the research takes place in the lab or the field, healthcare professionals must be aware of the many safety, resource, and ethical issues that can arise in research. They must consider how the research could impact their own health, their patients' health, and the environment.

Your Own Health. Ask yourself if the research requires you to change your work routine. If so, are the "usual" steps that you take to ensure your personal safety compromised? Is a new piece of equipment a potential tripping hazard? Are you exposed to potentially hazardous body fluids? Do you have the right personal protective equipment (safety glasses, gloves, lab coat)? If you are working with needles or blades, do you have a safe place (sharps container) to dispose of them? The questions you ask will depend on your situation, but it is important to anticipate the unexpected when thinking about safety.

Your Patient's Health. The research review process involves extensive consideration of potential risks to patients. Even a research project that has been reviewed and approved could present risks that the reviewers did not think of. Never hesitate to tell your supervisor if you have a concern about patient safety.

The Environment. Do the potential benefits of the research justify the environmental costs? Most human activities consume resources and generate waste products. Always try to find ways to minimize the resources needed and the waste created. Also look for ways to recycle resources. Be sure to follow proper procedures for disposing of waste materials.

Types of Research

Just as research occurs in many different settings, it takes many forms. For example, research projects can be descriptive, comparative, or experimental.

Descriptive research means accurately measuring "what's out there." This could mean measuring the height, weight, oral temperature, and age of each child who comes into the clinic. Or it could mean testing saliva samples from adults at the senior center for the presence of a newly discovered virus.

Comparative research involves making comparisons between one group and another. For example, you might want to compare the fitness of the students who take the bus to school to the fitness of those who walk or ride their bicycle to school.

Experimental research is more "active" than descriptive or comparative research. In experimental research, you do something and observe the results. For example, you might ask subjects to complete a math test 15 minutes after drinking coffee, and a week later have them do a similar math test without the coffee. Or you might do an experiment to see whether putting people on a program of regular exercise for two weeks improves their performance on tests of short-term memory.

In all cases, as researchers plan and implement their research, they ask questions and formulate testable hypotheses. They select the equipment and technology most appropriate for their particular investigation.

Taking It Further

1. Using the examples above, work in groups to plan and implement descriptive, comparative, and experimental investigations. Brainstorm, asking questions that lead to a testable hypothesis. Then select the appropriate equipment and technology for your investigation. Carefully record your method and your results, and present your report to the class.
2. Research OSHA requirements for safety practices. Then demonstrate your safety awareness by creating a poster that highlights what you believe are the most important safety precautions for both lab and field investigations. Include information about the use and conservation of resources and proper disposal and recycling of materials.

and refined as more research is conducted and new areas of science and new technologies are developed. Scientists use theories to advance scientific knowledge, to create new inventions, and to treat diseases.

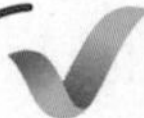

Check Your Understanding

1. What is the difference between a scientific theory and a hunch?
2. How can a hypothesis become a theory?

The Impact of Scientific Research: A Historic Journey

To appreciate the development of science, it is interesting to consider a brief historical perspective. The history of scientific research dates back to the dawn of civilization. One of the earliest topics of interest was the anatomy and physiology of humans.

Early Greek and Roman Anatomists

One of the first people to systematically study topics related to anatomy was the early Greek philosopher Aristotle (384–322 BCE). Aristotle studied and wrote about more than 540 species of animals in his anatomy book, *On the Parts of Animals*.

Another early anatomist and physiologist was the Roman physician, surgeon, and philosopher Galen (129–c.200 CE). While serving as the personal physician to several Roman emperors, Galen compiled numerous anatomical reports on his dissections of pigs and monkeys. During Galen's life, dissection of human cadavers was prohibited, so many of his assumptions about human anatomy were based on animal anatomy.

Based on his experiments, Galen was the first to advance the notion that the brain controls the muscles through signals from nerves. Galen also, however, advocated the notion that arteries carry the purest blood to the brain and lungs from the left ventricle of the heart, while veins carry blood to the other organs from the right ventricle. This notion is, of course, incorrect. For his belief to be true, some openings were needed in the walls of the ventricles, which Galen incorrectly claimed to have found.

Anatomists in the Renaissance

Spanning the mid-fourteenth to the mid-seventeenth centuries, the Renaissance was a period of significant cultural and scientific developments. Interest in science increased during this era, leading to new and exciting discoveries. Let's discuss some of the key anatomists of the Renaissance and the contributions they made to the study of anatomy and physiology.

Leonardo da Vinci

During the Renaissance period, the renowned artist Leonardo da Vinci (1452–1519) also distinguished himself as a scientist, engineer, and inventor. Among his many contributions was advancing knowledge of human anatomy and physiology.

To better understand the human body for his paintings, da Vinci was given permission to dissect human corpses at hospitals in Rome, Florence, and Milan. He was known to have dissected at least 30 corpses, including males and females of different ages. From his studies, he prepared a theoretical work on human anatomy with more than 200 drawings, including individual bones, muscles, tendons, ligaments, veins, and arteries.

The Vitruvian Man by da Vinci is one of the best known drawings in the world (**Figure 1.17**). This drawing represents what were considered to be the ideal proportions of man, and illustrates the blending of science and art that was an important trend during the Renaissance.

Andreas Vesalius

A Flemish physician, Andreas Vesalius (1514–1564) is regarded as the founder of modern human anatomy. Vesalius authored a comprehensive and influential work on human anatomy entitled *De Humani Corporis Fabrica (On the Structure of the Human Body)*.

In the course of his work, Vesalius proved that some views of human anatomy proposed by Aristotle and Galen were incorrect. Vesalius correctly observed, for example, that the human heart has four chambers, the liver has two lobes, and the blood vessels originate in the heart, not the liver. These findings were all in contrast to the assertions of Aristotle and Galen.

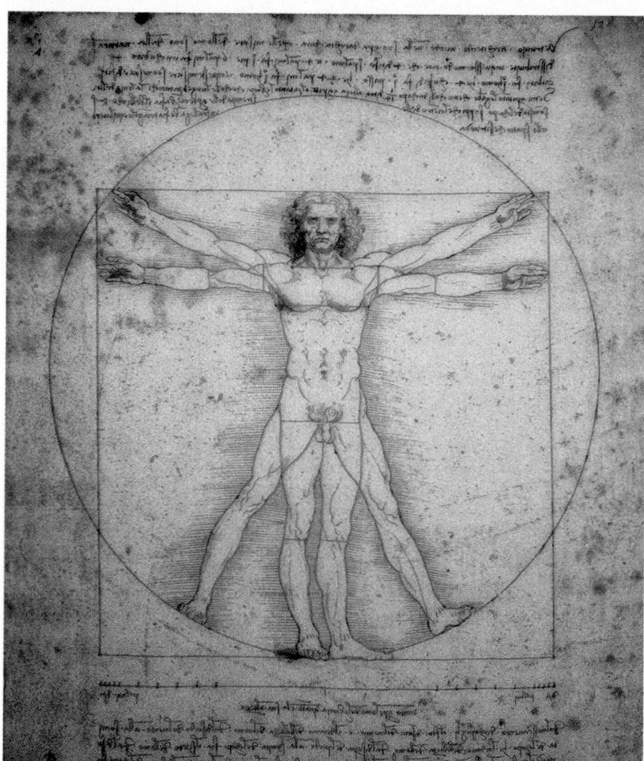

Reed/Shutterstock.com

Figure 1.17 Leonardo da Vinci's famous anatomical drawing, *The Vitruvian Man.*

Vesalius did, however, support Galen's views on bloodletting, which was the standard treatment of the day for most illnesses. The classical Greek procedure, advocated by Galen, was to drain blood from a site near the part of the body believed to be associated with an illness.

Using knowledge gained from dissecting human cadavers, Vesalius was able to construct anatomical drawings of the human body that were more detailed than other medical illustrations of the day. One of Vesalius' anatomical drawings is shown in **Figure 1.18**.

William Harvey

One of the first accurate descriptions of human physiology was provided by William Harvey (1578–1657), a physician to two kings of England. Harvey and his colleague Michael Servetus (1511–1553) were the first to understand that blood circulates continuously through the body, with the heart serving as the pump.

Robert Hooke and Antonie van Leeuwenhoek

Science took another large step forward thanks to the work of the Englishman Robert Hooke (1635–1703) and a Dutch textile merchant named Antonie van Leeuwenhoek (1632–1723). Hooke made a number of improvements to the microscopes of the day, which magnified only about 30 times (as opposed to modern microscopes, some of which can magnify up to 10 million times). Using his improved microscope, Hooke was the first to view and name cells. He published a book about microscopy called *Micrographia* in 1665.

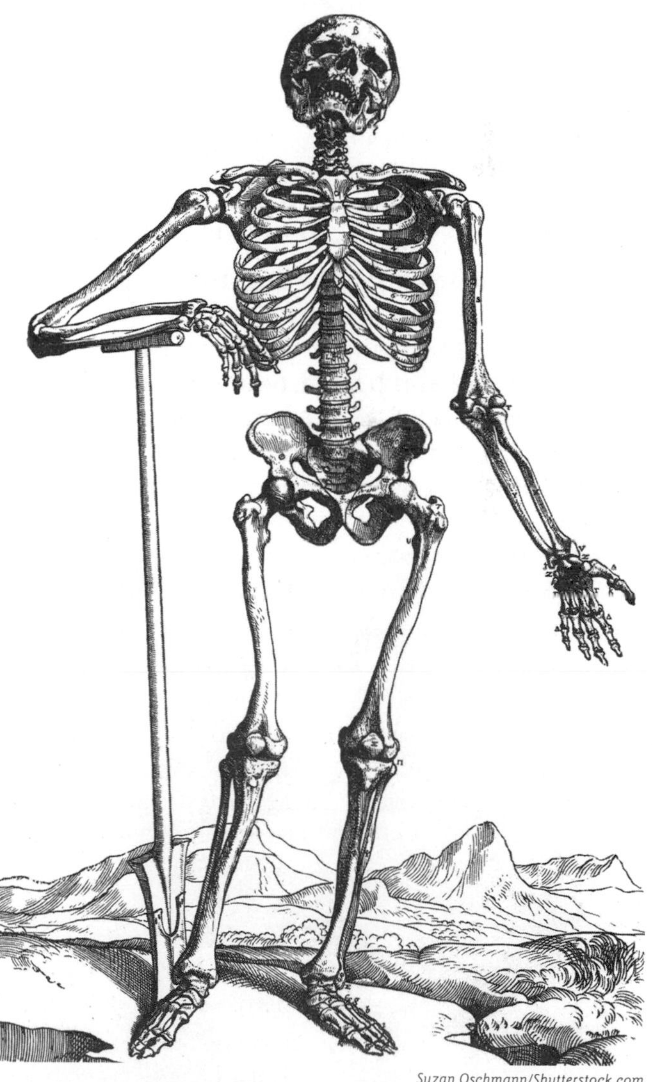

Suzan Oschmann/Shutterstock.com

Figure 1.18 An early anatomical drawing from Vesalius' 1543 text, *De Humani Corporis Fabrica.*

Leeuwenhoek further advanced the quality of the microscope, designing an instrument with a magnification of about 200 times for the purpose of close examination of the weave of fabrics. With the new power of his microscope, however, he was soon examining drops of water, blood, sperm, muscle tissue, and bacteria, and confirming that many biological materials are made of cells.

Looking Ahead

People have come a long way in advancing scientific knowledge since the discovery of cells. As is clear from reading about some of these early scientists, the prevailing views of human anatomy and physiology have changed greatly over time. This is true of all fields of science, and change continues today. As new discoveries are made and current assumptions are challenged, scientists continue to gain knowledge of many phenomena.

Today the scientific discoveries being made dramatically impact lives and improve the environment. Recent scientific breakthroughs as a result of research sponsored by the National Aeronautics and Space Administration (NASA) have contributed to the development of many new technologies and products related to human anatomy and physiology. Examples include memory foam for comfortable seating, LASIK surgery and scratch-resistant lenses to improve vision, cochlear implants and infrared ear thermometers, software for viewing partial blockages of the carotid artery, and automated insulin pumps. Research by NASA scientists has also improved the environment. They have made discoveries leading to technology for superior water filters and a compound called *emulsified zero-valent iron* that can be injected into groundwater to neutralize toxic chemicals.

Their research has also led to camera phones, wireless headsets, solar-powered appliances, improved insulation materials for residential and commercial buildings, and better fertilizer for plants. Many of these technological advances in turn enable scientists to expand their knowledge. In fact, science and technology, or "applied science," have a cyclical relationship, with each discovery enabling further advances (**Figure 1.19**).

Check Your Understanding

1. Who was the first person to assert that the brain controls muscles?
2. Why might accepted scientific principles change over time?

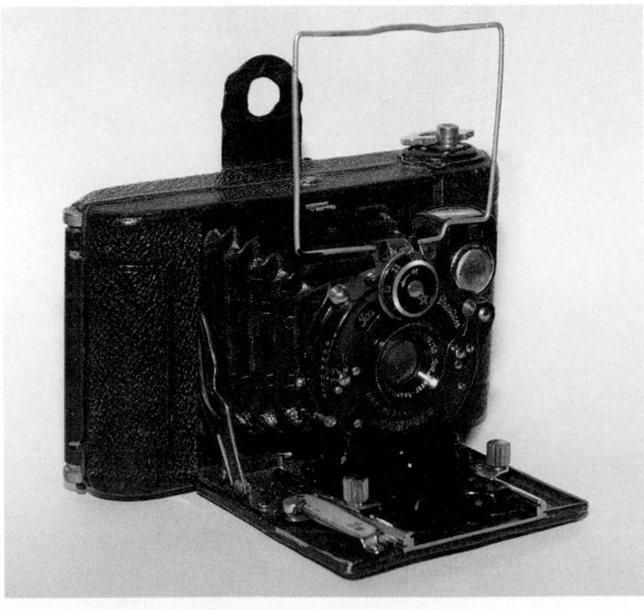

A

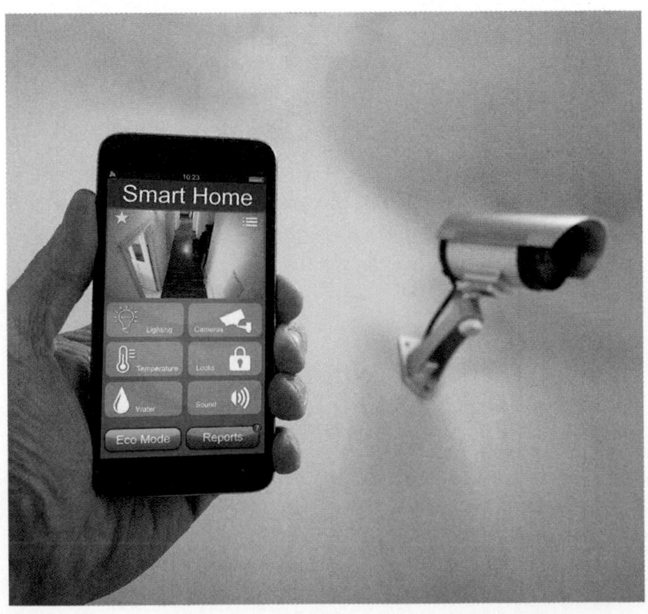

B

Albert H. Teich/Shutterstock.com, Andrey_Popov/Shutterstock.com

Figure 1.19 A—A state-of-the-art camera in the 1920s. B—Recently, applied science and technology enabled cameras in smartphones. Building on that idea, integrated systems have now been developed that allow people to control home security systems, as well as devices such as lamps and thermostats, from their phones.

LESSON 1.4 Review and Assessment

Mini Glossary

Make sure that you know the meaning of each key term.

data set systematically collected and recorded observations

hypothesis an educated guess about what the outcome of a study will be

research question a question to be answered or a problem to be solved in a research study

science a systematic process that creates new knowledge and organizes it into a form of testable explanations and predictions about an aspect of the universe

scientific method a systematic process that can be used to answer questions or find solutions to problems

scientific theory an explanation of some aspect of the natural world that is based on rigorously tested, repeatedly confirmed research

statistical inference the practice of generalizing the findings of a research study to a large population

statistical significance an interpretation of statistical data indicating that the results of a study can legitimately be generalized to the population represented in the study sample

Know and Understand

1. Elaborate on the definition of *hypothesis*. What are the characteristics of a testable research hypothesis?
2. List, in order, the steps of the scientific method.
3. On what is the strength of a scientific theory based?
4. Which famous artist was also a preeminent anatomist?
5. The improvement of which scientific tool in the 1600s produced significant advancements in the study of anatomy and physiology?

Analyze and Apply

6. Working with the definition of *science* and the information about science provided in this lesson, explain the limitations, if any, of science.
7. Give an example of a scientific theory that has been refined or improved since it was first established as a theory. Begin with a comprehensive list of the characteristics of a scientific theory. Be sure to show the difference between a hypothesis and a theory.
8. Assume that Aristotle and Galen had been able to dissect cadavers. How do you think that advancement in the study of anatomy might have been different?
9. Explain how Leonardo da Vinci's study of anatomy influenced the future of anatomical science and art.
10. How would you evaluate the impact of scientific research on a society and the environment in your city, state, or region of the country?
11. You may hear people talk about "scientific laws." Investigate the difference between a scientific law and a scientific theory. How is a law different from a theory? from a hypothesis?
12. This lesson mentions both molecules and compounds. What is the difference between a compound and a molecule?

IN THE LAB

13. Make a time line. Research scientific advancements and the scientists who brought about these changes. Create a 10-point time line from Aristotle through today showing significant milestones that have led to new discoveries and theories. Use the historical information in the text as a starting point. Describe your findings to the class.
14. Using the scientific method, investigate the following research question:

    With the advances of artificial intelligence and medical technology, what new body parts will be available for transplant in the near future, and how will they be procured?

    Perform your research using the internet and any other resources available to you. Create a research report in which you specify the steps you took to answer the question (your procedure), the data you obtained, and your interpretation or conclusions based on the data.
15. Think about the career opportunities available to people who understand human anatomy and physiology. Choose a career that interests you, and investigate the possibilities for job shadowing, community service projects, and other opportunities that may help you gain a better understanding of the career.

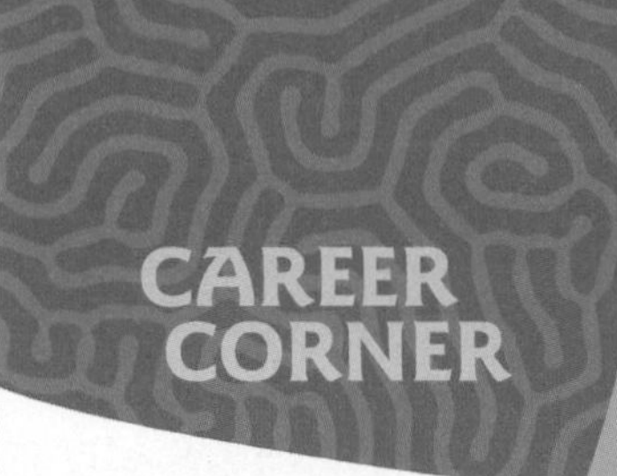

Anatomy & Physiology at Work

Studying anatomy and physiology provides a foundation of knowledge that you may use in an exciting and rewarding career in the future. The chapters in this book introduce you to a variety of related careers in the health professions. This first chapter discusses important general concepts related to identifying, qualifying for, and being hired as a professional in a health-related or healthcare profession.

Identifying the Right Job

The health professions offer an extensive array of jobs in different types of settings and with widely varying responsibilities. An important first step in determining a career you wish to pursue is recognizing your own capabilities and preferences. Are you willing to undergo many years of graduate or professional school training after getting a college bachelor's degree? Or would you prefer two years of technical training that enable you to start a job much sooner, possibly with lower pay? Would you enjoy a job that requires extensive interactions with people, or might you find it more satisfying to work in a laboratory environment? Do you prefer a job with regular hours during the day or would you be willing to work nights and weekends? There are many additional considerations, including job availability, salary range, location, setting, and level of responsibility.

Many resources provide information about health-related and healthcare professions. The *Occupational Outlook Handbook*, published by the US Department of Labor, provides current information on educational requirements and typical salaries for numerous professions. An internet search for a given occupation usually yields other information about job requirements. Of course, talking with healthcare professionals in person can provide more detailed descriptions, as well as invaluable insights into their daily tasks. Other opportunities for learning about different professions are through listening to guest speakers, participating in related community service activities, and job shadowing.

Planning for a Health-Related Career

Once you have acquired the education and skills necessary for the profession of your choice, you will need to apply and be chosen for a position. To be considered for a job you will need a compelling résumé and application letter.

Your *résumé* must be well-organized and professional in appearance. Colored paper and unusual print fonts are not appropriate. The content should focus on your professional preparation specific to the job for which you are applying. Personal information, such as your health status, religious preference, or the name of your spouse, is not appropriate. Samples and templates for résumés are available on the internet. However, be aware that the preferred format for a résumé varies with the type of position for which you are applying. It is advisable to ask knowledgeable professionals to review your résumé to ensure that it appropriately communicates your qualifications prior to submitting it for a job application.

A short, carefully written *application letter* should accompany your résumé. The letter should highlight the qualifications that make you a strong candidate for the advertised position. Refer to the qualifications listed in the position description and specifically identify the ways in which your own qualifications are a good match. It is appropriate to express enthusiasm. However, keep the content of the letter on a professional level. Do not suggest that this is a job you would like because of personal reasons such as the proximity to relatives, even though these may be relevant. It is vital that the letter be professional in appearance and content. Misspelled words or poorly constructed sentences will prevent consideration of your application.

If your résumé and application letter are viewed favorably, you may be offered an *interview*. It is important to prepare in advance for the interview. Make sure that you have thoroughly researched every aspect of the position so that you understand the expectations and opportunities associated with the job. Think about what questions you are likely to be asked and carefully plan how you will answer.

Of equal importance is preparing questions that you will ask during the interview. Asking good questions helps to demonstrate your strong interest in the job and can also give you insight into whether this position is a good fit for you. Remember that an interview is a two-way street. You are interviewing your prospective employers, just as they are interviewing you. If possible, do a practice interview with someone who is knowledgeable about the kind of job for which you are applying. This strategy can enhance the confidence that you will project during the real interview.

Finally, on the day of the interview, make sure that you appear clean and hygienic and dress professionally. Do not wear clothes that you would wear to a nightclub. Also keep in mind that it makes a good impression to model traits required for success in any workplace, including honesty, accountability, punctuality, and respect for diversity.

Characteristics of a Good Employee

Once you have landed a job, certain behaviors can help you keep it. Common traits valued in employees across many occupations include sound communication skills, including professional etiquette, and the ability to function as part of a team. Other valued employee behaviors are specific to health profession settings.

Communication and Teamwork

The importance of effective professional communication skills cannot be overemphasized. Remember that all communication is an interactive process. *Active listening* is the process of carefully listening to what someone is saying, asking clarifying questions, and then repeating what you believe has been said in your own words. This process helps to ensure that you truly understand what the other person is trying to communicate and can then respond appropriately. Taking the time to listen carefully to what your coworkers and supervisor are saying is the critical first step for effective communication.

In a professional setting, your speech and writing, including email communications, should be grammatical and appropriately formatted. You must have a command of the medical and technical terminology necessary for accurate communication specific to your professional environment. You should also develop the ability to determine the most appropriate type of communication in a given situation. Long, rambling emails are generally not the best way to deliver a complicated message. Information that is time-sensitive is usually best delivered in person or by phone. A large amount of information, especially if it involves questions or requires discussion, is usually best handled with a meeting.

When communicating in person, it is especially important to convey friendliness, respect, and empathy. *Empathy* is the ability to sense another person's emotions and to be able to imagine what the other person is thinking and feeling. Your tone of voice conveys information about what you are thinking. In-person communication also involves elements of *nonverbal communication*, such as your facial expression, degree of eye contact with the other person, and body position. These are all things to keep in mind when speaking with your coworkers and supervisor.

Many healthcare work environments involve coworkers functioning as a team. Healthcare professionals need to understand the roles and responsibilities of individual team members and the ways in which team members interact. Optimal teamwork involves interacting effectively and sensitively with all members of the healthcare team. Team members should be able to cooperate and collaborate to contribute optimally. Effective communication skills are essential for good teamwork.

Skills and Behaviors for Healthcare Professionals

There are a number of specific expectations for employees in healthcare settings:

- presenting a professional image through appearance and demeanor
- providing good customer service to patients
- employing critical thinking and problem-solving skills
- managing time effectively
- utilizing technology and specialized equipment competently
- keeping accurate records and other necessary documentation
- maintaining and upgrading skills through continuing education

Healthcare professionals must also understand the legal responsibilities, limitations, and implications of their actions within the healthcare delivery setting. They must also follow the provisions of the *Health Insurance Portability and Accountability Act (HIPAA)*. HIPAA is United States legislation to ensure data privacy and security provisions for safeguarding medical records, including strict requirements for the management and storage of all patient-related information.

CHAPTER 1 Review

>LESSON 1.1

The Language of Anatomy and Physiology

Key Points

- Anatomy and physiology are studied together because the structure of a cell, tissue, or organ is closely related to its function.
- Scientists use universal terminology for anatomical positions, planes, and directions to accurately describe body positions and movements.
- The metric system is used throughout the world in all fields of science to measure numerical quantities.

Key Terms

abdominal cavity
abdominopelvic cavity
anatomical position
anatomy
anterior (ventral) body cavity
conversion factor
cranial cavity
frontal plane
metric system
middle ear cavities
nasal cavity
oral cavity
orbital cavities
pelvic cavity
physiology
posterior (dorsal) body cavity
quadrant
sagittal plane
spinal cavity
thoracic cavity
transverse plane

>LESSON 1.2

Basic Physiological Processes

Key Points

- The human body is comprised of a hierarchy of structures, from atoms at the most basic unit to organ systems at the highest level.
- Although the human body is in a constant state of flux, it is kept in balance and healthy by maintaining homeostasis.
- Metabolism is the constant breaking down and building up of molecules to provide energy, create cells, and perform bodily functions needed to sustain life.

Key Terms

atoms
cells
control center
effector
homeostasis
homeostatic imbalance
homeostatic mechanisms
metabolic rate
metabolism
molecules
negative feedback
organ
organ system
positive feedback
receptor
tissues

>LESSON 1.3

How Forces Affect the Body

Key Points

- Kinetics is the study of forces on the human body. These forces include pressure, compression, torque, shearing, and stress.
- Forces can cause tissues to experience acceleration and deformation. Deformation may be either elastic or plastic.

Key Terms

acceleration
bending
combined loading
compression
deformation
elastic
force
kinetics
mass
net force
plastic
pressure
shear
stress
tension
torque
torsion
weight

› LESSON 1.4

Understanding Science

Key Points

- Scientific knowledge is increased via research conducted using the scientific method to ensure uniformity in experimentation.
- A scientific theory emerges from a hypothesis that has been rigorously and repeatedly researched and tested, when all evidence points to the accuracy of the theory in explaining a natural occurrence.
- Scientific knowledge has continued to grow over time with advancements in research methods and tools.

Key Terms

data set
hypothesis
research question
science
scientific method
scientific theory
statistical inference
statistical significance

Assessment

› LESSON 1.1

The Language of Anatomy and Physiology

Learning Key Terms and Concepts

1. Human _____ is the study of the functions of the human body.
   A. metabolism
   B. physiology
   C. homeostasis
   D. anatomy
2. The universal starting point for describing positions and movements of the human body is _____.
3. A cut that would divide the body into right and left parts is a _____ cut.
   A. sagittal
   B. transverse
   C. frontal
   D. coronal
4. The knee is _____ to the ankle.
   A. lateral
   B. posterior
   C. distal
   D. proximal
5. The _____ cavity contains the skull and brain.
6. The dorsal surface of a person or object is the _____ surface.
   A. superior
   B. inferior
   C. posterior
   D. anterior
7. Which of these organs is found in the thoracic cavity?
   A. heart
   B. stomach
   C. liver
   D. kidneys
8. Perform each of the following conversions. Round your answers to the nearest hundredth.
   A. Convert 4 inches to centimeters.
   B. Convert 0.7 inches to centimeters.
   C. Convert 16 pounds to kilograms.
   D. Convert 2 pounds to kilograms.

Thinking Critically

9. What plane(s) can the shoulder move in? Explain your answer.
10. Using the common directional terms for anatomy that you learned in lesson 1, provide a written description for the location of the index finger of the left hand.
11. Describe which planes the legs of a sprinter move in. Explain your answer.

› LESSON 1.2

Basic Physiological Processes

Learning Key Terms and Concepts

12. The smallest particle in the structural makeup of the human body is the _____.
13. Cells are composed of organized groups of _____.
    A. tissues
    B. organs
    C. proteins
    D. molecules
14. The next most complex level after the cellular level in organisms is the _____.
    A. organ
    B. tissue
    C. body system
    D. chemical
15. Which of the following is *not* one of the four main types of tissue in the body?
    A. muscle tissue
    B. connective tissue
    C. alveolar tissue
    D. nerve tissue
16. The lungs are part of the _____.
    A. circulatory system
    B. integumentary system
    C. endocrine system
    D. respiratory system
17. The body maintains a stable internal environment via _____.
    A. homeostasis
    B. transamination
    C. combined loading
    D. metabolism
18. _____ nerves carry a signal from the external environment to the control center.
    A. Elastic
    B. Effector
    C. Receptor
    D. Central
19. Which of the following is the *best* example of homeostasis?
    A. storage of food in the form of excess body fat
    B. sexual reproduction
    C. regulation of body temperature
    D. growth of underarm hair
20. The process in which complex molecules are broken down into simpler molecules is _____.
    A. anabolism
    B. catabolism
    C. metabolism
    D. homeostasis

Thinking Critically

21. You have a very muscular friend who needs to reduce his weight for wrestling. What advice would you give him about eating while trying to lose weight? Explain your answer.
22. It is a hot, dry day, and you are going to be running a race in the middle of the afternoon. What challenges does your body face in trying to maintain homeostasis while you run?

› LESSON 1.3

How Forces Affect the Body

Learning Key Terms and Concepts

23. _____ is the single force resulting from the summation of all forces acting on an object at a given time.
    A. Net mass
    B. Net force
    C. Net torque
    D. Net weight
24. The quantity of matter an object contains is its _____.
    A. weight
    B. force
    C. pressure
    D. mass
25. How is torque measured?
    A. the size of the force × perpendicular distance from the line of force application to the center of rotation
    B. the sum of all forces that are pushing or pulling on the object
    C. the size of the force divided by the area over which the force acts
    D. the amount of force distributed over a given area divided by net force
26. _____ is a force that, with enough energy, crushes tissue.
    A. Torque
    B. Shear
    C. Compression
    D. Tension

27. A bruise is caused by _____.
    A. compression
    B. tension
    C. shearing
    D. torque
28. _____ is a force that pulls or stretches the tissue.
    A. Acceleration
    B. Tension
    C. Pressure
    D. Torsion
29. _____ is a force that moves perpendicular to tissue.
    A. Torsion
    B. Compression
    C. Shear
    D. Pressure
30. _____ is caused by a combination of off-center forces.
    A. Pressure
    B. Torsion
    C. Deformation
    D. Bending
31. When a force is applied to an object, the change in the object's velocity is known as _____.
    A. deformation
    B. acceleration
    C. compression
    D. integration
32. A tissue's response to force is said to be _____ when a force is removed and the object returns to its original shape.
    A. plastic
    B. torqued
    C. efferent
    D. elastic

Thinking Critically

33. A football player's foot is planted, and he is in the process of turning when his knee is hit from the side, resulting in a serious injury to the ligaments of the knee. Which two forces acted on the knee to produce this injury?
34. Assume that your body is struck by a baseball and a basketball of the same weight traveling at the same speed. Which will exert more pressure on your body—the baseball or the basketball? Why?
35. Is skin or bone more elastic? Why?

› LESSON 1.4

Understanding Science

Learning Key Terms and Concepts

36. All research begins with the identification of a(n) _____.
37. Step 2 of the scientific method is _____.
    A. formulating a hypothesis
    B. planning the organization of the study
    C. identifying a research question
    D. collecting the data
38. The key to collecting data is that it must _____.
    A. be collected objectively using the same procedures every time
    B. be collected objectively and obtained in the largest quantities possible
    C. be collected subjectively using the same procedure every time
    D. be collected subjectively and obtained in the smallest possible quantities
39. When a hypothesis has been thoroughly investigated and found to accurately explain a natural or physical phenomenon, it becomes a _____.
    A. hunch
    B. guess
    C. hypothesis
    D. theory
40. Which of the following scientists did not contribute to increased understanding of anatomy during the Renaissance?
    A. Andreas Vesalius
    B. William Harvey
    C. Isaac Newton
    D. Robert Hooke

Thinking Critically

41. Create a measurable hypothesis about study time and its relationship to success on exams. Make precise, accurate measurements of both time and grades. What can you infer from your data? What trends can you predict? Communicate your conclusions to your classmates.
42. Suppose that a hypothesis is proven incorrect. Does this mean that the research was a waste of time? Defend your answer.

43. With the students in your anatomy and physiology class as the participants, research the impact of exercise on the homeostatic state of the respiratory system. Collect, organize, analyze, and evaluate both quantitative and qualitative data using appropriate tools. Will this population sample be considered statistically significant? Are there any possible sources of bias in your conclusions? If so, how could you restate your conclusions and evaluations to avoid bias? In what other ways could you improve this experiment?

Building Skills and Connecting Concepts

Analyzing and Evaluating Data

Instructions: The graph at the right shows the average number of steps (foot contacts) resulting in chronic injury, as they occur in groups of people in different weight categories. Use the graph in **Figure 1.20** to answer the following questions.

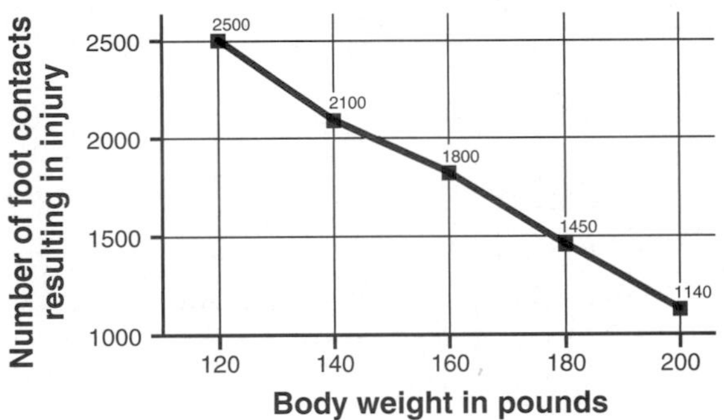

Figure 1.20

44. How many foot contacts is the group with a body weight of 160 pounds able to make before an injury occurs?
45. Which group is generating the most pressure per foot contact?
46. What prediction would you make about the number of foot contacts leading to injury for people in the 170- to 175-pound range?
47. Based on the data provided in the graph, write a hypothesis about body weight and foot contacts resulting in chronic injuries.

Communicating about Anatomy & Physiology

48. **Speaking and Listening** Working in small groups, create a poster that illustrates the anatomical planes and directional movements of the human body. Have a volunteer briefly stand before the class as a "visual aid" to help you accurately capture and represent anatomical position and directional relationships.

    First, draw a figure in anatomical position with the body erect, the arms at the sides, and the palms facing forward. Then, label the three anatomical planes: *sagittal*, *frontal* (coronal), and *transverse*. Within each of the planes, add labels to show the directional relationships among body parts and the different positions of movement: *superior* (cranial), *inferior* (caudal), *anterior* (ventral), *posterior* (dorsal), *medial*, *lateral*, and *proximal*. Use different-colored markers to outline and label each anatomical plane and directional relationship.

    As you work with your group, discuss the meaning of each term. If necessary, a member of your group might stand and demonstrate directional movements to confirm your understanding of the terms. Afterward, display your posters in the classroom as a convenient reference aid for discussions and assignments.

49. **Writing** Use the scientific method to answer this research question: *With the advances of artificial intelligence and medical terminology, what new body parts will be available for transplant in the near future, and how will we procure them?*

    Write a full report detailing your method and your findings. Be sure to include the references you used. Indicate the probable source of each body part (artificial, human, animal) and the improvement having this part would make in people's lives.

Lab Investigations

50. Working in groups of two or three students, create a three-dimensional anatomical man and label your creation using the terms that you have learned in this chapter. If you created a poster in the "Communicating" activity above, use it as a guide as you label your "anatomy man."

    Work with your group members to organize your project. Be creative in deciding what materials you will use to create your figure. Delegate responsibility to team members for bringing each of the needed materials. As much as possible, use materials that are readily available in your home (for example, boxes, string, balloons, plastic bottles, paper, tape, glue, or pipe cleaners). Do *not* use any sharp objects. Also refrain from using manufactured figures such as dolls, action figures, or stuffed animals.

    Incorporate into your anatomical man the directional and body cavity terms that you learned in this chapter. Include all the terms in **Figures 1.2** and **1.3**. You must be accurate in your placement of each term. You may use arrows, and you may create several layers on your anatomy man.

51. Work as a class for this lab. Increase your understanding of anatomical positions and directions by creating an index card for each key term in Lesson 1.1. Have the instructor or a classmate pin or tape a card to your back, without revealing the term on the card. Then walk around the room asking other students (who can see the term taped to your back) YES or NO questions, such as "Am I a plane?" "Am I a direction?" "Am I a cavity?" "Am I located in the abdomen?" After you correctly guess which anatomical term you are, take your seat. Which of the terms were hardest to guess: planes, directions, or cavities? Why was this difficult?

52. Conduct a class meeting in which you and your classmates discuss ways to test the effects of combined loads on the human body. Use proper meeting etiquette and parliamentary procedure to achieve an orderly, productive meeting. Develop and vote for approval on an appropriate testing protocol. After developing the protocol, conduct a class discussion on meeting etiquette and how following proper procedures can help produce efficient results.

Building Your Portfolio

53. Take digital photographs of the models you created and projects you worked on in this chapter. Create a document called "Foundations of Anatomy and Physiology" and insert the photographs, along with written descriptions of what the models or projects show and your reasons for creating and presenting them as you did. Add this document to your personal portfolio.

CHAPTER

2 Cells and Tissues

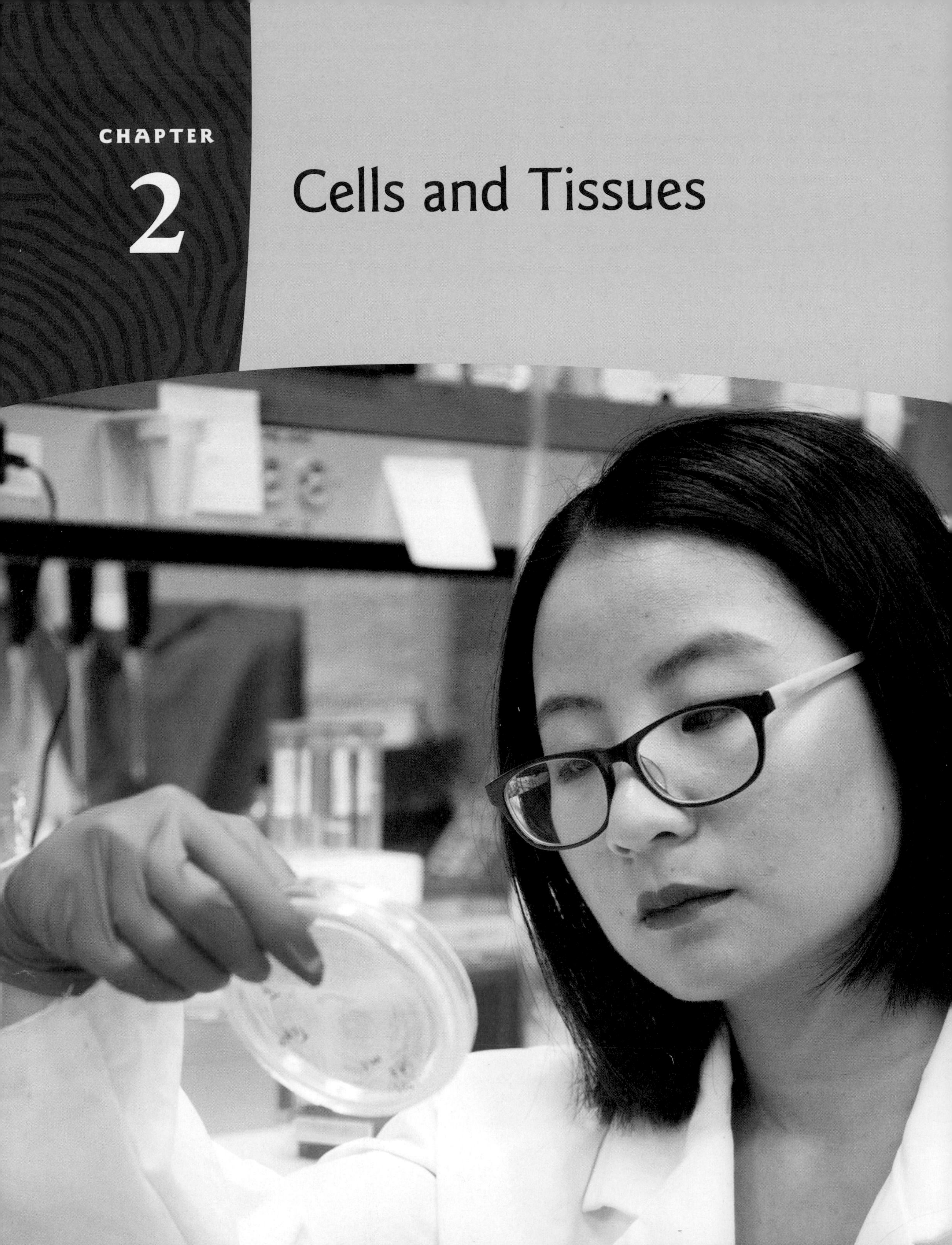

What will be the next breakthrough as scientists study human cells?

The human body is made of cells—20 to 40 trillion of them, not counting bacteria in the digestive tract. Although scientists have yet to come up with a satisfactory definition of life, it seems clear that the body's individual cells are alive. They reproduce and transmit information from one generation to the next. They transform energy from one form to another, and they use energy to maintain their internal environment.

Body cells cannot survive independently; they need one another to stay alive. Each cell is a specialist with its own job to do. Certain tasks, such as maintaining an internal environment, are performed by *all* cells. Other tasks, such as making ATP, are done by *most* cells. Some tasks, such as making antibodies, are done by *only one* type of cell.

To understand anatomy and physiology, you must first understand how cells work, and how they work together. An understanding of cells and the tissues made from cells is also necessary for understanding diseases and their treatment, because modern medicine relies more than ever on therapies targeted at cellular processes.

Chapter 2 Outline

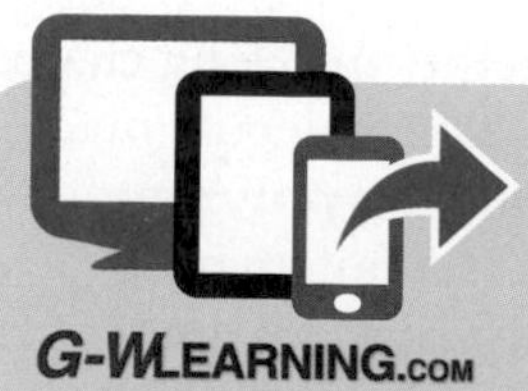

Click on the activity icon or visit www.g-wlearning.com/healthsciences/0202 to access online vocabulary activities using key terms from the chapter.

◂ SINITAR/Shutterstock.com

LESSON 2.1 Molecules of Life

Before You Read

Try to answer the following questions before you read this lesson.

- What are the four major types of large organic molecules in the human body?
- What molecule is the universal source of energy for cellular reactions?
- What properties of water make it essential for life?

Lesson Objectives

- List the types and functions of carbohydrates.
- Describe the structure and functions of proteins.
- Explain the properties of lipids, including fatty acids, glycerides, phospholipids, and steroids.
- Know the importance of DNA and RNA and the nucleotides of which they are composed, including ATP.
- Describe the polarity and pH of water.

Key Terms

adenosine triphosphate (ATP)	lipids
amino acids	nucleic acids
base pairs	nucleotides
chromosome	peptide bond
deoxyribonucleic acid (DNA)	pH
electrolytes	phospholipids
enzyme	polymer
fatty acid	polypeptide
gene	proteome
gene therapy	ribonucleic acid (RNA)
glucose	steroids
glycogen	triglycerides
human genome	

An almost countless number of different types of molecules exists in the human body. *Biochemistry* is the detailed study of the molecules of life, how they are made, how they interact, and how they are broken down. This lesson provides a short summary of the key molecules of life, the ones that will be important in your study of anatomy and physiology.

Most chemicals important for life are organic molecules. Organic molecules always contain carbon, hydrogen, and oxygen. In addition, they sometimes contain nitrogen, phosphorous, sulfur, and other elements. Major classes of large organic molecules in the body include carbohydrates, proteins, lipids, and nucleic acids. Important smaller molecules and atoms include ATP, sodium, potassium, chloride, calcium, phosphate, and, of course, water.

Carbohydrates

Carbohydrates, also known as *saccharides* (SAK-a-righdz), are "sugar and starch" molecules. Carbohydrates made of just one or two simple subunits are called *simple carbohydrates*, or sugars. **Glucose** ($C_6H_{12}O_6$) (**Figure 2.1**) is a monosaccharide (simple sugar) and is the main form of sugar that circulates in the blood. Sucrose (table sugar) is a disaccharide made of two monosaccharides: glucose and fructose.

MEMORY TIP

The name *carbohydrate* is derived from the elements that go together to make up a carbohydrate. The name also provides a clue to the atomic formula for carbohydrates. All carbohydrates are made of carbon, hydrogen, and oxygen atoms. The hydrogen and oxygen are usually present in a two-to-one ratio, like water (H_2O). *Hydrate* is a chemical term for water. So *carbohydrate* means "carbon and water."

Simple sugars can join together into long chains known as *complex carbohydrates*. A molecule made of many similar subunits is called a **polymer**. **Glycogen** (GLIGH-koh-jen) is a polymer of glucose and is found in animals; starch is a polymer of simple sugars and is found in plants.

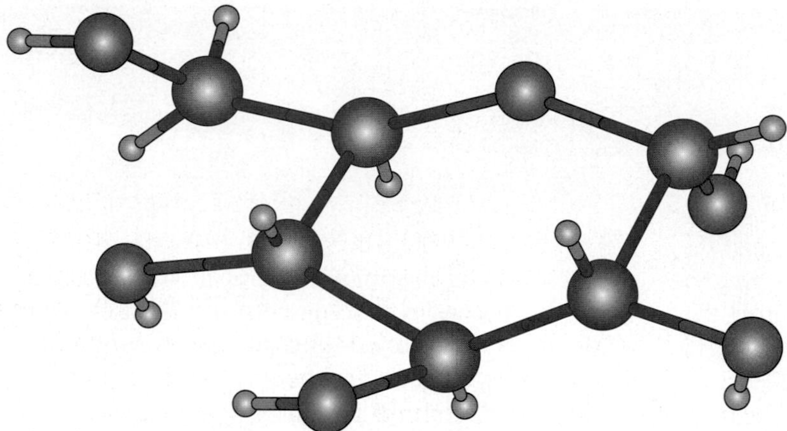

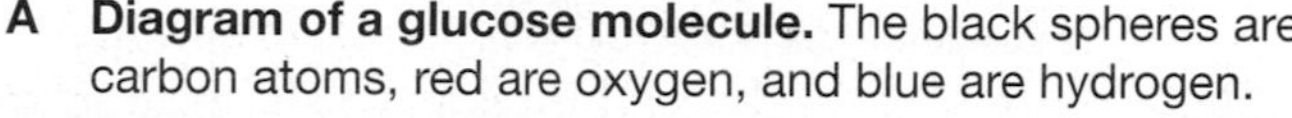

A Diagram of a glucose molecule. The black spheres are carbon atoms, red are oxygen, and blue are hydrogen.

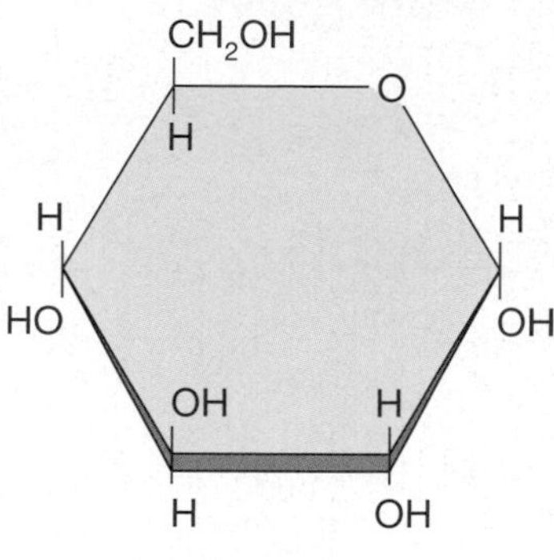

B Standard representation of a glucose molecule.

© Body Scientific International

Figure 2.1 Glucose, shown here in two ways, is an organic molecule. Notice the difference in the number of carbon atoms in A as opposed to B. The reason for this difference is that, in the standard method of representing the molecular structure of glucose (B), a carbon atom is assumed to be present at each unlabeled "corner" where two or more lines (bonds) meet.

Liver and muscle cells make glycogen molecules (**Figure 2.2**) from glucose. The glycogen polymer is a form of stored fuel. When a muscle cell needs fuel, it can break glucose subunits off of the glycogen and use the glucose for energy. If blood sugar becomes too low, liver cells break glucose off of the glycogen and release the glucose into the blood. A single glycogen molecule may contain hundreds of thousands of glucose subunits.

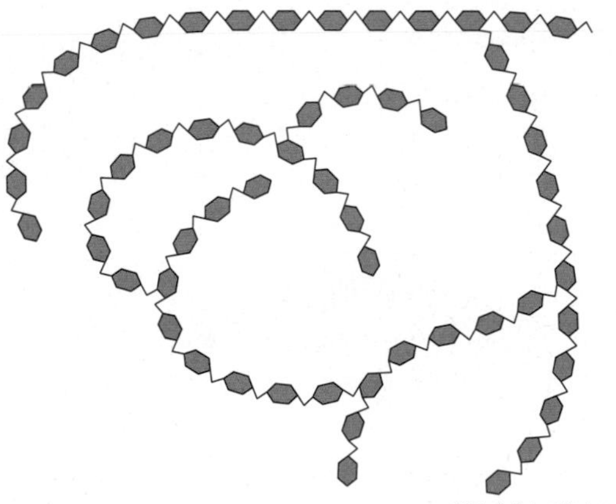

© Body Scientific International

Figure 2.2 Glycogen structure. Glycogen is a polysaccharide made of glucose subunits called *monomers*, which are shown here as hexagons. Glycogen has many branches. *What would you need to remove from this drawing to change the complex carbohydrate to many simple carbohydrates?*

MEMORY TIP

Polymer comes from the combining forms *poly*, meaning "many," and *mer*, meaning "unit." *Monomers* (*mono* means "one") are the building blocks from which polymers are made. Other "-mers" include *dimers* (two subunits), *trimers* (three subunits), and *tetramers* (four subunits).

The main function of carbohydrates in the body is to serve as a source of chemical energy, or fuel. The body can quickly utilize this fuel to make ATP, which you will learn about later in this chapter.

Check Your Understanding

1. What does the word *carbohydrate* mean?
2. What subunits form carbohydrates?
3. What is the term for simple sugars that join together in long chains?
4. Explain the relationship between polymers and complex carbohydrates.
5. Where in the body are glycogen molecules made from glucose?

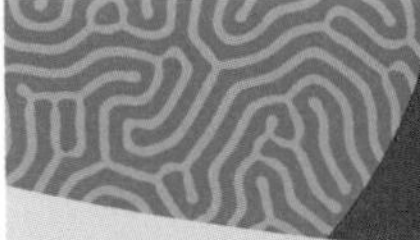

What Research Tells Us

...about Glycogen Storage Diseases

Glycogen storage diseases are a class of disorders in which either the formation or the breakdown of glycogen does not work properly (**Figure 2.3**). In healthy individuals, the liver and muscles perform two different processes involving glycogen and glucose. They synthesize glycogen from glucose, and they break down glycogen to release glucose. Glucose from the liver is released into the bloodstream. Glucose in muscle tissue is used to make ATP for energy.

In hepatic (liver) types of glycogen storage diseases, the liver does not release glucose into the blood as it should. The liver is often enlarged due to an abnormal accumulation of glycogen in its cells. In myopathic (muscle) types of glycogen storage diseases, the storage or breakdown of glycogen in muscles does not work properly. (The combining form *myo* means "muscle" and the combing form *path/o* means "sickness.")

Glycogen storage diseases are usually inherited. They are caused by genetic mutations that affect enzymes that catalyze biochemical reactions involving glycogen. There is no way to prevent or cure glycogen storage diseases, but in many cases, symptoms can be lessened by dietary changes, drugs, or a liver transplant.

Taking It Further

1. Conduct further research to investigate the types of disorders that are classified as glycogen storage diseases. What is the difference between hepatic and myopathic glycogen storage diseases?
2. Choose one specific glycogen storage disease and research its symptoms, causes, and treatment options.

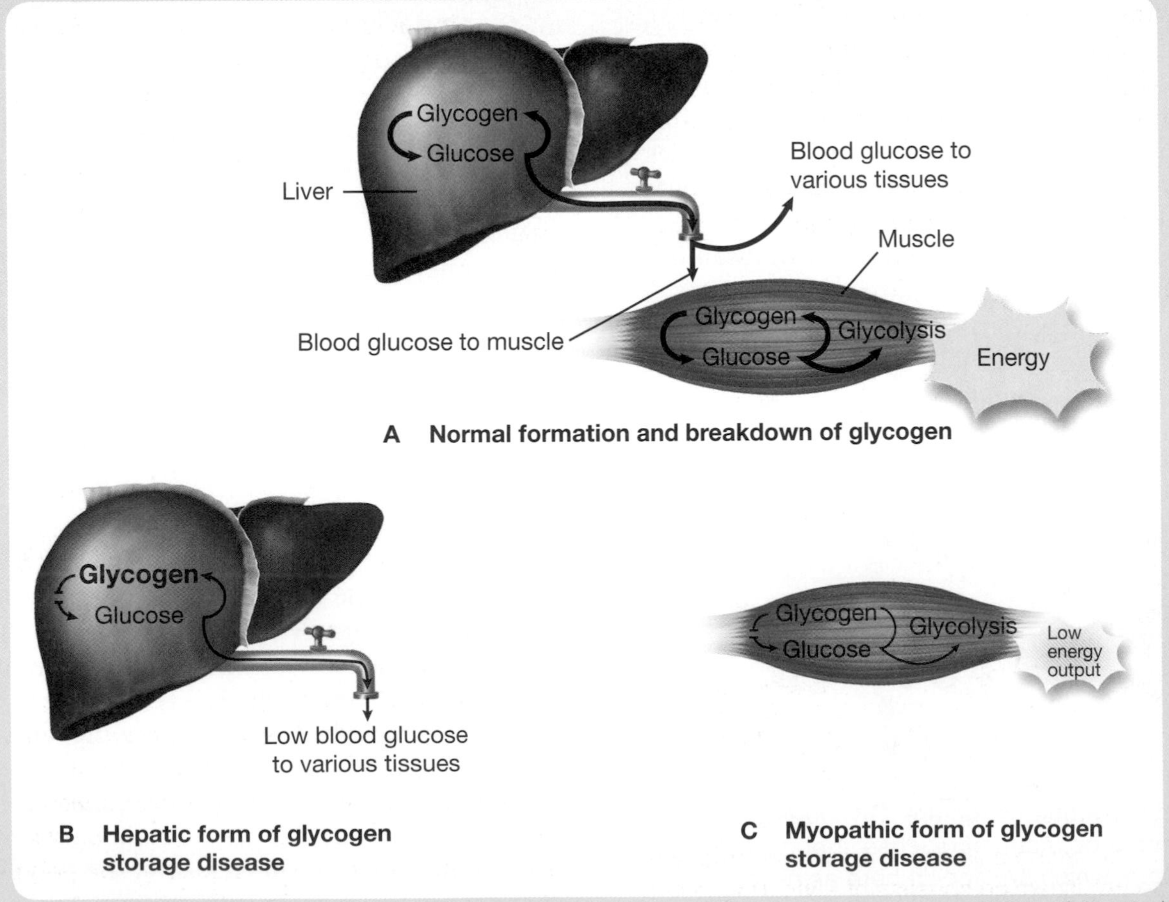

Figure 2.3 Glycogen storage disease. *If everything is working properly, does the liver turn glucose to glycogen, glycogen to glucose, or both?*

Proteins

Proteins are large molecules made of long chains of **amino acids**. Some proteins help form the structure of cells. Other proteins, called *enzymes*, catalyze (speed up) specific biological reactions. Still others (notably hemoglobin) act as carriers. For example, hemoglobin carries oxygen in red blood cells.

The relatively new term **proteome** refers to all the proteins that are expressed (made) by a particular cell or organism. The study of the proteins as an ensemble is called *proteomics*. A key goal of proteomics is to understand large-scale patterns and control mechanisms that govern which proteins are expressed in which cells under different conditions of health, disease, and development.

Amino Acids

Twenty amino acids make up the building blocks of proteins. All 20 amino acids share a common design: each has an identical "backbone" consisting of an amino group ($-NH_2$) and an acid group ($-COOH$), with a central carbon between them, as shown in **Figure 2.4**. The central carbon has a hydrogen atom and a variable group of atoms attached to it. The variable group is what varies from one amino acid to another. Biochemists call the variable group the *residual group*, so an R is used to indicate this group in **Figure 2.4**.

Glycine (GLIGH-seen), the simplest amino acid, has a residual group consisting of a single hydrogen atom. Tryptophan (TRIP-toh-fan) has the largest residual group (C_9H_4N). Some amino acids have residual groups that are acidic, some have residual groups that are basic, and two amino acids have residual groups that contain sulfur. The sulfur residual group is important because disulfide bonds, which connect sulfurs of different amino acids, are essential contributors to the structure of some proteins.

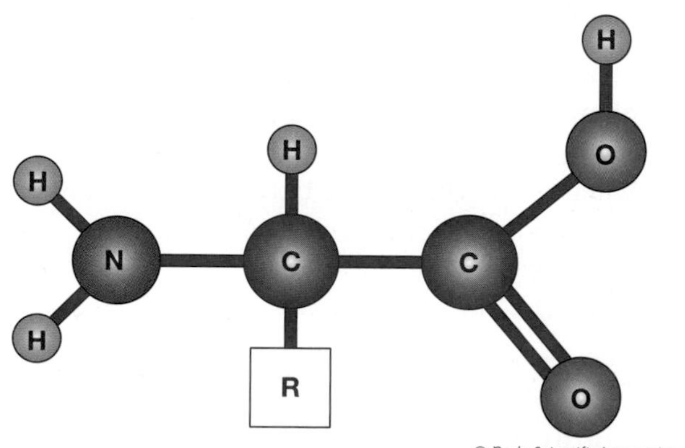

Figure 2.4 An amino acid has a "backbone" made of an amino group, which consists of $-NH_2$ (to the left in the drawing), a carboxylic acid group $-COOH$ (to the right), and a central carbon. A residual group (R) is attached to the central carbon. The residual group varies from one amino acid to another.

Peptide Bonds

Amino acids join together by forming a **peptide bond**, a bond linking the amino group of one amino acid to the acid group of another. Short chains of amino acids (fewer than 50) are often referred to as *peptides*. Examples include the octapeptide (8 amino acids) oxytocin (awk-see-TOH-sin), a hormone that is important in childbirth, and enkephalin (ehn-KEHF-uh-lin), a pentapeptide (5 amino acids) that acts in the brain to inhibit the perception of pain.

A longer chain of amino acids is called a **polypeptide**. Many proteins, such as actin (275 amino acids) and titin (more than 33,000 amino acids), are made of a single polypeptide chain. Both actin and titin are found in muscle tissue. Other proteins are made of multiple polypeptide chains. The oxygen-carrying protein hemoglobin (HEE-moh-gloh-bin) is made of four polypeptide chains, each containing between 140 and 150 amino acids.

Structure of Proteins

The structure, or shape, of a protein is determined by the sequence of amino acids it contains (**Figure 2.5**). The amino acid sequence is known as the *primary structure* of a protein.

The polypeptide chain folds up into a specific shape that is determined by its primary structure. This folding process allows the protein to reduce its potential energy. Just as a marble tends to roll downhill, a polypeptide tends to fold. The folding allows energetically favorable interactions of residual groups of amino acids with one another and with surrounding molecules, including water.

The first level of folding is called *secondary structure*. One common form of secondary structure is the alpha helix, in which part of the polypeptide chain assumes a spiral conformation. Another common form of secondary structure is the beta-pleated sheet, in which part of the chain assumes a "flat with slight folds" conformation.

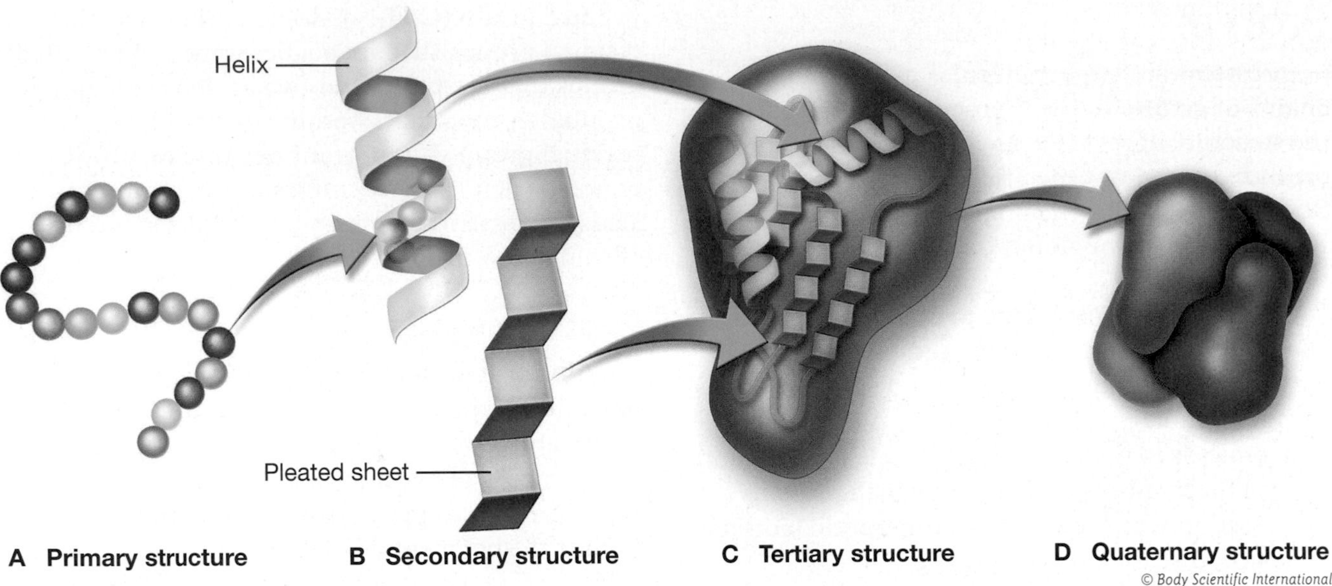

Figure 2.5 Levels of protein structure. How are these different levels of protein structure related to energy?

The next level of folding is called the *tertiary* (meaning "third level") *structure*. At this level, helical sections, pleated sheet sections, and other sections fold together into a three-dimensional whole. If the protein is made of a single polypeptide, the tertiary structure is the final level of protein structure. For proteins made of multiple subunits, the arrangement of subunits into a whole, or *quaternary* (meaning "fourth level") *structure*, is the final factor in determining the protein's shape.

Functions of Proteins

As mentioned earlier, proteins have many functions in the body, including acting as structural elements, enzymes, and carriers. Structural proteins are found both inside and outside the body cells. They hold cells in place, give strength to tissues, and help form physical barriers to protect the body from various threats. Collagen, which gives strength to ligaments and tendons, is an example of a protein that has a structural function.

An **enzyme** is a molecule that participates in a chemical reaction without being consumed or destroyed in the reaction. It allows a specific reaction to occur much faster than it would if the enzyme were not present. An enzyme does not alter the ultimate equilibrium for a chemical reaction, but it often helps the reaction reach equilibrium sooner than it would if the enzyme were not present.

Proteins that act as enzymes are sensitive to temperature, level of acidity, and local concentrations of ions. Therefore it is essential that these factors be kept within a narrow acceptable range, so that biochemical reactions in cells can proceed normally. The enzyme *salivary amylase*, found in saliva, is a protein that breaks down carbohydrate molecules into smaller sugar molecules. The enzyme myosin breaks down ATP (discussed below) and converts the chemical energy into mechanical energy. This will be discussed in more detail in Chapter 5.

Myoglobin (MIGH-oh-gloh-bin) and hemoglobin are examples of proteins that act as carriers. Myoglobin carries oxygen in muscle; hemoglobin carries oxygen in blood.

Check Your Understanding

1. What three components form the backbone of all 20 amino acids in proteins?
2. Name three functions of proteins in the body.
3. What is the difference between a peptide bond and a polypeptide?
4. What is an enzyme?

Lipids

Lipids are "fats and oils" and related molecules. They are rich in carbon and hydrogen, usually with a ratio of about two hydrogen atoms for every carbon atom. They also contain oxygen atoms and sometimes other types of atoms. Major types of lipids include fatty acids, glycerides, phospholipids, and steroids.

Lipid molecules do not get as big as the large proteins and carbohydrates, but they have a wide range of structures and functions. Most types of lipids do not dissolve well in water or blood; special proteins are needed to help carry lipids through the bloodstream.

Fatty Acids

A **fatty acid** is a hydrocarbon chain with a carboxylic acid group (–COOH) at one end. Fatty acids may have all single bonds, in which case they are called *saturated*. Fatty acids with one or more double bonds are called *unsaturated*. Stearic acid ($C_{18}H_{36}O_2$) and oleic acid ($C_{18}H_{34}O_2$) are examples of saturated and unsaturated fatty acids, respectively.

The presence of double bonds in a fatty acid often puts a "kink" in the molecule. Fatty acids in their pure form are not that common in the body, but they are key building blocks for other lipids, particularly glycerides and phospholipids (FAHS-foh-lip-idz).

Glycerides

Glycerides are composed of a glycerol molecule (a simple sugar) with one, two, or three fatty acids attached, to make mono-, di-, and **triglycerides** (trigh-GLIS-er-ighdz) (**Figure 2.6**). Glycerides are important energy storage molecules in the body. Most of the fat in fat cells is in the form of triglycerides.

Phospholipids

Phospholipids are similar to glycerides. The phosphate-bearing head of the phospholipid is *hydrophilic* (high-droh-FIL-ik), which means that it can form energetically favored hydrogen bonds with water molecules. The fatty acid tails

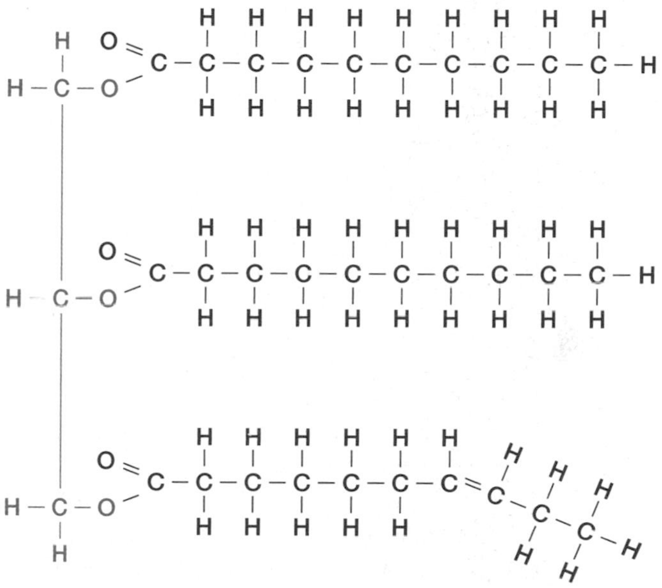

Figure 2.6 A triglyceride has a glycerol head (blue) and three fatty acid chains (red). The triglyceride shown here has two saturated fatty acids (top two chains) and one unsaturated fatty acid (bottom chain). *What is responsible for the bend in the unsaturated fatty acid?*

MEMORY TIP

The ability to carry a reserve fuel supply has a survival benefit if food becomes scarce. The body stores chemical energy for future use in the form of carbohydrates (especially glycogen) and fats (especially triglycerides). Which is the better way to store energy?

Each form of stored chemical energy has advantages and disadvantages. For example, glycogen can be turned into usable chemical energy more quickly than triglycerides, because glycogen provides glucose directly to cells. This glucose can then be used rapidly by virtually all body cells to make ATP (discussed later). The breakdown of triglycerides, however, yields fatty acids, which cannot be used by as many types of cells; in addition, they cannot be used as quickly as glucose.

Glycogen, but not triglycerides, can provide energy fast enough to sustain prolonged rigorous exercise—at least it can until the glycogen stores run out. It should be noted, however, that exercise does help consume unwanted fat because fat is used to some extent during exercise itself. Fat is also used during recovery from exercise to restock the body's storehouse of glycogen.

The big advantage of fat over glycogen is that it stores about twice as much energy per kilogram (or pound) as glycogen or other carbohydrates. A gram of glycogen stores about four to five kilocalories of chemical energy. A gram of fat stores about nine kilocalories of energy. There is obviously a benefit to carrying the same amount of energy reserves with fewer pounds. That is why, if one consumes more calories than are needed to meet the demands of living, the body stores the excess energy as fat.

are *hydrophobic* (high-droh-FOH-bik), which means they cannot form favorable hydrogen bonds with water. As a result, phospholipids in a watery environment tend to form bilayers, liposomes (LIGHP-oh-sohmz), or *micelles* (migh-SELZ) ("little spheres") with the heads facing the water and the tails adjacent to one another (**Figure 2.7**).

Steroids

Steroids are a class of lipids whose structure is very different from that of other lipids. All steroids have the same four-ring backbone but differ in the attached side groups. Three well-known steroid molecules—cholesterol, testosterone, and estrogen—are shown in **Figure 2.8**. Cholesterol is a component of cell membranes. Testosterone and estrogen are hormones that regulate the reproductive system.

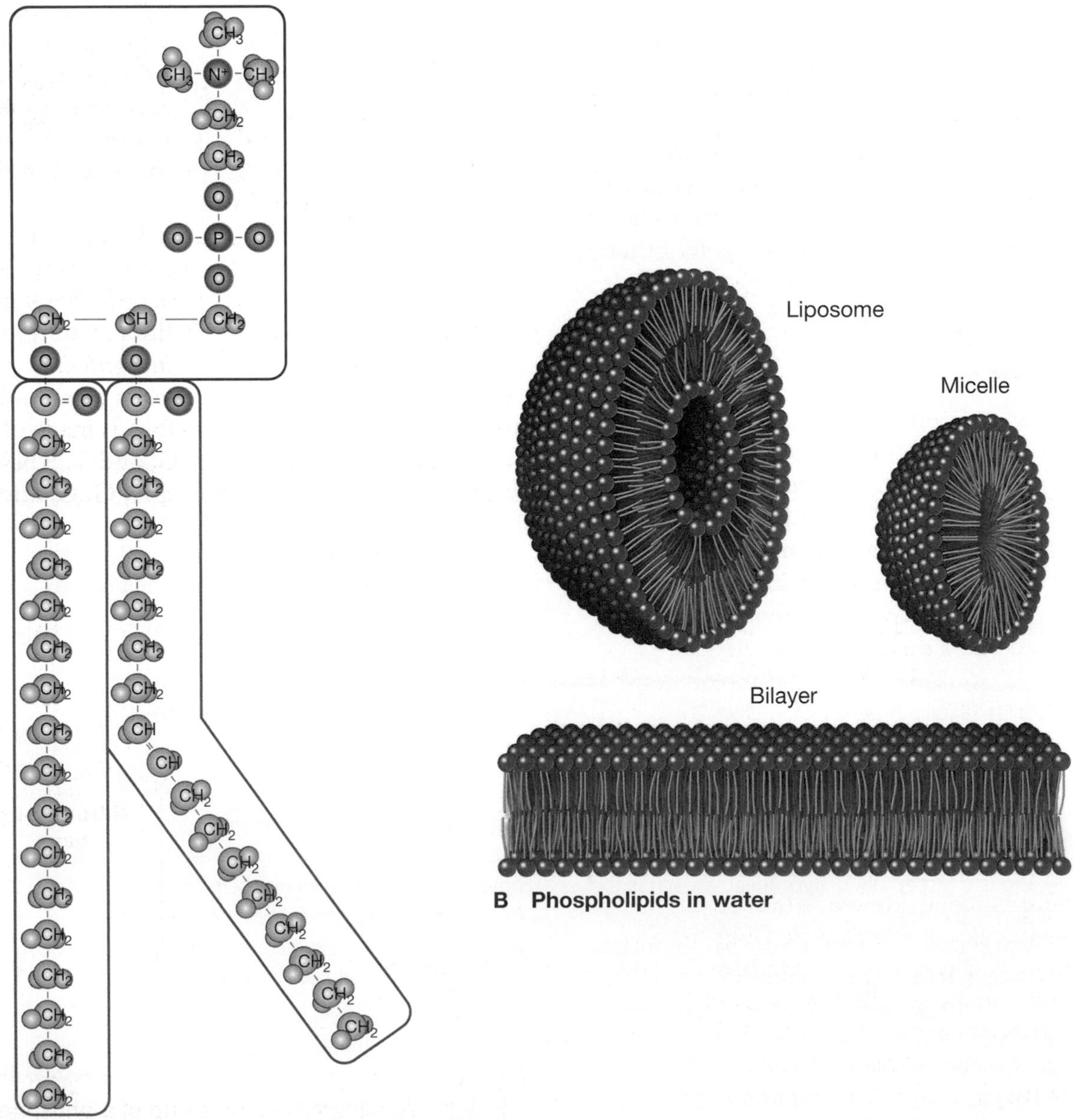

Figure 2.7 A—The atomic structure of a phospholipid includes a "head" (red outline) and two fatty acid tails (blue outline). The head is hydrophilic and the tails are hydrophobic. B—Phospholipids in water can form a bilayer, a liposome, or a micelle. In each of these arrangements, the hydrophilic phosphate heads face outward, toward water, and the hydrophobic tails face inward.

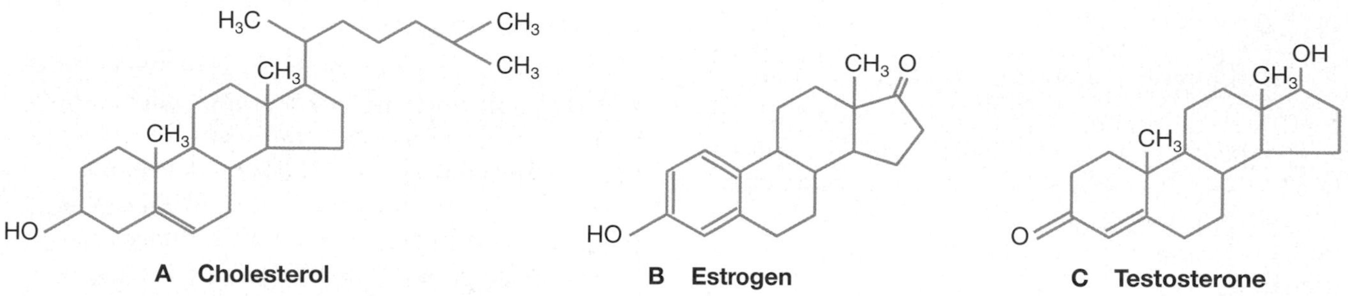

A Cholesterol

B Estrogen

C Testosterone

© Body Scientific International

Figure 2.8 Steroid molecules: cholesterol, estrogen, and testosterone.

MEMORY TIP

Molecules, and parts of molecules, differ in how well they bond with water. Molecules that easily bond with water are called *hydrophilic*, which means "water-loving." Molecules that do not bond well with water are called *hydrophobic*, or "water-fearing." Most lipids, including fatty acids, triglycerides, and steroids, are significantly hydrophobic. That is why oil and water do not mix. Phospholipids are different: they have hydrophilic heads and hydrophobic tails. This makes them ideally suited for making cell membranes, as shown in **Figure 2.7**.

Check Your Understanding

1. Identify the four types of lipids.
2. What are the two classes of fatty acids?
3. What is the difference between a hydrophilic molecule and a hydrophobic molecule?
4. Name two well-known steroid molecules that function as hormones.

Nucleic Acids and Nucleotides

Nucleic acids are key information-carrying molecules in cells. Some nucleic acids also function as enzymes. The two kinds of nucleic acids found in cells are ribonucleic acid (RNA) and deoxyribonucleic acid (DNA). Like proteins and complex carbohydrates, nucleic acids are polymers: they are large molecules composed of many subunits.

The subunits that make up nucleic acids are called **nucleotides** (NOO-klee-oh-tighdz). Each nucleotide is made of a phosphate group, a sugar group, and a nitrogenous (nitrogen-containing) base (**Figure 2.9**). Two nucleotides join together by forming a bond between the phosphate of one nucleotide and the sugar of another, with the bases "hanging off" to the side. A water molecule is produced and released in the process—as it is in the formation of a disaccharide and in the formation of a peptide bond.

Just as different side chains distinguish the various amino acids, different bases distinguish the nucleotides. However, there are only five kinds of nucleotides, as opposed to 20 different amino acids. The nucleotide bases are *adenine*, *guanine*, *cytosine*, *thymine*, and *uracil*, each of which is commonly abbreviated by its first letter. DNA is made of nucleotides containing A, G, C, and T. RNA is made of nucleotides containing A, G, C, and U.

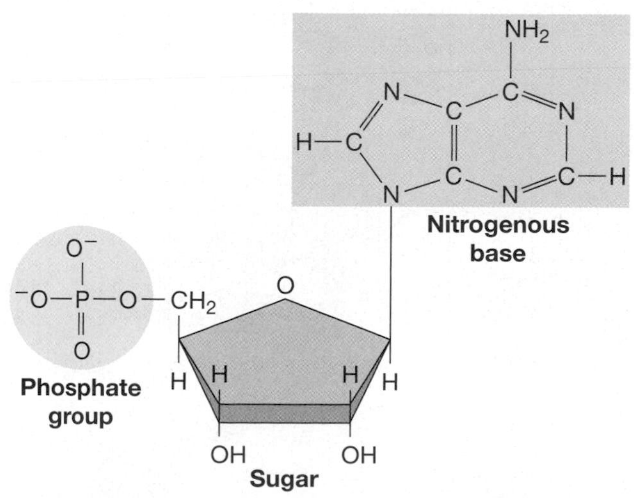

Figure 2.9 A nucleotide is made up of a phosphate group, a sugar group, and a nitrogenous base. The base shown here is adenine, and the entire molecule—base plus sugar plus phosphate—is called *adenosine monophosphate* because it contains a single phosphate group.

DNA

In **deoxyribonucleic acid (DNA)**, shown in **Figure 2.10**, two nucleotide chains coil around each other to form a double helix, which is similar in structure to a twisted ladder. The sugar and phosphate groups form the sides of the ladder. The bases from each side meet in the middle to form the rungs.

Each base can join with only one other base to form a rung: A and T form **base pairs**, and C and G form base pairs. Thus, if you know the base sequence of one strand, you can predict the base sequence of the complementary strand.

Base pairs are joined in the middle by hydrogen bonds, but the sugar-phosphate backbone is held together by covalent bonds. Because hydrogen bonds are weaker than covalent bonds, a DNA molecule can "unzip" down the middle with relative ease, while the backbone on each side remains intact. This ability of DNA to unzip is crucial for two processes: making a copy of the DNA before a cell divides and making transcripts of short segments of the DNA.

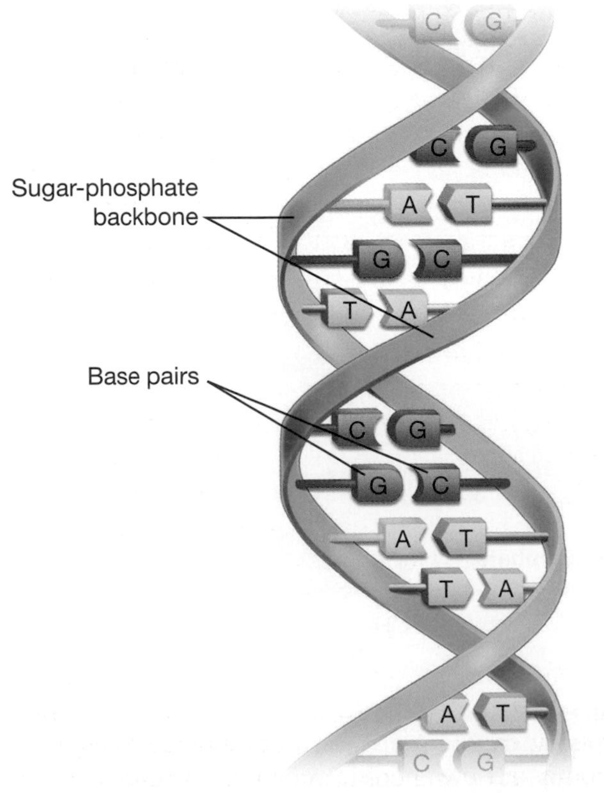

Figure 2.10 A DNA molecule. *What joins the base pairs, and how does this affect cell replication?*

Chromosomes

One DNA molecule and the proteins around which it coils make up one chromosome. Almost every human cell has 46 **chromosomes**—23 from each parent. There are 22 pairs of similar chromosomes (numbered 1 through 22), plus one X and one Y chromosome (in males) or two X chromosomes (in females).

Two exceptions to the 46-chromosomes-per-cell rule are sperm cells and egg cells, each of which has just 23 chromosomes. Another exception is red blood cells, which have neither nuclei nor chromosomes.

DNA is much bigger even than glycogen, which has a molecular weight in the tens of millions. Chromosome 1, with about 250 million base pairs, has a molecular weight of about 150 billion atomic units, which does not include the proteins that bind to it and help it coil. The 46 DNA molecules in a single cell, if laid out straight, would have a length of about 2 meters. The extreme thinness of DNA allows it to fit in a nucleus of 10 micrometers in diameter or smaller. This is similar to the ability of a fisherman to keep a quarter mile or more of fine fishing line (preferably on a spool) in a small tackle box.

Human Genomes

One set of 23 human chromosomes has about 3.2 billion base pairs. The DNA sequence of a human is referred to as the **human genome**. All humans (except identical twins, whose genomes are essentially the same) have very similar, but not quite identical, genomes. On average, about one base in every thousand bases is variable.

Certain base locations are much more likely to differ between individuals than other base locations. The base locations that tend to vary are called *single nucleotide polymorphisms*, or SNPs (pronounced "snips"). SNPs are the subject of much study given that they account for the genetic differences among individuals, including innate differences in athletic ability, disease susceptibility, and other inherited tendencies.

The Human Genome Project was an international research effort to determine the exact sequence of adenines, guanines, cytosines, and thymines that make up a "typical" human genome. The bulk of this effort was finished in 2003, but research on the genome continues. Scientists are hoping to understand the differences in sequences between individuals, and to understand the significance of those differences. Some differences in the genetic sequence appear to have no effect, but other differences can cause disease or have other effects.

Recent scientific advances make it possible to edit the genetic sequence of one or many cells. **Gene therapy** is the intentional alteration of a person's DNA in order to cure disease. In 2017, the US Food and Drug Administration (FDA) approved a gene therapy drug for the treatment of a form of inherited blindness. This was the first gene therapy approved by the FDA. Other forms of gene therapy are also showing promise. However, the ability to edit DNA also raises significant ethical questions if the technology is applied to egg or sperm cells or to embryos.

DNA Blueprints

It is interesting to note that cells can be very different even though they all contain the same DNA. For example, the bone cells, muscle cells, skin cells, and nerve cells in one person all contain complete and identical genetic blueprints, yet the cells are very different in structure and function. This brings up the subject of the information stored on the DNA.

DNA provides the blueprint for making proteins. The sequence of bases along DNA molecules specifies which amino acids to arrange in a particular order to make the proteins needed for life. It takes three bases of DNA to specify one amino acid in a protein. A set of three bases that specifies one amino acid in a protein is called a *codon*. A segment of DNA containing all the codons to make one polypeptide chain is called a **gene**.

RNA

Ribonucleic acid (RNA), like DNA, is a polymer of nucleotides. Its bases are adenosine, guanine, cytosine, and—instead of thymine, which is found in DNA—uracil. An RNA molecule is a single chain of nucleotides, as shown in **Figure 2.11**. In some RNA molecules, part of the chain forms a "hairpin" that doubles back on itself. When it does, the bases form pairs analogous to the pairs seen in the DNA double helix: C and G form pairs, and A and U form pairs.

There are several forms of RNA: messenger RNA (mRNA), transfer RNA (tRNA), ribosomal RNA (rRNA), and the most recently discovered and least well understood—regulatory RNA.

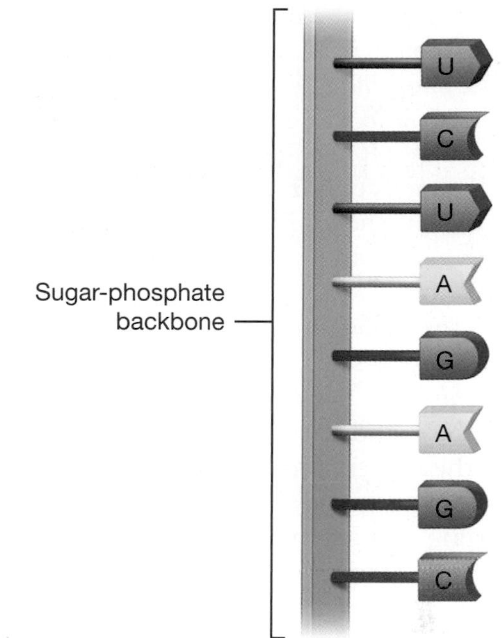

Figure 2.11 An RNA molecule is a chain of nucleotides. The four nucleotides—abbreviated A, C, G, and U—can occur in varying order. The chain can "fold up" in many possible ways, depending on the molecule's function.

Here is a brief description of the functions of each type of RNA:

- Messenger RNA functions as an information carrier in the manufacture of proteins.
- Transfer RNA assists in the manufacture of proteins.
- Ribosomal RNA forms ribosomes, large enzymes that act as catalysts for protein synthesis.
- Regulatory RNA helps regulate which proteins are produced.

The ability of RNA to function both as an information carrier (mRNA) and as an enzyme (rRNA) has led biologists to speculate that RNA may have been the first self-replicating molecule and, thus, a key molecule in the development of life. The functions of DNA and RNA are examined in more detail later in this chapter.

ATP

Adenosine triphosphate (ATP) (a-DEHN-oh-seen trigh-FAHS-fayt) is a nucleotide composed of an adenine base, a sugar, and three phosphate groups. ATP is a common energy source used in many cellular processes. A significant amount of chemical potential energy is stored in the bonds between the phosphates.

The energy in the bond between the last and middle phosphates in ATP can be released by splitting off the last phosphate. This process yields adenosine diphosphate (ADP) and inorganic phosphate, abbreviated P_i. (It is called inorganic phosphate because the molecular fragment contains no carbon.) This reaction is shown in **Figure 2.12** by the arrow on the left. ATP can be resynthesized by combining ADP and P_i and adding energy. This process is shown by the arrow on the right in **Figure 2.12**. These two processes are known collectively as *cellular respiration*.

To understand the role that ATP plays in cells, consider the role that money plays in the economy. If there were no money, people would have to trade certain items to get the things they need and want. If Alice raises goats, for example, she could trade goat's milk to get bread from Bob the bread maker. In an economy without money, Alice will have a hard time getting bread if Bob does not like goat's milk. In an economy with money, however, Alice can convert the goat's milk into money (by selling it), and she can use that money to get something that she wants. Money carries value and is accepted by everyone.

ATP plays a similar role in the energy economy of cells. Cells exchange the chemical potential energy stored in molecules (for example, in glucose or glycogen or triglycerides) for ATP by breaking down the energy-containing chemical (glucose, for example) and using the energy to make ATP. ATP is a carrier of energy that is accepted by all kinds of enzymes that need a source of energy. Those enzymes work by breaking down ATP to ADP plus P_i and using the energy obtained to accomplish some other energy-requiring process.

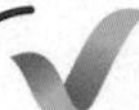

Check Your Understanding

1. Identify the three components of a nucleotide.
2. How many chromosomes does each parent contribute to its offspring?
3. What is the human genome?
4. Name the four forms of RNA.
5. What does ATP stand for and what is it composed of?

Water

Another molecule of life is dihydrogen oxide, more commonly known as *water*. All known life is water-based. Water makes up about two-thirds of the mass of the human body.

Polarity of Water

Water is a polar molecule, which means that it has a negatively charged region (the end of the oxygen atom that is situated away from the hydrogen atoms) and positively charged regions (at the far ends of the hydrogen atoms). The molecular configuration of water is shown in **Figure 2.13A**.

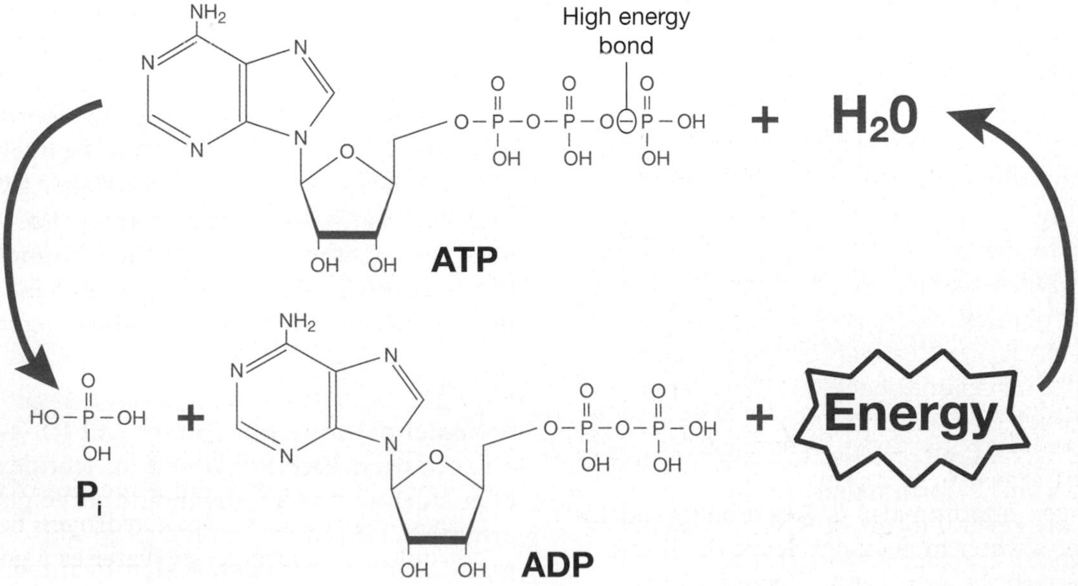

Figure 2.12 Breakdown and formation of ATP. ATP (top) can be broken down to yield ADP plus phosphate plus energy (bottom). *Why is ATP so important in the human body?*

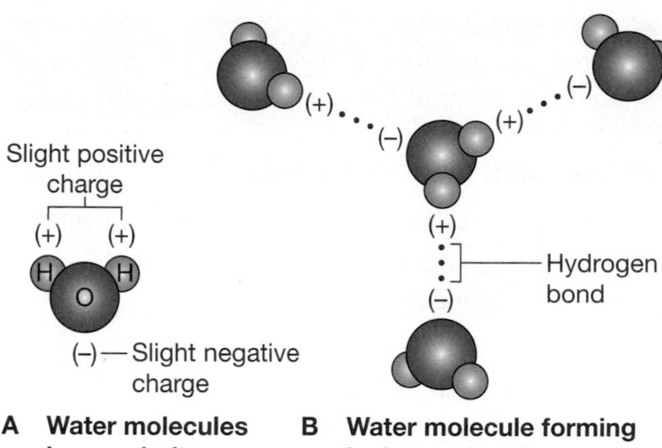

Figure 2.13 A—A water molecule is polar. That is, it has one side that is positively charged and one side that is negatively charged. B—A water molecule can form hydrogen bonds with other water molecules by orienting oppositely charged regions toward each other. In this diagram the central water molecule is forming hydrogen bonds with surrounding water molecules.

Hydrogen Bonding

The polarity of water molecules allows them to form hydrogen bonds with one another or with other charged or polar molecules. Hydrogen bonds are electrical interactions between the positive region around the hydrogen atom of a water molecule and the negatively charged region of another molecule.

Hydrogen bonds are relatively weak chemical bonds, but they are responsible for several biologically important properties of water. These properties include its high heat capacity, its relatively high boiling point, and its excellent solvent properties.

Water molecules also form short-lived hydrogen bonds with one another, as shown in **Figure 2.13B**. Hydrogen bonds in water quickly form, then break, and then reform as the molecules move around in a solution.

Hydrogen bonding gives water the ability to absorb or release a great deal of energy without much of a change in temperature. It is this property of water that creates the high heat capacity of water. Water's high heat capacity, and the fact that the human body is made mostly of water, means that body temperature doesn't change much when people gain or lose heat energy.

Hydrogen bonding also makes it energetically difficult for a water molecule to leave the liquid environment, because it cannot form hydrogen bonds in the gaseous state. Thus, water has a high heat of vaporization (it takes a lot of energy to boil water) and a high boiling point. This high heat of vaporization means that people can rid themselves of much heat when they sweat and water evaporates from the skin.

Water as a Solvent

The polar nature of water makes it a good solvent for many compounds. For example, ionic compounds, such as sodium chloride, dissolve well in water. This happens because the positively charged sodium ions are attracted to the negative parts of water molecules, and the negatively charged chloride ions are attracted to the positive parts of water molecules. Substances which dissolve into positively- and negatively-charged particles in water are called **electrolytes**. Examples of electrolytes include sodium chloride, calcium chloride, and sodium bicarbonate.

Other hydrophilic but uncharged compounds, such as glucose, have positive and negative regions. This means that they can interact favorably with opposite-charged parts of water molecules.

pH

A small fraction of water molecules in solution dissociates (comes apart) to make hydrogen ion (H^+) plus hydroxide ion (OH^-). A substance that, when added to water, increases its hydrogen ion concentration is called an *acid*. A substance that reduces the hydrogen ion concentration of a solution and increases its alkalinity is called a *base*. In short, acids are neutralized with bases, and bases are neutralized with acids. **pH** is a measure of the acidity or alkalinity of a solution.

Carbonic acid (H_2CO_3) is an important acid in the body. It dissociates to form H^+ and bicarbonate (HCO_3^-). It is considered a weak acid because, when added to water, not all of it dissociates. You may have the sodium salt of bicarbonate ($NaHCO_3$) in your kitchen. It is the white powder in the box labeled *baking soda*.

Check Your Understanding

1. What is a polar molecule?
2. Name three important properties of water that result from water's weak hydrogen bond.
3. Would you characterize water as a good or a poor solvent?
4. What does pH measure?

LESSON 2.1 Review and Assessment

Mini Glossary

Make sure that you know the meaning of each key term.

adenosine triphosphate (ATP) a nucleotide composed of an adenine base, a sugar, and three phosphate groups

amino acids the building blocks of proteins

base pairs pairs of complementary nucleic acid bases; that is, A and T or C and G

chromosome one DNA molecule and the proteins around which it coils

deoxyribonucleic acid (DNA) a polymer of nucleotides with the bases adenosine, guanine, cytosine, and thymine

electrolyte a substance that dissolves in water into particles with positive and negative charges

enzymes proteins that speed up specific biological reactions

fatty acid a hydrocarbon chain with a carboxylic acid group at one end

gene a segment of DNA containing all the codons to make one polypeptide chain

gene therapy the intentional alteration of a person's DNA in order to cure disease

glucose the main form of sugar that circulates in the blood

glycogen a polymer of glucose found in animals; stored form of glucose

human genome the DNA sequence of a human

lipids fatty molecules that dissolve poorly in water but dissolve well in a nonpolar solvent; fats and oils

nucleic acids key information-carrying molecules in cells

nucleotides subunits that make up nucleic acids

peptide bond the chemical bond that links two amino acids by connecting the amino group of one amino acid to the acid group of another

pH a measure of the acidity or alkalinity of a solution

phospholipids a lipid-containing phosphate group

polymer a molecule made of many similar subunits

polypeptide a long chain of amino acids

proteome all of the proteins that are expressed by (made by) a particular cell or organism

ribonucleic acid (RNA) one of two kinds of information-carrying nucleic acids found in cells

steroids a class of lipids with a structure that is different from other lipids; cholesterol, testosterone, and estrogen are three well-known steroids

triglycerides compounds composed of a glycerol molecule with three fatty acids attached

Know and Understand

1. Organic molecules always include what three elements?
2. The main purpose of carbohydrates in the body is to provide a source of _____.
3. The building blocks of proteins are _____.
4. Amino acids join together by forming a(n) _____ bond.
5. What does an enzyme do, and what happens to it in a chemical reaction?
6. Fats and oils in the body are known as _____.
7. The type of lipid that has both hydrophilic and hydrophobic areas is _____.
8. List the three nucleotides found in both DNA and RNA. Then identify the nucleotide found only in DNA and the one found only in RNA.
9. What is the purpose of gene therapy?
10. Describe the way ATP is used to create energy in the body.
11. What property of a water molecule allows it to form hydrogen bonds?
12. What property does pH measure?

Analyze and Apply

13. Is life possible without water? Why or why not?
14. Can body cells survive independently? Explain.
15. Find out more about the pH scale. What pH value is considered "neutral"? What values are considered acidic? What values are basic?

IN THE LAB

16. Working with a partner, create a model of ATP. Create the model so that the parts can be removed. Use your model to demonstrate to the class how ATP provides energy for body cells.
17. Verify that oil is hydrophobic; oil and water do not mix. Procedure: Take two large, clear cylinders of equal size. Fill one about one-third full with water and the other one-third full with cooking oil. Place three drops of red food coloring in the cylinder filled with water and mix by swirling. Pour the cooking oil into the cylinder filled with colored water. Swirl the cylinder. Why don't the molecules of colored water mix with the oil? Create a full lab investigation report to record your method, the materials you used, the results you observed, and your conclusions about those results.

LESSON 2.2

Cells

Before You Read

Try to answer the following questions before you read this lesson.

- How does a cell control what enters the cell and what comes out of it?
- How do cells move and change their shape?
- How do cells obtain and use energy to accomplish tasks?

Lesson Objectives

- Identify the major parts of a typical cell, including the plasma membrane, cytoskeleton, mitochondria, Golgi apparatus, ribosomes, endoplasmic reticulum, and nucleus.
- Explain the relationship among DNA, RNA, and proteins.
- Identify the phases and subphases in the life cycle of a cell.

Key Terms

active transport	extracellular matrix
centrioles	glycolysis
channel proteins	glycoproteins
cilia	Golgi apparatus
citric acid cycle	messenger RNA (mRNA)
codon	microvilli
cytokinesis	mitochondria
cytoplasm	mitosis
cytoskeleton	nucleus
diffusion	passive transport
endocytosis	plasma membrane
endoplasmic reticulum (ER)	ribosomes
exocytosis	transcription
extracellular fluid	transfer RNA (tRNA)

Inspection of a typical cell in the human body shows that the chemical reactions that are essential for life occur in different places within the cells. This lesson provides a "tour" of a typical cell that begins on the outside of the cell and works inward toward the middle. The lesson also examines the life cycle of a cell.

Anatomy and Physiology of a Cell

The cells of the human body are surrounded by **extracellular fluid**, which is mostly water, and an **extracellular matrix**. The extracellular matrix may be solid or gel-like and differs depending on the type of tissue. Structural molecules in the extracellular matrix, including proteins, connect cells to one another. These molecules also allow cells to migrate to the proper places during development, growth, maintenance, and recovery from injury. The **plasma membrane** defines the outer shell of a cell. Inside the membrane is the **cytoplasm** (SIGH-toh-plazm)—which contains everything except the nucleus—and the **nucleus** (**Figure 2.14**).

Plasma Membrane

The plasma membrane keeps the inside of the cell in and the outside of the cell out, and is *selectively permeable* (controls what passes through) (**Figure 2.15**). It is a phospholipid bilayer, as shown in **Figure 2.7**. In addition to phospholipids, the membrane contains cholesterol and a variety of proteins. The proteins include structural proteins, ion and water channels, and glycoproteins.

Proteins in the Plasma Membrane

Structural proteins such as cadherin, integrin, and spectrin connect the cell to neighboring cells, to the extracellular matrix, and to the cytoskeleton inside the cell. In this way these structural proteins form a link between the inside and the outside of the cell.

Channel proteins have a hollow central pore, or channel, that allows water or small, charged particles such as sodium, potassium, calcium, and chloride to pass into or out of the cell. These substances cannot enter or leave the cell without channels because their polarity, or charge, makes them unable to penetrate a lipid bilayer.

Channels are extremely selective about which substances they allow to cross the membrane, and when. For example, water channels, known as *aquaporins* (ah-kwah-POR-inz), let H_2O cross but do not let H^+ or OH^- cross, even though these two

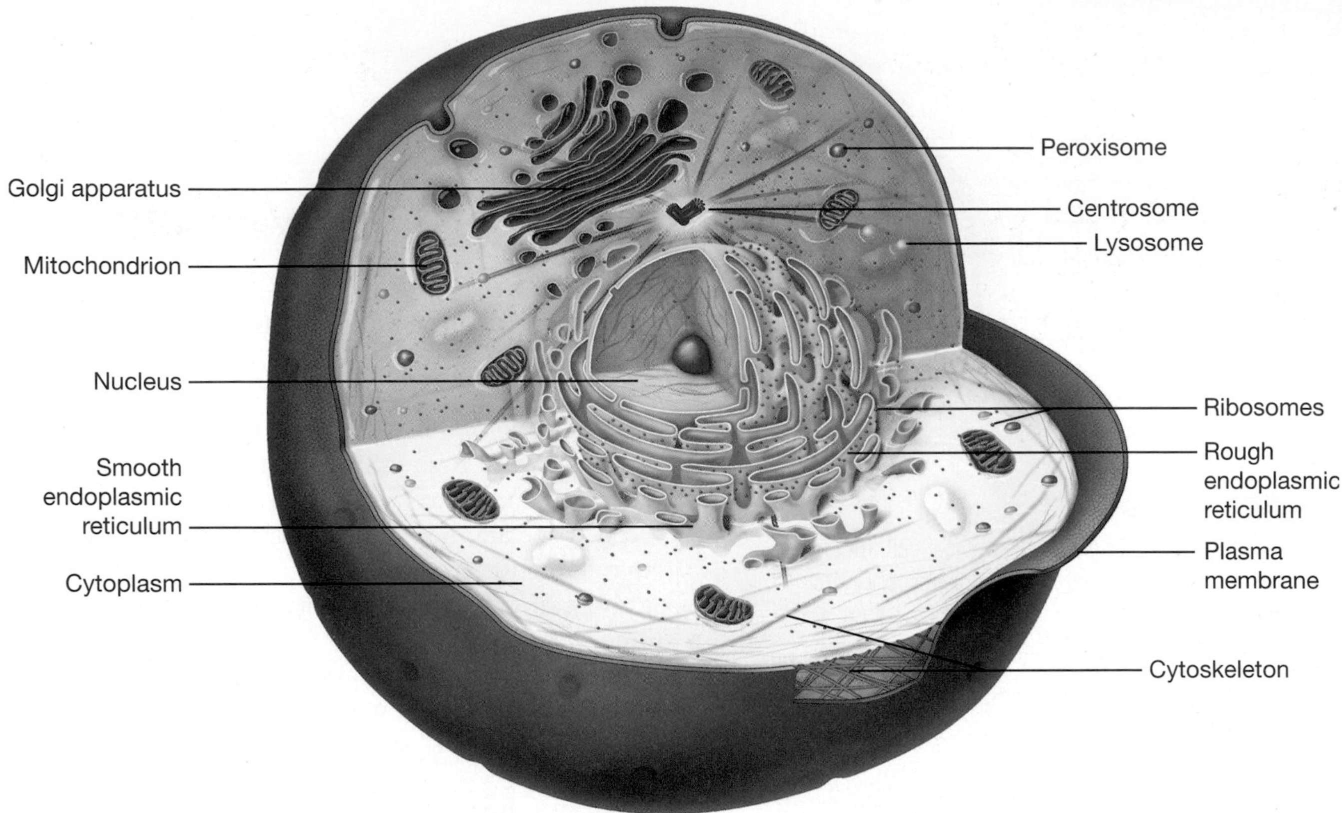

Figure 2.14 A typical cell. *If you were asked to label the area outside of this cell, what label would you use?*

substances are smaller. This selective property is important for controlling the cell's pH.

Other channels allow potassium ions to cross, but they do not let smaller sodium ions through. This ability of the channels to be selective is trickier than it might seem given that potassium and sodium ions are electrically similar (both have a single positive charge), but sodium ions are smaller. It is not obvious how one would design a channel that would let a large, similarly charged ion to pass through yet prevent a smaller ion from passing through.

Glycoproteins (GLIGH-koh-PROH-teenz) are proteins with carbohydrate groups attached. These proteins are usually found in the plasma membrane, with the carbohydrate group projecting into the extracellular fluid.

The layer of carbohydrate groups surrounding a cell is called the *glycocalyx* (GLIGH-koh-KAY-liks). The glycocalyx helps cells bind to extracellular substances, which is important for cell recognition. Immune system cells, for example, are always on the lookout for foreign cells and try to destroy those cells when they are found. The glycocalyx helps to identify the body's own cells as friend, not foe, to the immune system.

Membrane Transport

As you have just read, living cells take in substances (such as oxygen and glucose) and move out substances (such as carbon dioxide and other metabolic wastes). Membrane transport is the movement of these substances across the plasma membrane. Membrane transport can occur in one of two basic ways: by passive transport or active transport.

Passive transport does not require the expenditure of any extra energy. Passive transport usually involves **diffusion**—the movement of material from a place where it is concentrated to a place where it is less concentrated. For example, if you drop food coloring into a glass of water, the coloring is initially concentrated at the point where it hits the water. Gradually, however, the food coloring spreads and evens out—the result of diffusion.

Some small, non-polar molecules, such as oxygen and carbon dioxide, can diffuse directly through the cell membrane. This is called *simple diffusion*. Many other important molecules cannot penetrate the membrane, but they may diffuse by

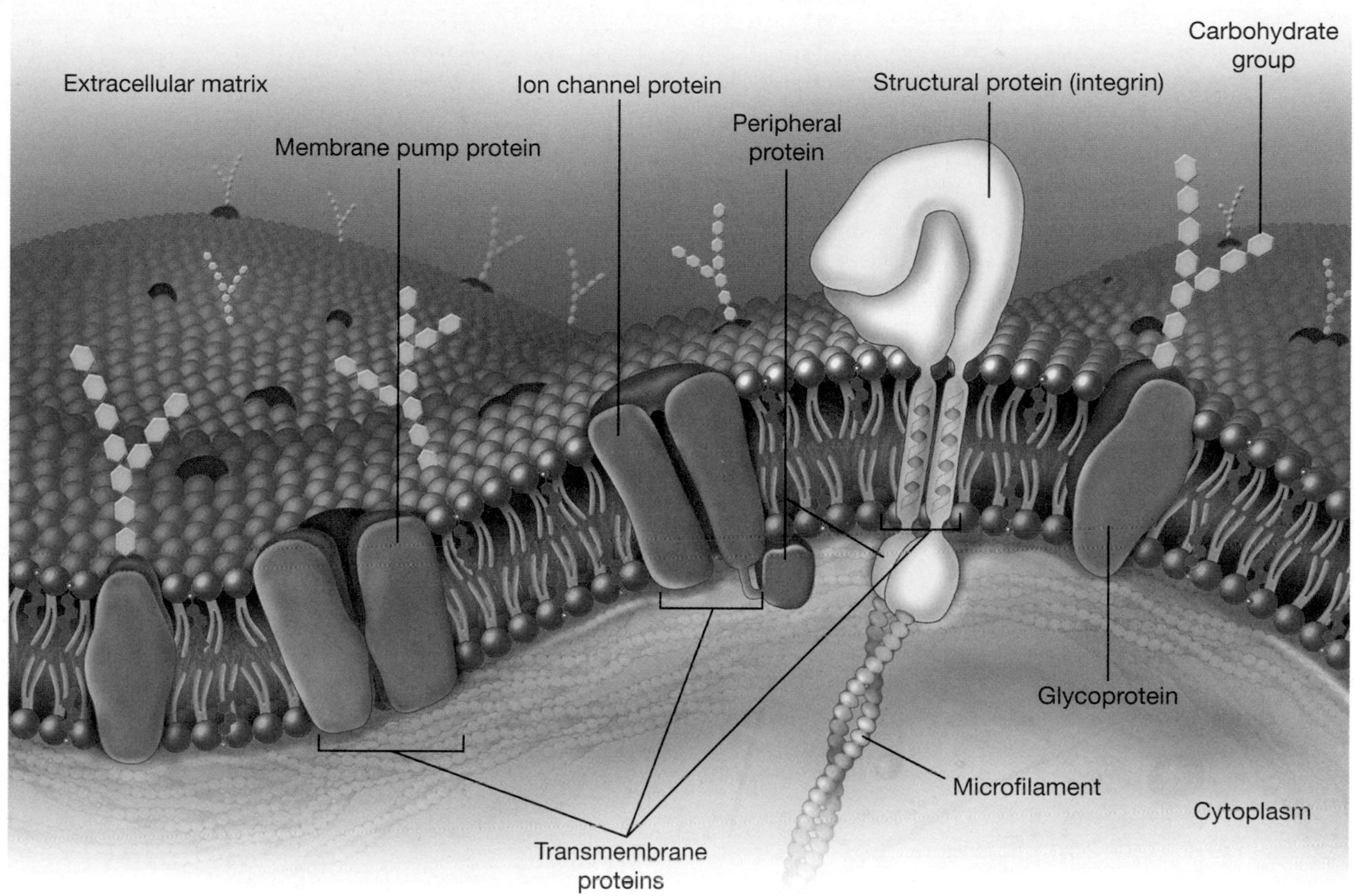

Figure 2.15 The plasma membrane. *What is the major purpose of the structural proteins in the plasma membrane?*

a process called *facilitated diffusion*. Proteins in the membrane that act as passive pores (channel proteins) or carriers allow facilitated diffusion of molecules including sodium, potassium, chloride, glucose, and many others. Aquaporin channels, for example, allow water to enter and leave cells by passive transport. The word *osmosis* is used by physiologists to refer to the movement of water by diffusion across cell membranes.

Active transport requires energy because it involves making a substance go where it "does not want to go": from areas of lower concentration to areas of higher concentration. The most important and widespread examples of active transport are the movement of sodium *out* of a cell and potassium *into* the cell. Because a resting cell has much less sodium inside than it does outside, energy is required to move the sodium out. Similarly, a cell with more potassium inside than outside needs energy to move potassium in. For this purpose, the cell membrane has a sodium-potassium pump protein. The pump breaks down the high-energy molecule ATP, and it uses the energy from the ATP to pump sodium out of the cell and potassium into the cell.

Endocytosis and exocytosis are other forms of active transport which are essential for cellular function. In **endocytosis**, a region of the cell membrane forms a pocket into the cell and then pinches off to form a membrane-bound sac, or vesicle, inside the cytoplasm. This brings with it anything that was bound to that piece of membrane, including small molecules dissolved in the extracellular fluid. **Exocytosis** is the opposite process: a small, membrane-bound vesicle in the cytoplasm fuses with the cell's membrane. This exports molecules that were inside the vesicle to the outside.

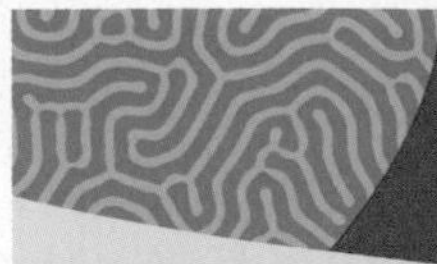

What Research Tells Us

...about Integrating Physical and Chemical Processes

As you know, different processes and control systems interact with one another to maintain homeostasis—ongoing balance within the body's internal environment. This happens even when the body faces extreme challenges. Examples include active and passive transport, equilibrium, pH balance, and biofeedback mechanisms.

Active and Passive Transport

Active and passive transport are inherently stable processes. "Inherently stable" means that small disturbances to the body's internal environment naturally tend to be corrected because of the way in which a process works.

The movement of potassium into and out of a muscle cell illustrates this point. Research has shown that during exercise a small amount of potassium leaves a muscle cell with each muscle twitch. During intense exercise the amount of potassium inside the cell may start to drop slightly, and the amount outside the cell may start to rise. This change in potassium balance across the cell membrane causes more potassium to enter the cell by passive transport because there is more potassium outside the cell and less inside the cell than usual. The passive transport process tends to bring the cell back to its normal, steady state.

The lower levels of potassium also cause the sodium-potassium pump, which actively transports sodium out of the cell and potassium into the cell, to run a bit faster. This active transport process, like the passive process, helps to correct the potassium imbalance.

You might think that pushing the sodium out of the cell would disrupt its sodium balance. This is not the case, however, because exercise also causes excess sodium accumulation inside the cell. Thus, speeding up the pump helps to fix the sodium imbalance as well as the potassium imbalance. In short, the active and passive transport processes, working together, naturally tend to correct temporary imbalances.

Equilibrium

A cell maintaining homeostasis is in a steady state, but it is *not* at equilibrium. The difference between a steady state and equilibrium is important. In fact, it is a matter of life and death.

Life is a nonequilibrium state of affairs. A living organism is not in equilibrium with its surroundings. However, an organism that is no longer living is, or soon will be, in a state of equilibrium.

Body temperature is a good example of this concept. Humans and other mammals are warm-blooded. The scientific term for this is *homeothermic* (from the Greek word for "same temperature"). The human nervous system and endocrine system are control systems that help to maintain a constant internal body temperature, which is in a steady state but not at equilibrium with the surroundings. If core body temperature starts to deviate from the norm, the nervous system and the endocrine system initiate responses that bring the temperature back to normal.

pH Balance

Like temperature, pH is a closely regulated internal property of the body. For example, the pH of arterial blood is about 7.35 to 7.45. Chemicals in the blood, especially bicarbonate ions (HCO_3) and circulating proteins, act as buffers that tend to prevent pH from changing. In addition, the respiratory system and the urinary system help to regulate blood pH via mechanisms that will be discussed in later chapters.

Biofeedback

The regulation of sodium concentration, body temperature, pH, and other physiological states occurs subconsciously, for most people, most of the time. In other words, you do not have to consciously think about the levels of these substances to control them. It is possible, however, to learn how to consciously control some of these variables. With training, some people have learned how to control their heart rate, blood pressure, and even body temperature. *Biofeedback* and *neurofeedback* both refer to the ability to control such variables. Biofeedback has been shown to be useful in treating certain medical conditions, including some types of headaches.

Taking It Further

1. In Lessons 2.1 and 2.2 you have read several examples of the integration of chemical and physical processes to achieve homeostasis. Select one of these examples or choose one of your own, do further research on the integrated processes, and then prepare a detailed description for your class.

Cytoskeleton

The **cytoskeleton** is a network of proteins that defines the shape of a cell and gives it mechanical strength (**Figure 2.16**). The cytoskeleton rearranges itself when necessary to change the shape of the cell or to allow the cell to move to a new location.

The cytoskeleton contains three types of long fibers that function as struts:

- Microfilaments, the thinnest of these fibers, are made of actin subunits. They are found in most cells and are especially prominent in muscle cells.
- Intermediate filaments are made of keratin. They extend across a cell and give the cell strength to resist external pulling forces.
- Microtubules (MIGH-kroh-TOO-byoolz) are the largest-diameter cytoskeletal fibers. They are composed of tubulin subunits that help separate and organize chromosomes during cell division. Motor proteins, such as kinesin and dynein, move along microtubules as they transport vesicles and other structures inside the cell (**Figure 2.16B**).

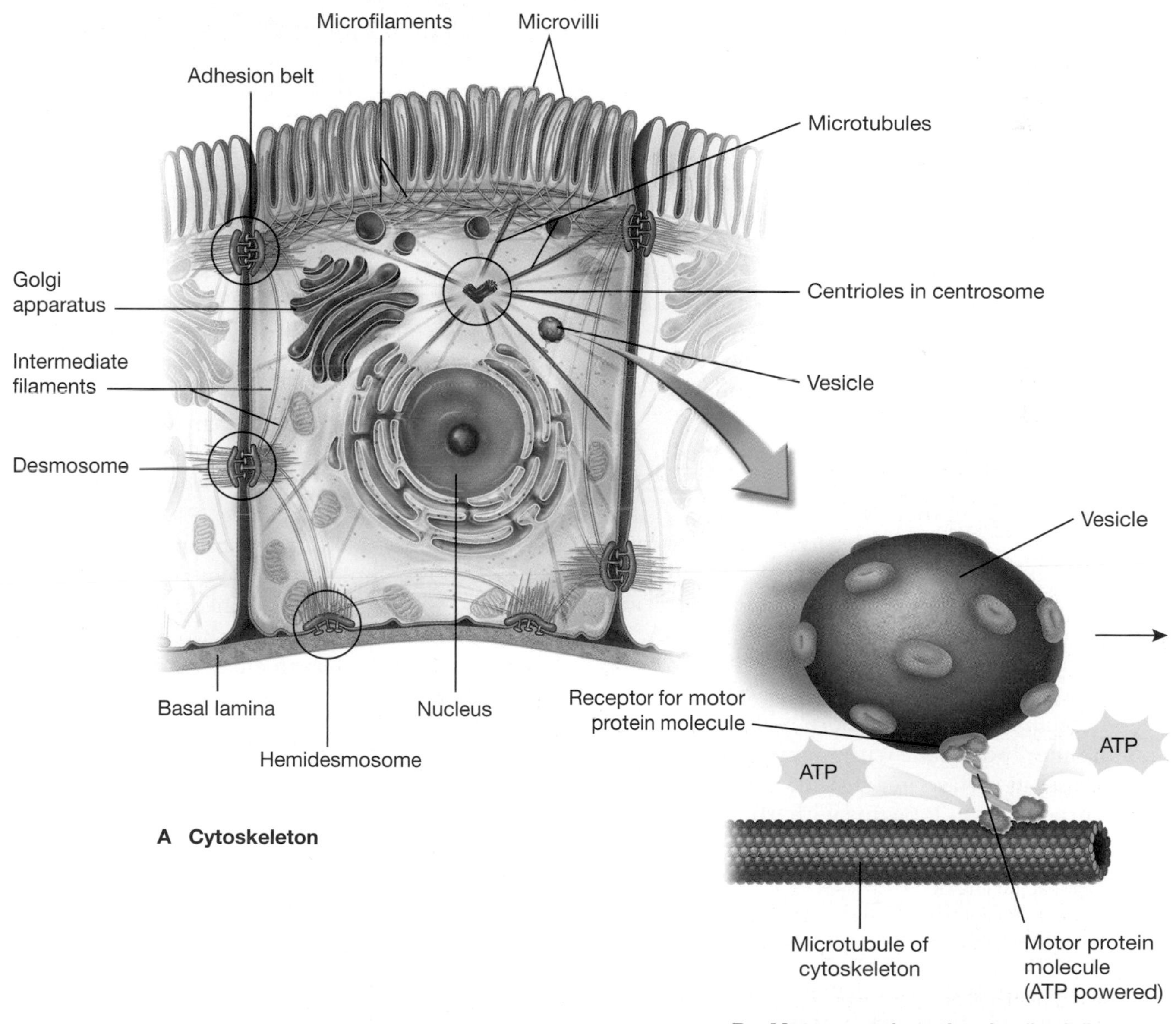

Figure 2.16 The cytoskeleton and the role of microtubules in cell division. *If you were to compare motor proteins and microtubules to automobiles and highways, which structure would be the automobile and which would be the highway?*

Some cells have **microvilli** (MIGH-kroh-vil-ee), finger-like extensions that increase the surface area of a cell. Microfilaments, the stringy proteins inside the microvilli, provide structural support.

Other cells have hair-like projections called **cilia** (SIL-ee-a), which are longer than microvilli. Cilia actively flex back and forth to move fluid or mucus across the outside of the cell. The active beating of cilia is caused by the microtubules inside them.

Most cells have a pair of **centrioles** (SEHN-tree-ohlz) in the centrosome (SEHN-troh-sohm), an area of the cell near the nucleus. Each centriole is a short cylinder made of nine triplets of parallel microtubules. The centrioles help guide the movement and separation of chromosomes during cell division.

Mitochondria and the Making of ATP

Mitochondria (migh-toh-KAHN-dree-a) are tubular-shaped organelles ("little organs") in the cytoplasm of cells. Mitochondria are responsible for making ATP. For this reason, mitochondria are often called the "powerhouses" of the cell. Cardiac muscle cells have abundant mitochondria to meet their large and unending demand for energy to drive muscular contraction. Cells with minimal energy needs have few mitochondria.

When a human egg is fertilized, the sperm contributes very few or zero mitochondria. Therefore the mitochondria in the zygote (fertilized egg) and in all subsequent cells are inherited from the maternal side. Mitochondria also have their own small loops of DNA. Some of the proteins in mitochondria are derived from genes on the mitochondrial DNA. The other proteins in mitochondria come from genes in the cell nucleus.

Mitochondria have a smooth outer membrane and an inner membrane with many cristae (folds) that increase its surface area, as shown in **Figure 2.17**. The synthesis of ATP begins with **glycolysis** (gligh-KAWL-i-sis), the breakdown of a glucose molecule into two pyruvate (PIGH-roo-vayt) molecules. Glycolysis occurs in the cytoplasm, outside the mitochondria.

The pyruvates pass from the cytoplasm into the mitochondrial matrix, the space inside the inner membrane. Enzymes in this space catalyze the reactions of the **citric acid cycle** (also known as the *Krebs cycle* or the *tricarboxylic acid cycle*). As a result of this chain of reactions, each pyruvate is

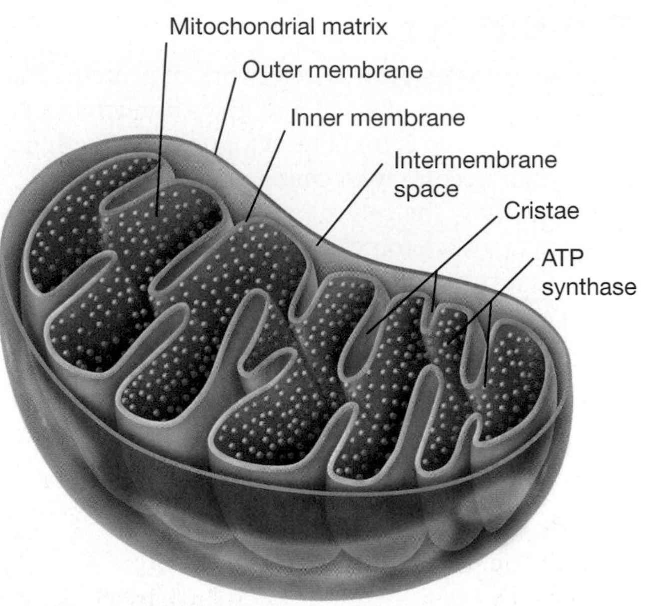

Figure 2.17 A mitochondrion. *Why is this structure called a "powerhouse"?*

broken down into individual carbon atoms, which combine with oxygen molecules to make CO_2.

The energy from pyruvate breakdown is used to pump hydrogen ions into the intermembrane space, which is, not surprisingly, the space between the inner and outer membrane of the mitochondrion. ATP synthase, an enzyme present in large numbers in the inner membrane, captures the energy from the hydrogen ions escaping from the intermembrane space. It then uses that energy to add inorganic phosphate to ADP, thus completing the synthesis of ATP (**Figure 2.12**). The newly formed ATP leaves the mitochondrion and enters the cytoplasm, where it can be used as an energy source for many different processes.

Golgi Apparatus

The **Golgi** (GOHL-jee) **apparatus**, or Golgi, is a set of membranous discs in the cytoplasm, usually between the endoplasmic reticulum and the plasma membrane of the cell (**Figure 2.14**). The Golgi produces small membranous spheres called *vesicles*.

Some of the vesicles deliver new membrane, sometimes with newly embedded proteins, to the cell's plasma membrane. Some vesicles are packed with proteins or glycoproteins that are destined for secretion from the cell. Other vesicles, called *lysosomes* (LIGH-soh-sohmz), are compartments in which reactions involving potentially dangerous enzymes and reactants can be conducted in isolation from the rest of the cytoplasm.

All the vesicles may need proteins, which are received at the inner side of the Golgi (the forming face) as transport vesicles from the endoplasmic reticulum. The proteins may be modified or sorted in the Golgi before they are released in vesicles from the outer side of the Golgi (the maturing face).

Ribosomes and Endoplasmic Reticulum

Ribosomes (RIGH-boh-sohmz) are very large enzymes that make polypeptides. A ribosome is made up of a small and a large subunit. Each subunit includes ribosomal RNA and protein subunits. Even the small subunit is large by molecular standards, with thousands of bases of RNA and dozens of protein subunits.

The small and large subunits are assembled separately in the nucleolus (part of the nucleus). They then move out to the cytoplasm, where they join to form a functional ribosome. Some ribosomes are found free in the *cytosol* (the liquid part of the cytoplasm); others are attached to the rough endoplasmic reticulum.

Endoplasmic reticulum (ER), shown in **Figure 2.18**, is a network of membranes in the cytoplasm. The ER is near, and connected to, the nuclear envelope (the membrane that defines the boundary of the cell nucleus). Rough ER, when viewed through an electron microscope, is (as the name implies) rough looking because it has ribosomes attached to it. It often has flattened or sheet-like chambers called *cisternae* (sis-TER-nee). Smooth ER does not have ribosomes attached to it, and it often has tubular cisternae.

The rough endoplasmic reticulum is a site for protein production and modification. Ribosomes on rough ER make polypeptides and secrete them into the cisternae of the rough ER. Here the polypeptides may join with other polypeptides to form a multi-subunit protein, or they may be modified by chemical reactions that alter their size or shape. Not all proteins are made on the rough ER, however. Free ribosomes in the cytoplasm also make many proteins.

Smooth ER makes “replacement” membrane for membranous structures in the cell, including the plasma membrane, the nuclear envelope, mitochondria, ER, and Golgi. It also produces steroid hormones in cells of the reproductive organs and triglycerides in adipocytes (fat cells) and hepatocytes (liver cells).

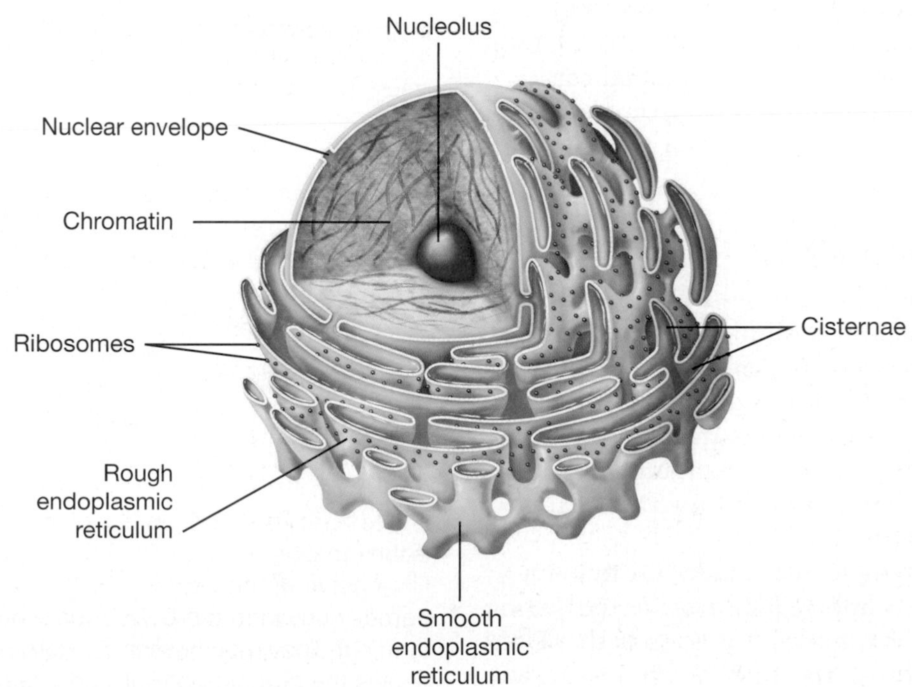

Figure 2.18 The nucleus and associated endoplasmic reticulum. *What creates the difference in appearance between smooth and rough endoplasmic reticulum?*

A cistern is a chamber or tank for holding water. The corresponding Latin words are *cisterna* (singular) and *cisternae* (plural). Besides referring to the interior of the endoplasmic reticulum, these words refer to the interior of the Golgi apparatus membrane compartments and to the interior of the sarcoplasmic reticulum in muscle.

The Nucleus: Home of DNA

The cell nucleus, shown in **Figure 2.14**, contains the cell's genetic information—its DNA. It also contains some, but not all, of the cell's RNA and many proteins that are involved with the coiling, uncoiling, copying, and maintaining of DNA.

The nuclear envelope is a lipid bilayer folded over to form a double membrane. It contains protein-lined pores that allow small molecules to pass in and out of the nucleus. The nucleolus is an area in the nucleus where ribosomal RNA is made and packaged with protein subunits to make the small and large ribosomal subunits. Nucleoli are not present in all cells all the time.

All of a cell's DNA resides in the nucleus. When a cell is neither dividing nor about to divide, the DNA is spread throughout the nucleus. It wraps around small proteins called *histones* (HIS-tohns). The mixture of DNA and associated protein is called *chromatin* (KROH-mah-tin).

When cell division is about to begin, the DNA becomes much more organized. It wraps into tight bundles called *chromosomes*. As described earlier, each chromosome contains one DNA molecule plus the many proteins that enable it to coil.

DNA, RNA, and Proteins

Three biological polymers—DNA, RNA, and proteins—are made up of similar but not identical subunits, which must be present in a specific order to work correctly. DNA and RNA are made of nucleotides, and proteins are made of amino acids. In each case, the order of subunits is a form of information; the use and continuation of this information is essential for life.

How are these molecules made? Or to put it another way, how is information transferred among the molecules? The quick explanation is that DNA is used to make RNA, and RNA is used to make protein. This fundamental concept is regarded as the core principle of molecular biology.

Making RNA from DNA

The sequence of bases in DNA contains the information essential for making the proteins and RNA needed for life. The production of RNA from DNA is shown in **Figure 2.19**. This process is called **transcription**.

RNA polymerase (pahl-IM-er-ays) is the enzyme that makes an RNA molecule complementary to a gene on DNA. RNA polymerase binds to a

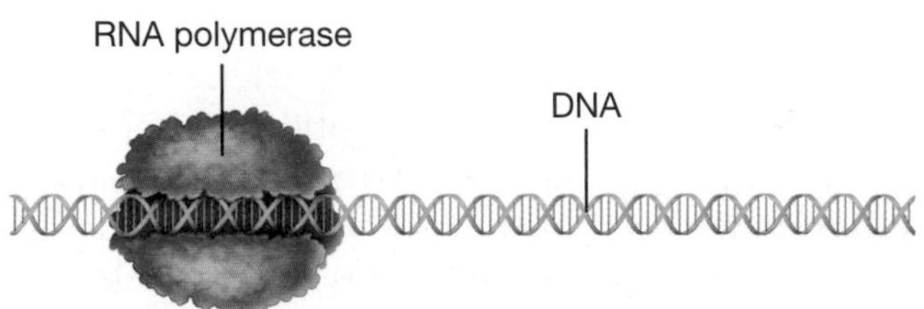

A RNA polymerase binds to DNA

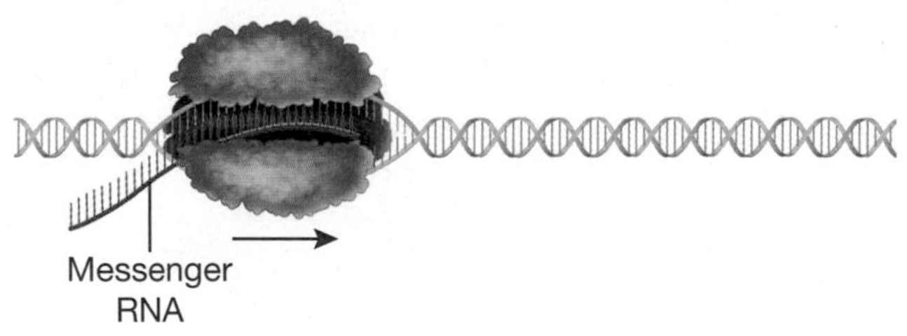

B RNA polymerase "unzips" the DNA and begins forming mRNA

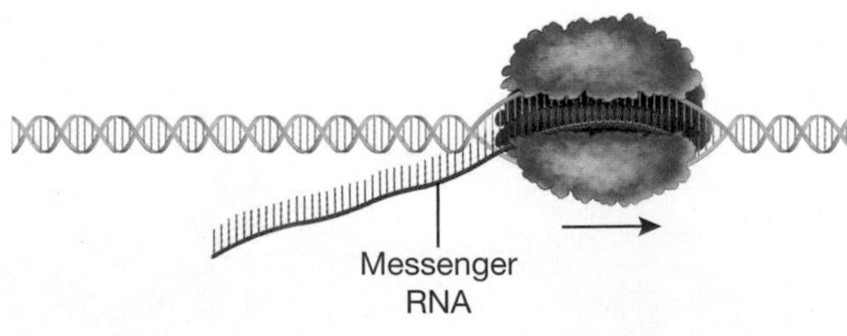

C RNA polymerase continues to form mRNA as it moves along the DNA

Figure 2.19 Transcription, which occurs in the nucleus, is the creation of a new RNA molecule. A—The enzyme RNA polymerase binds to DNA. B—RNA polymerase partially unwinds the DNA double helix and begins to form a molecule of messenger RNA (mRNA). The arrow shows the direction of RNA polymerase movement. C—RNA polymerase continues along the DNA, adding new bases to the growing mRNA molecule.

MEMORY TIP

Transcription and translation—which comes first, and what does each accomplish? It helps to remember that "DNA makes RNA makes protein" and to think of the everyday meaning of *transcribing* and *translating*.

Transcribing is copying words (or numbers) from one place to another, without changing them. Someone taking precise notes in class is transcribing the teacher's words. If you copy a line from a book into an email, you are transcribing. Likewise, when a cell makes RNA from DNA, it is simply copying, or transcribing, the information from one nucleic acid molecule to another.

Translating involves converting information from one language to another. In translating, the meaning is the same, but the words are not the same. When a cell makes protein from RNA, it is converting from the language of nucleotides to the language of amino acids.

So, transcription is making RNA from DNA, and translation is making protein from RNA.

region of DNA at the starting point of a gene. The DNA "unzips" in the region where the RNA polymerase binds. The RNA polymerase then starts moving along the DNA, one base at a time. As it moves, it generates an RNA strand whose nucleotides are complementary to the DNA nucleotides. RNA uses uracil (U) as the base complementary to adenine (A). In DNA, thymine (T) is the base complementary to A.

As the RNA polymerase moves along, the DNA strands reclose behind it. When the RNA polymerase encounters the end of the gene, it detaches from the DNA and releases the RNA strand. The RNA strand is called **messenger RNA (mRNA)** because it carries a message: the base sequence information that will be used to make a protein.

Making a Polypeptide from mRNA

The mRNA molecule made by transcription leaves the nucleus via a pore. Every three bases along the mRNA specifies, or codes for, one amino acid in the polypeptide. A **codon** (KOH-dahn) is a set of three bases in the mRNA that codes for one amino acid. It takes a 300-base (100-codon) mRNA strand to code for a protein 100 amino acids long. An mRNA molecule is like a blueprint for making a polypeptide.

In the cytoplasm, a small ribosomal subunit attaches to the beginning of the mRNA molecule. A **transfer RNA (tRNA)** molecule also binds to the mRNA-ribosome complex. Each tRNA can bind to one and only one amino acid, and each tRNA has a specific *anticodon*, a set of three bases that are complementary to a three-base codon on mRNA. The tRNA that binds to the ribosome and mRNA has its specific amino acid attached.

With the help of the ribosome, the tRNA aligns its three-base anticodon with the complementary three-base codon of the mRNA. Then the large ribosomal subunit binds, and a second tRNA arrives with a codon complementary to the next codon on the mRNA. This results in a complex incorporating mRNA, tRNA, and rRNA (in the ribosome).

The ribosome now catalyzes the formation of a peptide bond between the two amino acids of the two tRNAs. It also catalyzes the breaking of the bond connecting the first amino acid to its tRNA. Then the first tRNA detaches from the mRNA-ribosome complex, and the ribosome moves over by one codon on the mRNA.

Then another tRNA, complementary to the third codon of the mRNA and loaded with its amino acid, arrives at the complex and aligns its anticodon with the third codon of the mRNA. The ribosome joins the three amino acids to the 2:1 chain, and this process continues until the ribosome reaches the end of the mRNA. Then the large and small ribosomal subunits detach from one another and from the mRNA, and the complete polypeptide is released.

Check Your Understanding

1. Where are glycoproteins usually found?
2. How does the glycocalyx help the immune system?
3. What is the difference between active and passive transport?
4. What are two functions that the cytoskeleton performs for a cell?
5. What is the function of the mitochondria?
6. Where are ribosomes located?

The Life Cycle of a Cell

It may seem surprising that most cells in the human body have a life span that is considerably shorter than that of humans.

For example, the cells lining the intestines have a life span of just 2 to 7 days. Red blood cells live for about 120 days (4 months). Many of the neurons (nerve cells) in the brain, on the other hand, are as old as the individual.

Because most cells have shorter lives than people do, they must divide to make new cells for the body. Cell division includes two major phases of a cell's life cycle: *interphase* and the *mitotic phase*. During interphase, the cell performs its usual functions and prepares for cell division. It is during the mitotic phase that the cell actually divides. The diagram in **Figure 2.20** illustrates the phases and subphases in the life cycle of a cell.

Interphase

Interphase is divided into three subphases. It includes two "gap" phases, G_1 and G_2. Between the gap phases is a synthetic (S) phase.

Of these three subphases, the duration of G_1 varies the most among different cell types. G_1 is long—sometimes years long—in cells that have a long life span, and short in cells that have a brief life span. The other two phases of the cycle—G_2 and S—are usually short (just minutes or hours).

Each of the 46 chromosomes in a typical human cell is duplicated in the S phase. The synthesis of new DNA is what gives this phase its name. You might want to review the process of DNA replication (**Figure 2.19**).

After the S phase, the cell enters the second gap phase (G_2). During G_2 the cell completes its preparations for cell division.

Multiple "checkpoints" occur during interphase. At each checkpoint a cell verifies that it has successfully completed the appropriate steps

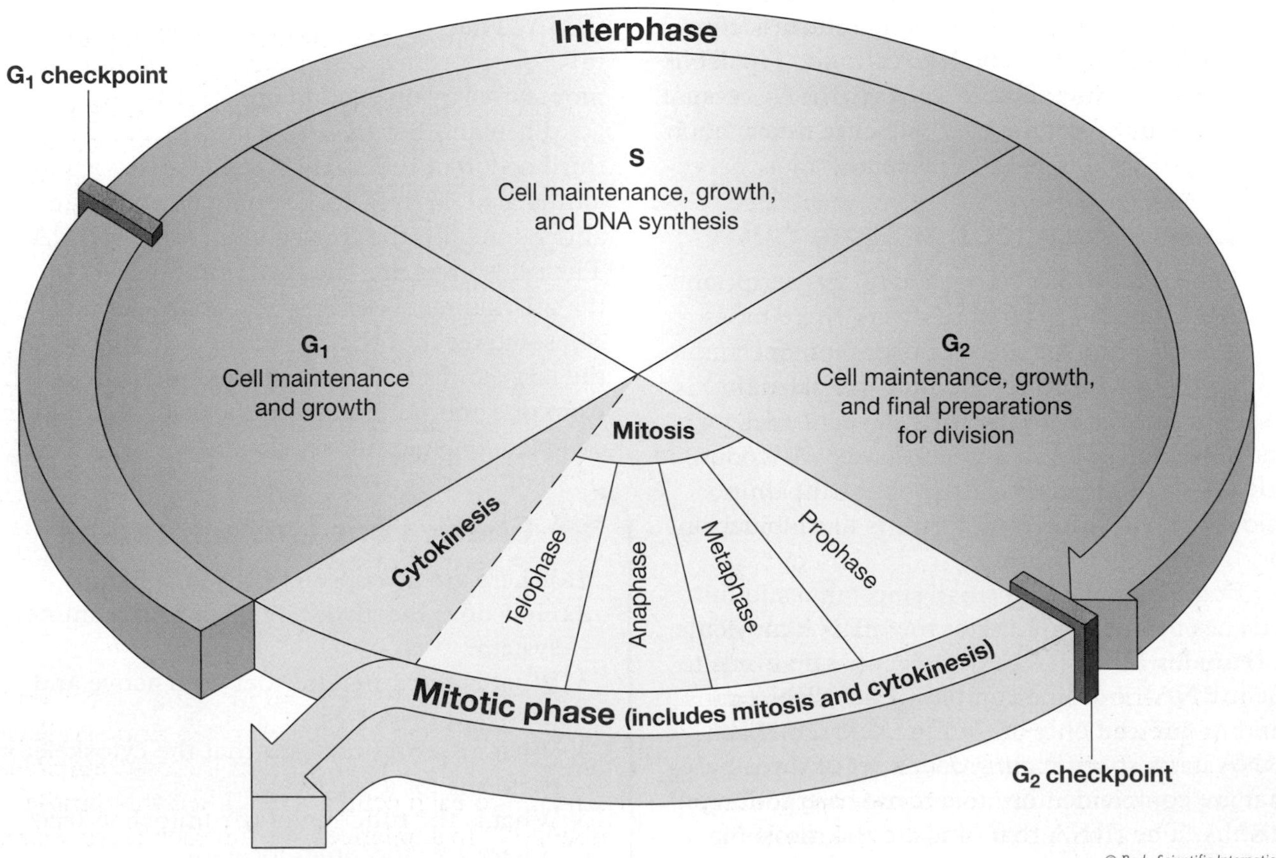

Figure 2.20 The two phases in the life cycle of a cell are interphase, when it is not dividing, and the mitotic phase, when it is dividing. Each of these phases is divided into subphases. *What is the last phase of mitosis?*

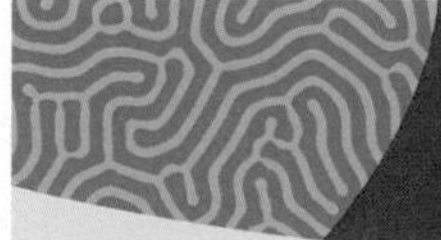

What Research Tells Us

... About Checkpoint Inhibitors

As explained in Lesson 2.2, a cell cycle checkpoint is a part of the cell's life cycle that regulates cell division. At each checkpoint, a cell will not proceed to the next phase of division if intracellular conditions such as significant DNA damage are detected. Damage to aspects of the checkpoint systems can increase the likelihood of cancer because cells with DNA damage are not prevented from dividing.

For example, the genes BRCA1 and BRCA2 code for proteins which play important roles in cell checkpoints. When these genes are damaged and the normal proteins are reduced or absent, the checkpoint systems may not work correctly. This increases the risk of cancer, including breast cancer, which is why the genes are called BRCA1 and BRCA2.

With that in mind, it may seem surprising that scientists looking for better cancer treatments would look for drugs to *inhibit* cell cycle checkpoints. It is true, however, and there is considerable excitement in the cancer care community about the potential of these drugs. To understand the role of checkpoint inhibitors in cancer therapy, you need to know a little about the immune system and cancer. T lymphocytes, also known as *T cells*, are white blood cells, which you will learn more about in Chapter 12. These immune cells attack foreign and abnormal cells.

T cells have unique cell cycle checkpoints that prevent them from attacking normal cells. Cancer cells often express many proteins that cause T cells to stop at the checkpoint. New drugs are available that inhibit the checkpoints in T cells. When the checkpoints are inhibited, T cells can be coaxed to attack tumors. At present, a half dozen immune checkpoint inhibitor drugs have been approved for cancer therapy by the US Food and Drug Administration, and more drugs are in the testing pipeline.

for that phase of the cycle and is ready to progress to the next phase. This verification process often involves checking for DNA damage and repairing any damage, if found, before clearing the checkpoint.

It should be noted that some cells never divide. Examples include red blood cells and most nerve cells in the brain. Cells such as these are said to be in *phase* G_0.

Mitotic Phase

The mitotic phase can be divided into two types of division: mitosis and cytokinesis. **Mitosis** is the division of a cell nucleus and chromosomes into two nuclei, each with its own set of identical chromosomes. **Cytokinesis** is the division of the cytoplasm. Mitosis followed by cytokinesis results in the formation of two identical daughter cells.

Mitotic cell division is the process by which a single fertilized egg cell develops into an adult made of trillions of cells. Meiosis, a different kind of nuclear division, will be discussed in Chapter 15. This chapter takes a closer look at mitosis—divided into prophase, metaphase, anaphase, and telophase—and cytokinesis (**Figure 2.21**). Keep in mind that when mitosis begins, the DNA has already been duplicated.

Prophase

In prophase, the chromatin (DNA plus associated proteins) "condenses" to form chromosomes, which are visible in the light microscope. Each chromosome is made of two identical DNA molecules, which are joined to each other at the centromere. As a result, each chromosome resembles a narrow X, and the centromere is the center of the X.

The two DNA molecules in a chromosome are called *sister chromatids*, and they form the two sides of each X-shaped chromosome. At the same time the chromosomes are forming, the nuclear membrane is breaking down, and the centrioles are migrating to opposite sides of the cell. Microtubules start to grow away from the centrioles, forming spindle fibers. The spindle fibers form *asters* (from the Latin for "star").

Metaphase

In metaphase, some spindle fibers "lock on" to the centromeres of the chromosomes. At least one spindle fiber from each of the two centrioles attaches to each centromere. Then the spindle fibers pull in a balanced way on each chromosome, causing all the chromosomes to be positioned along the midline of the cell.

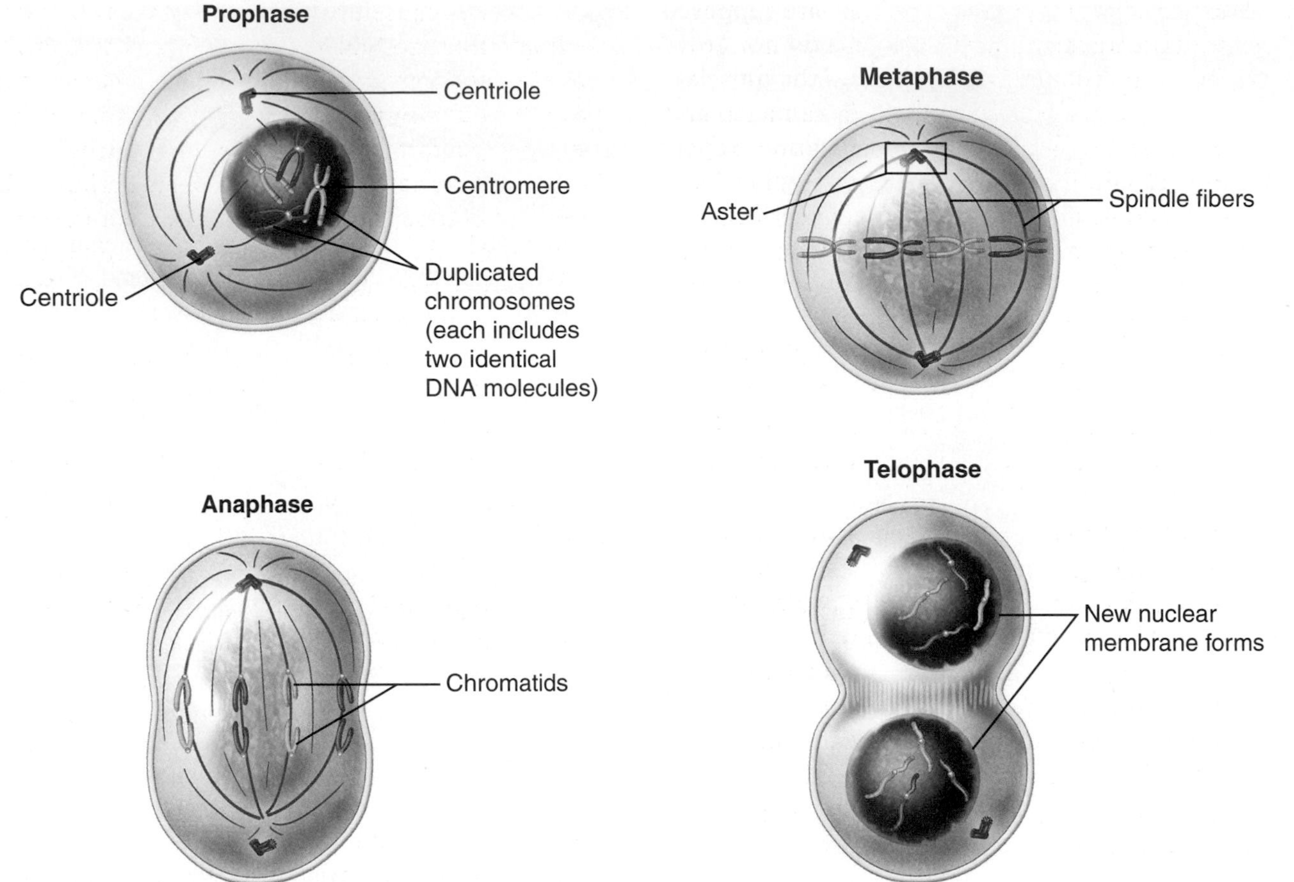

Figure 2.21 Mitosis. During telophase another process—cytokinesis—begins. *How many chromosomes would be shown if this were a human cell?*

Anaphase

In anaphase, the enzyme separase (sehp-a-RAYS), which functions like a molecular scissors, cuts each centromere in half. Now the sister chromatids are free to move apart. Each chromatid pulls itself along the spindle toward the centriole. As a result, 46 chromatids go to one side, and the other 46 chromatids go to the other side.

Telophase

In telophase, the chromosomes gather around each centriole, where they "decondense," which means that they spread out and are no longer visible in the light microscope. The spindles disappear, and a new nuclear membrane forms around the DNA. Mitosis is now complete. One nucleus has become two, and the DNA has been equally divided.

Cytokinesis

During telophase, cytokinesis begins. Cytokinesis is the division of the cytoplasm into two parts—the final step in cell division. A ring of actin microfilaments forms a circle around the cell. Myosin proteins pull on the actin filaments, making them shorten, much like what happens when you pull on a purse string. As a result of this pulling process, a *cleavage furrow*, or deepening groove, forms around the middle of the cell. The cleavage furrow gets tighter and tighter, until the cell splits into two daughter cells. Now cell division is complete.

Cancer

When the cell division process just described does not work properly, serious problems, such as cancer, occur. Cancer is the uncontrolled division and growth of abnormal cells. Normal cells divide just enough to allow people to grow when they are young, and just enough to replace dead or injured cells in adults.

Normal cells grow only where they are supposed to grow. This means that muscle cells do not grow in the brain, nor do brain cells grow in the muscles. A normal cell can detect if its DNA is damaged and tries to repair the damage. If the cell cannot repair the DNA, it will, in a sense, "commit suicide," a process called *apoptosis*. In general, cancer cells grow more than they should, they grow in places where they do not belong, and they do not destroy themselves when they should.

Cancer is caused by damage to a cell's DNA molecules. A mutation is damage to DNA that changes the genetic code—the pattern of As, Ts, Cs, and Gs. A mutation does not always, or even usually, cause cancer.

Certain mutations, however, can put a cell on the pathway to cancer. Mutations to genes that govern DNA repair, cell-cycle checkpoints, and apoptosis have all been implicated in cancer. For example, if a cell's DNA repair mechanism is damaged, more and more mutations tend to accumulate. If checkpoint-related genes suffer mutations, then a cell with damaged DNA does not stop at the checkpoint as it should. If apoptosis genes are damaged, a cell fails to self-destruct when it should.

Cancer is caused by damage to DNA, but what causes damage to DNA? Some mutations seem to occur by random chance, or for reasons whose cause is thus far unknown. Scientists do know that various chemicals, cigarette smoke, alcohol, sunlight, X-rays, and some viruses can cause mutations. This means, of course, that people can reduce their risk of cancer by not smoking, limiting alcohol intake, wearing sunscreen, and being vaccinated for human papillomavirus, for example.

Some chemicals that disrupt the cytoskeleton are useful in cancer treatment because they interfere with mitosis. For example, paclitaxel interferes with microtubules and, therefore, prevents cells from segregating their chromosomes during mitosis. Paclitaxel is used as a chemotherapy drug for cancers of the lung, breast, and other organs. You will learn more about various types of cancer in chapters throughout this text.

Check Your Understanding

1. Describe the transcription process.
2. Explain the life cycle of a cell, including all the phases and subphases.
3. What is the relationship between mutations and cancer?

LESSON 2.2 Review and Assessment

Mini Glossary

Make sure that you know the meaning of each key term.

active transport a process that requires energy to move against a concentration gradient, from an area of lower concentration to one of higher concentration

centrioles short cylinders made of nine triplets of parallel microtubules

channel proteins molecules with a hollow central pore that allows water or small, charged particles of certain substances to pass into or out of the cells

cilia hair-like projections that actively flex back and forth to move fluid or mucus across the outside of a cell

citric acid cycle a chain of reactions, catalyzed by enzymes in the mitochondrial matrix, in which pyruvate is broken down into individual carbon atoms, which combine with oxygen molecules to make CO_2

codon a set of three bases in DNA or RNA that codes for one amino acid

cytokinesis division of the cytoplasm during cell division

cytoplasm the part of the cell that contains all of the organelles inside the cell membrane except the nucleus

cytoskeleton a network of proteins that defines the shape of a cell and gives it mechanical strength

diffusion the movement of material from a place where it is concentrated to a place where it is less concentrated

endocytosis process in which a region of a cell membrane forms a pocket into the cell and then pinches off to form a membrane-bound sac, or vesicle, inside the cytoplasm

endoplasmic reticulum (ER) a network of membranes in the cytoplasm

exocytosis process in which a small, membrane-bound vesicle in the cytoplasm fuses with the cell's membrane to export molecules that were inside the vesicle to the outside

extracellular fluid the liquid—consisting mostly of water—that surrounds a typical cell

extracellular matrix the solid or gel-like substance that surrounds a typical cell

glycolysis the breakdown of a glucose molecule into two pyruvate molecules

glycoproteins proteins with carbohydrate groups attached

Golgi apparatus a set of membranous discs in the cytoplasm

messenger RNA (mRNA) single-strand RNA molecule whose base sequence carries the information needed by a ribosome to make a protein

microvilli finger-like extensions that increase the surface area of a cell

mitochondria organelles in the cytoplasm that make ATP

mitosis the division of a cell nucleus and chromosomes into two nuclei, each with its own set of identical chromosomes

nucleus a rounded or oval mass of protoplasm within the cytoplasm of a cell that contains the cell's DNA and is bounded by a membrane

passive transport a method of transport that does not require any energy

plasma membrane the membrane that defines the outer shell of a cell

ribosomes very large enzymes that make polypeptides

transcription the production of RNA from DNA

transfer RNA (tRNA) a molecule that binds to the mRNA-ribosome complex and helps assemble amino acids into polypeptides

Know and Understand

1. The material outside of and between cells is called _____.
2. What is a glycocalyx?
3. In what part of the cell can you find mitochondria?
4. Vesicles are produced in the _____, which is located in the cytoplasm of a cell.
5. DNA is contained in the _____ of a cell.
6. How does mRNA leave the nucleus?

Analyze and Apply

7. How might the human body be different if body cells had walls instead of membranes?
8. Explain the relationship between sodium and potassium in the sodium-potassium pump.
9. This lesson provided one example of diffusion: the dispersion of food coloring in water. Give two additional examples of diffusion.
10. Compare and contrast the body's skeleton to the cytoskeleton of body cells.
11. What process in a cell's life cycle could contribute to cancer?

IN THE LAB

12. Working with a partner, create a model of a typical cell. Include the following structures, making sure to place them properly: *centriole, channel protein* (just one as an example), *cilia, cytoplasm, endoplasmic reticulum, Golgi apparatus, microvilli* (just a small section as an example), *mitochondria, mRNA, nucleus, DNA, plasma membrane*, and *ribosomes*. Be creative in selecting materials for the various structures. Options include Jell-O with toothpicks for labels of structures, a shoebox with structures attached and labeled inside the box, or an opened beach ball with structures labeled inside.
13. If a microscope is available in your lab, view slides of cells in each stage of mitosis. Sketch what you see on each slide and write captions to explain what is happening.
14. Working in a team, find creative materials such as candy, string, pasta, clay, paper, toothpicks, Styrofoam, and so on, and use them to create a DNA model. Remember that DNA is the basic building block of life and contains all of the body's genetic material.
15. Working in a group of 4 students, find descriptions online of the four basic types of cellular reactions: synthesis, diffusion, single replacement, and double replacement. Condense the information about each type of reaction to create a simple formula or chemical word equation.
16. Conduct research to find out more about cell theory. Include a variety of sources, including scientific journals, news reports, and marketing and promotional materials. Evaluate the information from each source. Then write an essay briefly explaining current cell theory and its relationship to cell biology and life science theories.

LESSON 2.3

Tissues

Before You Read

Try to answer the following questions before you read this lesson.

- What are the major tissue types in the body?
- What are the functions of connective tissue?
- What does muscle tissue do that other types of tissue do not do?

Lesson Objectives

- Describe the various types and functions of epithelial tissue.
- Explain the properties and functions of different types of connective tissue.
- Identify the major types of muscle tissue.
- Describe the basic types and functions of nerve tissue.

Key Terms

adipose tissue	exocrine gland
areolar connective tissue	glands
cartilage	histology
chondroblasts	lumen
compressive strength	reticular connective tissue
connective tissue	simple epithelia
elasticity	stratified epithelia
endocrine gland	tensile strength
epithelial tissue	

Tissues are concentrations of cells with a similar structure that join together to accomplish a common function. The study of tissues is called **histology**. The many different tissues in the body have been classified into four main types: epithelial, connective, muscle, and nervous. Each of these has its own subtypes.

Organs and body systems are made of multiple types of tissues. Therefore, when one type of tissue is damaged by disease or trauma, the damage is usually accompanied by changes in nearby tissues. These changes can be helpful or harmful. For example, when epithelial cells of the skin are damaged by a first degree burn, blood flow beneath the damaged skin increases, and this promotes healing. On the other hand, when nerve tissue is damaged, the muscle tissue that the nerves stimulate tends to atrophy, or decrease in size, because the muscle is no longer receiving stimulatory nerve impulses.

Epithelial Tissue

Epithelial (EHP-i-THEE-lee-al) **tissue** includes epithelia and glands. *Epithelia* (singular: *epithelium*) are tissues that cover the body and line cavities within the body. Glands secrete chemicals, either to the outside world (exocrine glands) or within the body (endocrine glands). Epithelial tissues form the interface between the body and its surroundings. The design of epithelial tissues allows them to accomplish several functions:

- protecting the body from physical damage
- controlling what substances enter and leave the body
- providing sensory information
- secreting various substances

Epithelia: Inside and Outside

All epithelia have an inside and an outside, usually referred to as the *apical* (think *apex*, or *top*) and *basal* surface (think *base*). The apical surface faces the outside world, or the **lumen** (hollow inside portion) of a body cavity or tube, and the basal surface faces deeper body cells. For example, the surface of the skin is an epithelium that faces the outside world. It forms a barrier separating the inside of the body from the external environment.

Inside the body, however, it is not always obvious whether epithelial tissues separate the inside from the outside. In fact, most epithelia *do* separate inside from outside, if you define "outside" as a place that is connected to the external world, without any intervening tissues.

Figure 2.22 illustrates this concept of inside and outside. The figure shows the body as a rectangle penetrated by tubes that connect to the outside. The gastrointestinal tract (GI tract) runs through the body, from mouth to anus, so the lumen of the GI tract is all "outside." The

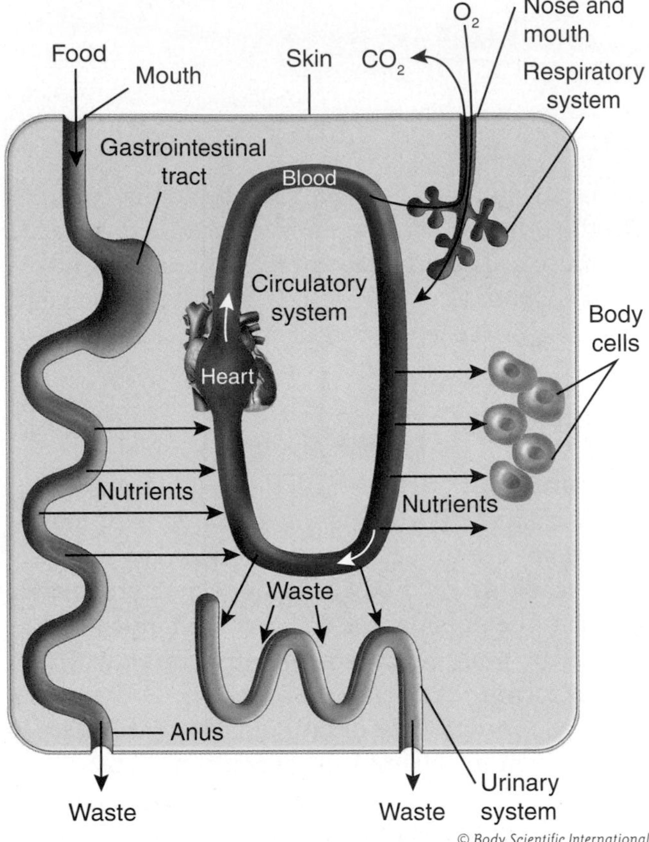

Figure 2.22 This diagram represents the human body's relationship to the outside world. *How do epithelial cells inside the body separate the internal environment from the external world?*

respiratory system, the urinary system, and the reproductive system (not shown) also connect to the outside. The only epithelia that do not separate outside from inside are the linings of the cardiovascular system and endocrine glands (which are not shown in the figure).

Epithelia: Cell Layers and Shapes

Epithelia are classified according to how many cell layers they have and the shape of those cells, as shown in **Figure 2.23**. **Simple epithelia** have a single layer of cells, and **stratified epithelia** have multiple layers of cells. The cell shapes include squamous (almost flat), cuboidal (height about equal to width), and columnar (tall and skinny). If an epithelium has multiple layers of cells that are not all the same shape, it is classified according to the shape of the most apical cells (that is, those on the top, facing outside).

Simple Epithelia

Simple squamous (SKWAY-muhs) *epithelia* have a single layer of flattened cells. The thinness of simple squamous epithelia allows rapid diffusion of substances. Examples of simple squamous epithelia in the body include:

- the gas-exchanging cavities (alveoli) of the lungs
- the lining of the abdominal cavity
- the endothelium, a single layer of cells that lines the blood vessels and the inside of the heart

Simple cuboidal epithelia have a single layer of cuboidal (roughly cube-shaped) cells. They surround tubules in the kidneys and are present in various secretory glands. They are typically involved with secretion or absorption.

Simple columnar epithelia have a single layer of columnar cells. They are found in the lining of some ducts in the kidneys and in the stomach and intestines, among other places. They sometimes have microvilli on their apical surfaces to increase surface area. **Figure 2.24** shows the simple columnar epithelium in the stomach. Like simple cuboidal epithelia, these epithelia have secretory and absorptive functions.

	Simple	Stratified
Squamous		
Cuboidal		
Columnar		

Figure 2.23 Types of epithelia. Some intermediate types, not shown, also exist.

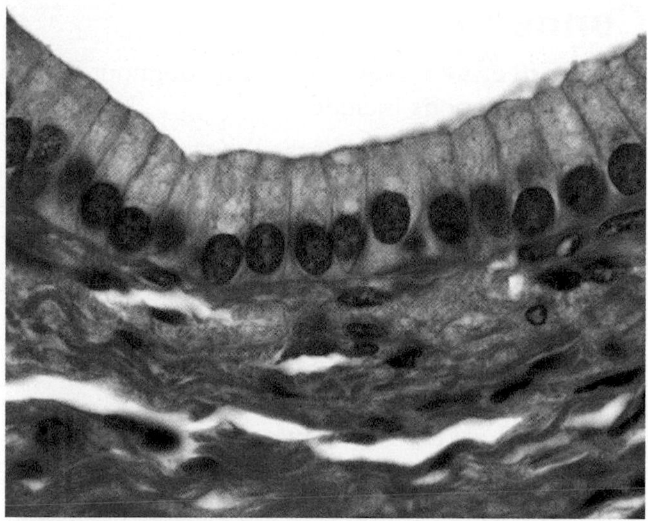

Jose Luis Calvo/Shutterstock.com

Figure 2.24 Light micrograph of a simple columnar epithelium. The purple ovals are cell nuclei.

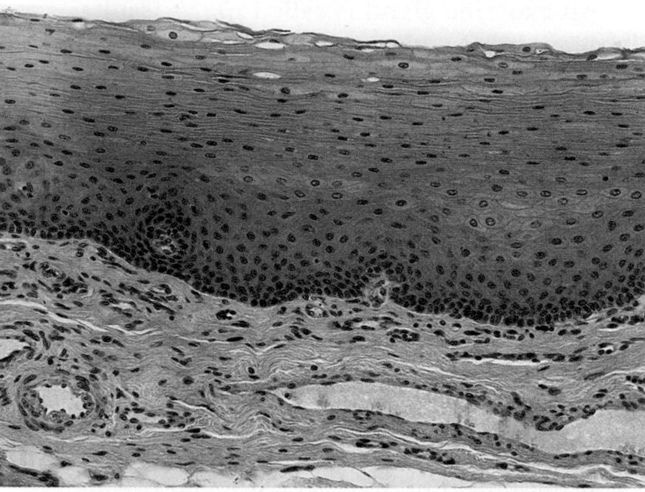

Jose Luis Calvo/Shutterstock.com

Figure 2.25 Light micrograph of stratified squamous epithelium. Here the epithelium extends from the surface, at the top, down to the basal cells, whose tightly packed nuclei form a dark layer. A lighter-staining layer of connective tissue lies below the epithelium. Dark circles are cell nuclei.

Stratified Epithelia

Stratified squamous epithelia are found where chemical and mechanical protection are most needed. The most familiar stratified squamous epithelium is the surface of the skin. Stratified squamous epithelia are also found in areas that are closely connected to the outside of the body, including the mouth, throat, anus, and rectum.

The most apical cells in the epithelium of the skin are actually dead and dying skin cells filled with the protein keratin (which also is a key component of hair and fingernails). The layer of keratinized cells helps prevent loss of water through the skin and provides additional protection. **Figure 2.25** shows the stratified epithelium of the esophagus.

Stratified cuboidal and stratified columnar epithelia are relatively rare. The stratified cuboidal epithelia are found in the ducts of some exocrine glands, including sweat glands. The stratified columnar epithelia line the ducts of the pancreas and salivary glands.

Other Epithelia

Some epithelia do not fit into the tidy classification scheme described so far. *Transitional epithelia*, for example, are stratified epithelia found in the lining of hollow organs that can stretch. For example, when the bladder is empty, or nearly so, it is relaxed, and the cells near the surface are rounded or cuboidal. When the bladder is full, however, the apical cells are stretched and have a more squamous appearance.

Glands

Epithelial cells that are organized to produce and secrete substances are called **glands**. A gland may have just a handful of cells, or it may be large and complex, with blood vessels and connective tissue, in which case it is considered a glandular organ.

An **exocrine gland** secretes its product to the outside world, as noted earlier. An **endocrine gland** secretes its product into the interstitial space. The secretion then diffuses from the interstitial space into the blood and is carried to the rest of the body. You will learn about the endocrine glands in Chapter 8.

Exocrine glands are classified by their structure. Unicellular (single-cell) exocrine glands are isolated secretory cells in an epithelium. In humans, unicellular exocrine glands are found in portions of the linings of the respiratory and digestive tracts. These cells secrete mucus, which forms a protective covering over the epithelial surface.

Multicellular exocrine glands (*multicellular* means "multiple cells") have two basic parts. One part is a secretory unit composed of cells that make and secrete a glandular product. The other part is a duct that connects the secretory unit to the surface of the epithelium.

An exocrine gland is called *simple* if it has a single, unbranched duct and *compound* if the duct branches as it travels from the surface to the secretory units. The secretory units of a gland may be tubular (tube-shaped) or alveolar, which is a more spherical shape. Some secretory units have both shapes and are therefore called tubuloalveolar (TOO-byool-oh-al-VEE-oh-lar). **Figure 2.26** shows examples of different types of exocrine glands.

Check Your Understanding

1. Where in the body are epithelial tissues found?
2. What are the two surfaces of an epithelium?
3. What four functions do epithelial tissues perform?
4. What is the difference between an exocrine gland and an endocrine gland?

Connective Tissue

Connective tissue is found throughout the body. Its functions include:

- giving the body and organs the strength to resist external forces, including gravity
- protecting internal organs
- maintaining the proper shape of organs (to keep the trachea, or windpipe, from collapsing, for example)
- providing a rigid framework on which muscle can pull, allowing movement

Connective tissue comprises several major classes: connective tissue proper, cartilage, bone, and blood. Blood connects distant body areas by circulating to all regions and carrying substances from place to place. You will learn about blood in more detail in Chapter 10.

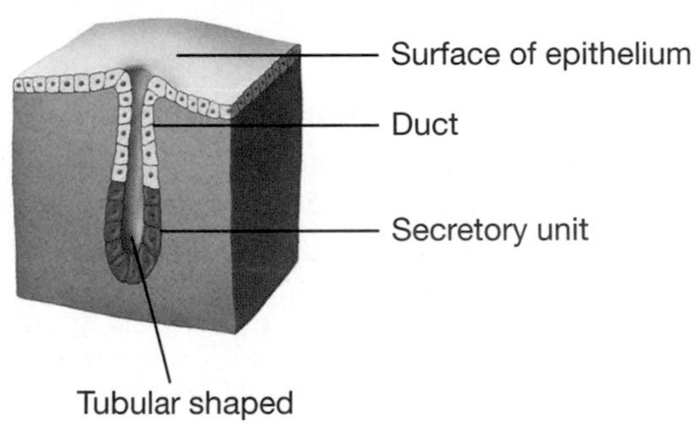

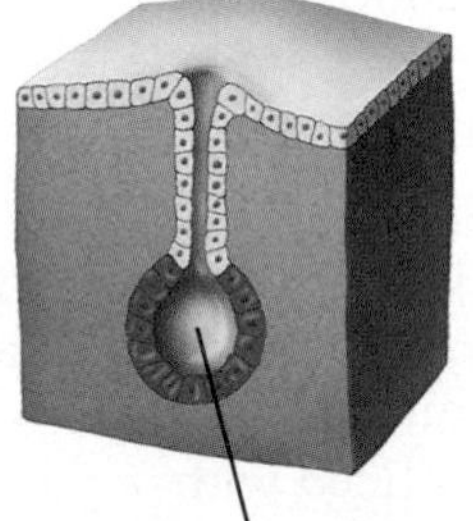

A Simple duct structure. A single duct to the secretory unit.

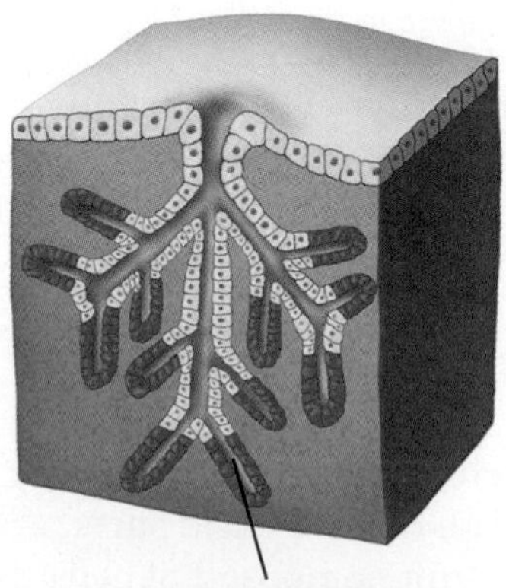

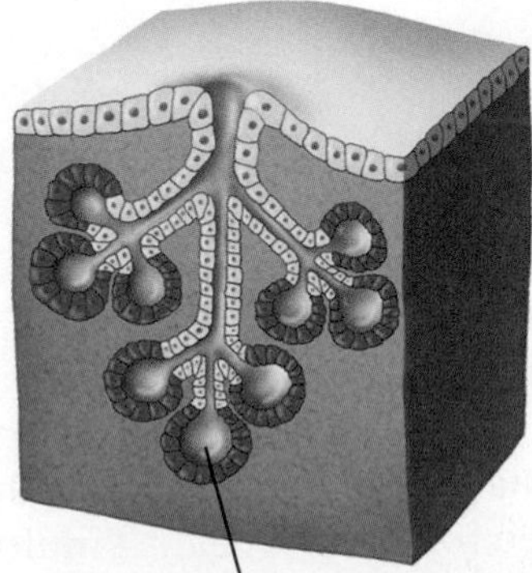

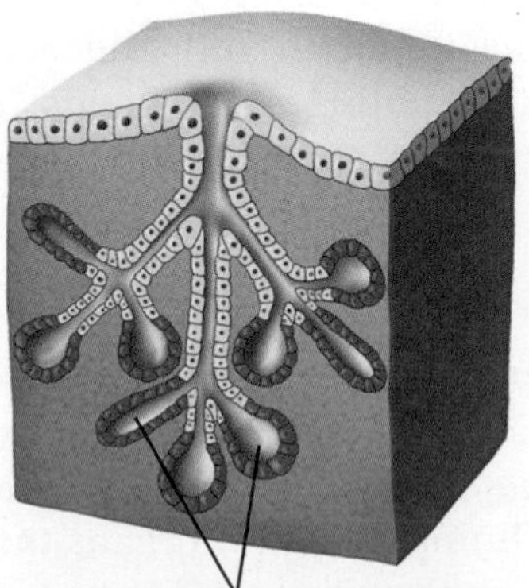

B Compound duct structure. The duct branches before reaching the secretory units.

Figure 2.26 The different structures of multicellular exocrine glands.

All forms of connective tissue include both cells and extracellular material that forms a matrix. The types of cells, and the nature of the extracellular matrix, differ among the major classes of connective tissue (**Figure 2.27**).

Extracellular fibers are an important part of connective tissue, helping to determine its mechanical properties (strength and elasticity, for example). Three types of fibers are found in connective tissue, although not all connective tissue has all types of fibers.

Collagen fibers are formed from tropocollagen (troh-poh-KAHL-a-jehn) proteins that link together. Collagen fibers are strong and resistant to stretch. They give **tensile strength** to tissue.

Reticular fibers are thinner and not as strong as collagen fibers. They help to provide a structural framework that keeps cells in place.

Elastic fibers can lengthen considerably when stretched, and then spring back to their original length when the stretching force is removed. Elastic fibers give springiness, or elasticity, to tissues.

Tension, Compression, and Elasticity

Before the word *tension* was used to describe an emotional state, it had, and still has, another meaning: a force that pulls something apart (which gives some insight into why it is now also a name for an emotional state). Tensile strength is the ability to withstand a pulling force without stretching much or breaking. The opposite of tension is *compression*: a force that pushes in. **Compressive strength** is the ability to withstand compression.

Major Classes of Connective Tissue

Class	Subclasses	Cells	Extracellular Matrix	Extracellular Fibers	General Features
Connective tissue proper	loose • areolar • reticular • adipose	fibroblasts adipocytes mast cells macrophages lymphocytes	loose includes fibers; areolar is gel-like; adipose has very little	all three subclasses: • collagen • reticular • elastic	variety of locations and functions; loose tissue provides support, strength, and elasticity; plays a role in immune defenses
	dense • regular • irregular • elastic		dense is mainly fibers; little else		dense fibers provide tensile strength and elasticity; resist stretching
Cartilage	hyaline elastic fibrocartilage	chondroblasts chondrocytes	secreted by chondroblasts; contains proteoglycan molecules, which blend to immobilize water molecules	collagen in all; elastic in some	provides support and flexibility; minimizes friction
Bone (osseous) tissue	cortical (compact) trabecular (spongy)	osteoblasts osteocytes (see Chapter 4 for more information)	secreted by osteoblasts	collagen	provides framework; protects organs; supports body
Blood	no major classes; see cell types in Chapter 10	red blood cells (erythrocytes); white blood cells (leukocytes); platelets	plasma	none	provides transportation, regulation and protection; carries oxygen and nutrients to cells; carries away wastes and carbon dioxide

Figure 2.27 Goodheart-Willcox Publisher

As an example of the difference between these two types of forces, consider a rope. When a rope is used in a tug-of-war, its tensile strength is evident. However, the rope does not have any significant compressive strength. If you try to compress a rope by pushing the ends together, it does not resist; it simply folds and buckles.

Elasticity is the ability to stretch when tension is applied, and then spring back to the original length when the tension is withdrawn. Elastic fibers give elasticity to skin. Unfortunately, elastic fibers in skin, like the elastic fibers in the waistband of a favorite pair of athletic shorts, tend to lose their elasticity as they get older. As a result, the skin (and the shorts) tend to get more baggy and wrinkly, and less elastic.

Connective Tissue Proper

Connective tissue proper includes loose and dense subtypes. Loose connective tissue has cells and an extracellular matrix with fibers running through it. Dense connective tissue has relatively few cells and an extracellular matrix composed mainly of fibers and little else.

Types of Loose Connective Tissue

Loose connective tissue includes areolar, reticular, and adipose connective tissue. **Areolar connective tissue** is found throughout the body, typically as a layer beneath epithelial tissues (**Figure 2.28**). It holds water in its gel-like extracellular matrix. Areolar connective tissue provides support, strength, and elasticity to overlying epithelia, thanks to collagen, reticular, and elastic fibers. It plays a role in inflammation and immune system defenses because it contains most of the cells—mast cells, macrophages, and the occasional white blood cells (lymphocytes)—involved in the inflammation process and immune system function.

Reticular connective tissue, which contains reticular fibers, is found in lymph nodes, bone marrow, and the spleen. In all these locations it provides a loose framework for blood-forming cells (in bone marrow) or immune system defenses (in the spleen and lymph nodes).

Adipose tissue consists almost entirely of cells—adipocytes, or fat cells—and very little extracellular matrix (**Figure 2.29**). It provides a reservoir of metabolic fuel as well as thermal insulation and cushioning for organs.

Types of Dense Connective Tissue

As mentioned earlier, dense connective tissue has few cells, and its extracellular matrix is made up primarily of fibers. Dense tissue can be of three types: regular, irregular, or elastic.

Regular dense connective tissue consists of collagen fibers that are mostly parallel to one another (**Figure 2.30**). It contains occasional fibroblasts, which secrete collagen. Regular dense connective tissue is found in tendons and ligaments. Its abundant collagen fibers give it great tensile strength, particularly when pulled parallel to the fiber direction.

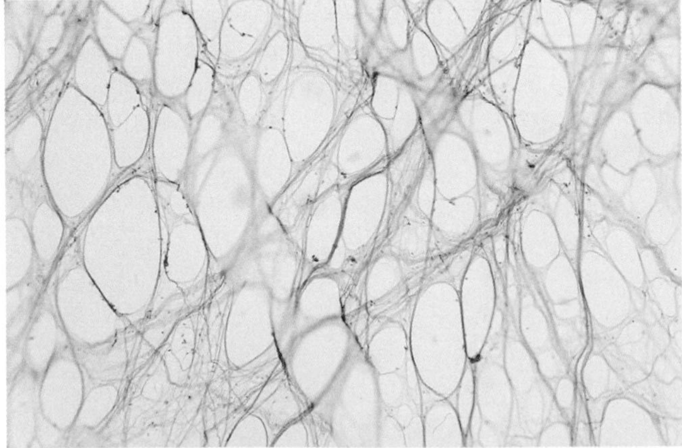

Choksawafdikom/Shutterstock.com

Figure 2.28 Areolar connective tissue is found below the epithelium of the skin and below the epithelial tissues of the respiratory and digestive tracts. In this image, cell nuclei appear as round or oval dark spots, and fibers appear as dark lines.

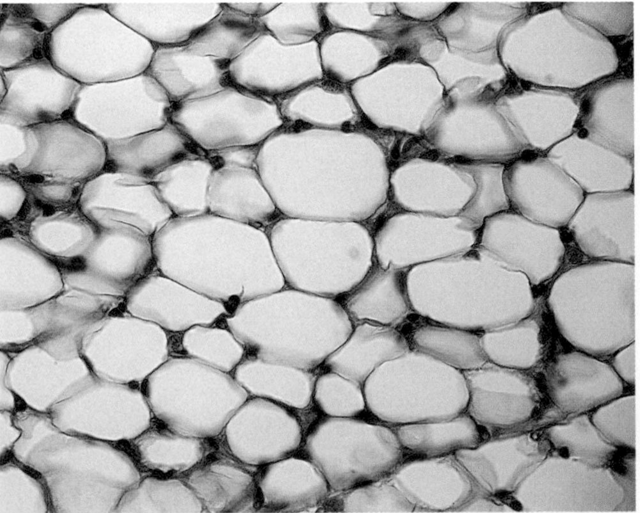

Jose Luis Calvo/Shutterstock.com

Figure 2.29 Light micrograph of adipose connective tissue.

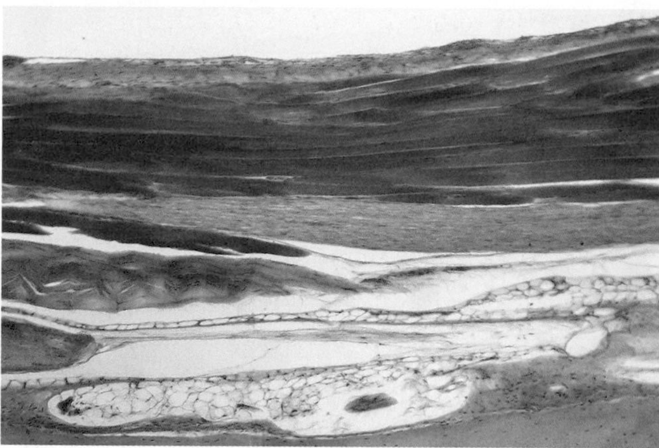
Kateryna Kon/Shutterstock.com

Figure 2.30 Regular dense connective tissue, seen in the upper part of this light micrograph, is found in ligaments and tendons

Irregular dense connective tissue (**Figure 2.31**), like regular dense connective tissue, is composed primarily of collagen fibers. However, the fibers run in all directions, unlike the parallel fibers in regular dense connective tissue. As a result, irregular dense connective tissue is good at resisting stretching forces from a variety of directions. It is found in the dermis, in the deep layer of the skin, and in the fibrous capsule around joints, among other places.

Dense elastic connective tissue has an extracellular matrix full of elastic fibers (**Figure 2.32**). Not surprisingly, it is highly elastic. It is found in the walls of airways and large arteries.

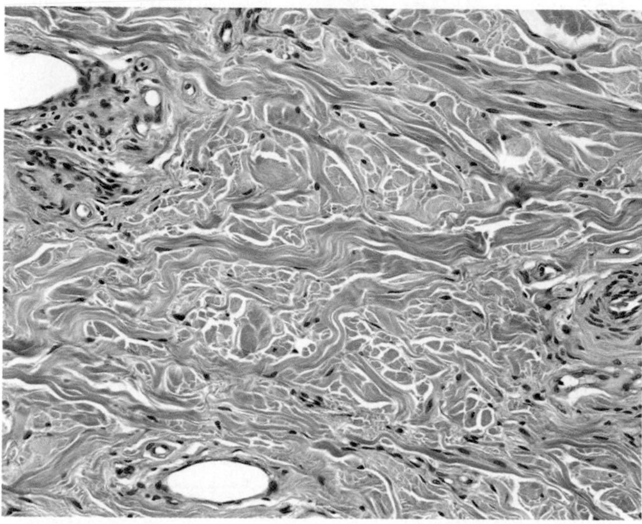
Jose Luis Calvo/Shutterstock.com

Figure 2.31 Irregular dense connective tissue. Collagen fibers stain pink, and cell nuclei stain dark purple. The large white ovals are blood vessels.

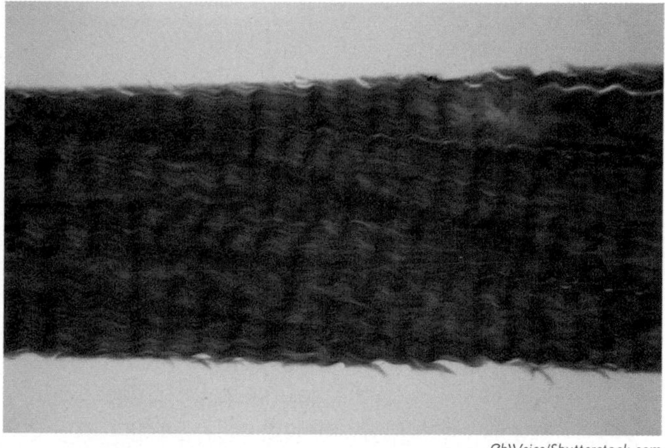
ChWeiss/Shutterstock.com

Figure 2.32 Light micrograph of dense elastic connective tissue.

Cartilage

Cartilage is part of the skeleton. It is found on the ends of bones and between bones. It provides support and flexibility, and it minimizes friction.

Chondroblasts (KAHN-droh-blasts) secrete the extracellular matrix of cartilage. The extracellular matrix contains collagen fibers and proteoglycan (PROH-tee-oh-GLIGH-kan) molecules (proteins with carbohydrates added), including hyaluronic acid and chondroitin (kawn-DROY-tin). These large molecules bind to and immobilize many water molecules. The high water content of cartilage helps to account for its high resistance to compression (given that water is incompressible) and for its low friction.

The most common form of cartilage is *hyaline* (HIGH-a-lin) *cartilage*, shown in **Figure 2.33**. The smooth, shiny substance at the end of a chicken or turkey leg bone is hyaline cartilage. Hyaline cartilage forms a smooth covering on the ends of long bones, and it forms the ends of

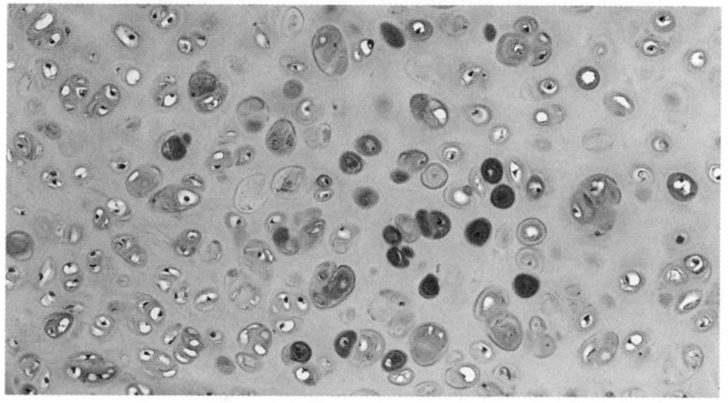
David Litman/Shutterstock.com

Figure 2.33 Light micrograph of hyaline cartilage.

MEMORY TIP

The combining forms *blast/o* and *-cyt/o* are used in cell names. The combining form *blast/o* is derived from the Greek word for "bud," and has been traditionally used to denote a precursor cell that can give rise to (precede) a variety of daughter cells. The words *blastula* and *blastocyst*, which refer to early stages in the development of an embryo, are based on this combining form.

Blast cells are sometimes called *stem cells*, which seems reasonable given the close relationship between buds and stems. Their descendant cells can branch out and develop into various subtypes of specialized mature cells.

The combining form *blast/o* has also come to be used, especially with regard to connective tissues, when referring to a cell that actively secretes components of the extracellular matrix. Fibroblasts secrete collagen (which is used to make fibers—hence the combining form *fibr/o*). Chondroblasts secrete proteoglycans in cartilage, and osteoblasts secrete osteoid, which hardens into bone.

The combining form *cyt/o* comes from the Greek word for "container" and is used to refer to cells in general. *Cytology* is the study of cells. When compared to the traditional use of *blast/o* to denote a stem cell, *cyt/o* usually denotes a mature cell that, unlike a blast cell, can only produce descendants that are just like the parent, or that cannot divide at all. For example, lymphoblasts give rise to lymphocytes, and erythroblasts give rise to erythrocytes. In connective tissue, *-cyt/o* is also used to denote a cell that is quiescent—that is, it does not actively secrete extracellular matrix content; thus *osteocytes*, *fibrocytes* (rare), and *chondrocytes*.

the ribs where they connect to the sternum, or breastbone. It is also found in the nose, trachea (windpipe), and larynx (voicebox).

Elastic cartilage is similar to hyaline cartilage but contains more elastic fibers. Its elastic fibers allow it to bend and spring back into its original shape. Elastic cartilage is found in the external ear and the epiglottis, a flap of tissue in the throat that prevents food and water from entering the lungs.

Fibrocartilage (figh-broh-KAR-ti-lij) has more collagen fibers than hyaline or elastic cartilage. Therefore, it has more tensile strength than other types of cartilage. It is found in the discs between vertebrae and in the discs in the knee joint.

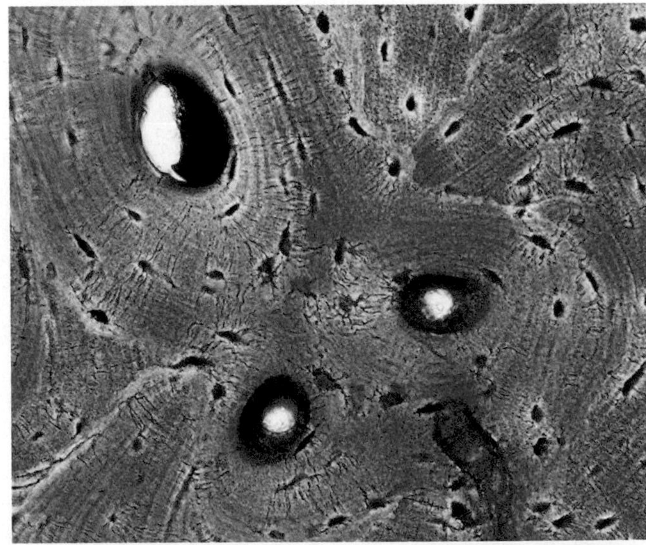

Choksawatdikom/Shutterstock.com

Figure 2.34 Cross section of a bone.

Bone

Bone, also known as *osseous* (AHS-ee-us) *tissue*, protects organs and supports the body, providing a rigid framework on which muscles can pull (**Figure 2.34**). Osteoblasts secrete the extracellular matrix of bone. The extracellular matrix contains collagen fibers, which give bone its tensile strength, and calcium salts, which make it hard and give it compressive strength. You will learn more about the structure and function of bone in Chapter 4.

Check Your Understanding

1. What four functions do connective tissues perform in the body?
2. What is the difference between loose connective tissue and dense connective tissue?
3. What is the function of chondroblasts?

Muscle Tissue

Muscle tissue allows the body to move. The distinguishing property of muscle is its ability to generate force on command. All muscle cells use intracellular filaments made of the proteins actin and myosin to generate force, and they all require ATP as fuel for contraction.

The three kinds of muscle tissue are skeletal, cardiac, and smooth muscle. Skeletal and cardiac muscle are both called *striated muscle* because they have striations, or stripes, when viewed through a light microscope. Following is a brief introduction to the types of muscle tissue. You will learn more about these tissues in various chapters throughout this textbook.

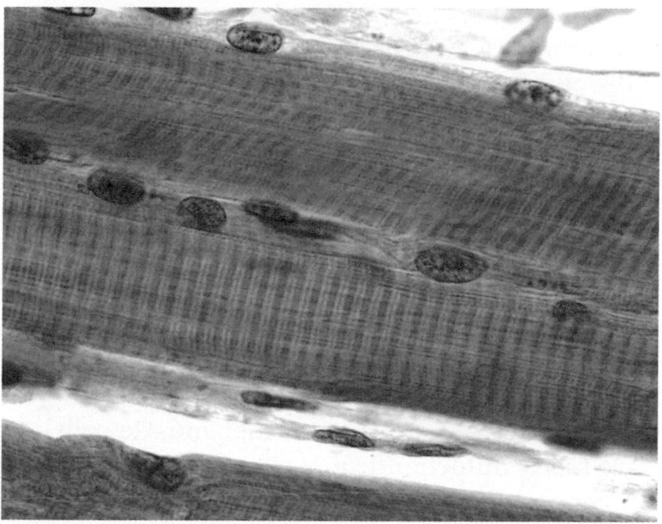

Jose Luis Calvo/Shutterstock.com

Figure 2.35 Skeletal muscle.

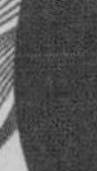

LIFE SPAN DEVELOPMENT: *Cells and Tissues*

Each human begins as a single fertilized egg cell, or zygote. The zygote completes its first mitotic division about 24 hours later. The two cells divide to make four cells, then eight. By the fourth day, there are 16 or more cells, and the cells have started to differentiate, or turn into different types of cells. As the ball of cells develops into an embryo and then a fetus, cells continue to differentiate, or specialize.

A *stem cell* is an undifferentiated cell that has the potential to divide repeatedly and to develop into different kinds of cells. In the early stages of development, fetuses have many stem cells. As development is completed, the number and variety of stem cells diminishes. Some scientists believe that many of the negative aspects of aging, such as slower healing processes and decrease in strength of bones and muscles, are due to the aging of stem cells. Old stem cells lose their ability to function as stem cells, and when they do, the tissues and organs lose their ability to maintain themselves through cellular regeneration.

A key finding in understanding aging at the cellular level was the discovery in the 1960s that normal human cells grown in tissue culture can divide 40 to 60 times, but after that they lose their ability to divide. This limit to cell division is known as the *Hayflick limit*, for its discoverer. Further study has indicated that a small amount of DNA is lost from the tips of chromosomes during each cycle of cell division. The chromosome tips, known as *telomeres*, do not code for proteins, so at first, the loss of chromosomal material does not interfere with cellular function. An enzyme, telomerase, rebuilds the lost ends of telomeres. However, telomerase activity diminishes in older cells, so the telomeres gradually shorten. Once the telomeres reach a critical shortness, the cell loses its ability to divide.

Interestingly, the enzyme telomerase stays active in sperm cells, and human egg cells stop dividing early in life. Therefore sperm and egg cells have full-length telomeres, which enables the next generation to have just as much potential for cell division as the preceding generation.

Cancer cells do not have a Hayflick limit. They can grow and divide in culture with no apparent limit. This is possible in part because telomerase remains active in cancer cells. Could physicians fight cancer by administering drugs that block telomerase? Maybe, but experiments so far show that this can have undesirable side effects, such as impaired wound healing and reduced immune function. Could enhancing telomerase activity help combat aging? Perhaps, but it could increase the risk of developing cancer. This remains an active area of research.

Life Span Review

1. Why do you think cells that can divide repeatedly to develop into many different kinds of cells are called *stem cells*?
2. What is the Hayflick limit?

Skeletal muscle is by far the most common type of muscle (**Figure 2.35**). Skeletal muscle pulls on bones to make the body move. Skeletal muscle cells are long and thin. They have multiple nuclei because they are formed from the merging of multiple embryonic cells. The striations in skeletal muscle are at right angles to the long axis of the cells.

Cardiac muscle is the major tissue of the heart. It is similar to skeletal muscle, but its cells are much shorter. Because the heart never stops working, cardiac muscle must generate ATP continuously. As a result, cardiac muscle cells have many mitochondria.

Smooth muscle is found in the walls of hollow organs, including the blood vessels, airways, gastrointestinal tract, bladder, and uterus. As its name implies, the cytoplasm of smooth muscle cells appears uniform, or smooth, under the light microscope.

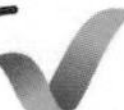

Check Your Understanding

1. What is the distinguishing property of muscle tissue?
2. Identify the three types of muscle tissue.
3. Which type of muscle has multiple nuclei? Why?
4. Which type of muscle has the most mitochondria? Why does it need so many?

Nerve Tissue

Nerve tissue is a class of tissue that has the unique ability to convey information by electrical signaling. Nerve tissue is concentrated in the brain and spinal cord, which comprise the central nervous system. However, nerves extend throughout the body.

The nerves outside the central nervous system comprise the *peripheral nervous system.* The peripheral nervous system has separate nerve fibers for sending out signals (motor commands to the muscles and glands) and for receiving incoming signals (sensory signals from the eyes, ears, skin, etc.).

Nerve tissue includes supporting cells, called *glial* (GLIGH-al) *cells* (from the root word for "glue"), and *neurons*, the nervous system cells that generate, transmit, and receive electrical signals. **Figure 2.36** shows neurons in the brain. Individual neurons have a compact cell body and extensions that carry electrical signals to their targets (muscles, glands, or other neurons, for example), and receive input from other neurons.

Check Your Understanding

1. What kind of signals does nerve tissue use to convey information?
2. Which two types of nerve fibers are located in the peripheral nervous system?
3. What is the purpose of glial cells?
4. Briefly describe a typical neuron.

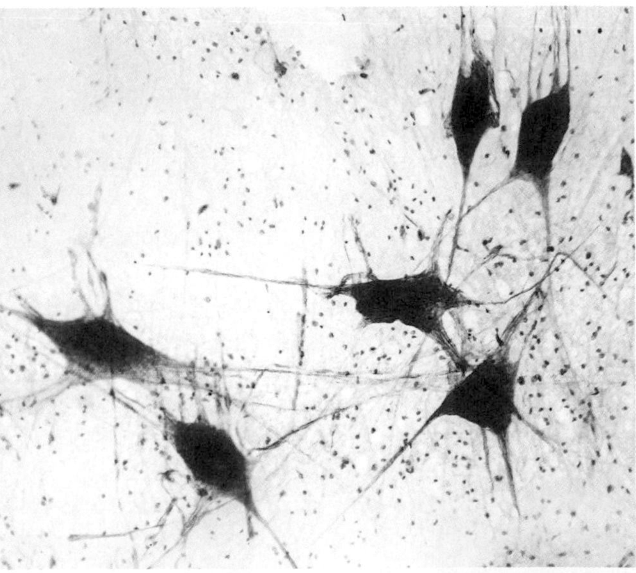

Kateryna Kon/Shutterstock.com

Figure 2.36 Light micrograph of a neuron. The dark-staining soma, or cell body, has dendrites and an axon extending from it.

LESSON 2.3 Review and Assessment

Mini Glossary

Make sure that you know the meaning of each key term.

adipose tissue tissue that consists almost entirely of adipocytes, or fat cells, with little extracellular matrix

areolar connective tissue connective tissue that has a gel-like extracellular matrix that holds water well and serves as a support for overlying epithelia

cartilage a connective tissue that provides support and flexibility to parts of the skeleton

chondroblasts cells that secrete the extracellular matrix of cartilage

compressive strength the ability of a material to withstand compression (inward-pressing force) without buckling

connective tissue supporting tissue, which consists mainly of an extracellular matrix

elasticity the ability of a material to spring back to its original shape after being stretched

endocrine gland a gland that secretes its product into the interstitial space

epithelial tissue a class of tissue that includes epithelia and glands

exocrine gland a gland that secretes its product to the outside world

glands epithelial cells that are organized to produce and secrete substances

histology the study of tissues

lumen the hollow inside portion of a body cavity or tube

reticular connective tissue a type of tissue that contains reticular fibers and is found in lymph nodes, bone marrow, and the spleen

simple epithelia epithelia that have a single layer of cells

stratified epithelia epithelia that have multiple layers of cells

tensile strength the ability to withstand tension (outward pulling force) without tearing or breaking

Know and Understand

1. What are the two types of glands and how do they differ?
2. What shape does an alveolar gland have?
3. What service do collagen fibers provide to tissues?
4. The most common type of cartilage is _____.
5. Bone is also known as _____ tissue.
6. Identify the two types of protein that make up the intracellular filaments in muscle.

Analyze and Apply

7. Compare and contrast skeletal and cardiac muscles. What do they have in common? How are they different?
8. What would be the consequences if the human body lacked internal epithelial tissues?
9. Assume that you are looking at cell cultures from the lining of the stomach, the wall of the heart, and a leg muscle, but the slides are not labeled. How can you identify each cell structure?
10. Why does the surface of the skin need chemical and mechanical protection?
11. Explain the difference between exocrine and endocrine glands. What substance(s) do endocrine glands secrete? What substance(s) do exocrine glands secrete?

IN THE LAB

12. Do some research to learn more about the effects of the aging process on body tissues. Select a type of tissue and create models to represent that tissue as it exists in a young person and in a senior citizen. Explain to the class how and why you have represented the tissue in the two different ways.
13. Using a microscope, view the three different types of muscle tissue: skeletal, cardiac, and smooth muscle. Sketch what you see on paper using colored pencils. Trade your sketch with a partner to see if he or she can determine which type of tissue you were drawing. If your partner is unable to tell which type of muscle tissue you illustrated, discuss what key elements were missing that would have helped your partner to identify the tissue correctly.

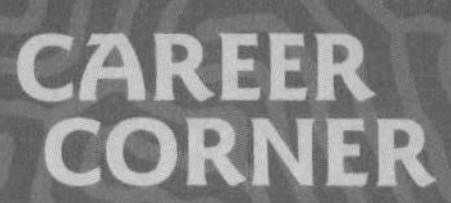

CAREER CORNER

Anatomy & Physiology at Work

A variety of career options are available to those interested in studying and working with human cells and tissues. Because modern medicine continues to develop new and improved diagnostic tests and technologies, career opportunities in this dynamic field are flourishing.

Cytotechnologist

A cytotechnologist (sigh-toh-tehk-NAHL-oh-jist) is a laboratory specialist who studies human tissues under a microscope for signs of abnormality or disease (**Figure 2.37**). In short, a cytotechnologist is a "cell detective" who works both independently and as part of a team to identify viral and bacterial infections, cancerous growths, and precancerous changes in cells.

A career as a cytotechnologist requires a high school diploma and completion of a four-year training program endorsed by the Commission on Accreditation of Allied Health Education Programs (CAAHEP), in conjunction with the Cytotechnology Programs Review Committee of the American Society of Cytopathology. Typically, students are admitted to a cytotechnology program in their junior or senior year of college. Although specific course requirements vary, it is recommended that students complete 20 semester hours of biological science, 8 semester hours of chemistry, and 3 semester hours of higher mathematics or statistics.

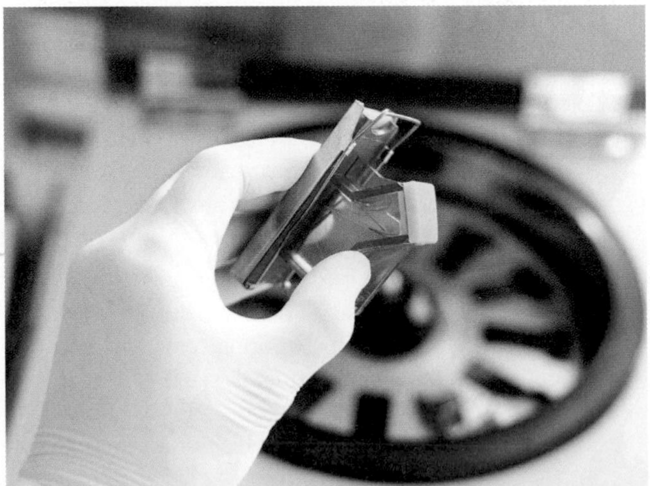

Komsan Loonprom/Shutterstock.com

Figure 2.37 Cytotechnologists routinely centrifuge and prepare specimens before examining them.

After completion of a CAAHEP-accredited program in cytotechnology, students must pass a national examination administered by the American Society for Clinical Pathology Board of Certification (ASCP BOC). With successful completion of this exam, a student has achieved entry-level proficiency and is recognized as a CT (ASCP), or certified cytotechnologist.

Cytotechnologists are typically employed in private medical laboratories, hospitals, university medical centers, government agencies, and industrial settings. Within these environments, cytotechnologists may have opportunities in education, supervision, and administration, some of which may require additional experience or education.

Pathologists' Assistant

A pathologists' assistant (PathA) is a health professional who prepares and examines human tissues under the direction and supervision of a pathologist (a medical doctor). Pathologists' assistants are responsible for tissue banking, examination of surgical pathology specimens, and assisting with complex surgeries and post-mortem examinations (**Figure 2.38**).

A career as a pathologists' assistant requires a bachelor's degree from a college or university program recognized by the National Accrediting Agency for Clinical Laboratory Sciences (NAACLS). The educational curriculum, which is rigorous, includes coursework in clinical anatomy, systemic pathology, autopsy pathology, and neuroscience. In addition, students must complete anatomic pathology clerkships in any of a number of medical specialties, such as neurosurgery, oncology, cardiothoracic surgery, and more.

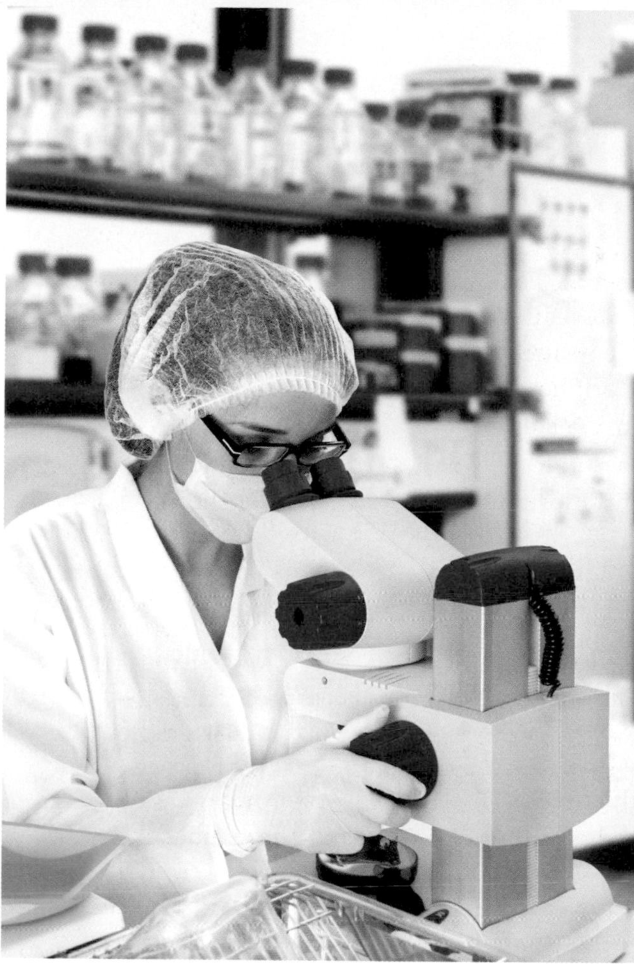
anyaivanova/Shutterstock.com

Figure 2.38 One of the pathologist's assistant's duties is to examine surgical specimens under a microscope.

Those with a bachelor's degree in the field and three years' continuous work experience can become an Affiliate member of the American Association of Pathologists' Assistants. As an Affiliate, a pathologists' assistant is eligible to take the certification examination given by the ASCP BOC. Upon successful completion of the exam, a pathologists' assistant achieves the status of a Fellow.

Pathologists' assistants work in community, government, and university hospitals; medical laboratories; medical schools; and within the Medical Examiner (ME) system. In the United States, the ME system partners with law enforcement to investigate unusual, suspicious, violent, and sudden and unexplained deaths that may pose a threat to public health.

Pathologists' assistants are qualified to teach courses in subjects such as anatomy and physiology, histology, gross pathology, and gross dissection skills for surgical and autopsy pathology.

Planning for a Health-Related Career

Do some research on the career of a cytotechnologist or pathologists' assistant. Alternatively, select a profession from the list of **Related Career Options**. Using the Internet or resources at your local library, find answers to the following questions:

1. What are the main tasks and responsibilities of the career that you have chosen to research?
2. What is the outlook for this career? Are workers in demand, or are jobs dwindling? For complete information, consult the current edition of the *Occupational Outlook Handbook*, published by the US Department of Labor. This handbook is available online or at your local library.
3. What special skills or talents are required? For example, do you need to be good at biology, chemistry, and anatomy and physiology? Do you need to thrive under the pressure of intense working conditions?
4. What personality traits do you think are needed to be successful in this job?
5. Does this career involve a great deal of routine, or are the day-to-day responsibilities varied?
6. Does the work require long hours, or is it a standard, "9-to-5" job?
7. What is the salary range for this job?
8. What do you think you would like about this career? Is there anything about it that you might dislike?

Related Career Options

- Clinical lab technologist
- Histotechnician
- Histotechnologist
- Medical laboratory technician
- Phlebotomy technician
- Specialist in cytotechnology
- Technologist in molecular biology

CHAPTER
2 Review

›LESSON 2.1
Molecules of Life

Key Points

- Carbohydrates, which always contain carbon and hydrogen, can be simple or complex.
- Proteins, which help form the structure of cells or speed up biological processes, are made up of long chains of amino acids.
- Lipids are fats and oils in the body; they store energy and regulate the reproductive system.
- DNA and RNA are nucleic acids that contain the body's genetic information and carry it from cell to cell.
- Water is essential to life, comprising about two-thirds of body mass.

Key Terms

adenosine triphosphate (ATP)
amino acids
base pairs
chromosome
deoxyribonucleic acid (DNA)
electrolytes
enzyme
fatty acid
gene
gene therapy
glucose
glycogen
human genome
lipids
nucleic acids
nucleotides
peptide bond
pH
phospholipids
polymer
polypeptide
proteome
ribonucleic acid (RNA)
steroids
triglycerides

›LESSON 2.2
Cells

Key Points

- Most body cells contain a plasma membrane, cytoskeleton, mitochondria, Golgi apparatus, ribosomes, endoplasmic reticulum, and nucleus.
- DNA is the template for making RNA, and RNA is the template for making protein; these three polymers contain information that is vital for life.
- The life cycle of a cell consists of two major phases—interphase and the mitotic phase—both of which are divided into several subphases. Cell division occurs in the mitotic phase.

Key Terms

active transport
centrioles
channel proteins
cilia
citric acid cycle
codon
cytokinesis
cytoplasm
cytoskeleton
diffusion
endocytosis
endoplasmic reticulum (ER)
exocytosis
extracellular fluid
extracellular matrix
glycolysis
glycoproteins
Golgi apparatus
messenger RNA (mRNA)
microvilli
mitochondria
mitosis
nucleus
passive transport
plasma membrane
ribosomes
transcription
transfer RNA (tRNA)

LESSON 2.3

Tissues

Key Points

- Epithelial tissues consist of epithelia, which include the skin and linings of internal body cavities, and glands, which secrete chemicals.
- Connective tissues protect the body and give it strength, help the body maintain its shape, and provide the structure against which muscles pull.
- Muscle tissues generate force to move the body.
- Nerve tissue conveys information through the body via electrical signals.

Key Terms

adipose tissue
areolar connective tissue
cartilage
chondroblasts
compressive strength
connective tissue
elasticity
endocrine gland
epithelial tissue
exocrine gland
glands
histology
lumen
reticular connective tissue
simple epithelia
stratified epithelia
tensile strength

Assessment

LESSON 2.1

Molecules of Life

Learning Key Terms and Concepts

1. The main type of sugar that circulates in the blood is _____.
2. *Carbohydrates*, as indicated by the word parts that make up the word, include both carbon and _____.
3. A molecule made of many similar subunits is called a(n) _____.
4. The amino acid _____ has the simplest residual group of all of the amino acids.
5. The type of bond that links the amino group of one amino acid to the acid group of another is a(n) _____ bond.
6. The four levels of protein structure are the primary, secondary, tertiary, and _____ structures.
7. The three types of glycerides are _____, diglycerides, and triglycerides.
8. DNA is formed in the shape of a(n) _____.
   A. double pleat
   B. double helix
   C. triple helix
   D. pleated helix
9. Adenosine triphosphate provides _____ for many cellular processes.
10. The _____, or relative charges, of water molecules allows them to form hydrogen bonds with other molecules.

Thinking Critically

11. Consider the enzymes discussed in this lesson. Which body functions might *not* be possible in their absence?
12. Using the information and figures in this lesson, analyze at least two different types of chemical reactions that provide the body with energy.
13. What might be the consequences of DNA damage in a person's cells?
14. Glycogen storage diseases are usually inherited. Research one of these diseases and share your research with your classmates.
15. One of the unique features of water that make it so useful in the human body and many other applications is its usefulness in more than one "state of matter." Investigate the three principle states of matter and list these states as they pertain to water. How does this information help you understand the role of water in the body?

> LESSON 2.2

Cells

Learning Key Terms and Concepts

16. Charged particles can only enter or leave a cell through _____.
    A. channel proteins
    B. microvilli
    C. the Golgi apparatus
    D. glycolysis
17. Glycoproteins are proteins with _____ groups attached.
    A. amino acid
    B. fatty acid
    C. phosphorus
    D. carbohydrate
18. The cytoskeleton does *not* include _____.
    A. cytofilaments
    B. intermediate filaments
    C. microfilaments
    D. microtubules
19. Located near the nucleus, the _____ help to guide the movement and separation of chromosomes during cell division.
    A. mitochondria
    B. ribosomes
    C. centrioles
    D. lysosomes
20. Because of their great need for energy to power muscle contractions, cardiac muscle cells have a high number of _____.
    A. centrosomes
    B. mitochondria
    C. glycoproteins
    D. ribosomes
21. The breakdown of a glucose molecule into two pyruvate molecules is called _____.
    A. glycolysis
    B. gluconeogenesis
    C. glycosylation
    D. gluconeolysis
22. Which of the following is a set of membranous discs in the cytoplasm?
    A. ATP
    B. endoplasmic reticulum
    C. Golgi apparatus
    D. vesicles
23. Which of the following does *not* describe a ribosome?
    A. It is a very large enzyme.
    B. It is found in the nucleus.
    C. It makes polypeptides.
    D. It includes a large and a small subunit.
24. Steroid hormones are produced by the _____ in the cytoplasm.
    A. mitochondria
    B. lysosomes
    C. smooth endoplasmic reticulum
    D. rough endoplasmic reticulum
25. The process of making RNA from DNA is known as _____.
    A. translation
    B. transduction
    C. transformation
    D. transcription
26. The enzyme that makes RNA, using DNA as a template, is _____.
    A. adenine
    B. transfer RNA
    C. adipocyte
    D. RNA polymerase
27. Two major phases of cell division are the mitotic phase and _____.
    A. anaphase
    B. interphase
    C. prophase
    D. telophase
28. The division of the cytoplasm during cell division, called _____, begins during telophase.
    A. cytokinesis
    B. interphase
    C. translation
    D. glycolysis

Instructions: Write the letter of the name of the cell structure on your answer sheet next to the corresponding number.

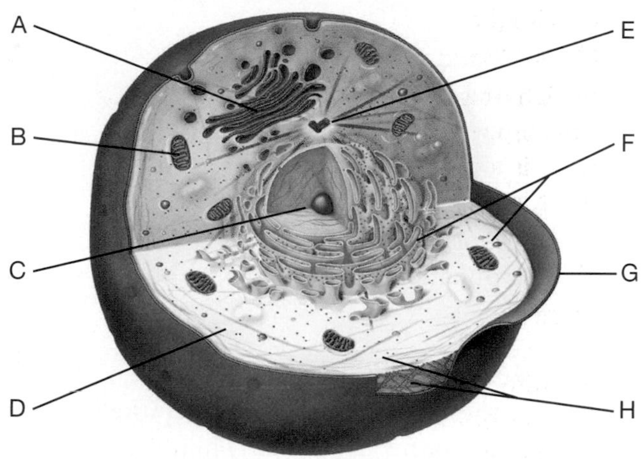

© Body Scientific International

29. Mitochondrion _____
30. Ribosomes _____
31. Golgi apparatus _____
32. Cytoskeleton _____
33. Centrosome _____
34. Nucleus _____
35. Plasma membrane _____
36. Cytoplasm _____

Thinking Critically

37. Compare and contrast microvilli and cilia.
38. Investigate the physical and chemical processes that contribute to homeostasis, including equilibrium, temperature, pH balance, chemical reactions, active and passive transport, and biofeedback. In an oral presentation, describe how these processes are integrated.
39. In what ways do you think the Human Genome Project has changed medicine in today's society?
40. Atoms and molecules that can gain or lose an electron to become ions (with a net positive or negative charge) are critical to many of the processes in the body that sustain life. Conduct research to find out what the difference is between a cation and an anion, and list common examples of both in the human body. Why is the charge important?

LESSON 2.3

Tissues

Learning Key Terms and Concepts

41. The study of tissues is called _____.
    A. physiology
    B. histology
    C. cytology
    D. pathology
42. Which of the following functions is *not* performed by epithelial tissue?
    A. provide a rigid framework for the body
    B. provide sensory information
    C. determine which substances enter and leave the body
    D. protect the body from physical damage
43. The apical and basal surfaces are the two sides of all _____ tissue.
    A. muscle
    B. nerve
    C. connective
    D. epithelial
44. The hollow inside portion of a body cavity or tube is called the _____.
    A. lumen
    B. cartilage
    C. codon
    D. alveolus
45. An exocrine gland is called _____ if its duct branches out as it travels from the surface to the secretory units.
    A. tubular
    B. alveolar
    C. unicellular
    D. compound
46. *True or False?* Blood is a type of connective tissue.
47. *True or False?* Collagen fibers are very elastic.
48. The fibers that provide a framework to keep cells in place are called _____ fibers.
    A. hyaline
    B. adipose
    C. reticular
    D. elastic

49. Which of the following is *not* a connective tissue?
    A. cartilage
    B. epithelia
    C. blood
    D. bone
50. _____ epithelia make up the alveoli in the lungs.
    A. Simple squamous
    B. Stratified squamous
    C. Simple columnar
    D. Transitional
51. Which of the following is *not* a form of loose connective tissue?
    A. adipose tissue
    B. areolar tissue
    C. columnar tissue
    D. reticular tissue
52. The three main types of cartilage are _____, elastic, and fibrocartilage.
    A. osseous
    B. hyaline
    C. choroidal
    D. reticular
53. Because skeletal and cardiac muscles have "stripes" when viewed through a microscope, they are considered _____ muscle.
    A. endoplasmic
    B. smooth
    C. nucleated
    D. striated
54. Two types of cells that make up nerve tissue are _____ and neurons.
    A. myocytes
    B. transport cells
    C. microfilaments
    D. glial cells

Thinking Critically

55. Review the general properties of epithelial tissue and connective tissue. Then explain why connective tissue is better suited than epithelial tissue for constructing cartilage.
56. Evaluate the cause and effect of cancer on the structure and function of cells, tissues, organs, and systems.
57. Describe the similarities and differences between cardiac muscles and skeletal muscles.

Building Skills and Connecting Concepts

Analyzing and Evaluating Data

Instructions: The chart in **Figure 2.40** lists 12 elements in order of their percentage of total body weight. Use the chart to answer the following questions.

58. Elements not shown in this chart that play a role in human physiology and contribute to total body weight are called *trace elements*. What percentage of body weight is made up of these trace elements? Round your answer to the nearest hundredth of a percent.
59. What percentage of your body weight is made up of the three elements contained in every organic molecule?
60. How much more nitrogen than potassium does your body contain?

Element	Percentage of total body weight
Oxygen	65%
Carbon	18%
Hydrogen	10%
Nitrogen	3%
Calcium	1.5%
Phosphorous	1%
Sulfur	0.25%
Potassium	0.20%
Sodium	0.15%
Chlorine	0.15%
Magnesium	0.05%
Iron	0.006%

Figure 2.40 Goodheart-Willcox Publisher

Communicating about Anatomy & Physiology

61. **Speaking and Reading** Lesson 2.1 explained that molecules, or parts of molecules, that bond easily with water are called *hydrophilic*, from the combining form *hydr/o* ("water") and *phil/o* ("loving"). By contrast, molecules that do not bond well with water are called *hydrophobic* (the suffix *-phobia* means "fearing").

    With a group of classmates, make a list of other words you know that contain the combining forms *hydr-*, *phil-*. and *phob-*. The words may be used in everyday language or in the fields of science or medicine. You may use a dictionary or online etymology resource to locate words that contain these combining forms.

    With your group, break each word into its combining form, practice pronouncing the word, and discuss its meaning. As a fun challenge, work together to compose a creative narrative using as many words as you can from your new list.
62. **Speaking and Listening** The Human Genome Project mapped the human genome and found that some differences in the genetic sequence can cause disease. Research one genetic disease, explain which chromosome is affected, and list 10 symptoms of that disease. Prepare a 2-minute oral presentation to convey your findings to the class.
63. **Writing** Look up information about the Salton Sea. What do you think the pH of the water might be? How does it compare with that of other sea water? Write a complete paragraph answering the following questions:
    A. Can you swim in the Salton Sea? Why or why not?
    B. Can anything live in the Salton Sea? Why or why not?

Lab Investigations

64. Working in groups of three or four students, build a clay model of one of the types of epithelial tissue listed below. Use modeling clay of various colors, index cards or paper and scissors, and transparent adhesive tape. Use the appropriate illustration(s) in this chapter as a guide while preparing your model.
    - Simple squamous
    - Simple cuboidal
    - Simple columnar
    - Stratified squamous
    - Stratified cuboidal
    - Stratified columnar

    When you have finished your model, create a label for the type of epithelial tissue that the model represents, and specify where the epithelial tissue is located in the body. Display your model in the classroom as a reference for discussion and study.
65. The study of cells and tissues depends heavily on the use of the light microscope. Conduct research to find out more about how the light microscope works. Create a sketch of a light microscope and label the parts. In an accompanying report, explain the function of each control.
66. Assume that you are a cytologist at a major university hospital. Using a microscope, observe tissue samples. In a lab notebook, describe what you see: color, patterns, and any other information you believe to be relevant. There is no one way to describe a slide. Be concise and write so the reader can understand what you are describing. Remember to use correct terminology. Return to your desk and see if you can label each slide based on your observations. Once you have identified the tissue, list three areas of the body in which you would find this tissue. Place your name on your paper and exchange it with another student. Can you identify the tissue your partner described?

Building Your Portfolio

67. Take digital photographs of the models you created as you worked through this chapter. Create a document called "Cells and Tissues" and insert the photographs, along with written descriptions of what the models show and your reasons for creating them using the materials and forms you chose. Add this document to your personal portfolio.

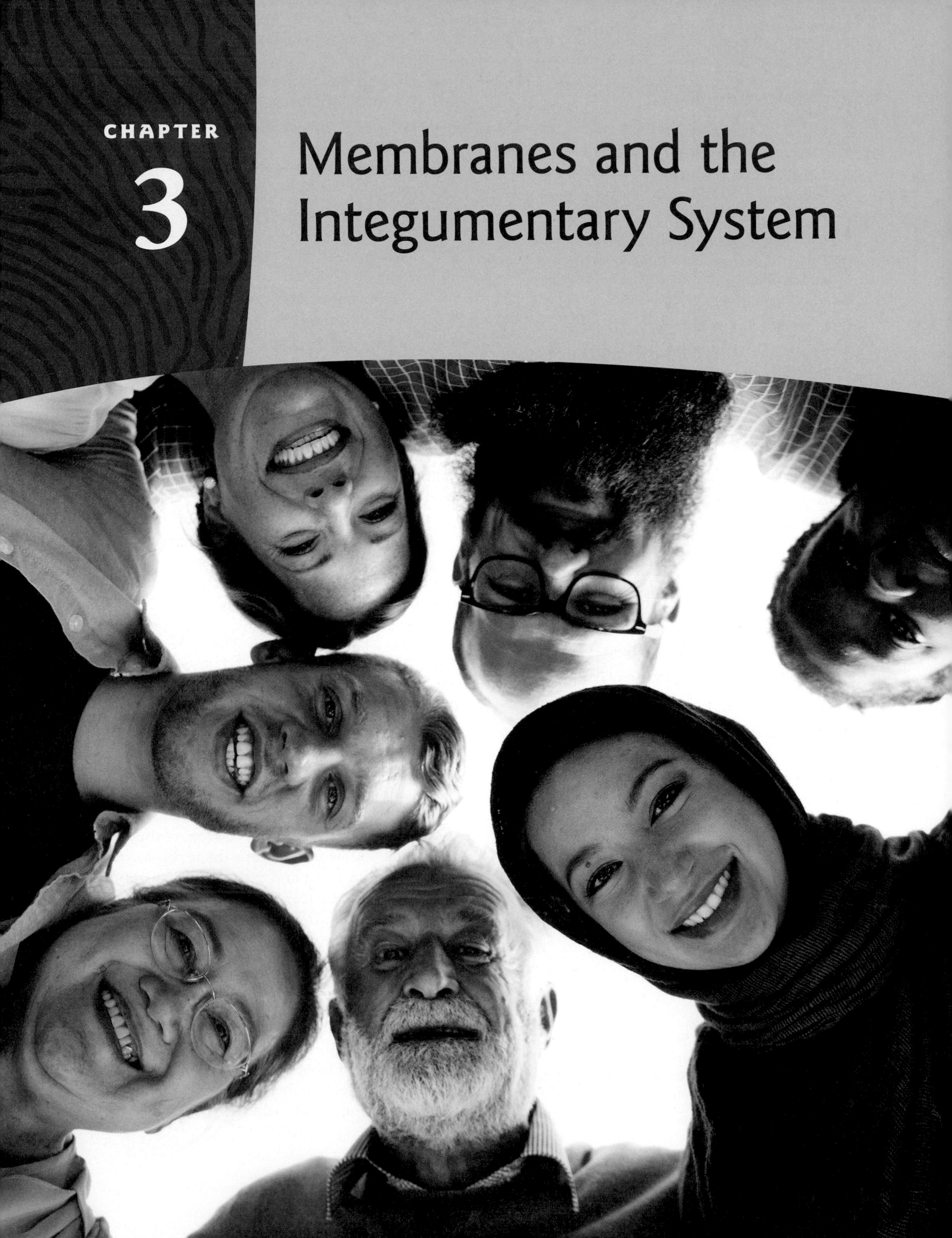

CHAPTER

3

Membranes and the Integumentary System

What determines whether people have straight, wavy, or curly hair?

People tend to think about their skin mainly when they are interested in getting a tan or avoiding sunburn. Consider, however, that the skin is actually a body organ like the heart or lungs. In fact, this organ called *skin* makes up approximately 15 percent of your total body weight!

The skin is quite a remarkable organ. It is far more than just an outer layer of covering. The skin contains glands and sensory receptors that perform specialized functions; it also grows hair and nails. For these reasons, the skin and its contents are considered a body system—the *integumentary system*.

This chapter examines the anatomy and functions of the integumentary system, including associated structures and membranes. It also discusses some of the common injuries and disorders of the skin and membranes, along with their symptoms and current treatments.

Chapter 3 Outline

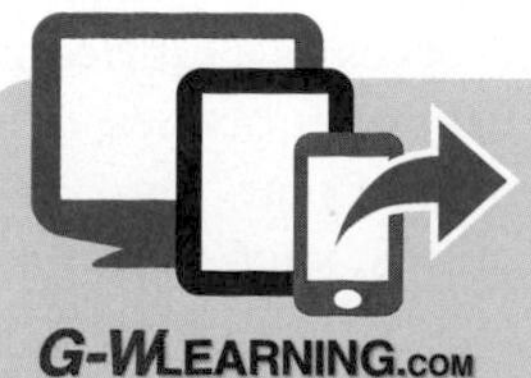

Click on the activity icon or visit www.g-wlearning.com/healthsciences/0202 to access online vocabulary activities using key terms from the chapter.

◄ Rawpixel.com/Shutterstock.com

LESSON 3.1 Body Membranes

Before You Read

Try to answer the following questions before you read this lesson.

- Do all membranes secrete some type of fluid?
- What is the common name for the cutaneous membrane?

Lesson Objectives

- Identify the differences among mucous, serous, and cutaneous membranes.
- Describe the structure and function of synovial membranes.

Key Terms

cutaneous membrane
epithelial membranes
membranes
mucous membranes
mucus
serous fluid
serous membranes
synovial fluid
synovial membrane

The **membranes** in the human body surround and help protect the body's surfaces. These surfaces include cavities that open to the outside world, internal cavities that house body organs, capsules that surround ball-and-socket synovial joints, and the skin. This lesson explores the similarities and differences among the membranes that cover these different body surfaces.

Epithelial Membranes

The **epithelial** (ehp-i-THEE-lee-al) **membranes** provide a lining, or covering, for the internal and external surfaces of the body. These membranes include both a sheet of epithelial cells and an underlying layer of connective tissue. There are several categories of epithelial membranes.

Mucous Membranes

The **mucous membranes** line the body cavities that open to the outside world (**Figure 3.1**). These cavities include all the hollow organs of the respiratory, digestive, urinary, and reproductive tracts. The mouth, nose, lungs, digestive tract, and bladder are examples of hollow organs lined with mucous membranes.

The structure of the mucous membranes comprises a layer of epithelium on top of loose connective tissue called *lamina propria*. The mucous membranes are all moist: the membranes of the digestive and respiratory tracts secrete mucus, and glands in the urinary tract add mucus there. **Mucus** is a slippery solution that protects the mucous membranes and aids in transporting substances.

Serous Membranes

Serous (SEER-us) **membranes** line body cavities that are closed to the outside world (**Figure 3.1**). Examples are the pleura (PLOO-ra), which encloses the lungs; the pericardium (per-i-KAR-dee-um), which surrounds the heart; and the peritoneum (per-i-toh-NEE-um), which lines the abdominal cavity.

The structure of serous membranes is an outer layer of simple squamous (flattened) epithelium on a thin layer of loose connective tissue. Each serous membrane forms a double lining with an outer lining and an inner lining. The outer lining of each body cavity is called the *parietal layer.* The inner lining that covers each organ within a body cavity is called the *visceral layer.*

Serous membranes secrete a thin, clear fluid called **serous fluid**. This fluid serves as a lubricant between the parietal and visceral membranes to minimize friction and "wear and tear" on organs that move within the linings, such as the beating heart.

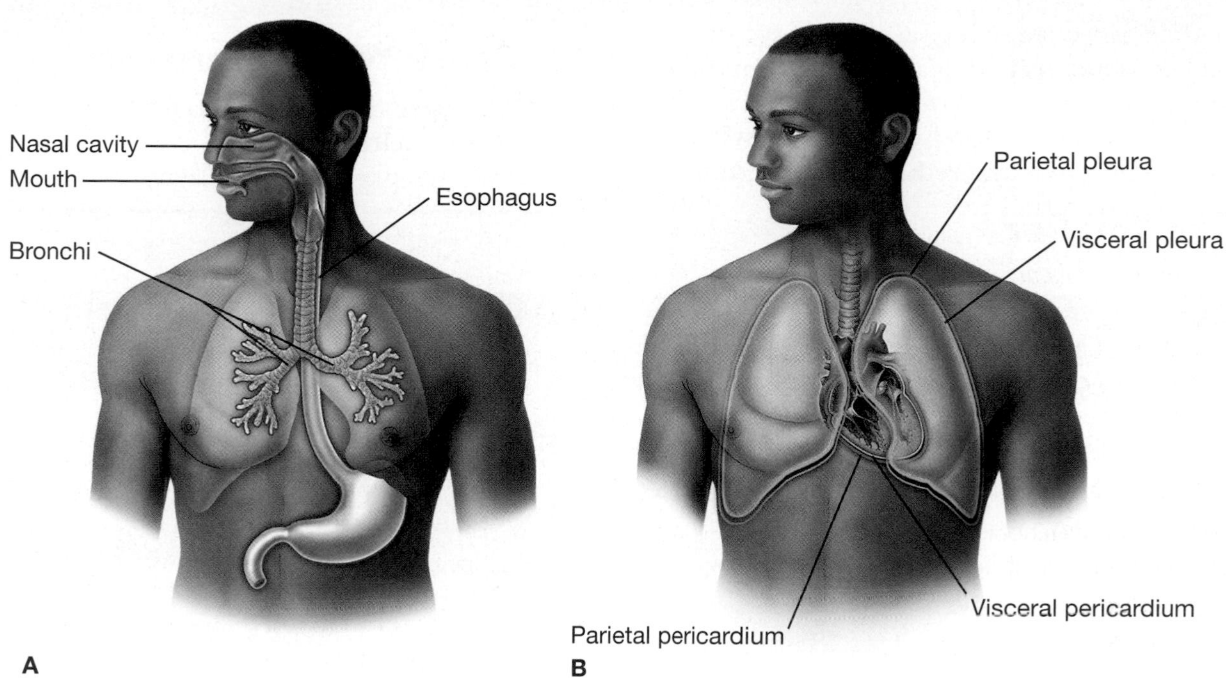

© Body Scientific International

Figure 3.1 Two classes of epithelial membranes. A—Mucous membranes line body cavities that open to the outside world. B—Serous membranes line body cavities that are closed to the outside world.

Cutaneous Membrane

The **cutaneous** (kyoo-TAY-nee-us) **membrane** is the anatomical name for the skin. The basic structure of skin is a keratinizing, stratified (layered) squamous epithelium over dense, fibrous connective tissue. Although the skin contains sweat glands, it is a dry membrane when sweat is not present. The integumentary system, which encompasses the skin and its related structures, is discussed in detail in the next lesson.

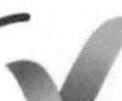

Check Your Understanding

1. Which two tissues make up epithelial membranes?
2. Where are epithelial membranes located? Name at least three locations for mucous membranes and three for serous.
3. What is the difference between mucous membranes and serous membranes?

Synovial Membranes

Synovial (si-NOH-vee-al) **membranes** are the only type of membrane in the body that are composed solely of connective tissue and include no epithelial cells. These membranes line the capsules that surround synovial joints, such as the shoulder and knee (**Figure 3.2**). They also line tendon sheaths (the connective tissue that surrounds tendons) as well as bursae,

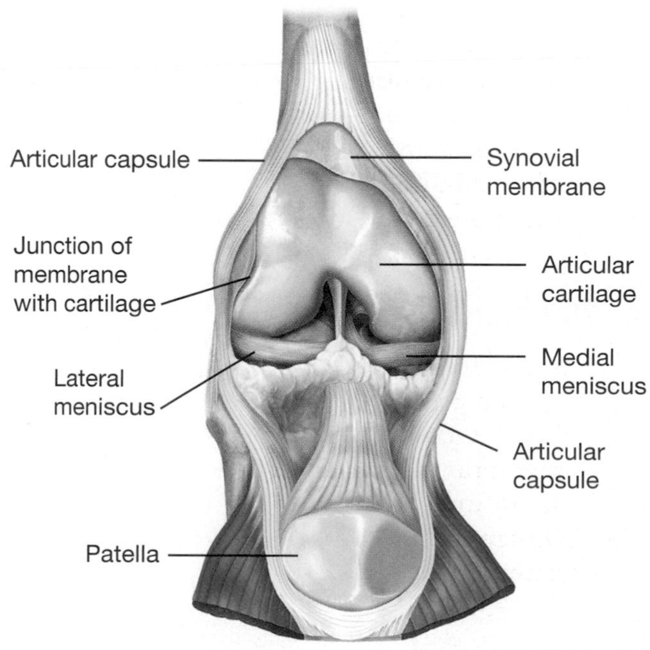

© Body Scientific International

Figure 3.2 Anterior view of a synovial joint.

the small, connective tissue sacs that serve as cushions for tendons and ligaments surrounding the joints. Synovial membranes in all these locations secrete a clear **synovial fluid**, which provides cushioning and reduces friction and wear on moving structures.

Check Your Understanding

1. Which type of body membrane contains no epithelial cells?
2. Name the two purposes of synovial fluid.

LESSON 3.1 Review and Assessment

Mini Glossary

Make sure that you know the meaning of each key term.

cutaneous membrane another name for skin

epithelial membranes thin sheets of tissue lining the internal and external surfaces of the body

membranes thin sheets or layers of pliable tissue

mucous membranes thin sheets of tissue lining the body cavities that open to the outside world

mucus a slippery solution that protects the mucous membranes and aids in transporting substances

serous fluid a thin, clear liquid that serves as a lubricant between parietal and visceral membranes

serous membranes thin sheets of tissues that line body cavities closed to the outside world

synovial fluid a clear liquid secreted by synovial membranes that provides cushioning for and reduces friction in synovial joints

synovial membrane the lining of the synovial joint cavity that produces synovial fluid

Know and Understand

1. List the two main categories of body membranes.
2. List the subcategories of the epithelial membranes.
3. Describe the basic structure of skin.
4. What type of tissue makes up synovial membranes?
5. Name three examples of serous membranes.
6. List the areas of the body in which mucous membranes are found.

Analyze and Apply

7. What is the primary purpose of the fluid that is produced by serous membranes?
8. If synovial fluid were not present, what would happen to the joints in the body?
9. Of what condition would dry mucous membranes in the body be a symptom, and how could this symptom be treated?
10. Serous membranes line and enclose several body cavities, where they secrete a lubricating fluid that reduces friction from the movement of what body tissue?
11. What is the main purpose of the cutaneous membrane, and how does it achieve its goal?

IN THE LAB

12. Using the information that you have learned about membranes, use a magnifying mirror to examine your mouth and nose. What do you see? What color is the skin that lines your mouth? Is it moist or dry? How would you describe the skin around your nose? Write a detailed description of the skin in your mouth and nose. Do the characteristics that you noted match the information presented in this lesson?
13. Search online for pictures of laboratory slides of each type of tissue discussed in this chapter: epithelial, mucous, serous, cutaneous, and connective tissue. Print and paste the pictures to 3×5 cards to create flash cards. On the back of each card, write the name and function of the tissue. With a partner, use these cards to study the various types of tissue. Practice pronouncing any terms with which you are not familiar.

LESSON 3.2

The Integumentary System

Before You Read

Try to answer the following questions before you read this lesson.

- What causes differences in skin color, and what causes tanning?
- What causes people to have straight, wavy, or curly hair?

Lesson Objectives

- Describe the functions of the integumentary system.
- Identify the layers of the skin.
- Explain the purpose and functions of the appendages of the human skin.

Key Terms

apocrine glands	Merkel cells
dermis	papillary layer
eccrine glands	reticular layer
epidermal dendritic cells	sebaceous glands
epidermis	sebum
hypodermis	stratum basale
integumentary system	stratum corneum
keratin	stratum granulosum
keratinocytes	stratum lucidum
lipocytes	stratum spinosum
melanin	subcutaneous fascia
melanocytes	sudoriferous glands

The skin is the major organ of the **integumentary** (in-tehg-yoo-MEHN-ta-ree) **system**. The term *integumentary* comes from the Latin word *integumentum*, which means "covering." However, the integumentary system is not simply a membrane like those discussed in the previous lesson. It is an entire system that includes a cutaneous membrane, sweat and oil glands, and nails and hair. Working together, these structures perform critically important functions that are not only convenient but also essential for life.

Functions of the Integumentary System

The skin forms a protective cover that serves a variety of purposes. When you sustain a cut or an abrasion, your skin acts as the first line of defense in protecting the underlying tissues. The skin's outermost layer contains **keratin** (KER-a-tin), a tough protein also found in hair and nails that adds structural strength. In addition, keratin helps to protect the skin against damage from harmful chemicals.

Keratin and naturally occurring oils in the skin also act as a water barrier. The skin substantially lessens the evaporation of water and the loss of essential molecules that the water carries from inside the body. Furthermore, keratin prevents water from entering the body during bathing or swimming.

The skin is also critically important in regulating body temperature, due to the extensive array of tiny capillaries and sweat glands that lie near the surface of the skin. When the body is overheated, the capillaries dilate (expand), enabling body heat to dissipate. Likewise, during hot conditions, the sweat glands become active, producing sweat that evaporates and has a cooling effect on the skin. When the environment is cold, the capillaries constrict (tighten), and blood flow moves to deeper vessels away from the skin to minimize heat loss.

Skin is also involved in certain chemical processes in the body. Specialized cells in the skin called **melanocytes** (MEHL-a-noh-sights) produce **melanin**, a pigment that helps protect the body against the harmful effects of ultraviolet ray damage from sunlight. Exposure to the ultraviolet-B (UVB) rays from sunlight causes the conversion of modified cholesterol molecules called *provitamin D3* in the skin to vitamin D. Vitamin D is essential for bone health. In addition, during the process of sweating, the body eliminates chemical waste products, including urea, uric acid, and salts. And, because the fluid secreted by the sweat glands is acidic, it helps to protect the body against bacterial infections.

Finally, the skin contains specialized sensory receptors that are part of the nervous system. These receptors transmit nerve signals that contain information about the environment, including touch, pressure, vibration, pain, and temperature. The table in Figure 3.3 summarizes the functions of the integumentary system.

Check Your Understanding

1. What elements in the skin act as a water barrier?
2. How do sweat glands protect against bacterial infections?

Anatomy of the Skin

The skin has two layers—an outer **epidermis** (ehp-i-DERM-is) and an underlying **dermis** (Figure 3.4). A blister is produced when a burn or friction causes these two layers to separate, forming a fluid-filled pocket. The epidermis and dermis are thick over areas such as the soles of the feet and thin in delicate areas such as the eyelids.

MEMORY TIP

The word *dermis* means "true skin." The prefix *epi-* means "upon" or "over." The prefix *hypo-* means "below," or "under." Thus, the epidermis lies above the dermis, and the hypodermis lies below the dermis.

Beneath the dermis is the **hypodermis**, or **subcutaneous fascia**, which serves as a storage repository for fat. The hypodermis is not part of the skin, but it connects the skin to the underlying tissues. It also provides cushioning and insulation against extreme external temperatures.

Epidermis

The outer layer of skin, the epidermis, is the visible skin. The epidermis contains five layers of tissue (Figure 3.5). From superficial to deep (the outside going in), these are named the **stratum corneum**, **stratum lucidum**, **stratum granulosum**, **stratum spinosum**, and **stratum basale**.

All epidermal layers consist of cells, but they do not include a blood supply that provides nutrients to the skin. The innermost layer, the stratum basale, absorbs nutrients from the underlying dermis. The cells in the stratum basale are constantly producing new skin cells. As new cells germinate, they are pushed toward the surface and away from nutrients. Eventually, they die.

Most of the cells within the epidermis are **keratinocytes** (keh-RAT-i-noh-sights), which produce keratin. Moving up through the stratum spinosum and stratum granulosum, cells become progressively flatter and more filled with keratin, which makes them tough and water-resistant. The stratum lucidum is a clear layer of thick skin found only on the palms of the hands, fingers, soles of the feet, and toes.

Functions of the Integumentary System

Function	Mechanisms
Protection	Tough keratin protects against mechanical injury and chemical damage. Melanocytes produce melanin to protect against UV ray damage. Acidic sweat protects against bacterial infections.
Water barrier	Keratin and oils in the skin reduce water loss through evaporation and form a barrier against water infusion.
Temperature regulation	Capillaries dilate to dissipate heat and constrict to conserve heat. Sweat evaporation provides a cooling effect.
Vitamin D production	Sunlight converts modified cholesterol molecules to vitamin D, which is essential for bone health.
Waste elimination	Urea and uric acid are eliminated in sweat.
Sensory perception	Receptor cells transmit information about touch, pressure, vibration, pain, and temperature to the nervous system.

Goodheart-Willcox Publisher

Figure 3.3

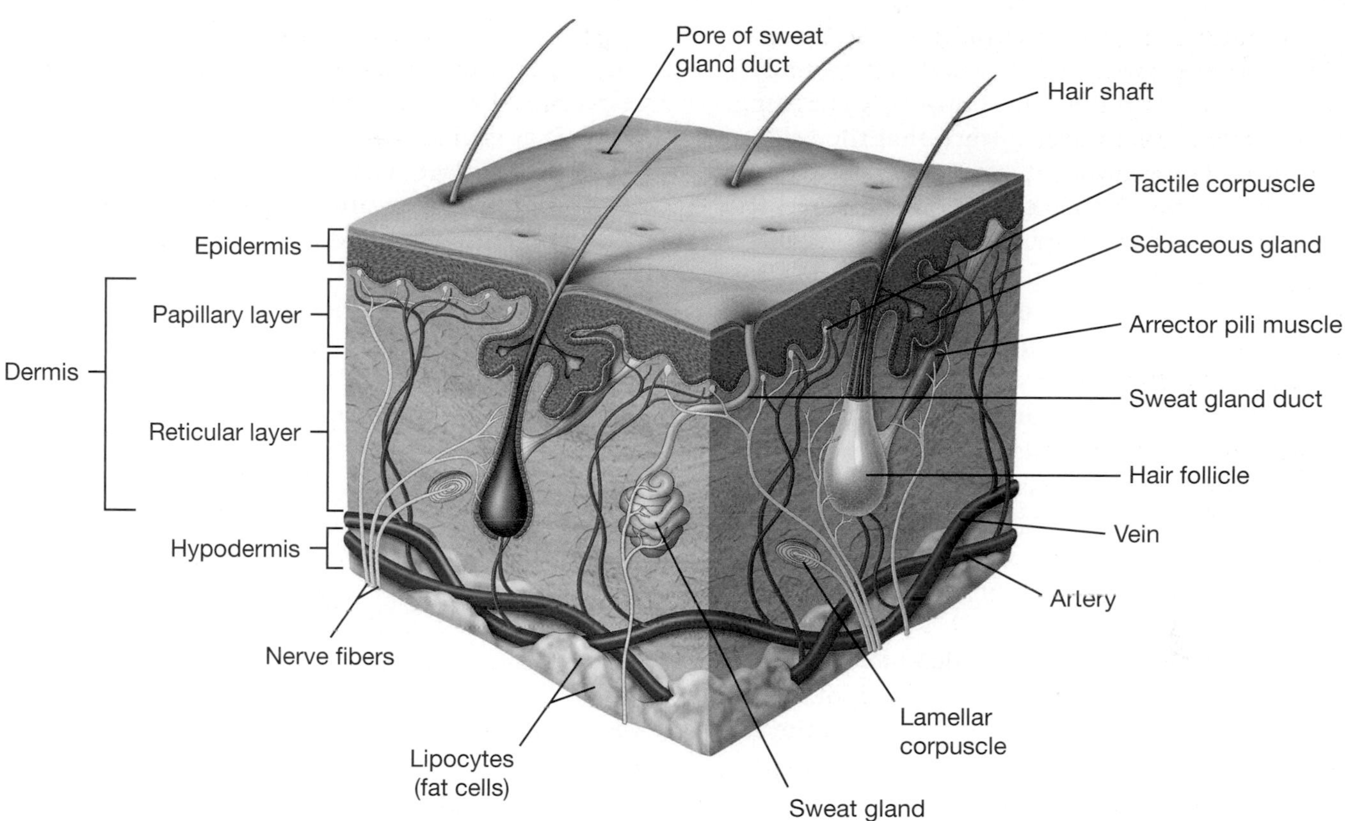

Figure 3.4 The layers and structures of the integumentary system.

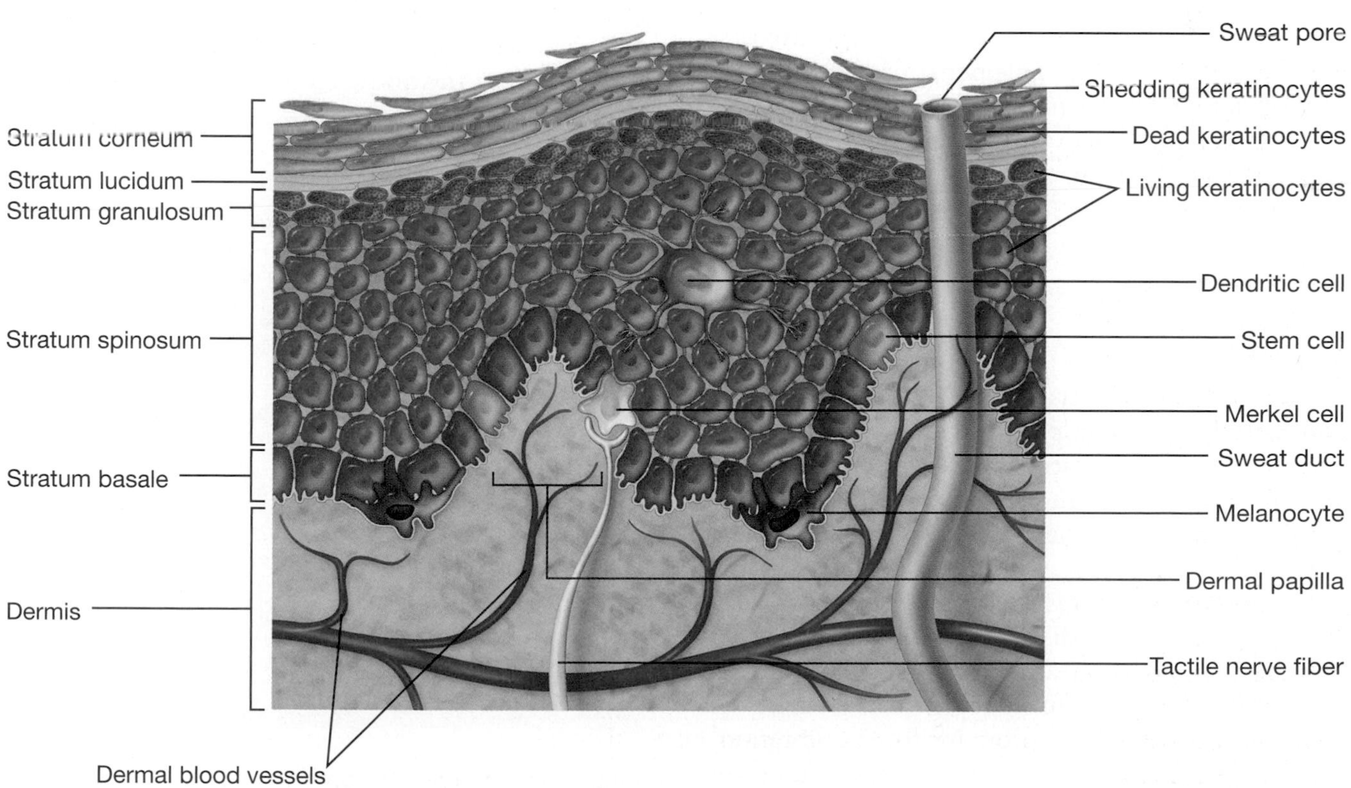

Figure 3.5 The layers of the epidermis. *Which layer continually produces new cells?*

The outer layer of the epidermis, the stratum corneum, consists of dead cells that are totally filled with keratin and are continually shedding. You might be surprised to learn that the epidermis completely replaces itself every 25 to 45 days.

The stratum basale contains melanocytes. As you may recall, these specialized cells produce the pigment melanin. Melanin, which ranges in color from reddish yellow to brown and black, is primarily responsible for human skin color. Exposure to sunlight causes melanocytes to produce more melanin. As melanin granules are pushed out into the neighboring skin cells, the result is tanning.

The presence of extra melanin in the skin functions as a sunscreen, which is why sunburn is more likely to affect individuals with light skin. Sunburn is also less likely once a light-skinned person has a tan.

An inherited condition called *albinism* (AL-bi-nizm) prevents the normal production of melanin. Albinism produces very little pigment in the skin, hair, and eyes. Individuals with albinism have extremely pale skin and white hair.

The epidermis contains specialized cells associated with the immune and nervous systems. **Epidermal dendritic cells** respond to the presence of foreign bacteria or viruses by initiating an immune system response, which brings in other specialized cells to attack the foreign invaders. There are as many as 800 dendritic cells per square millimeter of skin to help ward off infections.

Merkel cells (also called *Merkel-Ranvier cells*), located in the stratum basale, function as touch receptors. These cells form junctions with sensory nerve endings that relay information about touch to the brain.

Dermis

The dermis, or "true skin," is a dense, fibrous connective tissue composed of collagen and elastic fibers. The collagen fibers provide toughness and also bind with water molecules to help keep the inner skin moist. The elastic fibers are what keep the skin looking young, without wrinkles or sagging.

The dermis has a rich supply of blood vessels, which, as previously discussed, dilate or constrict to help dissipate or retain body heat, respectively. Also present throughout the dermis is a variety of specialized sensory receptors for touch, vibration, pain, and temperature. These receptors communicate with nerve endings to transmit information to the brain about what the body is sensing. Specialized white blood cells called *phagocytes* (FAG-oh-sights), which are distributed throughout the dermis, are responsible for ingesting foreign material, including bacteria as well as dead cells.

The outer layer of the dermis is the **papillary** (PAP-i-lar-ee) **layer**, after the *dermal papillae* (pa-PIL-ee) that protrude from its surface up into the epidermis (**Figure 3.6**). Some of the dermal papillae contain capillaries that supply nutrients to the epidermis. Other dermal papillae contain nerve endings involved in sensing touch and pain. These papillae form genetically determined, ridged patterns on the palms of the hands, fingers, toes, and soles of the feet. It is from the papillae patterns on the fingers that each person's unique fingerprints are derived.

Underneath the papillary layer lies the **reticular layer** of the dermis. The collagen and elastic fibers in this region have an irregular arrangement. The reticular layer includes blood and lymphatic vessels, sweat and oil glands, involuntary muscles, hair follicles, and nerve endings.

Hypodermis

The hypodermis, or subcutaneous fascia, includes fibrous connective tissue and adipose (fatty) tissue. It is within the hypodermis that **lipocytes** (LIP-oh-sights), or fat cells, reside. Some amount of body fat is important for padding and insulating the interior of the body. Fat also serves as a source of energy.

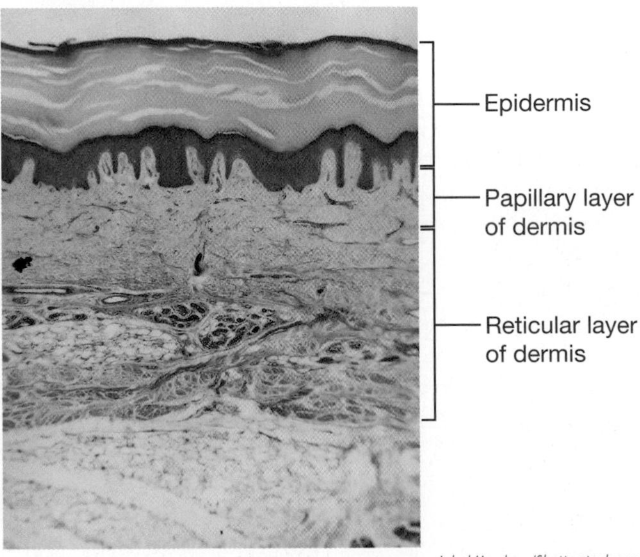

Jubal Harshaw/Shutterstock.com

Figure 3.6 Light micrograph showing the two regions of the dermis below the epidermis. *Why do you think the dermis is called the "true skin"?*

Check Your Understanding

1. What are the two layers of skin?
2. Where does the body store fat?
3. What specialized cells are responsible for human skin color?

Appendages of the Skin

The integumentary system includes several appendages, or accessory structures, that help the skin perform its functions. Structures considered to be appendages of the skin include the sudoriferous glands, sebaceous glands, hair, and nails.

Sudoriferous Glands

Sudoriferous (soo-doh-RIF-er-us) **glands** are sweat glands. They are distributed in the dermis over the entire body, with larger concentrations in the axilla (under the arms), on the palms of the hands and soles of the feet, and on the forehead. Each person has approximately 2 to 3 million sweat glands. The two types of sweat glands are eccrine glands and apocrine glands (**Figure 3.7**).

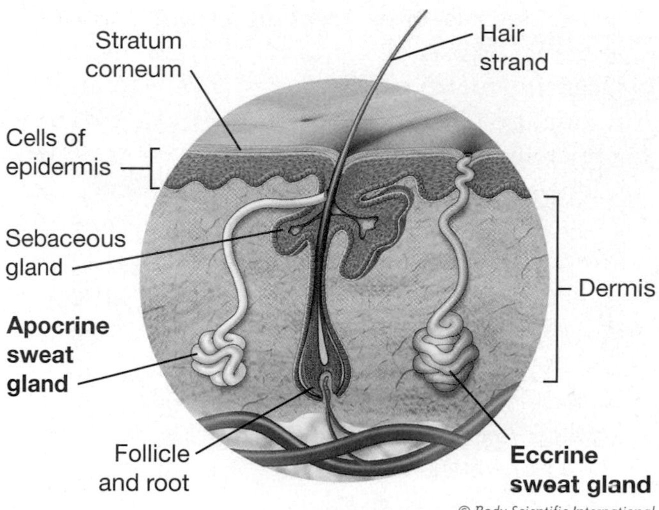

Figure 3.7 The eccrine and apocrine sweat glands. *What is the difference between the eccrine and the apocrine glands?*

The **eccrine** (EK-rin) **glands** are the major sweat glands of the body. They cover most of the body and open directly onto the skin. The sweat secreted by eccrine glands is a clear, acidic fluid that consists of approximately 99% water, but it also contains waste products such as urea, uric acid, salts, and vitamin C.

LIFE SPAN DEVELOPMENT: *The Integumentary System*

The integumentary system develops through a series of events, beginning before birth and continuing throughout life. Following birth, these changes are brought about by the normal aging process and are influenced by genetic, environmental, and lifestyle-related factors.

In the developing fetus, the beginnings of the epidermis and dermis are present by the end of the first month. Keratinocytes start developing at 9 weeks, and at 13 weeks differentiation of the skin layers is noticeable. Hair follicles originate at 14 weeks, sebaceous glands at 18 weeks, and eccrine glands at 23 weeks. By 34 weeks, the keratinocytes are mature and flattened. During the third trimester, a protective covering called the *vernix caseosa* is secreted by the sebaceous glands. This white substance, composed of lipids, protein, and water, surrounds and protects the fetal skin.

At birth, a baby's skin transitions from continuous immersion in the mother's amniotic fluid to exposure to the air. This causes an initial dehydration of the skin, followed by increasing hydration for up to three months as the skin adapts. The increased skin hydration lasts for approximately the first year of the baby's life. Although at birth, the skin in full-term infants includes all five layers, the skin continues to develop functional capabilities over the first year. Infant skin is in a constant state of flux with changes in hydration, lipid content, and skin acidity.

The next developmental period lasts from infancy to puberty. The skin of both males and females thickens continuously during this stage, although the epidermal and dermal layers of males thickens more than that of females.

With the onset of puberty, hormones exert significant influence on the glands in the skin. Androgens (steroids) stimulate the sebaceous glands, which increase the oiliness of the skin and hair and may cause acne (**Figure 3.8A**). Females accumulate a layer of subcutaneous fat, which is absent in males. Males begin a gradual thinning of their thick epidermal and dermal layers. In females, these layers maintain a constant thickness throughout adolescence and adulthood until menopause. Beginning with puberty, both genders experience a decrease in skin collagen content that progresses with age.

Characteristic skin changes occur for both genders in older adulthood. Thinning of the skin with the loss of collagen eventually results in translucence, with the blood vessels

(continued)

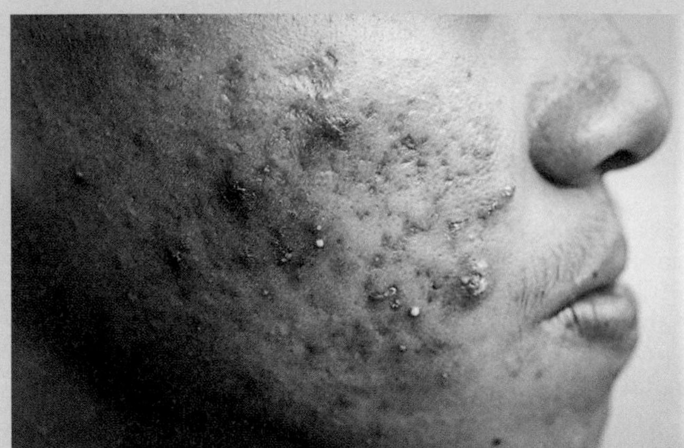

A

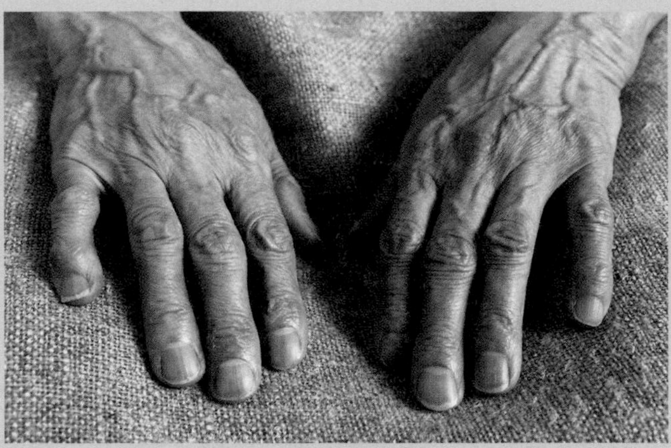

B

Bangkoker/Shutterstock.com, Alex75/Shutterstock.com

Figure 3.8 Characteristic skin changes throughout the life span. A—In puberty, hormonal changes increase the oiliness of the skin, which may result in acne. B—As a person ages, wrinkling and sagging of the skin result from loss of subcutaneous fat, combined with lower collagen levels and decreased elasticity.

clearly showing through (**Figure 3.8B**). Loss of subcutaneous fat, coupled with the decrease in collagen and elastic fibers, creates the wrinkling and sagging of the skin commonly seen in old age. Because females have lower collagen density than males, they appear to age earlier than males. The skin and hair become drier, and the skin's dermal blood vessels become fewer and more fragile. The remaining fragile vessels are easily damaged, so bruising becomes more frequent and more severe. These changes in the blood vessels and sweat glands, along with the loss of subcutaneous fat, combine to make body temperature regulation a challenge. Thus, elderly people are more prone to hypothermia in cold weather and heat stroke in hot weather.

The hair also undergoes characteristic changes with aging. Hair follicles produce less melanin, which results in the graying of hair. In some people, graying may begin as soon as the early 30s. The rate of hair color change is primarily determined by genetics. The hair strands also become finer, and fewer follicles produce new hairs. By the age of 50, most people have a reduction of approximately a third in functioning hair follicles. Male-pattern baldness is the common, large absence of hair on the top of the head. The less common female-pattern baldness involves significant thinning of the hair to the point that the scalp readily shows through.

With aging, the nails grow more slowly and may become dull or yellowed and brittle. The nails, particularly the toenails, may become thicker and may develop lengthwise ridges.

Although many of these described changes to the integumentary system are a function of aging and genetic makeup, environment and lifestyle are also factors. The strongest accelerator of facial wrinkling is smoking. The nicotine in cigarettes causes narrowing of the blood vessels in the skin. With less blood flow, the skin receives less oxygen and important nutrients. Many of the chemicals in tobacco smoke also damage collagen in the skin, causing premature wrinkling and sagging. Skin damage from smoking becomes noticeable after about 10 years. The more cigarettes you smoke and the longer you smoke, the more skin wrinkling is accentuated.

Aging of the skin is also accelerated by exposure to the sun. Over time, exposure to the ultraviolet rays in sunlight can damage collagen, making the skin less elastic and leading to wrinkling. Skin may even become thickened and leathery. The more sun exposure you have, the earlier your skin ages. Wearing sunscreen, protective covering, and avoiding excessive sun exposure can slow the onset of the characteristic changes associated with aging skin.

Life Span Review

1. Why does a newborn's skin become dehydrated during the first three months after birth?
2. What factors, other than age, can contribute to the "aging" of the skin?

Sweat is odorless, but if it is left on the skin, bacteria can chemically change it to produce an unpleasant odor. Sweat glands contain nerve endings that cause sweat to form when body temperature or external temperature is elevated. Evaporation of sweat from the skin's surface is very effective in dissipating body heat. However, during periods of physical activity in a hot environment, the body can lose as much as a liter of liquid per hour in the process of sweating. In such circumstances, it is important to drink appropriate amounts of fluids to avoid serious, potentially life-threatening conditions.

The **apocrine** (AP-oh-krin) **glands**, which begin to function during puberty, are located in the genital and axilla (armpit) areas. The apocrine glands are larger than the eccrine glands. They secrete a milky fluid consisting of sweat, fatty acids, and proteins. Unlike the eccrine gland ducts, which open directly onto the skin, the apocrine gland ducts empty into hair follicles.

Sebaceous Glands

Sebaceous (seh-BAY-shus) **glands**, located all over the body except for the palms of the hands and soles of the feet, produce an oily substance called **sebum** (SEE-bum). Most sebaceous glands empty into a hair follicle, although some secrete directly to the skin. Sebum helps to keep the skin and hair soft and also contains chemicals that kill bacteria. Because the sebaceous glands are particularly active during adolescence, teenagers' skin tends to be oily.

Hair

Hair follicles (FAHL-i-kuhlz) are bulb-shaped structures in the dermis that produce hair (**Figure 3.9**). The base of the follicle is "invaded" by a papilla of connective tissue containing a rich capillary blood supply, which provides nourishment for hair cell formation. In the matrix, or growth zone, within the base of the follicle are specialized cells that divide and generate living hair cells. But, like the epithelial cells generated in the stratum basale, as these cells are pushed up toward the scalp, they become filled with keratin and die. Most of a shaft of hair is, therefore, nonliving material composed mainly of protein.

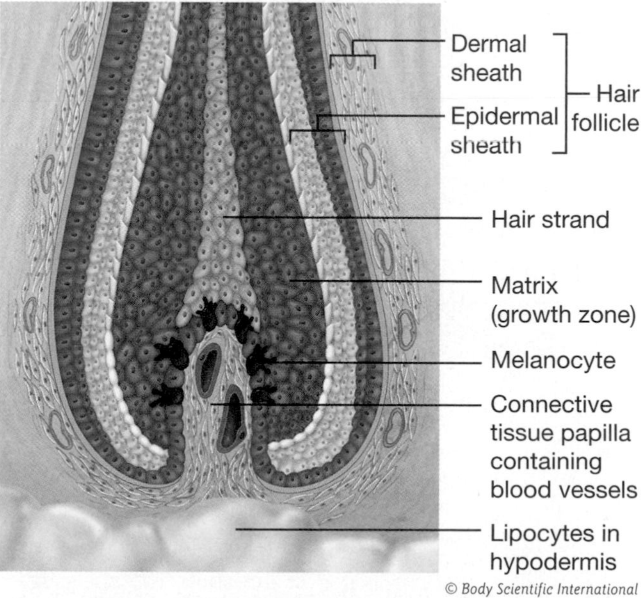

Figure 3.9 The base of a hair follicle—longitudinal section view. *If you were to ask a stylist or barber to trim all the "dead ends" from your hair, you would be practically bald. Why?*

What gives a person's hair a particular color and texture (straight, wavy, or curly)? Melanocytes within the follicle produce the pigment melanin that gives hair its color. As a person ages, the melanocytes produce less pigment, resulting in gray or white hair.

The shape of the hair follicle is genetically determined. A round hair follicle produces straight hair; an oval follicle causes hair to be wavy; and a flat follicle produces curly hair.

What causes the familiar "goose bumps" that are part of an involuntary reaction when you are cold or frightened? Tiny muscles called *arrector pili* (ah-REHK-tor PIGH-ligh) connect both sides of the hair follicle to the epidermis. When stimulated, these muscles contract, pulling the hair upright and causing the appearance of goose bumps on the skin. The erect hair traps a layer of air close to the skin, which adds insulation and helps to warm the body.

Nails

Underlying each nail is a specialized region of the stratum basale known as the *nail bed*. The proximal end of the nail bed is a thickened region called the *nail matrix*, or growth zone. Nail growth occurs within the matrix, with new cells rapidly becoming keratinized and dying.

Nails are transparent, but they appear pinkish in color because of the capillary blood supply beneath the stratum basale. The white, crescent moon-shaped region at the base of the nail, which is positioned over the thickened nail matrix, is called the *lunule* (LOO-nyool). The word *lunule* gets its name from the Latin word *luna*, which means "moon." The lunule has a curved shape like that of a crescent moon.

Check Your Understanding

1. Name four body structures that are considered to be appendages of the skin.
2. What are the two main types of sudoriferous glands?
3. What is the purpose of sebum?

LESSON 3.2 Review and Assessment

Mini Glossary

Make sure that you know the meaning of each key term.

apocrine glands sweat glands located in the genital and armpit areas that secrete a milky fluid consisting of sweat, fatty acids, and proteins

dermis layer of skin between the epidermis and hypodermis; includes nerve endings, glands, and hair follicles

eccrine glands sweat glands located over the majority of the body that produce a clear, acidic fluid that consists of approximately 99% water, but it also contains waste products such as urea, uric acid, salts, and vitamin C.

epidermal dendritic cells skin cells that initiate an immune system response to the presence of foreign bacteria or viruses

epidermis the outer layer of skin

hypodermis the layer of tissue beneath the dermis, which serves as a storage repository for fat

integumentary system enveloping organ of the body that includes the epidermis, dermis, sudoriferous and sebaceous glands, and nails and hair

keratin a tough protein found in the skin, hair, and nails

keratinocytes cells within the epidermis that produce keratin

lipocytes fat cells

melanin a pigment that protects the body against the harmful effects of ultraviolet ray damage from the sun

melanocytes specialized cells in the skin that produce melanin

Merkel cells touch receptors in the skin

papillary layer the outer layer of the dermis

reticular layer the layer of skin superficial to the papillary layer

sebaceous glands glands located all over the body that produce sebum

sebum an oily substance that helps to keep the skin and hair soft

stratum basale the deepest layer of the epidermis

stratum corneum the outer layer of the epidermis

stratum granulosum a layer of somewhat flattened cells lying just superficial to the stratum spinosum and inferior to the stratum lucidum

stratum lucidum the clear layer of thick skin found only on the palms of the hands, fingers, soles of the feet, and toes

stratum spinosum the layer of cells in the epidermis superior to the stratum basale and inferior to the stratum granulosum

subcutaneous fascia the tissue that connects the skin to underlying structures; the hypodermis

sudoriferous glands sweat glands that are distributed in the dermis over the entire body

Know and Understand

1. List the important features of the epidermal dendritic cells and Merkel cells of the epidermis.
2. What is the purpose of collagen fibers?
3. Describe elastic fibers and list the areas of the body in which they are located.
4. Describe two ways in which skin helps to protect the body.
5. What is the other name for sweat glands?
6. What are the two types of sweat glands? Describe them both.
7. Where does hair and nail growth occur?

Analyze and Apply

8. The epidermis completely replaces itself every 25 to 45 days. Describe the process of skin shedding and how the body constantly supplies nutrients to the outer layers of the skin.
9. In the summer months, exposure to extreme temperatures can be life threatening, but glands close to the surface of the skin help to keep the body cool. What are these glands and how do they help to regulate body temperature?
10. The skin is involved in chemical processes. Which vitamin is essential to bone health, and what role does the skin play in producing that vitamin?
11. In previous chapters, you read about homeostasis. Relate what you have previously read to the function of the skin in regard to regulating the body's temperature.
12. If a person has albinism, does the person's epidermis function normally? Explain.

IN THE LAB

13. Using the information that you have learned about the layers of skin, examine your hands, arms, and feet. Describe what the skin looks like on these areas. Does the skin of your hands and feet have a different color, thickness, or design than that of your arms? Describe in detail why this is or is not the case.
14. Assume that you are a forensic scientist who has been asked to help solve a murder using a few strands of hair that were caught in the victim's hand. Using a few strands of your own hair, follow this procedure:
    1. Place a drop of water on a clean microscope slide.
    2. Place several strands of hair on the drop of water.
    3. Use forceps to place a coverslip on top.
    4. Examine the slide under low and high power.
    5. In your lab notebook, record the color and structure of the hair. Be specific.

LESSON 3.3 Injuries and Disorders of the Skin

Before You Read

Try to answer the following questions before you read this lesson.

- Why are the worst skin burns not painful?
- Which common viral infection never completely goes away?

Lesson Objectives

- Describe common injuries of the skin and how they are treated.
- List common viral, fungal, and bacterial infections of the skin.
- Describe common inflammatory conditions of the skin and membranes.
- Explain the difference between benign and malignant tumors.

Key Terms

ABCD rule
basal cell carcinoma
cellulitis
decubitus ulcers
first-degree burns
fourth-degree burns
herpes simplex virus type 1 (HSV-1)
herpes simplex virus type 2 (HSV-2)
herpes varicella
herpes zoster
human papillomavirus (HPV)
impetigo
melanoma
peritonitis
plantar warts
pleurisy
psoriasis
rule of nines
second-degree burns
squamous cell carcinoma
third-degree burns
tinea

As the first "line of defense" in protecting the body from the external environment, the skin is routinely subject to minor injuries and is exposed to a variety of common infections. Fortunately, the skin is a multilayered system with a remarkable capacity for self-healing.

CLINICAL CASE STUDY

Joe plays left wing on his school's club ice hockey team. At a recent team practice, he realized that he had forgotten his uniform pants, so he borrowed a pair from a teammate who is about the same size. Two days later, Joe has developed a red, itchy rash on his upper, inner thighs. When questioned by his doctor about this, Joe reveals that he has not had recent sexual activity. As you read this section, try to determine which of the following conditions Joe most likely has.

A. Herpes simplex type 2
B. Genital warts
C. Tinea cruris
D. Impetigo

Skin Injuries

The skin commonly sustains minor cuts, abrasions, and blisters that tend to heal quickly. This healing is aided by the skin's normal self-renewal process. Every 25 to 45 days, new epithelial cells reach the surface of the skin.

With all minor skin injuries, infection is a major concern. Injuries to the skin that penetrate the underlying tissues are more complicated, and infection is still the most significant concern.

Decubitus Ulcers

Decubitus (deh-KYOO-bi-tus) **ulcers** are pressure ulcers. Often inaccurately called *bedsores*, decubitus ulcers are skin injuries caused by an area of localized pressure that restricts blood flow to one or more areas of the body. Without the normal blood supply to provide nutrients and oxygen, the skin cells die. These skin injuries typically occur in people who undergo prolonged bed rest. When a bedridden patient is not turned often enough, sustained pressure over an area can result in a decubitus ulcer. Decubitus ulcers can occur anywhere on the body, but most form over bony areas such as the lower back, coccyx (tailbone), hips, elbows, and ankles.

A decubitus ulcer begins as an area of reddened skin, but as cells start to die, small cracks or openings appear in the skin. As the condition progresses, the tissue continues to degenerate and an open ulcer forms. If not treated, tissue degeneration can progress all the way to the bone and eventually can be fatal.

Decubitus ulcers can develop in any situation in which the blood supply to the tissues is restricted. People who use wheelchairs, for example, can develop decubitus ulcers over pressure points. Individuals with numbness in parts of the body from a spinal injury or diabetes mellitus must be particularly careful to avoid remaining in the same position for prolonged periods.

Treatment for decubitus ulcers includes prescription of oral antibiotics to address or prevent infection. Removal of damaged tissues is another component of treatment. Because dead tissue prevents healing, it must be removed for proper healing to occur.

There are two approaches to removing ulcer-damaged tissues: debridement and vacuum-assisted closure. Debridement is the removal of dead tissue using a surgical or chemical procedure. In vacuum-assisted closure, a vacuum tube is attached to the wound. The vacuum draws moisture from the ulcer, thereby shortening the healing process and reducing the risk of infection.

Proper nutrition is an important factor in both the prevention and healing of decubitus ulcers. Vitamins A, B, C, and E and the minerals magnesium, manganese, selenium, and zinc all contribute to skin health. Sufficient amounts of dietary protein are also important.

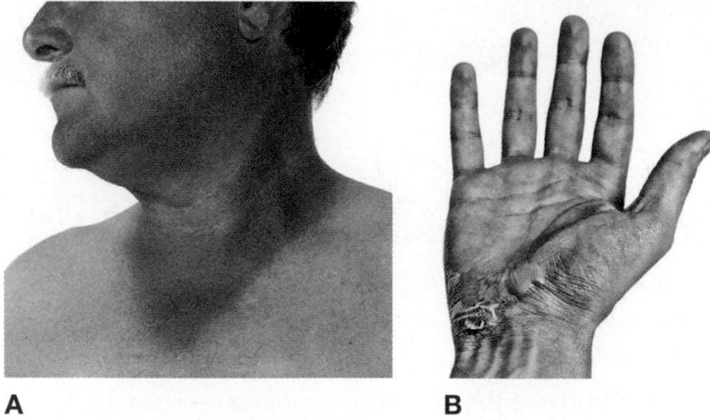

A B

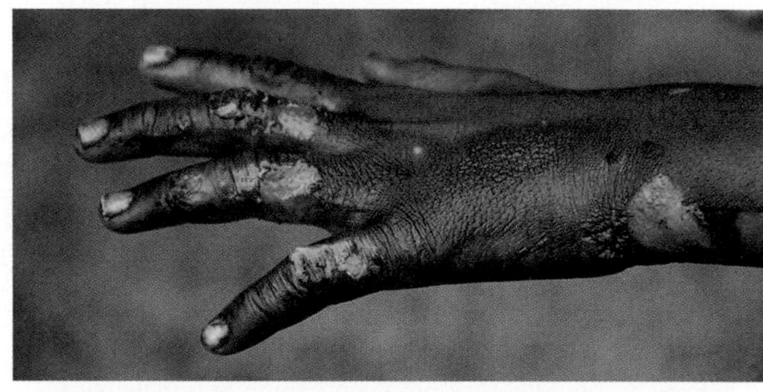

C

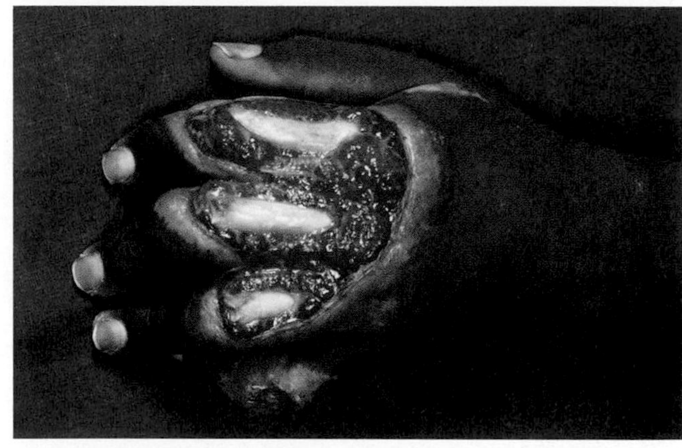

D

Suzanne Tucker/Shutterstock.com, JTeffects/Shutterstock.com, Naiyyer/Shutterstock.com, Dr. M.A. Ansary/Science Source

Figure 3.10 Different types of burns. A—First-degree burn. B—Second-degree burn. C—Third-degree burn. D—Fourth-degree burn.

Burns

Burns are injuries that can arise from exposure to excessive heat, corrosive chemicals, electricity, or ultraviolet radiation (from sunburn, for example). Burns, which vary considerably in severity, cause tissue damage and cell death.

First-degree burns affect only the epidermal layer of skin (**Figure 310A**). These burns involve reddening of the skin and mild pain, and they tend to heal in less than a week. Most types of sunburn are first-degree burns.

Second-degree burns involve damage to both the epidermis and the upper portion of the underlying dermis (**Figure 3.10B**). Second-degree burns are characterized by blisters, fluid-filled pockets that form between the epidermal and dermal layers. These burns are painful and take longer to heal than first-degree burns. An even longer period of healing is required for larger blisters.

Third-degree burns destroy the entire thickness of the skin (**Figure 3.10C**). For this reason, they are also called *full-thickness burns*. (First- and second-degree burns are called *partial-thickness burns*.) The area affected by a third-degree burn appears grayish-white or blackened. Although a third-degree burn is a serious injury, it is initially not painful because the nerve endings in the skin have been destroyed. Later, scarring and pain will occur. A third-degree burn cannot heal on its own because the stratum basale, which generates new skin cells, has been destroyed. Treatment involves grafting skin over the damaged area.

The most serious burns are **fourth-degree burns**, which destroy all layers of skin, and also some of the underlying tissues (**Figure 3.10D**). These may include nerve endings, muscle, tendon, ligament, and bone. Reconstruction of these underlying tissues may be required, as well as the grafting of new skin.

When a large region of skin has been burned, clinicians use the **rule of nines** to estimate the extent of burned tissue. **Figure 3.11** illustrates the rule of nines. According to this rule, the percentage of total body surface area covered by burns is approximated as follows:

- 9% for both the anterior (front) and posterior (back) of the head and neck;
- 18% for the anterior and 18% for the posterior of the torso;
- 9% for both the anterior and posterior of each arm;
- 18% for both the anterior and posterior of each leg; and
- 1% for the genital region.

Using this approach for both the anterior and posterior surface areas of the body, the total is 100%. For example, if the anterior of the torso and the anterior of one arm were burned, the affected surface area would be approximately 23% (4.5% for the anterior of the arm and 18 percent for the anterior of the torso).

The descriptions of the various diseases and disorders throughout this textbook include information about the following aspects of each:

- The etiology (cause) of the disease
- Strategies for prevention
- Pathology (clinical characteristics)
- Diagnosis (keys for identifying the condition)
- Common treatments

Each type of skin injury is diagnosed and treated according to accepted, or standard, practices. The etiology, strategies for prevention, pathology, diagnosis, and common treatments for these injuries of the skin are summarized in **Figure 3.12**.

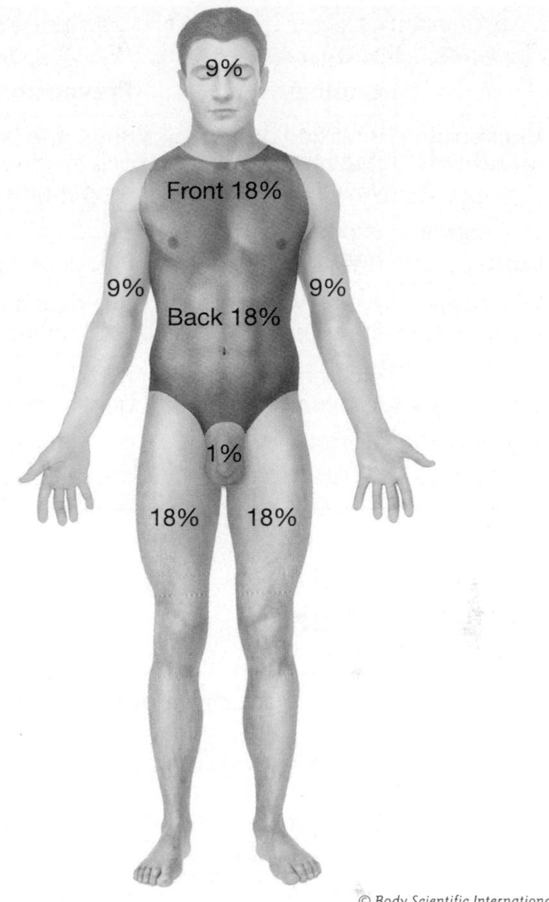

© Body Scientific International

Figure 3.11 The rule of nines. *How is the rule of nines useful in helping a physician determine how to treat a patient with burns on his body?*

Check Your Understanding

1. What causes decubitus ulcers?
2. Where on the body do decubitus ulcers commonly occur?
3. What is the difference between a first-degree and second-degree burn?

Infections of the Skin and Membranes

Skin infections can be caused by contact with an infectious agent that is present on another person or a surface. They can also be caused by airborne particles such as viruses or bacteria or by contamination introduced by a foreign object into a penetrating wound.

Injuries of the Skin					
	Etiology	**Prevention**	**Pathology**	**Diagnosis**	**Treatment**
Decubitus ulcer	localized pressure that reduces blood flow to the skin	changing body position frequently, proper nutrition	reddened area of skin progresses to an open ulcer	visual observation and case history	oral antibiotics, removal of dead tissue
1st-degree burn	exposure to sun or heat source	avoidance of sun or heat	reddening of skin, mild pain	visual observation	topical analgesic
2nd-degree burn	prolonged exposure to sun or heat	avoidance of heat source	damage to epidermis, blisters	visual observation	topical analgesic
3rd- and 4th-degree burns	prolonged exposure to extreme heat	avoidance of heat source	destruction of all skin layers, including nerve endings; 4th-degree also damages underlying tissues	visual observation	skin grafting, antibiotics

Figure 3.12 Goodheart-Willcox Publisher

Viral Infections

Many people think of viruses as the cause for respiratory illnesses, such as flu or the common cold. However, viruses can also cause infections in many body systems, including the integumentary system.

Herpes

Herpes is a viral infection that produces small, painful, blister-like sores. Once a herpes infection is present, it lasts for the rest of a person's life. Fortunately, herpes infections tend to stay dormant most of the time, with no noticeable sign of infection. Occasional flare-ups do occur, however; the resurgence of symptoms usually accompanies periods of stress or sickness. Several different varieties of the herpes virus are known to exist.

Herpes varicella (vair-i-SEHL-a), better known as *chickenpox*, is a common childhood disease. Because chickenpox is highly contagious, it tends to spread quickly and widely. The fluid-filled blisters caused by chickenpox are extremely itchy. They can spread over most of the body, or they can be limited in scope. A vaccine is available for chickenpox that decreases the chance of infection or reduces the seriousness of the virus if infection does occur. Treatment is a topical ointment or spray to reduce itching.

Once a person infected with chickenpox has recovered, the virus lies dormant. In an adult, the virus can recur as **herpes zoster** (ZAHS-ter), commonly known as *shingles* (**Figure 3.13A**). Shingles involves an extremely painful, blistering rash accompanied by headache, fever, and a general feeling of unwellness. The shingles virus may

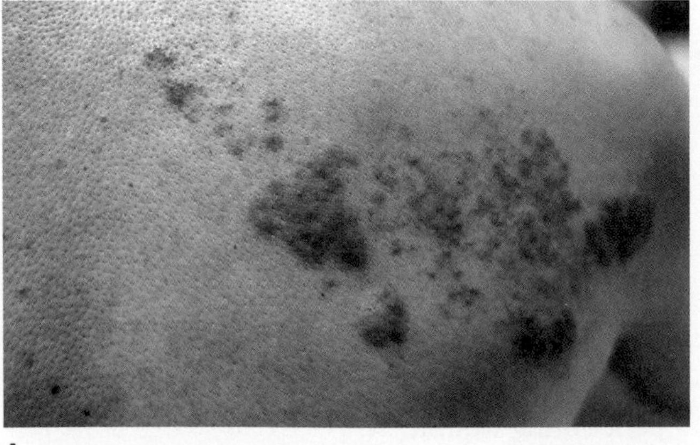

A

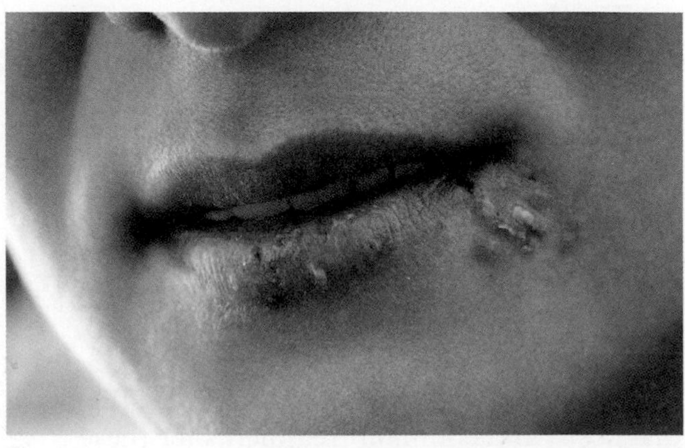

B

Mumemories/Shutterstock.com, Cherries/Shutterstock.com

Figure 3.13 Two different types of herpes infections. A—Herpes zoster (shingles) infection. B—Herpes simplex (cold sore) infection.

trigger more serious symptoms, such as chronic nerve pain. In the United States, approximately 50% of people older than 80 years of age have had shingles at least once. A vaccine for shingles is recommended for adults older than 60 years of age. Treatments include an antiviral medication and analgesic.

Herpes simplex virus type 1 (HSV-1), sometimes associated with the common cold, generates "cold sores" or "fever blisters" around the mouth (**Figure 3.13B**). **Herpes simplex virus type 2 (HSV-2)** is the genital form of herpes. Both types of the herpes simplex virus are highly contagious and can be transmitted to the mouth or genital area through physical contact with an infected person. In the United States, about one in six people has genital herpes.

Transmission of the herpes simplex virus from an infected male to a female partner occurs with greater ease than from an infected female to a male partner. Thus, more women than men are infected with the virus.

During the first outbreak of genital herpes, a person may experience flu-like symptoms such as fever, body aches, and swollen glands. Repeat outbreaks are common, particularly during the first year of infection. Symptoms during repeat outbreaks are usually shorter in duration and less severe than those in the first outbreak. As with all herpes infections, once a person has been infected by a herpes simplex virus, it remains dormant, with the potential to reactivate, throughout the remainder of the person's life. However, the number of outbreaks tends to decrease over time.

What Research Tells Us

...about High-Risk HPVs and Cancer

The human papillomavirus (HPV) infects epithelial cells on the skin and in the membranes that line areas such as the genital tract and anus. When an HPV enters an epithelial cell, the virus begins making specialized proteins. Two of these proteins initiate cancer by interfering with the cell's normal functions, enabling the cell to grow in an uncontrolled manner and resist cell death (**Figure 3.14**).

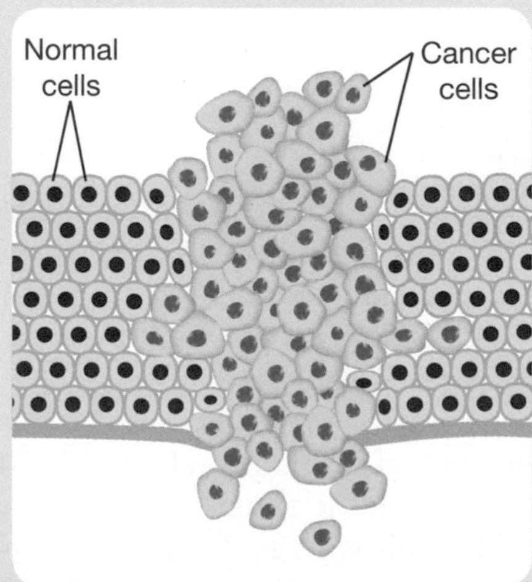

Alila Sao Mai/Shutterstock.com

Figure 3.14 Development of cancer cells. *Explain how HPV-infected cells can develop into a tumor.*

When the immune system recognizes HPV-infected cells, it attacks and attempts to destroy them. When the immune system fails, however, these infected cells continue to grow, and infection takes root. As the cells multiply, they can develop mutations that further promote cell growth, sometimes leading to tumor development.

Researchers believe that some 10 to 20 years can pass between the initial HPV infection and tumor formation. They estimate, however, that less than 50% of high-grade HPV infections lead to cancer. Fortunately, because HPVs do not enter the bloodstream, an HPV infection in one part of the body should not spread to other parts of the body.

Taking It Further

1. Working with a group of classmates, design a brochure to raise HPV awareness. Your brochure should address these questions: What is HPV? How do people become infected with this virus? How is HPV diagnosed? What treatments are available? What is the link between HPV and certain cancers? How can HPV be prevented? You might include separate discussions for HPV in women and HPV in men. Share your brochure with the rest of the class.

Human Papillomavirus (HPV)

Warts are raised, typically painless growths on the skin that vary in shape and size. Warts can spread from one part of the body to another. Less commonly, warts can spread from one person to another. All types of warts are caused by the **human papillomavirus (HPV)**.

HPVs are a group of more than 150 related viruses. Common warts typically appear on the hands or fingers and tend to disappear without treatment. It is important, however, to make sure that a wart-like growth on an adult is not a form of skin cancer. **Plantar warts**, which develop on the soles of the foot, grow inward and can become painful. When warranted, warts can be removed by surgery, cryotherapy (freezing), and topical medications such as salicylic acids (**Figure 3.15**).

Genital warts caused by HPV infections are the most common sexually transmitted infections in the United States. More than 40 of the HPVs can be easily spread through direct, skin-to-skin contact during vaginal, anal, and oral sex. More than 50% of all sexually active people are infected with an HPV at some point during their life.

There are two major categories of HPVs: low risk and high risk. Low-risk HPVs can cause warts on the skin around the genital area and anus but are not known to cause cancer. High-risk HPV infections, however, do cause nearly all cervical cancers, which is why some healthcare professionals advocate the papillomavirus vaccine for teenage girls and boys. High-risk HPV infections also cause most anal cancers and about 50% of all vaginal, vulvar, and penile cancers. In addition, HPV infections cause cancer of the soft palate, the base of the tongue, and the tonsils. High-risk HPVs account for about 5% of all cancers. Information about the HPVs and other viral infections of the skin described in this chapter is summarized in **Figure 3.16**.

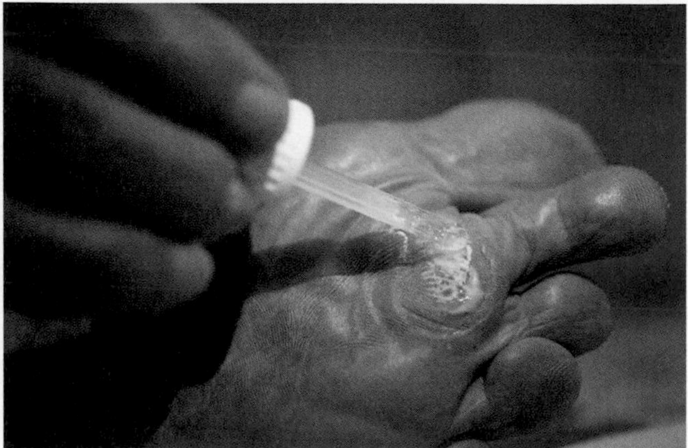

SURKED/Shutterstock.com

Figure 3.15 Salicylic acid is commonly used to treat plantar warts.

Fungal Infections

Fungal infections, or **tinea** (TIN-ee-a), tend to occur in areas of the body that are moist. They therefore tend to be more prevalent during warm weather, and they are more common in individuals whose work or sporting activities involve frequent periods of sweating.

Athlete's Foot

Tinea pedis (athlete's foot) is the most common fungal infection. It is characterized by cracked, flaky skin between the toes or on the side of the foot. The skin may also be red and itchy. Because tinea pedis is highly contagious, it spreads rapidly on locker room and shower floors. Treatment and prevention include keeping the feet clean and dry, especially between the toes, and using over-the-counter, antifungal powder or cream that contains clotrimazole, miconazole, or tolnaftate.

Jock Itch

Tinea cruris, or jock itch, is an itchy, red rash on the genitals, inner thighs, or buttocks that primarily affects males. It is caused by the combination of prolonged sweating and friction from clothes. It can be spread through direct contact with infected skin or unwashed clothing. Tinea cruris typically is treated by keeping the skin clean and dry, wearing loose clothing, and applying a topical antifungal or drying powder that contains clotrimazole, miconazole, or tolnaftate.

Ringworm

Tinea corporis, more commonly known as *ringworm*, does not actually involve any type of worm. However, the characteristically red, ring-shaped rash with a pale center somewhat resembles the shape of a worm (**Figure 3.17**).

Tinea corporis is especially common in children. It is highly contagious and can be spread through direct contact with the fungus on a person, pet, or contaminated items such as clothes or bedding. Treatment involves keeping the skin clean and dry and applying an over-the-counter, antifungal cream that contains clotrimazole, miconazole, ketoconazole, or oxiconazole.

Viral Infections of the Skin

	Etiology	Prevention	Pathology	Diagnosis	Treatment
Herpes varicella (Chickenpox)	spread by coughing, sneezing, and direct contact	vaccination	itchy, fluid-filled blisters over part or most of the body, fever	confirmed by visual observation	topical treatment for itching, (no aspirin)
Herpes zoster (Shingles)	herpes varicella lies dormant and reoccurs as herpes zoster	vaccination for adults over age 60	painful, blistering rash accompanied by headache and fever	visual observation can be confirmed with biopsy in lab	antiviral medication and analgesic
Herpes simplex (Type 1: oral herpes) (Type 2: genital herpes)	physical contact with the herpes infection on another person	avoid contact with an infected person	type 1: blister on lips type 2: blistering rash on genital area, flu-like symptoms	visual observation can be confirmed with biopsy in lab	medication to relieve pain and shorten duration
Human Papillomavirus (HPV): Low risk	physical contact with the HPV on another person or object	avoid contact or sharing objects with an infected person	small skin growths on the hands (common warts), on the soles of the feet (plantar warts), in the genital area (genital warts)	visual observation can be confirmed with biopsy in lab	if necessary, can be removed with surgery or topical treatments
Human Papillomavirus (HPV): High risk	vaginal, anal, or oral sexual contact with an infected person	vaccination prior to onset of sexual activity	can cause cancer of the cervix, vulva, vagina, penis, anus or back of the throat, including the tongue and tonsils	visual observation can be confirmed with biopsy in lab	topical treatments; cancer treatments if cancer occurs

Figure 3.16

Goodheart-Willcox Publisher

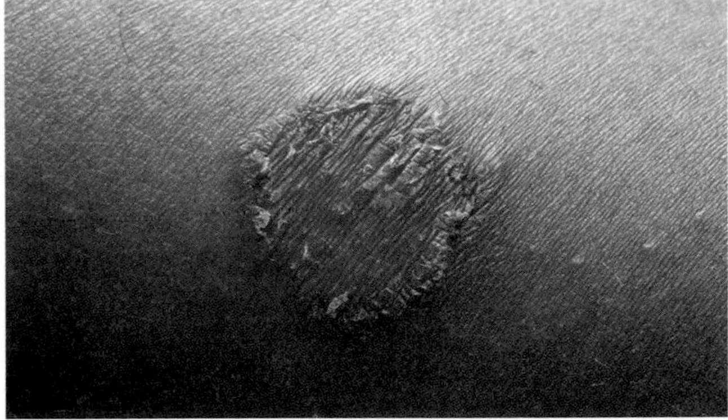

frank60/Shutterstock.com

Figure 3.17 Tinea corporis, or ringworm.

Toenail Fungus

Tinea unguium is a fungal infection under the nails of the fingers or toes. It causes discoloration and thickening of the infected nail. In general, over-the-counter antifungal creams do not help this condition. A prescription antifungal medication must be taken orally for several weeks.

Bacterial Infections

Impetigo (im-peh-TIGH-goh) is a highly contagious staphylococcus infection common in elementary school children. Its symptoms are pink, blister-like bumps, usually on the face around the mouth and nose, that develop a yellowish crust before they rupture. Antibiotic ointment is used to treat impetigo.

Cellulitis (sehl-yoo-LIGH-tis), another staphylococcus infection, is characterized by an inflamed area of skin that is red, swollen, and painful. The origin of cellulitis often is an open wound or ulceration that most commonly occurs on the lower legs but can occur anywhere on the body. Cellulitis is a serious condition that can become life threatening if not treated with antibiotics.

The etiology, strategies for prevention, pathology, diagnosis, and common treatments for fungal and bacterial infections of the skin are summarized in **Figure 3.18**.

Fungal and Bacterial Infections of the Skin					
	Etiology	**Prevention**	**Pathology**	**Diagnosis**	**Treatment**
Tinea pedis (athlete's foot) **Tinea cruris (jock itch)** **Tinea corporis (ringworm)**	contact with the fungus on a person, clothing, or object	avoid contact with fungus; keep body area clean and dry	T. pedis: cracked, flaky skin on the feet T. cruris: itchy, red rash on the genitals, inner thighs, and buttocks T. corporis: ring-shaped, red rash that spreads outward from the center	observation with a black light, in which the fungus glows	antifungal powder or cream
Tinea unguium (toenail fungus)	contact with the fungus on a person or object	avoid contact with fungus; keep body area clean and dry	discoloration and thickening of the infected nail of the hand or foot	observation with a black light, in which the fungus glows	prescription oral medication
Impetigo	contact with a person or object infected with the impetigo staphylococcus bacteria	avoid contact with infected people; wash frequently	red sores that quickly rupture, ooze for a few days, and then form a yellowish-brown crust	confirmed by visual observation	antibiotic ointment
Cellulitis	staphylococcus bacteria invades an open wound, often in the lower leg	keep skin wounds clean and protected from infection	red, swollen, painful area; can be accompanied by a fever	visual observation can be confirmed with blood test	oral antibiotic

Figure 3.18

Goodheart-Willcox Publisher

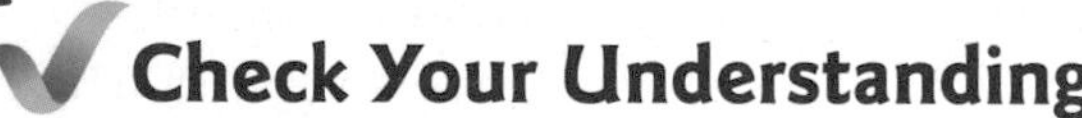

Check Your Understanding

1. Which type of herpes is responsible for "fever blisters"?
2. What causes warts?
3. What are the most common sexually transmitted infections in the United States?
4. What is impetigo?

Inflammatory Conditions of the Skin and Membranes

Inflammation is a general response of body tissue to any injury or disease that damages cells. It is a protective response that involves increased blood flow to the distressed area, along with marshalling of specialized cells that attack infectious agents and destroy dead tissue. The increased blood flow causes redness; major inflammation also causes pain and swelling. Although most infections and disorders of the skin and membranes provoke an inflammatory response, those discussed in this section are specific inflammatory conditions that may have different causes. The etiology, strategies for prevention, pathology, diagnosis, and common treatments for these inflammatory conditions of the skin and membranes are summarized in **Figure 3.19**.

Pleurisy

Pleurisy (PLOOR-i-see) is an inflammation of the pleura, the membrane that lines the thoracic (chest) cavity and lungs. It can be caused by an infection, such as pneumonia or tuberculosis. It can also be caused by cancer, rheumatoid arthritis, lupus, injury to the chest, a blockage in the blood supply to the lungs, or the harmful presence of inhaled asbestos.

Pleurisy causes the normally smooth surfaces of the pleura to become rough. With each breath, the pleura lining the chest cavity and the pleura lining the lungs rub against each other, producing a grating sound called a "friction rub" that can readily be heard with a stethoscope (**Figure 3.20**).

Inflammatory Conditions of the Skin and Membranes

	Etiology	Prevention	Pathology	Diagnosis	Treatment
Pleurisy	inflammation of pleura caused by infection, cancer, or injury	no specific strategy	chest pain that worsens with inhalation or coughing	exam with stethoscope, X-ray	anti-inflammatory drugs; other treatment depends on cause
Peritonitis	inflammation of the peritoneum caused by infection	no specific strategy	abdominal pain and tenderness, fever, nausea, fatigue, shortness of breath, rapid heartbeat, decreased urine and stool output	physical exam, X-ray	surgery to repair abdominal damage; strong antibiotics
Psoriasis	skin condition possibly caused by an autoimmune disorder	no specific strategy	overproduction of skin cells, resulting in thick, red skin with silver-white scales that itch and burn	physical exam; can be confirmed with biopsy	topical treatments, light therapy, systemic medications

Figure 3.19

Goodheart-Willcox Publisher

The primary symptom of pleurisy is chest pain that sharpens with inhalation or coughing. The pain may radiate to one or both shoulders. Pleurisy can cause an accumulation of fluid in the thoracic cavity. This fluid accumulation can make breathing difficult and may cause a bluish skin color (due to reduced oxygen circulation in the blood), shortness of breath, rapid breathing, and coughing.

The course of treatment for pleurisy depends on the cause. Bacterial infections are treated with antibiotics. When fluid has accumulated in the chest cavity, it can be drained through a surgical procedure. Anti-inflammatory drugs can help control the pain caused by pleurisy.

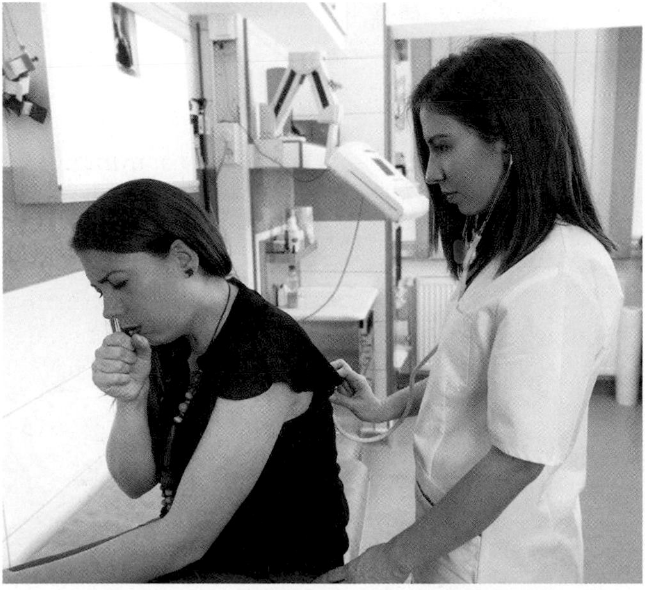

Marius Pirvu/Shutterstock.com

Figure 3.20 Doctor examining patient. *Why will the doctor be able to determine whether or not the patient has pleurisy?*

Peritonitis

Peritonitis (per-i-toh-NIGH-tis) is an inflammation of the peritoneum, the membrane that lines the inner wall of the abdomen and covers the abdominal organs. Peritonitis can result when a bacterial or fungal infection is introduced into the abdominal cavity through a rupture in the abdominal wall or a surgical procedure. Symptoms include abdominal pain and tenderness that may worsen with movement or touch. The abdomen may also be swollen. Other symptoms may include fever and chills, nausea and vomiting, fatigue, shortness of breath, rapid heartbeat, and decreased urine and stool output (**Figure 3.21**).

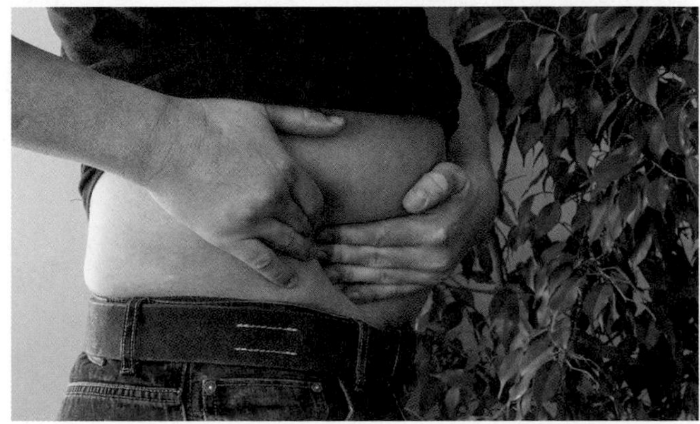

Shidiovski/Shutterstock.com

Figure 3.21 Peritonitis, like many other intestinal conditions, can result in painful swelling of the abdomen.

Peritonitis is a serious, potentially life-threatening condition. Medical treatment typically involves surgery to repair the internal damage that caused the condition, along with a course of strong antibiotics.

Psoriasis

Psoriasis (soh-RIGH-a-sis) is a common skin disorder that speeds up the life cycle of skin cells. It causes cells to build up rapidly on the surface of the skin. The extra skin cells form regions of thick, red skin with flaky, silver-white patches called *scales* that itch, burn, crack, and sometimes bleed (**Figure 3.22**).

According to the prevailing hypothesis, psoriasis has its roots in an autoimmune disorder, an inappropriate immune response to a substance or tissue that is present in the body. In the case of psoriasis, the body's immune system causes skin cells to be produced too quickly. Psoriasis is not contagious and may be hereditary. It typically develops between 15 and 35 years of age and can progress quickly or slowly. It may disappear and return, or it may persist indefinitely. Outbreaks of psoriasis most commonly affect the elbows, knees, and trunk region, although they can occur anywhere on the body.

A variety of conditions can trigger or exacerbate psoriasis. These conditions include bacterial or viral infections, minor injuries to the skin, dry skin, stress, too little or too much sunlight, excessive alcohol consumption, and certain medications. Psoriasis is also worsened by a weakened immune system due to AIDS, chemotherapy, or autoimmune disorders such as rheumatoid arthritis.

The goal of psoriasis treatment is to control symptoms and prevent infection. Three treatment approaches are available: topical treatments, systemic treatments, and light therapy. Topical treatments include special skin lotions, ointments, creams, and shampoos that are applied to the affected area. Systemic treatments, which treat the whole body, include medications that can be injected or taken orally.

Light therapy, also called *phototherapy*, is a medical treatment in which the skin is carefully exposed to ultraviolet light. The UVB in natural sunlight is an effective treatment for psoriasis. It penetrates the skin and hinders the growth of skin cells affected by the condition. In light therapy, the skin is exposed at regular intervals to a source that delivers artificial UVB (**Figure 3.23**).

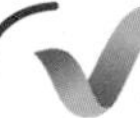

Check Your Understanding

1. What causes the redness associated with inflammation?
2. What is pleurisy?
3. What skin disorder is characterized by regions of thick, red skin with flaky, silver-white patches?

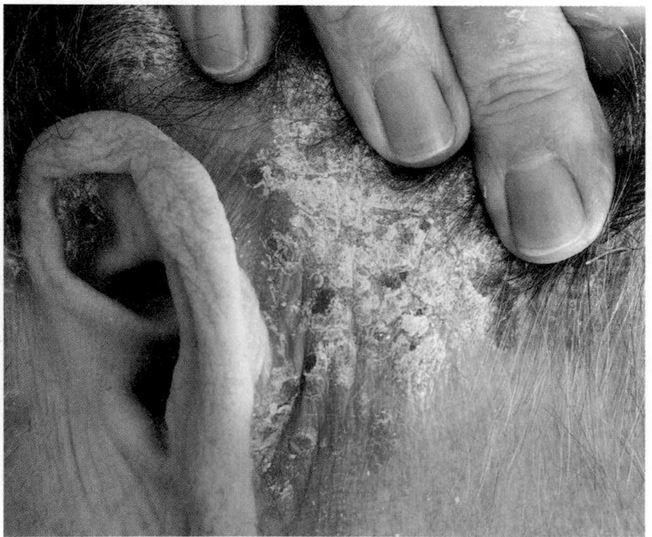

Lipowski Milan/Shutterstock.com

Figure 3.22 Psoriasis.

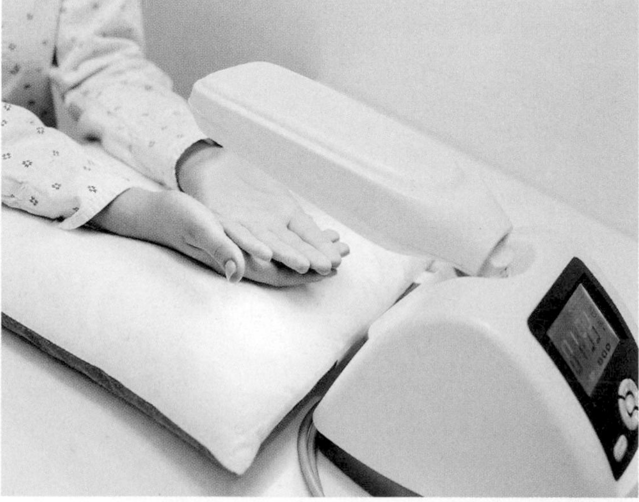

Eugeniy Kalinouskiy/Shutterstock.com

Figure 3.23 Phototherapy is a form of treatment that exposes psoriatic skin to UBV light in controlled doses.

Cancers of the Skin

As described earlier in this lesson, many skin conditions involve bumps or small, noncancerous lesions. Common warts are an example. Thus far, the conditions described have been benign—that is, they involve tumors that do not *metastasize*, or spread, to remote regions of the body.

When a tumor is malignant, or cancerous, it tends to metastasize to other body parts. Skin cancer is the most common type of cancer in the United States; at some point, about one-fifth of the population experiences skin cancer. Overexposure to the sun is a major risk factor. The three most common forms of skin cancer are basal cell carcinoma, squamous cell carcinoma, and melanoma.

Basal cell carcinoma (kar-si-NOH-ma) is the most common form of skin cancer and, fortunately, is also the least malignant (**Figure 3.24**). It is caused by overproduction of cells in the stratum basale that push upward, forming dome-shaped bumps. These bumps most often appear on areas of the head or neck that have been exposed to the sun. Slow-growing basal cell carcinomas are usually noticed and surgically removed before they can spread and become dangerous.

Squamous cell carcinoma is caused by overproduction of cells in the stratum spinosum layer of the epidermis. These cancers appear as a scaly, reddened patch that progresses to an ulcer-like mass with a raised border (**Figure 3.25**). The most commonly affected locations are the scalp, ears, lower lip, and backs of the hands among fair-skinned people. Dark-skinned people typically develop this condition in areas not exposed to the sun, such as the legs or feet. Squamous cell carcinomas grow rapidly and can easily spread to nearby lymph nodes. With early removal by surgery or radiation treatment, these cancers can be completely cured.

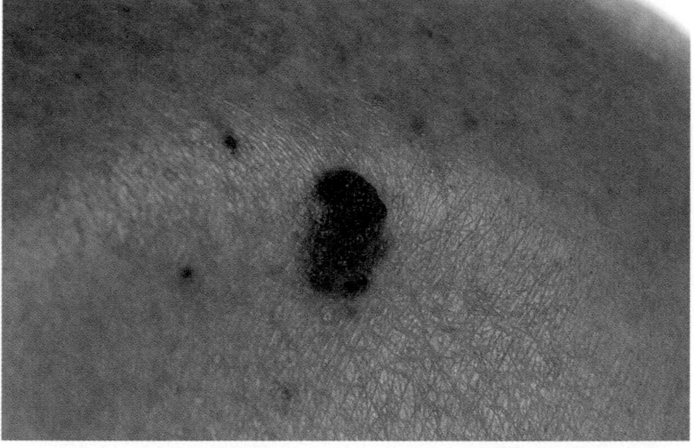

Sergei Primakov/Shutterstock.com

Figure 3.25 Squamous cell carcinoma.

The most serious form of skin cancer is **melanoma** (mehl-a-NOH-ma), so named because it is a cancer of the melanocytes (**Figure 3.26**). Melanoma can also form in the eyes and, rarely, in internal organs, such as the intestines.

Although typically dark colored and irregular in shape, a melanoma can appear pink, red, or "fleshy." Change in the size, shape, color, or elevation of a mole are typical warning signs of a malignant melanoma.

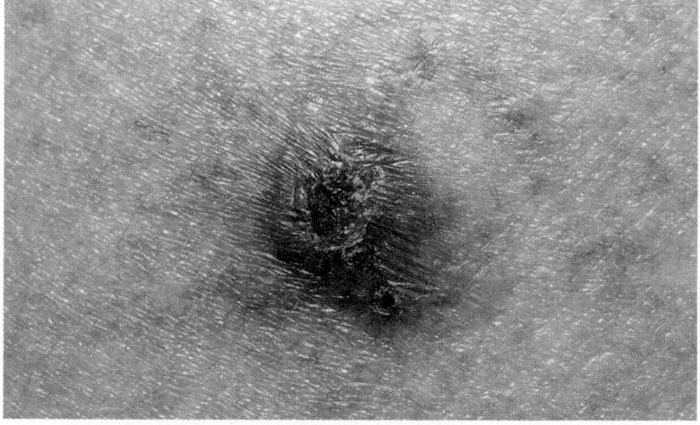

jax10289/Shutterstock.com

Figure 3.24 Basal cell carcinoma. *How are slow-growing basal cell carcinomas often treated?*

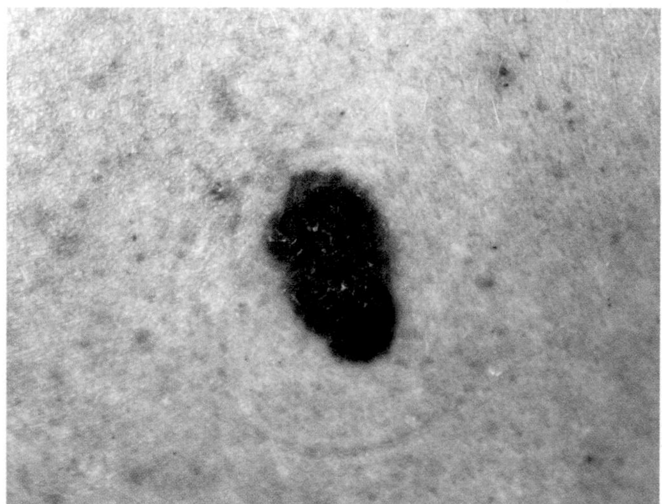

Nasekomoe/Shutterstock.com

Figure 3.26 Melanoma. *What is the ABCD rule for determining the presence of a melanoma?*

The American Cancer Society advocates the **ABCD rule** for determining the presence of melanoma:

Asymmetry: The shape of the mole is irregular.
Border irregularity: The outside borders are not smooth.
Color: More than one color is present. Melanomas may contain different shades of black and brown, blues, reds, or pinks.
Diameter: The mole size is larger than about one-quarter of an inch in diameter, or larger than the diameter of a pencil.

It is important to see a healthcare provider immediately if melanoma is suspected. Although these cancers comprise only about 5% of all skin cancers, they can be deadly. Use of indoor tanning beds, booths, or sun lamps has been shown to increase the incidence of melanoma and all other skin cancers. For this reason, a number of states and other countries have banned all forms of indoor tanning. The etiology, strategies for prevention, pathology, diagnosis, and common treatments for cancers of the skin are summarized in **Figure 3.27**.

Check Your Understanding

1. Squamous cell carcinoma is an overproduction of cells in which layer of the epidermis?
2. What is the ABCD rule for detecting melanoma?

Cancers of the Skin

	Etiology	Prevention	Pathology	Diagnosis	Treatment
Basal cell carcinoma	overproduction of cells in the stratum basale caused by overexposure to UV rays	avoid excessive sun exposure and tanning beds; use sunscreen and protective clothing	dome-shaped bumps appearing in areas of skin exposed to sun	physical exam, biopsy	surgical procedure or freezing
Squamous cell carcinoma	overproduction of cells in the stratum spinosum layer of the epidermis	avoid excessive sun exposure and tanning beds; use sunscreen and protective clothing	scaly, reddened patch that progresses to an ulcer-like mass with a raised border	physical exam, biopsy	surgical procedure or freezing
Melanoma	cancer in the melanocytes, which produce melanin	avoid excessive sun exposure and tanning beds; use sunscreen and protective clothing	a growth with asymmetry, border irregularity, more than one color present, and more than a quarter-inch in diameter	physical exam, biopsy	surgical removal followed by cancer treatments, as needed

Figure 3.27

Goodheart-Willcox Publisher

LESSON 3.3 Review and Assessment

Mini Glossary

Make sure that you know the meaning of each key term.

ABCD rule The American Cancer Society's rule for determining the presence of melanoma

basal cell carcinoma the most common form of skin cancer and the least malignant type

cellulitis a bacterial infection characterized by an inflamed area of skin that is red, swollen, and painful

decubitus ulcers ulcers caused by an area of localized pressure that restricts blood flow to one or more areas of the body

first-degree burns burns that affect only the epidermal layer of skin

fourth-degree burns full-thickness burns that destroy both the skin and underlying tissues including muscles, tendons, ligaments, and bone

herpes simplex virus type 1 (HSV-1) the form of herpes that generates cold sores or fever blisters around the mouth

herpes simplex virus type 2 (HSV-2) the genital form of herpes

herpes varicella (chickenpox) a highly contagious, common childhood disease that is characterized by extremely itchy, fluid-filled blisters

herpes zoster (shingles) a disease that involves a painful, blistering rash accompanied by headache, fever, and a general feeling of unwellness

human papillomavirus (HPV) a group of approximately 150 viruses that cause warts

impetigo a bacterial infection common in elementary school children that is characterized by pink, blister-like bumps, usually on the face

malignant melanoma cancer of the melanocytes; the most serious form of skin cancer

peritonitis inflammation of the peritoneum, the membrane lining the inner wall of the abdomen and covering the abdominal organs

plantar warts warts that develop on the soles of the foot, grow inward, and can become painful

pleurisy inflammation of the pleura, the membrane that encases the lungs

psoriasis a common skin disorder that involves redness, irritation, and scales (flaky, silver-white patches) that itch, burn, crack, and sometimes bleed

rule of nines a method used in calculating body surface area affected by burns

second-degree burns burns that involve damage to both the epidermis and the upper portion of the underlying dermis; characterized by blisters

squamous cell carcinoma a type of rapidly growing cancer that appears as a scaly, reddened patch of skin

third-degree burns burns that destroy the entire thickness of the skin

tinea a fungal infection that tends to occur in areas of the body that are moist

Know and Understand

1. Describe how the skin regenerates.
2. Name two interventions that can help to reduce a bedridden patient's risk for developing decubitus ulcers.
3. Describe each of the four types of skin burns.
4. Name two types of skin infections common in school-age children.
5. List the medical treatments for warts.
6. Briefly describe four common fungal infections.

Analyze and Apply

7. Why are third-degree burns not painful? Why are they not able to heal on their own?
8. What is the connection between herpes varicella and herpes zoster?
9. Wrestlers tend to get ringworm at a higher rate than any other type of athlete. Why do you think this might be, and what would you suggest be done to prevent it?
10. Why might tanned or dark-skinned people tend to be diagnosed with skin cancer in later stages than people who have lighter skin?

IN THE LAB

11. Go to the Centers for Disease Control (CDC) website and search *herpes varicella, herpes zoster, herpes simplex type 1,* and *herpes simplex type 2*. What characteristics are similar among all of these herpes viruses? What characteristics, if any, are different? Prepare a short written report of the differences and present your report to the class.
12. Using the rule of nines, calculate the percentage of total body surface area covered by burns for each of the following burn victims:
    A. burns on one leg: all of the front, half of the back
    B. burns in the genital area and all of the lower limbs
    C. burns to just the front of the body: the head, right arm, and torso
    D. burns over the entire body except for the head

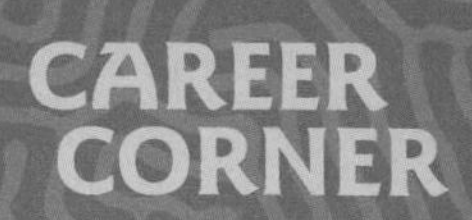

CAREER CORNER

Anatomy & Physiology at Work

Dermatology is the field of medicine that deals with the anatomy, functions, and diseases of the skin. A career in dermatology can be challenging, profitable, and rewarding.

Dermatology Assistant/Technician

A dermatology assistant or dermatology technician usually provides patient support and performs specialized technical tasks for a licensed dermatology practice. Some dermatology technicians, however, choose to work independently in salons or spas, providing services such as hair removal, facials, and skin-care treatments. Because dermatology assistants and technicians work directly with patients or clients and handle a variety of duties, they must have strong communication skills and the ability to multitask.

In some states, the educational requirements for dermatology technicians is higher than those for dermatology assistants. In these areas, assistants may perform general office duties, while technicians perform basic client services. At a minimum, dermatology assistants and technicians must have a high school diploma or GED, although most businesses prefer candidates who have earned a certificate or associate's degree in medical assisting. Community colleges offer certificate and associate's degree programs in medical assisting accredited by the Commission on Accreditation of Allied Health Education Programs (CAAHEP) or the Accrediting Bureau of Health Education Schools (ABHES). In addition, most college programs offer internships beyond traditional coursework.

Medical Assistant Certificate

A one-year medical assistant certificate program prepares students for clinical and administrative duties in a variety of healthcare settings. Coursework typically includes medical terminology, anatomy, dermatology, and pharmacology. Administrative subjects include clerical functions, basic accounting, and insurance billing.

Associate of Applied Science for Medical Assistants

An associate's degree program in medical assisting takes 18 to 24 months to complete. Most programs include externships in a clinical setting in which students are trained in drawing blood, giving injections, preparing and maintaining patients' medical records, and using appropriate telephone techniques. Coursework covers computer software applications, medical office procedures, biology, microbiology, and hematology.

Dermatologist

A dermatologist is a medical doctor (MD) who specializes in treating diseases and disorders of the skin through medicine and surgery (**Figure 3.28**). Many dermatologists also perform cosmetic procedures.

To become a dermatologist, one must earn a college degree and complete four years of medical school followed by a residency in dermatology. In the United States, residency training typically

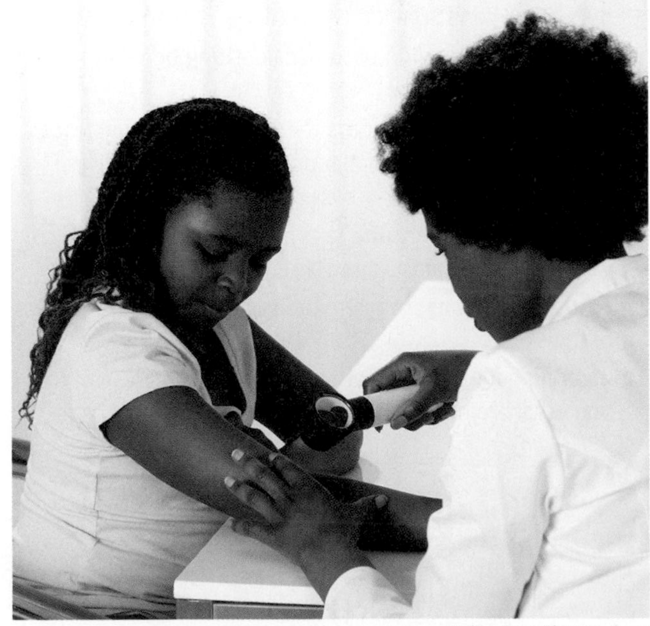

Andrey_Popov/Shutterstock.com

Figure 3.28 A dermatologist evaluates a patient's skin for melanoma.

takes four years to complete. The first year of residency usually consists of a supervised internship in medicine or surgery. During the following three years, residents receive specialized training in dermatology. Further specialization can be acquired through an additional two-year fellowship.

The following specialized procedures are generally performed by dermatologists:

- Photodynamic therapy for treatment of skin cancer and precancerous growths
- Cryosurgery for treatment of warts and skin cancers
- Laser therapy for management of unwanted birthmarks or tattoos and for cosmetic resurfacing
- Hair removal
- Hair transplantation
- Injections of cosmetic filler substances
- Liposuction
- Allergy testing for allergies caused by skin contact
- Topical therapies for various skin conditions

Veterinary Dermatology Technician

Do you love animals? If so, you may be interested in becoming a veterinary dermatology technician (**Figure 3.29**) These technicians assist veterinarians in the care of domestic or wild animals with various skin conditions or diseases. They may be asked to provide medicated baths, apply various topical medications, and even assist in veterinary surgery.

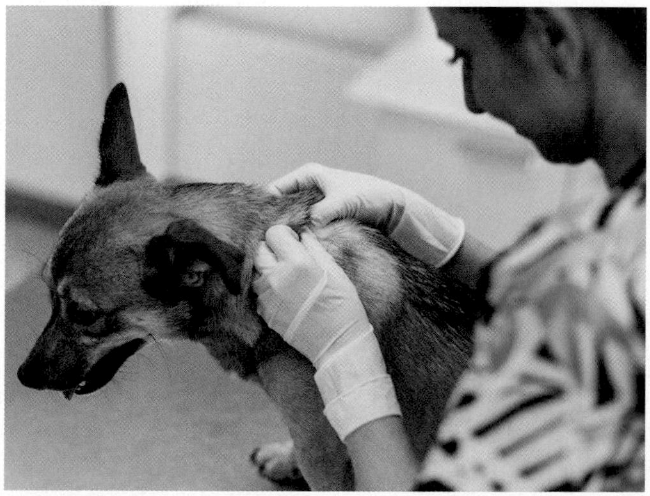

ShutterDivision/Shutterstock.com

Figure 3.29 Veterinary dermatology technicians assist veterinarians in providing skin care to various animals.

The educational requirements are similar to those for a general dermatology technician. An employer may also require special courses in veterinary subjects or require on-the-job training.

Planning for a Health-Related Career

Do some research on the career of a dermatologist or dermatology technician. Alternatively, select a profession from the list of related career options. Using the Internet or resources at your local library, find answers to the following questions:

1. What are the main responsibilities of the career that you have chosen to research?
2. What is the outlook for this career? Are workers in demand, or are jobs dwindling? For complete information, consult the current edition of the *Occupational Outlook Handbook*, published by the US Department of Labor. This handbook is available online or at your local library.
3. What special skills or talents are required? For example, do you need to be good at biology and anatomy? Do you need to enjoy interacting with other people?
4. What personality traits do you think are needed to be successful in this job? For example, a dermatology career involving laboratory research requires collaboration with other people. Do you enjoy teamwork?
5. Does this career involve a great deal of routine, or do the day-to-day responsibilities vary?
6. Does the work require long hours, or is it a standard "9-to-5" job?
7. What is the salary range for this job?
8. What do you think you would like about this career? Is there anything about it that you might dislike?

Related Career Options

- Dermatology assistant
- Dermatology technician
- Medical assistant
- Dermatologist
- Immunodermatologist
- Medical aesthetician
- Pediatric dermatologist
- Teledermatologist
- Veterinary dermatologist

CHAPTER 3 Review

LESSON 3.1
Body Membranes

Key Points

- Epithelial membranes, including the mucous, serous, and cutaneous membranes, line or cover the internal and external surfaces of the body.
- Synovial membranes are the only membranes that do not include epithelial cells; they consist entirely of connective tissue.

Key Terms

cutaneous membrane
epithelial membranes
membranes
mucous membranes
mucus
serous fluid
serous membranes
synovial fluid
synovial membrane

LESSON 3.2
The Integumentary System

Key Points

- The integumentary system protects the body against damage from harmful chemicals and ultraviolet rays from sunlight, serves as a water barrier, and helps to regulate body temperature.
- The two layers of the skin are the epidermis (outer layer) and the dermis (underlying layer).
- The appendages of the skin include the sweat glands, the sebaceous glands, hair, and nails.

Key Terms

apocrine glands
dermis
eccrine glands
epidermal dendritic cells
epidermis
hypodermis
integumentary system
keratin
keratinocytes
lipocytes
melanin
melanocytes
Merkel cells
papillary layer
reticular layer
sebaceous glands
sebum
stratum basale
stratum corneum
stratum granulosum
stratum lucidum
stratum spinosum
subcutaneous fascia
sudoriferous glands

LESSON 3.3
Injuries and Disorders of the Skin

Key Points

- Common injuries to the skin include decubitus, or pressure, ulcers and burns.
- Infections of the skin and membranes may be caused by viruses, fungi, or bacteria.
- Common inflammatory conditions of the skin and membranes include pleurisy, peritonitis, and psoriasis.
- The three types of skin cancer are basal cell carcinoma, squamous cell carcinoma, and melanoma.

Key Terms

ABCD rule
basal cell carcinoma
cellulitis
decubitus ulcers
first-degree burns
fourth-degree burns
herpes simplex virus type 1 (HSV-1)
herpes simplex virus type 2 (HSV-2)
herpes varicella
herpes zoster
human papillomavirus (HPV)
impetigo
melanoma
peritonitis
plantar warts
pleurisy
psoriasis
rule of nines
second-degree burns
squamous cell carcinoma
third-degree burns
tinea

Assessment

➤ LESSON 3.1

Body Membranes

Learning Key Terms and Concepts

1. *True or False?* The body membranes surround and help to protect the body's surfaces.
2. Which of the following surfaces is *not* surrounded and protected by membranes?
   A. ball-and-socket synovial joints
   B. internal cavities housing organs
   C. fingernails and toenails
   D. cavities open to the outside world
3. _____ membranes line or cover the internal and external surfaces of the body.
4. *True or False?* The epithelial membranes line or cover the internal surfaces of the body only.
5. The _____ membranes line the body cavities that open to exterior surfaces.
6. The mucous membranes line which of the following body cavities?
   A. digestive tract
   B. heart
   C. lungs
   D. abdominal cavity
7. *True or False?* Mucous membranes tend to be dry.
8. The pleura, pericardium, and peritoneum are all examples of which type of membranes?
9. *True or False?* The visceral layer is the outer lining of each serous membrane.
10. *True or False?* Cutaneous membrane is another name for skin.
11. Which type of membrane is composed only of connective tissue and includes no epithelial cells?

Thinking Critically

12. Compare and contrast the characteristics of a mucous membrane and a serous membrane. Give examples of both types of membranes in your answer.
13. Assume that someone challenges you when you tell them that skin is a membrane. Explain why the person might think that but why he or she would be wrong.
14. Describe what you would see if you looked at the visible mucous membranes of a person who is severely dehydrated.
15. The oral cavity is often referred to as the "mirror of the body" because the mucous membranes in the mouth change depending on many different diseases. What diseases or conditions might a dry mouth indicate?

➤ LESSON 3.2

The Integumentary System

Learning Key Terms and Concepts

16. Which type of protein, found in the outermost layer of the skin, adds structural strength to the skin?
17. _____ receptors transmit nerve signals containing information from the skin about the environment, including touch, pressure, vibration, pain, and temperature.
18. The skin is made up of which two layers?
    A. epidermis and hypodermis
    B. epidermis and dermis
    C. hypodermis and dermis
    D. hypodermis and underlying tissues
19. *True or False?* The epidermis completely replaces itself every 25 to 45 days.
20. *True or False?* Keratin is primarily responsible for human skin color.
21. Collagen and elastic fibers make up the dense, fibrous connective tissue called _____.
22. Which of the following are considered to be appendages of the skin?
    A. eyes
    B. nerves
    C. hair
    D. muscles
23. The _____ muscles are responsible for "goose bumps" on the skin.

Instructions: Write the letter of the integumentary system structure on your answer sheet next to the corresponding number.

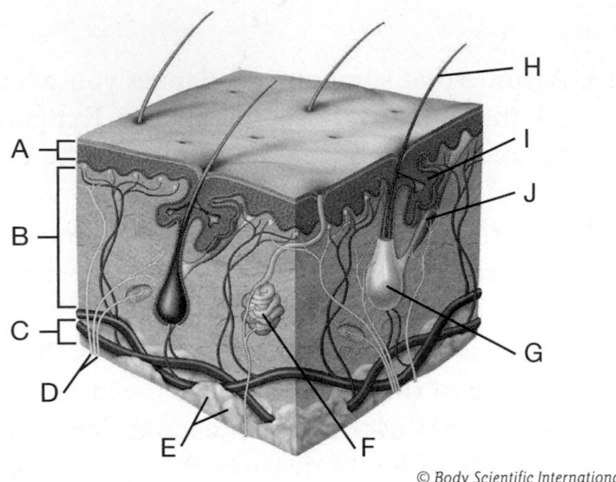

© Body Scientific International

24. lipocytes _____
25. hypodermis _____
26. sebaceous gland _____
27. arrector pili muscle _____
28. dermis _____
29. hair follicle _____
30. epidermis _____
31. sweat gland _____
32. hair shaft _____
33. nerve fibers _____

Thinking Critically

34. Explain the skin's function in regulating body temperature. Compare and contrast the ways in which the skin helps the body cool to the way it helps the body warm.
35. Explain to an imaginary person why his or her hair color and texture (straight, wavy, or curly) have developed as they have.
36. The skin is described as keratinizing stratified squamous epithelial tissue. Describe what each of these terms means in relationship to the structure and function of the skin. (You may need to refer to the discussion in Chapter 2 on types of epithelial tissue.)
37. In what way does the skin protect the body from damage due to ultraviolet rays from the sun? What would happen to your body if you did not have this protection?

➤ **LESSON 3.3**

Injuries and Disorders of the Skin

Learning Key Terms and Concepts

38. Decubitus ulcers may form on the body when _____ is restricted.
39. *True or False?* Burns can be caused by exposure to electricity.
40. *True or False?* First-degree burns damage the epidermis and parts of the underlying dermis.
41. A(n) _____, also referred to as a full-thickness burn, destroys the entire skin, leaving underlying tissues intact.
42. The most common fungal infection in humans is athlete's foot, also called _____.
43. _____ is a highly contagious staphylococcus infection that is common in elementary school children.
44. *True or False?* Psoriasis is a highly contagious disease characterized by scaly skin patches that itch, burn, crack, and sometimes bleed.
45. _____ is a common skin disorder characterized by regions of thick, red skin with flaky, silver-white patches.
46. Which of the following is *not* a type of viral infection?
    A. herpes
    B. psoriasis
    C. plantar warts
    D. genital warts
47. The most serious type of skin cancer is _____.

Thinking Critically

48. What is the difference between chickenpox and shingles?
49. Compare and contrast HSV-1 and HSV-2.
50. Name seven potential causes of pleurisy.
51. Name the two major categories of HPVs and explain how they differ.
52. Compare and contrast tinea and impetigo. Mention how they look, what causes them, and how they are treated.

Building Skills and Connecting Concepts

Analyzing and Evaluating Data

Instructions: Using the information that you learned in this chapter about skin burns and the rule of nines, answer the following questions.

53. What percentage of burned tissue would you assign to a patient who suffered burns to the anterior and posterior portions of the head and the anterior portion of both arms?
54. What percentage would you assign to a patient who suffered burns to the anterior portion of the left leg and the anterior portion of the torso?
55. What percentage would you assign to a patient who suffered burns to the anterior and posterior right leg, the anterior portion of the torso, and the posterior portion of the right arm?

Communicating about Anatomy & Physiology

56. **Writing** Go to the Centers for Disease Control (CDC) website and research skin injuries and disorders that commonly occur in the work environment. List steps that you can take to prevent possible dermal exposure to yourself. Develop a plan that could be used to help people in the event of dermal exposure at work. Use key terms from this chapter to explain how the exposure could occur. Write your plan and present it to the class. If you do not have an actual workplace, specify a place you would like to work.
57. **Writing** Research the effects of chemicals on the skin. Then write a three-paragraph summary about how a worker in a chemical plant might be exposed to chemicals through the different layers of the skin.
58. **Speaking** After researching emergency first aid for burns, teach a mini-lesson to your peers on how to treat first-, second-, third-, and fourth-degree burns.

Lab Investigations

59. Working in a small group, design a laboratory experiment to test a hypothesis developed by your group. Specific procedures will vary depending on the hypothesis that you test.

    Reminders:
    - List the steps in your experiment.
    - The experiment must be repeatable.
    - Your directions must be very clear so that someone else could repeat the experiment exactly as your group did.
    - The data collected must be measurable.

    On a sheet of paper, summarize the procedure that your group used. Record your observations as accurately and in as much detail as possible. Then summarize the results of your experiment.
    - Was your hypothesis supported?
    - What problems did you encounter?
    - What did you learn from this experiment?
60. The tissue that lines the inside of the mouth is known as the basal mucosa and is composed of squamous epithelial cells. In this lab, view your own cells under a microscope. **Materials:** microscope, slides and coverslips, methyl blue stain, gloves, paper towels, cotton swab. **Procedure:** Put on gloves and gently scrape the inside of your mouth with the tip of the cotton swab. Smear the cotton swab on the center of the slide for 2 to 3 seconds. Add a drop of methylene blue solution and place a coverslip on the slide. Place the slide under the microscope and examine it under low and high power. Describe your observations in your lab book.

Building Your Portfolio

61. Take digital photographs of the models you created as you worked through this chapter. Create a document called "Cells and Tissues" and insert the photographs, along with written descriptions of what the models show and your reasons for creating them using the materials and forms you chose. Add this document to your personal portfolio.

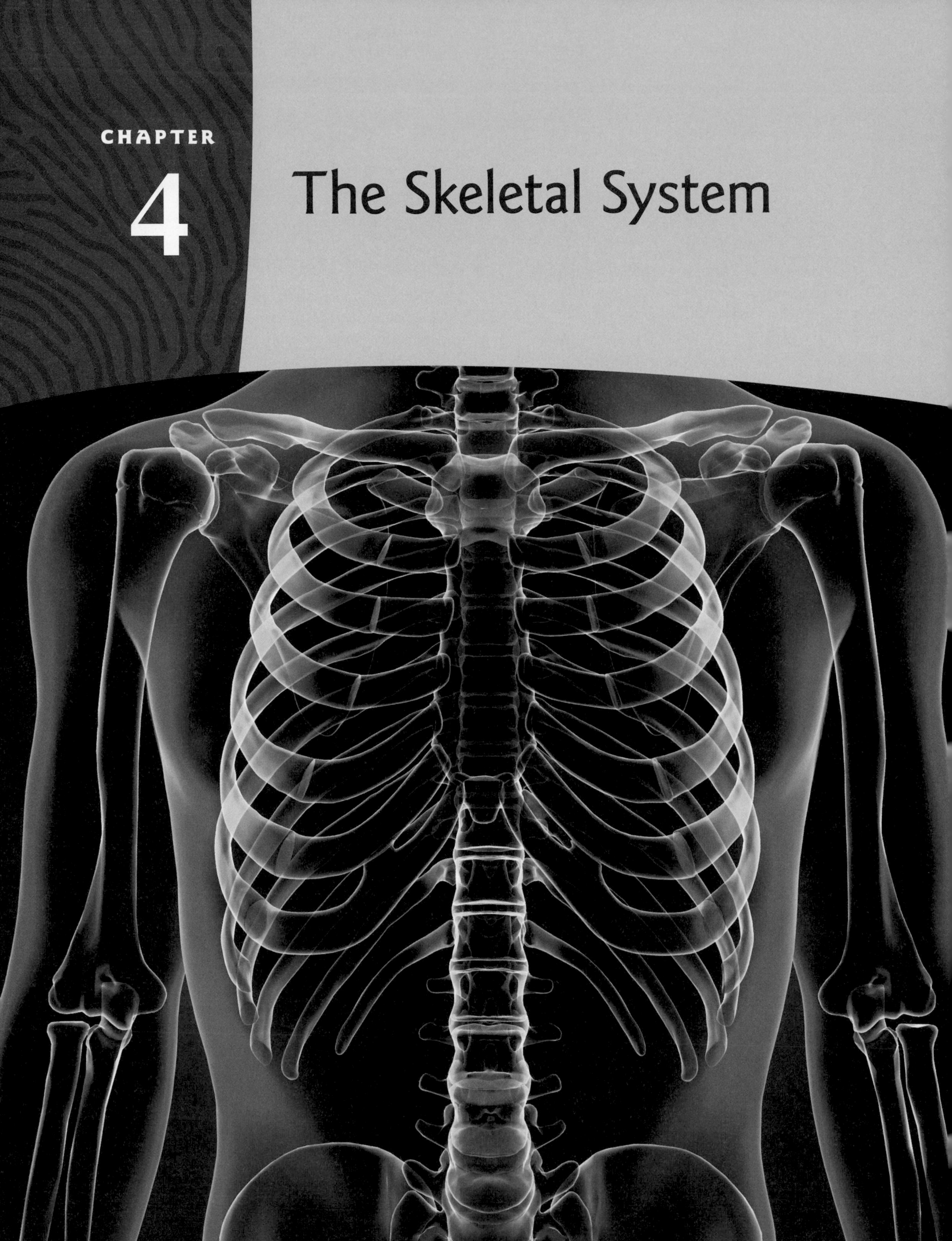

CHAPTER

4 The Skeletal System

Why are bones considered "living tissue"?

People tend to think of bone as a hard, dried-up chunk of mineral that a dog would enjoy chewing. While this is true of dead bone, the living bones inside the human body are made up of amazing, complex living tissues. Bones are not only hydrated (containing water), but also very dynamic, continually changing in size, shape, and strength over time.

How and why do these processes of change occur? This chapter explores the characteristics of living bone and describes the well-tailored functionality of the major bones and joints in the human skeleton. It also discusses some of the common injuries and disorders of the bones and joints, how these problems tend to occur, and how their likelihood can be reduced.

Chapter 4 Outline

Click on the activity icon or visit www.g-wlearning.com/healthsciences/0202 to access online vocabulary activities using key terms from the chapter.

◂ Life science/Shutterstock.com

LESSON 4.1

Bone as a Living Tissue

Before You Read

Try to answer the following questions before you read this lesson.

- Do all bones have the same internal structure?
- When and why do bones stop growing?
- What practices can make bones stronger or weaker?

Lesson Objectives

- Describe the functions of the skeletal system.
- Describe the anatomical structure of the various types of bones.
- Discuss bone remodeling, including the cells responsible and the practices and environments that can dramatically influence remodeling.

Key Terms

articular cartilage	medullary cavity
bone marrow	ossification
cortical bone	osteoblasts
diaphysis	osteoclasts
endosteum	osteocytes
epiphyseal plate	osteon
epiphysis	perforating (Volkmann's) canals
Haversian canals	periosteum
Haversian system	remodeling
hematopoiesis	trabecular bone
lacunae	

The approximately 206 individual bones comprising the human skeleton come in many different sizes and shapes, each uniquely well designed to serve a particular function. This lesson describes the structure and function of human bones, as well as their development and maintenance throughout a person's lifetime.

Functions of the Skeletal System

The skeletal system performs several important functions. These functions are summarized in this section.

Support

It is hard to imagine humans without bones because, like the wooden framework of a house, bones form the internal support system that provides shape and structural support to the body's trunk and limbs. The bones in your legs enable you to stand upright, and your ribs support your chest cavity.

Protection

Bones surround and support the body's delicate internal organs. For example, the ribs serve as bony protectors of critical organs such as the heart and lungs nestled in the thoracic cavity. Equally important, the skull provides protection for the brain, and the vertebral column surrounds and protects the delicate spinal cord.

Movement

What produces human movement? Movement is generated by muscles, which attach to bones. When muscles contract or shorten, they pull on the attached bones, causing movement.

The design of the skeletal system, with bones able to rotate or glide in certain ways around joints, is extraordinarily functional. This amazing design enables walking, running, jumping, pushing, pulling, and throwing, as well as all of the routine activities that people take for granted every day.

A joint such as the shoulder allows movement in multiple directions, while movement at the knee is largely constrained to one direction. These movement capabilities are favorably designed for the ways in which humans move. You will learn more about the muscles and how they work in the next chapter.

Storage

Bones also serve as a storage repository for minerals, notably phosphorus and calcium. Phosphorus plays a vital role in the development and maintenance of healthy bones and teeth, and it also plays a role in the chemical reactions that release energy from stored fat in the body. Calcium is essential for normal functioning of the neuromuscular system, as well as for blood clotting. Through a chemical balancing procedure known as homeostasis (hoh-mee-oh-STAY-sis), discussed in Chapter 1, the body can draw upon the stored phosphorus or calcium in bone if the levels of these minerals in the bloodstream fall below normal. This process is under hormonal control. See Chapter 8 for more information about hormonal control of calcium.

Another storage site in the skeletal system is the **medullary** (MEHD-yoo-lair-ee) **cavity**, a central hollow space inside most of the long bones, such as those of the arms and legs. The medullary cavity is also known as the *marrow cavity* because it stores **bone marrow**, a flexible tissue found inside bones.

There are two types of bone marrow—yellow and red. Both types contain a rich blood supply. Yellow marrow, found within the medullary cavity, is a major storehouse for fat in the body. Red marrow is found in the cavities of many bones, including flat and short bones, bodies of the vertebrae, sternum, ribs, and articulating ends of long bones.

Blood Cell Formation

It is in the red marrow that the critically important function of **hematopoiesis** (hee-ma-toh-poy-EE-sis), or blood cell formation, occurs. As you will discover in Chapters 10 and 11, blood cells deliver oxygen to tissues throughout the body and also transport waste in the form of carbon dioxide to the lungs, where it can be breathed out.

Check Your Understanding

1. List the five functions of the skeletal system.
2. What are two functions of bone marrow?

Structures and Classification of Bones

The composition and structure of bone make it remarkably strong and resilient, given its relatively light weight. Beyond this, bones assume specialized shapes in accordance with their specific functions.

Composition of Bones

Cells are the structural building blocks of bone, as they are in other kinds of tissues in the body. **Osteocytes** are mature bone cells.

Bones have both organic and inorganic content. One factor that distinguishes bone from other tissues is that 60%–70% of a bone's mass comes from its mineral, or inorganic, content—primarily calcium carbonate and calcium phosphate. The remaining 30%–40% of bone mass comes from water and collagen, a protein that provides the bone with flexibility. Collagens and other proteins in bone are considered organic content. Both the mineral and water content contribute to bone strength. The bones of children tend to be more flexible than the bones of adults due to higher collagen and water content.

Organization of Bones

Bone is structurally organized into two different types of tissue—cortical (compact) and trabecular (cancellous) bone. Whereas **cortical** (KOR-ti-kal) **bone** tissue is relatively dense, **trabecular** (tra-BEHK-yoo-lar) **bone** tissue, also known as *spongy* bone, is relatively porous, with a honeycomb structure (**Figure 4.1**). Cortical bone is stiffer due to its higher mineral content, so it is generally stronger than trabecular bone. Trabecular bone, with its spongy structure, is more flexible than cortical bone.

Most bones include both cortical and trabecular tissue. The function of a given bone determines whether it is composed mostly of cortical or trabecular bone. The outer layer of a bone is always composed of hard, protective cortical bone, with spongy trabecular bone present to varying degrees in the interior.

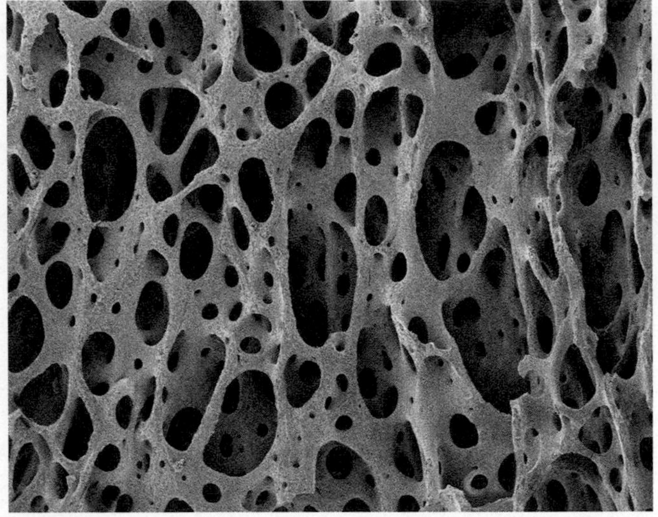
A

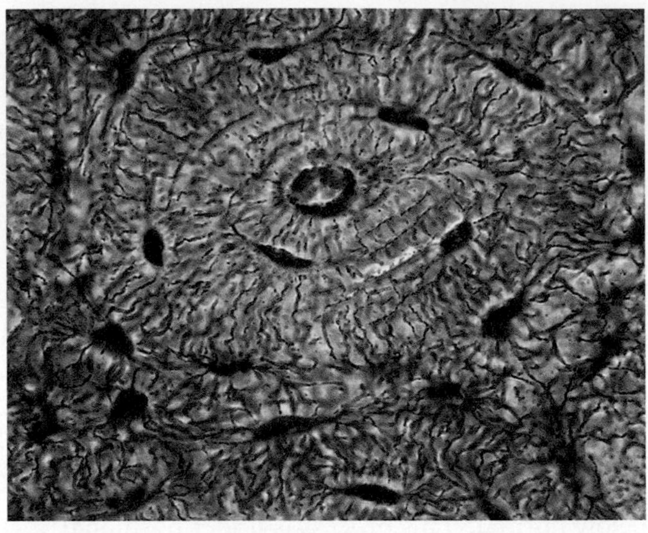
B

Susumu Nishinaga/Science Source, Jose Luis Calvo/Shutterstock.com

Figure 4.1 A—A micrograph of trabecular bone tissue. B—Cortical bone tissue. *How would you describe the difference between trabecular and cortical bone to someone who knew nothing about these two types of bone tissue?*

The long bones in the arms and legs are primarily composed of strong cortical bone tissue, although there is trabecular bone inside the ends. The bones in the spinal column contain a large amount of trabecular bone inside their cortical encasings, giving them a certain amount of shock-absorbing capability. **Figure 4.2** compares the properties of these two types of bone tissue.

MEMORY TIP

The word *cortical* (coming from *cortex*) pertains to the outer layer of something. For example, the outer layer of the brain is known as the *cerebral cortex*. The outer layer of many structures and objects, including a plant stem or even a rock, is also known as its *cortex*. The type of bone tissue forming the outer layer of bone is therefore called *cortical* bone.

Shape Categories of Bones

Because of the large variety of sizes and shapes of the bones in the human skeleton, for purposes of discussion bones are traditionally divided into five categories (**Figure 4.3**):

- *Long bones* have a long, somewhat round shaft made of cortical bone, with bulbous knobs of trabecular bone encased in cortical bone at both ends. The shafts enclose the central hollow medullary cavity or canal. The major bones of the arms and legs are long bones.
- *Short bones* are shaped like a cube and are composed mainly of trabecular bone. The bones of the wrists and ankles are short bones.

Properties of the Two Types of Bone Tissue

	Cortical Bone	**Trabecular Bone**
Structure	dense	porous (honeycomb structure)
Mineral content	relatively high	relatively low
Strength	relatively high	low
Flexibility	low	relatively more
Shock-absorbing ability	low	relatively more
Primary locations	outer surface of all bones, long bones of limbs	interior of vertebrae, femoral neck, wrist, and ankle bones

Figure 4.2

Goodheart-Willcox Publisher

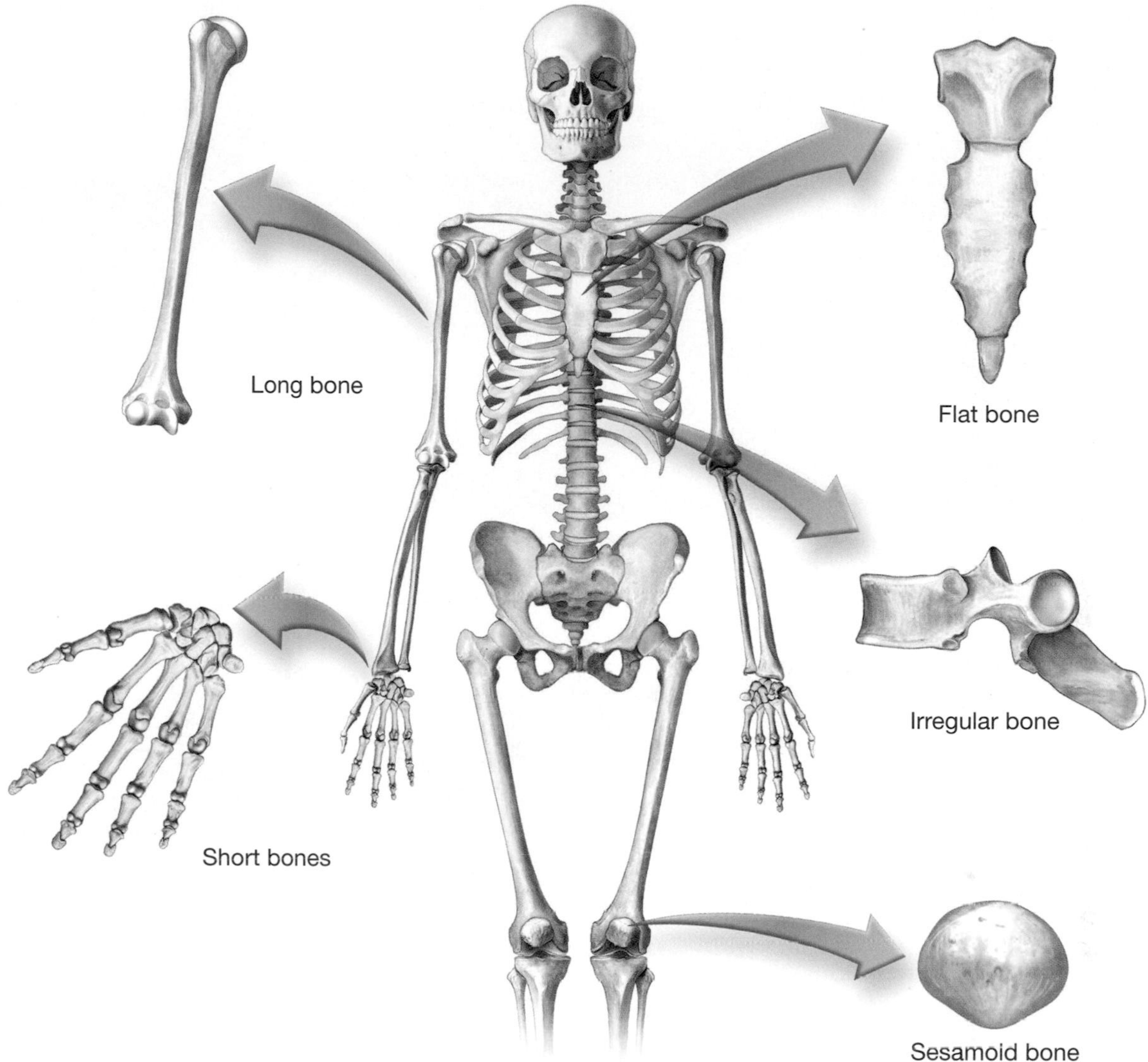

Figure 4.3 The five categories of bones.

- *Flat bones* are thin, relatively large in surface area, and generally curved to some extent. Structurally, they consist of two thin layers of cortical bone with a layer of trabecular bone in between. These bones protect underlying organs and also provide large areas for muscle attachments. The scapula and the bones of the skull are considered flat bones.
- *Sesamoid bones* are bones that are formed within tendons. The patella (at the front of the knee) is an example of a sesamoid bone.
- *Irregular bones* are all those bones that do not fit into one of the preceding categories. They have individualized shapes to fulfill specific functions. The bones of the spinal column and hip girdle are in this category.

Check Your Understanding

1. What percentage of bone mass comes from its mineral content?
2. What is collagen?
3. Where is cortical bone typically found?
4. Where is trabecular bone typically found?
5. List the five shape categories of bone.

Anatomical Structure of Long Bones

The **diaphysis** (digh-AF-i-sis) of a long bone is the hollow shaft of the bone composed of cortical bone (**Figure 4.4**). A fibrous connective tissue membrane called the **periosteum** (per-ee-AHS-tee-um) surrounds and protects the diaphysis. The periosteum contains blood and lymph vessels,

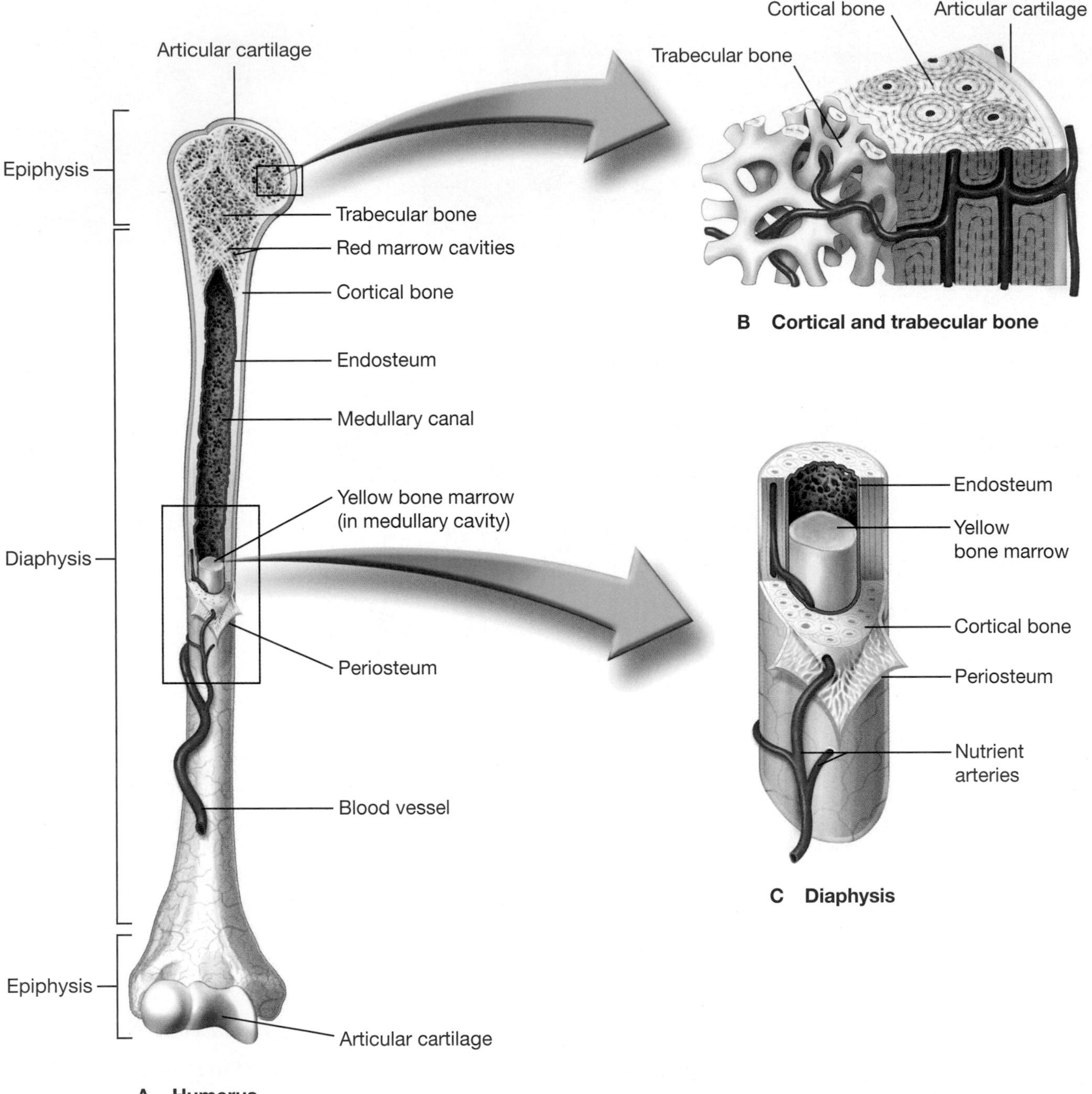

Figure 4.4 The anatomical structure of a long bone. A—Anterior view of the humerus with the interior of the top half exposed. B—Cortical and trabecular bone of the epiphysis. C—Enlargement of the diaphysis.

as well as nerves. It is involved in bone growth, repair, and nutrition.

The hollow center of the diaphysis is the medullary cavity, or canal. Beginning when a person is about five years old, this cavity is filled with yellow bone marrow, which has a rich supply of blood vessels and is a storehouse for fat. The medullary cavity is lined by a membrane known as the **endosteum** (ehn-DAHS-tee-um).

The bulbous endings of the long bones are known as **epiphyses** (eh-PIF-i-seez). These regions are composed of trabecular bone that contains red marrow, which participates in the formation of red blood cells, or erythrocytes (e-RITH-roh-sights), and some white blood cells, or leukocytes (LOO-koh-sights). Each epiphysis is surrounded by a protective covering of **articular** (ar-TIK-yoo-lar) **cartilage**. You may have noticed the shiny white

LIFE SPAN DEVELOPMENT: *Bones*

Over the course of the life span from birth through old age, some parts of the human body grow, while others tend to shrink. Knowledge of the processes by which bones grow and develop is key to understanding why these phenomena occur.

Osteoblasts and Osteoclasts

Specialized bone cells called **osteoblasts** (AHS-tee-oh-blasts) carry out the work of building new bone tissue. When there is a need to resorb or eliminate weakened or damaged bone tissue, that work is accomplished by other specialized cells called **osteoclasts** (AHS-tee-oh-klasts).

Bone growth clearly involves more osteoblast activity than osteoclast activity. However, both osteoblasts and osteoclasts remain extremely busy over the course of a normal person's life. In healthy adult bone, the activity of osteoblasts and osteoclasts is balanced.

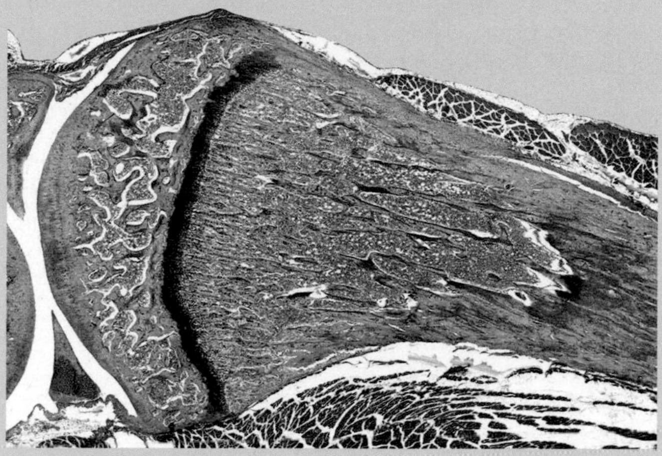

MicroScape/Science Source

Figure 4.5 Bones grow in length at the epiphyseal plates (the dark blue area). *When will this plate dissolve?*

MEMORY TIP

Osteoblast and *osteoclast* are similar-sounding names for these specialized bone cells. An easy way to avoid confusing them is to remember the "b" in *osteoblast* is the same as the "b" in *build*. Similarly, the "cl" in *osteoclast* is the same as the "cl" in *clear*. Osteoblasts *b*uild bone and osteoclasts *cl*ear away old or damaged bone.

Bone Formation

Bone modeling is the process in which new bone is created through osteoblast activity during the formation and growth of immature bones. The skeleton of early-developing embryos is composed mainly of a flexible tissue called *hyaline cartilage*. By the end of the eighth week there is a rapid replacement of cartilage with bone in the developing fetus.

The process of bone formation is called **ossification** (ahs-i-fi-KAY-shun). Before birth, this occurs in two phases. During the first phase, a bone matrix shell covers the hyaline cartilage through the activity of osteoblasts. Next, osteoclasts resorb the enclosed hyaline cartilage, creating a medullary cavity within the bony superstructure.

Longitudinal Growth

Bones grow in length at the **epiphyseal** (ehp-i-FIZ-ee-al) **plates**, located close to the ends of long bones (**Figure 4.5**). During childhood growth, osteoblasts on the central side of the epiphyseal plate produce new bone cells, resulting in an increase in bone length. At the end of the growth period, occurring during or shortly after adolescence, the plate dissolves and the bone on either side of the plate fuses, ending the longitudinal growth of the bone.

Circumferential Growth

Although most bone growth occurs during childhood, bones actually grow in diameter, or width, throughout most of life (**Figure 4.6**). Osteoblasts in the internal layer of the periosteum build concentric layers of new bone on top of existing ones. To understand the process, it helps to visualize the way in which the rings on a cross-cut tree stump reveal the tree's growth.

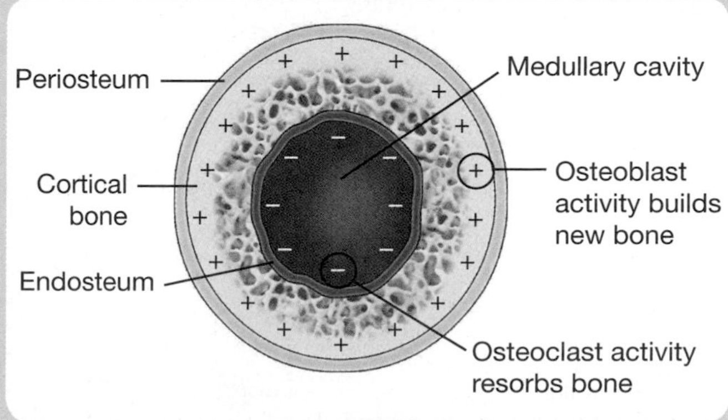

© Body Scientific International

Figure 4.6 Cross section of a long bone showing normal bone throughout life. *Is it the circumference or the length of bones that continues to grow throughout life?*

(continued)

At the same time that the osteoblasts are doing their work, the osteoclasts resorb layers of bone inside the medullary cavity, causing the diameter of the cavity to be progressively enlarged. This beautifully engineered process occurs in such a way that a healthy bone remains optimally functional, lightweight, and strong enough to resist daily stresses.

Adult Bone Development

As people age, there is a progressive loss of collagen and a subsequent increase in bone brittleness. This means that children are often able to sustain falls and other accidents without harm, while older adults tend to be increasingly vulnerable to bone fractures.

Bone mineral normally peaks in women at about 25 to 28 years of age and in men at about 30 to 35 years of age. Thereafter, bone mass is progressively lost. Because women tend to have smaller bones than men, the loss of bone mass and bone mineral density is generally more problematic for women.

Life Span Review

1. During which parts of life are osteoblasts and osteoclasts active?
2. How and why is the medullary cavity in bone enlarged?
3. What is the importance of the epiphyseal plate?
4. Why are elderly individuals more prone to bone fractures?

covering of articular cartilage over the ends of the bone in chicken drumsticks.

How does living bone receive nourishment and get rid of waste products? Bone has what you might think of as its own subway system. An intricate array of passageways exists at a microscopic level inside the mineralized part of bone. Blood vessels and nerves course through these tiny tunnels (**Figure 4.7**). Major passageways running lengthwise through the bone are called **Haversian** (ha-VER-zhen) **canals**. Tiny cavities called **lacunae** (la-KOO-nee) are

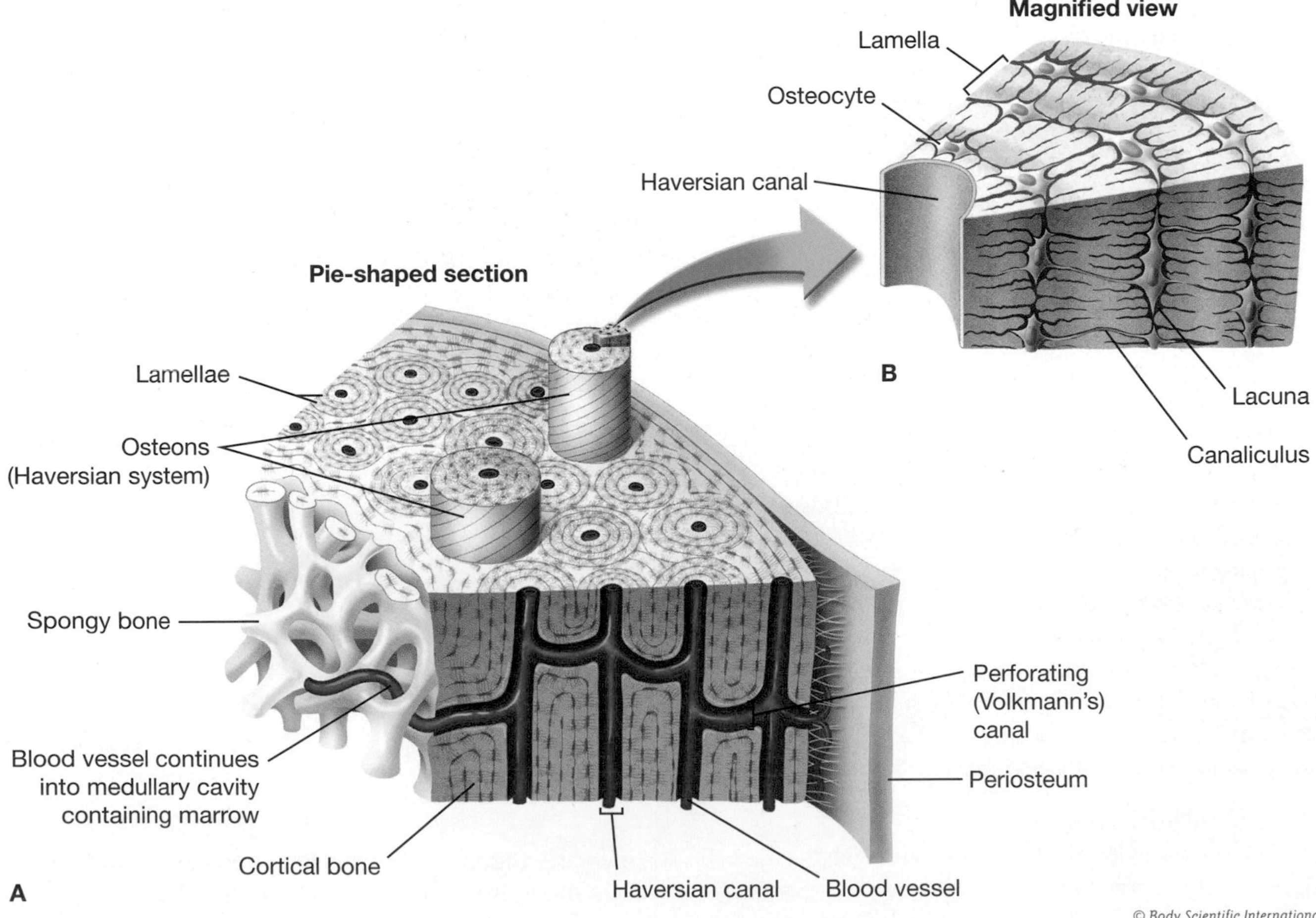

Figure 4.7 A—A microscopic view of the inside of bone tissue. B—An even more magnified view. *Why might someone compare the inside of living bone to a subway system?*

What Research Tells Us

...about Physical Activity and Bones

There are many documented examples of bone remodeling, and hypertrophy (enlargement), in response to regular physical activity. Sports that require repeated, forceful use of a certain limb promote not only muscle hypertrophy, but also bone hypertrophy, in the stressed area. For example, clinical case studies have shown increased bone mass, circumference, and mineralization in the dominant forearm of professional tennis players and in the dominant upper arm of baseball players.

It also appears that the larger the forces habitually encountered, the more dramatic the effect. In one interesting study, researchers measured the density of the femur among 64 nationally ranked athletes from different sports. The densest femurs were those of the weight lifters, followed by hammer and discus throwers, runners, soccer players, and swimmers. As you might expect from this research, the size of the regularly acting forces on the body is one factor that appears to be related directly to bone mass.

The other important factor contributing to increased bone mineral density is absorption of repeated impacts, such as those routinely encountered during running and landings from jumps (**Figure 4.8**). In an investigation involving collegiate female athletes, those participating in high-impact sports (basketball and volleyball) were found to have much higher bone mineral densities than the swimmers, with the soccer and track athletes having intermediate values. Another study compared the bone mineral densities of trained runners and cyclists to those of sedentary individuals of the same age. Not surprisingly, the runners were found to have increased bone density, but the cyclists did not.

On the whole, the evidence suggests that physical activity involving impact forces is necessary for maintaining or increasing bone mass. One need not be an athlete, however, to exercise for bone health—even vigorous walking generates bone-building impact forces.

Competitive swimmers, who spend a lot of time in the water where the buoyant force counteracts gravity, may have even less bone mineral density than sedentary individuals. It is important for competitive swimmers to also participate in activities such as weight training and running to maintain normal bone density.

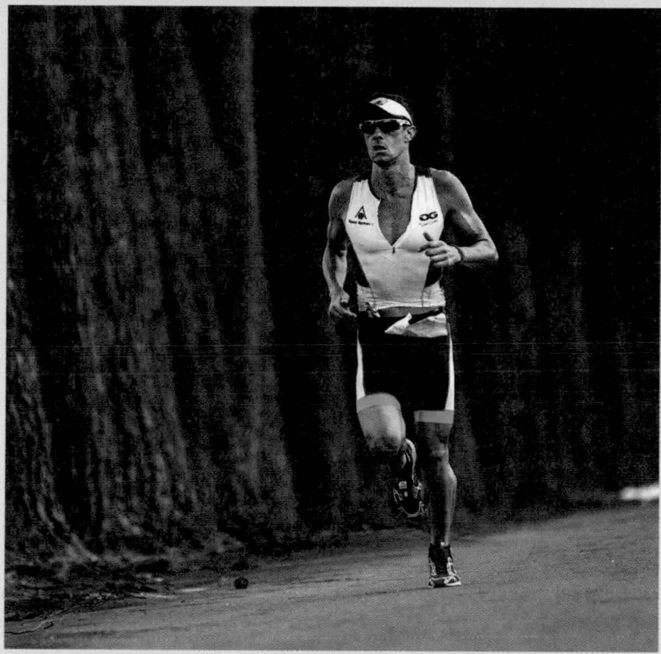

Fernanda Paradizo/Shutterstock.com

Figure 4.8 *Why is running especially good for bones?*

Taking It Further

1. Explain in your own words the relationship between physical activity, bone remodeling, and hypertrophy.
2. Create a continuum, placing activities that negatively impact bone mass, such as swimming, on one end and those that increase bone mass (for example, basketball and volleyball) on the other end. Plot your daily activities on the continuum. Could you change your routine in a way that would increase your ability to build bone mass?

laid out in concentric circles called *lamellae* (la-MEHL-ee) around the Haversian canals, and it is the lacunae that house the osteocytes.

Each Haversian canal, with its surrounding layers of lacunae, forms a structural unit called an **osteon**, or **Haversian system**. Within the system are tiny sideways canals called *canaliculi* (kan-ah-LIK-yoo-ligh). The canaliculi connect with the lacunae, forming a comprehensive transportation matrix for supply of nutrients and removal of waste products throughout the Haversian system. The multiple Haversian systems are joined by **perforating (Volkmann's) canals**, also running sideways, that connect the Haversian canals.

Check Your Understanding

1. What is the periosteum? Name at least three functions of the periosteum.
2. Where is the endosteum found? Is it inside or outside the periosteum?
3. What covers the ends of long bones?
4. Describe the functions of osteoblasts and osteoclasts.
5. Describe and analyze the effects of less elasticity on the body as people age.

Remodeling of Bones

Living adult bone is a very active tissue, always changing at a microscopic level in bone mineral content (and thereby strength) and sometimes in size or shape. This occurs through osteoblast and osteoclast activity during a process called **remodeling**.

Forces, such as gravitational force, muscle forces, forces received when you push or pull on something, and impact forces when you bump into something, all influence bones. The remodeling process converts the size and direction of the forces acting on bone to changes in bone mineral density. (Refer to Chapter 1 for more information about the effects of forces on the body.) In some circumstances, the remodeling process also causes changes in the size or shape of bone.

Hypertrophy of Bones

Generally, when bone is subjected to larger (stronger) forces, it tends to *hypertrophy* (high-PER-troh-fee), with increases in density and growth at the sites of force application (often muscle attachments). As a result, the bones of people who are physically active are usually denser and stronger than the bones of people who are sedentary.

Because gravity is also a force that continuously acts on bones, people who are heavier tend to have greater bone mass and density than people who are lightweight for their height. Dynamic activities such as running and jumping involve landing impacts, which cause motion of fluid within the bone matrix. This motion is particularly effective at triggering the actions of osteoblasts to build bone.

Altogether, bones account for only about 15% of body weight. This tends to be true whether a person is underweight, of average weight, or overweight. No one is overweight because of heavy bones, however. Being overweight is almost always the result of carrying excess body fat.

Atrophy of Bones

People who are subject to reduced forces are prone to bone *atrophy*, or loss of bone mineral density and strength. This has been observed, for example, in individuals who are bedridden for long periods of time.

Somewhat surprisingly, bone atrophy has also been observed in elite swimmers who spend hours a day training in a swimming pool. Swimming involves a large amount of muscle activity, but the buoyancy of the water counteracts much of the force of gravity. So, while swimmers are in the water, their bones are subjected to greatly reduced stresses.

Loss of bone mass and strength is an even more significant problem for astronauts, who spend time completely out of the earth's gravitational field. The loss of bone in astronauts in space is so rapid that it is currently one of the major factors preventing a manned space mission to Mars.

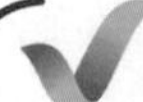

Check Your Understanding

1. What factors can cause bone to hypertrophy, increasing mass, density, and sometimes circumference?
2. What factors can cause bone to atrophy, losing mass and mineralization?

LESSON 4.1 Review and Assessment

Mini Glossary

Make sure that you know the meaning of each key term.

articular cartilage dense, white, connective tissue that covers the articulating surfaces of bones at joints

bone marrow material with a rich blood supply found within the marrow cavity of long bones; yellow marrow stores fat, and red marrow is active in producing blood cells

cortical bone dense, solid bone that covers the outer surface of all bones and is the main form of bone tissue in the long bones

diaphysis the shaft of a long bone

endosteum membrane lining the medullary cavity

epiphyseal plate growth plate near the ends of long bones where osteoblast activity increases bone length

epiphysis the bulbous end of a long bone

Haversian canals major passageways running in the direction of the length of long bones, providing paths for blood vessels

Haversian system a single Haversian canal along with its multiple canaliculi, which branch out to join with lacunae, forming a comprehensive transportation matrix for supply of nutrients and removal of waste products; also called an *osteon*

hematopoiesis process of blood cell formation

lacunae tiny cavities laid out in concentric circles around the Haversian canals

medullary cavity central hollow in the long bones

ossification process of bone formation

osteoblasts specialized bone cells that build new bone tissue

osteoclasts specialized bone cells that resorb bone tissue

osteocytes mature bone cells

osteon a Haversian system

perforating (Volkmann's) canals large canals that connect the Haversian canals; also known as *perforating canals*; oriented across bones and perpendicular to Haversian canals

periosteum fibrous connective tissue membrane that surrounds and protects the shaft (diaphysis) of long bones

remodeling process through which adult bone can change in density, strength, and sometimes shape

trabecular bone interior, spongy bone with a porous, honeycomb structure

Know and Understand

1. List each of the five functions of the skeletal system and describe how they benefit the body.
2. Explain the differences between cortical bone and trabecular bone.
3. Describe where the diaphysis of a long bone is in relation to the epiphysis, and where the periosteum is in relation to the endosteum.
4. Briefly describe the process of remodeling.

Analyze and Apply

5. Compare and contrast osteoblasts and osteoclasts and explain how they work together to reshape and remodel bones.
6. Explain why a physician might be worried about a child who broke a long bone close to the epiphyseal plate.
7. Keeping in mind the properties of cortical and trabecular bone tissue, describe the structure of a bone and why the two bone tissue types are found where they are in bones (outside or inside).
8. An elderly woman and her young granddaughter are involved in an automobile accident. The woman sustained several broken ribs, but her granddaughter did not have any injuries. In terms of bone mineralization, why might the older woman have sustained injuries, while her granddaughter did not?
9. Explain why someone whose job involves manual labor, such as construction, roofing, or carpentry, would have noticeably larger and stronger upper body bones than someone who has a different occupation.

IN THE LAB

10. Before reading further in this chapter, make labels for all the bones that you can name. Quickly research the bones identified on your labels. Taking turns with your classmates, place your labels on the correct bones of the classroom skeleton and tell what category (long, short, flat, sesamoid, irregular) each bone belongs to.
11. Draw or trace a cross-section picture of a long bone. Label the outside parts: epiphysis, diaphysis, and articular cartilage. Using different colors, draw and label the inside parts: trabecular bone, endosteum, yellow bone marrow, medullary cavity, and red marrow. On a separate piece of paper, describe each part that you have labeled.

LESSON 4.2 The Axial Skeleton

Before You Read

Try to answer the following questions before you read this lesson.

- Why is the skull composed of multiple bones?
- Why is the spine curved instead of straight?

Lesson Objectives

- Identify the bones of the cranium and face and describe their locations.
- Describe the structure of a typical vertebra and explain how the atlas, axis, and other cervical, thoracic, and lumbar vertebrae are specialized for their specific functions.
- Discuss the structure and functional importance of the thoracic cage.

Key Terms

atlas
axial skeleton
axis
cervical region
coccyx
cranium
facial bones
fontanel
intervertebral discs
lumbar region
mandible
maxillary bones
process
sacrum
skull
sternum
sutures
thoracic cage
thoracic region
vertebrae
vomer

Anatomists divide the body into the axis, consisting of the head and trunk, and the appendages—the arms and legs (**Figure 4.9**). Consequently, the major bones of the axis are known as the **axial skeleton**, which includes three major parts—the skull, vertebral (spinal) column, and thoracic cage. The axial skeleton is designed to provide stability to the core of the body. This lesson discusses the axial skeleton. Lesson 4.3 describes the appendicular skeleton.

The Skull

The 22 bones of the **skull** are divided into two groups: the cranial and the facial bones (**Figure 4.10**). The thin, curved bones of the **cranium** surround and protect the delicate brain. The round shape of the cranium is structurally strong in resisting impact forces and tends to absorb less force than if it were composed of flat surfaces. The **facial bones** protect the front of the head, give people's faces their individual shapes, protect and orient the eyes, and allow chewing of food.

Most of the bones of the skull and face are joined together by irregularly shaped, interlocking, and immovable joints called **sutures**. A suture is a joint in which bones of the skull are bound together by strong, tiny fibers. The sutures permit a very small amount of movement, which contributes to the compliance (ability to change size and shape in response to force) and elasticity of the skull. The one exception is the mandible, or jawbone, which is attached to the skull by a movable joint (for obvious reasons!).

The skull of a newborn infant is quite different from the adult skull. Compared to adults, babies have big heads relative to the size of their bodies. Whereas the skull of an adult accounts for about one-eighth of total body height, the skull of a newborn represents about one-fourth of body height.

As previously discussed, the skeletal system of children includes regions of hyaline cartilage. The sutures of the skull in infants are composed of this soft, connective tissue, which will ossify (turn to bone) in early childhood. In regions of the infant skull where several bones join together, there are openings connected only by pockets of fibrous membranes. Because the baby's pulse can be felt through these "soft spots," they have been given the name **fontanel** (fahn-ta-NEHL), which is French for "little fountain."

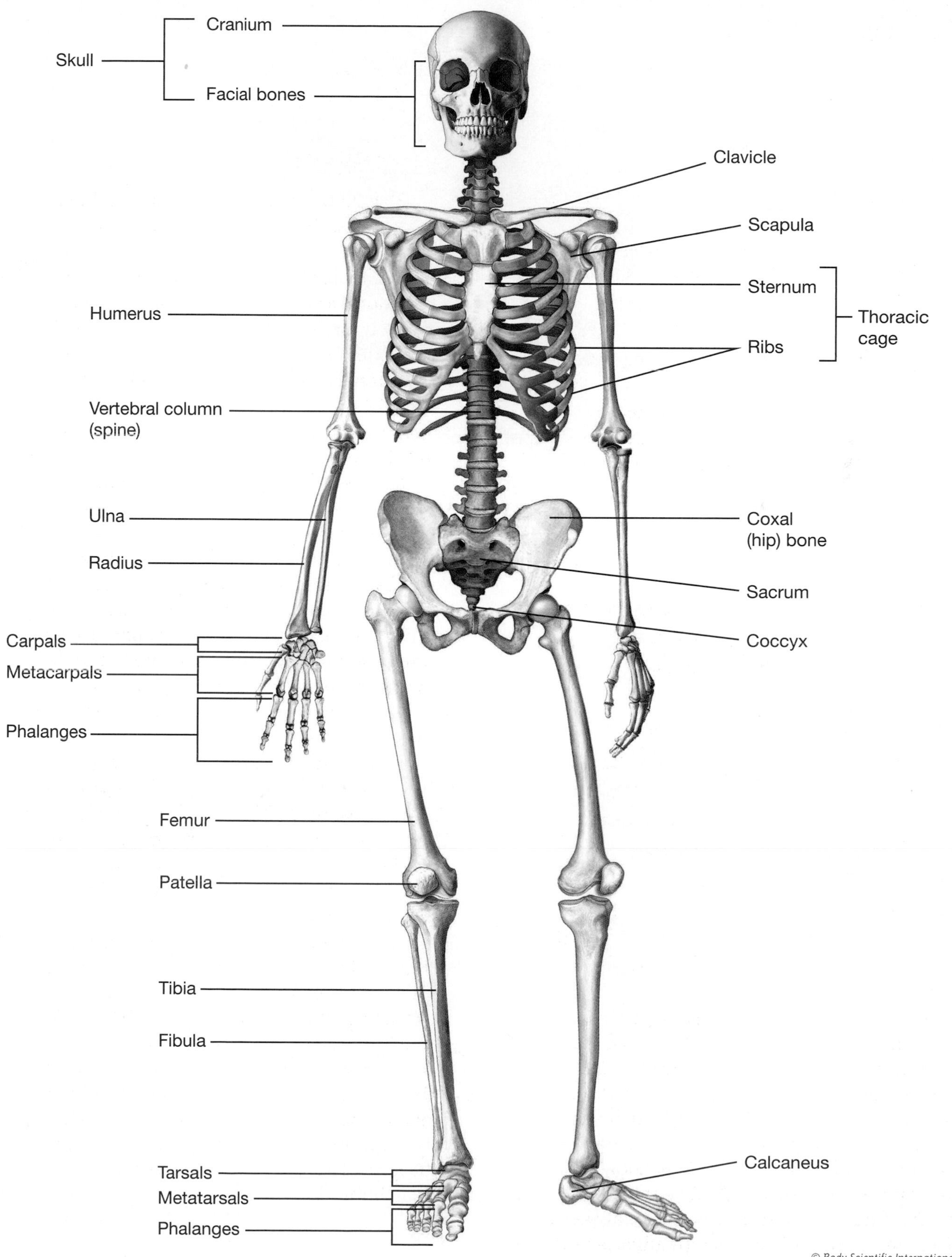

Figure 4.9 The axial skeleton (shown in a reddish color) and the appendicular skeleton.

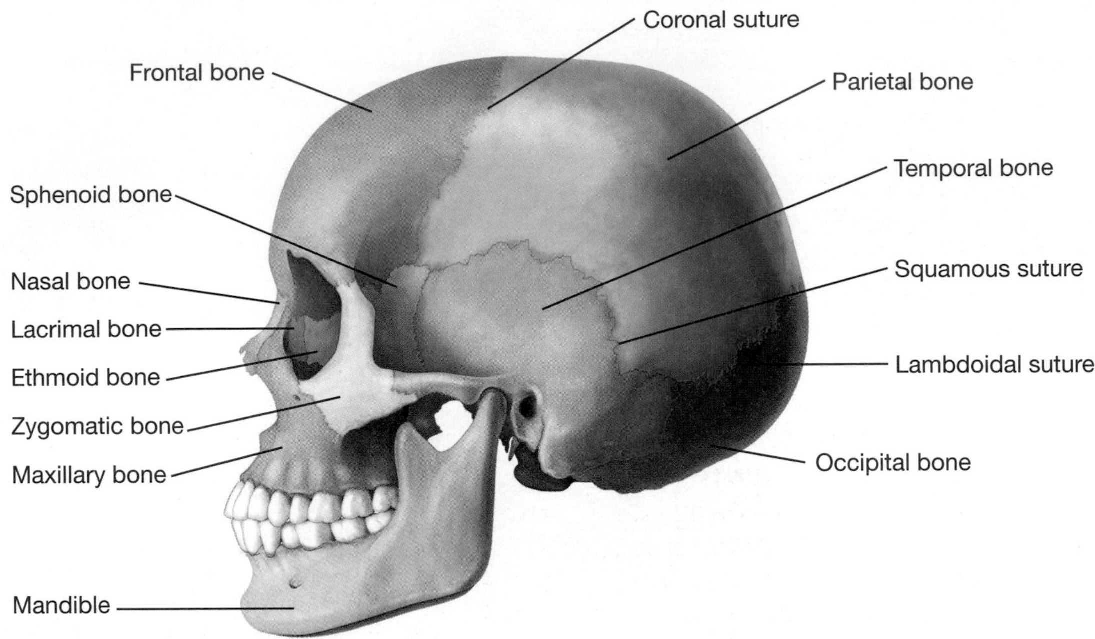

A Side view

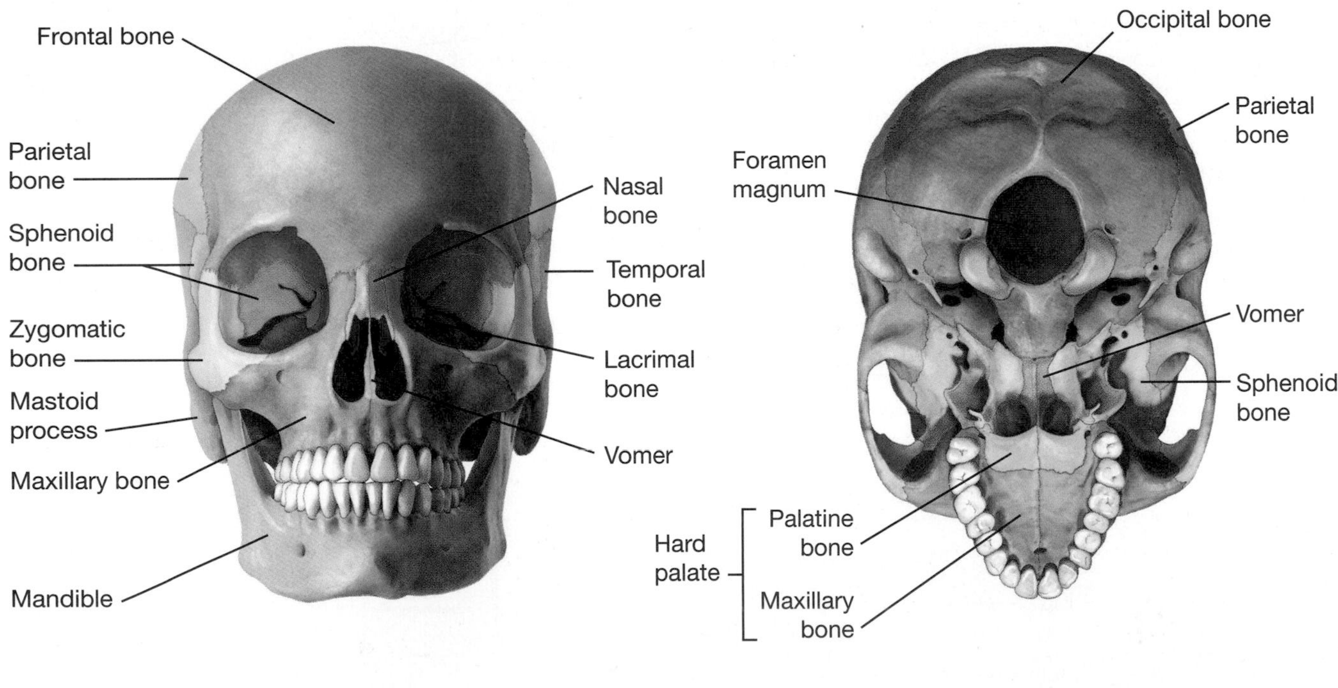

B Front view

C Base of the skull

Figure 4.10 Bones of the skull. *How many bones go together to make up the skull? What type of joints hold these bones together?*

The soft sutures and fontanels serve two important functions. They enable some compression of the skull (the largest part of the body) during birth. Equally important, they enable brain growth during late pregnancy and early infancy. The fontanels ossify to bone by 22 to 24 months following birth.

The Cranium

The cranium includes eight bones. There are two sets of paired (left and right side) bones; the rest are single bones. The bones that make up the cranium include:

- the *frontal bone*, which forms the forehead
- the two paired *parietal* (pah-RIGH-eh-tal) *bones*, which form the majority of the top and sides of the skull
- the two paired *temporal* (TEHM-poh-ral) *bones*, which surround the ears
- the *occipital* (ahk-SIP-i-tal) *bone*, which forms the base and lower back portions of the skull
- the *ethmoid* (EHTH-moyd) *bone*, which forms part of the nasal septum
- the *sphenoid* (SFEE-noyd) *bone*, which is butterfly shaped and centrally located within the skull. The sphenoid bone supports part of the base of the brain, forms part of the orbits of the eyes, and is connected to all of the other bones of the skull.

The Facial Bones

A total of fourteen bones form the face, including the mandible (MAN-di-buhl), vomer (VOH-mer), and six pairs (left and right) of bones. The facial bones include:

- the two fused **maxillary** (MAK-si-lair-ee) **bones**, which form the upper jaw, house the upper teeth, and connect to all other bones of the face, with the exception of the mandible
- the two *palatine* (PAL-a-tighn) *bones*, which form the posterior part of the hard palate, or roof of the mouth
- the two *zygomatic* (zigh-goh-MAT-ik) *bones*, or cheekbones, which also form much of the sides of the orbits, or eye sockets
- the two *lacrimal* (LAK-ri-mal) *bones*, tiny bones connecting to the orbits and surrounding the tear ducts
- the two *nasal bones*, forming the bridge of the nose
- the **vomer** (plow-shaped) bone, comprising most of the bony nasal septum
- the two *inferior concha* (KAHN-ka) *bones*, forming the sides of the nasal cavity
- the **mandible**, or lower jawbone, which is the largest facial bone, as well as the only movable facial bone.

Check Your Understanding

1. Scientists often divide the human skeleton into two parts. What are these parts called?
2. What holds the bones of the skull together? Is movement possible at these joints? Why is this important?
3. List the two functions of the fontanels in a baby's skull.
4. List the eight cranial bones and tell where each is found.
5. List the fourteen facial bones and tell where each is found.

The Vertebral Column

Although the word *spine* suggests a straight, rigid bar, the human spine, or vertebral column, is anything but straight and rigid. The human vertebral column is well designed to perform its functions of protecting the extremely delicate spinal cord, while supporting the weight of the trunk and allowing flexibility in multiple directions.

Thirty-three stacked, individual bones called **vertebrae** (VER-teh-bray) comprise the spine. The vertebrae differ in size and shape in the different regions of the spine to best fulfill their respective functions (**Figure 4.11**).

Regions of the Spine

There are five named sections of the spine:

1. The **cervical** (SER-vi-kal) **region** (neck) includes the upper seven vertebrae that enable nodding the head up and down, as well as rotation to the right and left. The first cervical vertebra, the **atlas**, is specialized to provide the connection between the occipital bone of the skull and the spinal column (**Figure 4.12**). The second cervical vertebra, the **axis**, is also specialized, with an upward projection called the *odontoid process*, on which the atlas rotates.
2. The **thoracic** (thoh-RAS-ik) **region** encompasses the next 12 vertebrae, which extend through the chest region and articulate (connect) with the ribs.

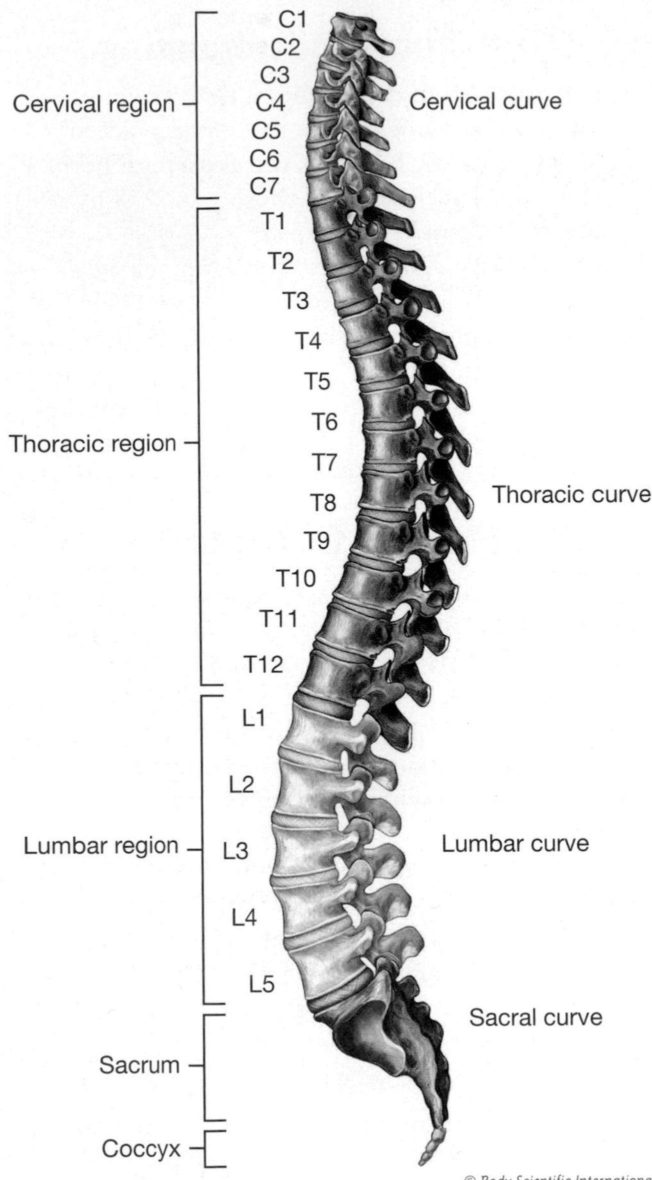

Figure 4.11 The vertebral column (spine). *How many bones make up the sacrum? The coccyx? How do these bones differ from the bones of the other three regions of the vertebral column?*

3. The **lumbar** (LUM-bar) **region** includes the five vertebrae found in the lower back.
4. The **sacrum** (SAY-krum) consists of five fused vertebrae that form the posterior portion of the pelvic girdle.
5. The **coccyx** (KAHK-siks), or tailbone, located at the bottom of the spine, includes four fused vertebrae.

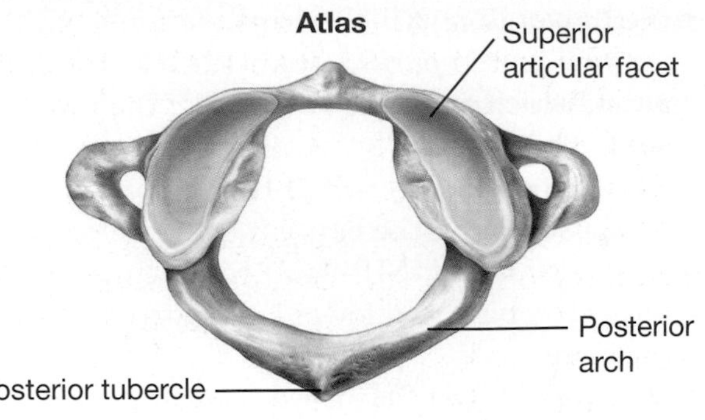

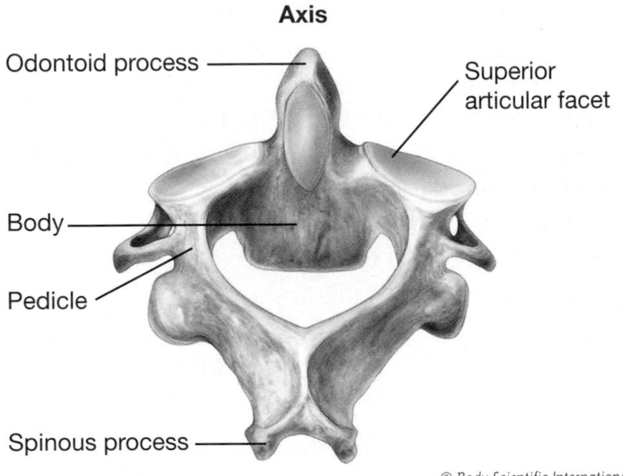

Figure 4.12 The first and second cervical vertebrae, the atlas and the axis.

Structures of the Vertebrae

Although no two vertebrae are exactly alike, most of the vertebrae have several structural features in common (**Figure 4.13**):

- The *vertebral body* is the thick, disc-shaped portion that bears weight and forms the anterior portion of the vertebra.
- The *vertebral arch* is the round projection of bone on the posterior aspect of the vertebra. It surrounds a hole known as the *vertebral foramen* (foh-RAY-mehn), through which the spinal cord passes.
- The *transverse processes* are bony projections on the lateral sides of the vertebral arch. In anatomy, a **process** is a projection on a bone or other tissue.
- The *spinous process* is a bony projection that extends posteriorly.

- The *superior* and *inferior articular processes* are indentations or facets where a vertebra articulates, or joins, with the vertebrae immediately above and below. These articulations are called *facet* (FAS-eht) *joints*.

Vertebral size increases progressively from the cervical region down through the lumbar region (**Figure 4.14**). This gradual size increase serves a functional purpose.

When the body is in an upright position, each vertebra must support the weight of all of the body parts positioned above it. Think about what this means. While a cervical vertebra supports only the weight of the head and neck, a lumbar vertebra supports the weight of the head, neck, arms, and all of the trunk positioned above that vertebra.

The size and angulation of the vertebral processes also vary throughout the spinal column. This changes the orientation of the facet joints, which connect the vertebrae and limit range of motion in the different spinal regions.

The Spinal Curves

The characteristic shapes of the vertebrae in the different spinal regions also form the normal spinal curves. As **Figure 4.11** shows, the cervical and lumbar curves are posteriorly concave, while the thoracic, sacral, and coccyx curvatures are anteriorly concave. These alternating curves make the spine stronger and better able to resist potentially injurious forces than if it were straight.

The thoracic and sacral curves are known as *primary spinal curves* because they are present at birth. The lumbar and cervical curves are referred to as *secondary spinal curves*. They develop after the baby begins to raise the head, sit, and stand, as increased muscular strength enables the young child to shift body weight to the spine.

Abnormal spinal curvatures can develop due to genetic or congenital abnormalities or when the spine is habitually subjected to asymmetrical forces (**Figure 4.15**). Exaggeration of the lumbar curve is termed *lordosis* (lor-DOH-sis), accentuation of the thoracic curve is called *kyphosis* (kigh-FOH-sis), and any lateral deviation of the spine is known as *scoliosis* (skoh-lee-OH-sis).

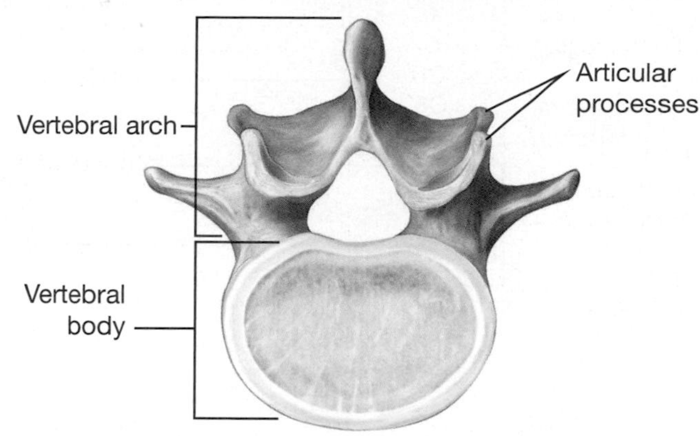

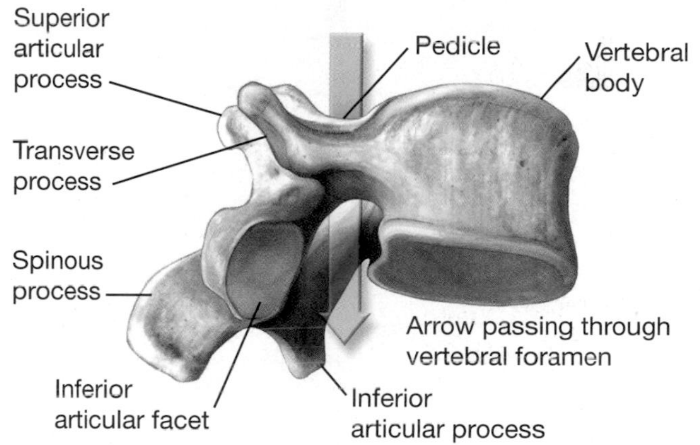

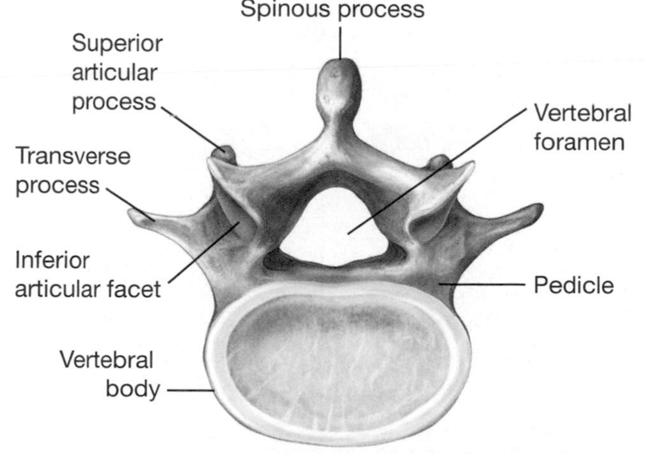

Figure 4.13 Three views of a typical vertebra. *What are the names of the indentations on the articular processes?*

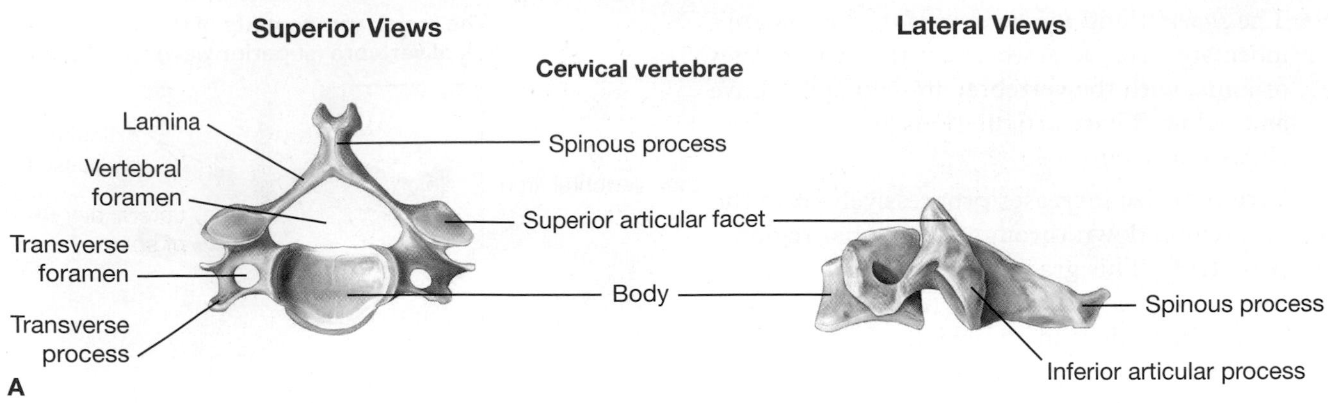

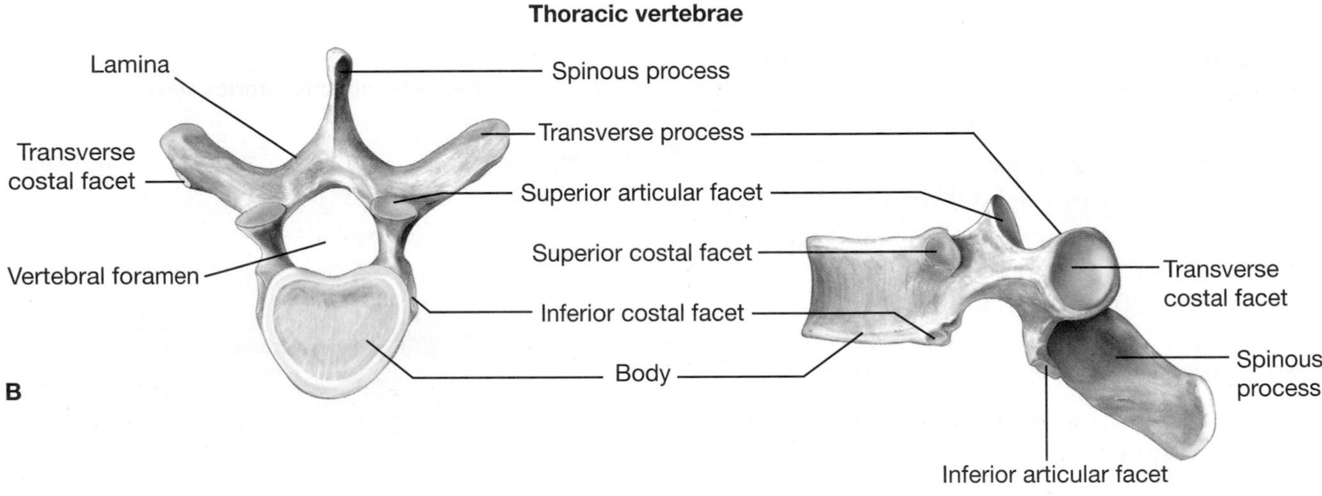

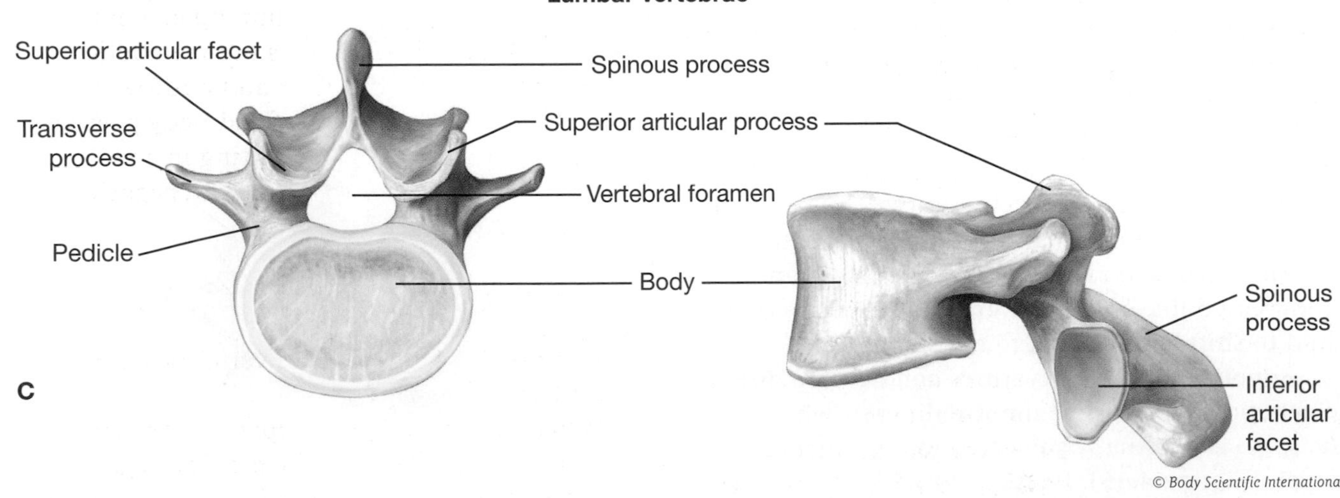

Figure 4.14 Superior and left lateral views of typical vertebrae. A—cervical vertebra. B—thoracic vertebra. C—lumbar vertebra.

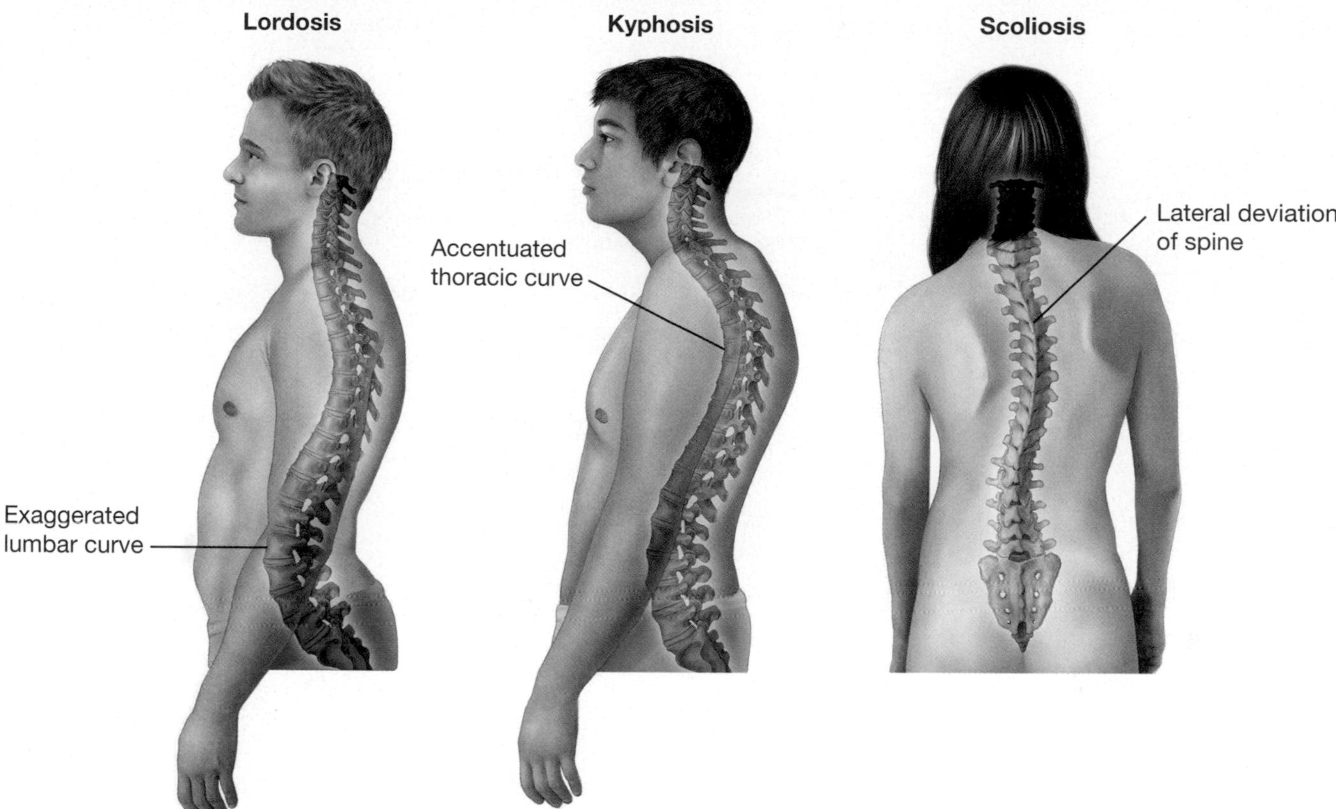

Figure 4.15 Three types of abnormal spinal curvature. *What are some causes of abnormal curvature?*

The Intervertebral Discs

Intervertebral (in-ter-VER-teh-bral) **discs** composed of fibrocartilage provide cushioning between all of the articulating vertebral bodies except those that are fused. These discs serve as shock absorbers and allow the spine to bend. The differences in the anterior and posterior thicknesses of these discs produce the normal cervical, thoracic, and lumbar curves.

In a normal adult, the discs account for approximately one-quarter of the height of the spine. When a person is lying in bed during overnight sleep, the discs absorb water and expand slightly. During periods of upright standing and sitting, when the discs are bearing weight, they lose a small amount of fluid and are compressed. For this reason, people are as much as three-fourths of an inch taller when they first arise in the morning. Injury and progressive aging reduce the water retention capability of the discs, accounting for diminished standing height in elderly individuals.

Because the discs receive no blood supply, they must rely upon changes in posture and body position to produce a pumping action that brings in nutrients and flushes out metabolic waste products with an influx and outflow of fluid. Because maintaining a fixed body position curtails this pumping action, sitting in one position for a long period of time can negatively affect disc health.

Check Your Understanding

1. List the five regions of the vertebral column, from upper to lower.
2. What is the functional purpose of the vertebrae increasing in size from the cervical region down to the lumbar region?
3. What is the function of the intervertebral discs?

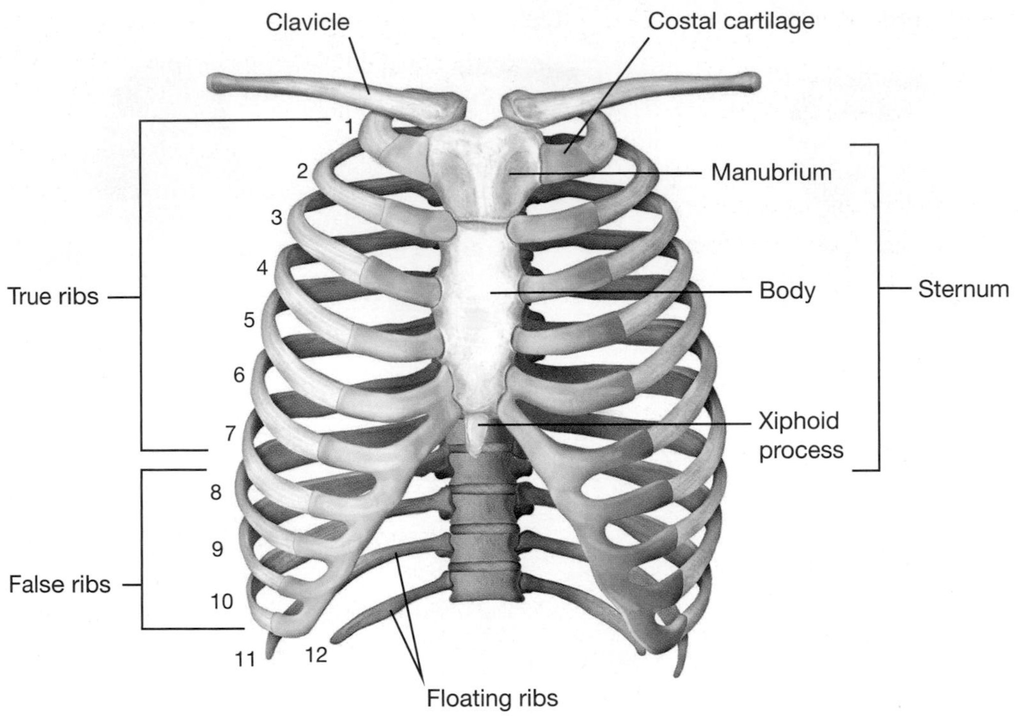

Figure 4.16 The thoracic cage. *Why are the false ribs called false ribs?*

The Hyoid Bone

Technically not part of the cranium, spine, or thoracic cage, the hyoid bone is considered part of the axial skeleton. It is located at the base of the mandible and helps with movements of the tongue, larynx, and pharynx.

The Thoracic Cage

The ribs, sternum, and thoracic vertebrae are collectively known as the **thoracic cage**, or *bony thorax*. Why are these bones given this name? It is because together they form a protective, bony "cage" that surrounds the heart and lungs in the thoracic cavity, as shown in **Figure 4.16**. The **sternum** (STER-num), or breastbone, includes three regions:

- The *manubrium* (ma-NOO-bree-um) is the upper portion of the sternum. It has articulations to the left and right bones of the clavicle, or collarbone, as well as to the first and second ribs.
- The remainder of the bony portion of the sternum is the body of the sternum.
- At the lower end of the sternum is a projection called the *xiphoid* (ZIGH-foyd) *process.*

There are 12 pairs of ribs in the thoracic cage, as shown in **Figure 4.16**.

- The first seven pairs (1–7) attach directly to the sternum and are, therefore, called *true ribs*.
- The next three pairs of ribs (8–10) are called *false ribs* because they have cartilaginous (kar-ti-LAJ-i-nuhs) attachments to the cartilage of the seventh rib, rather than attaching directly to the sternum.
- The lowest two pairs of ribs (11–12) are known as *floating ribs*, because they do not attach to bone or cartilage in front of the body.

Check Your Understanding

1. Which bones make up the thoracic cage?
2. List the three regions of the sternum.
3. How many pairs of ribs are in the thoracic cage?

LESSON 4.2 Review and Assessment

Mini Glossary

Make sure that you know the meaning of each key term.

atlas the first cervical vertebra; specialized to provide the connection between the occipital bone of the skull and the spinal column

axial skeleton central, stable portion of the skeletal system, consisting of the skull, spinal column, and thoracic cage

axis the second cervical vertebra; specialized with an upward projection called the *odontoid process*, on which the atlas rotates

cervical region the first seven vertebrae, comprising the neck

coccyx four fused vertebrae at the base of the spine forming the tailbone

cranium fused, flat bones surrounding the back of the head

facial bones bones of the face

fontanel openings in the infant skull through which a baby's pulse can be felt; these openings enable compression of the skull during birth and brain growth during late pregnancy and early infancy

intervertebral discs fibrocartilaginous cushions between vertebral bodies that allow bending of the spine and help to create the normal spinal curves

lumbar region low back region of the spine composed of five vertebrae

mandible jawbone

maxillary bones two fused bones that form the upper jaw, house the upper teeth, and connect to all other bones of the face, with the exception of the mandible

process an outgrowth or projection on a bone or other body tissue

sacrum five fused vertebrae that form the posterior of the pelvic girdle

skull the part of the skeleton composed of all of the bones of the head

sternum breastbone

sutures joints in which irregularly grooved, articulating bone sheets join closely and are tightly connected by fibrous tissues

thoracic cage bony structure surrounding the heart and lungs in the thoracic cavity; composed of the ribs, sternum, and thoracic vertebrae

thoracic region the 12 vertebrae in the middle of the back

vertebrae the bones making up the spinal column

vomer a plow-shaped bone that comprises most of the bony nasal septum

Know and Understand

1. Explain the function of the axial skeleton and which parts of the skeleton are included in it.
2. The bones of the skull are often divided into two groups. Name those two groups.
3. Which bone of the skull is freely movable?
4. Describe how sutures and fontanels relate to each other.
5. List the five named sections of the spine and tell how many vertebrae are included in each of these sections.
6. Name five structural features common to most vertebrae.

Analyze and Apply

7. Why is it important to protect and cradle a baby's head when you are holding the baby?
8. Compare and contrast the conditions of lordosis, kyphosis, and scoliosis.
9. How does the structure of an intervertebral disc (made of fibrocartilage) relate to its function?
10. Explain the different ways in which ribs are attached to the sternum.
11. What are the primary and secondary spinal curves? Explain why and distinguish between them.

IN THE LAB

12. Using different colors of clay, construct a model of the axial skeleton. Be sure to label all of the bones included. You will add to this skeleton in a later lesson in this chapter.
13. Work with a team of one or two classmates. On a Styrofoam mannequin head, draw in all of the sutures of the skull and outline them in black marker. Draw in all of the bones of the cranium and face and color each a different color using markers or crayons. Label each suture and bone with a number and then create a key listing the name of each suture and bone to correspond with the number label.

LESSON 4.3

The Appendicular Skeleton

Before You Read

Try to answer the following questions before you read this lesson.

- Why are there two bones in the forearm?
- What are the best and worst design features of the hip joint?

Lesson Objectives

- Discuss the joints of the shoulder girdle, arms, wrists, and hands, including the names of the articulating bones, their locations, and their functions.
- Identify the bones of the pelvis, legs, ankles, and feet, and explain their functions.

Key Terms

appendicular skeleton	pectoral girdle
carpal bones	pelvis
clavicle	phalanges
femur	radius
fibula	scapula
humerus	tarsal bones
lower extremity	tibia
metacarpal bones	ulna
metatarsal bones	upper extremity
patella	

The **appendicular skeleton**, as the name suggests, includes the body's appendages. These include both the bones of the **upper extremity** (the shoulder complex, arms, wrists, and hands) and those of the **lower extremity** (the pelvic girdle, legs, ankles, and feet). Altogether, there are approximately 126 bones in the appendicular skeleton. The appendicular skeleton is built for motion.

The Upper Extremity

The upper extremity is well designed for all of the tasks that people routinely ask it to perform. The muscles, bones, and joints of the upper extremity enable movements as diverse as carrying a load, throwing a ball, and threading a needle. The different movements of hammering a nail, texting on a smartphone, and performing a handspring are also made possible by this unique design.

The Pectoral Girdle

The bones surrounding the shoulder are referred to as the **pectoral** (PEHK-toh-ral) **girdle**, or *shoulder girdle*, and include a left and right **clavicle**, or collarbone, and a left and right **scapula** (SKAP-yoo-la, plural *scapulae*), or shoulder blade (**Figure 4.17**). These bones serve as sites for attachment of the numerous muscles that enable motion of the arms at the shoulders in so many different directions.

As **Figure 4.18** shows, there are two bony projections on the scapula, known as the *acromion* (a-KROH-mee-ahn) and the *coracoid* (KOR-a-koyd) *process*. The lateral end of the clavicle attaches to the acromion process to form the *acromioclavicular* (a-kroh-mee-oh-kla-VIK-yoo-lar) *joint* (**Figure 4.17**). The medial end of the clavicle attaches to the sternum to form the *sternoclavicular* (ster-noh-kla-VIK-yoo-lar) *joint*.

The acromioclavicular joint primarily allows you to raise your arm so that you can perform movements overhead. The sternoclavicular joint enables you to move your clavicle and scapula for motions such as shrugging the shoulders, raising your arms, and swimming.

The clavicle serves as a brace for positioning the shoulder laterally away from the trunk. Although there are no bony articulations between the scapulae and the posterior aspect of the trunk, the region between each scapula and the underlying tissues is sometimes referred to as the *scapulothoracic* (skap-yoo-loh-thoh-RAS-ik) *joint*.

The *glenoid* (GLEE-noyd) *fossa* of the scapula is a relatively shallow indentation that articulates, or joins, with the head of the **humerus** (HYOO-mer-us), the bone in the upper arm, to form the *glenohumeral joint*, or shoulder joint. Because the glenoid fossa (socket) is less curved than the humeral head, the humerus is able to glide against the glenoid fossa, in addition

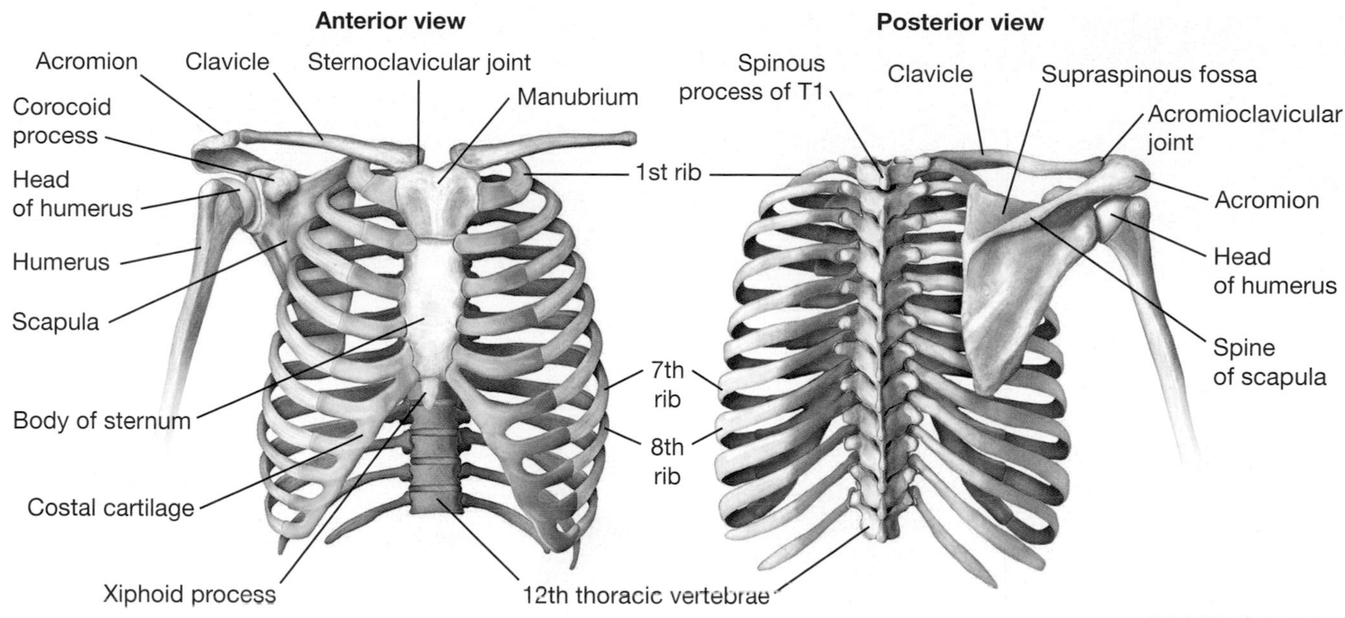

Figure 4.17 Anterior and posterior views of the shoulder girdle, ribs, and humerus.

to rotating. As a result, the glenohumeral joint allows motion in more directions than any other joint in the body.

The glenohumeral joint, along with the bones and joints of the pectoral girdle, are referred to as the *shoulder complex*. Together these joints provide the significant range of motion present in a healthy shoulder. This large degree of mobility, however, comes at the cost of instability: the shoulder is one of the most frequently dislocated joints in the human body. **Figure 4.19** summarizes the joints of the shoulder complex.

The Arm

The single bone of the upper arm is the humerus (**Figure 4.20**). The humerus is a large, strong bone, second in size only to the major bone of the

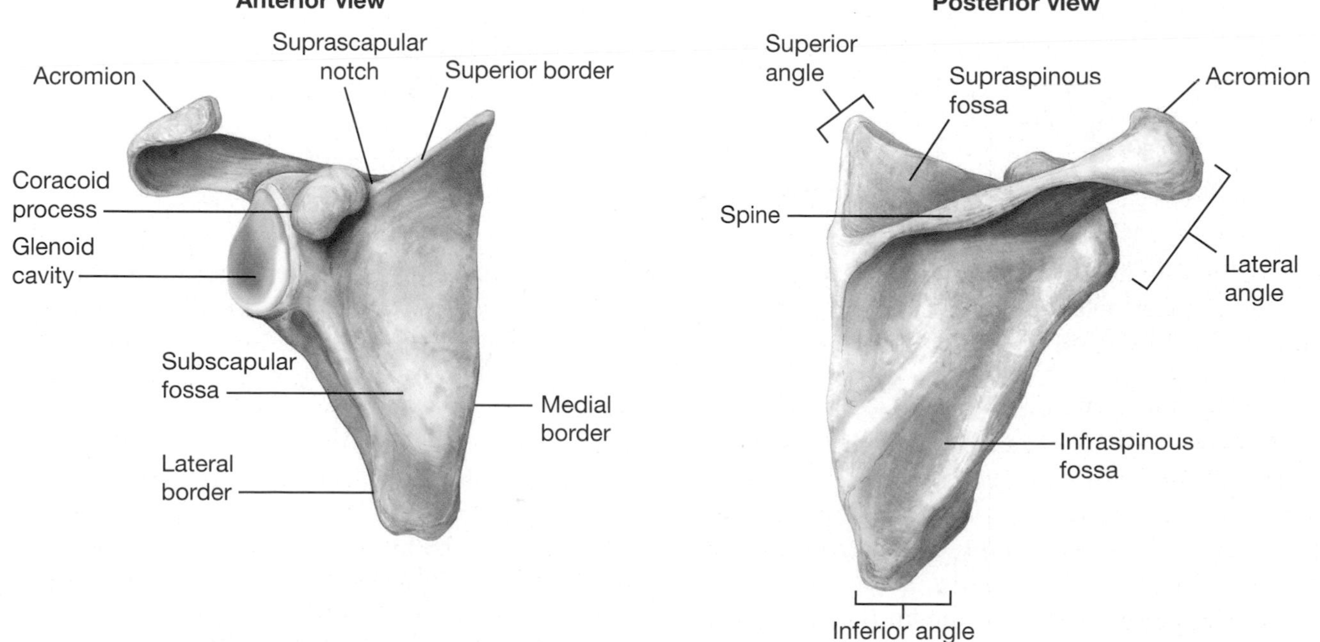

Figure 4.18 Anterior and posterior views of the scapula.

Articulating Bones of the Shoulder Complex		
Joint	**Notched Bone**	**Joining Bone or Region**
acromioclavicular joint	acromion of the scapula	clavicle
sternoclavicular joint	sternum	clavicle
scapulothoracic joint	scapula	thorax
glenohumeral joint	glenoid fossa of the scapula	humerus

Figure 4.19 Goodheart-Willcox Publisher

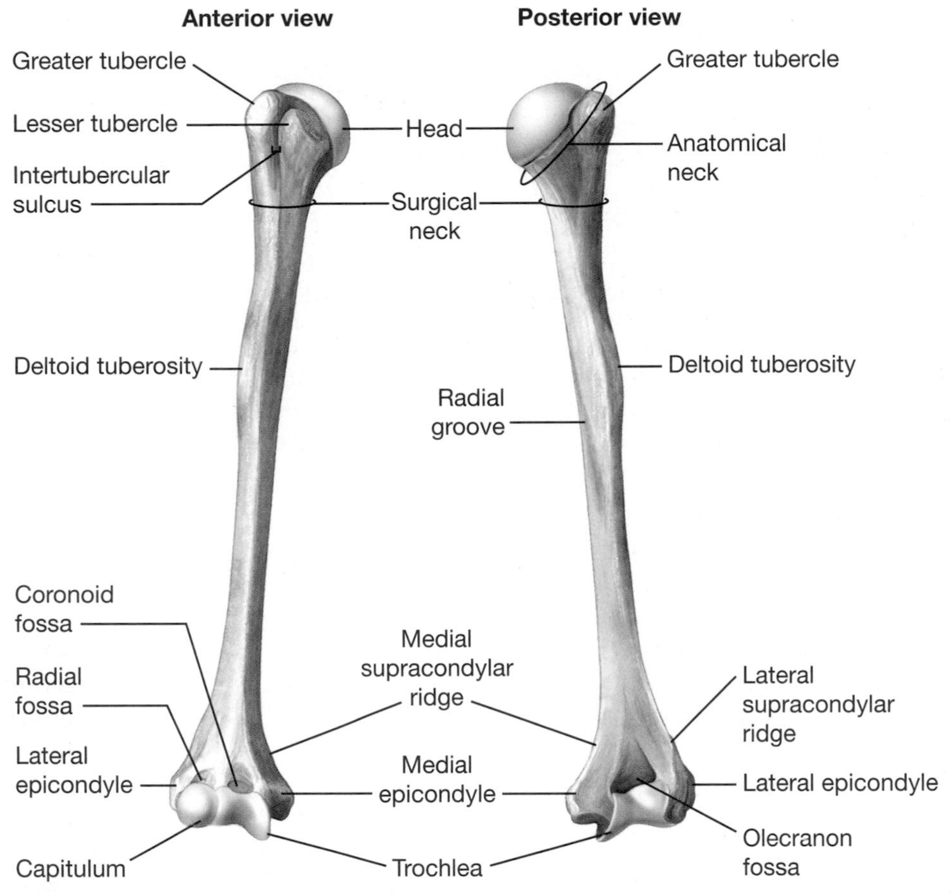

Figure 4.20 Anterior and posterior views of the humerus.

upper leg. The upper end of the humerus forms a rounded head, which, as mentioned, articulates with the glenoid fossa of the scapula to form the glenohumeral joint.

As **Figure 4.21** shows, the framework for the forearm consists of two bones—the **radius** (RAY-dee-us) and **ulna** (UHL-nuh). The radius is the bone that articulates with the wrist on the thumb side. The name *radius* comes from the ability of this bone to "radially" rotate around the ulna. This radial rotation is the familiar motion that enables the forearm and hand to rotate freely.

The ulna is larger and stronger than the radius, and it articulates with the humerus at the humeroulnar (hyoo-mer-oh-UHL-ner) joint at the elbow. The ulna attaches to the wrist on the "little finger" side. The bony projection at the upper end of the ulna, called the *olecranon* (oh-LEHK-ra-nahn) *process*, is what people refer to as the *elbow*.

The radius and ulna are connected along their entire lengths by an *interosseus* (in-ter-AHS-ee-us) *membrane*. The two bones articulate at both ends, and these joints are known as the *proximal* and *distal radioulnar* (ray-dee-oh-UHL-nar) *joints*.

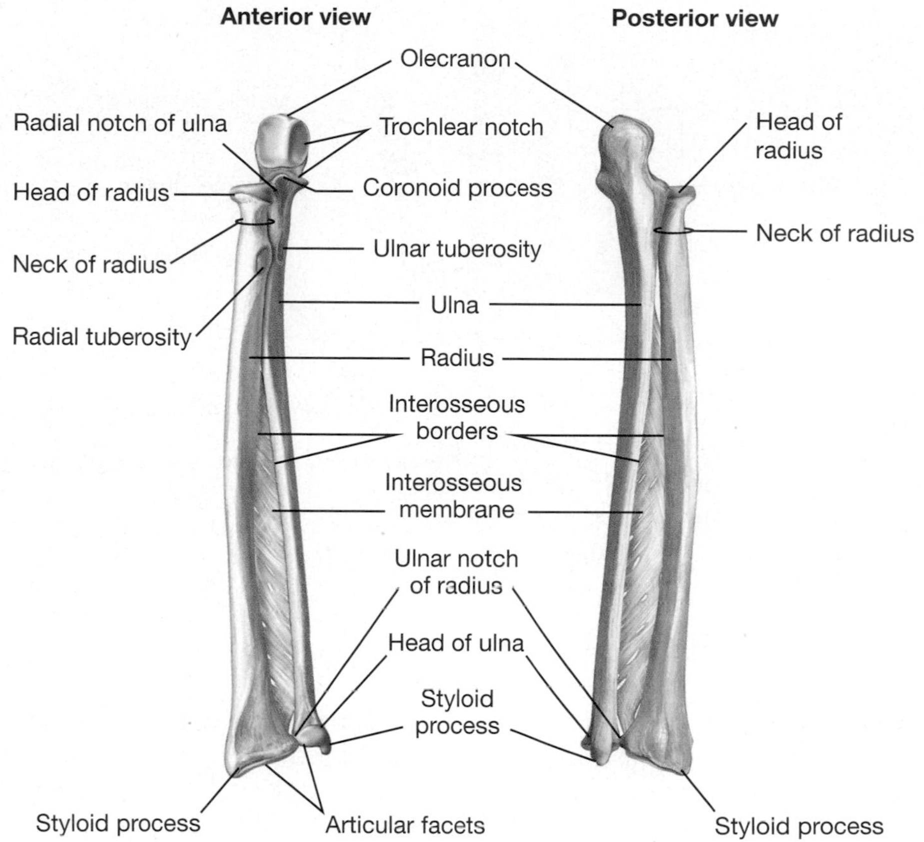

Figure 4.21 Anterior and posterior views of the radius and ulna. *Which of these two bones allows your forearm and hand to rotate freely?*

At the distal (lower) ends of both the radius and ulna are *styloid* (STIGH-loyd) *processes* that are easy to see and feel with your fingers. The distal end of the radius unites with several of the carpal bones of the wrist to form the *radiocarpal* (ray-dee-oh-KAR-pal) *joint* (**Figure 4.22**).

The Wrist and Hand

Collectively, the wrists and hands contain 54 bones—27 on the left and 27 on the right. This large number of bones enables a wide range of precise movements, along with the important ability to grasp objects.

The wrist includes eight **carpal** (KAR-pal) **bones** that are roughly arranged in two rows (**Figure 4.23**). The carpal bones are bound together by ligaments that allow a small amount of gliding motion at the intercarpal joints. However, the main function of the carpals is to provide a base for the bones of the hand.

Five **metacarpal** (meht-a-KAR-pal) **bones** in each hand articulate with the carpal bones in each wrist. There are 14 **phalanges** (fa-LAN-jeez)—the bones in the fingers. Each of the four fingers has proximal, medial, and distal phalanges, but the thumb has only two.

Articulating Bones of the Arm and Wrist		
Joint	**Notched Bone**	**Joining Bone**
humeroulnar (elbow) joint	humerus	ulna
radioulnar joints (proximal and distal)	radius	ulna
radiocarpal (wrist) joint	radius	three carpal bones

Figure 4.22

Goodheart-Willcox Publisher

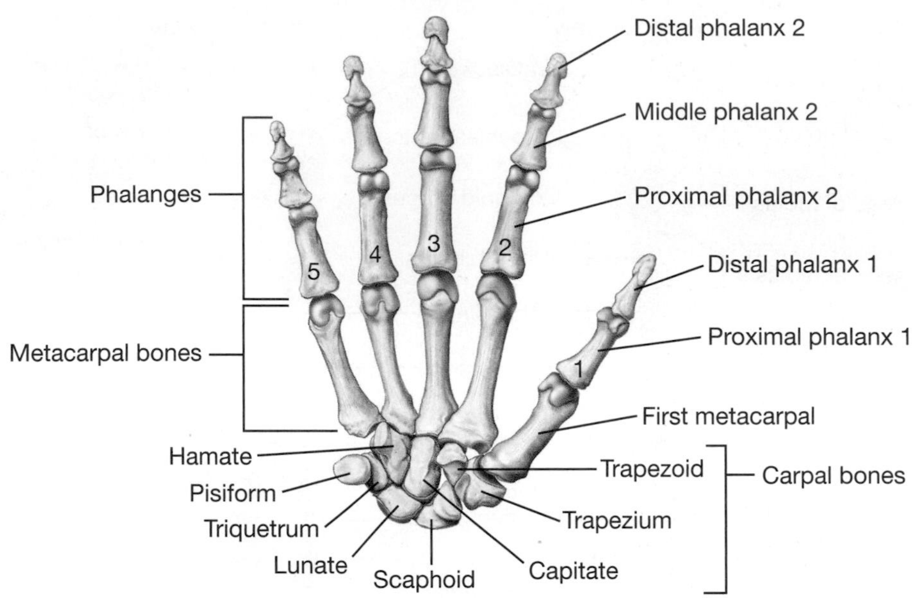

Figure 4.23 Anterior view of the bones of the right hand.

Whereas the joints of the fingers permit motion in only one plane, the thumb has the ability to freely rotate and to stretch across the palm of the hand. This capability, known as an *opposable thumb*, is shared only by humans and other primates.

Check Your Understanding

1. Which bones make up the appendicular skeleton?
2. Which bones are included in the shoulder complex?
3. Which forearm bone enables rotation of the hand around the longitudinal axis of the arm?
4. How many bones are in each wrist and hand?

The Lower Extremity

The lower extremity is well designed for its functions of weight bearing and gait, including walking and running. During sporting activities, the muscles, bones, and joints of the lower extremity also enable movements involved in jumping, skating, surfing, skiing, and dancing, for example.

The Pelvic Girdle

As the name suggests, the pelvic girdle is a bony encasement of the pelvic region that shelters the reproductive organs, bladder, and part of the large intestine. It is formed by two large, strong *coxal* (KAHK-sal) *bones* (hip bones, also known as the *os coxa*) and the sacrum (**Figure 4.24**). These three bones, with the addition of the coccyx, comprise the **pelvis**. The female pelvis is wider than the male pelvis to enable pregnancy and childbirth. The pelvis is one of the hallmark differences that allows classification of a skeleton as male or female.

Each coxal bone is formed by the fusion of the ilium, ischium, and pubis. During childhood these are three separate bones.

The *ilium* (IL-ee-um) comprises most of each coxal bone, connecting posteriorly to the sacrum at the *sacroiliac* (sa-kroh-IL-ee-ak) *joint*. The prominent upper edge of the ilium, which can usually be palpated (examined or felt by touch), is called the *iliac crest*.

The *ischium* (IS-kee-um), which forms the inferior portion of each coxal bone, is the bone that supports the weight of the upper body during sitting. Within each coxal bone lies an *acetabulum* (as-eh-TAB-yoo-lum): a deep, bony socket that receives the head of the thigh bone.

The *pubis* (PYOO-bis) is the anterior portion of each coxal bone. The two pubic bones fuse in the center front of the body at the *pubic symphysis* (PYOO-bik SIM-fi-sis), where the bones are joined by a disc of hyaline cartilage.

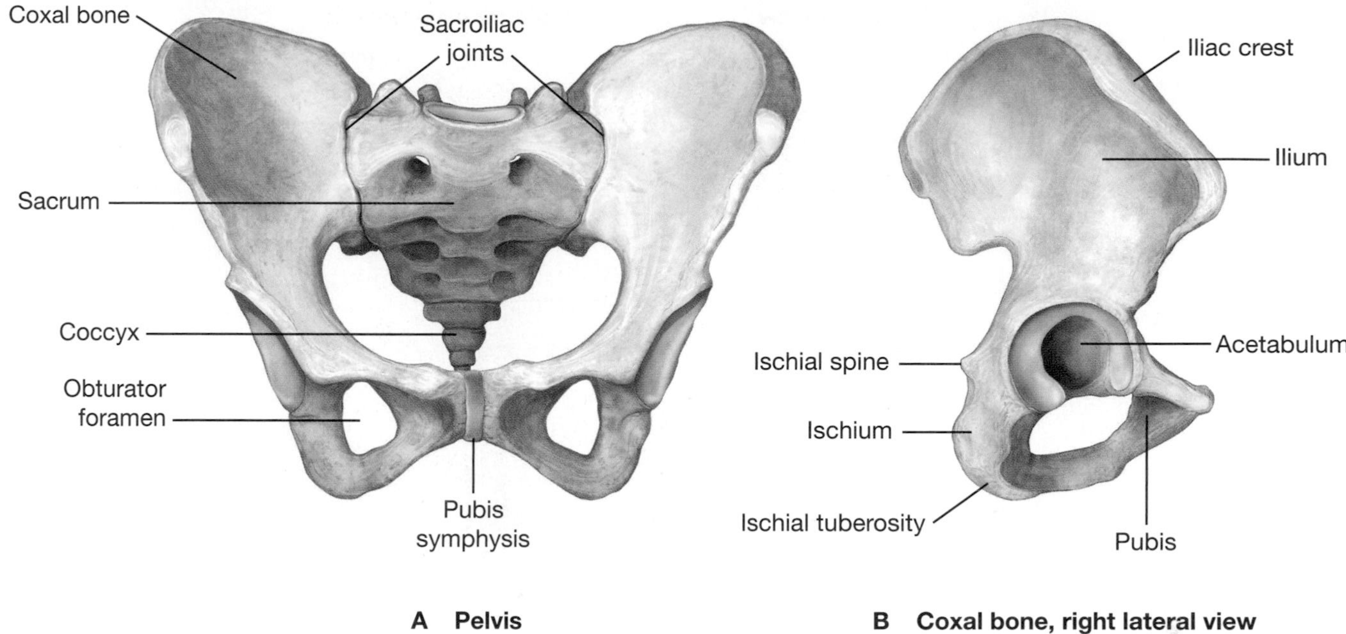

Figure 4.24 Bones of the pelvis. *Why are these bones important when classifying skeletons?*

The Leg

The single bone of the upper leg, or thigh, is the **femur** (FEE-mer), which is the longest and strongest bone in the body. **Figure 4.25** shows the anatomical features of the femur. The head of the femur fits snugly into the acetabulum of the hip, making the joint extremely stable. The most vulnerable part of the femur is the neck, which is the site where most hip fractures occur.

The lower leg has two bones: the tibia and fibula (**Figure 4.26**). The thick, strong **tibia** (TIB-ee-a)—or shinbone—is the bone that bears most of the weight of the body above it.

Unlike the radius in the forearm, the **fibula** (FIB-yoo-la) has no special motion capability and serves primarily as a site for muscle attachments. The fibula is not part of the articulation with the femur at the knee joint, but the distal end of the fibula has a bony prominence called the *lateral malleolus* (mal-LEE-oh-lus), which you can readily touch and feel on the lateral (outer) side of the ankle.

Like the radius and ulna in the forearm, the tibia and fibula are connected along their lengths by an interosseous membrane, and they articulate at both ends of the fibula. The **patella** (pa-TEHL-a), or kneecap, is a small, flat, triangular-shaped bone that protects the front of the knee. The articulations of the bones of the leg and ankle are summarized in **Figure 4.27**.

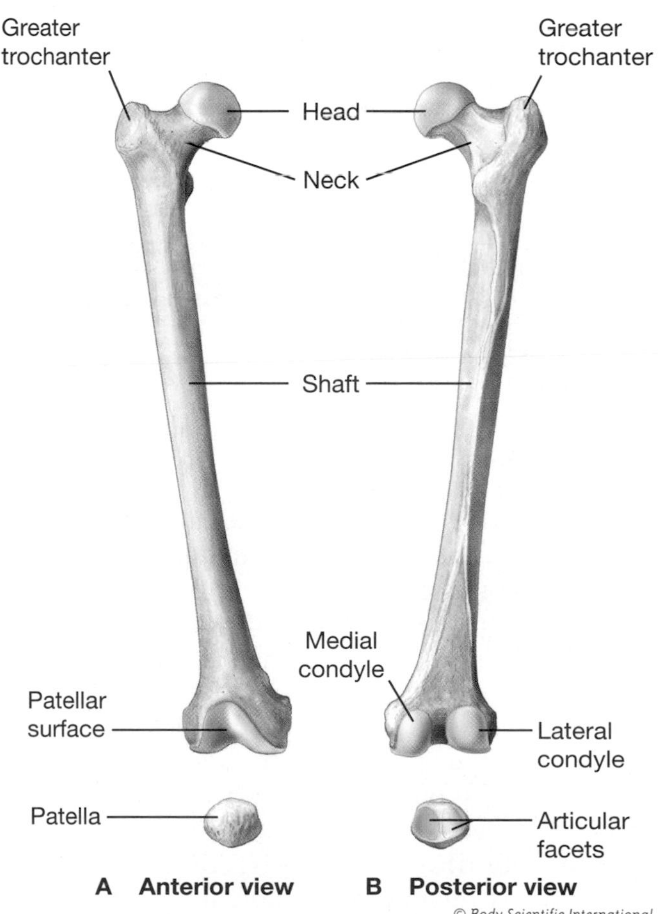

Figure 4.25 The right femur and the patella. *Although the femur is the strongest bone in the body, one part is vulnerable to fracture. What is the most vulnerable part of the femur?*

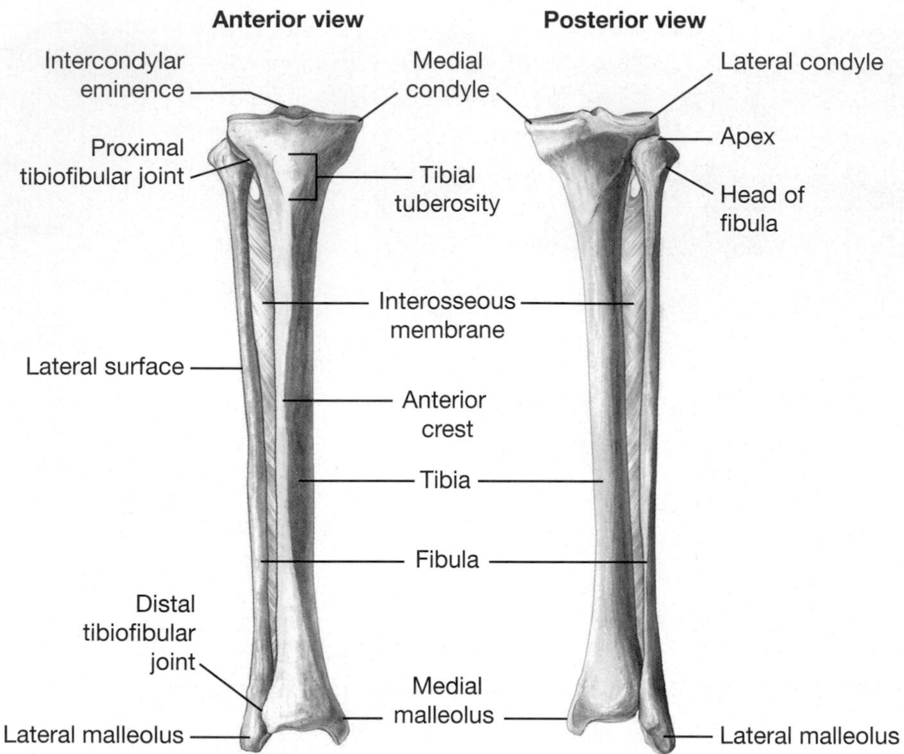

© Body Scientific International

Figure 4.26 The right tibia and fibula, anterior and posterior views.

Articulating Bones of the Leg and Ankle		
Joint	**Notched Bone or Socket**	**Joining Bone or Region**
iliofemoral (hip) joint	acetabulum	femur
tibiofemoral (knee) joint	tibia	femur
patellofemoral joint	patella	anterior knee
tibiofibular joints (proximal and distal)	tibia	fibula

Figure 4.27

Goodheart-Willcox Publisher

The Ankle and Foot

The ankle and foot serve the critically important functions of supporting body weight and enabling locomotion. The foot is so well designed that it assists with walking and running by acting like a spring that stores and releases energy.

The hindfoot is constructed of **tarsal** (TAR-sal) **bones**, with the two largest, the *talus* (TAY-lus) and *calcaneus* (kal-KAY-nee-us)—or heel bone—bearing most of the weight of the body (**Figure 4.28**). The five **metatarsal** (meht-a-TAR-sal) **bones** that support the midfoot region are similar to the metacarpals of the hand. Like the fingers, each toe is comprised of three phalanges, and like the thumb, the big toe has only two phalanges. The toes function by increasing the area of the foot during weight-bearing activities such as walking and running—thereby increasing body stability.

The configuration of the metatarsal bones forms two important arches (**Figure 4.29**). The *longitudinal arch* runs lengthwise from the calcaneus to the heads of the metatarsals. The *transverse arch* runs sideways (perpendicular to the longitudinal arch), and in most people causes

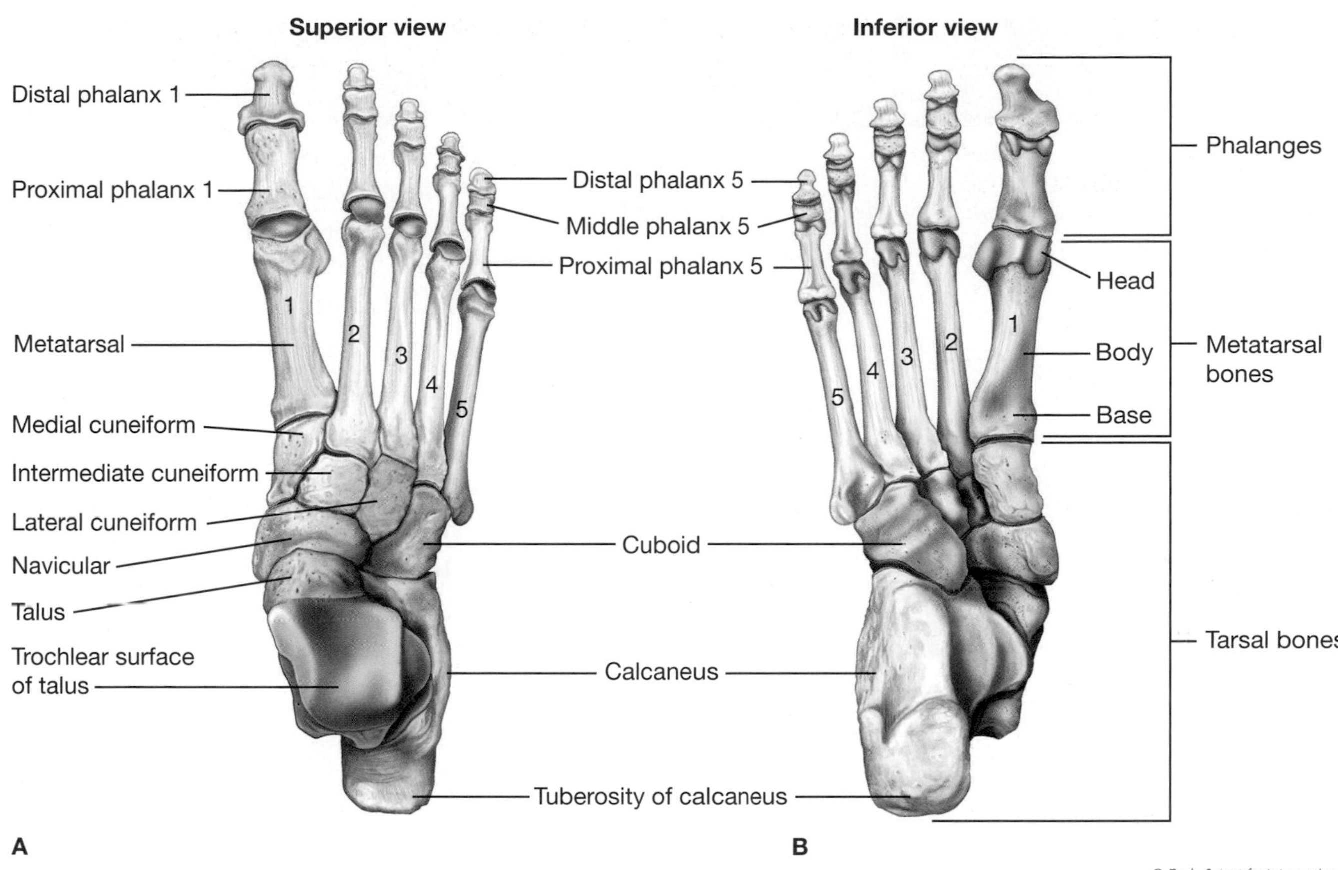

Figure 4.28 Superior (A) and inferior (B) views of the bones of the right foot.

the medial center of the bottom of the foot to be slightly elevated. It is these arches that compress somewhat during the weight-bearing phase of your gait, but then act as springs when they rebound to their original shape during the propulsive (push-off) phase of the gait.

Check Your Understanding

1. Which bones make up the pelvic girdle?
2. Which three bones fuse to form each coxal bone?
3. What is the longest and strongest bone in the body?
4. Although relatively small bones, the bones of the toes serve what important function?
5. What is the purpose of the two arches formed by the metatarsal bones?

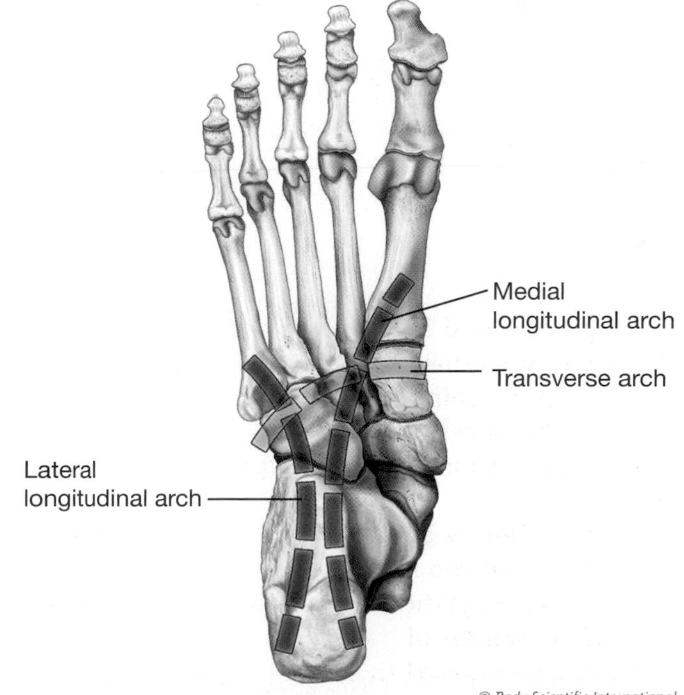

Figure 4.29 Arches of the foot, inferior view. *How do these arches contribute to the ability to walk with a smooth, easy gait?*

LESSON 4.3 Review and Assessment

Mini Glossary

Make sure that you know the meaning of each key term.

appendicular skeleton the bones of the body's appendages; the arms and legs

carpal bones bones of the wrist

clavicle doubly curved long bone that forms part of the shoulder girdle; the collarbone

femur thigh bone

fibula bone of the lower leg; does not bear weight

humerus major bone of the upper arm

lower extremity bones of the hips, legs, and feet

metacarpal bones the five interior bones of the hand, connecting the carpals in the wrist to the phalanges in the fingers

metatarsal bones small bones of the ankle

patella kneecap

pectoral girdle bones surrounding the shoulder, including the clavicle and scapula

pelvis bones of the pelvic girdle and the coccyx at the base of the spine

phalanges bones of the fingers

radius smaller of the two bones in the forearm; rotates around the ulna

scapula shoulder blade

tarsal bones bones of the ankle

tibia major weight-bearing bone of the lower leg

ulna larger bone of the lower arm

upper extremity bones of the shoulders, arms, and hands

Know and Understand

1. Explain how the bones of the pectoral girdle, along with various muscles and joints, allow movement in many different directions.
2. Which bone of the forearm is larger and stronger than the other?
3. What is the common name for the olecranon process?
4. How many bones are present in your left wrist and hand?
5. Why is the pelvis of a female wider than the pelvis of a male?
6. What is the name of the part of the coxal bone that receives the head of the femur?
7. Which bone of the lower leg is the stronger bone that bears most of the weight of the body above it?
8. What is the anatomical name for the heel bone?
9. What is the purpose of the two arches in the foot?
10. Compare the motions allowed by the sternoclavicular joint with those allowed by the acromioclavicular joint. Explain how both joints contribute to the motions needed at the shoulder.

Analyze and Apply

11. Functionally, why does the pectoral girdle have much more range of motion than the pelvic girdle?
12. Why are there two bones in the forearm rather than just one?
13. Why would you not be able to walk properly if you had a fracture in one of the metatarsals or phalanges?
14. The finger joints allow movement in only one plane, but the thumb can rotate freely. How is this beneficial in everyday life?
15. Why are there two bones in the lower leg rather than just one? Explain how those two bones work together.
16. Find out the difference between intramembranous and endochondral ossification. Name your sources.

IN THE LAB

17. Using different colors of clay, construct a model of the appendicular skeleton, labeling all of the bones included. Attach your appendicular skeleton to the axial skeleton you constructed in Lesson 4.2. When you have finished, analyze the strengths and weaknesses of your model. Does it adequately represent the human skeleton? What are the limitations of the model?
18. Using clay, construct models of a male pelvis and a female pelvis. Research the normal size of each coxal bone in each gender and write a short report detailing the size differences in the male and female models. Further explain how this information is helpful to forensic scientists.

LESSON 4.4

Joints

Before You Read

Try to answer the following questions before you read this lesson.

- Some joints permit little to no movement; what is the purpose of these joints?
- What prevents damage to joints from frictional wear over time?

Lesson Objectives

- Describe the general structures and functions of the three major categories of joints.
- Explain the functions of articular tissues such as cartilage, tendons, and ligaments.

Key Terms

amphiarthrosis	pivot joint
articular fibrocartilage	saddle joint
ball-and-socket joint	symphysis
bursae	synarthrosis
condyloid joint	synchondrosis
diarthrosis	syndesmosis
gliding joint	synovial joint
hinge joint	tendon
ligaments	tendon sheaths

The joints of the human body govern the extent and directions of movement of the bones that articulate (come together) at the joint. Although the range of motion at a given joint is affected by the tightness of the soft tissues crossing that joint, it is the structure of the bony articulation that determines the directions of motion permitted.

Types of Joints

Anatomists classify joints in different ways based on joint complexity, the number of axes present, joint structure, and joint function. Joint function determines movement capability and is the most easily remembered; therefore, this classification is used in this lesson.

There are three main categories of joints with regard to function: the immovable joints, the slightly movable joints, and the freely movable joints. Most of the joints of the body appendages are freely movable, because moving is the function of the arms, hands, legs, and feet. The joints of the axial skeleton are primarily immovable or slightly movable, because stability and protection of vital organs are their functions.

Immovable Joints

The immovable joints are called **synarthroses** (sin-ar-THROH-seez). The prefix *syn-* means "together" and the root word *arthron* means "joint." Synarthroses are fibrous joints that can absorb shock but permit little or no movement of the articulating bones. The two types of immovable joints are sutures and syndesmoses.

Sutures, which you read about earlier in this chapter, are joints in which irregularly grooved, articulating bone sheets join closely and are tightly connected by fibrous tissues. The fibers begin to ossify (turn to bone) in early adulthood and are eventually replaced completely by bone. The only sutures in the human body are the sutures of the skull.

Syndesmoses (sin-dehz-MOH-seez), meaning "held by bands," are joints in which dense, fibrous tissue binds the bones together, permitting extremely limited movement. Examples include the coracoacromial (kor-a-koh-a-KROH-mee-al) joint and the distal tibiofibular (tib-ee-oh-FIB-yoo-lar) joints.

Slightly Movable Joints

The **amphiarthroses** (am-fee-ar-THROH-seez)—the prefix *amphi-* means "on both sides"—are joints that permit only slight motion. These cartilaginous joints allow more motion of the adjacent bones than do the synarthrodial joints and are therefore somewhat better able to absorb shock. The two types of amphiarthroses are synchondroses and symphyses.

Synchondroses (sin-kahn-DROH-seez), meaning "held by cartilage," are joints in which the articulating bones are held together by a thin layer of hyaline cartilage. Examples include the sternocostal joints (between the sternum and the ribs) and the epiphyseal plates in the long bones.

Symphyses (SIM-fi-seez) are joints in which thin plates of hyaline cartilage separate a disc of fibrocartilage from the bones. Examples include the vertebral joints and the pubic symphysis.

Freely Movable Joints

Freely movable joints are called **diarthroses** (digh-ar-THROH-seez). They are also referred to as **synovial** (si-NOH-vee-al) **joints** because each joint is surrounded by an articular capsule with a synovial membrane lining that secretes a lubricant known as *synovial fluid* (**Figure 4.30**). Each of the six different types of diarthroses is structured to permit different types of motion (**Figure 4.31**).

At **gliding joints** the articulating bone surfaces are nearly flat. The only movement permitted is gliding.

In **hinge joints**, one articulating bone surface is convex (curved outward), and the other is concave (curved inward). Strong ligaments restrict movement to a planar, hingelike motion, similar to the hinge on a door.

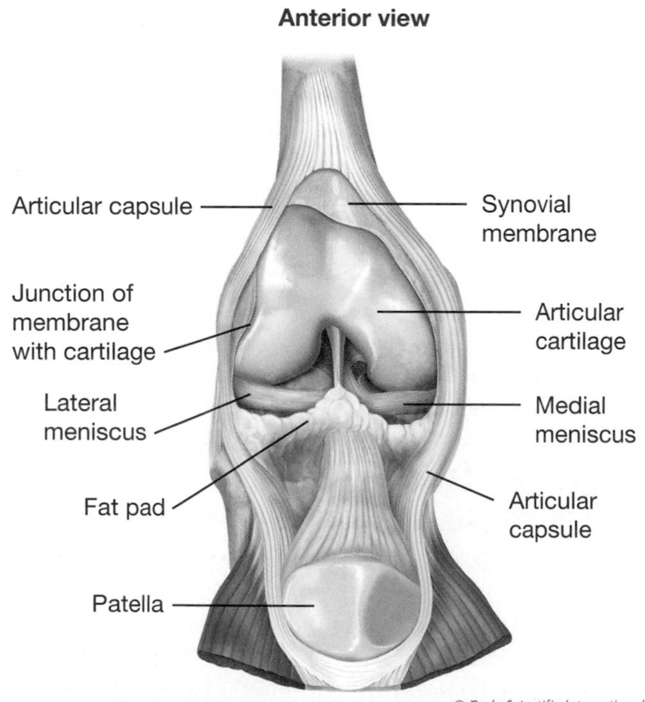

Figure 4.30 Anterior view of the knee, which is a synovial joint.

Pivot joints permit rotation around only one axis. (Think about moving around your stationary pivot foot in basketball.)

At **condyloid** (KAHN-di-loyd) **joints**, one articulating bone surface is an oval, convex shape, and the other is a reciprocally shaped concave surface. Flexion, extension, abduction, adduction, and circumduction are permitted.

Saddle joints are so named because their articulating bone surfaces are both shaped like the seat of a riding saddle. Movement capability is the same as that of the condyloid joint but greater range of movement is allowed.

Ball-and-socket joints are the most freely movable joints in the body. In these joints the surfaces of the articulating bones are reciprocally convex and concave, with one bone end shaped like a "ball" and the other like a "socket." Rotation is permitted in all three planes of movement. In cases in which the joint socket is relatively shallow, such as in the shoulder, a large range of motion is permitted, but at the sacrifice of joint stability. Alternatively, the deep socket of the hip joint maximizes stability but allows much less of a range of motion than at the shoulder.

Two structures often associated with diarthrodial joints are bursae and tendon sheaths. **Bursae** (BER-see) are small capsules lined with synovial membranes and filled with synovial fluid that cushion the structures they separate. Most bursae separate tendons from bone, reducing the friction on the tendons during joint motion.

Tendon sheaths are double-layered synovial structures surrounding tendons that are subject to friction because they are close to bones. These sheaths secrete synovial fluid to promote free motion of the tendon during joint movement. Many long muscle tendons crossing the wrist and finger joints are protected by tendon sheaths.

Check Your Understanding

1. Which types of joints are most prevalent in the axial skeleton? Why?
2. What are the two main types of synarthroses?
3. What are the two main types of amphiarthroses?

Gliding joint (intercarpal)

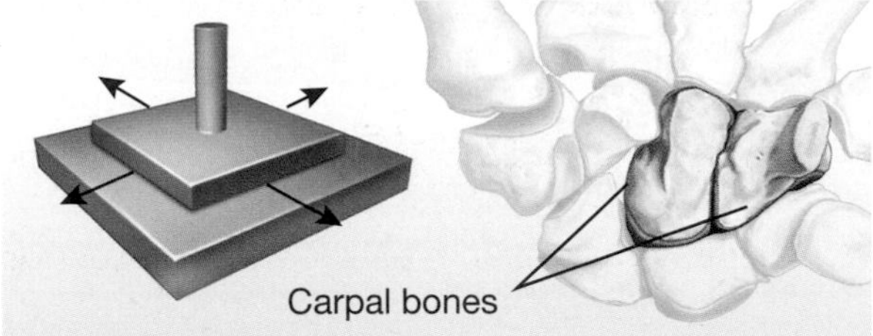

Hinge joint (humeroulnar)

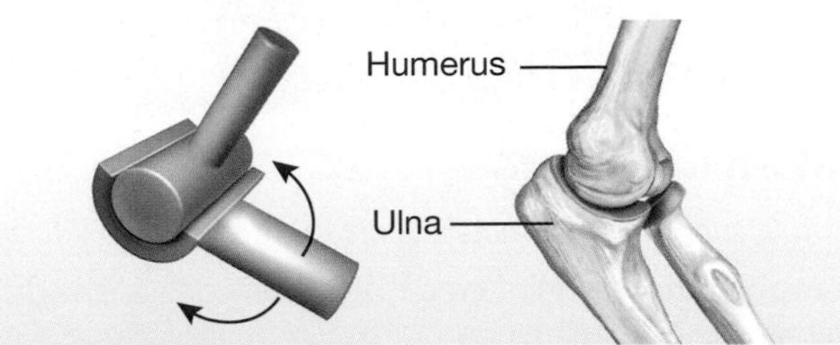

Pivot joint (radioulnar)

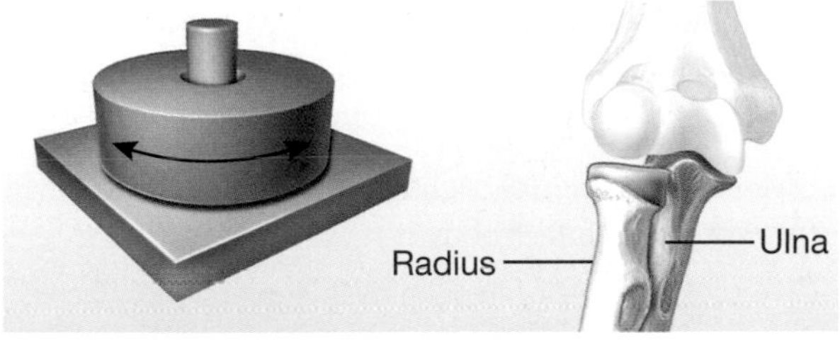

Condylar joint (metacarpophalangeal)

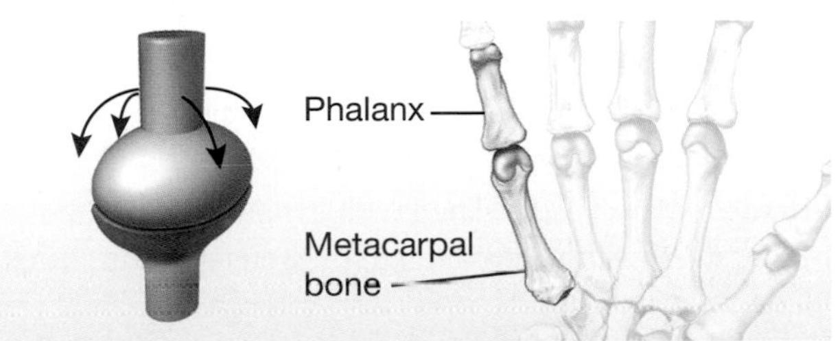

Saddle joint (trapeziometacarpal)

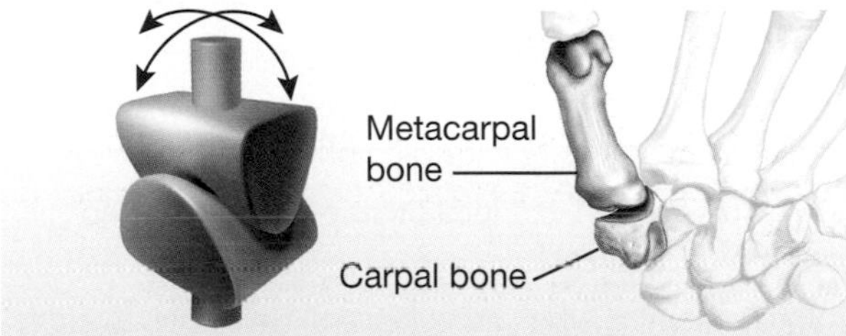

Ball-and-socket joint (humeroscapular)

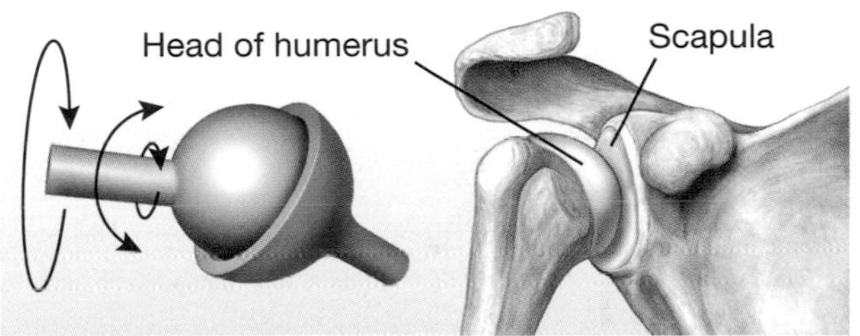

Figure 4.31 Examples of the six different types of diarthroses. *Which of these six types of joints is the most freely movable?*

Articular Tissues

The joints of any mechanical device must be properly lubricated if the movable parts are to move freely and not wear against each other. In the human body, articular cartilage covers the ends of bones at diarthrodial joints and provides a protective lubrication. Articular cartilage cushions the joint and reduces friction and wear.

At some joints, **articular fibrocartilage**, shaped like a disc or a partial disc called a *meniscus*, is also present between the articulating bones. The intervertebral discs and the menisci of the knee are examples. These discs and menisci help to distribute forces evenly over the joint surfaces and absorb shock at the joint.

Tendons, which connect muscles to bones, and **ligaments**, which connect bones to other bones, are also present at the diarthrodial joints. Composed of collagen and elastic fibers, these tissues are slightly elastic and will return to their original length after being stretched, unless overstretched to the point of injury. The tendons and ligaments crossing a joint play an important role in joint stability. The hip joints, in particular, are crossed by a number of large, strong tendons and ligaments.

Check Your Understanding

1. What is the purpose of articular fibrocartilage?
2. In functional terms, what is the difference between a tendon and a ligament?

LESSON 4.4 Review and Assessment

Mini Glossary

Make sure that you know the meaning of each key term.

amphiarthrosis joint type that permits only slight motions

articular fibrocartilage tissue shaped like a disc or partial disc called a *meniscus* that provides cushioning at a joint

ball-and-socket joint synovial joint formed between one bone end shaped roughly like a ball and the receiving bone reciprocally shaped like a socket

bursae small capsules lined with synovial membranes and filled with synovial fluid; they cushion the structures they separate

condyloid joint type of diarthrosis in which one articulating bone surface is an oval, convex shape, and the other is a reciprocally shaped concave surface

diarthrosis freely movable joints; also known as *synovial joints*

gliding joint type of diarthrosis that allows only sliding motion of the articulating bones

hinge joint type of diarthrosis that allows only hingelike movements in forward and backward directions

ligaments bands composed of collagen and elastic fibers that connect bones to other bones

pivot joint type of diarthrosis that permits rotation around only one axis

saddle joint type of diarthrosis in which the articulating bone surfaces are both shaped like the seat of a riding saddle

symphysis type of amphiarthrosis joint in which a thin plate of hyaline cartilage separates a disc of fibrocartilage from the bones

synarthrosis fibrous joint that can absorb shock, but permits little or no movement of the articulating bones

synchondrosis type of amphiarthrosis joint in which the articulating bones are held together by a thin layer of hyaline cartilage

syndesmosis joint at which dense, fibrous tissue binds the bones together, permitting extremely limited movement

synovial joint a diarthrodial joint

tendon tissue band composed of collagen and elastic fibers that connects a muscle to a bone

tendon sheaths double-layered synovial structures surrounding tendons subject to friction given their position close to bones; secrete synovial fluid to promote free motion of the tendons during joint movement

Know and Understand

1. What does it mean to say that bones articulate with each other?
2. Give two examples of immovable joints and where they are found in the body.
3. Give two examples of slightly movable joints and where they are found in the body.
4. Give six examples of freely movable joints and where they are found in the body.
5. What is the purpose of articular fibrocartilage?

Analyze and Apply

6. Why is it important to have a layer of cartilage between bones that articulate with each other?
7. Why do people need joints that permit little or no skeletal movement?
8. What happens when articular cartilage begins to erode from excessive wear and stress on a joint?
9. Why does the human skeleton need freely movable joints?
10. Functionally, how does a torn meniscus change the knee joint?

IN THE LAB

11. Obtain (or draw) a picture of a skeleton. Label the areas on the skeleton where these types of joints are located: sutures, syndesmoses, synchondroses, symphyses, gliding, hinge, pivot, condyloid, saddle, and ball-and-socket. Be prepared to explain to the class the kind of movement that each type of joint allows.
12. Obtain a model of a skeleton, or use the clay skeleton you made earlier in this chapter. Pick two each of the immovable joints, slightly movable joints, and freely movable joints, and find them on the skeleton model. Explain to the class why those joints are found where they are, relating structure to function.

LESSON 4.5

Common Injuries and Disorders of the Skeletal System

Before You Read

Try to answer the following questions before you read this lesson.

- What is the female athlete triad, and why is it potentially deadly?
- What is osteoarthritis, and how might it possibly be prevented?

Lesson Objectives

- Identify the different types of bone and epiphyseal injuries, and in each case explain the types of forces that can cause these injuries.
- Discuss osteoporosis, including contributing factors, groups at risk, consequences, and prevention strategies.
- Describe the common types of joint injuries, including the structures affected and symptoms.
- Describe specific types of arthritis, including symptoms.

Key Terms

amenorrhea	female athlete triad
anorexia nervosa	fracture
apophysis	osteoarthritis
arthritis	osteopenia
avulsion	osteoporosis
bulimia nervosa	rheumatoid arthritis
bursitis	sprain
dislocation	stress fracture

CLINICAL CASE STUDY

Joan is an outside hitter on her high school varsity volleyball team. Recently the shoulder of her hitting arm has been stiff and somewhat achy when she first wakes up in the morning. After a long, hard team practice the shoulder is quite painful. Joan does not recall having done or experienced anything unusual to injure her shoulder. As you read this section, try to determine which of the following conditions Joan most likely has.

A. Stress fracture
B. Sprain
C. Bursitis
D. Arthritis

Injuries and disorders of the skeletal system include problems with bones, joints, and the articular tissues. This lesson discusses many of the most common disorders.

Common Bone Injuries

Considering all of the important functions performed by bone, bone health is a vital part of general health. Bone health can be diminished by injuries and pathologies. The etiology, strategies for prevention, pathology, diagnosis, and common treatments for these common bone injuries and disorders are summarized in **Figure 4.32** and are discussed further in this lesson.

Fractures

A **fracture** is a break or a crack in a bone. The nature of a fracture depends on the size, direction, and duration of the injurious force, as well as the health and maturity of the bone.

Fractures are classified as *simple* when the bone ends remain within the surrounding soft tissues, and *compound* when one or both bone ends protrude from the skin. When the bone is splintered, the fracture is classified as *comminuted*. See **Figure 4.33**.

An **avulsion** is a fracture caused when a tendon or ligament pulls away from its attachment to a bone, taking a small chip of bone with it. Explosive throwing and jumping movements may cause avulsion fractures of the medial epicondyle (ehp-i-KAHN-dighl) of the humerus and the calcaneus.

Forceful bending and twisting movements can produce spiral fractures of the long bones. A common example occurs during downhill skiing. When a ski is planted in one direction, and the skier rotates while falling in a different direction, a spiral fracture of the tibia can result.

Common Bone Injuries and Disorders					
	Etiology	**Prevention**	**Pathology**	**Diagnosis**	**Treatment**
Fractures	a force strong enough to cause a partial or complete break in a bone	Be careful!	swelling, tenderness, bruising, deformity, bone protrudes through skin if a compound fracture	physical exam, X-ray	cast immobilization, functional cast or brace, traction, external fixation
Stress fractures	repetitive activity that overwhelms a bone's ability to self-repair	avoid dramatic increase in activity, running or landing on a hard surface, and poorly cushioned shoes	pain with activity	X-ray, CT scan, MRI	cease the activity that caused the stress fracture until healing occurs
Osteochondrosis (Osgood-Schlatter disease)	overuse of the quadriceps in adolescent athletes	avoid excessive, repetitive physical activity involving the quadriceps	pain and swelling over the anterior tibial growth plate that worsens with physical activity	physical exam, X-ray	cease the activity that caused the injury, stretching exercises, medication
Osteoporosis	abnormally low bone mineralization and strength due to aging or the female athlete triad	regular weight-bearing exercise, adequate intake of calcium and vitamin D; avoid excessively low body weight	daily activity results in bone fractures, with associated pain and deformity	physical exam, X-rays, bone densitometry, specialized laboratory tests	estrogen replacement therapy, prescribed medications to increase bone mass
Herniated disc	rupture in an intervertebral disc	regular exercise, healthy weight, good posture	arm or leg pain, numbness, weakness	physical exam, imaging, nerve tests	exercise, medication, physical therapy

Figure 4.32

Goodheart-Willcox Publisher

The bones of children contain relatively larger amounts of collagen than do the bones of adults. For this reason, children's bones are more flexible and are generally less likely to fracture than adult bones. Consequently, greenstick fractures, or incomplete fractures, are more common in children than in adults. A greenstick fracture is an incomplete fracture caused when a bone bends or twists but does not break all the way through.

Bone fractures are diagnosed and treated as appropriate for the nature of the injury. Symptoms of a simple fracture typically include swelling and

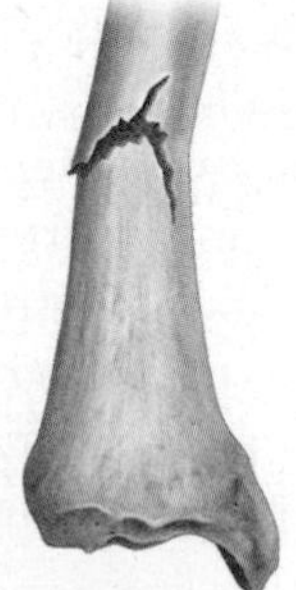

A A *greenstick fracture* is incomplete. The break occurs on the convex surface of the bend in the bone.

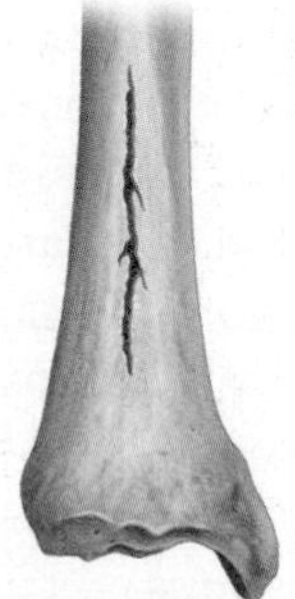

B A *stress fracture* involves an incomplete break.

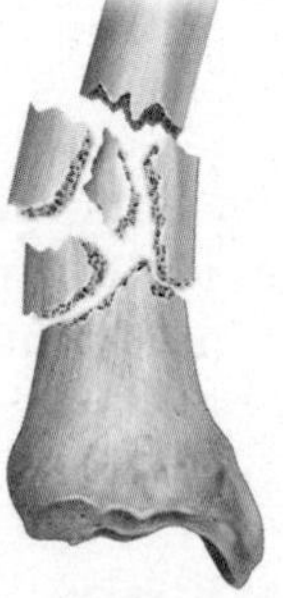

C A *comminuted fracture* is complete and splinters the bone.

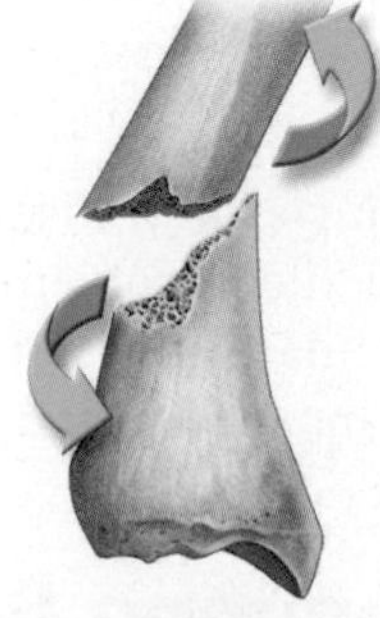

D A *spiral fracture* is caused by twisting a bone excessively.

© Body Scientific International

Figure 4.33 Types of fractures.

tenderness around the fracture site. There may also be bruising, and in the case of a complete fracture, the limb may look deformed or out of place. A compound fracture, with a bone fragment protruding through the skin, is accompanied by bleeding and extreme pain. The most common treatment is application of a plaster or fiberglass cast to completely immobilize the fracture after the doctor has properly aligned the bone.

Avulsions and incomplete fractures may be treated with a functional cast or brace, such as a walking boot. If the doctor cannot readily align the bone ends, traction may be applied to gently pull on opposite ends of the fractured bone to achieve proper realignment. With more serious, complicated fractures the doctor may elect to use external fixation. This is a surgical procedure in which metal pins or screws are placed into the broken bone above and below the fracture site. The pins or screws are connected to a metal bar outside the skin to hold the bones in the proper position while they heal. **Figure 4.34** displays a variety of bone fractures.

Stress fractures are tiny, painful cracks in bone that result from overuse. Under normal circumstances, bone responds to stress-related injury by remodeling. Osteoclasts resorb the damaged tissue, and osteoblasts deposit new bone at the site, resulting in repair of the injury. However, with repeated overuse, the remodeling process cannot keep up with the damage being done by the overuse. When this happens, the condition progresses to a stress fracture.

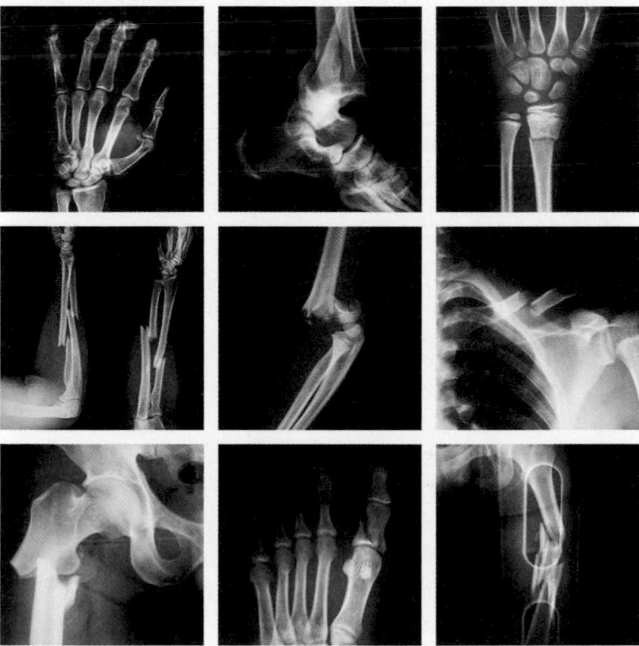

Puwadol Jaturawutthichai/Shutterstock.com

Figure 4.34 X-rays are an important diagnostic tool for finding bone fractures.

Runners and athletes in sports such as soccer, basketball, gymnastics, and tennis are prone to stress fractures, particularly in the tibia and the metatarsals. Common causes are increasing running mileage or playing time too abruptly, running or repetitive landing on a hard surface, and wearing shoes with inadequate cushioning.

Diagnosis of stress fractures is not always as straightforward as diagnosis of other types of fractures. The primary symptom is pain with activity. X-rays are the first tool for diagnosing a stress fracture. However, very small stress fractures may only be visible with a computed tomography (CT) scan or magnetic resonance imaging (MRI). The treatment for a stress fracture is rest. Resuming activity too soon can prevent healing.

Epiphyseal Injuries

Epiphyseal injuries include injuries to the epiphyseal plate, articular cartilage, and apophysis. An **apophysis** (a-PAHF-i-sis) is a site where a tendon attaches to a bone. Both acute and overuse-related injuries can damage the growth plate, potentially resulting in premature closure of the epiphyseal junction and termination of bone growth.

Osteochondrosis (ahs-tee-oh-kahn-DROH-sis), also known as *Osgood-Schlatter disease*, is inflammation of the apophysis and growth plate at the superior end of the tibia. This apophysis is the site where the powerful quadriceps muscle group on the front of the thigh attaches to the tibia through a tendon extending down from the patella. The apophysis is positioned over the tibial growth plate. When the quadriceps is used a lot in running, jumping, and other sports activities during the adolescent growth spurt, the tibial growth plate and apophysis can become inflamed, swollen, and painful.

Osteochondrosis is common in adolescents who play soccer, basketball, and volleyball, and who participate in gymnastics, with more boys affected than girls. The primary symptom is a painful region of swelling at the muscle attachment site, which can occur on one or both legs, as shown in **Figure 4.35**. The pain worsens with physical activity.

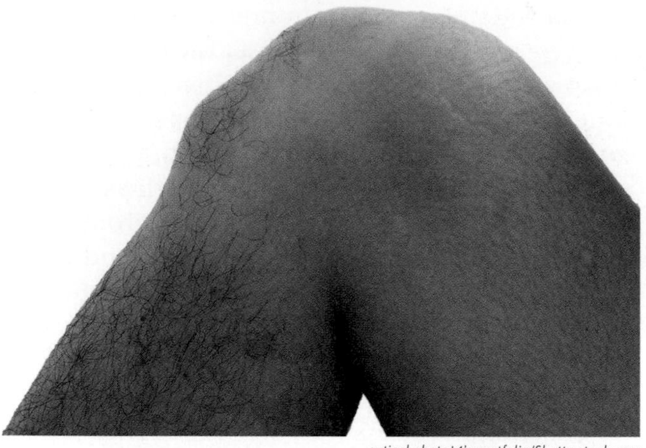

sutisakphoto14's portfolio/Shutterstock.com

Figure 4.35 Note the prominent swelling below the knee. This is characteristic of Osgood-Schlatter disease.

A physical exam and X-ray can confirm the diagnosis of osteochondrosis. The primary treatment is cessation of the activity believed to have been the cause. Stretching exercises for the thigh muscles can also help to relieve the strain on the tibial apophysis. Oral anti-inflammatory drugs can be prescribed to help address the pain and swelling. In severe cases, a physician may apply a cast to ensure complete rest of the knee.

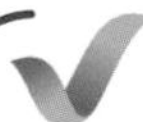

Check Your Understanding

1. List and describe the following types of fractures: simple, compound, comminuted, avulsion, spiral, greenstick, and stress.
2. Explain osteochondrosis.
3. Why is it important for children to avoid activities that could cause damage to an epiphyseal plate?

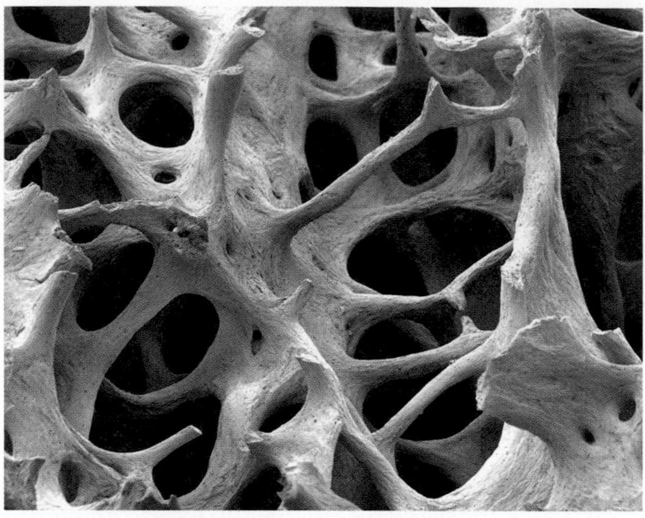

A

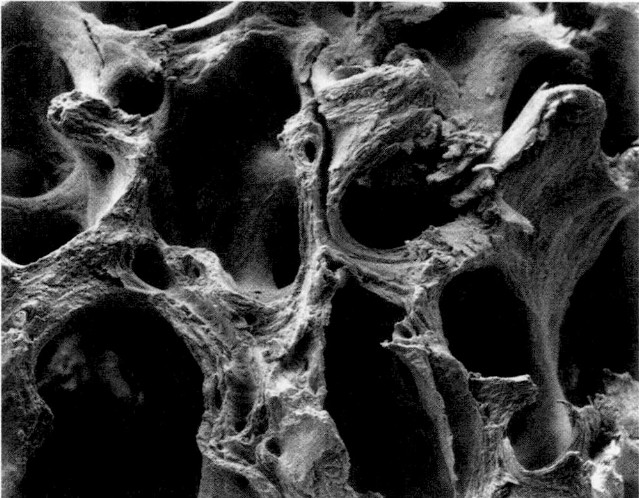

B

Steve Gschmeissner/Science Source, Dee Breger/Science Source

Figure 4.36 Compare the normal trabecular bone (A) with the brittle, degraded bone (B) characteristic of osteoporosis. The yellowish, underlying tissue in B is visible because the surface of the bone (orange colored) has worn away. As the bone becomes more brittle, it is more likely to fracture. *Which groups of people are most likely to suffer from osteoporosis?*

Osteoporosis

Osteoporosis (ahs-tee-oh-poh-ROH-sis) is a condition in which bone mineralization and strength are so abnormally low that regular, daily activities can result in painful fractures. With its honeycomb structure, trabecular bone is most commonly the site of osteoporotic fractures (**Figure 4.36**).

Age-Related Osteoporosis

Osteoporosis occurs in most elderly individuals, with earlier onset in women. The condition begins as **osteopenia** (ahs-tee-oh-PEE-nee-a), reduced bone mass without the presence of a fracture. The osteopenia often progresses to osteoporosis, with fractures present. Although once regarded as primarily a health issue for women, with the increasing age of the population, osteoporosis is now also becoming a concern for older men.

With type I osteoporosis, also known as *postmenopausal osteoporosis*, fractures usually begin to occur about 15 years post-menopause; the femoral neck, vertebrae, and wrist bones are the most common fracture sites. Type II osteoporosis, also called *age-associated osteoporosis*, affects most women and also affects men over 70 years old. After 60 years of age, the majority of fractures in both men and women are osteoporosis-related. In the elderly population, fractures of the femoral neck, in particular, often trigger a downward health spiral that leads to death.

The most common symptom of osteoporosis, however, is back pain derived from crush-type fractures of the weakened trabecular bone of the vertebrae. These fractures can be caused by activities as simple as picking up a bag of groceries or a bag of trash. These vertebral crush fractures frequently cause reduction of body height and tend to accentuate the kyphotic curve in the thoracic region of the spine. This disabling deformity is known as *dowager's hump*.

A diagnosis of osteoporosis is confirmed with X-rays, bone densitometry, and specialized laboratory tests. Treatments can include estrogen replacement therapy and prescribed medications to increase bone mass.

The Female Athlete Triad

Unfortunately, osteoporosis is not confined to the elderly population. It can also occur in female athletes at the high school and collegiate levels who strive to maintain an excessively low body weight.

What Research Tells Us

...about Preventing Osteoporosis

Osteoporosis is not inevitable with advancing age. It is typically the result of a lifetime of habits that are erosive to the skeletal system. Simply stated, it is easier to prevent osteoporosis than it is to treat it.

The single most important strategy for preventing or delaying the onset of osteoporosis is maximizing bone mass during childhood and adolescence. Weight-bearing exercise such as running, jumping, and even walking is particularly important prior to puberty because of the high level of growth hormone present during this period (**Figure 4.37**). Growth hormone makes exercise particularly effective in increasing bone density.

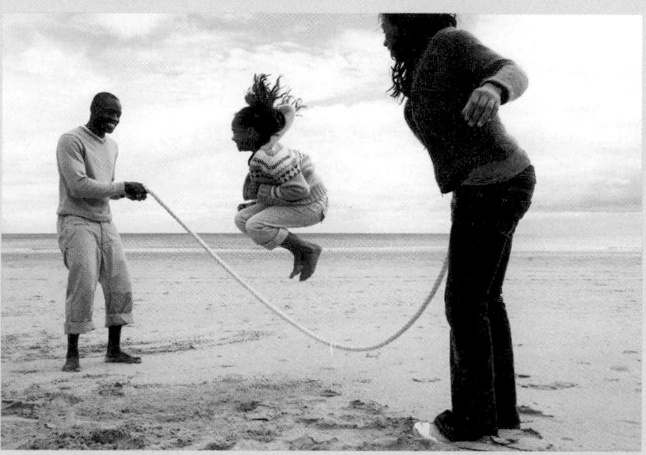

oliveromg/Shutterstock.com

Figure 4.37 *How can this activity help prevent osteoporosis in later life?*

Diet also plays an important role in bone health. Physicians now recognize that a predisposition for osteoporosis can begin in childhood and adolescence when a poor diet interferes with bone mass development. Adequate dietary calcium is particularly important during the teenage years, but unfortunately the typical American girl falls below the recommended daily intake of 1,200 mg per day by 11 years of age. A modified diet or calcium supplementation can be critically important for the development of peak bone mass among adolescent females who have this dietary deficiency.

The role of vitamin D is also important, because vitamin D enables bone to absorb calcium. In North America, more than 50% of women being treated for low bone density also have a vitamin D deficiency.

Other lifestyle factors also affect bone mineralization. Risk factors for developing osteoporosis include a sedentary lifestyle, weight loss or excessive thinness, and smoking tobacco. To help prevent later development of osteoporosis, young women are encouraged to engage in regular physical activity and to avoid the lifestyle factors that negatively affect bone health.

Taking It Further

1. Make a list of activities that you can engage in now that will increase your chances of preventing or delaying the onset of osteoporosis. Share your list with classmates.
2. What foods might you recommend for bone health in young teenage girls?

In females, striving for an extremely low weight can cause a dangerous condition known as the **female athlete triad**. This condition involves a combination of disordered eating, **amenorrhea** (ah-men-oh-REE-a)—having no period or menses—and osteoporosis. Because this triad can cause negative health consequences ranging from irreversible bone loss to death, friends, parents, coaches, and physicians need to be alert to the signs.

Female athletes participating in endurance or appearance-related sports are most likely to be affected by the female athlete triad. Disordered eating can take the form of anorexia nervosa or bulimia nervosa.

Symptoms of **anorexia nervosa** in girls and women include a body weight that is 15% or more below the minimal normal weight range, extreme fear of gaining weight, an unrealistic body image, and amenorrhea. **Bulimia nervosa** involves a minimum of two eating binges per week for at least three months; an associated feeling of lack of control; use of self-induced vomiting, laxatives, diuretics, strict dieting, or exercise to prevent weight gain; and an obsession with body image.

Although the incidence of osteoporosis among female athletes is unknown, the consequences of the female athlete triad are potentially tragic. Amenorrheic, premenopausal female athletes are known to have an elevated rate of stress fractures. More important, the loss of bone that occurs may be irreversible, and osteoporotic wedge fractures of the vertebrae can ruin posture for life.

Female athletes who are extremely thin and are missing menstrual periods, may have disordered eating, or experience stress fractures should be evaluated by a medical professional to check for bone density. Treatment for the female athlete triad often requires a team of medical professionals. The team may include a primary care provider, gynecologist, nutritionist, and psychological counselor.

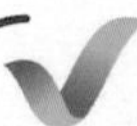

Check Your Understanding

1. How does osteoporosis differ from osteopenia?
2. What two eating disorders are common in women diagnosed with the female athlete triad?

Common Joint Injuries

The freely movable joints of the human body are subject to significant wear over the course of a lifetime. Both acute and overuse injuries affect the joints. The etiology, strategies for prevention, pathology, diagnosis, and common treatments for these common joint injuries and disorders are summarized in **Figure 4.38**.

Sprains

Sprains are injuries caused by abnormal motion of the articulating bones that results in overstretching or tearing of ligaments, tendons, or other connective tissues crossing a joint. The most common site of sprain is the ankle, and the most common mechanism is injury to the lateral ligaments. Lateral ankle sprains occur frequently because the ankle is a major weight-bearing joint and because there is less ligamentous support on the lateral than on the medial side of the ankle.

Pain and swelling are the symptoms of joint sprains. Immediate self-treatment should include R.I.C.E.:

Rest. (Avoid activities that exacerbate the pain.)

Ice. (Apply an ice pack as soon as possible for 15–20 minutes and repeat every two to three hours while you are awake for the first few days after the injury.)

Compression. (Use an elastic bandage to gently compress the joint until the swelling stops. Be careful not to tighten the bandage to the point of stopping circulation.)

Elevation. (Elevate the injured joint above the level of your heart, especially at night, which allows gravity to help reduce swelling.)

Over-the-counter pain medications can also be taken. Serious sprains should be evaluated by a physician, who may ask for an MRI to determine whether a ligament or tendon has been completely ruptured. Such cases may require surgical repair.

Dislocations

When one of the articulating bones is displaced from the joint socket, the injury is called a **dislocation** of that joint. Dislocations usually result from falls or forceful collisions. Common dislocation sites are the shoulders, fingers, knees, elbows, and jaw.

Common Joint Injuries and Disorders					
	Etiology	**Prevention**	**Pathology**	**Diagnosis**	**Treatment**
Sprains	motion causing overstretching of ligaments and tendons	Be careful!	swelling and pain that is exacerbated with use of the joint	physical exam, MRI to check for complete rupture of a ligament or tendon	R.I.C.E. (Rest, intermittent Icing, Compression with an elastic bandage, Elevation), surgical repair if necessary
Dislocations	force that dislodges a bone from its normal position in a joint	Be careful!	visible joint deformity, pain, swelling, some loss of movement capability	physical exam, X-ray or MRI to assess joint damage	may include immobilization with a splint or sling, surgical repair if necessary
Bursitis	overuse of a joint	avoid excessive, repetitive joint motion	joint aching, stiffness, pain with motion, swelling	physical exam	cease the activity that caused the injury, rest the joint
Lyme disease	borrelia bacteria is transmitted in the bite of a deer tick	avoid wooded or grassy areas, insecticide, prompt removal of any ticks	bull's-eye shaped rash, fever, head-ache, fatigue; if untreated can cause joint pain and other problems	physical exam, blood test for presence of antibodies to the bacteria	oral or injected antibiotics
Rheumatoid arthritis	the body's immune system attacks the synovial membranes	no known prevention	inflammation and thickening of synovial membranes leading to destruction of the joint over time	physical exam, blood tests for inflammation, imaging tests to track joint destruction	anti-inflammatory drugs, steroids, disease-modifying anti-rheumatic drugs
Osteoarthritis	wearing away of articular cartilage	no known prevention	pain, tenderness, loss of flexibility, and joint stiffness	physical exam, imaging tests	anti-inflammatory medications, joint injections of cortisone or hyaluronic acid, joint replacement

Figure 4.38 *Goodheart-Willcox Publisher*

Signs and symptoms include visible joint deformity, pain, swelling, and some loss of movement capability. Treatment involves first reducing the dislocation, which means restoring the displaced bone to its correct anatomical location. A physician may order an X-ray or MRI to assess the damaged joint. Depending on the nature of the damage, a splint or sling may be used to immobilize the joint for a time. Surgical repair may be necessary if tendons or ligaments have ruptured.

Bursitis

Bursitis is the inflammation of one or more bursae, the fluid-filled sacs that provide cushioning of the moving tissues around a joint. Bursitis is an overuse injury that produces irritation and inflammation of the bursae due to friction. The most common locations are the shoulder, elbow, and hip. Symptoms of bursitis may include aching and stiffness of the joint, pain with joint motion, and sometimes swelling. Treatment consists of simply resting the joint until symptoms disappear.

Check Your Understanding

1. Which structures are affected when a joint is sprained?
2. What types of actions may result in dislocations?
3. What are the causes and symptoms of bursitis?

Arthritis

Arthritis is a common pathology associated with aging. It is characterized by joint inflammation accompanied by pain, stiffness, and sometimes swelling. Arthritis is not a single condition but a large family of pathologies. More than 100 different types of arthritis have been identified.

Rheumatoid Arthritis

Rheumatoid arthritis is a chronic inflammatory disorder in which the body's own immune system attacks the healthy membranes that surround synovial joints (**Figure 4.39**). The progression includes inflammation and thickening of the synovial membranes followed by breakdown of the joint structures over time. The result is extremely limited joint motion and, in extreme cases, complete fusing of the articulating bones. Associated symptoms include tenderness, warmth, and swelling of the joints, with stiffness that is usually worse in the mornings and after inactivity.

Fatigue, fever, and weight loss may also occur. This is the most debilitating and painful form of arthritis. It is more common in adults but occasionally occurs in children (juvenile rheumatoid arthritis).

The cause of rheumatoid arthritis is unknown, although genetics may play a role. Diagnosis is difficult in the early stages because the symptoms are like those of many other diseases. Blood tests can reveal the presence of inflammation in the body and imaging tests can help to detect progression of the disorder. There is no cure for rheumatoid arthritis. Treatment may include anti-inflammatory drugs, steroids, and a class of drugs called *disease-modifying anti-rheumatic drugs (DMARDs)*. These drugs can slow the progression of rheumatoid arthritis and save the joints and other tissues from permanent damage.

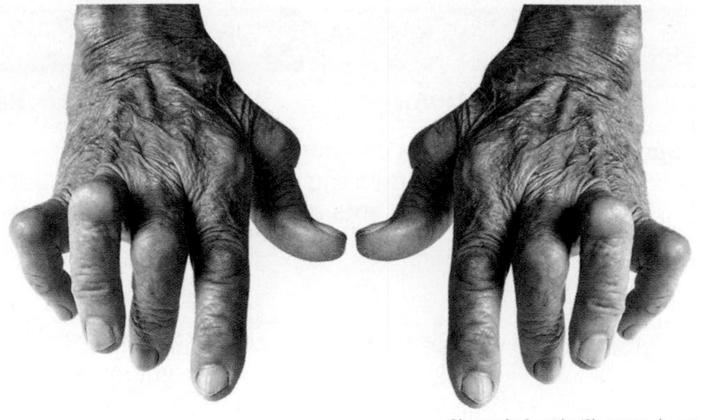

Chaowalit Seeneha/Shutterstock.com

Figure 4.39 This person's hands have been disfigured by rheumatoid arthritis. Most patients take medication for the intense pain.

Osteoarthritis

Arthritis also takes a noninflammatory form as **osteoarthritis**, a degenerative disorder of articular cartilage. Onset of osteoarthritis is characterized by progressive roughening of the normally smooth joint cartilage, with the cartilage eventually wearing away completely. The most commonly affected joints are in the hands, knees, hips, and spine, although any joint can be affected.

Pain, tenderness, loss of flexibility, and stiffness are all symptoms, with the pain typically relieved by rest and joint stiffness improved by activity. Bone spurs may form around affected joints, causing a grating sound with joint motion. Diagnosis is achieved with physical examination and imaging tests. Treatments include anti-inflammatory medications and injections into the joint of cortisone or hyaluronic acid (a joint lubricant). When the condition becomes too painful, joint replacement is warranted.

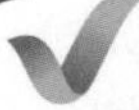

Check Your Understanding

1. What are the general symptoms associated with all forms of arthritis?
2. What is believed to be the cause of rheumatoid arthritis?

LESSON 4.5 Review and Assessment

Mini Glossary

Make sure that you know the meaning of each key term.

amenorrhea absence of a menstrual period in women of reproductive age

anorexia nervosa condition characterized by body weight 15% or more below the minimal normal weight range, extreme fear of gaining weight, an unrealistic body image, and amenorrhea

apophysis site at which a tendon attaches to bone

arthritis family of more than 100 common pathologies associated with aging, characterized by joint inflammation accompanied by pain, stiffness, and sometimes swelling

avulsion a fracture caused when a tendon or ligament pulls away from its attachment to a bone, taking a small chip of bone with it

bulimia nervosa disordered eating that involves a minimum of two eating binges a week for at least three months; an associated feeling of lack of control; use of self-induced vomiting, laxatives, diuretics, strict dieting, or exercise to prevent weight gain; and an obsession with body image

bursitis inflammation of one or more bursae

dislocation injury that involves displacement of a bone from its joint socket

female athlete triad a combination of disordered eating, amenorrhea, and osteoporosis

fracture any break or disruption of continuity in a bone

osteoarthritis degenerative disease of articular cartilage, characterized by pain, swelling, range-of-motion restriction, and stiffness

osteopenia reduced bone mass without the presence of a fracture

osteoporosis condition in which bone mineralization and strength are so abnormally low that regular, daily activities can result in painful fractures

rheumatoid arthritis autoimmune disorder in which the body's own immune system attacks healthy joint tissues; the most debilitating and painful form of arthritis

sprain injury caused by abnormal motion of the articulating bones that results in overstretching or tearing of ligaments, tendons, or other connective tissues crossing a joint

stress fracture tiny, painful crack in bone that results from overuse

Know and Understand

1. What is an avulsion?
2. At what point in a person's life is osteochondrosis most likely to occur?
3. What is the most common symptom of osteoporosis?
4. Which joint in the skeleton is the most commonly sprained?
5. What happens to healthy joint tissue in a person with rheumatoid arthritis?

Analyze and Apply

6. Explain how the remodeling of a bone and a stress fracture are related.
7. Why are females who participate in certain sports more vulnerable to the condition known as *female athlete triad*?
8. A 17-year-old soccer player has sustained several fractures to different parts of her body. When her bone density was tested, she was found to be on the low end of the normal range. What would you suggest that she do to increase her bone strength?
9. Why are epiphyseal injuries especially worrisome in children?
10. Keeping in mind the description in this chapter of mineral content and structure of the two types of bone tissue, explain why fractures in someone with osteoporosis occur most often in trabecular bone.

IN THE LAB

11. You are a healthcare worker, and you have a patient with one of the following conditions: osteoporosis, osteopenia, rheumatoid arthritis, bursitis, or osteoarthritis.

    Decide which condition your patient has and then create a treatment plan for the patient. Your plan should include a description of the disorder; age groups typically affected by the disorder; medications to ease pain and inflammation, if any; foods to help minimize the progression of the disorder; foods to omit from the diet; physical activities to add to or increase in the daily routine; and a workout schedule for each day of the week.

    Create your treatment plan in the form of a presentation. Share the presentation with the class, as though the class were your patient. Ask for and answer any questions that your "patient" might have.
12. You are a research scientist studying the effects of lifestyle choices (regarding diet and exercise) on the risks of developing osteoporosis. Your task is to create a lifestyle plan to educate people of all ages on the things they can do to lower or possibly even eliminate their risk for developing osteoporosis later in life.

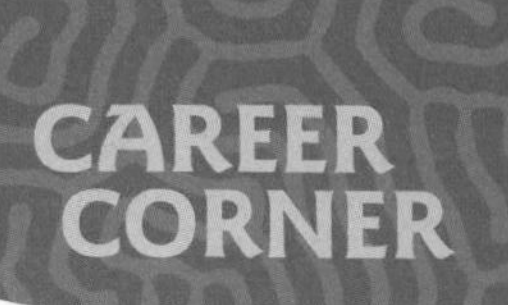

Anatomy & Physiology at Work

Orthopedics is a field of medical science that specializes in treating injuries, disorders, and diseases of the bones and joints. Many different health professionals, however, are involved in helping patients overcome skeletal injuries and improve the health of their bones and joints.

Physician

When bone and joint injuries or age-related conditions arise, which healthcare professionals team up to take care of these problems? The person injured should usually seek help first from a family physician, general practitioner, or other primary care provider who offers comprehensive healthcare for people of all ages.

Family physicians have either the MD (Doctor of Medicine) degree or the DO (Doctor of Osteopathic Medicine) degree. The family physician can examine the patient and, as appropriate, administer a series of tests to determine whether referral to an orthopedic surgeon is warranted for more specialized care.

Orthopedic surgeons have specialized training beyond the MD or DO degree in the care of bone and joint injuries and pathologies. The orthopedic surgeon most likely will want to see an X-ray and sometimes an MRI (magnetic resonance image) to determine whether surgery is warranted, and what other follow-up care may be appropriate.

Radiographer

Radiographers use imaging techniques, such as radiographs (X-rays) and MRI scans, to capture pictures of injured or pathological tissues. These professionals, also called *medical radiation technologists*, provide the images to doctors, who evaluate the images to determine the most effective treatment for the patient.

These technologists are trained in positioning patients to get the best kinds of images for evaluation (**Figure 4.40**). Radiographers may specialize in mammography, fluoroscopy, computed tomography, ultrasound, or MRI. The education required to become a radiologic technologist typically is a bachelor's degree that includes training in radiography.

Orthotist/Prosthetist

Sometimes the best way to treat an orthopedic injury is with a customized device. Such devices, called *orthotics*, include custom shoe inserts and leg braces. For more serious injuries, a patient's limb may need to be replaced with a prosthetic one. A *prosthetic* is a fabricated substitute developed to assist a damaged body part or replace one that is missing. A person who treats patients with orthotics or prosthetics is called an orthotist/prosthetist (OR-tha-tist/PRAHS-theh-tist), or O&P professional.

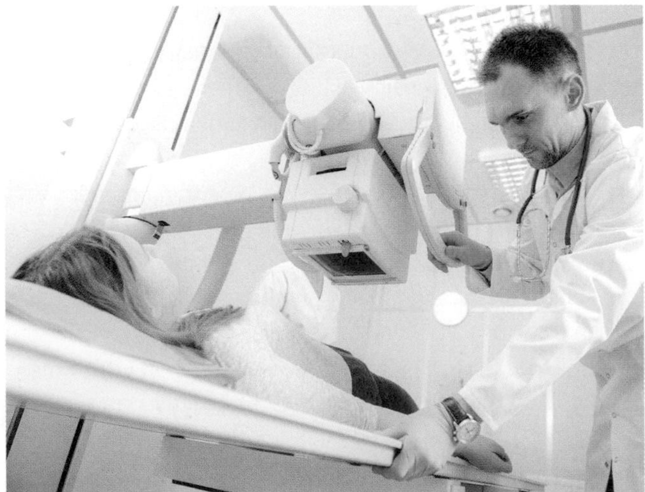

Poznyakou/Shutterstock.com

Figure 4.40 A radiographer needs to know how to operate the many types of imaging equipment used to help diagnose patient injuries.

O&P professionals have a master's degree in orthotics and prosthetics, and they have passed a certification exam administered by the American Board for Certification in Orthotics, Prosthetics and Pedorthics (ABC). O&P professionals may specialize in both orthotics and prosthetics, or only one of these fields. To be certified in both fields, candidates must complete one year of residency in each specialty and pass the required ABC exams.

Orthotists and prosthetists meet with patients to evaluate their needs, measure patients for custom design and fitting of medical devices, and design their patients' devices and repair or update them as needed (**Figure 4.41**). They also instruct patients in the proper use and care of their devices. O&P professionals are employed in small, private offices or in larger medical facilities, and they often work in the shops where orthotics and prosthetics are made.

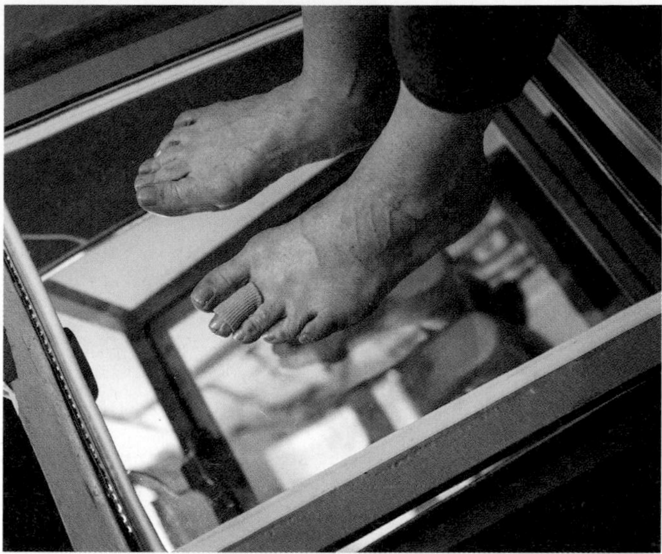

fotoliza/Shutterstock.com

Figure 4.41 Orthotists may use a digital foot scan to provide the basis for custom shoe insoles.

Planning for a Health-Related Career

Research the career of an orthopedic surgeon, a radiographer, or an orthotist/prosthetist. Alternatively, select a profession from the list of related career options. Using the internet or resources at your local library, find answers to questions such as the following:

1. What are the main tasks and responsibilities of the career you are researching?
2. What is the outlook for this career? Are workers in demand, or are jobs dwindling? For complete information, consult the current edition of the *Occupational Outlook Handbook*, published by the US Department of Labor. This handbook is available online or at your local library.
3. What special skills or talents are required? For example, do you need to be good at biology and chemistry? Do you need to enjoy interacting with other people?
4. What personality traits do you think are needed to be successful in this job? For example, a career as a surgeon requires directing other people. Are you comfortable with giving directions to others?
5. Does this career involve a great deal of routine, or are the day-to-day responsibilities varied?
6. Does the work require long hours, or is it a standard, "9-to-5" job?
7. What is the salary range for this job?
8. What do you think you would like about this career? Is there anything about it that you might dislike?

Related Career Options

- Family practitioner
- Magnetic resonance (MR) technologist
- Orthotist/prosthetist
- Physical therapist
- Physician assistant
- Podiatrist
- Surgical nurse

CHAPTER 4 Review

LESSON 4.1

Bone as a Living Tissue

Key Points

- The five functions of the skeletal system are support, protection, movement, storage, and blood cell formation.
- The five categories (by shape) of bones are long bones, short bones, flat bones, sesamoid bones, and irregular bones.
- Remodeling of bones continues throughout life to keep bones strong.

Key Terms

articular cartilage
bone marrow
cortical bone
diaphysis
endosteum
epiphyseal plate
epiphysis
Haversian canals
Haversian system
hematopoiesis
lacunae
medullary cavity
ossification
osteoblasts
osteoclasts
osteocytes
osteon
perforating (Volkmann's) canals
periosteum
remodeling
trabecular bone

LESSON 4.2

The Axial Skeleton

Key Points

- The skull contains eight cranial bones and fourteen facial bones.
- The five sections of the vertebral column, or spine, are the cervical region, thoracic region, lumbar region, sacrum, and coccyx.
- The thoracic cage, which protects the heart and lungs, is made up of the ribs, sternum, and thoracic vertebrae.

Key Terms

atlas
axial skeleton
axis
cervical region
coccyx
cranium
facial bones
fontanel
intervertebral discs
lumbar region
mandible
maxillary bones
process
sacrum
skull
sternum
sutures
thoracic cage
thoracic region
vertebra
vomer

LESSON 4.3

The Appendicular Skeleton

Key Points

- The upper extremity includes the pectoral girdle, arms, wrists, and hands; the pectoral girdle includes the clavicles and scapulae.
- The lower extremity, which includes the pelvic girdle, legs, ankles, and feet, is designed for weight-bearing and gait.

Key Terms

appendicular skeleton
carpal bones
clavicle
femur
fibula
humerus
lower extremity
metacarpal bones
metatarsal bones
patella
pectoral girdle
pelvis
phalanges
radius
scapula
tarsal bones
tibia
ulna
upper extremity

›LESSON 4.4

Joints

Key Points

- The three main categories of joints, with regard to function, are the immovable joints (synarthroses), the slightly movable joints (amphiarthroses), and the freely movable joints (diarthroses).
- Articular tissues include articular fibrocartilage, tendons, and ligaments.

Key Terms

amphiarthrosis
articular fibrocartilage
ball-and-socket joint
bursae
condyloid joint
diarthrosis
gliding joint
hinge joint
ligament
pivot joint
saddle joint
symphysis
synarthrosis
synchondrosis
syndesmosis
synovial joint
tendon
tendon sheath

›LESSON 4.5

Common Injuries and Disorders of the Skeletal System

Key Points

- Common bone injuries include fractures, or breaks, and epiphyseal injuries.
- Osteoporosis is a condition in which bone mineralization and strength are critically low, often leading to fractures.
- Sprains, dislocations, and bursitis are common joint injuries and disorders.
- The signs and symptoms of arthritis include joint inflammation, pain, stiffness, and sometimes swelling.

Key Terms

amenorrhea
anorexia nervosa
apophysis
arthritis
avulsion
bulimia nervosa
bursitis
dislocation
female athlete triad
fracture
osteoarthritis
osteopenia
osteoporosis
rheumatoid arthritis
sprain
stress fracture

Assessment

›LESSON 4.1

Bone as a Living Tissue

Learning Key Terms and Concepts

1. The five functions of the skeletal system are blood cell formation, movement, support, storage, and _____.
2. The term for blood cell formation is _____.
   A. osteocyte
   B. hematopoiesis
   C. osteogenesis
   D. osteoblast
3. The strong, dense type of bone tissue is called _____.
   A. trabecular bone
   B. coxal bone
   C. cortical bone
   D. hard bone

4. The five shape categories of bones are irregular, short, flat, long, and _____.
5. The shaft of a bone is called the _____; the ends of a bone are called the epiphyses.
6. Specialized bone cells that build new bone are called _____.
   A. osteocytes
   B. osteoclasts
   C. osteoblasts
   D. osteopaths
7. Specialized bone cells that break down bone are called _____.
   A. osteocytes
   B. osteoclasts
   C. osteoblasts
   D. osteopaths

Thinking Critically

8. The microscopic structure of long bones can be compared to a city. Using the following terms, describe what each type of long bone could be compared to in your city (a building, streets running through the city, or a water tower, for example): Haversian canal, lacunae, lamellae, canaliculi. Draw a picture to illustrate.
9. Write a short story about the development of a bone from when it was created and continuing into adulthood. The bone is the main character in the story. Have the bone describe the changes that occur after its development. Include anatomical terms from this chapter in your story.
10. Compare and contrast hypertrophy and atrophy of bones. Include a person's level of activity in your discussion, and explain what is happening on a cellular level.
11. Remembering the shape categories of bones, discuss their cortical-trabecular bone ratios and relate structure to function.

LESSON 4.2

The Axial Skeleton

Learning Key Terms and Concepts

12. The three major parts of the axial skeleton are the vertebral column, the thoracic cage, and the _____.
13. The immovable joints that connect the bones of the skull and face are known as _____.
14. Which thoracic region includes the vertebrae of the neck?
    A. thoracic
    B. lumbar
    C. sacral
    D. cervical
15. Which thoracic region connects to the ribs?
    A. thoracic
    B. lumbar
    C. sacral
    D. cervical
16. Which condition causes a lateral (sideways) curvature of the spine?
    A. osteopenia
    B. kyphosis
    C. scoliosis
    D. lordosis
17. Which of the following is part of the thoracic cage?
    A. the fibula
    B. the zygomatic bones
    C. the sternum
    D. the pelvic girdle
18. Which of the following is true about the false ribs?
    A. They do not attach directly to the sternum.
    B. They do not attach directly to the vertebrae.
    C. They do not attach directly to anything.
    D. They do not exist.

Thinking Critically

19. Given your knowledge of the intervertebral discs, what activities should a person avoid to promote disc health? Name at least two activities and explain why each should be avoided.
20. The bones of the cranium form a solid case to allow maximum protection for the brain. Would this solid structure be more beneficial to the lungs and offer more protection than the thoracic cage, with its open spaces between each rib? Why or why not?
21. Discuss the five spinal curves and tell why each of the spinal curves is the shape it is.
22. Explain why people who have led sedentary lives tend to "shrink" as they age.

➤ LESSON 4.3

The Appendicular Skeleton

Learning Key Terms and Concepts

23. Which structures are part of the appendicular skeleton?
    A. the head
    B. the spinal column
    C. the legs
    D. the trunk
24. The pectoral girdle consists of the right and left scapula and the right and left _____.
25. The bone in the forearm that attaches on the "little finger" side is the _____.
26. There are _____ bones in each wrist and hand.
27. The _____ is the prominent, upper edge of the hip bone.
28. The longest, strongest bone in the body is the _____.
29. Which of the following is the heel bone?
    A. talus
    B. femur
    C. patella
    D. calcaneus

Thinking Critically

30. If a forensic scientist finds skeletal remains after a house fire, how will she determine whether the individual was a male or female?
31. Using the internet, research the origin of the word *appendicular*. Then explain why the bones of the appendicular skeleton are so named and how they relate to the axial skeleton.
32. In terms of functionality, why does it make sense that there is only one bone in the upper arm but two in the forearm?
33. How would the function of the body be different if the foot had no arches?

➤ LESSON 4.4

Joints

Learning Key Terms and Concepts

34. Another term for freely movable joints is _____.
35. The two main types of immovable joints are sutures and _____.
36. The vertebral joints are examples of _____ movable joints.
37. _____ are small sacs filled with synovial fluid that cushion the structures they separate.
38. Three functions of the _____ tissues are to cushion the joints and reduce friction and wear on them.
39. Ligaments connect bone to bone, while _____ connect muscle to bone.

Thinking Critically

40. Give reasons why you either would or would not want all of your joints to be ball-and-socket joints.
41. What would be the effect on human function if the bursae and tendon sheaths were not present?
42. In terms of function, explain why tendons and ligaments are made of elastic fibers instead of a more rigid tissue.

➤ LESSON 4.5

Common Injuries and Disorders of the Skeletal System

Learning Key Terms and Concepts

43. A(n) _____ fracture is one in which the ends of a bone protrude from the skin.
44. A(n) _____ fracture is more common in children than in adults because children's bones are more flexible than those of adults.
45. _____ fractures are tiny, painful cracks in a bone that result from overuse.
46. The site where a tendon attaches to a bone is known as the _____.
47. Injuries to which of the following can stop the growth of a long bone?
    A. intervertebral disc
    B. meniscus
    C. epiphyseal plate
    D. sutures
48. A condition that involves reduced bone mass but no fractures is _____.
49. A combination of amenorrhea, disordered eating, and _____, called the female athlete triad, is a dangerous condition that may occur in females who participate in endurance or appearance-related sports.

50. In the acronym R.I.C.E. for self-treatment of sprains, the *C* stands for _____.
51. _____ is an autoimmune disorder in which the body's own immune system attacks healthy joint tissues.

Thinking Critically

52. A 10-year-old boy and his 42-year-old father were building a tree house when the branch they were standing on broke away from the tree. The father sustained two broken ribs, but the boy had only a few bruises. Explain.
53. Explain how a stress fracture can happen, in terms of osteoblasts and osteoclasts. Further explain why stress fractures are particularly common in the tibia and metatarsals, given the functions of those bones.
54. Compare and contrast rheumatoid arthritis and osteoarthritis. In your own words, explain anatomically and physiologically what is occurring in each condition.

Building Skills and Connecting Concepts

Analyzing and Evaluating Data

Instructions: The astronaut in **Figure 4.42** is exercising on a special treadmill system in the International Space Station. Without this type of resistance training, he could lose 1% to 2% bone mass per month. Consider this information as you answer the following questions.

55. If the astronaut spends three months in space and never exercises, what percentage of his bone mass might he lose?
56. You read in this chapter that bones account for about 15% of human body weight. If this astronaut weighs 170 pounds, how much do his bones weigh?
57. If he fails to exercise for six months in space, how much weight might this astronaut lose in bone mass?
58. If this astronaut spends 12 months in space, but only exercises for 3 months, what percentage of bone mass will he lose?

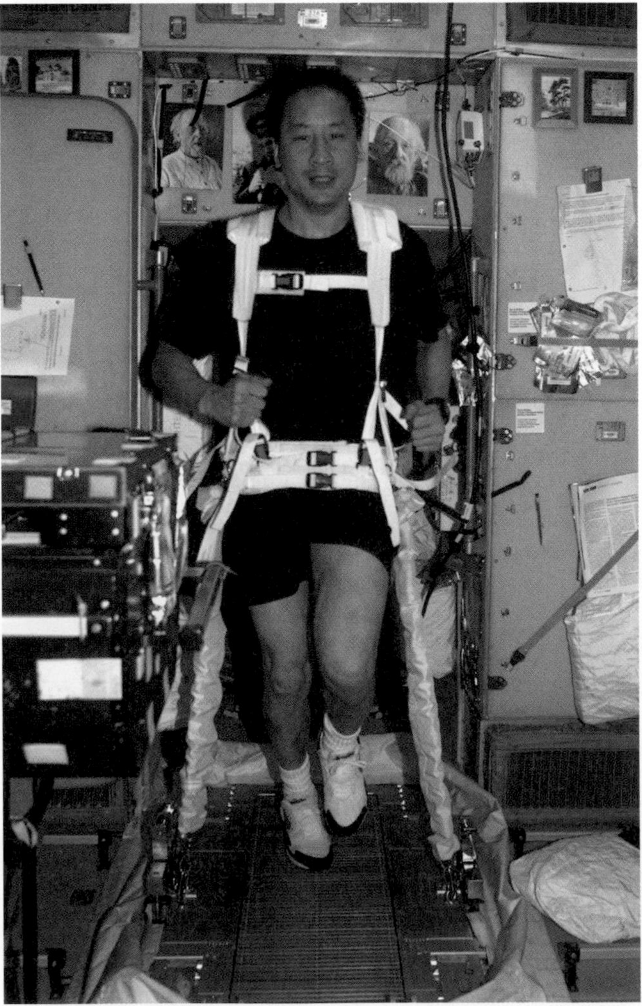

Figure 4.42 NASA/JSC

Communicating about Anatomy & Physiology

59. **Speaking** Divide into groups of four or five students. Each group should choose one of the following topics: anorexia nervosa, bursitis, dislocation, female athlete triad, fracture, osteoporosis, rheumatoid arthritis, sprain, or stress fracture.

    Using your textbook as a starting point, research your topic and prepare a report on causes and treatments. As a group, deliver your presentation to the rest of the class. Take notes while other students give their reports. Ask questions about any details that you would like clarified.
60. **Listening** Take notes while other students give their reports for the previous question. Ask questions about any details that you would like clarified.
61. **Writing** Write an "osteostory" about a superhero who helps someone in distress. Be creative and find ways to mention the following bones in your story: skull, sternum, femur, humerus, tibia, calcaneus, tarsals, carpals, metatarsals, metacarpals, ribs, clavicle, scapula, mandible, and patella. Try to work into the story reasons for describing the locations of these bones in the body.

Lab Investigations

62. Construct a skeleton of an animal of your choice using toothpicks and glue. Your animal can be real or imaginary. Draw the outline for your animal and then use the toothpicks to make the bones of the animal's skeleton. When you are finished, use labels to identify the bones. Include a label for the name and species of your animal. At a minimum, include these bones in your skeleton: carpals, cervical vertebrae, coxal bones, femur, fibula, humerus, lumbar vertebrae, mandible, maxilla, metacarpals, metatarsals, patella, phalanges, radius, ribs, scapula, skull, sternum, tarsals, thoracic vertebrae, tibia, ulna.
63. People with bone fractures, especially to the lower limbs, often require assistive devices while they are recovering. Examples of assistive devices include crutches, walkers, and canes. Assistive devices must be used correctly in order to be effective. Choose a specific assistive device and conduct research on its proper use for various types of injuries. Obtain or borrow the device and provide a demonstration for your class on its proper use. Identify incorrect usage, as well as limitations of the device and abnormalities that may prevent a patient from using the device effectively.
64. Conduct research to find out what range-of-motion exercises are commonly used in physical therapy sessions to help people who are recovering from injuries to regain their full range of motion. Find out the difference between active and passive range-of-motion exercises. Perform a demonstration of active and passive exercises for the class. Include exercises for the shoulders, arms, wrists, knees, and ankles. As you demonstrate, explain the purpose of each exercise.
65. Conduct research on the internet to find out the basic steps involved in repairing a fracture of a long bone. Be sure to use good internet etiquette and follow safety guidelines for working on the internet. Write a summary report, and list your sources.
66. Using medical textbooks and other biological resources, gather information about bone matrix, various types of bone cells, and glycoproteins, such as osteocalcin and alpha-glycoprotein. Identify bone minerals and explain how they can change bone cells during bone development. Prepare a written report, and include your sources.

Building Your Portfolio

67. Take digital photographs of the models and projects you created as you worked through this chapter. Create a document called "The Skeletal System" and insert the photographs, along with written descriptions of what the models show and your reasons for creating them using the materials and forms you chose. Add this document to your personal portfolio.

CHAPTER

5 The Muscular System

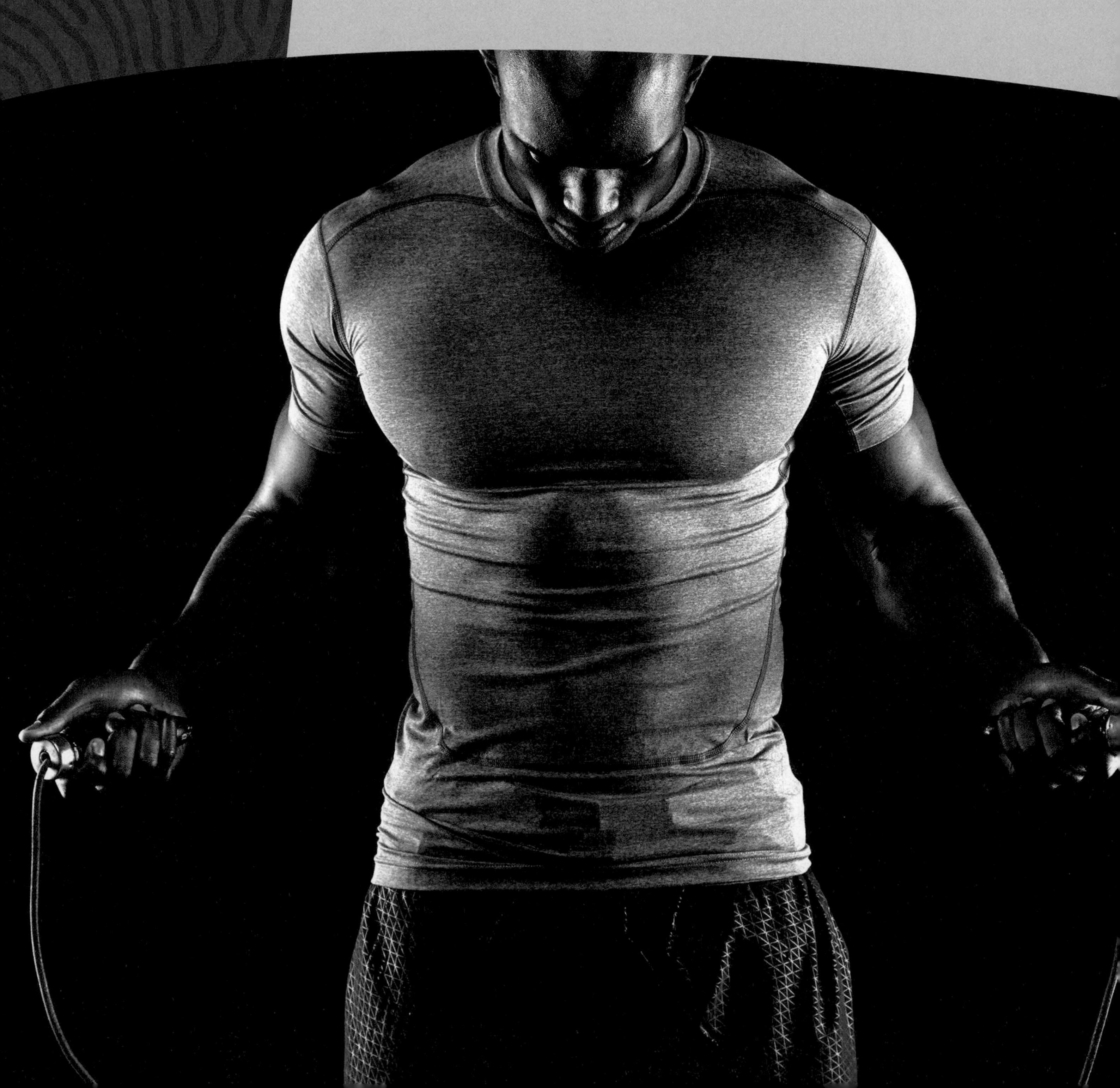

Which is most important for an athlete—muscular strength, power, or endurance?

Muscle is the only human tissue capable of shortening, or contracting. This unique ability is what makes purposeful body movements possible.

Without muscle the powerful movements required in athletic performance would be impossible, as would the finely tuned, graceful movements needed to send a text message or play a musical instrument. Muscles also control the movements of the eyes, the movement of food through the digestive system, and the beating of the heart.

What enables muscle to be so versatile? This chapter looks at the different types, properties, and structures of muscle, and examines the effects of different kinds of physical training on skeletal muscle. It also discusses some of the common injuries and disorders of muscles, how these problems tend to occur, and how their likelihood, in some cases, can be reduced.

Chapter 5 Outline

Click on the activity icon or visit www.g-wlearning.com/healthsciences/0202 to access online vocabulary activities using key terms from the chapter.

◂ Jacob Lund/Shutterstock.com

LESSON 5.1

Muscle Tissue Categories and Functions

Before You Read

Try to answer the following questions before you read this lesson.

- Why are some muscles controlled involuntarily?
- When a skeletal muscle is stimulated to contract, what three types of actions can occur?

Lesson Objectives

- Discuss the structural and functional characteristics of each of the three categories of muscle.
- Describe the behavioral characteristics common to all muscle tissue and the additional functional roles of skeletal muscle.

Key Terms

agonist	extensibility
antagonist	fascicle
aponeurosis	irritability
concentric	isometric
contractility	muscle fiber
eccentric	perimysium
elasticity	peristalsis
endomysium	sarcolemma
epimysium	

Muscles can be categorized according to both their type, or structure, and their functional and behavioral properties. This lesson describes the major muscle categories and their functions.

Muscle Categories

The three major categories of muscle fibers are skeletal, smooth, and cardiac muscle. This section examines the important structural and functional differences among these three types of muscle fibers.

Skeletal Muscle

The skeletal muscles attach to bones and are responsible for voluntary body movements. Skeletal muscle is also known as *striated muscle* due to the prominent cross-stripes, or striations, that can be seen when examining this tissue under a microscope (**Figure 5.1A**). A third name, *voluntary muscle*, is an appropriate name because this type of muscle is stimulated by consciously directed nerve activity.

An individual skeletal muscle cell is referred to as a **muscle fiber** because of its thread-like shape. Muscle fibers include many nuclei and vary considerably in length and diameter. Some fibers run the entire length of a muscle; others are much shorter.

As **Figure 5.2** shows, skeletal muscle is highly organized. The cell membrane of the muscle fiber is called the **sarcolemma** (sar-koh-LEHM-a). Over the sarcolemma of each muscle fiber is a fine, protective sheath of connective tissue called an **endomysium** (ehn-doh-MIZ-ee-um). Groups of muscle fibers are bundled together by a strong fibrous membrane called a **perimysium** (per-i-MIZ-ee-um) into a unit known as a **fascicle** (FAS-i-kuhl).

All of the fascicles in a muscle are enclosed by a thick, tough connective tissue called an **epimysium** (ehp-i-MIZ-ee-um). The epimysium connects at both ends of the muscle either with a cordlike tendon composed of extremely strong connective tissue or with a flat, sheetlike **aponeurosis** (ap-oh-noo-ROH-sis).

Tendons and aponeuroses directly connect each muscle to a bone, cartilage, or other connective tissue. Recall from Chapter 4 that tendons differ from ligaments in that ligaments connect bone to bone.

Smooth Muscle

In contrast to skeletal muscle fibers, smooth muscle cells are small, spindle-shaped, and nonstriated. They are involuntary (not under

Skeletal muscle tissue. The skeletal muscles move the body.

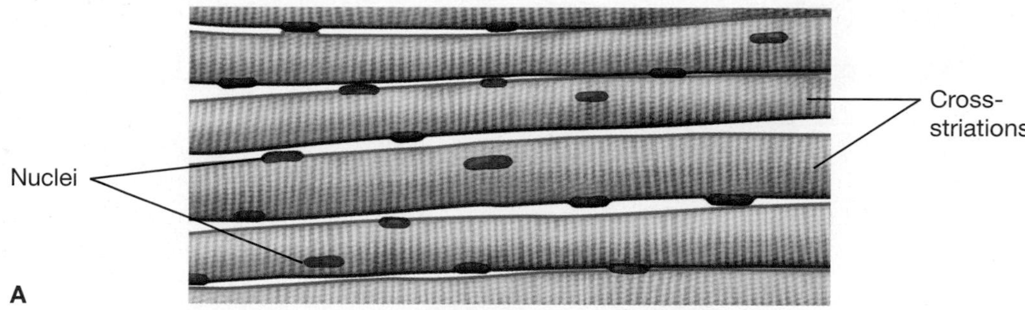

Smooth muscle tissue. The smooth muscles move food through the digestive system and perform other important involuntary functions.

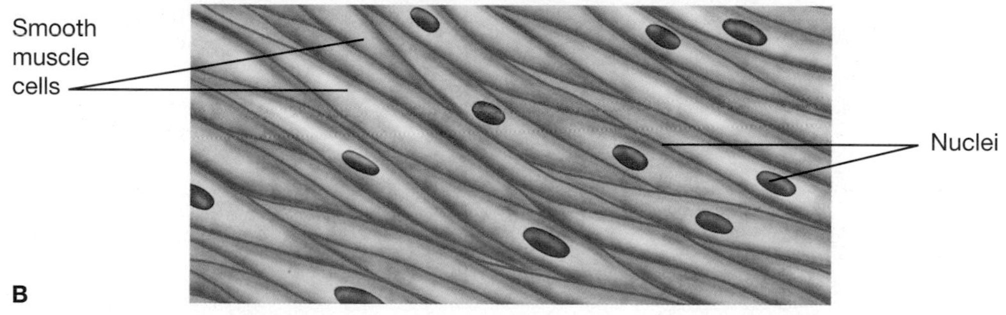

Cardiac muscle tissue. Cardiac muscle is found only in the heart.

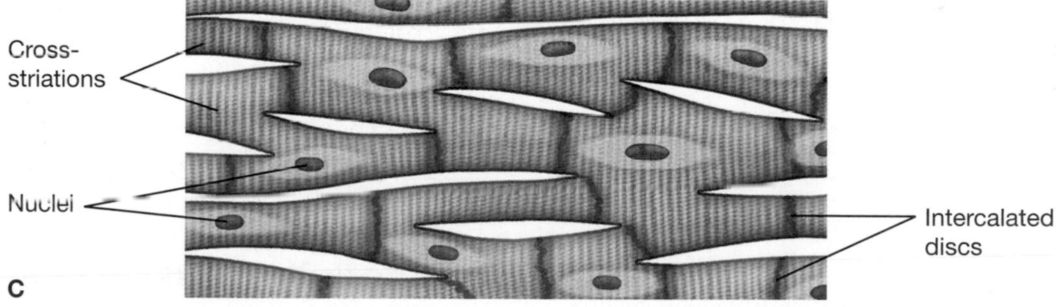

Figure 5.1 The three primary types of muscle tissue. *What are two additional names for skeletal muscle?*

conscious control), and they have a single nucleus (**Figure 5.1B**). Also known as *visceral muscle*, this type of muscle is found in the walls of many internal organs, such as the stomach, intestines, urinary bladder, and respiratory passages.

Smooth muscle cells are arranged in layers, with one layer running lengthwise and the other surrounding the organ in which the muscles are contained. The coordinated, alternate contracting and relaxing of these layers changes the size and shape of the organ and can aid in moving the contents of the organ. Moving food through the digestive system, emptying the bladder, and changing the diameter of the blood vessels are examples of the important functions of these muscles. During digestion, food is propelled along by a wave of symmetrical squeezing of the walls of the digestive tract. This process, called **peristalsis**, is described further in Chapter 13.

The autonomic (automatic) nervous system controls smooth muscle activity. Unlike the skeletal muscles, smooth muscles can sustain contraction for long periods of time without becoming fatigued.

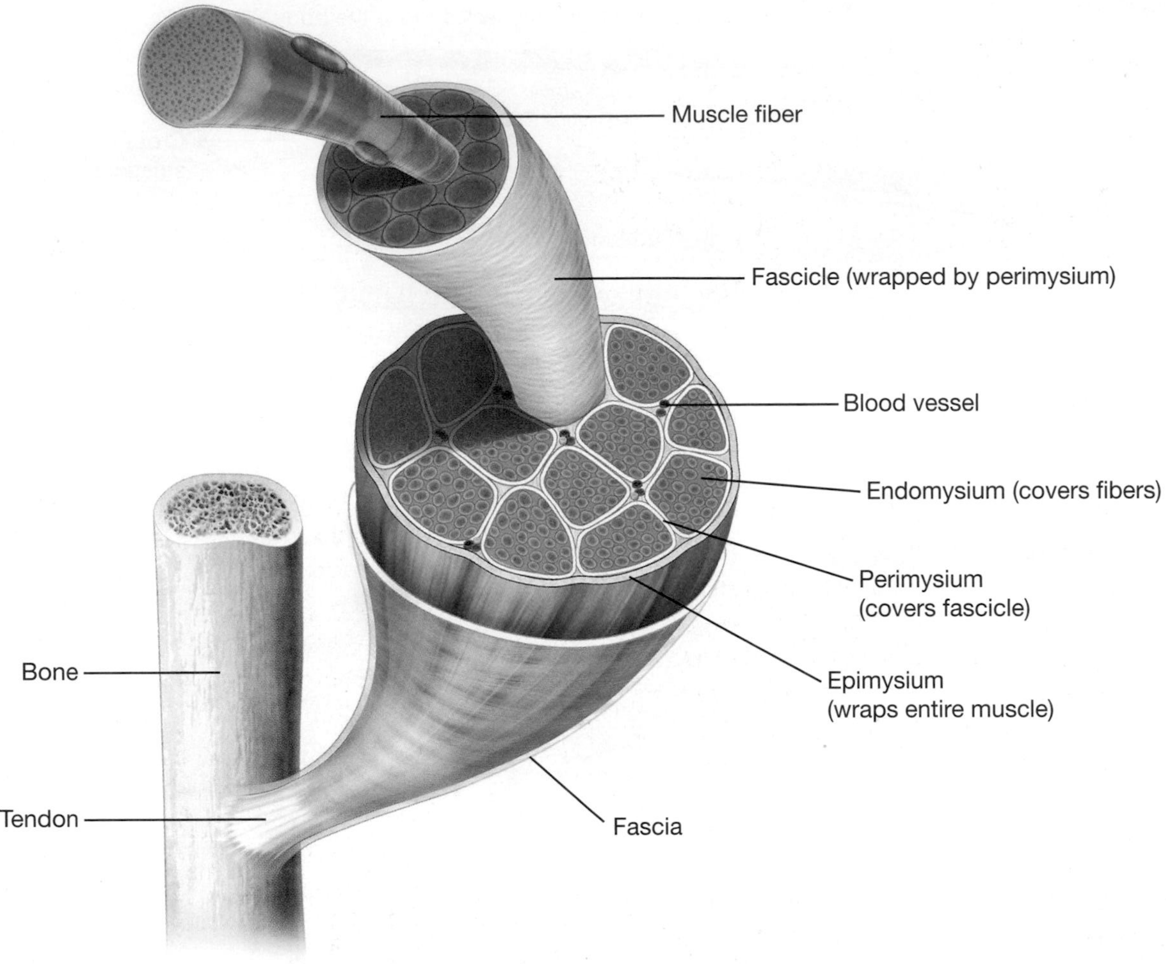

Figure 5.2 The organization of skeletal muscle. The sarcolemma (membrane of muscle fiber) is not shown in this view.

Cardiac Muscle

As the name suggests, cardiac muscle is located solely in the walls of the heart. Cardiac muscle cells are branched, cross-striated, and involuntary—they are under the control of the autonomic nervous system (**Figure 5.1C**). Cardiac cells are arranged in an interconnected network of figure-eight or spiral-shaped bundles that join together at structures called *intercalated* (in-TER-kah-lay-tehd) *discs*. This arrangement enables the coordinated contraction of neighboring cells to produce the heartbeat.

The table in **Figure 5.3** summarizes the major features of the three categories of muscle tissue. Although all three types are important and, in fact, essential for human life, this chapter focuses primarily on the skeletal muscles.

Check Your Understanding

1. What is the difference between voluntary and involuntary muscles?
2. Categorize each muscle type as voluntary or involuntary.
3. What are the three layers of tissue that run the length of a skeletal muscle?

Muscle Functions

Despite the different properties of the three types of muscle, certain behavioral characteristics are common to all muscle tissue. In the case of skeletal muscles, there are also certain functional roles that muscles can play in contributing to different movements of the body.

Muscle Categories			
Characteristic	**Skeletal**	**Smooth**	**Cardiac**
Cell structure	varying lengths, thread-shaped, striated	short, spindle-shaped, no striations	branching interconnected chains, striated
Nucleus	multinucleate	one nucleus	one nucleus
Control	voluntary	involuntary	involuntary
Location	most attach to bones; some facial muscles attach to skin	walls of internal organs other than the heart	walls of the heart

Figure 5.3 *Goodheart-Willcox Publisher*

Behavioral Properties

All muscle tissue has four behavioral characteristics in common: irritability, extensibility, elasticity, and contractility. Two of these—**extensibility**, the ability to be stretched, and **elasticity**, the ability to return to normal length after a stretch—are common not just to muscle, but to many types of biological tissues. For example, when a muscle group such as the hamstrings (on the posterior side of the thigh) is stretched over a period of time, the muscles lengthen, and the range of motion at the hip increases, making it easier to touch the toes. The stretched muscles do not return to resting length immediately, but shorten over a period of time.

Another behavioral characteristic common to all muscle is **irritability**, or the ability to respond to a stimulus. Muscles are routinely stimulated by signals from the nerves that supply them. Muscles can also be irritated by a mechanical stimulus, such as an external blow to a muscle. The response to all forms of stimuli is muscle contraction.

As mentioned in the chapter introduction, **contractility** (sometimes called *flexibility*), the ability to contract or shorten, is the one behavioral characteristic unique to muscle tissue. Most muscles have a tendon attaching to a bone at one end and a tendon attaching to another bone at the other end. When a muscle contracts, it pulls on the bones at the attachment sites. This pulling force is called a *tensile force*, or *tension*. The amount of tension developed is constant throughout the muscle, tendons, and attachment sites.

Tension and Types of Skeletal Muscle Contraction

Although people commonly use the term *contraction* (which implies shortening) to mean that tension has developed in a muscle, muscles do not always shorten when they develop tension. When a skeletal muscle develops tension, one of three actions can happen: the muscle can shorten, remain the same length, or actually lengthen.

The biceps and triceps, which are the large muscle groups on the anterior and posterior sides of the upper arm, provide examples of these three different types of tension. When the biceps muscle develops tension and shortens, the hand moves up toward the shoulder (**Figure 5.4A**). This is called a **concentric** (kun-SEHN-trik), or shortening, contraction of the biceps.

In this example, the biceps is performing the role of **agonist** (AG-un-ist), or prime mover, and the opposing muscle group, the triceps, is playing the role of **antagonist** (an-TAG-un-ist). The antagonist muscles may be completely relaxed or may develop a slight amount of tension, depending on the requirements of the movement.

You might wonder if a muscle can lengthen while developing tension, and if so, how it can lengthen. Suppose someone were to place in your hands a very heavy weight that was too heavy for you to hold in position. At first, your biceps would develop tension in an effort to hold the weight in place. But if the weight were too heavy to manage, causing you to lower the weight, your biceps would lengthen. This type of action is known as an **eccentric** (ehk-SEHN-trik), or lengthening, contraction (**Figure 5.4B**). In this case the force of gravity (not the triceps) acting on the weight causes the weight to lower. Both concentric and eccentric contractions are also known as *isotonic contractions*.

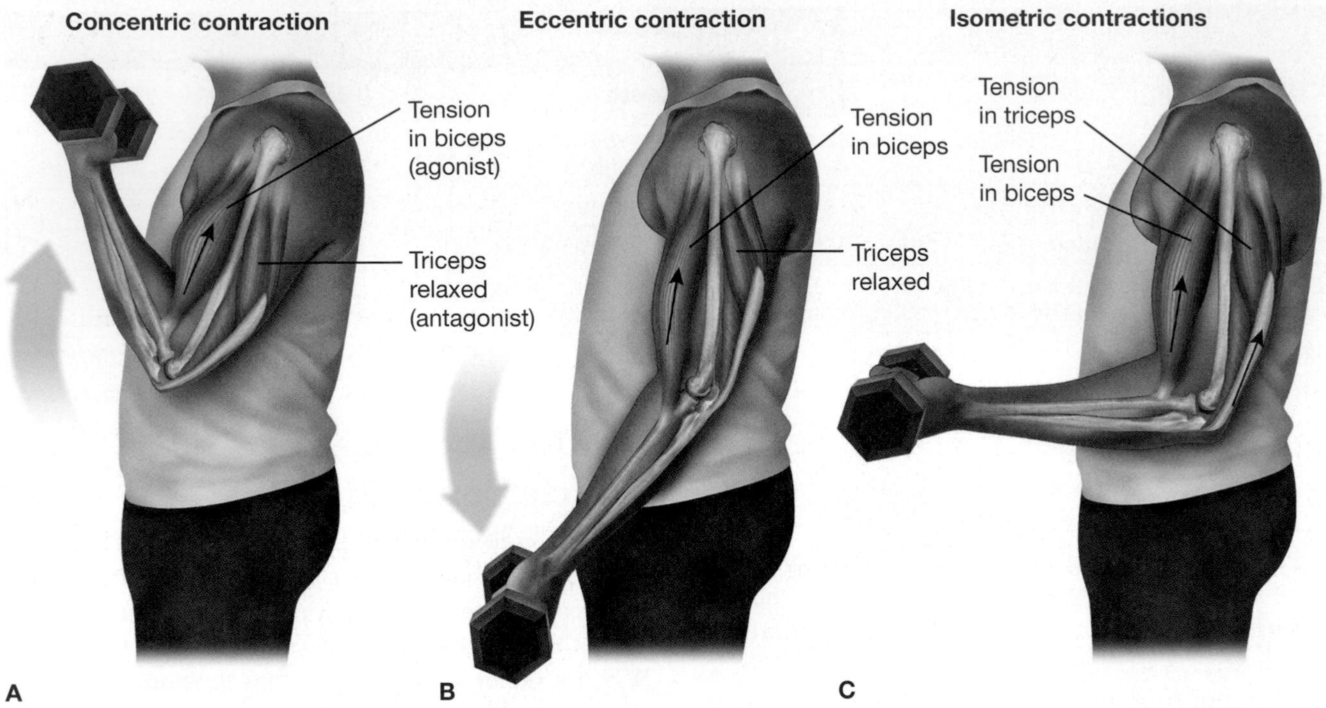

Figure 5.4 A—In this depiction of concentric contraction, the agonist biceps contracts and the antagonist triceps relaxes. B—The biceps is eccentrically contracting (lengthening) while serving as a brake to control the downward motion of the weight. C—Isometric contractions involve both the biceps and triceps developing tension, but neither muscle shortens, and there is no motion. *If you push against an immovable object, such as a wall, as hard as you can, do your muscles contract? If so, what kind of contraction occurs?*

In a third scenario (**Figure 5.4C**) you "flex" the muscles in your arm, developing tension in both the biceps and triceps, but there is no movement. This is called an **isometric** (igh-soh-MEHT-rik) contraction of both the biceps and triceps. With an isometric contraction, no change in muscle length occurs.

It is the versatility of the arrangements of human muscles in agonist and antagonist pairs around joints that enables the different movements of the human body. These versatile arrangements also help to stabilize joints and maintain body posture.

The Production of Heat

You probably know that vigorous exercise is typically accompanied by an increase in body temperature and sweating. Do you know why this happens? It happens because the working muscles generate heat. But even when you are not exercising, the muscles, typically comprising at least 40% of body mass, generate heat, and this heat helps maintain normal body temperature.

How does this happen? Muscles require energy in the form of adenosine triphosphate (ATP) to function. You may recall from your study of Chapter 2 that ATP is generated within muscle cells. The ATP is then released to provide energy when the muscle is stimulated, generating heat in the process.

Check Your Understanding

1. Explain contractility and how it creates movement.
2. What chemical substance in the body provides energy for muscles?

LESSON 5.1 Review and Assessment

Mini Glossary

Make sure that you know the meaning of each key term.

agonist role played by a skeletal muscle to cause a movement

antagonist role played by a skeletal muscle acting to slow or stop a movement

aponeurosis a flat, sheetlike fibrous tissue that connects muscle or bone to other tissues

concentric a type of contraction that results in shortening of a muscle

contractility the ability to contract or shorten

eccentric contraction accompanied by lengthening of a muscle

elasticity the ability to return to normal length after a stretch

endomysium a fine, protective sheath of connective tissue around a skeletal muscle fiber

epimysium the outermost sheath of connective tissue that surrounds a skeletal muscle

extensibility the ability to be stretched

fascicle a bundle of muscle fibers

irritability the ability to respond to a stimulus

isometric a type of contraction that involves no change in muscle length

muscle fiber an individual skeletal muscle cell

perimysium a connective tissue sheath that envelops each primary bundle of muscle fibers

peristalsis a wave of symmetrical squeezing of the digestive tract walls that occurs during digestion

sarcolemma the delicate membrane surrounding each striated muscle fiber

Know and Understand

1. Starting with a muscle fiber and working from the inside out, name each part of the skeletal muscle structure.
2. Describe the role of each type of muscle tissue (cardiac, smooth, and skeletal).
3. What is the difference between extensibility and elasticity?
4. Explain the difference between irritability and contractility.

Analyze and Apply

5. Give three examples of how you use isometric contractions during a typical day.
6. Compare and contrast the three types of muscles.
7. What do you think would happen if your antagonist muscles no longer functioned?
8. Muscles contribute to many types of body movement, for various purposes. One purpose is to move the bones. Name at least two other purposes for muscle movements.
9. Compare and contrast the three different types of muscle tissue.

IN THE LAB

10. Using spaghetti and plastic wrap, create a muscle that includes muscle fibers, fascicles, endomysium, perimysium, and the epimysium. Work in groups and verbally describe which part of the muscle you are constructing as you assemble it.
11. Do a full push-up (up then down). Determine when the triceps experienced concentric contractions and when they experienced eccentric contractions.
12. Dissect a chicken leg and identify the muscle, tendon, aponeurosis, and epimysium.
13. Standing in front of a wall, holding a piece of tape, place the tape as high on the wall as you can reach. Next, assume a jumping position, with your arms stretched behind you and your knees bent. Jump up and place a second piece of tape as high as you can reach. Finally, jump again, but from a standing position. Measure the distance from the floor to each piece of tape. Explain why the jump from the jumping position was different from the jump from the standing position.
14. Conduct research to discover the role of fixators and synergists in muscle movement. How do they help the agonists and antagonists? Create a model that shows how agonists, antagonists, fixators, and synergists work together to create muscle movement.

LESSON 5.2

Skeletal Muscle Actions

Before You Read

Try to answer the following questions before you read this lesson.

- Do sprinters and distance runners have different types of skeletal muscle fibers?
- What factors influence how rapidly a muscle fatigues?

Lesson Objectives

- Describe a motor unit and explain the functional differences between motor units that contain large and small numbers of muscle fibers.
- Explain the various types of skeletal fiber architecture.
- Discuss the concepts of muscular strength, power, and endurance.

Key Terms

acetylcholine	motor unit
action potential	neuromuscular junction
all-or-none law	parallel
axon	pennate
axon terminals	sarcomeres
cross bridges	slow-twitch
fast-twitch	synaptic cleft
motor neuron	

The development of tension in a skeletal muscle is influenced by a number of variables. Among these variables are signals from the nervous system, the properties of the muscle fibers, and the arrangement of fibers within the muscle. This lesson describes the effects of these influences. The lesson also explains how muscle actions contribute to muscular strength, power, and endurance.

The Motor Unit

Muscle tissue cannot develop tension unless stimulated by one or more nerves. Because of the dependent relationship of the muscular system on the nervous system, the two are often referred to collectively as the *neuromuscular system*.

A nerve that stimulates skeletal muscle, which is under voluntary control, is known as a **motor neuron**. A single motor neuron and all of the muscle cells that it stimulates is known as a **motor unit** (**Figure 5.5**). The motor unit is considered to be the functional unit of the neuromuscular system.

One motor neuron may connect to anywhere between 100 to nearly 2,000 skeletal muscle fibers, depending on the size and function of the muscle. The small muscles responsible for finely tuned movements, such as those in the eyes and fingers, have small motor units with few fibers per motor unit. Large, powerful muscles, such as those surrounding the hips, have large motor units with many fibers. Motor units are typically contained within a portion of a muscle, but may also be interspersed with the muscle cells of other motor units.

Generating Action Potentials

How does the motor neuron communicate with the muscle cells in the motor unit to stimulate them? A long, thin fiber called an **axon** connects the motor neuron cell body with the muscle fibers included in the motor unit. Close to the fibers, the axon branches into **axon terminals** which in turn branch out to individual muscle fibers. The link between each axon terminal and muscle fiber is called the **neuromuscular junction**. The axon terminal and fiber are separated by a tiny gap known as the **synaptic cleft**, which is filled with interstitial fluid (**Figure 5.6**).

When a nerve impulse reaches the end of an axon terminal, a chemical called a *neurotransmitter* discharges and diffuses across the synaptic cleft to attach to receptors on the muscle fiber sarcolemma. The neurotransmitter that stimulates muscle is **acetylcholine** (a-see-til-KOH-leen).

The effect of acetylcholine is to make the sarcolemma temporarily permeable. Channels open that allow positive sodium ions (Na^+) to rapidly invade the fiber at the same time that positive potassium ions (K^+) rush out of the fiber. Because more Na^+ enters than K^+ exits, the net effect is the creation of a positive charge inside the muscle fiber.

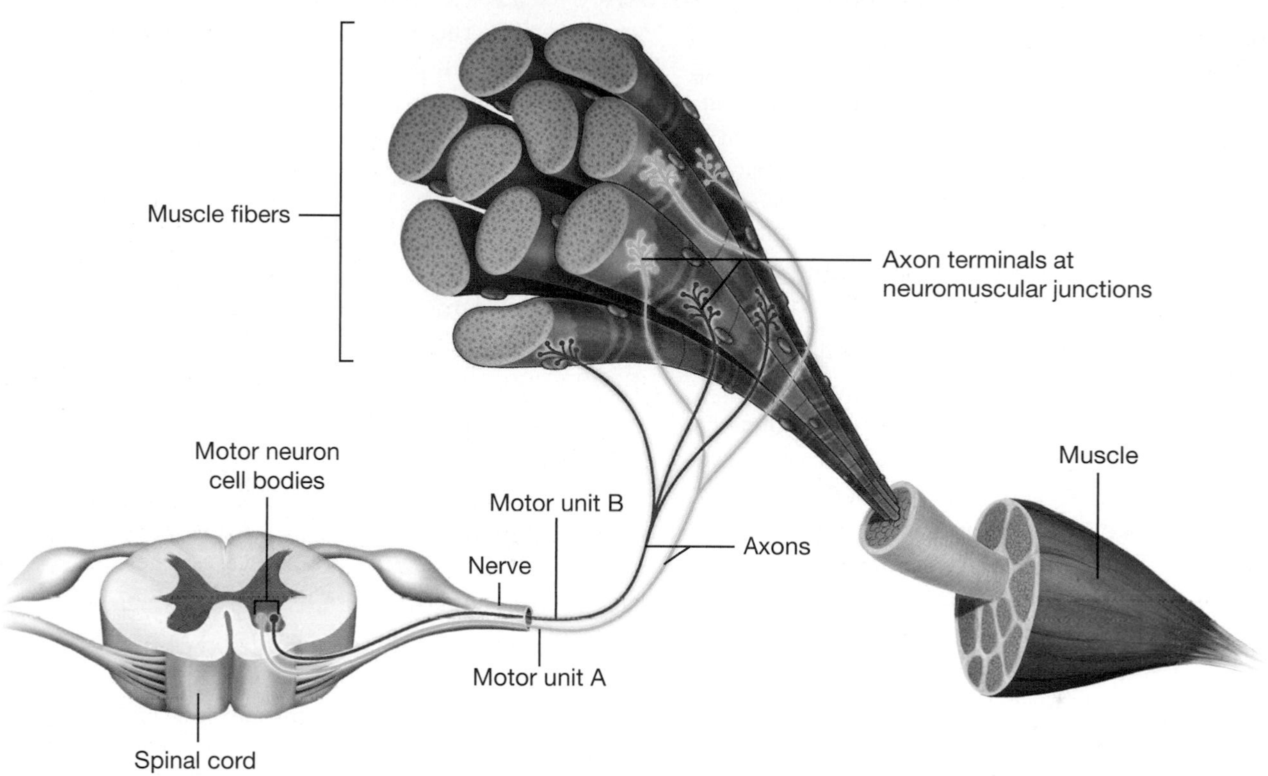

© Body Scientific International

Figure 5.5 Each motor unit includes a motor neuron and all the muscle fibers it activates. *How does a motor neuron activate muscle fibers?*

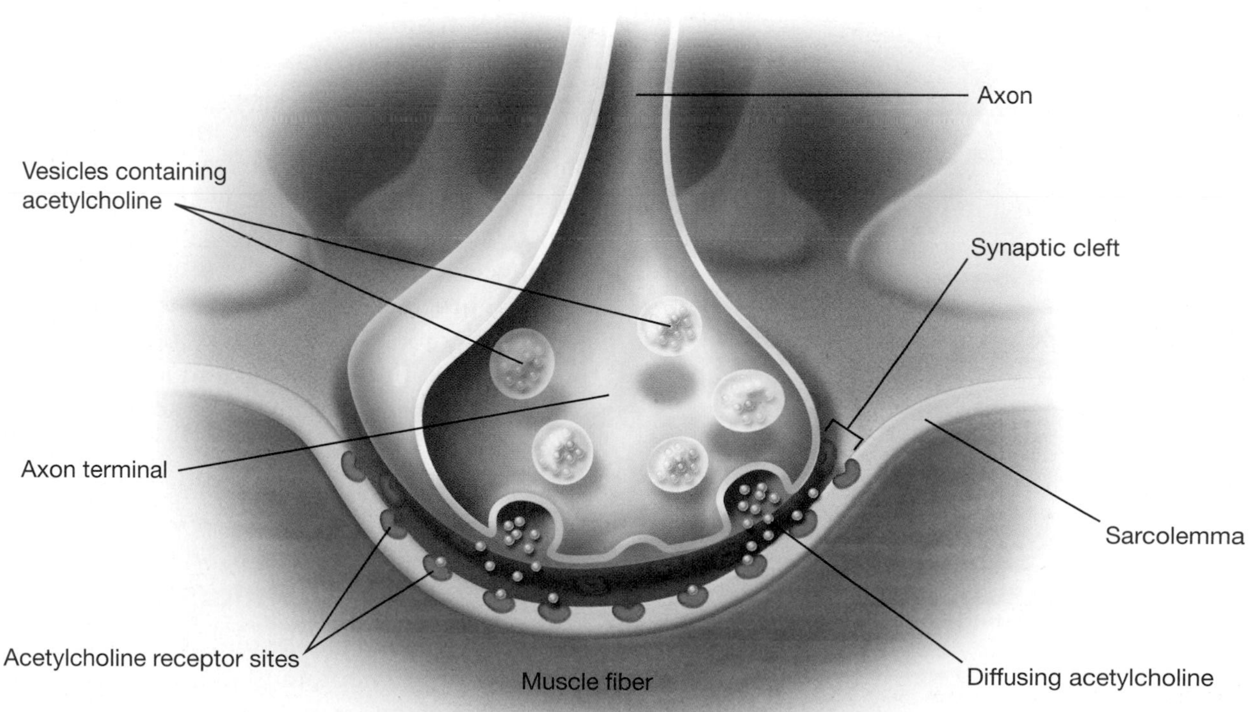

© Body Scientific International

Figure 5.6 The neuromuscular junction, the site at which nerve impulses are transmitted to muscle. *Which chemical labeled in this drawing is a neurotransmitter?*

This reversal of electrical charge is known as *depolarization*. Depolarization triggers the opening of additional channels in the fiber membrane that allow entry of additional Na^+ only. This flood of positive ions into the fiber generates an electrical charge called an **action potential**.

Contractions of the Sarcomeres

Glucose stored in the form of glycogen within the muscle cell provides the energy for creating the action potential. Phosphocreatine within the cell enables the transfer of energy to the protein filaments actin and myosin. Actin and myosin are contractile proteins that reside in functional units called **sarcomeres** (SAR-koh-meerz) inside the muscle fiber. The release of calcium ions (Ca^{++}) triggers the sliding of the actin filaments over the myosin filaments, resulting in a contraction of the sarcomere (**Figure 5.7**).

What causes the actin filaments to slide over the myosin filaments? Notice in **Figure 5.7** that the myosin filaments are encircled by small protrusions called *heads*. When the sarcomere is activated by an action potential, these heads attach to receptor sites on the actin filaments, forming **cross bridges**. The cross bridges contract, pulling the actin filaments toward the center of the sarcomere. During the process of sarcomere contraction, these cross bridges attach, pull, and release multiple times. The Ca^{++} ions released with the arrival of the action potential enable the attachments of the myosin heads to the actin filaments.

The neuromuscular system can produce slow, gentle movements as well as fast, forceful movements. This ability to produce different kinds of movements and force is accomplished by regulating the number and frequency of action potentials. Only a small number of action potentials are needed for slow, gentle movements. Fast or forceful movements require a large number of action potentials, released rapidly.

Relaxed

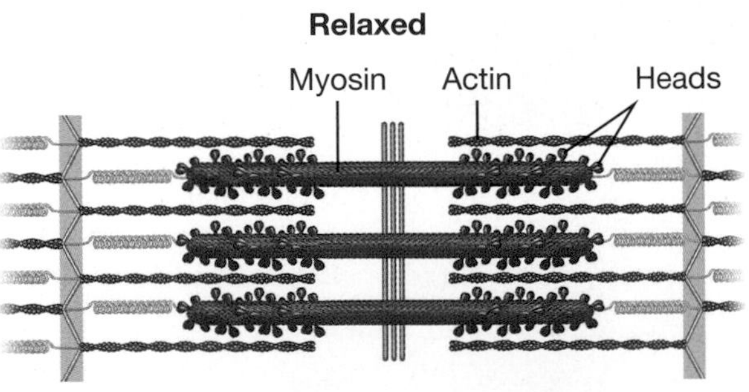

Contracted

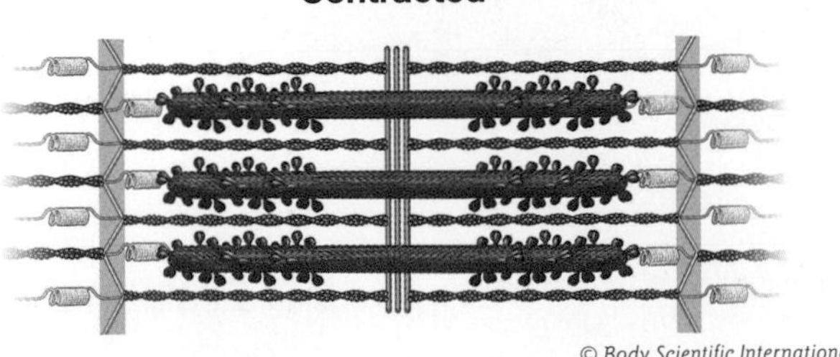

Figure 5.7 The sarcomere is the contractile unit of muscle. When the muscle is stimulated, the actin filaments slide together, producing contraction of the sarcomere.

Maximum Tension and Return to Relaxation

When receiving an action potential, a given motor unit always develops maximum tension, a physiological principle known as the **all-or-none law**. But because each whole muscle includes multiple motor units, simultaneous activation of many motor units is required for the muscle to develop maximum tension. The diagram in **Figure 5.8** displays the relationship between number and frequency of action potentials and the development of tension in the muscle. With high-frequency stimulation, the muscle develops a sustained, maximal level of tension called *tetanus*.

Almost all skeletal motor units develop tension in a twitch-like fashion, generating maximum tension very briefly and then immediately relaxing. After the action potential has traveled the length of the muscle fiber, chemical processes return the fiber to its resting state. Sodium ions diffuse back out of the cell into the interstitial fluid, and calcium ions return to storage sites within the cell. The actin filaments slide back to their original positions as the cross bridges release them, and the muscle fiber returns to a state of relaxation.

Check Your Understanding

1. What structures make up a motor unit?
2. Describe the neuromuscular junction.
3. What is an action potential?
4. Explain the all-or-none law.
5. How do muscles relax?

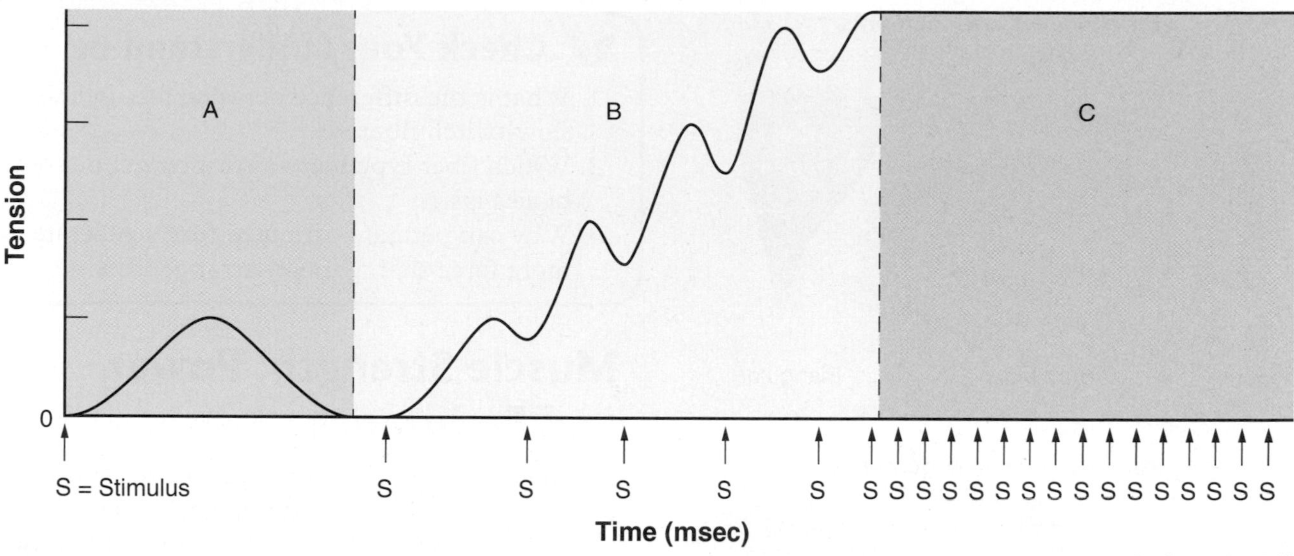

Goodheart-Willcox Publisher

Figure 5.8 Tension developed in a muscle. A—Tension in response to a single stimulus. B—Tension in response to repetitive stimulation. C—Tension in response to high-frequency stimulation, or tetanus. *Does this graph represent the activation of one or many motor units? Explain.*

Skeletal Fiber Types

Why are some athletes especially good at events or tasks that require endurance, whereas others excel at activities that require explosive strength or speed? The answer may have something to do with the ways in which these individuals train, but that is only a small part of the explanation. In fact, a big part of why certain people are better at particular activities and sports may relate to the characteristics of their skeletal muscle fibers.

Skeletal muscle fibers may be divided into two umbrella categories—**slow-twitch** (Type I) and **fast-twitch** (Type II). As the names suggest, the fast-twitch fibers contract much faster than slow-twitch fibers.

Because sufficient variation exists among the fast-twitch fibers, they too have been divided into two categories—Type IIa and Type IIb. The Type IIa fibers are intermediate in contraction speed between the slow-twitch fibers and the classic fast-twitch fibers, which are Type IIb. The Type IIb fibers contract very rapidly, in about one-seventh the time required for slow-twitch fibers to contract. As a result, the Type IIb fibers also fatigue rapidly. Although all of the muscle fibers in a motor unit are of the same type, most skeletal muscles include motor units of both fast-twitch and slow-twitch fibers. The fast-twitch/slow-twitch ratio varies from muscle to muscle and from person to person.

Fiber Architecture

Another factor that affects the ways in which skeletal muscles function is fiber architecture. Fiber architecture refers to the ways in which fibers are arranged within the muscle. The two major categories of muscle fiber arrangement are parallel and pennate.

Parallel Fiber Architecture

In **parallel** fiber architecture, the fibers run largely parallel to each other along the length of the muscle. As **Figure 5.9** shows, these parallel fiber arrangements may result in muscle shapes that are fusiform (wide in the middle and tapering on both ends), bundled, or triangular. Examples of muscles with this type of architecture are the biceps brachii (fusiform), rectus abdominis (bundled), and pectoralis major (triangular).

The individual fibers in the parallel architecture typically do not run the entire length of the muscle. Instead, the individual parallel fibers have interconnections with neighboring fibers. These interconnections promote contraction when the muscle is stimulated. This fiber arrangement enables shortening of the muscle and the ability to move body segments through large ranges of motion.

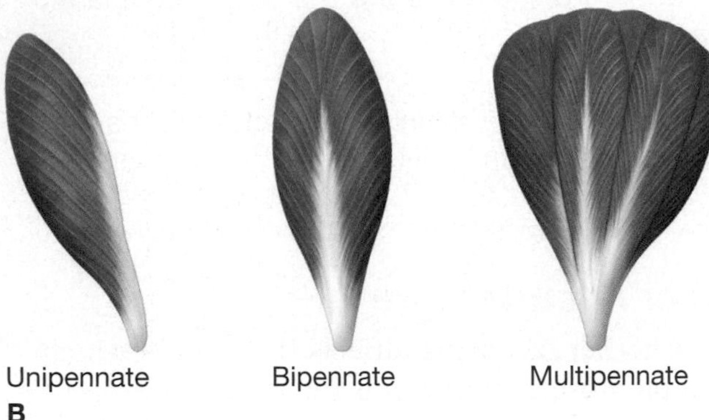

Figure 5.9 Fibers within a muscle may be arranged so that they are largely parallel or pennate (feathered). *Can you identify a muscle with parallel fiber arrangement? With pennate fiber arrangement?*

Pennate Fiber Architecture

In a **pennate** fiber arrangement, each fiber attaches obliquely to a central tendon, and sometimes attaches to more than one tendon:

- Fibers that are aligned in one direction to a central tendon are *unipennate.*
- Fibers that attach to a central tendon are *bipennate.*
- Fibers that attach to a central tendon in more than two directions are *multipennate.*

Certain muscles of the hand are unipennate, the rectus femoris (a member of the quadriceps group in the thigh) is bipennate, and the deltoid is multipennate.

With a pennate fiber arrangement, the muscle does not shorten as much upon contraction as a muscle with a parallel fiber arrangement. However, the pennate arrangement makes it possible to pack more fibers into the muscle. This means that the muscle can generate more force.

Check Your Understanding

1. What is the difference between fast-twitch and slow-twitch fibers?
2. Which fiber type helps a sprinter get out of the blocks fast?
3. Why can pennate-arranged fibers generate more force than parallel-arranged fibers?

Muscle Strength, Power, and Endurance

In everyday conversation people sometimes use *strength* and *power* interchangeably. However, muscular strength and power are quite different concepts, as discussed in this section. This section also examines what it means to have muscle fatigue, along with the related concept of muscular endurance, which is a little more complicated.

Muscular Strength

It may be tempting to think that muscular strength is the amount of force a given muscle can produce. It is impossible, however, to measure muscle force directly without penetrating the body. So, to avoid invasive procedures, external measures (such as the amount of resistance a person can move) are used to establish an indirect measure of muscle strength.

Remember that most joints in the human body are crossed by more than just one muscle. Additionally, many exercises involve more than one joint. This means that an index-of-strength measure such as maximum bench press actually assesses the collective work of several muscles that cross the shoulder and elbow (**Figure 5.10**).

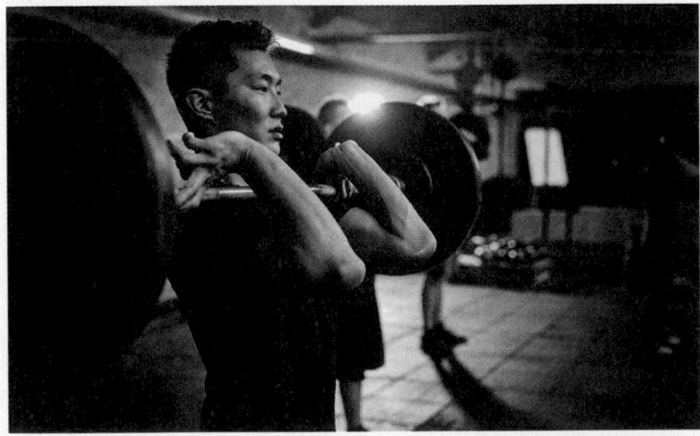

Figure 5.10 The amount of weight this man is lifting is an indirect measure of his muscle strength.

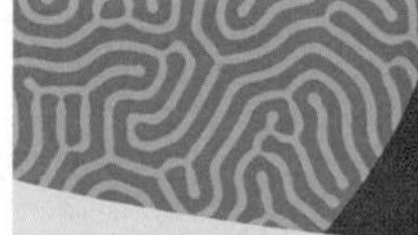

What Research Tells Us

...about Fast- and Slow-Twitch Muscles

Researchers have taken muscle biopsies (small, needle-sized plugs of muscle tissue) from elite athletes in a variety of sports. They have found that individuals specializing in events that require explosive strength or speed have unusually high proportions of fast-twitch (FT) fibers, and that elite endurance athletes tend to have very high proportions of slow-twitch (ST) fibers.

It may be the case that many of those who are able to achieve athletic success at the highest levels are simply born with high percentages of either FT or ST fibers. Once these individuals have experienced success in a particular sport or event, it is likely that they gravitate toward that sport or event (**Figure 5.11**).

Of course, certain individuals within the general population of untrained people also have high percentages of FT or ST muscles. The distribution of FT/ST ratios among the general population is represented in the normal, bell-shaped curve (**Figure 5.12**).

We also know from research that FT fiber types can change over time. FT fibers can be converted to ST fibers with years of endurance training. No evidence exists, however, that any form of training can convert ST fibers to FT fibers. A progressive loss of FT motor units and fibers occurs as people age, although this loss can be minimized by regular, high-intensity exercise throughout life.

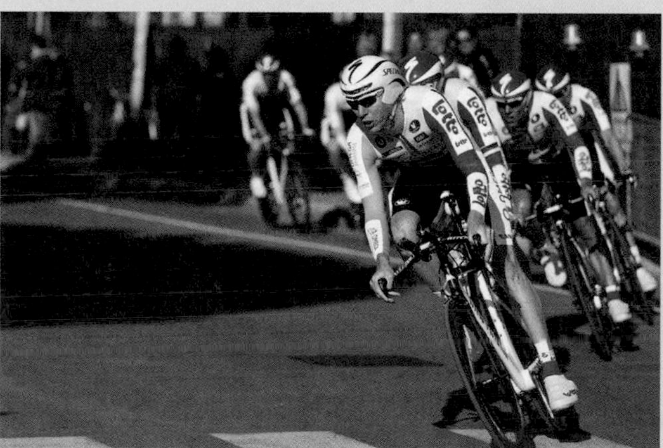

Claudio Bertoloni/Shutterstock.com

Figure 5.11 Elite sprint cyclists tend to have high percentages of fast-twitch muscle fibers. *Aside from sprint cycling, what are some sports in which athletes with high percentages of fast-twitch muscle fibers would be particularly successful?*

Taking It Further

1. Why do FT muscle fibers affect strength and speed? Why do ST muscle fibers provide increased endurance?
2. Why might regular exercise minimize the natural loss of FT muscle fibers with age?

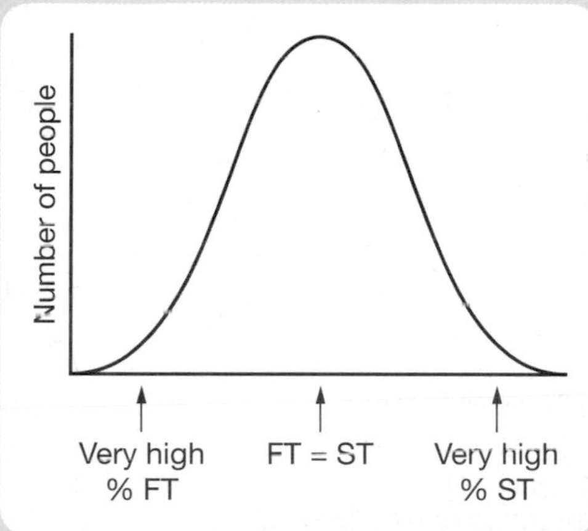

Goodheart-Willcox Publisher

Figure 5.12 The percentages of fast-twitch (FT) and slow-twitch (ST) fibers in the general population are normally distributed.

The main muscles that work during execution of a bench press include the pectoralis major, pectoralis minor, anterior deltoid, and triceps brachii.

A more precise assessment of the strength of a muscle group at a given joint is the amount of torque (TORK), or rotary force, that the muscles can generate. Torque is the product of the size of a force and the perpendicular distance of that force from an axis of rotation. For the joint shown in **Figure 5.13**, the torque produced by a muscle is the product of muscle force and the perpendicular distance from the muscle attachment to the center of rotation at the joint.

The more torque a muscle generates at a joint, the greater the tendency for movement of the bones at the joint. Machines called *dynamometers*

Calculating Muscle Force

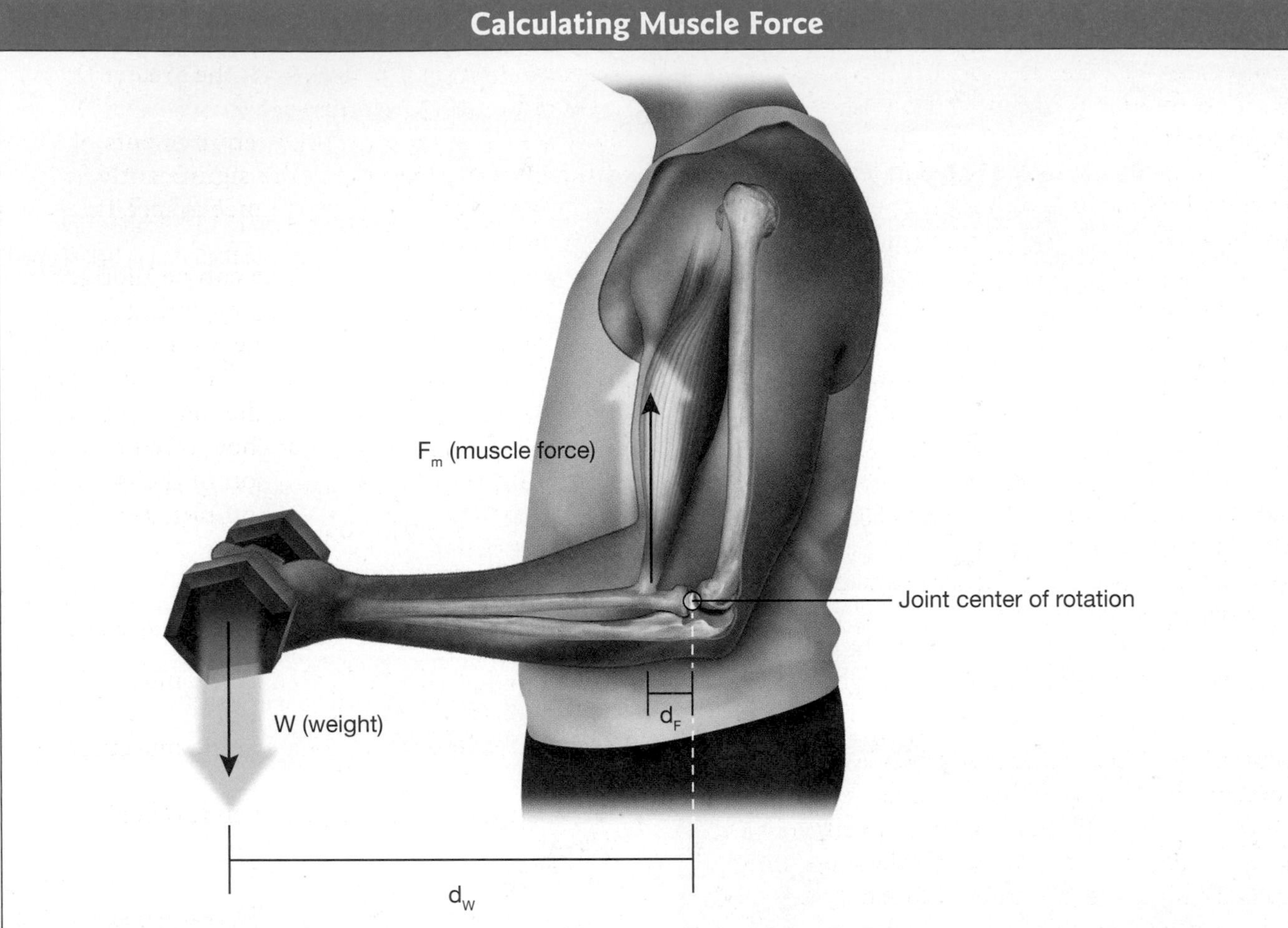

Do you know how much force your muscle must generate to hold a 5-pound weight in the position shown in the illustration? To hold the weight in this position, the torque at the elbow joint generated by the muscle (muscle torque) must balance the torque produced by the weight (weight torque) at the elbow.

Muscle torque is the product of muscle force and the perpendicular distance of that force from the center of rotation at the joint. The formula is:

$$T_m = F_m \times d_F$$

where T_m = muscle torque, F_m = muscle force, and d_F = the perpendicular distance.

Weight torque is the product of the weight and the perpendicular distance of that weight from the center of rotation at the joint. This formula is:

$$T_W = W \times d_W$$

where T_W = weight torque, W = weight, and d_W = the perpendicular distance.

Suppose that the weight in the illustration is 5 pounds, and that it is being held at a distance (d_W) of 12 inches from the center of the joint. The distance of the muscle attachment from the joint center (d_F) is 1 inch. How much force must the muscle produce to support the weight?

$$T_m = T_W$$
$$F_m \times d_F = W \times d_W$$
$$F_m \times 1'' = 5 \text{ lb} \times 12''$$
$$F_m = 60 \text{ lb}$$

Are you surprised? To support just 5 pounds in the hand, the muscle must generate 60 pounds of force. Because muscles attach so closely to joints, the human musculoskeletal system is designed more for movement speed than for strength.

Now you try: Suppose that the weight (W) in this picture is 10 pounds, the d_W is 15 inches, and the d_F is 1 inch. What is the F_m?

Figure 5.13

Goodheart-Willcox Publisher

measure joint torque. Joint torque, which is used as a measure of strength, is based solely on the resistance moved or matched. The speed with which a resistance is moved is not relevant to the strength measurement.

Some athletes and body builders have succumbed to the temptation to take drugs to increase muscle size, strength, and power production. Anabolic androgenic steroids are synthetic versions of the male hormone testosterone. These dangerous drugs can cause severe, long-lasting, and sometimes irreversible negative effects on health, including baldness, liver damage, and severe depression. In males they can also cause breast development, shrinking of testicles, and impotence. In females they can cause irreversible deepening of the voice, male pattern hair growth, and abnormal menstrual cycles.

Muscular Power

The variable that does involve speed is muscular power. *Mechanical power* is defined as force multiplied by velocity (force × velocity). *Muscular power*, then, is defined specifically as muscle force multiplied by muscle-shortening velocity during contraction. Notice, however, that neither muscle force nor shortening velocity can be measured from outside the body. Research dynamometers have the ability to generate estimates of muscular power based on the resistance moved and movement speed.

Like muscular strength, muscular power is typically generated by several different muscles working collectively. Sprinting, along with the jumping and throwing events in track and field, are good examples of activities that require muscular power. Because force production and movement speed contribute equally to muscular power, the sprinter with the greatest leg strength may not necessarily be the fastest.

Muscle Endurance

Muscle endurance is the ability of a muscle to produce tension over a period of time. The tension may be constant (for example, when a gymnast holds a motionless handstand), or it may vary cyclically (for example, during running, cycling, or rowing). Generally, the longer the physical activity is maintained, the greater the required muscular endurance (**Figure 5.14**). Because the force and speed requirements of different movements can vary significantly, the definition of muscular endurance is specific to each physical activity.

In general, muscle fatigue can be thought of as the opposite of muscular endurance. The faster a muscle fatigues, the less endurance it has. A variety of factors affect the rate at which a muscle fatigues, including the nature of the work or exercise being done, how often the muscle is used, the composition of the muscle fibers, and the temperature and humidity of the environment.

Check Your Understanding

1. What is measured to determine muscular strength?
2. What is measured to determine muscular power?
3. What influences muscular endurance?

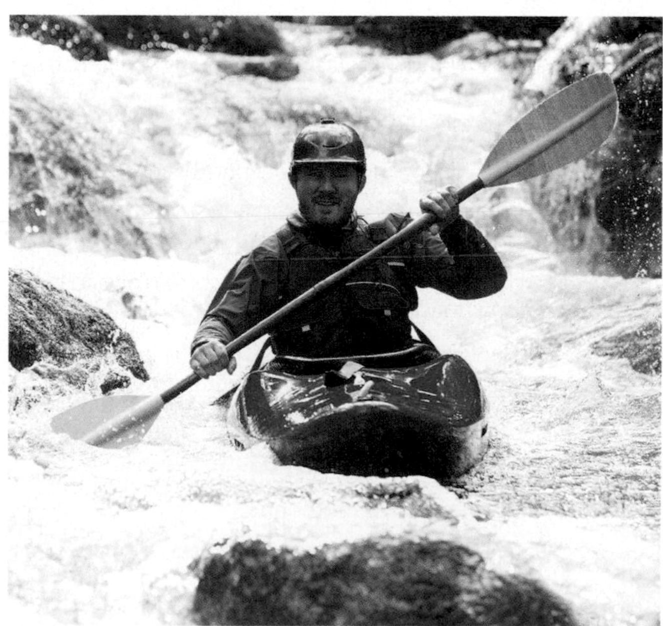

Collin Quinn Lomax/Shutterstock.com

Figure 5.14 Muscle endurance is a measure of how long a muscle can perform a specific task before fatiguing. *Which muscles need endurance when you are kayaking?*

LESSON 5.2 Review and Assessment

Mini Glossary

Make sure that you know the meaning of each key term.

acetylcholine a neurotransmitter chemical that stimulates muscle

action potential the electric charge produced in nerve or muscle fiber by stimulation

all-or-none law the rule stating that the fibers in a given motor unit always develop maximum tension when stimulated

axon a long, thin fiber connected to the motor neuron cell body

axon terminals offshoots of the axon that branch out to connect with individual muscle fibers

cross bridges connections between the heads of myosin filaments and receptor sites on the actin filaments

fast-twitch type of muscle that contracts quickly

motor neuron a nerve that stimulates skeletal muscle tissue

motor unit a single motor neuron and all of the muscle fibers that it stimulates

neuromuscular junction the link between an axon terminal and a muscle fiber

parallel a type of muscle fiber arrangement in which fibers run largely parallel to each other along the length of the muscle

pennate a type of muscle fiber arrangement in which each fiber attaches obliquely to a central tendon

sarcomeres units composed of actin and myosin that contract inside the muscle fiber

slow-twitch type of muscle that contracts slowly and is fatigue resistant

synaptic cleft the tiny gap that separates the axon terminal and muscle fiber

Know and Understand

1. Describe the parts of a motor unit.
2. Discuss the differences between a large and small motor unit and their functions.
3. Explain the role of acetylcholine in muscle contractions.
4. What chemical change causes a muscle cell to relax?
5. What is the role of the sarcomere in muscle contraction?
6. Describe parallel and pennate fiber patterns.

Analyze and Apply

7. Which fiber types contribute to each of the following: muscular strength, power, and endurance? Explain your reasoning.
8. What would happen if you had no Na+ in your body? No Ca++?
9. Why do temperature and humidity increase the rate of muscle fatigue?
10. Do you think a soccer player has more fast-twitch or slow-twitch muscle fibers? Why?
11. Explain why several different exercises would be needed to improve endurance throughout the body.

IN THE LAB

12. Try an experiment. Get into and then hold a squatting position for as long as you can while a partner times you. Allow five minutes to rest; then continually move into and out of a squatting position for as long as possible, again with your partner timing you. Did you fatigue more quickly holding a squatting position or while moving up and down in a squatting motion? Why? Now reverse roles with your partner.
13. Work in groups of three, taking on the following roles: recorder, counter, and demonstrator. The demonstrator squeezes a tennis ball as many times as possible within 60 seconds. The counter counts how many squeezes occur every 10 seconds, and the recorder records the numbers. Then rotate positions until all three of you have been demonstrators. Then create a graph to display your results. When did fatigue occur for each person? How can you increase your endurance?
14. Conduct research if necessary to discover the characteristics of the three major types of levers. Create a poster using various joints in the human body to illustrate the lever types. Are all three types of levers present in the human body?

LESSON 5.3 The Major Skeletal Muscles

Before You Read

Try to answer the following questions before you read this lesson.

- Which muscles are responsible for breathing?
- What important functions do the neck and trunk muscles contribute beyond movement capabilities?

Lesson Objectives

- Describe and give examples of the types of body motions that occur in the sagittal, frontal, and transverse planes.
- Identify the locations and functions of the muscles of the head and neck, trunk, and upper and lower limbs.

Key Terms

abduction	lateral rotation
adduction	medial rotation
circumduction	myocytes
dorsiflexion	opposition
eversion	origin
extension	plantar flexion
flexion	pronation
hyperextension	radial deviation
insertion	supination
inversion	ulnar deviation

The human body contains more than 650 skeletal muscles. This lesson presents only the most important muscles from the standpoint of functional movement. Almost all of these muscles are arranged in agonist-antagonist pairs, causing opposing actions at one or more joints.

Directional Motions

To understand the movement of muscles, you must first understand more about muscle attachments. It will also be helpful to review some directional terms from Chapter 1.

Skeletal muscles attach at either end of the muscle; the most common attachments are tendon connections to bone. The end of a muscle that attaches to a relatively fixed structure is called the **origin**. The end of a muscle that attaches to a bone that typically moves when the muscle contracts is called the **insertion**.

For an example of origin and insertion, consider the brachialis muscle, which crosses the anterior side of the elbow. Its origin is on the humerus, and its insertion is on the ulna in the forearm. When the brachialis contracts, the forearm (ulna) is pulled toward the upper arm, while the upper arm (humerus) remains stationary.

Remember, when stimulated to develop tension, muscles can only pull. They are incapable of pushing. In addition, remember from Chapter 1 that to describe the human body and its movements, scientists refer to three major planes that pass through the center of the body:

- The *sagittal* plane is in line with forward and backward motions.
- The *frontal* plane is in line with sideways movement.
- Rotational movements occur in the *transverse* plane.

Also recall from Chapter 1 that the frame of reference for all movement is the anatomical position. In this position the human body is erect with the hands at the sides and the palms facing forward.

Sagittal Plane Movements

The primary sagittal plane (forward/backward) movements are **flexion** (FLEHK-shun), **extension**, and **hyperextension** (Figure 5.15). Flexion describes forward-bending motion of the head, trunk, upper arm, forearm, hand, and hip; and backward motion of the lower leg at the knee. In flexion movements, body surfaces are coming together. Extension returns body segments from a position of flexion to anatomical position. Hyperextension continues the extension motion past anatomical position.

Two movements of the foot also occur primarily in the sagittal (SAJ-i-tal) plane. Bringing the top of the foot toward the lower leg is called **dorsiflexion** (DOR-si-flehk-shun), and moving the foot in the opposite direction, away from the lower leg, is called **plantar flexion**.

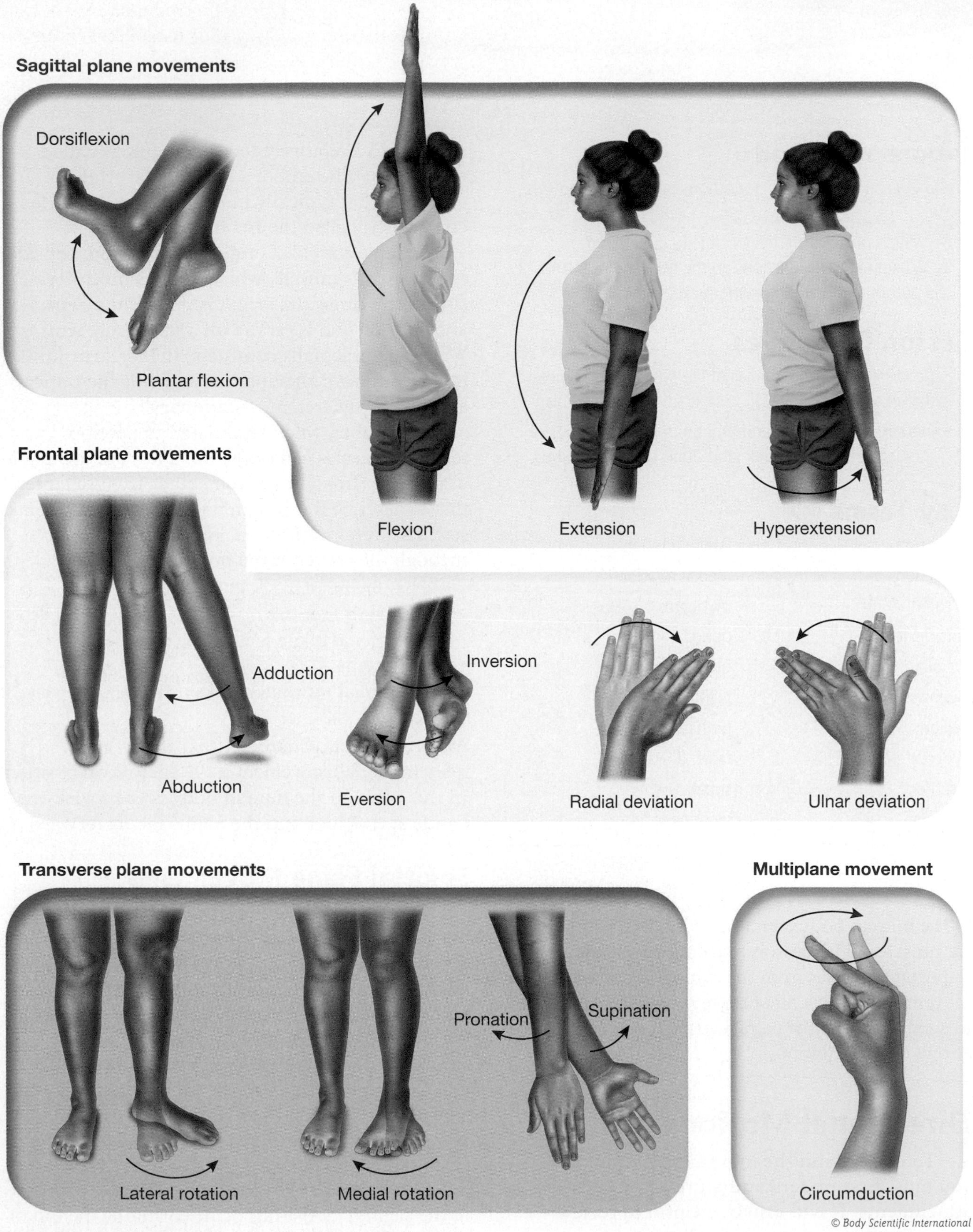

Transverse plane movements

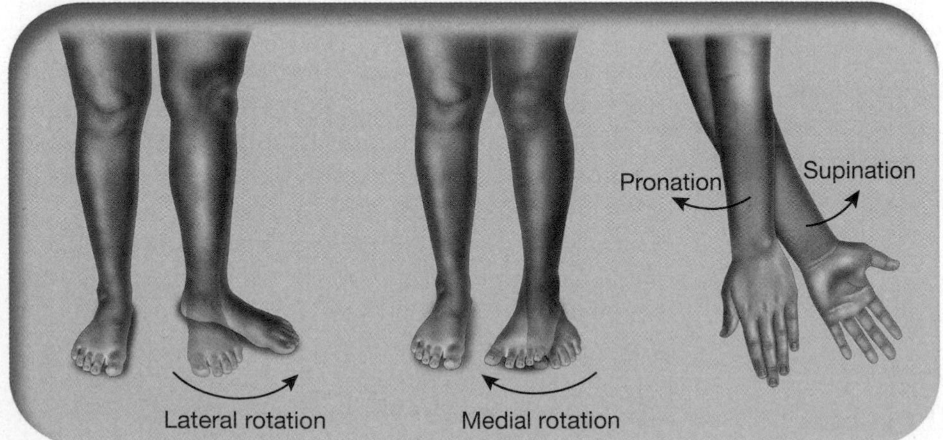

Multiplane movement

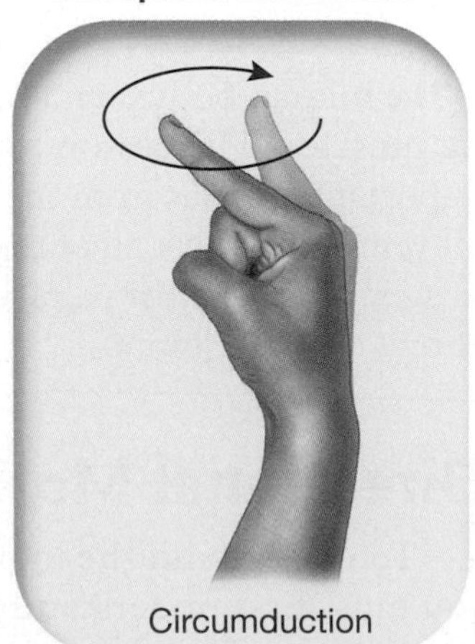

Figure 5.15 Directional movement terminology.

MEMORY TIP

Planting the ball of the foot is the motion involved in *plantar* flexion.

Frontal Plane Movements

Common movements in the frontal plane include **abduction** and **adduction** (**Figure 5.15**). Movements at the shoulder and hip that take the arm and leg away from the midline of the body are called *abduction*. Movements that bring the arm and leg closer to the midline of the body are called *adduction*.

MEMORY TIP

Just as *abduct* means "to take away," abduction takes a body segment away from the body. Just as *add* means "to bring back," adduction returns a body segment closer to the body.

Movements of the foot that occur mainly in the frontal plane are **inversion** and **eversion**. Rolling the sole of the foot inward is inversion, while rolling the sole of the foot outward is eversion (**Figure 5.15**).

Frontal plane movements of the hand at the wrist are called **radial deviation** and **ulnar deviation**. Recall from Chapter 4 that the forearm has two bones—the radius and the ulna. The radius is on the thumb side of the hand, and the ulna is on the "little finger" side. From the anatomical position, with the palms facing forward, abduction of the hand toward the thumb is called *radial deviation*, and adduction of the hand toward the little finger is called *ulnar deviation*.

Trunk and neck motions away from anatomical position in the frontal plane are called *lateral flexion* and *side bending*. Return from a position of lateral flexion to the anatomical position is called *lateral extension*.

Transverse Plane Movements

Transverse plane movements mostly involve rotation around the long axis of a body segment. When the head or trunk rotate from side to side, the movement is simply called *left* or *right rotation*. Rotation of an arm or a leg in the transverse plane is called **medial rotation** if the rotation is directed medially, or inward, and **lateral rotation** if the movement is directed laterally, or outward (**Figure 5.15**). The special terms used for rotation of the forearm are **pronation** for medial (palm down) rotation and **supination** (soo-pi-NAY-shun) for lateral (palm up) rotation.

Multiplanar Movements

A few movements of body segments do not fall within a single plane. If you have ever purchased running shoes, you may have heard the terms *pronation* and *supination* used to describe motions of the foot occurring specifically at the subtalar joint (where the heel and ankle bones meet). Pronation at the subtalar joint is a combination of eversion, abduction, and dorsiflexion. Supination at this joint includes inversion, adduction, and plantar flexion. Moving a finger, arm, or leg in a rotational manner such that the end of the segment traces a circle is called **circumduction** (ser-kum-DUK-shun), which you can see in **Figure 5.15**. And, finally, touching any of your four fingers to the thumb is known as **opposition**. Having an opposable thumb gives you the all-important ability to grasp objects.

Check Your Understanding

1. Which end of the muscle typically moves?
2. In what direction are movements guided on the sagittal plane?
3. What special movements occur on the frontal plane at the hand? The foot?
4. Describe circumduction.
5. Explain the difference between medial and lateral rotation.

Skeletal Muscle Groups

Muscles can be grouped loosely according to where they are in the body, because different body areas have different overall functions. Organizing the muscles in this way can help you understand the functional groups and remember the major muscles in each group.

Head and Neck Muscles

The muscles of the head and neck can be divided into three groups: facial muscles, chewing muscles, and neck muscles. The difference between facial muscles and most other muscles is that facial muscle insertions connect them to other muscles or skin. When these muscles contract, pulling on the skin, they produce an array of facial expressions.

With the exception of the orbicularis oris, which encircles the mouth, and the sheetlike platysma on the front and sides of the neck, all of the other head and neck muscles are paired—one on the right and one on the left. The head and neck muscles are displayed in **Figure 5.16**, and their locations and functions are summarized in **Figure 5.17**.

Trunk Muscles

The trunk muscles provide stability for the vertebral column. They are also responsible for maintaining upright posture. American football players train to strengthen the neck and trunk muscles in an effort to maximize spinal stability and minimize risk of injury to the delicate spinal cord and internal organs (**Figure 5.18**). Conversely, female gymnasts train to enhance the flexibility of the spine and are capable of extraordinary spinal hyperextension, especially during balance-beam and floor-exercise routines.

Collectively, the trunk muscles enable flexion, extension, hyperextension, lateral flexion, and rotation of the head and trunk. From a functional perspective, the anterior abdominal muscles also assist with urination, defecation, forced expiration during breathing, and childbirth. The all-important diaphragm muscle helps regulate breathing. The trunk muscles also serve as a protective sheath for the organs of the thoracic and abdominal cavities. The major muscles of the anterior and posterior trunk are shown in **Figure 5.19**. The locations and primary functions of these muscles are summarized in the table in **Figure 5.20**.

Upper Limb Muscles

Because the shoulder is a ball-and-socket joint and the most freely movable joint in the human body, the movement capabilities of the upper limb are impressive. To achieve this large range of motion, the bone structure of the glenohumeral (gleh-noh-HYOO-mer-al) joint provides little to no stability, rendering it susceptible to dislocation. Therefore, it is up to the large, powerful muscles surrounding the shoulder to maintain the stability and integrity of the joint.

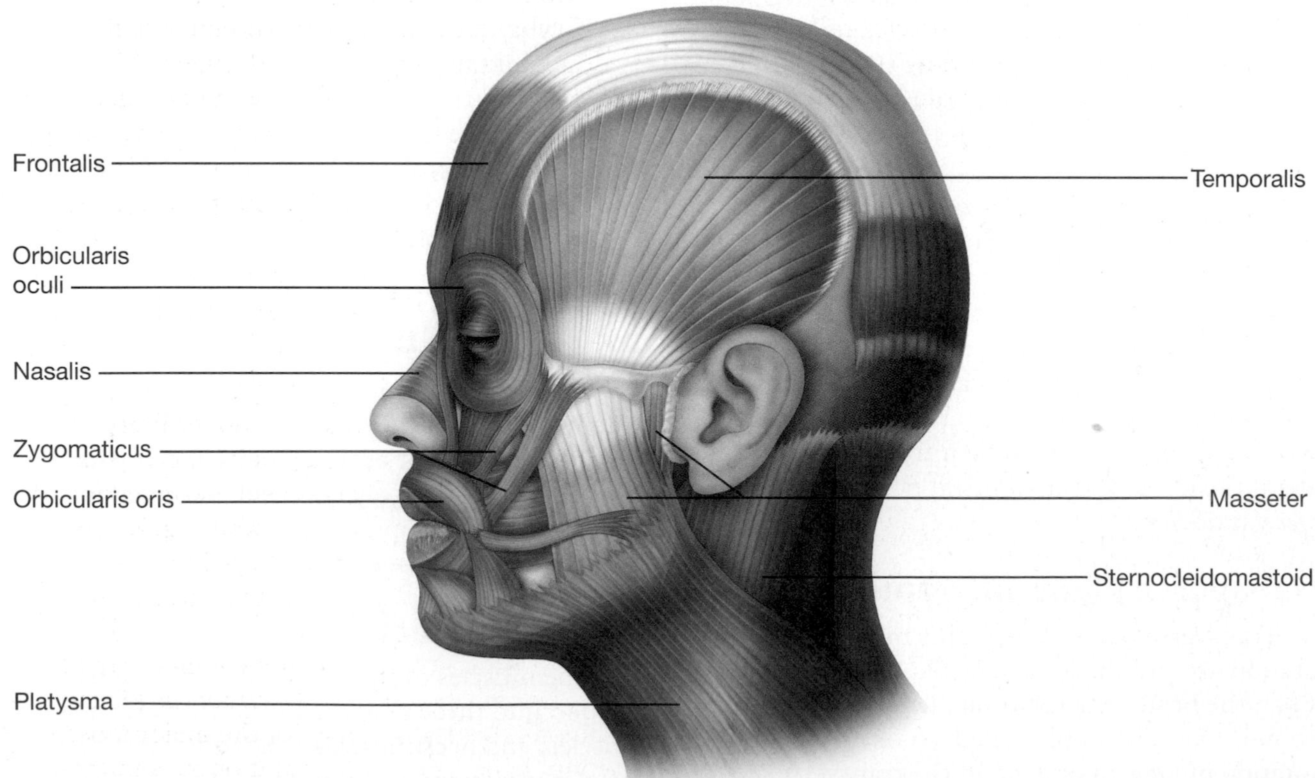

Figure 5.16 Major muscles of the head and neck. *Which muscle is referred to as the "smiling" muscle?*

Muscles of the Head and Neck		
Muscle	**Location**	**Primary Functions**
Facial Muscles		
Frontalis	forehead; connects cranium to skin above eyebrows	raises eyebrows, wrinkles forehead
Orbicularis oculi	encircles the eyes	closes eyes, enables squinting
Nasalis	nose	modifies size of nostrils
Orbicularis oris	encircles mouth	closes lips, produces kissing motion
Zygomaticus	connects cheekbones to corners of mouth	the "smiling" muscle
Platysma	front and sides of neck	pulls corners of mouth down, opens mouth wide
Chewing Muscles		
Masseter	connects temporal bone to mandible	closes the jaw
Temporalis	fan-shaped muscle over temporal bone	assists masseter with closing the jaw
Neck Muscles		
Sternocleidomastoid	sides of neck	flexion of head, rotation of head toward opposite side of contraction

Figure 5.17

Goodheart-Willcox Publisher

The arm muscles enable strong, controlled movements in sports such as gymnastics, rowing, and archery, as well as fast, powerful movements in weightlifting, boxing, and throwing. The dexterity of the finger muscles enables precise movements, such as typing, texting, knitting, and playing musical instruments.

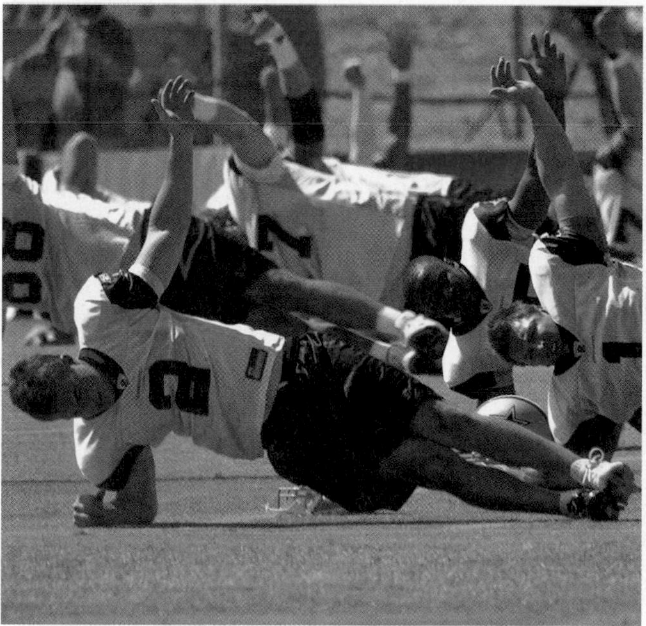

Arthur Eugene Preston/Shutterstock.com

Figure 5.18 Football players conditioning. *Why is it critically important for football players to strengthen their neck and trunk muscles?*

The joints of the upper limb include those of the shoulder, elbow, wrist, and fingers. This lesson includes information about the major muscles that cross the shoulder and elbow joints. The nine muscles that cross the wrist and the ten muscles within the hand (some of which branch out to several of the fingers) are not discussed. **Figure 5.21** shows the major muscles of the upper limb, and **Figure 5.22** summarizes their locations and functions.

Lower Limb Muscles

While the structure of the upper limb lends itself well to activities that involve large ranges of motion, the lower limb is well designed for its primary jobs of standing and walking. Running, jumping, kicking, climbing, skipping, hopping, and dancing are just a few of the additional capabilities of the lower limb.

The lower limb includes the joints of the hip, knee, and ankle, along with numerous joints in the foot. This lesson includes the major muscles of the hip, knee, and ankle, but it omits a number of small muscles that play assistive roles. **Figure 5.23** shows the major muscles of the lower limb. The table in **Figure 5.24** outlines the locations and primary functions of these muscles.

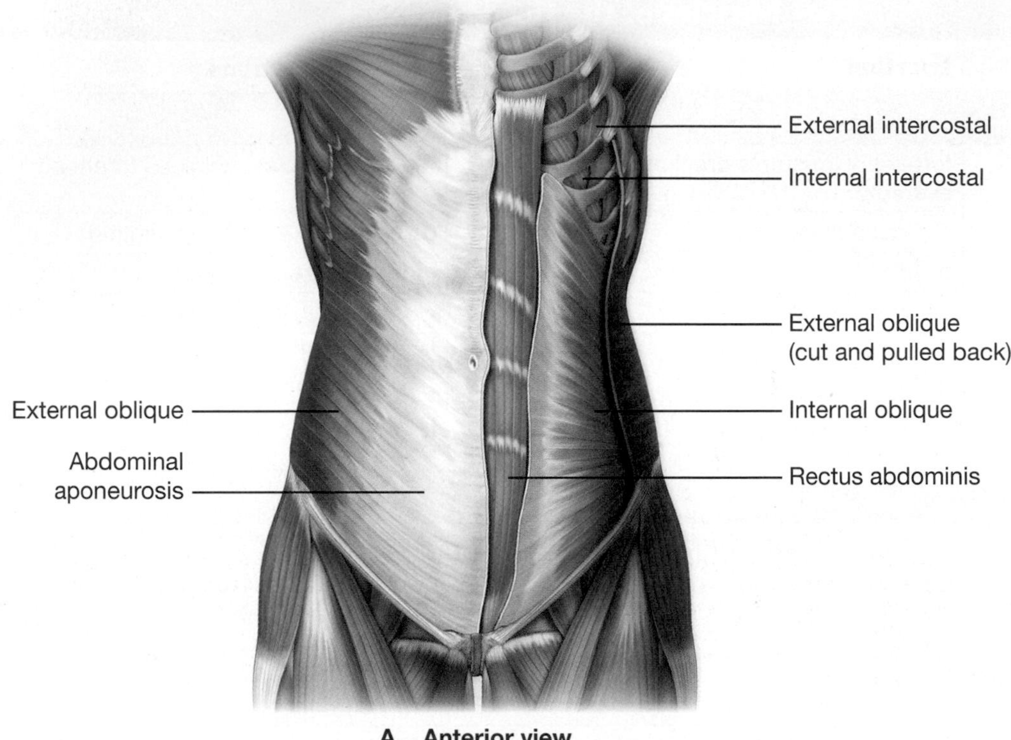

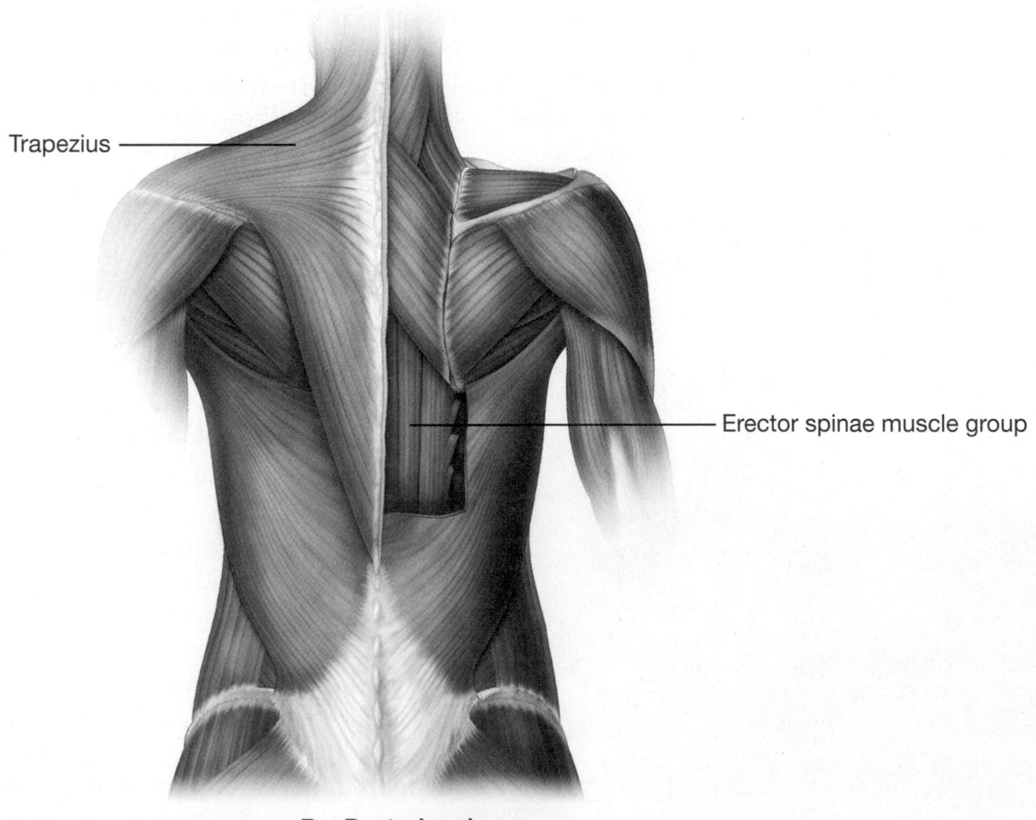

Figure 5.19 Major muscles of the trunk. *What are some basic functions that the muscles of the trunk assist with, in addition to movement of the trunk and the head and protection of the organs?*

Muscles of the Trunk		
Muscle	**Location**	**Primary Functions**
Anterior Muscles		
Pectoralis major	upper chest; connects sternum, shoulder girdle, and upper ribs to proximal humerus	adduction and flexion of arm
Rectus abdominis	center front of abdomen; connects ribs to pubic crest	flexion and lateral flexion of trunk
External oblique	front of abdomen; connects lower eight ribs to anterior iliac crest	flexion, lateral flexion, and rotation to opposite side of trunk
Internal oblique	front of abdomen beneath the external obliques; connects lower four ribs with the iliac crest	flexion, lateral flexion, and rotation to same side of trunk
Posterior Muscles		
Trapezius	upper back and neck; connects skull and thoracic vertebrae to clavicle and scapula	extension and hyperextension of head
Erector spinae	length of vertebral column; connects adjacent vertebrae	extension, lateral flexion, and rotation to opposite side of vertebral column
Muscles for Breathing		
Diaphragm	dome-shaped muscle separating thoracic and abdominal cavities	enlarges thoracic cavity for inhalation
Internal intercostals	connect the ribs; located between them	decrease thoracic cavity during forced expiration
External intercostals	connect the ribs; located between them	help enlarge thoracic cavity for inhalation

Figure 5.20

Goodheart-Willcox Publisher

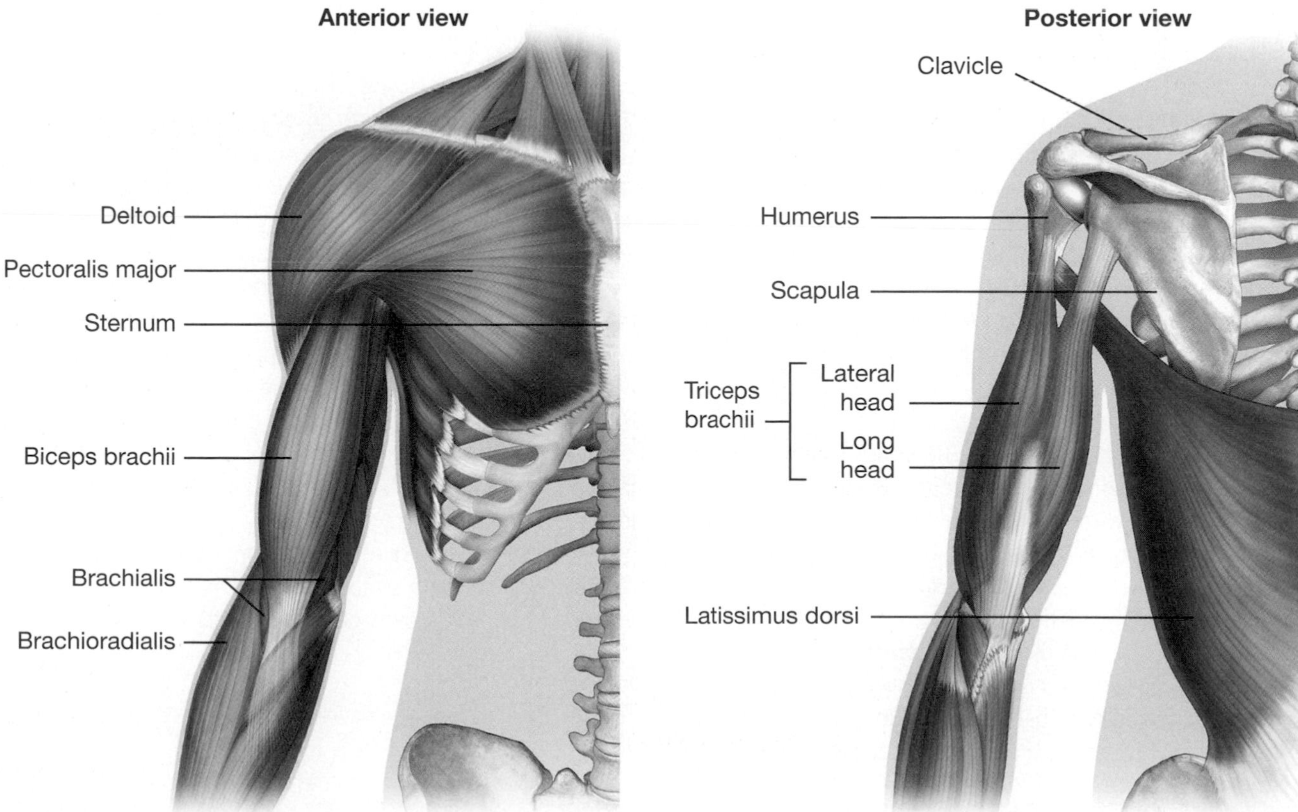

© Body Scientific International

Figure 5.21 Muscles of the upper limb.

Muscles of the Upper Limb		
Muscle	**Location**	**Primary Functions**
Shoulder Muscles		
Pectoralis major	upper chest; connects sternum, shoulder girdle, and upper ribs to proximal humerus	adduction and flexion of arm
Deltoid	covers external shoulder; connects scapula and clavicle to humerus	abduction, flexion, extension, and rotation of arm
Latissimus dorsi	midback and lower back; connects lower vertebral column and lower ribs to the humerus	extension, adduction, and medial rotation of arm
Elbow Muscles		
Biceps brachii	anterior arm; connects scapula to radius	flexion, and assists with supination of forearm
Brachialis	connects upper arm to forearm (humerus to ulna)	flexion of forearm
Brachioradialis	connects upper arm to forearm (humerus to radius)	flexion of forearm
Triceps brachii	posterior arm; connects scapula and humerus to ulna	extension of forearm

Figure 5.22

Goodheart-Willcox Publisher

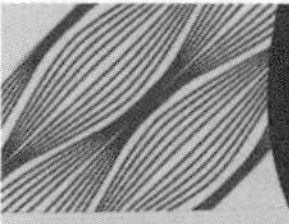

LIFE SPAN DEVELOPMENT: *Muscle*

Human muscle tissue begins to form from dividing stem cells in the embryo in a process known as *myogenesis*. The embryonic stem cells destined to become muscle cells are called *myoblasts*. The myoblasts fuse into *myotubes* that contain multiple nuclei. These myotubes mature into muscle cells, or **myocytes**. The myocytes are specialized as skeletal, cardiac, or smooth muscle cells, that then organize into tissues and organs. By the 16th week of pregnancy, the muscles are sufficiently developed that fetal movements can be felt.

The number of muscle fibers in each person is genetically determined, and does not change with age, except for occasional loss of fibers resulting from injury. Although fiber number does not change, the skeletal muscle fibers grow in length and diameter from birth to adulthood.

An infant's ability to make purposeful movements depends on the development of the nervous system, as well as the development of muscular strength. Because of this interrelationship between the nervous and muscular systems, they are often referred to collectively as the *neuromuscular system*. Neuromuscular development in the infant and toddler proceeds in a superior to inferior direction through the body. Babies can raise their heads before they can sit and can sit before beginning to crawl. The ability to stand and walk requires the ability to balance in an upright position, as well as sufficient leg strength and motor control.

During childhood, neuromuscular control continues to develop. Generally, gross motor skills are acquired before fine motor skills. A task such as tying a shoe is challenging for a young child but is readily mastered once the neuromuscular system has reached a sufficient level of maturity. Peak development of motor control is acquired during adolescence.

The strength of boys and girls is essentially equal during preadolescence, increasing as muscle mass increases. With the onset of puberty, strength development accelerates in boys, while girls continue to develop strength at approximately the same rate as during the preadolescent years. In the absence of strength training, peak strength is attained at approximately age 20 in women and between the ages of 20 and 30 in men.

As people age, they experience an associated loss of muscle mass and strength known as *sarcopenia*. Beginning in the 30s, skeletal muscle mass and strength decline in a linear fashion, with up to 50% of muscle mass being lost by age 70. Sarcopenia is brought on by a complex host of factors, including hormonal changes, decline in neuromuscular functionality, and fatty infiltration of muscle, all exacerbated by physical inactivity. Interventions to address the condition include exercise and proper nutrition. Adults of any age can increase muscle fiber diameter and strength by resistance training with just a few repetitions of heavy loads on a regular basis over time.

Life Span Review

1. Briefly describe the development of cells into myocytes in the embryo and fetus.
2. What can people do as they age to minimize the effects of sarcopenia?

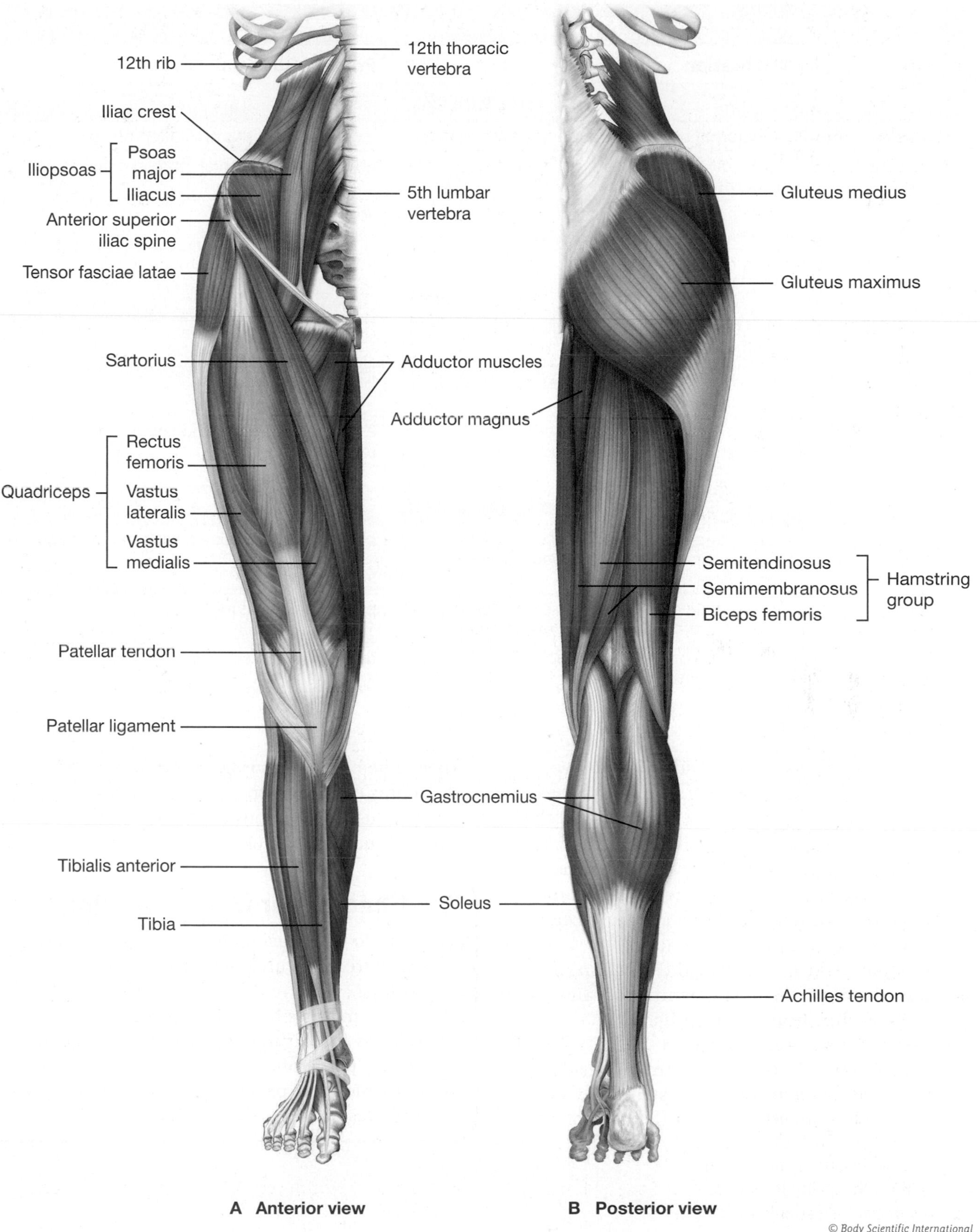

Figure 5.23 Major muscles of the lower limb. *Are the hamstring muscles part of an anterior or posterior muscle group?*

Muscles of the Lower Limb		
Muscle	**Location**	**Primary Functions**
Hip Muscles		
Gluteus maximus	external buttocks; connects pelvis to femur	extension and lateral rotation of leg
Gluteus medius	directly under maximus; connects ilium of pelvis to femur	abduction and medial rotation of leg
Iliopsoas	anterior groin; connects ilium and lower vertebrae to femur	flexion of leg at hip
Adductor muscles	anterior-medial thigh	adduction and medial rotation of leg
Knee Muscles		
Quadriceps	anterior thigh; connects ilium and proximal femur to tibia	extension of leg at knee
Hamstrings	posterior thigh; connect ischium to tibia and fibula	flexion of leg at knee
Sartorius	long, straplike muscle that crosses anterior thigh obliquely; connects ilium to distal tibia	assists with flexion, abduction, and lateral rotation of thigh
Ankle/Foot Muscles		
Gastrocnemius	prominent muscle on posterior calf; connects femur to calcaneus (heel bone) via Achilles tendon	plantar flexion of foot, flexion of leg at knee
Soleus	underlies gastrocnemius on posterior calf; connects fibula and tibia to calcaneus	plantar flexion of foot
Tibialis anterior	anterior lower leg; connects tibia to tarsal and metatarsal bones of foot	dorsiflexion and inversion of foot

Figure 5.24

Goodheart-Willcox Publisher

Notice in **Figures 5.23** and **5.24** the two muscle groups on the anterior side and posterior side of the thigh. The anterior group, called the *quadriceps*, includes the rectus femoris, vastus lateralis, vastus medialis, and vastus intermedius, which lies under the rectus femoris. These four muscles are often referred to as a group because they all attach to the patellar tendon.

The posterior group, called the *hamstrings*, includes the biceps femoris, semimembranosus (sehm-ee-mehm-bray-NOH-suhs), and semitendinosus (sehm-ee-tehn-di-NOH-suhs). What these muscles have in common, besides their general location, is strong, stringlike tendons that can be felt on either side of the back of the knee. The name *hamstrings* comes from the fact that hams consist of thigh and hip muscles, and butchers use the tendons of these muscles to hang the hams for smoking.

Check Your Understanding

1. How do the attachments for facial muscles differ from the attachments for other muscles?
2. Which muscles help with posture?
3. What is sacrificed at the shoulder to allow greater range of motion?
4. For which two primary functions is the lower limb designed?

LESSON 5.3 Review and Assessment

Mini Glossary

Make sure that you know the meaning of each key term.

abduction movement of a body segment away from the body in the frontal plane

adduction movement of a body segment closer to the body in the frontal plane

circumduction rotational movement of a body segment such that the end of the segment traces a circle

dorsiflexion movement of the top of the foot toward the lower leg

eversion movement in which the sole of the foot is rolled outward

extension movement that returns a body segment to anatomical position in the sagittal plane

flexion forward movement of a body segment away from anatomical position in the sagittal plane

hyperextension backward movement of a body segment past anatomical position in the sagittal plane

insertion muscle attachment to a bone that tends to move when the muscle contracts

inversion movement in which the sole of the foot is rolled inward

lateral rotation outward (lateral) movement of a body segment in the transverse plane

medial rotation inward (medial) movement of a body segment in the transverse plane

myocytes mature muscle cells

opposition touching any of your four fingers to your thumb; this movement enables grasping of objects

origin muscle attachment to a relatively fixed structure

plantar flexion downward motion of the foot away from the lower leg

pronation medial rotation of the forearm (palm down)

radial deviation rotation of the hand toward the thumb

supination lateral rotation of the forearm (palm up)

ulnar deviation rotation of the hand toward the little finger

Know and Understand

1. What are the directions of movement for the sagittal, frontal, and transverse planes?
2. Describe hyperextension.
3. Describe the difference between abduction and adduction.
4. What types of movements are enabled by the muscles of the trunk?
5. Using the drawings and tables in this lesson, identify the agonist/antagonist pairs for abduction/adduction of the hip and plantar flexion/dorsiflexion of the ankle.

Analyze and Apply

6. What type of motor units do you think the forearm and hands have? Why?
7. Compare and contrast inversion and eversion of the foot and supination and pronation of the hand.
8. Which joints in the upper and lower limbs can perform flexion and extension?
9. What position are you in if all of your joints that can perform flexion do so at the same time?
10. A patient is diagnosed with sarcopenia. How could you explain sarcopenia to the patient, and what suggestions might you make?
11. The rotator cuff is a combination of muscles and tendons located in the shoulder that allow for stable movements of the shoulder and upper arm. Find out more about the rotator cuff. Which muscles are included? What is the function of each muscle?
12. One of the adductor muscles in the thigh is the gracilis muscle. What are the attachments of this muscle, and what is its purpose?

IN THE LAB

13. Try writing the answers to one of the questions in this lesson review without using your thumb. Why is opposition important?
14. In a push-up, what movements are happening at the shoulder and elbow when you are moving up? Which muscles are performing these movements? What movements occur when you move down? Which muscles cause these movements?
15. Demonstrate the position that would result if all of your joints that can perform flexion did so at the same time.
16. Develop a graphic that identifies the name of the muscle, the directional motion, location, and function of each of the major muscle groups in the body.

LESSON 5.4

Common Muscle Injuries and Disorders

Before You Read

Try to answer the following questions before you read this lesson.

- What causes muscle cramps?
- Which individuals are at greatest risk for developing low back pain?

Lesson Objectives

- Explain the causes of common muscle injuries.
- Describe the causes and symptoms of muscular dystrophy and hernias.

Key Terms

contusion
delayed-onset muscle soreness (DOMS)
hernia
muscle cramps
muscle strain
muscular dystrophy (MD)
myositis ossificans
shin splint
tendinitis
tendinosis

CLINICAL CASE STUDY

As a freshman, Stella competes for her high school junior varsity swim team in the freestyle and butterfly events. She has enjoyed swimming since early childhood, but prior to starting high school she had not swum competitively. Recently, her shoulders have become painful following team practices. On weekends when she can rest, the pain subsides. As you read this section, try to determine which of the following conditions Stella most likely has.

A. muscle strain
B. muscle cramp
C. muscle contusion
D. tendinitis, specifically swimmer's shoulder

Although most problems with muscles are due to injury, some disorders are inherited or congenital (present at birth). This lesson describes some of the common muscle injuries and disorders.

Common Muscle Injuries

Although common, most muscle injuries are relatively minor. Fortunately, the healthy human body has considerable ability to self-repair a variety of injuries, including those to muscles. The etiology (cause), strategies for prevention, pathology (clinical characteristics), diagnosis (keys for identifying the condition), and common treatments for these muscle injuries are summarized in **Figure 5.25**.

Strains

A **muscle strain** happens when a muscle is stretched beyond its usual limits. Someone who has a large degree of flexibility at a particular joint is at much lower risk of straining those muscles than someone with extremely "tight" muscles crossing that same joint.

Another factor in muscle strains is the speed with which the muscles are stretched. Many strains to the hamstrings, for example, result from participating in activities in which the individual is running, accelerating, and changing direction all at the same time. When the muscle group is overstretched, a strain results.

Strains are classified as Grade I, II, or III:

- Grade I (mild): muscle tightness the day after the injury, but nothing more
- Grade II (moderate): pain caused by a partial tear in the muscle; associated weakness and temporary loss of function may also occur
- Grade III (severe): significantly greater damage and symptoms than in Grades I and II; involve a tearing of the muscle, loss of function, internal bleeding, and swelling

Common Muscle Injuries					
	Etiology	**Prevention**	**Pathology**	**Diagnosis**	**Treatment**
Muscle strain	overstretching of a muscle-tendon unit	stretching and strengthening exercises	ranges from muscle tightness to loss of function, internal bleeding, swelling	physical exam, ultrasound	R.I.C.E. (rest, ice, compression, and elevation)
Myositis ossificans	error in healing of a deep muscle contusion causes calcium to form within muscle	wear appropriate padding for contact sports	warmth, swelling, a lump at the injury site, decreased range of motion	physical exam, imaging test	R.I.C.E.
Muscle cramps	unknown; possibly electrolyte imbalance, deficiency in calcium, magnesium, or potassium; dehydration	maintain hydration during physical activity	pain and muscle spasm	physical exam	rehydration, rest
Whiplash injuries	abnormal motion of the cervical spine, typically from being rear-ended in an automobile accident	Be careful!	neck muscle pain; pain or numbness in shoulders, arms, and hands; headache	physical exam, imaging to check for fracture	rest, pain medication, stretching exercises for neck muscles
Fibromyalgia	pain, sleep problems, fatigue, memory loss	none	general musculoskeletal pain, fatigue, cognitive issues	widespread pain for >3 months with no other cause	medication, exercise, stress reduction, therapy

Figure 5.25 *Goodheart-Willcox Publisher*

Strains of the hamstrings are a frequent problem for athletes because these injuries are slow to heal and tend to recur. One-third of all hamstring strains recur within the first year of returning to a sport or an activity.

A regular program of stretching and strengthening exercises can help prevent muscle strains. This is especially important for a muscle that has been previously strained. For more severe strains, a physician will perform a physical exam and possibly an ultrasound to make the diagnosis. Treatment for a strain typically consists of R.I.C.E. (rest, ice, compression, and elevation). Extremely serious strains involving significant tearing of a muscle or tendon may require surgical repair.

Contusions and Myositis Ossificans

A **contusion** is a bruise or bleeding within a muscle, resulting from an impact. Sometimes when a hard impact causes a deep muscle contusion, a more serious condition, called **myositis ossificans** (migh-oh-SIGH-tis ah-SIF-i-kanz), can develop.

Myositis ossificans involves the formation of a calcium mass within the muscle over a period of three to four weeks. Due to an error in the healing process, muscle cells are replaced by immature bone cells at the site of the injury After six or seven weeks, the mass usually begins to dissolve and is resorbed by the body. In some cases, a bony lesion may remain in the muscle.

The symptoms of myositis ossificans may include warmth, swelling, a lump at the injury site, and decreased range of motion. As healing progresses there may also be an increase, rather than the usual decrease, in pain.

Physicians use imaging tests to detect the presence of calcium within a muscle. When myositis ossificans is detected, treatment consists of R.I.C.E along with gentle stretching.

Cramps

Muscle cramps involve moderate to severe muscle spasms that cause pain. The cause of cramps is unknown; in fact, there may be numerous causes. Some of the possible causes include an electrolyte imbalance; deficiency in calcium, magnesium, or potassium; and dehydration.

Whiplash Injuries

Whiplash injuries to the neck are common, often resulting from automobile accidents in which the victim's car was rear-ended. Such injuries result from abnormal motion of the cervical vertebrae, accompanied by rapid, forceful contractions of the neck muscles as the neuromuscular system attempts to stabilize and protect the spine. Symptoms include neck muscle pain; pain or numbness extending down the shoulders, arms, and hands; and headache. Treatment includes rest, followed by stretching exercises for the neck muscles, and medication or injections for pain.

Check Your Understanding

1. Describe the differences among the three classifications of muscle strains.
2. Why are athletes more likely than others to have problems with strains?
3. What causes contusions? Give an example.
4. What are possible causes of cramps?
5. What is the role of the neuromuscular system in whiplash injuries?

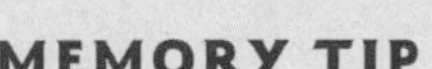

MEMORY TIP

The suffix *-itis* means "inflammation." You will learn about numerous conditions that involve inflammation of a part of the body. The names for all of those conditions contain the *-itis* suffix.

Overuse Injuries

Some muscle injuries are specifically related to overuse. The same action that may be perfectly normal when taken occasionally may injure a muscle if the action is repeated or taken to an extreme. The table in **Figure 5.26** describes common muscle overuse injuries.

Delayed-Onset Muscle Soreness

Muscle soreness is common and typically arises shortly after unaccustomed activity. **Delayed-onset muscle soreness (DOMS)** follows participation in a particularly long or strenuous activity, with the soreness typically beginning 24 to 72 hours after the activity. Eccentric exercise, in which the muscles are being stretched as they contract, is especially likely to cause the condition. DOMS involves multiple, microscopic tears in the muscle tissue and causes inflammation, pain, swelling, and stiffness. Rest and massage are the usual treatments.

Common Muscle Overuse Injuries

	Etiology	Prevention	Pathology	Diagnosis	Treatment
Delayed-onset muscle soreness (DOMS)	unaccustomed activity causes microscopic tears in the muscle	avoid a dramatic increase in exercise	inflammation, pain, swelling, and stiffness	physical exam	rest, massage
Tendinitis and tendinosis	acute and overuse injuries to tendons, facilitated by aging, diabetes, and rheumatoid arthritis	avoid overuse of muscles	tendinitis: inflammation, pain, swelling tendinosis: pain	physical exam	rest, ice, pain medication
Shoulder rotational injuries	repetitive, forceful overhead motions at the shoulder	condition the shoulder muscles, use proper motion mechanics	pain and stiffness of shoulder muscles	physical exam	rest, ice, surgical repair if necessary
Elbow overuse injuries	repetitive motions of the wrist and hand that overload the muscles crossing the elbow	stretching and strengthening of the forearm muscles	pain and inflammation on the medial or lateral side of the elbow	physical exam	rest, pain medication

Figure 5.26 Goodheart-Willcox Publisher

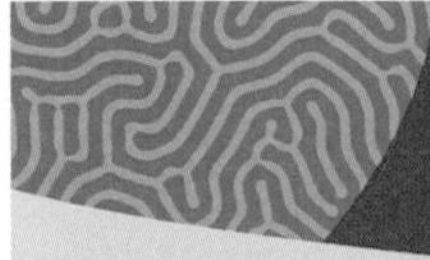

What Research Tells Us

...about Low Back Pain (LBP)

Low back pain (LBP) is a major health problem. Approximately 80%–85% of people experience it at some time during their lives.

In addition, back injuries are the most common and most expensive of all worker's compensation claims. Second only to the common cold in causing absences from work, the incidence of LBP has steadily increased in the United States for the past 15 years. This is likely due, in part, to the increasing proportion of overweight and obese individuals. LBP is significantly associated with excess weight in both men and women of all ages.

Nearly 30% of children in the United States also experience LBP. The likelihood that children will experience LBP increases with age. By age 16, the percentage of children with LBP is similar to that of adults. Children who are more physically active tend to incur LBP more often than sedentary children.

Athletes of all ages have a much higher incidence of LBP than nonathletes. In fact, more than 9% of college athletes receive treatment for LBP. Gymnasts (particularly those who are female) have much higher incidences of LBP. Studies show that as many as 85% of competitive gymnasts experience this health problem (**Figure 5.27**).

What causes LBP? Although injuries and certain disorders may cause LBP, 60% of LBP is of unknown origin. Low back muscle strains, resulting in soreness and stiffness, can be one source of LBP. In almost all cases of LBP, the low back muscles are sore and painful.

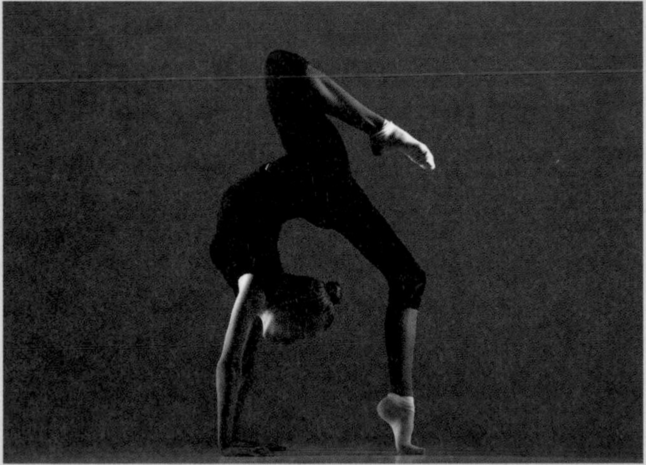

fizkes/Shutterstock.com

Figure 5.27 Repeated, extreme lumbar hyperextension increases the likelihood that female gymnasts will develop low back pain.

In some cases this pain is caused by muscle injury. In many cases, however, the pain may be due to what is called a *sympathetic contraction* of the low back muscles. This means that the muscles involuntarily contract as the body attempts to stabilize an underlying injury of the spinal column.

Fortunately, most LBP is self-limiting—75% of patients are back to normal within three weeks. Approximately 90% have recovered within two months, with or without medical treatment.

What can you do to avoid developing LBP? Known risk factors for LBP include the following:

- sitting for prolonged periods
- standing for long periods in an unchanging position
- working in an unnatural posture
- working with one hand
- encountering sudden or unexpected motions
- performing heavy manual labor

Taller and heavier individuals are at increased risk for developing LBP. Cigarette smoking is also associated with increased risk of LBP, most likely because habitual smoking can contribute to degeneration of the intervertebral discs.

Taking It Further

1. Why do you think LBP is so common? Based on what you have read about LBP, do you think a higher or lower percentage of people will have LBP in the future? Explain your reasoning.
2. What do you think *self-limiting* means? Do some research, write a definition, and then give some examples of self-limiting behavior.
3. Conduct a survey among people you know to find out who has and who has not experienced LBP. Include males and females, athletes and nonathletes, and people of various ages in your survey. What conclusions can you draw from your survey about the occurrence of LBP?
4. One common treatment for low back pain is transcutaneous electrical nerve stimulation (TENS). Find out more about this treatment. How does it help? What are its limitations?

Tendinitis and Tendinosis

Tendons are the bands of tough, fibrous connective tissue that connect muscles to bones. **Tendinitis** is inflammation of a tendon, usually accompanied by pain and swelling.

Both acute and overuse injuries can cause tendinitis. The condition can also occur with aging, as the tendon wears and elasticity decreases. Diseases such as diabetes and rheumatoid arthritis can also promote the development of tendinitis. Tendinitis can occur in any part of the body, but common sites involving injury include the shoulder, elbow, wrist, and the Achilles tendon of the heel.

Treatment of tendinitis includes rest and application of heat or cold. Pain relievers such as aspirin and ibuprofen can reduce pain and inflammation. In severe cases, steroid injections into the tendon can help control pain. Once the pain is reduced, physical therapy to stretch and strengthen both muscle and tendon promotes healing and can help prevent reinjury.

If untreated, chronic tendinitis can progress to **tendinosis**. Tendinosis, or degeneration of a tendon, is believed to be caused by microtears in the tendon connective tissue that decrease the tendon's strength. This weakened condition increases the likelihood that the tendon will rupture.

Although the condition is painful, no inflammation is present, unlike with tendinitis. Once tendinosis has developed, recovery takes months to years of minimal use. In many cases physical therapy can help.

Rotational Injuries of the Shoulder

Repetition of forceful overhead motions at the shoulder (as in throwing, spiking in volleyball, and serving in tennis) can lead to tendinitis or tears of the muscles and muscle tendons surrounding the shoulder (**Figure 5.28**). A similar condition among competitive swimmers is known as *swimmer's shoulder.*

Improper motion mechanics increases the likelihood of these types of shoulder injuries. The symptoms are pain and stiffness with overhead or rapid movements. If not treated, the pain can become constant. Treatment includes application of ice, rest, and, when necessary, surgical repair.

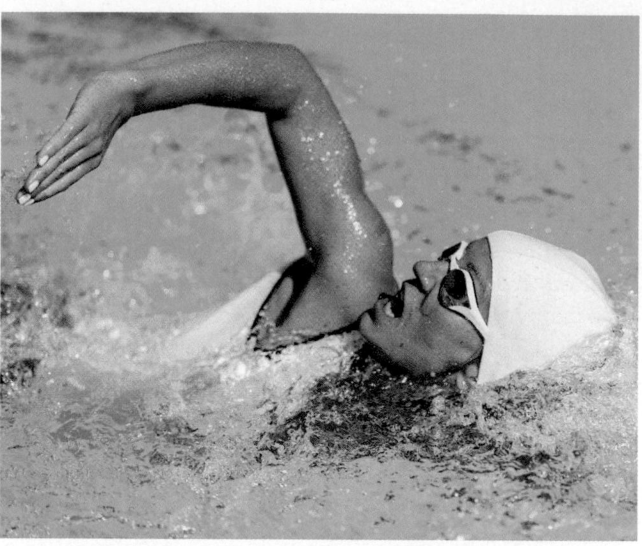

Microgen/Shutterstock.com

Figure 5.28 Sports such as swimming can sometimes lead to overuse injuries of the shoulder muscles. *What other activities can cause injuries to the shoulder muscles?*

Overuse Injuries of the Elbow

Epicondylitis (ehp-ih-kahn-di-LIGH-tis) is a painful condition resulting from tendinitis and sometimes microtearing of the muscle tendons that cross the lateral and medial epicondyles of the elbow. It is caused by repetitive motions of the wrist and hand that overload the muscles crossing the elbow. If unchecked, the condition can worsen, leading to swelling and scarring of the tendons near the elbow. Lateral epicondylitis, which is reported in 30%–40% of tennis players, is known as *tennis elbow,* although it also occurs in activities such as swimming, fencing, and repetitious hammering. Medial epicondylitis, known as *Little Leaguer's elbow,* can result from repeated throwing, especially with improper pitching mechanics. Both lateral and medial epicondylitis commonly occur among amateur golfers.

Rest and over-the-counter pain medications are commonly used to treat epicondylitis. A physical therapist can also prescribe exercises to stretch and strengthen the forearm muscles.

Shin Splints

The term **shin splint** is often used to describe pain localized along the medial, anterior aspect of the tibia, or shin bone. The medical term for this injury is *medial tibial stress syndrome*. The condition is an overuse injury that typically arises from running or dancing—particularly running on a hard surface or uphill. The cause of the pain is believed to be microdamage to the muscle tendons that attach to the tibia or inflammation of the periosteum of the tibia. The muscles potentially involved include the soleus, tibialis anterior, and extensor digitorum.

Rest and ice application can be used to treat shin splints. Wearing well-cushioned shoes and avoiding dramatic increases in activity can help to avoid recurrence of shin splints.

Check Your Understanding

1. What is the difference between tendinitis and tendinosis?
2. What causes swimmer's shoulder?
3. What is the difference between tennis elbow and Little Leaguer's elbow?
4. What strategies can help to prevent shin splints?

Muscle Disorders

In addition to injuries, the muscular system is subject to a variety of disorders and conditions. Two of the more common disorders are discussed in this section. The etiology, strategies for prevention, pathology, diagnosis, and common treatments for these muscle disorders are summarized in **Figure 5.29**.

Muscular Dystrophy

Muscular dystrophy (MD) is a group of similar, inherited disorders characterized by progressively worsening muscle weakness and loss of muscle tissue. In muscular dystrophy, genetic abnormalities interfere with the production of proteins needed to form healthy muscle. Depending on the specific type, the onset of MD may occur during either childhood or adulthood, and the symptoms vary.

Some forms of MD affect only certain muscle groups, whereas other forms affect all of the muscles. The primary sign of MD is progressive muscle weakness. The more severe types of MD begin in childhood; symptoms may include intellectual disability, delayed development of motor skills, frequent falling, drooling, and drooping of the eyelids. Some forms of MD also affect the heart muscle, resulting in an irregular heartbeat.

Common Muscle Disorders

	Etiology	Prevention	Pathology	Diagnosis	Treatment
Muscular dystrophy	inherited through genetics	none	progressive muscular weakness; other symptoms may include intellectual disability, delayed development of motor skills, frequent falling, drooling, drooping of the eyelids, irregular heartbeat	physical exam, blood test for enzyme levels and genetics, electromyography test for muscle function, muscle biopsy, tests for heart and lung function	medications, physical and occupational therapy, surgical and other procedures
Hernia	no specific cause, but can be caused by any activity or medical problem that increases pressure inside the abdominal cavity	none	a balloon-like section of the abdominal cavity lining protrudes through a hole or weakened section of the muscles in the abdomen	physical exam	surgery, as required

Figure 5.29 *Goodheart-Willcox Publisher*

There are no known cures for the various muscular dystrophies; the goal of treatment is to control symptoms. Some types of muscular dystrophy lead to a shortened life; others cause little disability, allowing for a normal life span (**Figure 5.30**).

Depending on symptoms, physicians employ an array of tests to assist with diagnosis and proper treatment of muscular dystrophy. These include blood tests for enzyme levels and genetics, an electromyography test for muscle function, a muscle biopsy, and tests for heart and lung function (**Figure 5.31**). Treatments include medications, physical and occupational therapy, and surgical or other procedures, as appropriate.

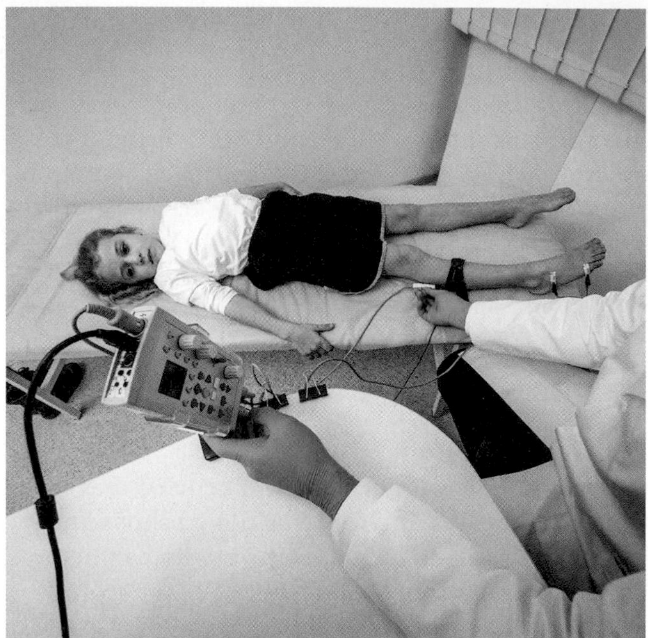

Romaset/Shutterstock.com

Figure 5.31 Electromyography is often used to diagnose and monitor patients who have muscular dystrophy.

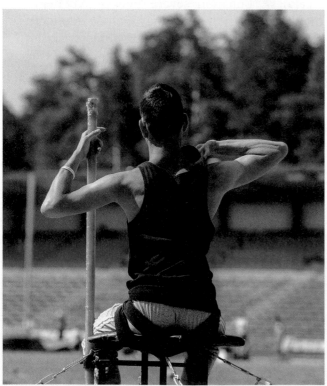

sportpoint/Shutterstock.com

Figure 5.30 People with some forms of muscular dystrophy are able to adapt partly or fully to lead active lives.

Hernia

A **hernia** is a balloon-like section of the abdominal cavity lining that protrudes through a hole or weakened section of the muscles in the abdomen. A hernia can be caused by heavy lifting or by any activity or medical problem that increases pressure inside the abdominal cavity. In most cases, however, no specific cause is evident. Some hernias are present at birth, and some occur in infants and children. A hernia that is present at birth may not become noticeable until later in life.

Most hernias produce no symptoms, although some are accompanied by discomfort or pain that intensifies with heavy lifting or other activities that produce abdominal strain. A large hernia may "strangulate," or cut off the blood supply to the tissue inside the hernia. A strangulated hernia requires immediate surgery.

Small hernias that cause no symptoms do not necessarily require treatment. Larger hernias and those that cause discomfort can be permanently remedied with surgery.

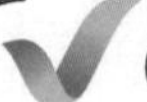

Check Your Understanding

1. What are the characteristics of MD?
2. What are the different forms that MD may take?
3. What causes a hernia?

LESSON 5.4 Review and Assessment

Mini Glossary

Make sure that you know the meaning of each key term.

contusion the bruises or bleeding within a muscle that result from an impact

delayed-onset muscle soreness (DOMS) muscle pain that follows participation in a particularly long or strenuous activity; begins 24–73 hours later, and involves multiple, microscopic tears in the muscle tissue that cause inflammation, pain, swelling, and stiffness

hernia a balloon-like section of the lining of the abdominal cavity that protrudes through a hole or weakened section of the muscles

muscle cramps moderate to severe muscle spasms that cause pain

muscle strain an injury that occurs when a muscle is stretched beyond the limits to which it is accustomed

muscular dystrophy (MD) a group of similar, inherited disorders characterized by progressively worsening muscle weakness and loss of muscle tissue

myositis ossificans a condition in which a calcium mass forms within a muscle three to four weeks after a muscle injury

shin splint the name for pain localized to the anterior lower leg

tendinitis inflammation of a tendon, usually accompanied by pain and swelling

tendinosis degeneration of a tendon believed to be caused by microtears in the tendon connective tissue

Know and Understand

1. What causes a muscle strain?
2. What can you do to help avoid muscle strains?
3. What is myositis ossificans?
4. What do common shoulder, elbow, and shin injuries have in common?
5. What is the main cause of DOMS?
6. Why is it important to treat chronic tendinitis?
7. What is believed to be the main cause of shin splints?
8. Name an activity often associated with hernias.

Analyze and Apply

9. If obesity is a major cause of LBP, why would gymnasts experience this health problem?
10. How do poor mechanics contribute to overuse injuries such as swimmer's shoulder and tennis elbow? Describe and analyze the effect of torque in these injuries.
11. What types of muscle can be affected by muscular dystrophy?
12. Explain the differences between a physical therapist and an occupational therapist.

IN THE LAB

13. Interview a physical therapist or an athletic trainer. Ask the person to describe a typical day at work. Here are some questions you might ask:
    - What is the work environment like?
    - What are the job duties?
    - What kinds of injuries are dealt with?
    - What other types of professionals does he or she work with?

    Report your findings to the class, giving reasons why you would or would not want to pursue a career similar to that of the person you interviewed. You may want to incorporate additional research from the Career Corner activity on the next two pages into your report.
14. Research shin-splint taping. Determine its purpose and how it helps the athlete.
15. With a partner, research American Red Cross guidelines for splinting muscle injuries. Demonstrate an anatomic splint on your partner. Be sure to follow the guidelines. Explain what you are doing and why as you do it. Next, demonstrate a rigid splint on your partner, following the guidelines. Explain what you are doing and why.
16. Back injuries are the most common and most expensive of all Worker's Compensation claims. Conduct research to find out which occupations have the highest incidence of back injuries. Why might these occupations put people at greater risk for back injury?

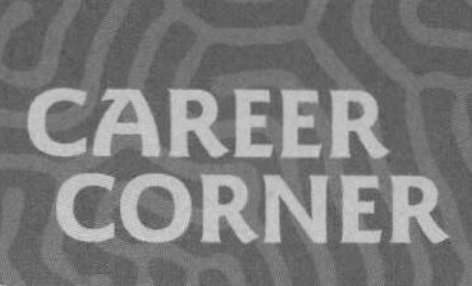

Anatomy & Physiology at Work

Many challenging and rewarding careers involve treating and rehabilitating the muscles of the body. Two common career options are physical therapist and athletic trainer.

Physical Therapist

Physicians often prescribe physical therapy for patients with muscle injuries. Frequently employed in physical therapy clinics, physical therapists and related professionals treat each patient's condition with appropriate exercise, stretching, and other therapeutic protocols (**Figure 5.32**). Treatment at a physical therapy clinic can last from a few visits to a series of visits over a period of months, depending on the severity of the condition being treated.

Prescribed exercise and stretching regimens are typically progressive in nature, beginning with a relatively easy routine that grows increasingly challenging. All patient activity in the clinic is closely supervised by a physical therapist to ensure that all movements are carried out in the correct directions and through appropriate ranges of motion.

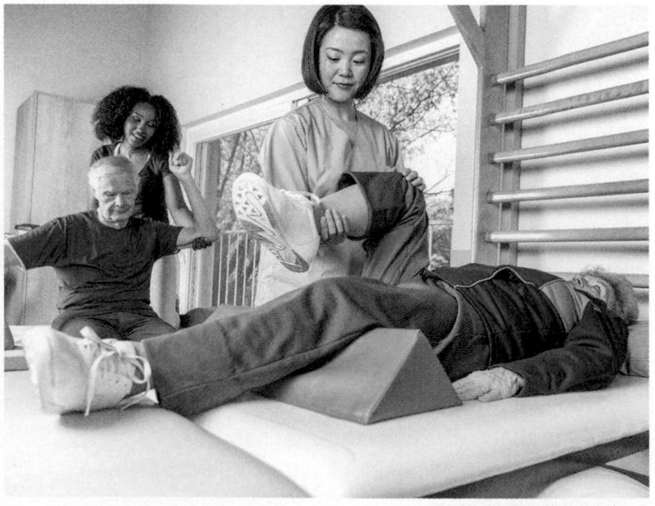

Gagliardilmages/Shutterstock.com

Figure 5.32 Physical therapists assist patients with exercises for range of motion.

The academic degree that physical therapists must earn is the DPT, or Doctor of Physical Therapy. Nationwide, entry into DPT programs is highly competitive. To qualify, students must possess a bachelor's degree and must also have completed prerequisite courses in biology, chemistry, physics, calculus, and human anatomy and physiology, among others. When applying to a DPT program, candidates must provide documentation showing that they have a substantial amount of experience (paid or unpaid) assisting patients in a physical therapy clinic. This documentation ensures that applicants are appropriately familiar with the field of physical therapy. Most DPT programs take approximately three years to complete and require supervised clinical rotations as well as academic coursework. Physical therapists are employed by schools and universities, as well as in hospitals and other clinical environments.

Athletic Trainer

If an injury is related to a sport played at the high school or collegiate level, the first professional to examine the patient will likely be an expert in athletic training (**Figure 5.33**). Athletic trainers are knowledgeable first responders who are trained to apply advanced first aid, as well as to know when immediate referral to emergency care, a physician, or a specialist is necessary.

Athletic trainers are also well qualified to administer rehabilitative treatments when appropriate, typically after the injured athlete has been seen by a physician. Athletic trainers work with active individuals of all ages and physical abilities in industrial settings, gyms, fitness centers, youth athletic leagues, the Special Olympics, and anywhere that people are active.

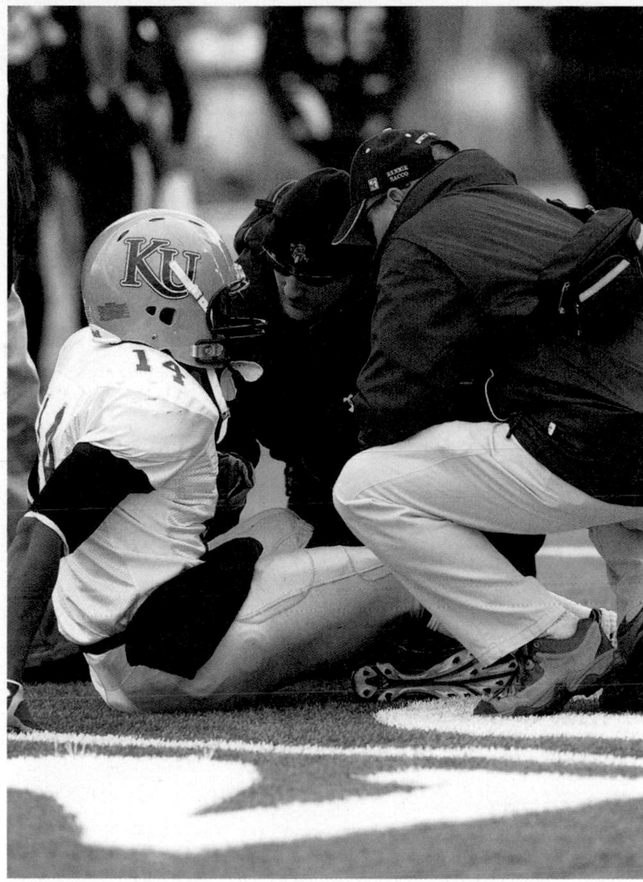

Aspen Photo/Shutterstock.com

Figure 5.33 Athletic trainers work with student athletes to prevent, treat, and rehabilitate injuries.

To become an ATC, or Certified Athletic Trainer, students must complete a master's degree in athletic training and then pass a national certification examination. Programs of study in athletic training include a number of basic science courses, human anatomy and physiology, and in-depth lecture/laboratory courses that cover prevention and treatment of athletic injuries to all parts of the body. Athletic trainers are employed in high schools, colleges and universities, hospitals, and clinics.

Planning for a Health-Related Career

Do some research on career opportunities for physical therapists or athletic trainers. Keep in mind the different levels of education and certifications that are required.

You may want to select a profession from the list of related career options. Using the Internet or resources at your local library, find answers to the following questions:

1. What are the main tasks and responsibilities of an athletic trainer or a physical therapist?
2. What is the outlook for these careers? Are workers in demand, or are jobs dwindling? For complete information, consult the current edition of the *Occupational Outlook Handbook*, published by the US Department of Labor. This handbook is available online or at your local library.
3. What special skills or talents are required? For example, do you need to be capable of lifting? Are you comfortable looking at injuries that may be severe?
4. What personality traits do you think are needed to be successful in these jobs? For instance, both athletic trainers and physical therapist must work closely with their patients. Do you enjoy working with others?
5. Do these careers involve a great deal of routine, or are the day-to-day responsibilities varied?
6. Does the work require long hours, or are these standard, "9-to-5" jobs?
7. What is the salary range for these jobs?
8. What do you think you would like about each career? Is there anything about them that you might dislike?

Related Career Options

- Massage therapist
- Occupational therapist
- Physical therapist assistant
- Recreational therapist
- Rehabilitation counselor

CHAPTER 5

Review

›LESSON 5.1

Muscle Tissue Categories and Functions

Key Points

- The three major categories of muscle fibers are smooth, cardiac, and skeletal (striated), each with a different function.
- Muscles have four common behavioral characteristics: extensibility, elasticity, irritability, and contractility.

Key Terms

agonist
antagonist
aponeurosis
concentric
contractility
eccentric
elasticity
endomysium
epimysium
extensibility
fascicle
irritability
isometric
muscle fiber
perimysium
peristalsis
sarcolemma

›LESSON 5.2

Skeletal Muscle Actions

Key Points

- The motor unit is the functional unit of the neuromuscular system and is made up of the neuron and the muscle fibers that the neuron stimulates. The location at which the neurons and the fibers come together is known as the *neuromuscular junction*.
- Skeletal muscle fibers are divided into fast-twitch fibers, which are powerful and fatigue quickly, and slow-twitch fibers, which are fatigue resistant.
- Muscular strength is determined by measuring torque, muscular power is defined as force × velocity, and muscular endurance is how long a muscle fiber can continuously contract before it fatigues.

Key Terms

acetylcholine
action potential
all-or-none law
axon
axon terminals
cross bridges
fast-twitch
motor neuron
motor unit
neuromuscular junction
parallel
pennate
sarcomeres
slow-twitch
synaptic cleft

›LESSON 5.3

The Major Skeletal Muscles

Key Points

- Directional motions are described using movements in the sagittal, frontal, and transverse planes; some movements are multiplanar.
- The muscles of the head and neck include facial muscles, chewing muscles, and neck muscles.
- Trunk muscles provide stability for the vertebral column and help maintain upright posture.
- Upper limb muscles include the muscles of the shoulder, arm, wrist, and hand.
- Lower limb muscles are designed for standing and walking.

Key Terms

abduction
adduction
circumduction
dorsiflexion
eversion
extension
flexion
hyperextension
insertion
inversion
lateral rotation
medial rotation
myocytes
opposition
origin
plantar flexion
pronation
radial deviation
supination
ulnar deviation

➤ LESSON 5.4

Common Muscle Injuries and Disorders

Key Points

- Common muscle injuries include strains, contusions, myositis ossificans, muscle cramps, and whiplash injuries.
- Overuse muscle injuries include delayed-onset muscle soreness (DOMS), tendinitis, tendinosis, rotational shoulder injuries, overuse injuries of the elbow, and shin splints.
- Muscular dystrophy (MD) and hernia are examples of disorders related to the muscles.

Key Terms

contusion
delayed-onset muscle soreness (DOMS)
hernia
muscle cramps
muscle strain
muscular dystrophy (MD)
myositis ossificans
shin splint
tendinitis
tendinosis

Assessment

➤ LESSON 5.1

Muscle Tissue Categories and Functions

Learning Key Terms and Concepts

1. An individual skeletal muscle cell is referred to as a muscle _____.
   A. aponeurosis
   B. neuron
   C. fiber
   D. axon
2. The three layers of muscle tissue, from the inside out, are the _____.
   A. endomysium, perimysium, epimysium
   B. epimysium, endometrium, perimysium
   C. perimysium, epimysium, endometrium
   D. epimysium, endomysium, perimysium
3. Skeletal muscle is connected to bone by either _____ or aponeuroses.
   A. ligaments
   B. tendons
   C. fascicles
   D. sarcomeres
4. _____ muscle is found in organs and blood vessels.
   A. Cardiac
   B. Skeletal
   C. Striated
   D. Smooth
5. The heart is made up of _____ muscle cells.
   A. cardiac
   B. smooth
   C. striated
   D. skeletal
6. The ability of a muscle and other tissue to be stretched is the behavioral characteristic known as _____.
   A. extensibility
   B. elasticity
   C. irritability
   D. contractility
7. The ability of a muscle to respond to stimuli is the behavioral characteristic known as _____.
   A. extensibility
   B. elasticity
   C. irritability
   D. contractility

Thinking Critically

8. Discuss in depth the differences between concentric, isometric, and eccentric contractions and provide examples of how each one is used in daily life.
9. Describe the pros and cons of body organs being made up exclusively of voluntary muscle (no involuntary muscle). Provide specific examples and some pros and some cons for each.
10. Describe the structure of skeletal muscle.
11. Given what you learned about ATP in this and other chapters, explain how energy is stored and moved around to meet the body's energy needs.

LESSON 5.2

Skeletal Muscle Actions

Learning Key Terms and Concepts

12. A nerve that stimulates skeletal muscle is called a _____.
    A. motor unit
    B. sensory unit
    C. motor neuron
    D. sensory neuron
13. The functional unit of the neuromuscular system is the _____.
    A. motor unit
    B. sensory unit
    C. motor neuron
    D. sensory neuron
14. A(n) _____ is an electrical charge that creates tension within a muscle fiber.
    A. action potential
    B. sarcolemma
    C. cross bridge
    D. antagonist
15. Which type of muscle fibers contract powerfully but fatigue quickly?
    A. fast-twitch
    B. cross bridge
    C. slow-twitch
    D. junctional
16. In _____ muscle fiber architecture, each fiber attaches obliquely to a central tendon, and sometimes attaches to more than one tendon.
    A. parallel
    B. perpendicular
    C. straight
    D. pennate
17. The ability of a muscle to produce tension over a period of time is called muscle _____.
    A. force
    B. strength
    C. endurance
    D. torque

Thinking Critically

18. Discuss muscle fiber arrangements that contribute to the force a muscle can generate.
19. How do you think slow-twitch muscle fibers are usually arranged? Give reasons for your answer.
20. Who generates more power: an Olympic weight lifter who must lift 400 pounds from the ground to a position over his head very rapidly, or a power lifter who must squat down and stand up with 800 pounds on his back? Defend your answer.
21. Discuss how torque is used to measure the strength of a muscle group at a specific joint.

LESSON 5.3

The Major Skeletal Muscles

Learning Key Terms and Concepts

Instructions: Refer to **Figure 5.34**. Write the letter of the name of the muscle on your answer sheet next to the corresponding number.

22. Deltoid _____
23. Abdominal aponeurosis _____
24. Biceps brachii _____
25. Rectus femoris _____
26. Temporalis _____
27. Pectoralis major _____
28. Tibialis anterior _____
29. External oblique _____

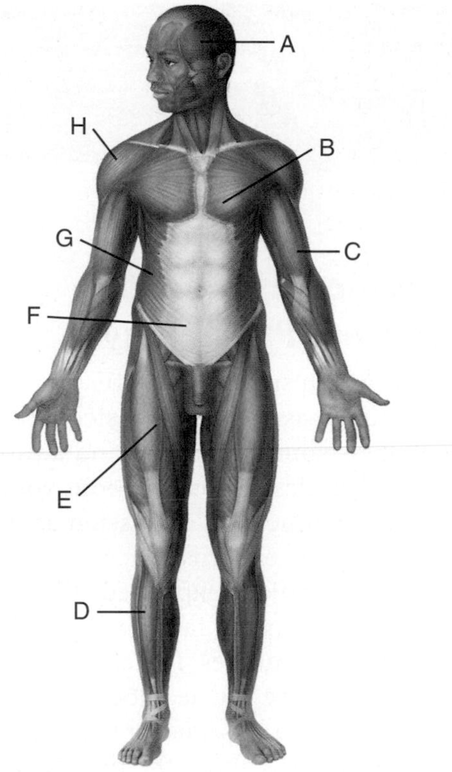

Figure 5.34 © Body Scientific International

Thinking Critically

30. Compare and contrast the sagittal and frontal planes and discuss the movements that occur in each plane.
31. In circumduction, which planes does the limb move through and what actions are used to make the conical/circular motion?
32. Do agonists and antagonists have to perform their actions in the same plane? Why?
33. The strength of males and females is roughly equal during preadolescence. Why does this change with puberty?

LESSON 5.4

Common Muscle Injuries and Disorders

Learning Key Terms and Concepts

34. Muscle _____ may be classified as Grade I, Grade II, or Grade III.
    A. sprain
    B. fatigue
    C. strain
    D. atrophy
35. A _____ is a bruise or bleeding within a muscle.
    A. contusion
    B. hernia
    C. cramp
    D. strain
36. A complication that can arise from a contusion is _____, or the formation of a calcium mass within a muscle.
    A. tendinitis
    B. tendinosis
    C. myositis ossificans
    D. muscular dystrophy
37. The role of the neuromuscular system in a whiplash injury is _____.
    A. an inhibitory response that causes the muscles to relax and the head to move freely
    B. a strong, fast series of contractions that attempt to stabilize the head
    C. not present because the movement is so intense that muscles do not have time to contract
    D. dependent on whether the movement is mediolateral or anteroposterior
38. Lateral epicondylitis is also known as _____.
    A. Little Leaguer's elbow
    B. swimmer's shoulder
    C. jumper's knee
    D. tennis elbow
39. In _____, genetic abnormalities interfere with the production of proteins needed to form healthy muscle.
    A. muscular dystrophy
    B. DOMS
    C. epicondylitis
    D. tendinitis

Thinking Critically

40. If being active is considered healthy, why do active people and athletes have a significantly higher incidence of LBP than inactive, sedentary people?
41. Compare and contrast the responsibilities of physical therapists and athletic trainers. How are they similar? How are they different? Which job seems more appealing to you and why?
42. One common cause of hernia is heavy lifting. What are some other causes?

Building Skills and Connecting Concepts

Analyzing and Evaluating Data

Instructions: Use the bar graph in **Figure 5.35** to answer the following questions.

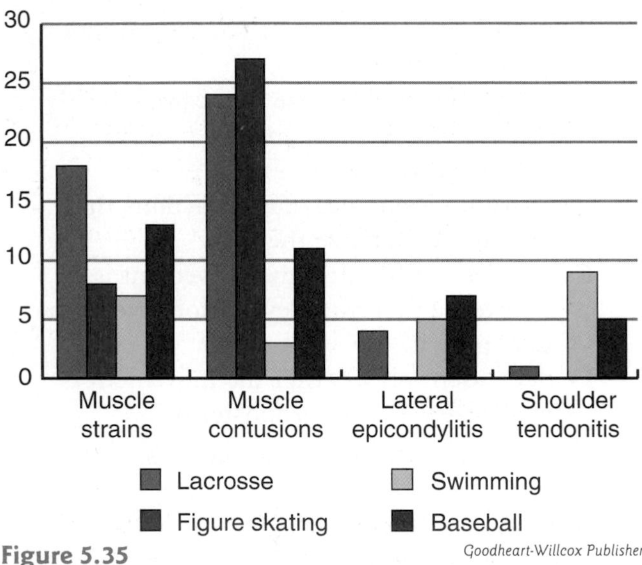

Figure 5.35 Goodheart-Willcox Publisher

43. Which sport involves the most muscle strains?
44. Which sport involves the most muscle contusions?
45. What percentage of swimming injuries is attributed to muscle strains?
46. Overall, which sport has the highest incidence of muscle injuries? Show your work.
47. What is the approximate ratio of muscle contusions in figure skating to muscle contusions in baseball? Show your work.
48. What percentage of lacrosse injuries were due to muscle contusions? Show your work.
49. Compare the total number of swimming injuries with the total number of figure skating injuries.

Communicating about Anatomy & Physiology

50. **Listening** In small groups discuss with your classmates—in basic, everyday language—your knowledge and awareness of your muscles as you go about your daily routine. Conduct this discussion as though you had never read this chapter. Take notes on the observations expressed. Then review the points discussed, factoring in your new knowledge of muscles. Develop a summary of what you have learned about muscles and present it to the class, using the terms that you have learned about the muscular system in this chapter.
51. **Speaking** Pick a figure in this chapter, such as Figure 5.1, 5.4, or 5.6. Working with a partner, tell and then retell the important information being conveyed by that figure. Through your collaboration, develop what you and your partner believe is the most interesting verbal description of the importance of the chosen figure. Present your narration to the class.
52. **Writing** Create a trifold brochure explaining what myositis ossificans is and how to prevent and treat it. Include pictures to clarify the information.
53. **Speaking** Conduct research to find out how many types of muscular dystrophy have been identified. Create an electronic presentation that describes each type, along with its symptoms and any specific treatments. Present your presentation to the class, and be prepared to answer any questions your classmates may have.

Lab Investigations

54. Do a push-up starting in the "up" position. Go down. Which muscles are experiencing concentric contractions? Which muscles are experiencing eccentric contractions? Which muscles are experiencing isometric contractions? Which plane(s) is the shoulder moving through? What actions are occurring at the shoulder, elbow, and wrist? Record your observations and then compare them with those of your classmates in a class discussion.
55. Make a working model of a joint that includes both the agonist and the antagonist muscles. Write a brief explanation of how they work together to produce movement.
56. Try to switch the common (what people think of as normal) origin and insertion points of as many muscles as you can. Focus on the most frequent, everyday movements. Make a list and describe what you did to switch them. Hint: Compare origin and insertion points when doing straight-leg sit-ups and straight-leg leg lifts.
57. With a partner, demonstrate each of the movements listed below and identify the plane they are working in as you demonstrate. Then have your partner perform a return demonstration of the same movements, but in a different plane. Continue until you have run out of planes to demonstrate. Were there any planes in which you could not demonstrate movement? If so, explain. Movements: abduction, adduction, circumduction, dorsiflexion, eversion, extension, flexion, hyperextension, inversion, lateral rotation, medial rotation, opposition, plantar flexion, pronation, radial deviation, supination, ulnar deviation.
58. Consider a patient who is 75 years old and is suffering from sarcopenia. Based on the symptoms listed in this chapter, create a hypothesis about what this patient might be feeling. Test your hypothesis by placing ankle weights and wrist weights on your ankles and wrists. Go for a walk while wearing the weights. Then write a synopsis of your findings. What did it feel like? Compare your answers with your hypothesis.
59. Anyone who has ever had a cast on a broken long bone, such as an arm or leg bone, has probably noticed what happens to the muscles beneath the cast. The muscles atrophy, becoming less flexible and resilient, and they take on a withered appearance because the muscles have not been used for a period of several weeks. Find out more about muscle atrophy. What exactly is the physiological effect of disuse on a muscle? How can this effect be reversed? Create a model with movable parts to show the effect of atrophy on a muscle and how the muscle can be restored.

Building Your Portfolio

60. Take digital photographs of the models and projects you created as you worked through this chapter. Create a document called "The Muscular System" and insert the photographs, along with written descriptions of what the models show and your reasons for creating them using the materials and forms you chose. Add the reports from your laboratory experiments and add this document to your personal portfolio.

CHAPTER

6 The Nervous System

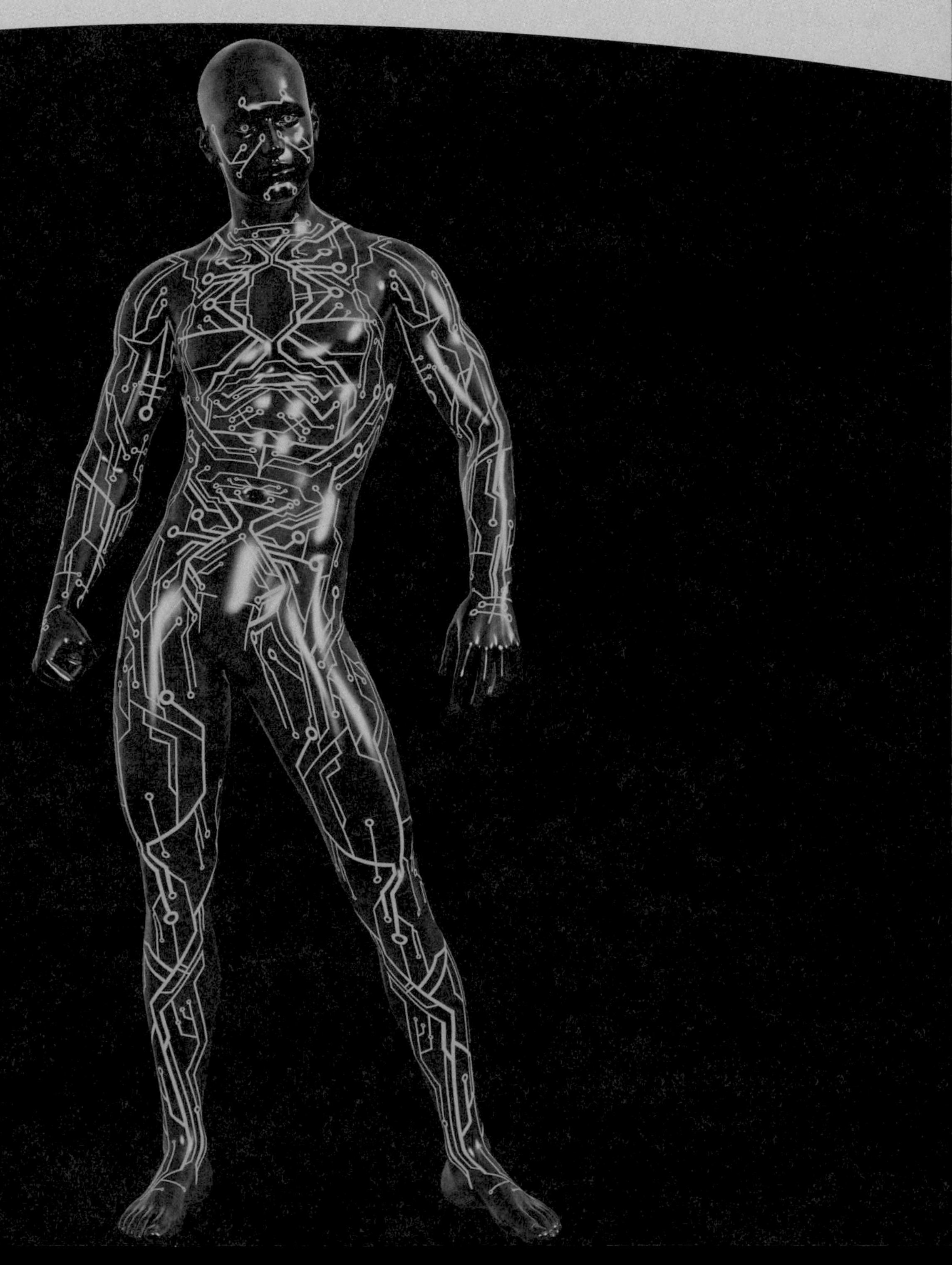

Did you know that the human nervous system runs on electricity?

To understand the nervous system, start by thinking of your body as a biological machine that runs on electricity. In fact, this is true; your body does run on electricity! Your brain is the control center of your biological machine and sends and receives electrical impulses, or signals, throughout your body. The sophisticated communication system that delivers these electrical signals to and from the brain is your nervous system.

With all this electrical activity going on, what keeps the body from lighting up? The answer is that the electrical charges within the human body are very tiny. In the eighteenth century, Italian scientist Luigi Galvani discovered that muscle produces a detectable electric current, or voltage, when developing tension. It was not until the twentieth century, however, that technology became sophisticated enough to detect and record the extremely small electrical charges that move through the nervous system.

What enables the nervous system to perform these various functions so efficiently? This chapter explains the anatomical structures and the functions of the nervous system. It also discusses some common injuries and disorders of the nervous system, along with their symptoms and treatments.

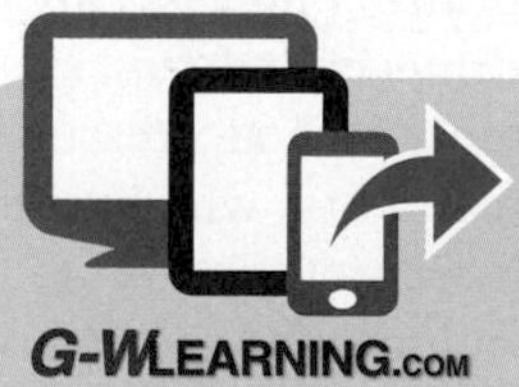

Click on the activity icon or visit www.g-wlearning.com/healthsciences/0202 to access online vocabulary activities using key terms from the chapter.

Chapter 6 Outline

◄ rick eppedio/Shutterstock.com

LESSON 6.1 Overview of the Nervous System

Before You Read

Try to answer the following questions before you read this lesson.

- Why are some body functions under involuntary control?
- Why is the myelin sheath around nerve axons so important?

Lesson Objectives

- Explain the general organization of the nervous system.
- Describe the categories of tissue that make up the nervous system.

Key Terms

afferent nerves
astrocytes
autonomic nervous system
central nervous system (CNS)
dendrites
efferent nerves
ependymal cells
interneurons
microglia
myelin sheath
neuroglia
neurotransmitters
oligodendrocytes
peripheral nervous system (PNS)
satellite cells
Schwann cells
somatic nervous system
synapse

The human nervous system is amazing in its ability to simultaneously direct a whole host of different functions. The nervous system not only controls voluntary movement by activating skeletal muscle, but it also directs the involuntary functions of smooth muscle in internal organs and cardiac muscle in the heart. By automatically controlling the functions of smooth muscle and cardiac muscle, the nervous system ensures that these life functions can occur without conscious thought.

At the same time that your heart is beating and your last meal is making its way through your digestive tract, you may be talking to a friend, walking to a class, or even reading this book. Your senses—the ability to see, hear, smell, taste, feel pressure, and feel pain—all depend on sensory electrical input from specialized receptors.

For the purpose of discussion, the nervous system is organized into structural and functional subdivisions. This organization makes it easier to learn about the activities directed by the various parts of the nervous system, and how these parts interact.

Organization of the Nervous System

The human body's nervous system has two major divisions: the central nervous system and the peripheral nervous system. The peripheral nervous system is further subdivided. **Figure 6.1** illustrates these major divisions and subdivisions.

This section looks at the organization of the nervous system. The structure and function of the two major divisions of the nervous system are examined in greater detail later in the chapter.

Two Major Divisions

The **central nervous system (CNS)** includes the brain and spinal cord. The CNS directs the activity of the entire nervous system. Injuries to either the brain or the spinal cord have serious consequences and can be life threatening. Fortunately, these delicate structures are well protected inside the skull and vertebral column.

The parts of the nervous system other than the brain and spinal cord make up the **peripheral nervous system (PNS)**. The PNS includes spinal nerves that transmit information to and from the spinal cord and cranial nerves that transmit information to and from the brain. The PNS also includes specialized nerve endings called *sensory receptors*, which respond to stimuli such as pressure, pain, or temperature. These receptors, which send information to the CNS for interpretation and further action, are critical to maintain homeostasis in the body. Refer to Chapter 1 for more information about homeostasis.

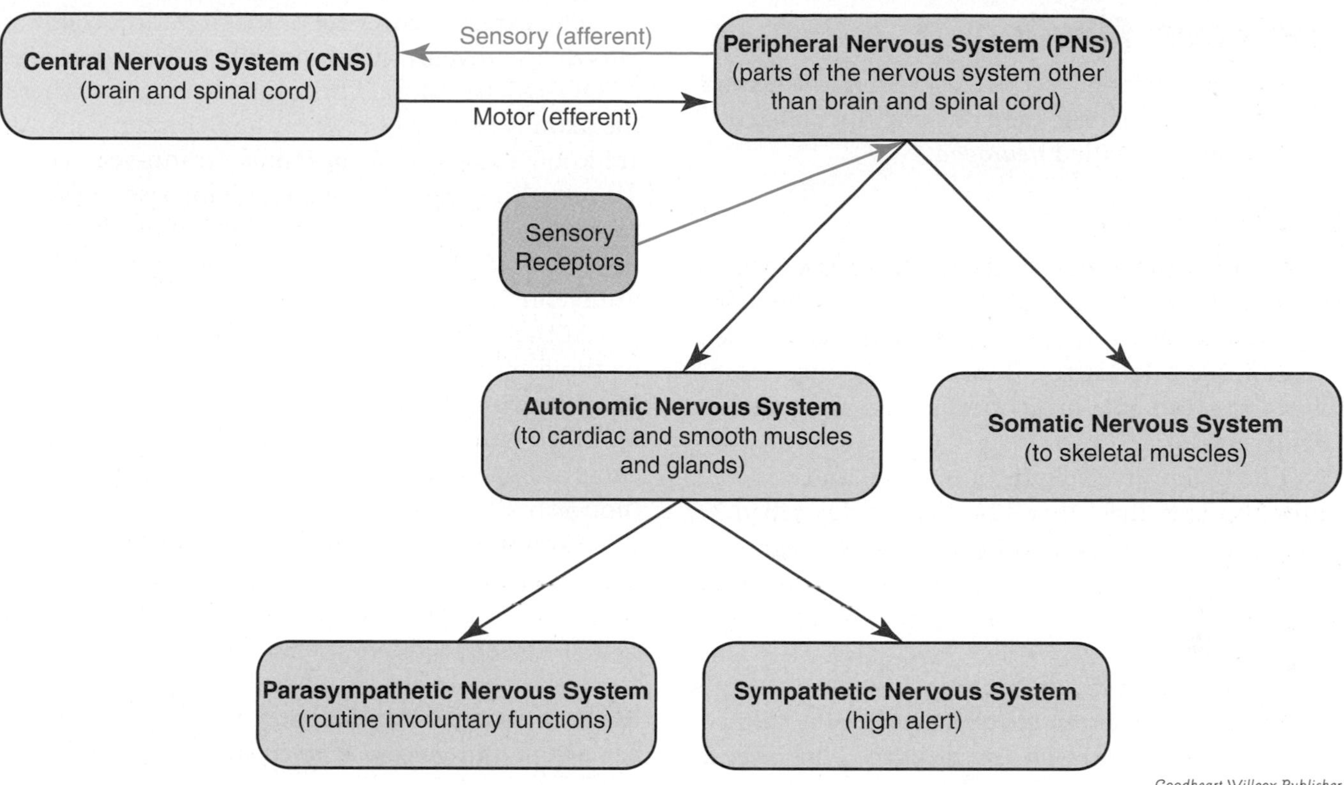

Figure 6.1 This diagram represents the organization of the nervous system and summarizes the relationships among the subdivisions. *If you were asked to put the word* voluntary *into one of the six boxes above and* involuntary *into another one of the boxes, where would you put each word?*

Nerves that transmit impulses from the sensory receptors in the skin, muscles, and joints to the CNS are known as **afferent** (sensory) **nerves**. Those that carry impulses from the CNS out to the muscles and glands are **efferent** (motor) **nerves**.

MEMORY TIP

Afferent nerves tell the body how it is being *affected* by stimuli such as light, heat, and pressure.

Efferent nerves stimulate muscles to produce *effort*.

Types of Efferent Nerves

The efferent, or motor, nerves have two functional subdivisions. The **somatic** (voluntary) **nervous system** stimulates the skeletal muscles, causing them to develop tension. The **autonomic** (involuntary) **nervous system** controls the cardiac muscle of the heart and the smooth muscles of the internal organs. The autonomic nervous system prompts the heart to beat faster when you exercise and causes the smooth muscle activities that move food through the digestive system.

Thanks to your autonomic nervous system, you do not have to think about everyday body functions that sustain life. And under certain circumstances, such as when you inadvertently touch a hot surface, the efferent neurons can trigger involuntary action of the skeletal muscles through a reflex arc. The autonomic nervous system includes *sympathetic* and *parasympathetic* branches, which you will learn about in Lesson 6.4.

Becoming aware of these various subdivisions of the nervous system will help you learn and understand the different functional capabilities of the nervous system. Keep in mind, however, that the nervous system as a whole is a single, remarkably coordinated, functioning unit.

Check Your Understanding

1. Which structures make up the CNS?
2. Which structures make up the PNS?
3. For which function is the somatic nervous system responsible?
4. For which functions is the autonomic nervous system responsible?

Nervous Tissues

Two categories of tissues exist within the nervous system. These include neurons and specialized supporting cells called *neuroglia*.

Neurons

Neurons are nerve cells that transmit information in the form of nerve impulses throughout the body. A typical neuron consists of a cell body surrounded by branching dendrites. The typical neuron also has a long, tail-like projection called an *axon* (**Figure 6.2**).

The cell body includes a nucleus and mitochondria, like all cell bodies, as described in Chapter 2. The **dendrites** (DEHN-drights) collect stimuli and transport them to the cell body. Axons (AK-sahns) transmit impulses away from the cell body.

Within the PNS, the **Schwann** (shwahn) **cells** wrap around the axon, covering most of it with a fatty **myelin** (MIGH-eh-lin) **sheath**. The myelin sheaths serve an important purpose: insulating the axon fibers, which increases the rate of neural impulse transmission. Bundles of nerve fibers (axons) are called *tracts* when they are located in the CNS. In the PNS, bundles of nerve fibers are called *nerves*.

The external covering of the Schwann cell, outside the myelin sheath, is called the *neurilemma* (NOO-ri-LEHM-a). The uninsulated gaps, where the axon is exposed between the Schwann cells, are known as the *nodes of Ranvier* (rahn-vee-AY). The myelin sheaths are white, giving rise to the term *white matter* to describe tracts of myelinated fibers within the CNS. *Gray matter* is the term for unmyelinated nerve fibers.

At the terminal end of each axon, there can be thousands of axon terminals that connect with other neurons or muscles. The axon terminals are filled with tiny sacs, or vesicles, that contain chemical messengers called **neurotransmitters** (noo-roh-TRANS-mit-erz).

Axon terminals do not actually touch adjacent neurons or muscles. Instead, they are separated by a microscopic gap called the *synaptic cleft*. This intersection, including the synaptic cleft, is known as the **synapse** (SIN-aps). A synapse between an axon terminal and a muscle fiber is called the *neuromuscular junction*, as you learned in Chapter 5.

When classified by their function, there are three types of neurons:

- Sensory (afferent) neurons carry impulses from the skin and organs to the spinal cord and brain, providing information about the external and internal environments.

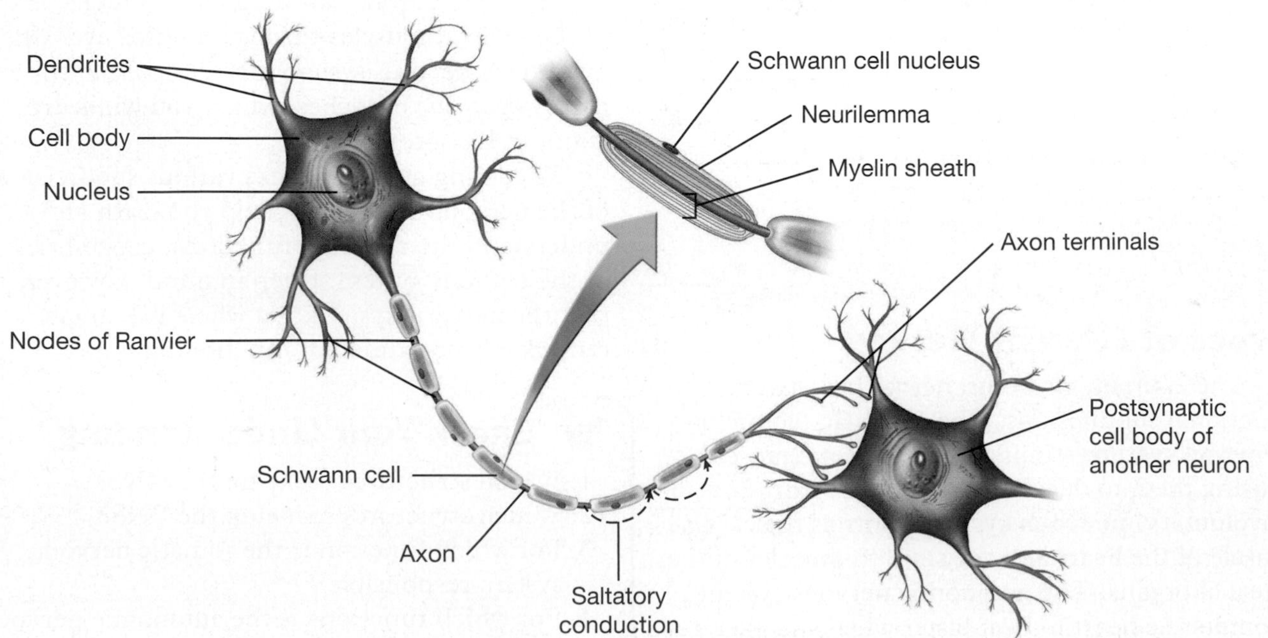

Figure 6.2 A typical neuron. *Why do neural impulses travel faster through myelinated axons than through nonmyelinated axons?*

- Motor (efferent) neurons transmit impulses from the brain and spinal cord to the muscles and glands, directing body actions.
- Neurons that form bridges to transmit impulses between other neurons are called **interneurons** (inter-NOO-rahnz), or *association neurons*.

As shown in **Figure 6.3**, there are also three different neuron structures:

- *Bipolar neurons* have one axon and one dendrite. These are sensory processing cells found in the eyes and nose.
- *Unipolar neurons* have a single axon with dendrites on the peripheral end and axon terminals on the central end. The peripheral process carries impulses to the cell body, and the central process carries impulses to the central nervous system. Some of the sensory neurons in the PNS are unipolar.
- *Multipolar neurons* have one axon and multiple dendrites. All motor neurons and interneurons are multipolar.

Neuroglia

The **neuroglia** (ner-ROHG-lee-a), also known as *glial* (GLIGH-al) *cells*, are a category of specialized cells that perform support functions for neurons (**Figure 6.4**). Within the CNS are four types of glial cells:

- **Astrocytes** (AS-troh-sights) are positioned between neurons and capillaries. Astrocytes link the nutrient-supplying capillaries to neurons and control the chemical environment to protect the neurons from any harmful substances in the blood. The astrocytes are so numerous that they account for nearly half of all neural tissue.
- **Microglia** (migh-KROHG-lee-a) absorb and dispose of dead cells and bacteria.
- **Ependymal** (eh-PEHN-di-mal) **cells** form a protective covering around the spinal cord and central cavities within the brain.
- **Oligodendrocytes** (ohl-i-goh-DEHN-droh-sights) wrap around nerve fibers and produce a fatty insulating material called *myelin*.

The PNS includes two forms of glial cells:

- **Schwann cells** form the fatty myelin sheaths around nerve fibers in the PNS.
- **Satellite cells** serve as cushioning support cells.

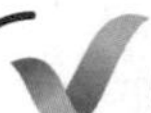

Check Your Understanding

1. List the four types of glial cells in the CNS and state their functions.
2. List the two types of glial cells in the PNS and state their functions.
3. What is the purpose of a myelin sheath?

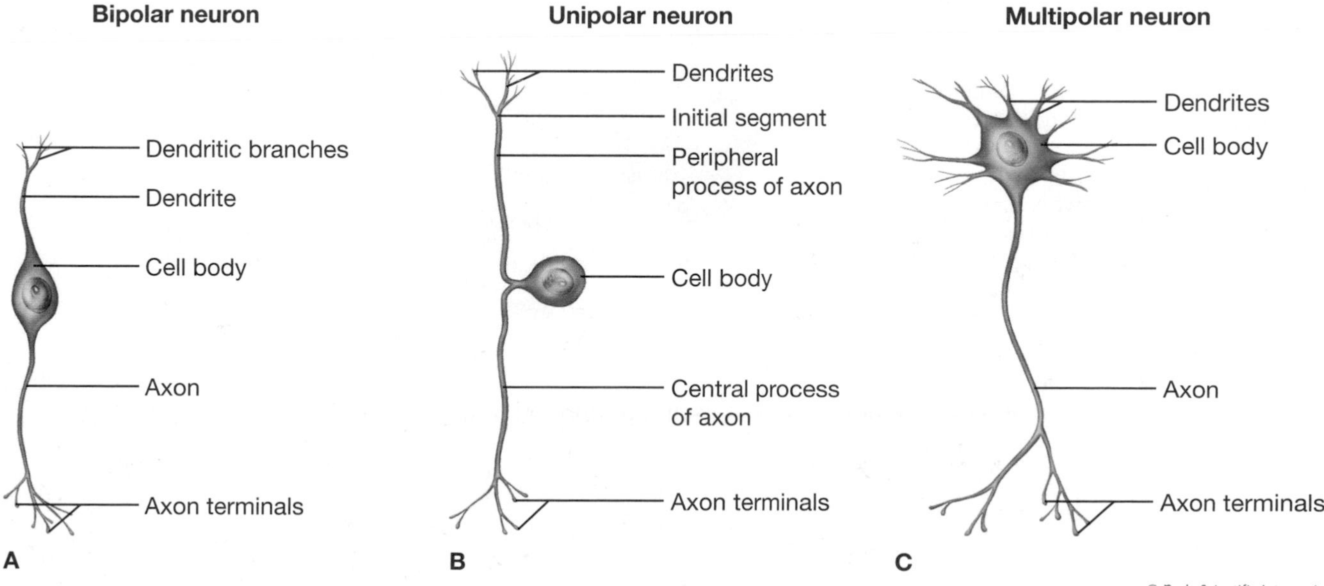

Figure 6.3 Neuron structures. A—Bipolar neurons have two processes: an axon and a dendrite. B—Unipolar neurons have a single axon process, with the cell body in the middle and to the side. C—Multipolar neurons have a single axon and multiple dendrites.

CNS glial cells

Capillary
Astrocyte (links capillaries to neurons)
Neuron cell bodies
Central canal of spine
Ependymal cells (line canal or cavity)
Microglia (remove debris)
Myelinated axons
Oligodendrocyte (produces myelin)

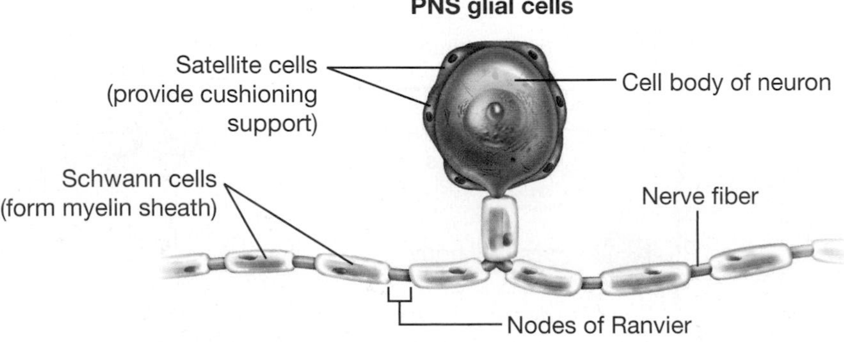

Figure 6.4 The glial cells of the central nervous system and peripheral nervous system.

LESSON 6.1 Review and Assessment

Mini Glossary

Make sure that you know the meaning of each key term.

afferent nerves sensory transmitters that send impulses from receptors in the skin, muscles, and joints to the central nervous system

astrocytes glial cells that link neurons to capillaries and control the chemical environment to protect the neurons from any harmful substances in the blood

autonomic nervous system branch of the nervous system that controls involuntary body functions

central nervous system (CNS) the brain and spinal cord

dendrites branches of a neuron that collect stimuli and transport them to the cell body

efferent nerves motor transmitters that carry impulses from the central nervous system out to the muscles and glands

ependymal cells glial cells that form a protective covering around the spinal cord and central cavities within the brain

interneurons neurons that form bridges to transmit nerve impulses between afferent and efferent neurons

microglia glial cells that absorb and dispose of dead cells and bacteria

myelin sheath the fatty bands of insulation surrounding axon fibers

neuroglia non-neural tissue that forms the interstitial or supporting elements of the CNS; also known as *glial cells*

neurotransmitters chemicals that act as messengers between an axon of one neuron and a dendrite on another, or between an axon and a muscle fiber

oligodendrocytes glial cells that wrap around nerve fibers and produce a fatty insulating material called myelin to insulate some neurons

peripheral nervous system (PNS) all parts of the nervous system external to the brain and spinal cord

satellite cells glial cells that serve as cushioning support cells within the PNS

somatic nervous system branch of the nervous system that stimulates the skeletal muscles

Schwann cells glial cells that wrap around the axons of some neurons in the PNS, providing them with a myelin sheath that speeds up their rate of transmission

synapse the intersection between a neuron and another neuron, a muscle, a gland, or a sensory receptor

Know and Understand

1. Explain how the nervous system is organized, including subdivisions of each component.
2. What is a sensory receptor?
3. Which nerves—the afferent nerves or efferent nerves—are also referred to as motor nerves? Why are they called motor nerves?
4. List the three parts of a typical neuron and state the function of each part.
5. What do the tiny sacs inside axon terminals contain?
6. Explain the difference between bipolar, unipolar, and multipolar neurons.
7. What is the purpose of microglia?

Analyze and Apply

8. Describe a synapse. In your description, use at least three terms that you learned in this lesson.
9. Explain the negative effects on a neuron when the myelin sheath is damaged or destroyed by a demyelinating disorder.
10. Discuss the difference between afferent and efferent nerves. Include the direction in which they transmit impulses and in which division of the nervous system each are found.
11. Describe the structural and functional differences among the three types of neurons.
12. Describe how the CNS and PNS work together to coordinate communication throughout the body. Could either system work without the other? Explain.

IN THE LAB

13. Using clay, or a substitute material, create a model of a typical neuron as described in the lesson. Include all of the different parts mentioned. Label the parts and list the functions of those parts.
14. Make a poster that depicts the organization of the nervous system. Include all of the subdivisions and branches and the function of each. Use a different color for each subdivision.

LESSON 6.2 Transmission of Nerve Impulses

Before You Read

Try to answer the following questions before you read this lesson.

- How fast do nerve impulses travel?
- How can muscles contract without the brain being involved?

Lesson Objectives

- Explain what an action potential is and how it is generated.
- Explain the factors that influence the speed of neural impulse transmission.
- Describe the three types of reflexes and explain how they work.

Key Terms

action potential	refractory period
autonomic reflexes	repolarization
conductivity	saltatory conduction
depolarized	sodium-potassium pump
polarized	somatic reflexes
reflexes	

Neurons have one behavioral property in common with muscle: irritability (the ability to respond to a stimulus). Neurons, however, have an aspect of irritability that muscles do not have: the ability to convert a stimulus into a nerve impulse. **Conductivity**, the other behavioral property of neurons, is the ability to transmit nerve impulses.

What, exactly, is a nerve impulse? It is a tiny electrical charge that transmits information between neurons. This lesson explores the processes by which nerve impulses are created and spread throughout the nervous system.

Action Potentials

When a neuron is inactive or at rest, there is a higher concentration of potassium (K^+) ions inside the cell and a higher concentration of sodium (Na^+) ions outside the cell membrane. Although both of these ion types have a positive charge, the overall distribution of ions is such that the inside of the membrane is more negatively charged than the outside. Because of this difference in electrical charge, the cell membrane is said to be **polarized**. The electrical potential associated with this polarized state is known as the *resting membrane potential*.

Many different stimuli can activate a neuron. A bright light in the eyes, a bitter taste on the tongue, and other sensory inputs are all potential stimuli. More commonly, however, the stimulus is the reception of neurotransmitter chemicals from another neuron. A relatively weak stimulus triggers a local electrical current known as a *graded potential* in the neuron. Graded potentials are so-named because they vary in magnitude, or are "graded," proportional to the magnitude of the stimulus. A graded potential lessens with distance from the stimulation site. It does not travel the length of the neuron, subsides over time, and does not provoke any action.

When a stimulus exceeds a critical voltage, however, hundreds of gated sodium channels in the cell membrane briefly open at the stimulus site. Because the concentration of sodium outside is much greater than that inside the neuron, sodium ions rapidly diffuse into the neuron. As a result, the electrical charge inside the membrane becomes more positive and the neuron membrane at the site becomes **depolarized**.

The depolarization of the neuron membrane successively opens more gated ion channels along the membrane, generating a wave of depolarization through the length of the neuron. This electrical charge is known as a nerve impulse, or **action potential**, and it executes in an all-or-none fashion. This means that the electrical charge of the action potential is always the same size, and once initiated, it always travels the full length of the axon.

Within a few milliseconds following the discharge of the action potential, the membrane becomes impermeable to sodium ions, but permeable to (or accepting of) potassium ions, which rapidly diffuse out of the cell. This begins the process of restoring the membrane to its original, polarized resting state, a process called **repolarization**. Until the cell membrane is repolarized, it cannot respond to another stimulus. The time between the completion of the action potential and repolarization is called the **refractory** (ree-FRAK-toh-ree) **period**. During the refractory period, the neuron is temporarily "fatigued."

Following repolarization, the membrane is restored to its initial resting state. This occurs through activation of the **sodium-potassium pump**. The pump is an enzyme powered by ATP to pump sodium ions out of the cell and potassium ions into the cell, with both moving against their concentration gradients. For every ATP molecule the pump uses, three sodium ions are exported and two potassium ions are imported. The pump operates until the original resting concentrations of sodium and potassium are present. Like the transmission of the action potential, repolarization and restoration of resting state progress along the nerve axon in a sequential fashion. **Figure 6.5** illustrates the transmission of a nerve impulse.

Check Your Understanding

1. What is meant when a cell membrane is said to be polarized?
2. Do action potentials occur when neuron cell membranes are polarized or depolarized?

Impulse Transmission

Two factors—the presence or absence of a myelin sheath and the diameter of the axon—have a major impact on the speed at which a nerve impulse travels. Because the fatty myelin sheath is an electrical insulator, action potentials in a myelinated

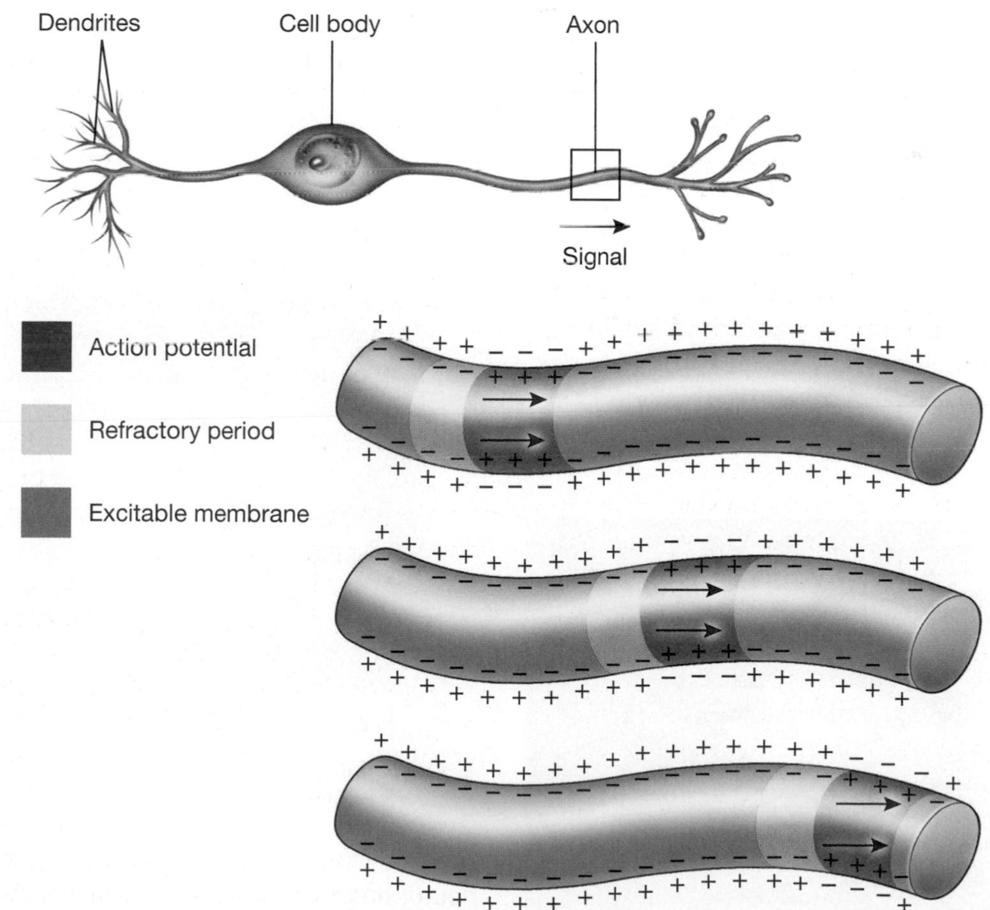

Figure 6.5 Propagation of an impulse along the axon proceeds in a wave-like fashion. The refractory period, in which the cell membrane is undergoing repolarization and is temporarily unable to respond to another stimulus, follows immediately after the action potential.

axon "jump over" the myelinated regions of the axon. Depolarization occurs only at the nodes of Ranvier, where the axon is exposed (**Figure 6.2**). This process, known as **saltatory** (SAWL-ta-toh-ree) **conduction**, results in significantly faster impulse transmission than is possible in nonmyelinated axons.

Impulse conduction is much faster in nonmyelinated axons with larger diameters than in those with smaller diameters. The larger the axon, the greater the number of ions it has to conduct current. This is somewhat like a large-diameter pipe versus a small-diameter pipe when transferring water from one place to another. In a given amount of time and at a given flow rate, more water can move through the large-diameter pipe than through the small-diameter pipe.

A third factor influencing conduction speed is body temperature. Warmer temperatures increase ion diffusion rates, whereas local cooling, which occurs when holding an ice cube, for example, decreases ion diffusion rates.

Speed of Transmission

So how fast do nerve impulses travel? Impulses that signal limb position to the brain travel extremely fast—up to 119 meters per second (m/s). Information or impulses from the objects that you touch travel more slowly, at around 76 m/s (**Figure 6.6**). The sensation of pain moves even more slowly, at less than 1 m/s. Thought signals, which are happening right now as you are reading, transmit at 20–30 m/s. For a nerve to transmit impulses at speeds greater than 1 m/s, it must have a myelinated axon.

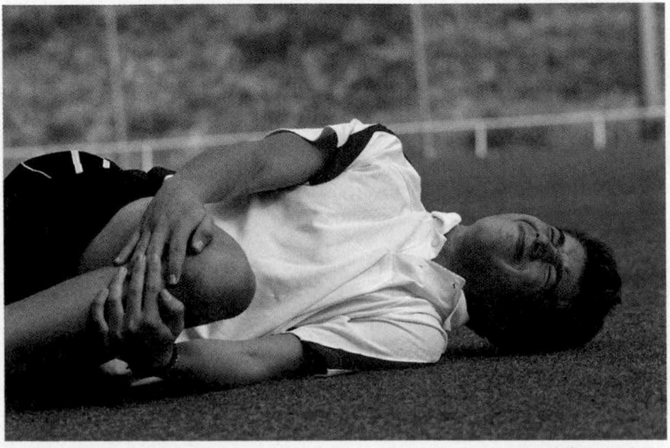

Fresnel/Shutterstock.com

Figure 6.6 Although it may seem as though you feel pain instantly, nerve impulses communicating pain travel more slowly than other nerve impulses.

Transmission at Synapses

Communication between some cells occurs through direct transfer of electrical charges within specialized sites called *gap junctions*. The intercalated discs between cardiac muscle fibers, for example, serve as gap junctions.

Communication between neurons, however, occurs at the synapse. Because the action potential is electrical, and what occurs at the synapse is chemical, transmission of nerve impulses is called an *electrochemical event*.

When an action potential reaches an axon terminal, the terminal depolarizes, calcium gates open, and calcium (Ca^{++}) ions flow into the terminal. The axon terminal is filled with tiny vesicles containing neurotransmitters (**Figure 6.7**). The influx of calcium causes these vesicles to join to the cell membrane adjacent to the synaptic cleft. Pores then form in the membrane, allowing the neurotransmitter to diffuse across the synapse to receptors on the membrane of the joining neuron or muscle fiber.

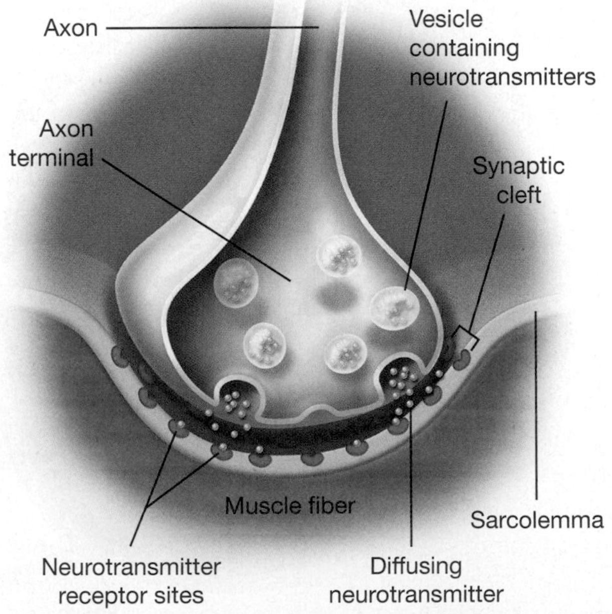

© Body Scientific International

Figure 6.7 The synapse is the site at which the neurotransmitter is released from the nerve axon terminal. The neurotransmitter then diffuses across the synaptic cleft to receptor sites on the next nerve cell body, or to a muscle fiber, as shown here. *What two decidedly different effects can neurotransmitters have on the receiving cells?*

Neurotransmitters can have an excitatory effect or an inhibitory effect on the receiving cell. An example of an excitatory neurotransmitter is acetylcholine (ah-see-til-KOH-leen), the chemical that activates muscle fibers. Endorphins (en-DOR-finz) are neurotransmitters released to inhibit nerve cells from discharging more pain signals.

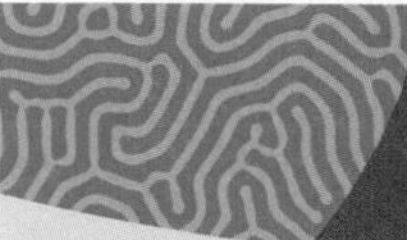

What Research Tells Us

...about Measuring Nerve Impulses

How do scientists and clinicians measure the speed and function of nerve impulses? One common method is the use of a nerve conduction velocity (NCV) test.

Conducting and Interpreting NCV Tests

The NCV test begins with the attachment of three small, flat, disc-shaped electrodes to the skin. One electrode is attached over the nerve being studied and another electrode over the muscle supplied by the nerve. The third electrode is attached over a bony site, such as the elbow or ankle, to serve as an electrical ground.

The technician then administers short, tiny electrical pulses to the nerve through the first electrode and records the time it takes for the muscle to contract (as sensed by the second electrode). Computer software calculates the NCV as the distance between the stimulating and sensing electrodes divided by the elapsed time between stimulation and contraction.

Placing stimulating electrodes at two or more different locations along the same nerve makes it possible to determine the NCV across different segments of the nerve. To test for sensory neuron function, the stimulating electrode is placed over a region of sensory receptors such as a fingertip. The recording electrode is then placed at a distance up the limb.

How are the results of a clinical NCV test interpreted? An NCV that is significantly slower than normal suggests that damage to the myelin sheath is likely. Alternatively, if NCV is slow but close to the normal range, damage to the axons of the involved neurons is suspected. Evaluation of the overall pattern of responses can serve as a diagnostic tool in helping a clinician determine the likely pathology involved in an abnormal NCV.

Microneurography

Scientists have used a similar but more sophisticated procedure called *microneurography* (migh-kroh-noo-RAHG-ra-fee) to record electrical activity from single sensory fibers. **Figure 6.8** shows that the technique involves the direct insertion of fine-tipped needle electrodes into the nerve being studied.

The use of microneurography has helped develop scientists' current understanding of the sympathetic nervous system. Topics studied include various reflexes, interactions within the sympathetic nervous system, metabolism, hormones, and the effects of drugs or anesthesia during operative procedures. Sympathetic recordings have also been used to study the effects of performance at high altitudes, as well as in space.

Taking It Further

1. Working with a partner, research nerve damage further. Develop a report for the class on the more common causes.
2. Investigate and report to the class on technologies, in addition to NCV tests, that are used for diagnostic and therapeutic purposes to treat nerve disorders.

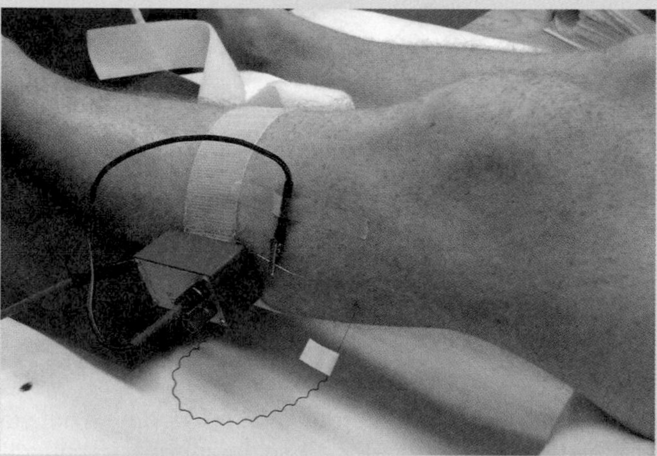

Courtesy of Dr. Bill Farquhar

Figure 6.8 Microneurography is a technique involving insertion of fine wire electrodes into a nerve for direct recording of electrical impulse activity.

The final step in communication between nerves at a synapse is the removal of the neurotransmitter, usually by an enzyme, to prevent ongoing stimulation of the receptor cell. Acetylcholine, for example, is deactivated by the enzyme acetylcholinesterase (a-see-til-koh-lin-EHS-ter-ays).

Reflexes

Reflexes are simple, rapid, involuntary, programmed responses to stimuli. The transmission of impulses follows a *reflex arc* that includes both PNS and CNS structures (**Figure 6.9**). There are two categories of reflexes.

Somatic reflexes are those that involve stimulation of skeletal muscles. For example, have you ever withdrawn your hand quickly from something hot, even before you realized that it was hot? If so, you were experiencing a somatic reflex. In such a situation the motion of your hand occurs so quickly because a motor nerve has been directly stimulated by a sensory neuron, by way of an interneuron in the spinal cord. The signal between neurons is so fast because it did not have to travel to the brain and back.

Autonomic reflexes are those that send involuntary stimuli to the cardiac muscle of the heart and the smooth muscle of internal organs. Digestion, elimination, sweating, and blood pressure are all activities that are regulated by autonomic reflexes.

Check Your Understanding

1. What three factors influence the speed at which a nerve impulse travels?
2. Give an example of both an excitatory neurotransmitter and an inhibitory neurotransmitter.
3. Why is the transmission of nerve impulses often referred to as an electrochemical event?
4. What are the two types of reflexes discussed in this lesson?

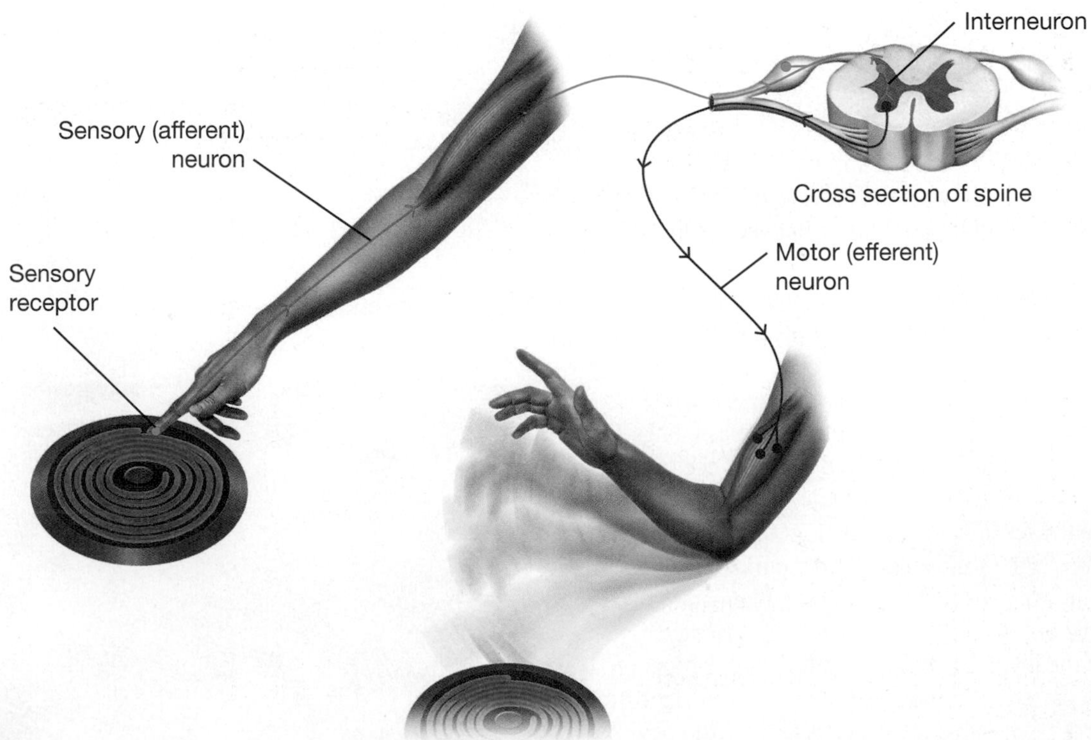

Figure 6.9 A sensory receptor is stimulated by a hot surface, sending an afferent signal to the spinal cord. The signal is then transferred by an interneuron directly to a motor neuron, stimulating quick removal of the hand from the hot surface.

LESSON 6.2 Review and Assessment

Mini Glossary

Make sure that you know the meaning of each key term.

action potential nerve impulse caused by a wave of depolarization along the length of a neuron

autonomic reflexes involuntary stimuli transmitted to cardiac and smooth muscle

conductivity the ability of a neuron to transmit a nerve impulse

depolarized a condition in which the inside of a cell membrane is more positively charged than the outside

polarized a condition that occurs when the inside of a cell membrane is more negatively charged than the outside

reflexes simple, rapid, involuntary, programmed responses to stimuli

refractory period the time between the completion of the action potential and repolarization

repolarization the reestablishment of a polarized state in a cell after depolarization

saltatory conduction the rapid skipping of an action potential from node to node on myelinated neurons

sodium-potassium pump a pumping mechanism powered by ATP molecules that actively transports potassium and sodium ions into and out of the cell, respectively, against their gradients in order to accomplish repolarization of the cell

somatic reflexes involuntary stimuli transmitted to skeletal muscles from neural arcs in the spinal cord

Know and Understand

1. Name two behavioral properties of a nerve impulse.
2. Briefly describe how a graded potential works and explain what has to happen in order for a graded potential to result in depolarization of a neuron.
3. Describe a neuron at rest compared to a neuron activated by a stimulus.
4. What has to happen before a cell membrane can respond to a second stimulus?
5. Why is ATP required to activate the sodium-potassium pump that restores a membrane to its resting state?
6. What is the effect of myelin sheaths on nerve impulses?
7. How does body temperature affect the conduction speed of an electrical impulse?
8. What are the two categories of reflexes? Name a body part that would be affected by each of the two types.

Analyze and Apply

9. How would submerging a person in a tub of cold water affect the conduction speeds of the person's nerve impulses?
10. Is conduction of nerve impulses always faster in axons with a larger diameter, compared to axons with a smaller diameter? Explain.
11. Why is it impossible for a neuron to transmit an impulse during its refractory period?

IN THE LAB

12. Using a toothpick and a piece of ice, test a fellow student's sensory impulse reaction. Gently poke the student's ventral forearm (the part of the forearm closer to the wrist) with the toothpick and note the length of time it takes for your partner to sense pain. Then place a piece of ice on the same spot on the student's ventral forearm for one minute. Remove the ice and again gently poke the forearm. Note the length of time and amount of pressure required before the student senses pain. Explain your results.
13. Create a bar graph to show the relative speeds of the different types of nerve impulses mentioned in this section. Choose a scale that maximizes the impact of the speed differences for people viewing the graph. Arrange the bars in order from slowest to fastest. Be sure to label both axes of the graph, as well as the individual bars, to make it easier to understand.
14. Conduct research to find out how physicians evaluate cranial nerves by testing reflexes. Create a chart showing the various tests and listing normal and abnormal responses.

LESSON 6.3

Functional Anatomy of the Central Nervous System

Before You Read

Try to answer the following questions before you read this lesson.

- Is brain size related to intelligence?
- Which brain structure functions particularly well in athletes?

Lesson Objectives

- Describe the location and functions of the brain and its supporting structures.
- Identify the location and functions of the spinal cord.

Key Terms

cerebellum	meninges
cerebrospinal fluid (CSF)	midbrain
cerebrum	occipital lobes
corpus callosum	parietal lobes
diencephalon	pons
epithalamus	primary motor cortex
fissures	primary somatic sensory cortex
frontal lobes	spinal cord
hypothalamus	temporal lobes
lobes	thalamus
medulla oblongata	

The central nervous system includes numerous anatomical structures with specialized functions. Using sophisticated imaging techniques, scientists have been able to identify which structures control or contribute to many physiological processes and actions.

The Brain

As you might expect, given its all-important role in directing the activity of the entire nervous system, the brain is structurally and functionally complex. The adult human brain weighs between 2¼ and 3¼ pounds and contains approximately 100 billion neurons and even more glial cells. Recent research indicates that the size of a person's brain does have some relationship to intelligence; about 6.7% of individual variation in intelligence is attributed to brain size. The four major anatomic regions of the brain are the cerebrum, diencephalon, brainstem, and cerebellum.

Cerebrum

The left and right cerebral (seh-REE-bral) hemispheres are collectively referred to as the **cerebrum** (seh-REE-brum), which makes up the largest portion of the brain. The outer surface of the cerebrum, called the *cerebral cortex*, is composed of nonmyelinated gray matter. The internal tissue is myelinated white matter, with small, interspersed regions of gray matter called *basal nuclei*.

As you can see in **Figure 6.10A**, the surface of the brain is not smooth; instead, it is convoluted. Each of the curved, raised areas is called a *gyrus* (JIGH-rus), and each of the grooves between the gyri is called a *sulcus* (SUL-kus). Together, these structures are referred to as *convolutions*. No two brains look exactly alike in their pattern of convolutions. However, the major sulci are arranged in the same pattern in all human brains.

The sulci divide the brain into four regions called **lobes**. The four lobes of the brain are the frontal, parietal, occipital, and temporal lobes.

Like the sulci, **fissures** are uniformly positioned, deep grooves in the brain. The longitudinal fissure runs the length of the brain and divides it into left and right hemispheres. As a result, the lobes are paired on the left and right sides of the body. The left and right hemispheres of the brain are connected by the **corpus callosum**, a large, myelinated tract containing more than 200 million axons. Neural communications to and from the right side of the body are controlled by the left brain, and communications with the left side of the body are controlled by the right brain.

The **frontal lobes**, located behind the forehead in the most anterior portion of the brain, are sectioned off from the rest of the brain by the central sulcus (**Figure 6.10B**). Within the frontal lobes and just anterior to the central sulcus is the **primary motor cortex**, which sends neural impulses to the skeletal muscles to initiate and control the development of muscle tension and voluntary movement of body parts.

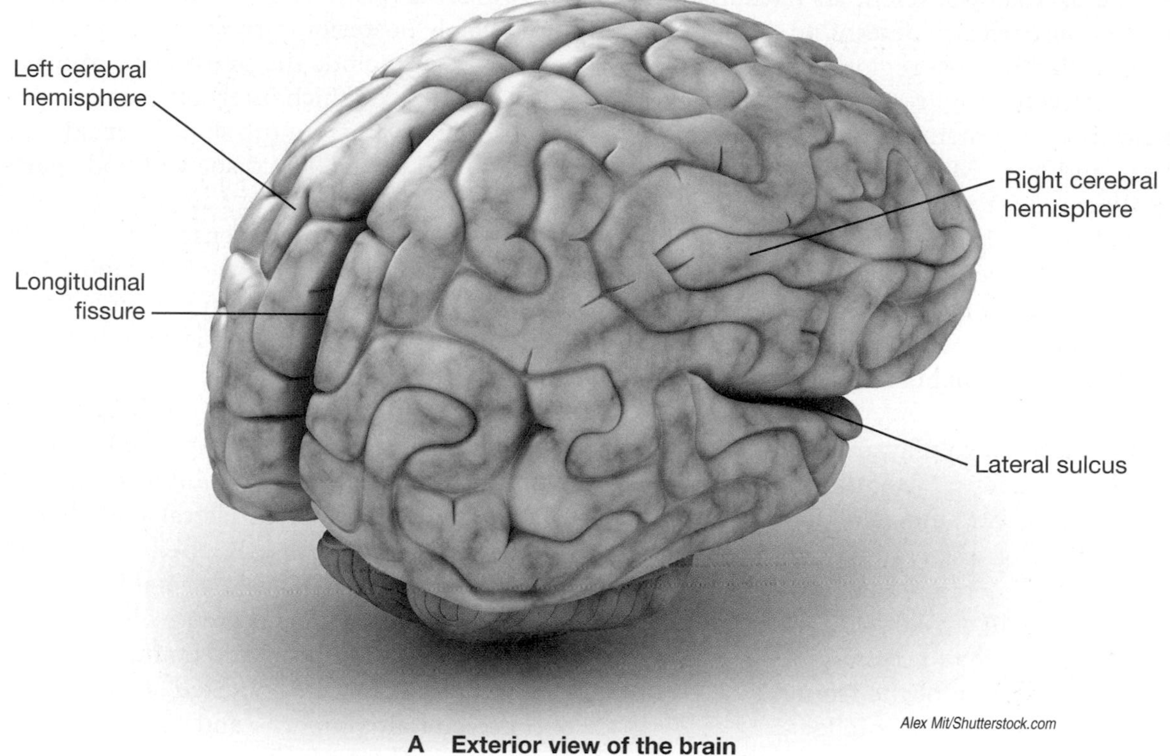

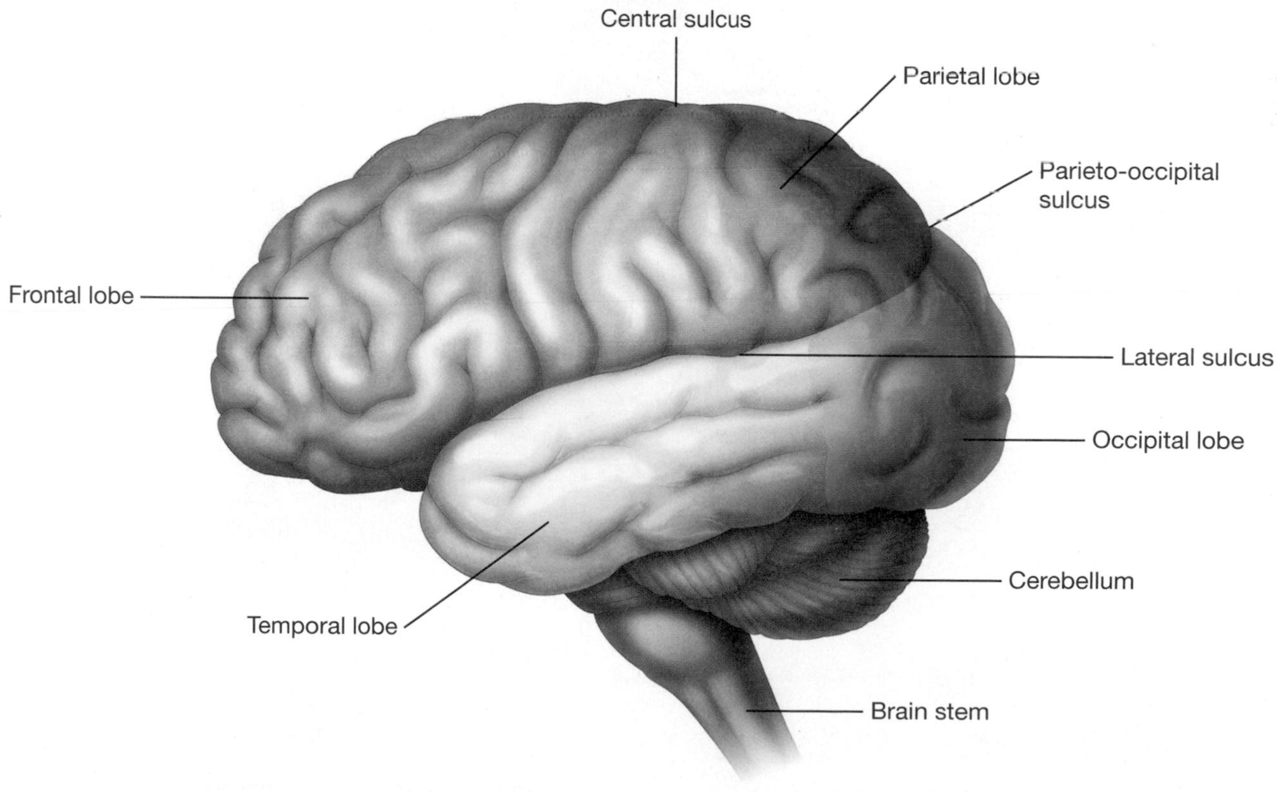

© Body Scientific International

Figure 6.10 A—The hemispheres of the cerebrum. B—The four lobes of the cerebrum (shown in contrasting colors) are separated by indentations called *sulci*.

As **Figure 6.11** shows, scientists have mapped the primary motor cortex to determine which body parts are controlled in each region of the cortex. Notice that relatively small regions of the cortex control major body segments, such as the trunk, pelvis, thigh, and arm. Much larger regions of the cortex are allocated for control of smaller body segments, such as the hands, lips, and tongue.

Why is this the case? If you think about it, the body parts associated with larger areas of the motor cortex are the ones capable of the more fine-tuned movements. Such movements require the activation of more nerves.

The frontal lobes also play an important role in higher order intellectual functioning, including planning, reasoning, and memory. The left frontal lobe also includes *Broca's area*, which controls the tongue and lip movements required for speech. Damage to this area in stroke patients produces difficulty with speaking. The *association cortex* on the most anterior portion of the frontal lobe is believed to be responsible for intellect.

The **parietal** (pa-RIGH-eh-tal) **lobes** are immediately posterior to the frontal lobes. The parietal lobes include the **primary somatic sensory cortex**, which interprets sensory impulses received from the skin, internal organs, muscles, and joints. The display of body parts in the somatic sensory part of **Figure 6.11** represents the density, or amount, of sensory neural input received from different parts of the body. Notice that the fingertips and lips, in particular, have a lot of sensory receptors. This is why they occupy large portions of the sensory cortex.

The **occipital** (ahk-SIP-i-tal) **lobes**, posterior to the parietal lobes, are responsible for vision, including both reception and interpretation of visual sensory inputs. The lateral sulci divide the **temporal** (TEHM-poh-ral) **lobes**, the most inferior lobes, from the frontal and parietal lobes above them. The temporal lobes are involved in speech, hearing, vision, memory, and emotion. The region responsible for speech is located at the intersection of the occipital, temporal, and parietal lobes.

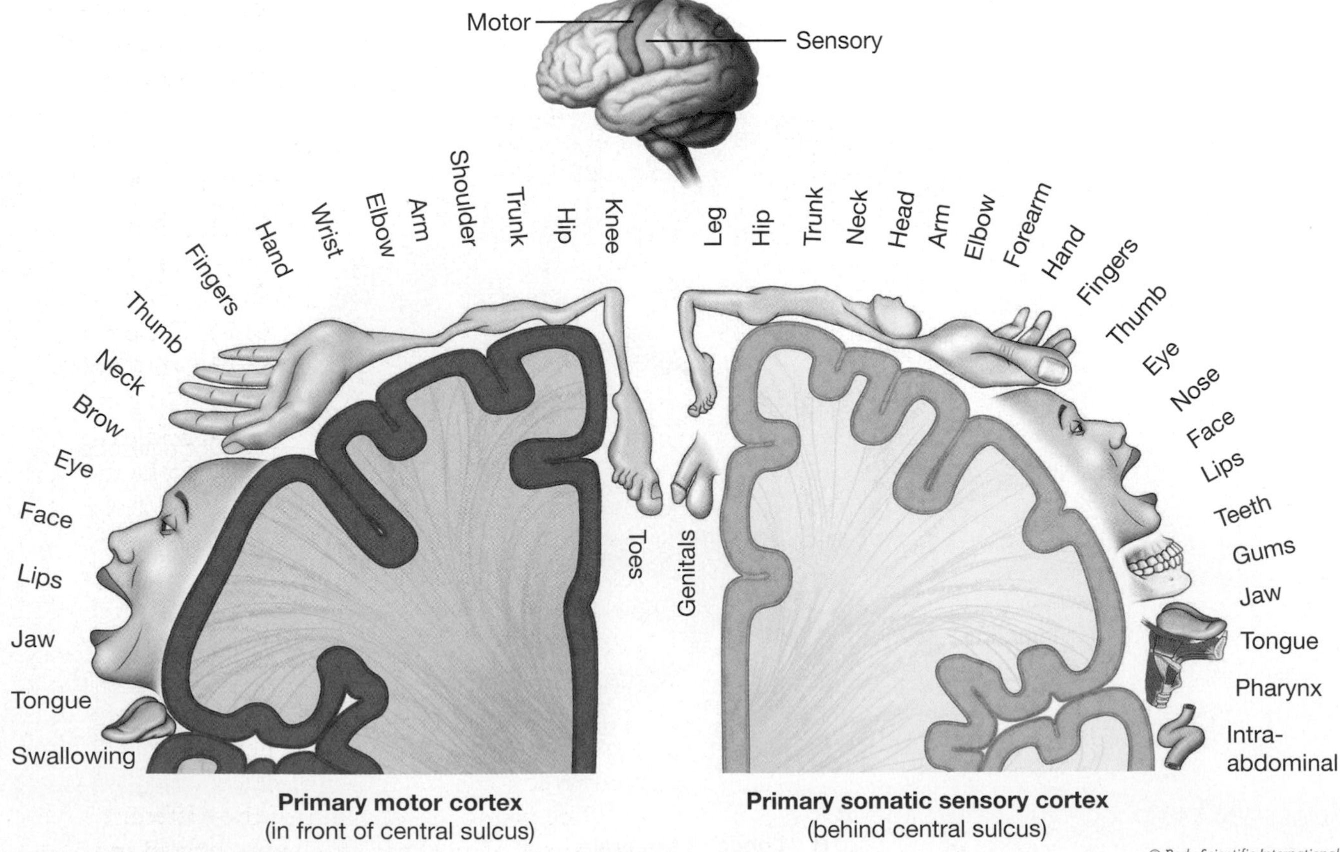

Figure 6.11 The primary motor and somatic sensory cortexes, with mapped regions of motor output and sensory input depicted. *Why do smaller areas of the body, such as the fingers or lips, require more nerves than larger areas, such as the shoulder or trunk?*

Diencephalon

The **diencephalon** (digh-ehn-SEHF-uh-lahn), also known as the *interbrain*, is located deep inside the brain, enclosed by the cerebral hemispheres (**Figure 6.12**). It includes several important structures—the thalamus, hypothalamus, and epithalamus.

- The **thalamus** (THAL-uh-mus) serves as a relay station for communicating both sensory and motor information between the body and the cerebral cortex. It also plays a major role in regulating the body's states of arousal, including sleep, wakefulness, and high-alert consciousness.
- Only about the size of a pearl, the **hypothalamus** (high-poh-THAL-uh-mus) is a key part of the autonomic nervous system, regulating functions such as metabolism, heart rate, blood pressure, thirst, hunger, energy level, and body temperature. The centers for sex, pain, and pleasure also lie within the hypothalamus.
- The **epithalamus** (ehp-i-THAL-uh-mus) includes the pineal gland and regulates the sleep-cycle hormones secreted by this gland.

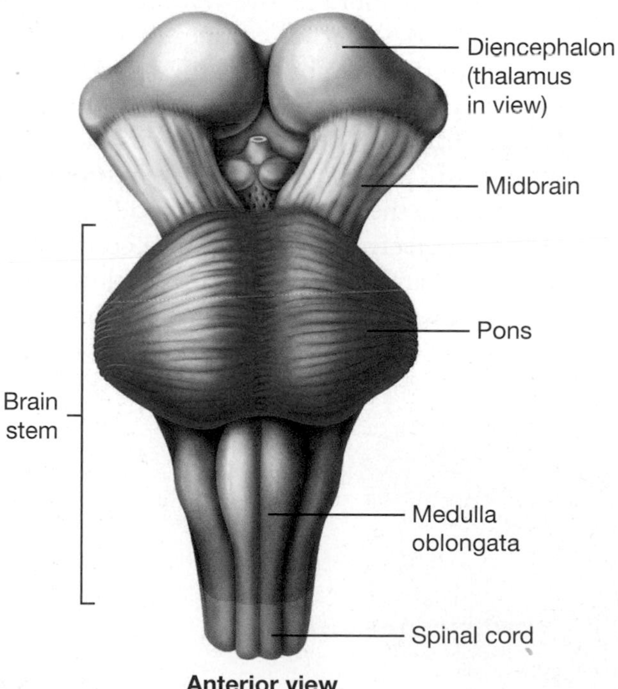

Figure 6.12 The diencephalon includes the thalamus (exterior), and the hypothalamus and epithalamus (both interior). The brainstem includes the midbrain, pons, and medulla oblongata. *Which area of the brain identified above controls your sneezing reflex?*

Brainstem

Approximately the size of a thumb, the brainstem is shaped somewhat like a plant stem and includes three structures: the midbrain, pons, and medulla oblongata (**Figure 6.12**).

- The **midbrain** on the superior end of the brainstem serves as a relay station for sensory and motor impulses. Specifically, it relays information concerning vision, hearing, motor activity, sleep and wake cycles, arousal (alertness), and temperature regulation.
- The **pons** (pahnz), located immediately below the midbrain, plays a role in regulating breathing.
- Inferior to the pons, the **medulla oblongata** (meh-DOOL-a ahb-lawn-GAH-tah) regulates heart rate, blood pressure, and breathing, and controls the reflexes for coughing, sneezing, and vomiting.

The *reticular* (reh-TIK-yoo-lar) *formation* is a collection of gray matter that extends the length of the brainstem. The reticular formation regulates waking from slumber, as well as heightened states of awareness. Individuals with severe brain injuries can continue to live as long as the brainstem remains functional and they receive sufficient hydration and nutrition.

Cerebellum

The **cerebellum** (ser-eh-BEHL-um), found below the occipital lobe, looks similar to the cerebrum with its outer gray cortex, convolutions, and dual hemispheres (**Figure 6.10**). The cerebellum serves the important role of coordinating body movements, including balance.

To coordinate body movements and maintain balance, the cerebellum receives input from the eyes, inner ears, and sensory receptors throughout the body. It also continuously monitors body segment positions and motions. If the body's positions and motions are not what the cerebellum intended them to be, it sends out signals to make adjustments. The cerebellums of accomplished athletes have been found to be well-developed in terms of size and numbers of neural connections, compared to those of non-athletes.

The primary functions of the different structures of the brain are summarized in the table in **Figure 6.13**. Keep these functions in mind as you read about the brain's supporting structures and the rest of the CNS.

Functions of the Brain	
Part of Brain	**Primary Functions**
Cerebral Lobes	
Frontal lobe	memory, intelligence, behavior, emotions, motor function, smell
Parietal lobe	somatic sensations (pain, touch, hot/cold), speech
Occipital lobe	vision, speech
Temporal lobe	hearing, smell, memory, speech
Diencephalon	
Thalamus	relays sensory impulses up to the sensory cortex
Hypothalamus	autonomic center regulating metabolism, heart rate, blood pressure, thirst, hunger, energy level, and body temperature
Epithalamus	regulates hormones secreted by pineal gland
Brainstem	
Midbrain	relays sensory and motor impulses
Pons	assists with regulation of breathing
Medulla oblongata	regulates heart rate, blood pressure, and breathing, and controls the reflexes of coughing, sneezing, and vomiting
Reticular formation	regulates waking from slumber and heightened states of awareness
Cerebellum	coordinates body movements and balance

Figure 6.13

Goodheart-Willcox Publisher

Meninges

Three protective membranes, the **meninges** (meh-NIN-jeez), surround the brain and spinal cord (**Figure 6.14**). The outer membrane, the *dura mater* (DOO-rah MAY-ter), a Latin term meaning "hard mother," is a tough, double-layered membrane that lies beneath the skull and surrounds the brain. The inner layer of the dura mater continues down to enclose the spinal cord.

The middle membrane, the *arachnoid mater* (ah-RAK-noyd MAY-ter), is composed of weblike tissue. Beneath this membrane is the subarachnoid space, filled with **cerebrospinal** (seh-ree-broh-SPIGH-nal) **fluid (CSF),** which cushions the brain and spinal cord. The composition of cerebrospinal fluid is similar to the plasma in the blood, but it has a different electrolyte balance and contains more vitamin C and less protein. It is produced by the choroid plexus in the ventricles of the brain.

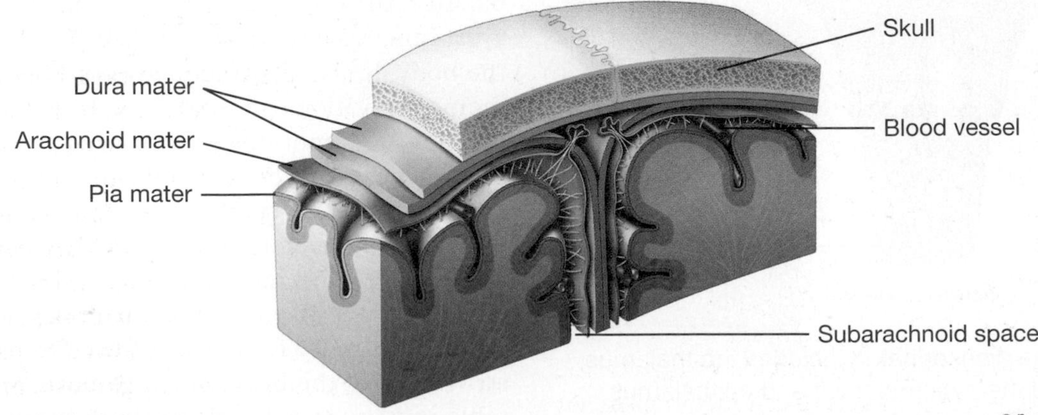

© Body Scientific International

Figure 6.14 The three meninges (the protective linings of the brain and spinal cord) include the double-layered dura mater, the arachnoid mater, and the pia mater. *What is the function of each of the meninges?*

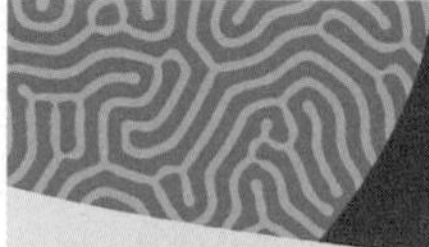

What Research Tells Us

...about Studying the Brain

An increasing variety of approaches is available for studying the functional roles of different parts of the central nervous system. As technology advances, more sophisticated techniques emerge.

fMRI Scans

One procedure extremely useful for both scientific and clinical evaluation of the brain is called *functional magnetic resonance imaging (fMRI)*. This technology creates images of changes in blood flow to activated brain structures. This is made possible by the slightly different magnetic properties of oxygenated and deoxygenated blood. The images show which brain structures are activated and the amount of time they are activated during performance of different tasks. The individual undergoing the brain scan is presented with certain tasks that can cause activation (increased blood flow) to the regions of the brain responsible for perception, thought, and a stimulated motor action, such as raising an arm or smiling (**Figure 6.15**).

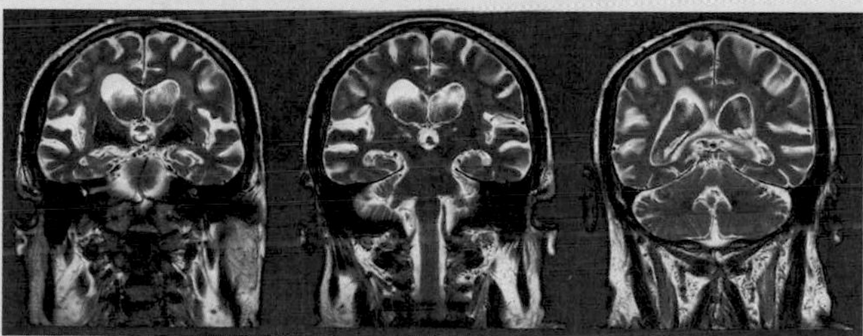

MriMan/Shutterstock.com

Figure 6.15 Functional magnetic resonance imaging (fMRI) scans of the brain show different areas of activation.

Increasingly, physicians are using fMRI to diagnose disorders and diseases of the brain. With a fine sensitivity to changes in blood flow, fMRI is particularly useful for evaluating patients who may have suffered a stroke. Early diagnosis of stroke is important because treatment can be significantly more effective the earlier it is given.

PET Scans

Another approach for studying brain function involves positron emission tomography (toh-MAHG-ra-fee), or PET. This procedure tracks the locations of radioactively labeled chemicals in the bloodstream. PET scans can show blood flow, oxygen absorption, and glucose absorption in the active brain, indicating where the brain is active and inactive. Although fMRI has largely replaced PET for the study of brain activation patterns, PET scans still provide the advantage of showing where particular neurotransmitters are concentrated in the brain. PET scans are also still widely used in diagnosing various forms of brain disease because they can be analyzed and interpreted more quickly than fMRI scans.

Taking It Further

1. How is an fMRI used to help diagnose disease and disorders?
2. Why is the blood-flow pattern to the brain a revealing factor in the diagnosis of a particular brain disease or disorder?
3. In what situations might a doctor prefer to use an fMRI or PET scan?

The innermost layer of the meninges attaches directly to the surface of the brain and spinal cord. This layer is the delicate *pia mater* (PIGH-ah MAY-ter), meaning "gentle mother."

Blood-Brain Barrier

A rich network of blood vessels supplies the brain. Like all tissues of the body, the brain depends on a circulating blood supply to provide nutrients and carry away the waste products of cell metabolism. At any given time, roughly 20%–25% of the blood in your body is circulating in the region of the brain. The capillaries supplying the brain, however, are different from other capillaries in the body. They are impermeable to many substances that freely diffuse through the walls of capillaries in other body regions. This property of impermeability has given rise to the term *blood-brain barrier.*

The blood-brain barrier protects the brain against surges in concentrations of hormones, ions, and some nutrients. Substances allowed to pass through the capillaries include water, glucose, and essential amino acids. Other substances that can penetrate the blood-brain barrier are bloodborne alcohol, nicotine, fats, respiratory gases, and anesthetics.

Check Your Understanding

1. List the four major anatomic regions of the brain.
2. Describe the relationship between gyri and sulci.
3. List the four lobes of the brain and state their locations.
4. Name the three structures that make up the brainstem and state the function of each.
5. Where is the cerebellum located and what is its function?

The Spinal Cord

The **spinal cord** extends from the brainstem down to the beginning of the lumbar region of the spine. It serves as a major pathway for relaying sensory impulses to the brain and motor impulses from the brain. It also provides the neural connections involved in reflex arcs. Like the brain, the spine is surrounded and protected by the three meninges and cerebrospinal fluid.

When viewed in cross section, the exterior of the spinal cord is myelinated white matter, with butterfly-shaped gray matter, composed of neuron cell bodies and interneurons, located centrally (**Figure 6.16**). The regions of the white and gray matter in the spinal cord are named after their locations—ventral (anterior), lateral, or dorsal (posterior). The dorsal columns of white matter carry sensory impulses to the brain, and the lateral and ventral columns transmit both sensory and motor impulses. The dorsal, lateral, and ventral projections of gray matter are called *horns*. The central canal containing cerebrospinal fluid runs through the middle of the gray matter.

Check Your Understanding

1. What are the three regions of white and gray matter in the spinal cord?
2. What is the name of the projections of gray matter in the spinal cord?

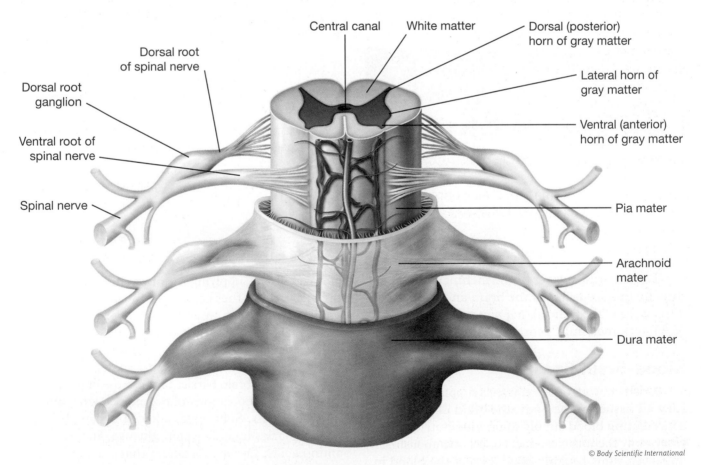

Figure 6.16 Layers and regions of the spinal cord. *Which is shaped like a butterfly—the layers and regions of the spinal cord, the gray matter, or the white matter?*

LESSON 6.3 Review and Assessment

Mini Glossary

Make sure that you know the meaning of each key term.

cerebellum section of the brain that coordinates body movements, including balance

cerebrospinal fluid (CSF) fluid in the subarachnoid space that cushions the brain and spinal cord

cerebrum the largest part of the brain, consisting of the left and right hemispheres

corpus callosum a large, myelinated tract connecting the left and right hemispheres of the brain; contains more than 200 million axons

diencephalon area of the brain that includes the epithalamus, thalamus, and hypothalamus; also known as the interbrain

epithalamus the uppermost portion of the diencephalon; includes the pineal gland and regulates sleep-cycle hormones

fissures the uniformly positioned, deep grooves in the brain

frontal lobes sections of the brain located behind the forehead

hypothalamus a portion of the diencephalon that regulates functions such as metabolism, heart rate, and blood pressure

lobes the four regions of the brain—frontal, parietal, occipital, and temporal

medulla oblongata the lower portion of the brainstem; regulates heart rate, blood pressure, and breathing, and controls several reflexes

meninges three protective membranes that surround the brain and spinal cord

midbrain relay station for sensory and motor impulses; located on the superior end of the brainstem

occipital lobes sections of the brain located behind the parietal lobes; integrate sensory information from the skin, internal organs, muscles, and joints

parietal lobes sections of the brain located behind the frontal lobes; integrate sensory information from the skin, internal organs, muscles, and joints

pons the section of the brain that plays a role in regulating breathing

primary motor cortex outer region of the brain in the frontal lobes that sends neural impulses to the skeletal muscles

primary somatic sensory cortex outer region of the brain in the parietal lobes that interprets sensory impulses received from the skin, internal organs, muscles, and joints

spinal cord a column of nerve tissue that extends from the brainstem to the beginning of the lumbar region of the spine

temporal lobes the most inferior portions of the brain; responsible for speech, hearing, vision, memory, and emotion

thalamus the largest portion of the diencephalon; communicates sensory and motor information between the body and the cerebral cortex

Know and Understand

1. What is the difference between gray matter and white matter in the brain? Where is each found?
2. Are major body segments, such as the trunk and pelvis, controlled by large or small regions of the brain's primary motor cortex?
3. What area of the brain has probably been damaged if a stroke patient has difficulty speaking?
4. Name the three structures that make up the diencephalon and state their functions.
5. In what way are the capillaries in the brain different from the capillaries in other parts of the body?
6. Like the brain, the spinal cord has gray and white matter. Identify the responsibility of both the gray and white matter in the spinal cord.

Analyze and Apply

7. Explain why someone might say that the brain is convoluted.
8. Compare and contrast the three protective membranes surrounding the brain and spinal cord. Discuss their structures and functions.
9. Which general area of the brain—the anterior or posterior region—is associated with more sophisticated functions? Explain.
10. A person with a traumatic brain injury may still remain living as long as which part of the brain remains active? Explain the reason for this.

IN THE LAB

11. Obtain a model or picture of a human brain. Color-code the different lobes and structures on the model or picture and then list the functions and body processes that each area controls.
12. Using different colors of clay, construct a lateral (side) view of the brain. Include these structures: frontal lobe, parietal lobe, temporal lobe, occipital lobe, cerebellum, and brainstem.

LESSON 6.4

Functional Anatomy of the Peripheral Nervous System

Before You Read

Try to answer the following questions before you read this lesson.

- What is in a nerve besides nerve tissue?
- What are the similarities and differences between the sympathetic and parasympathetic nervous systems?

Lesson Objectives

- Describe the basic structure of a nerve.
- Explain the organization of the cranial nerves, the spinal nerves, the dorsal and ventral rami, and the plexuses.
- Differentiate between the functions of the sympathetic and parasympathetic branches of the autonomic nervous system.

Key Terms

cranial nerves	perineurium
craniosacral branch	plexuses
dorsal ramus	postganglionic neuron
endoneurium	preganglionic neuron
epineurium	spinal nerves
ganglion	thoracolumbar branch
norepinephrine	ventral ramus
paravertebral ganglia	

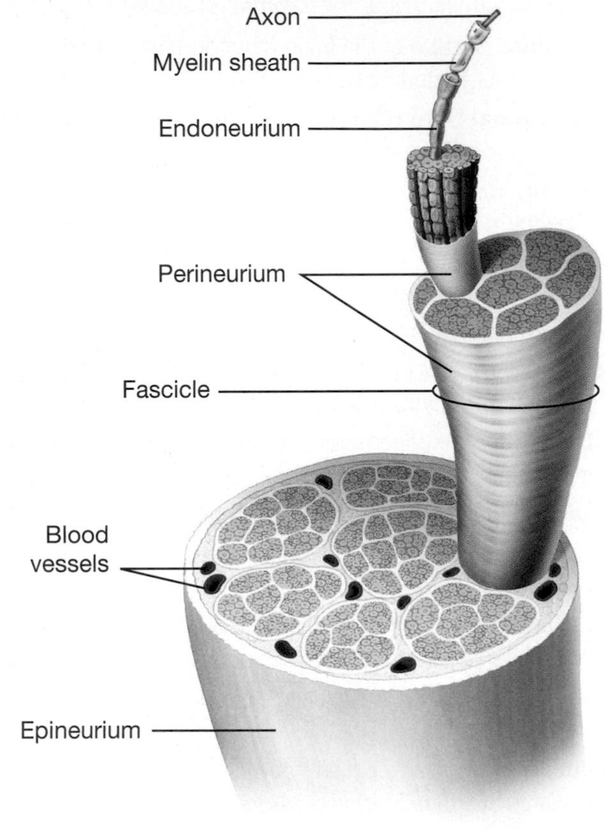

Figure 6.17 Structure of a nerve showing the protective, fibrous tissue sheaths. *How does the structure of a nerve help to protect it from injury?*

The peripheral nervous system (PNS) transmits information to the CNS and carries instructions from the CNS. It achieves these functions through a network of nerves outside of the CNS.

Nerve Structure

Each nerve consists of a collection of axons (nerve fibers) and nutrient-supplying blood vessels, all bundled in a series of protective sheaths of connective tissue. As shown in **Figure 6.17**, each axon is covered by a fine **endoneurium** (ehn-doh-NOO-ree-um). In myelinated axons, the endoneurium surrounds the myelin sheath as well as the nodes of Ranvier.

Groups of these sheathed axons are bundled into fascicles surrounded by a protective **perineurium** (per-i-NOO-ree-um). Finally, groups of fascicles and blood vessels are encased in a tough **epineurium** (ehp-i-NOO-ree-um). This structural arrangement provides a cordlike strength that helps the nerve resist injury.

Cranial Nerves

Twelve pairs of **cranial nerves** relay impulses to and from the left and right sides of the brain. These pairs are referred to by both a name and a number (**Figure 6.18**). The functions of the cranial nerves are summarized in the table in **Figure 6.19**. The names of these nerves indicate their functions.

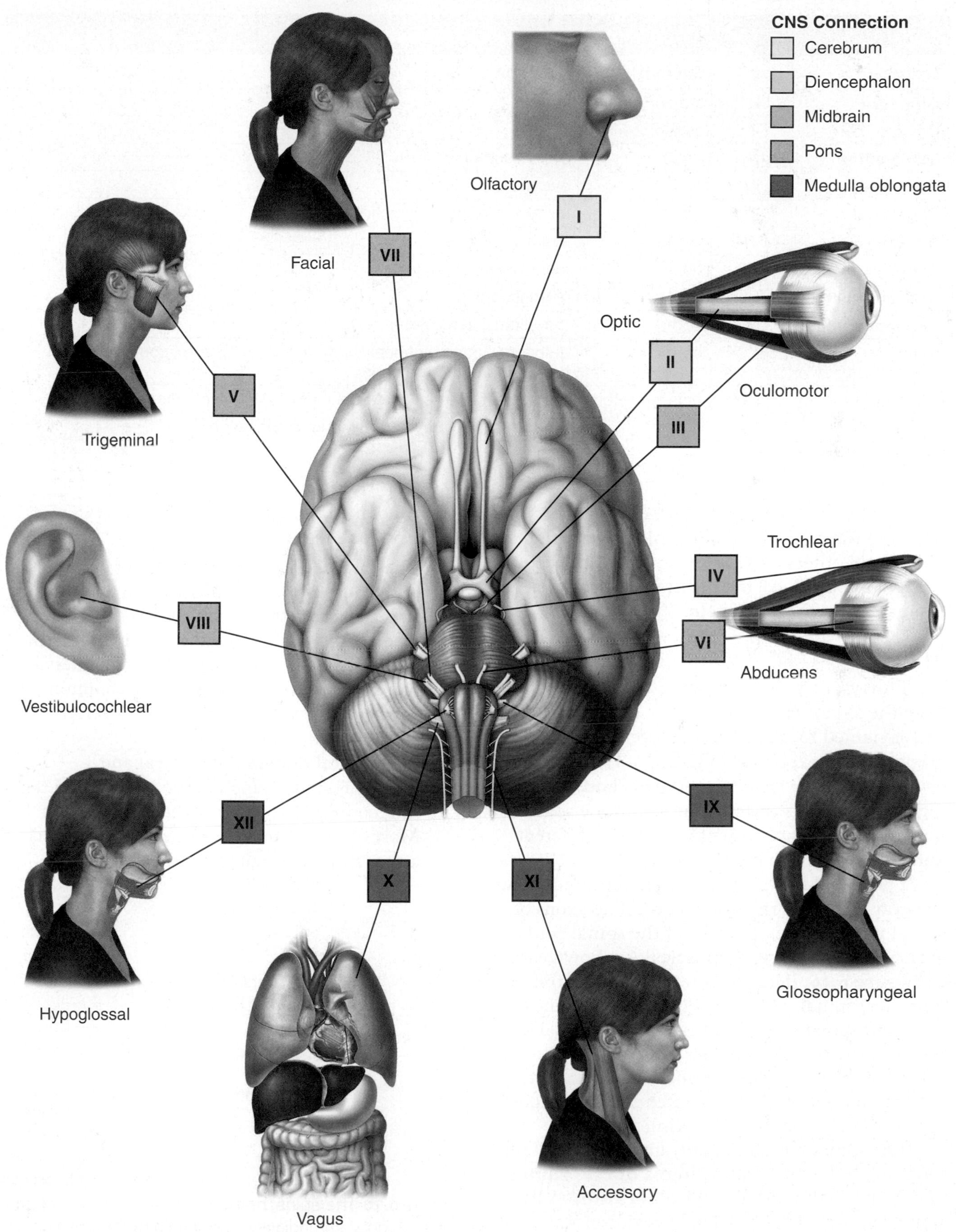

Figure 6.18 The cranial nerves. *Name at least two organs that receive impulses from the vagus nerve.*

Functions of the Cranial Nerves			
Nerve	**#**	**System**	**Function**
Olfactory	I	sensory	smell
Optic	II	sensory	sight
Oculomotor	III	both	eye movements
Trochlear	IV	both	eye movements
Trigeminal	V	both	facial sensation, jaw motion
Abducens	VI	both	eye movements
Facial	VII	both	facial movements, taste
Vestibulocochlear	VIII	sensory	hearing, balance
Glossopharyngeal	IX	both	throat muscle movements, taste
Vagus	X	both	autonomic control of heart, lungs, digestion, taste, communication between brain and organs
Accessory	XI	mostly motor	trapezius movements, sternocleidomastoid movements
Hypoglossal	XII	both	tongue muscle movements, tongue sensation

Figure 6.19

Goodheart-Willcox Publisher

Some cranial nerves contain only afferent (sensory) fibers, some contain only efferent (motor) fibers, and others—the *mixed nerves*—carry both kinds of impulses. All but the first two cranial nerves emanate from the brainstem.

Spinal Nerves and Nerve Plexuses

Thirty-one pairs of **spinal nerves** branch out from the left and right sides of the spinal cord. Each pair is named for the vertebral level from which it originates. As explained in Chapter 4, the vertebral levels include the cervical, thoracic, and lumbar regions, as well as the sacrum. All of the spinal nerves are mixed nerves, carrying both afferent and efferent information.

The spinal nerve cell bodies are located within the gray matter of the spinal cord. The axons of spinal nerve cells extend out of the spinal cord and eventually connect with muscles. As shown earlier in **Figure 6.16**, dorsal (posterior) and ventral (anterior) spinal nerve roots unite to form the left and right spinal nerves that exit at each spinal level. Because the spinal cord does not extend the entire length of the vertebral column, the spinal nerves at the inferior end of the cord extend for a way down the vertebral canal before exiting.

The spinal nerves are only about one-half inch long, immediately dividing into a **dorsal ramus** (DOR-sal RAY-mus) and **ventral ramus** (VEHN-tral RAY-mus) (**Figure 6.20**). The dorsal and ventral rami carry nerve impulses to the muscle and skin of the trunk.

All of the rami are mixed nerves, carrying both afferent and efferent signals.

- The small dorsal rami transmit motor impulses to the posterior trunk muscles and relay sensory impulses from the skin of the back.
- The ventral rami in the thoracic region of the spine (T_1–T_{12}) become the intercostal nerves (running between the ribs). They communicate with the muscles and skin of the anterior and lateral trunk.
- The ventral rami in the cervical and lumbar regions branch out to form complex interconnections of nerves called **plexuses**. Most of the major efferent nerves in the neck, arms, and legs originate in the plexuses.

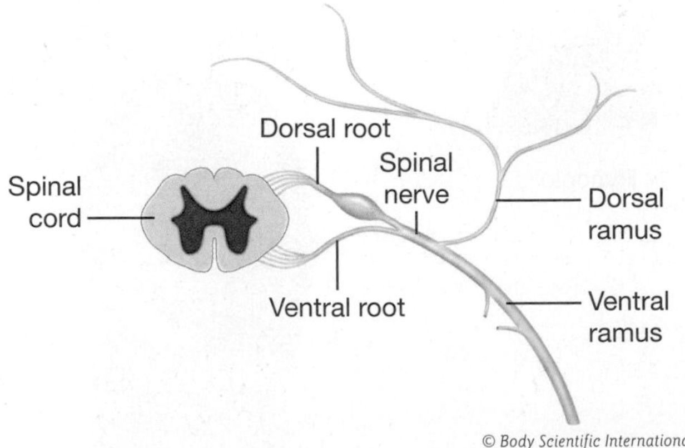

© Body Scientific International

Figure 6.20 The spinal nerves, formed from dorsal and ventral roots, immediately branch into dorsal and ventral rami. *What motor impulses do the dorsal and ventral rami transmit? What sensory nerve impulses do they transmit?*

The four plexuses in the body are summarized in **Figure 6.21**. To see how the major nerves branch out from the lower three plexuses, refer to **Figure 6.22**.

Check Your Understanding

1. How many pairs of cranial nerves does the body have?
2. What kind of impulses do mixed nerves carry?
3. How many pairs of spinal nerves does the body have?

Autonomic Nervous System

As described in Lesson 6.1, the peripheral nervous system has two divisions—the somatic nervous system and the autonomic, or involuntary, nervous system. The somatic nervous system sends impulses to activate the skeletal muscles, whereas the autonomic nervous system is programmed by the CNS to activate the heart, smooth muscles, and glands.

Within the autonomic system, two nerves connect the CNS to the organs supplied. The cell body of the first nerve originates in the gray matter of the brain or spinal cord. The autonomic cell bodies that originate in the spinal cord reside in the lateral horn. The axons of these nerves terminate with a synapse to a second neuron in an enlarged junction called a **ganglion** (GAYNG-glee-ahn). The second neuron then courses from the ganglion to the cardiac muscle, smooth muscle, or gland.

As you might suspect, the first neuron in the sequence just described is called the **preganglionic** (pree-gayng-glee-AHN-ik) **neuron**. The second is called the **postganglionic** (pohst-gayng-glee-AHN-ik) **neuron**. The autonomic nervous system has two branches: the sympathetic and parasympathetic branches. Both branches contain both preganglionic and postganglionic neurons.

Sympathetic Nerves

The sympathetic nerves activate the fight-or-flight response by stimulating the adrenal gland to release epinephrine, also known as *adrenaline*. Supposedly in primitive times, when a person was confronted by a predator, the fight-or-flight response—characterized by increased heart and breathing rates and sweating—prepared the individual either to fight or run. In modern times the sympathetic response is physiologically the same, but it can be triggered by any type of

Spinal Nerve Plexuses

Plexus	Spinal nerves	Exiting nerves	Region supplied
Cervical	C_1–C_5	phrenic	diaphragm, skin and muscles of neck and shoulder
Brachial	C_5–C_8 and T_1	axillary	skin and muscles of shoulder
		radial	skin and muscles of lateral and posterior upper arm and forearm
		median	skin and flexor muscles of forearm, some hand muscles
		musculocutaneous	skin of lateral forearm, elbow flexor muscles
		ulnar	skin of hand, flexor muscles of forearm, wrist, and some hand muscles
Lumbar	L_1–L_4	femoral	skin of medial and anterior thigh, anterior thigh muscles
		obturator	skin and muscles of medial thigh and hip
		saphenous	skin of the medial thigh and medial lower leg
Sacral	L_4–L_5 and S_1–S_4	sciatic	two of the hamstrings (semimembranosus, semitendinosus), adductor magnus
		tibial	muscles of knee flexion, plantar flexion, and toe flexion; skin of the posterior lower leg and sole of the foot
		common fibular	biceps femoris, tibialis anterior, muscles of toe extension, skin of the anterior lower leg, superior surface of foot, and lateral side of foot
		superior and inferior gluteal	gluteal muscles
		posterior femoral cutaneous	skin of posterior thigh and posterior lower leg

Figure 6.21 *Goodheart-Willcox Publisher*

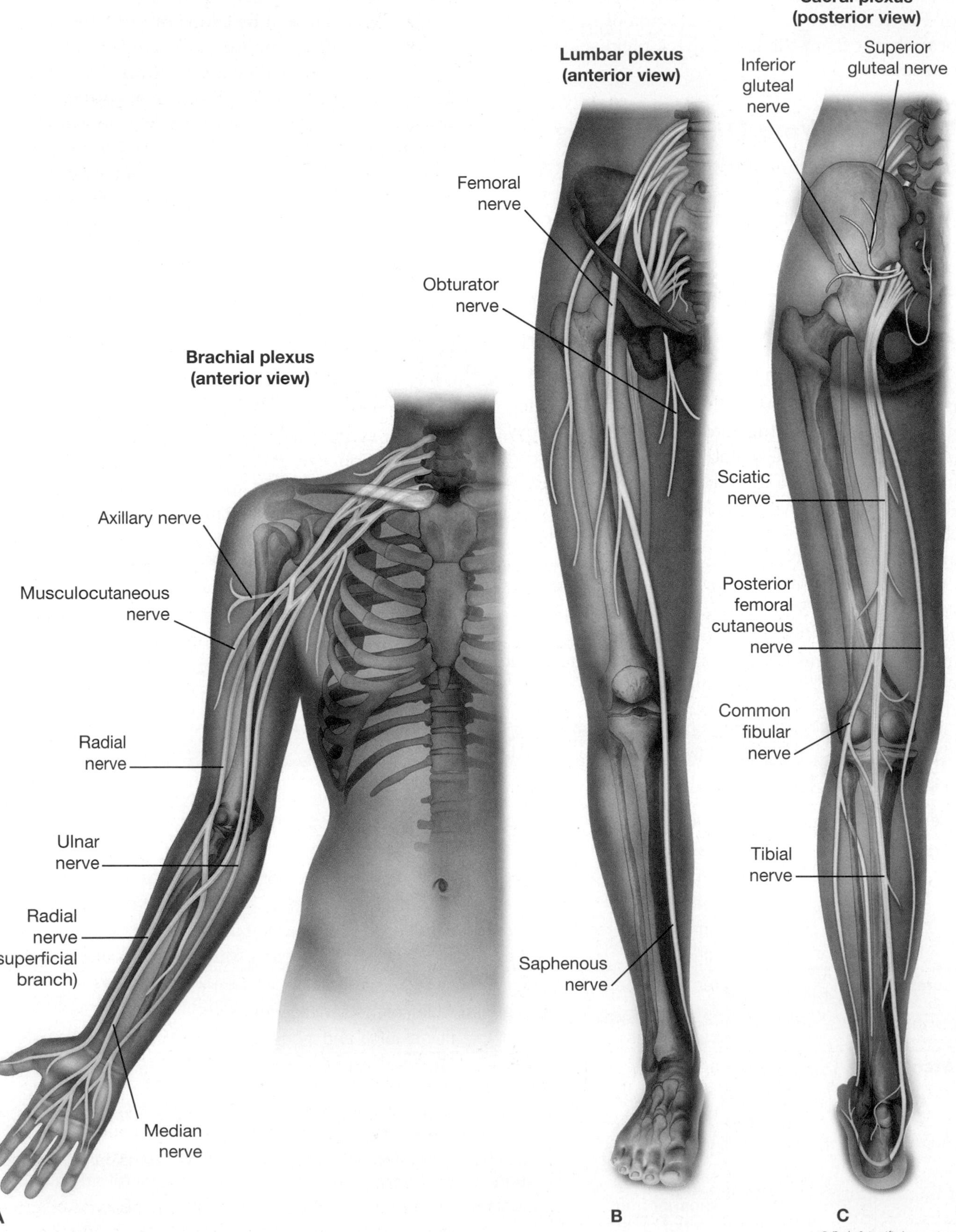

Figure 6.22 Major nerves emanate from the brachial, lumbar, and sacral plexuses.

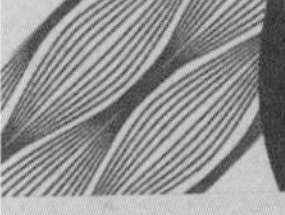

LIFE SPAN DEVELOPMENT: *The Nervous System*

Neural stem cells, known as *neural progenitor cells*, in the developing human embryo are responsible for producing all the different cells that make up the brain and central nervous system. During weeks 3 through 8 in the developing human embryo, the basic structures of the brain and spinal cord are formed. At the beginning of week 7, neurons begin to form. As the neurons are generated, they travel to different areas of the brain and begin organizing into primitive neural networks. The human brain contains billions of neurons, most of them having been produced by the midpoint of the pregnancy.

During the fetal period, beginning with week 9 and extending through birth, the gyri and sulci form in the brain. The first fissure to form is the longitudinal fissure that separates the two cerebral hemispheres.

Brain development continues for an extended period after birth. The brain's volume increases by a factor of four by age 6, at which time it is approximately 90% the size of an adult brain. During childhood and adolescence there are structural changes in the gray and white matter in the brain and spinal cord, with a dramatic increase in myelination of the neurons. These changes in structure are accompanied by changes in functional organization that enable progressively more neuromuscular control and adult-like behavior. The formation and distribution of glial cells also continues throughout childhood.

The progressive development of the nervous system during infancy and childhood is reflected in a number of reflexes that first emerge at different stages. Many reflexes, such as constriction of the pupils of the eyes in the presence of bright light, are present at birth and persist through life. Others appear and disappear with development. For example, the *Babkin reflex*, in which pressure applied to the baby's palm causes opening of the mouth and closing of the eyes, is present at birth but disappears within 2 to 4 months. The *Landau reflex*, in which suspending the infant in a horizontal, prone position and flexing the head against the trunk causes the legs to flex against the trunk, appears at approximately 3 months and disappears between the ages of 1 and 2 years. Doctors run a series of reflex tests on newborns in the delivery room to check for normal neural function.

The brain reaches full size in young adulthood. During the rest of life, the brain and spinal cord lose volume and weight, as neurons are damaged and die. After a certain age, which varies from person to person, brain function tends to decline. Different aspects of brain function are affected at different times. Short-term memory, which affects the ability to learn new information, tends to be one of the first functions to diminish. Verbal abilities, including vocabulary and word choice, may begin to decline at about age 70. Intellectual capacity, or the ability to process information, is usually maintained until at least age 80 if no diseases or disorders influence it. The peripheral nerves may conduct impulses more slowly, resulting in decreased sensation, longer reaction time, and slower movement speed. However, regular physical exercise has been shown to postpone all these effects of aging on the nervous system.

Life Span Review

1. What cells are responsible for the origination of the nervous system in the developing human embryo?
2. What structures in the nervous system continue to develop after birth?
3. Why does brain function tend to diminish with aging?

situation that is perceived to be stressful. You will learn more about the fight-or-flight response in Chapter 8, *The Endocrine System*.

The preganglionic neurons in the sympathetic branch arise from the spinal segments extending from T_1 to L_2. For this reason, the sympathetic system is also called the **thoracolumbar** (thoh-rah-koh-LUM-bar) **branch**. These neurons secrete acetylcholine to stimulate the postganglionic neurons in the **paravertebral ganglia** (pair-a-VER-teh-bral GAYNG-glee-a). The paravertebral ganglia are named after their location; they lie parallel to the vertebrae. The postganglionic neurons release the neurotransmitter **norepinephrine** (nor-ehp-i-NEHF-rin).

Parasympathetic Nerves

In contrast to the sympathetic branch, the parasympathetic branch of the autonomic nervous system controls all of the automatic, day-in-and-day-out functions of the circulatory, respiratory, and digestive systems. For these reasons it is sometimes called the *resting and digesting system*. In addition, after a fight-or-flight situation, the parasympathetic nervous system produces a calming effect that returns the body to a normal state.

Preganglionic parasympathetic neurons originate in one of two separate regions—the brainstem or the sacral region of the spinal cord. For this reason, the parasympathetic system is also known as the

craniosacral (kray-nee-oh-SAY-kral) **branch**. Activation of both preganglionic and postganglionic nerves in this branch triggers the release of the neurotransmitter acetylcholine. Although acetylcholine stimulates skeletal muscle, it also inhibits activity in cardiac and smooth muscle.

Check Your Understanding

1. List the two branches of the autonomic nervous system.
2. Which nerves—sympathetic or parasympathetic—activate the fight-or-flight response?

LESSON 6.4 Review and Assessment

Mini Glossary

Make sure you that know the meaning of each key term.

cranial nerves 12 pairs of nerves that originate in the brain and relay impulses to and from the PNS

craniosacral branch the parasympathetic branch of the autonomic nervous system, in which nerves originate in the brainstem or sacral region of the spinal cord

dorsal ramus posterior spinal nerves that transmit motor impulses to the posterior trunk muscles and relay sensory impulses from the skin of the back

endoneurium a delicate, connective tissue that surrounds each nerve fiber

epineurium the tough outer covering of a nerve

ganglion a mass of nervous tissue composed mostly of nerve cell bodies

norepinephrine a neurotransmitter released by postganglionic neurons in the sympathetic nervous system

paravertebral ganglia mass of nerve cell bodies close to the spinal cord

perineurium a protective sheath that surrounds a bundle of nerve fibers

plexuses complex interconnections of nerves

postganglionic neuron the second neuron in a series that transmits impulses from the CNS

preganglionic neuron the first neuron in a series that transmits impulses from the CNS

spinal nerves neural transmitters that branch from the left and right sides of the spinal cord

thoracolumbar branch the sympathetic nerves that lie near the thoracic and lumbar regions of the spine

ventral ramus anterior spinal nerves that communicate with the muscle and skin of the anterior and lateral trunk

Know and Understand

1. Explain the function of the peripheral nervous system.
2. What is the combined purpose of the endoneurium, perineurium, and epineurium?
3. How would you describe cranial nerves in terms of sensory and motor fibers?
4. From where do the majority of cranial nerves emanate?
5. Are spinal nerves efferent, afferent, or mixed?
6. Which division of the peripheral nervous system sends impulses to the heart?
7. Explain the difference between a preganglionic neuron and a postganglionic neuron.
8. Why is the parasympathetic nervous system also known as the *craniosacral division*?

Analyze and Apply

9. Explain how the structure of a nerve decreases the chances of nerve damage.
10. Describe the fight-or-flight response activated by sympathetic nerves and explain how it could be a lifesaver.
11. Neurons meet at junctions called *ganglions*. Explain the purpose of a ganglion and how these structures help transmit nerve impulses throughout the body.
12. Explain how the function of a cranial nerve might determine whether it is a sensory or motor fiber, or both.
13. Explain how the parasympathetic branch of the autonomic nervous system can restore calm to the body after a fight-or-flight situation has been activated by the sympathetic nervous system.

IN THE LAB

14. Using clay, create a model of a nerve. Use different colors for the different parts of the nerve. Begin with a simpler structure, such as an axon, and continue until you have a more complex structure (complete nerve). Use the illustrations in this lesson to guide you in constructing your model.
15. Using clay, construct a cross section of the spinal cord and the nerves that originate from it. Label the different parts of the nerves. Include this terminology in your labels: dorsal root, ventral root, dorsal ramus, ventral ramus. Also show where each part of the nerve transmits impulses.

LESSON 6.5

Injuries and Disorders of the Nervous System

Before You Read

Try to answer the following questions before you read this lesson.

- What are the important first steps to take—and actions not to take—when someone may have an injury to the brain or spinal cord?
- What are the symptoms of early and advanced Alzheimer's disease?

Lesson Objectives

- Describe the symptoms and recovery strategies for someone who has suffered a traumatic brain or spinal cord injury.
- Identify common diseases and disorders of the nervous system.

Key Terms

acute flaccid myelitis (AFM)
Alzheimer's disease (AD)
cerebral palsy (CP)
dementia
epilepsy
meningitis
multiple sclerosis (MS)
paraplegia
Parkinson's disease (PD)
quadriplegia
traumatic brain injury (TBI)

CLINICAL CASE STUDY

Jeremy enjoys spending time with his grandparents, who live nearby. In particular, he loves going fishing with his granddad on weekends during the early fall when the fish are biting. Lately Jeremy has noticed that his granddad seems to walk more slowly and that there is a tremor in his hands when he casts his fishing line. Mentally, his granddad seems perfectly fine. As you read this section, try to determine which of the following conditions Jeremy's granddad most likely has.

A. Cerebral palsy
B. Multiple sclerosis
C. Parkinson's disease
D. Alzheimer's disease

Given the critical roles played by the central nervous system, injuries and disorders of the CNS can have potentially serious consequences. This lesson describes some of the more common injuries and disorders of the CNS.

Injuries to the Brain and Spinal Cord

The brain and spinal cord are well protected. They are encased, respectively, in the skull and vertebral column, and both are surrounded by the three meninges and cerebrospinal fluid. Unfortunately, violent injuries can still cause mild to severe damage to these CNS structures. The etiology (cause), strategies for prevention, pathology (clinical characteristics), diagnosis (keys for identifying the condition), and common treatments for these injuries to the brain and spinal cord are summarized in **Figure 6.23**.

Traumatic Brain Injury

Traumatic brain injury (TBI) can occur during violent impacts to the head, particularly when the skull is pierced or fractured and bone fragments penetrate the brain. These injuries are classified as mild, moderate, or severe, with increasing levels of damage to the nervous system, particularly the cells and tissues of the brain.

With mild TBI, a person may remain conscious or may lose consciousness for a short time. Symptoms may include any of the following: headache, confusion, dizziness, disturbed vision, ringing in the ears, bad taste in the mouth, fatigue, abnormal sleep patterns, behavioral changes, and trouble with intellectual functions.

Symptoms of moderate to severe TBI include all of those listed above, and may also involve more serious symptoms such as prolonged headache, repeated nausea or vomiting, convulsions or seizures, inability to awaken from sleep, dilation

Injuries to the Brain and Spinal Cord					
	Etiology	**Prevention**	**Pathology**	**Diagnosis**	**Treatment**
Traumatic Brain Injury	violent impact to the head	Be careful!	mild: headache, confusion, dizziness, disturbed vision, ringing in the ears, bad taste in the mouth, fatigue, abnormal sleep patterns, behavioral changes, trouble with intellectual functions severe: repeated nausea, dilation of pupils, weakness in the extremities, loss of coordination, agitation	physical exam, imaging tests	individualized rehabilitation program
Cerebral Palsy	brain damage before or during birth	none	tight muscles and joints, muscle weakness, gait abnormalities; may include learning disabilities, problems with speech, hearing, sight, swallowing, digestion; seizures, pain, slowed growth, drooling, breath irregularities, and incontinence	brain imaging; tests for reflexes, muscle tone, posture, coordination	steps to promote quality of life
Spinal Cord Injury	fractures or displacement of the vertebrae	steps to avoid high-speed impacts	complete severing: paralysis below the injury site incomplete severing: some degree of sensory and motor function below the injury	physical exam, imaging	surgery when warranted, rehabilitation program

Figure 6.23

Goodheart-Willcox Publisher

of one or both pupils of the eyes, slurred speech, weakness or numbness in the extremities, loss of coordination, confusion, and agitation. Cases of moderate and severe TBI require immediate medical care, with the goal of preventing further brain injury. X-rays and imaging tests may be performed to help assess the nature and extent of the damage. Maintaining proper blood pressure and a constant flow of oxygenated blood to the brain and throughout the body are priorities. About 50% of severe TBI cases require surgical repair.

Case Study: Phineas Gage

A miraculous story of survival from a significant TBI is the case of Phineas Gage, a railroad construction foreman who was injured in 1848 at 25 years of age. Gage and his crew were blasting rock to make way for railroad construction outside the town of Cavendish, Vermont, when a 3½-foot iron rod was accidentally blasted through Gage's skull. The iron rod entered below the left cheekbone and exited through the top of the skull. The blast was of such force that the rod landed approximately 80 feet away.

Amazingly, within a few minutes Gage was able to speak, walk, and ride upright in a cart back to his home, where he received medical attention. Gage's recovery was slow, with advances and declines, including time spent in a coma due to brain swelling. Nevertheless, his physical recovery was complete.

Accounts of Gage's mental recovery vary, but they suggest that his personality was negatively altered. Gage survived for 12 years after the accident. He began to suffer a series of increasingly severe seizures that eventually resulted in his death. The case of Phineas Gage is still discussed in medical and neurology classes.

Treating and Preventing TBI

Today, follow-up care for TBI involves individualized rehabilitation programs that may include physical, occupational, and speech language therapies; psychiatry; and social support. The prognosis for those who have suffered from a traumatic brain injury varies greatly, with potential for lingering problems with intellectual functioning, sensation, and behavior. Serious head injuries can result in an unresponsive state or a coma.

What Research Tells Us

...about Concussions

The most common form of traumatic brain injury is a concussion. Symptoms include headache as well as problems with concentration, memory, judgment, balance, and coordination. Fortunately, these effects are usually temporary. Although a concussion *can* cause a loss of consciousness, most concussions do not. Thus, many people experience mild concussions without realizing it.

The most common cause of concussion is a blow to the head. However, concussions can also occur when the head and upper body are violently shaken. In fact, the word *concussion* comes from the Latin *concutere*, which means "to shake violently."

Concussions in Sports

Injuries that produce concussions are of particular concern for participants in American football, boxing, and soccer, although they also occur in other sports. According to the CDC, as many as 3.8 million sports- and recreation-related concussions occur in the United States each year. Concussions also result from car and bicycle accidents, work injuries, and falls.

Because all concussions injure the brain to some extent, it is crucial that these injuries have time to heal. Healing time is particularly important for athletes in contact sports, which involve higher risks of reinjury to the brain. For this reason, researchers are focusing attention on the consequences of repeated concussions (**Figure 6.24**).

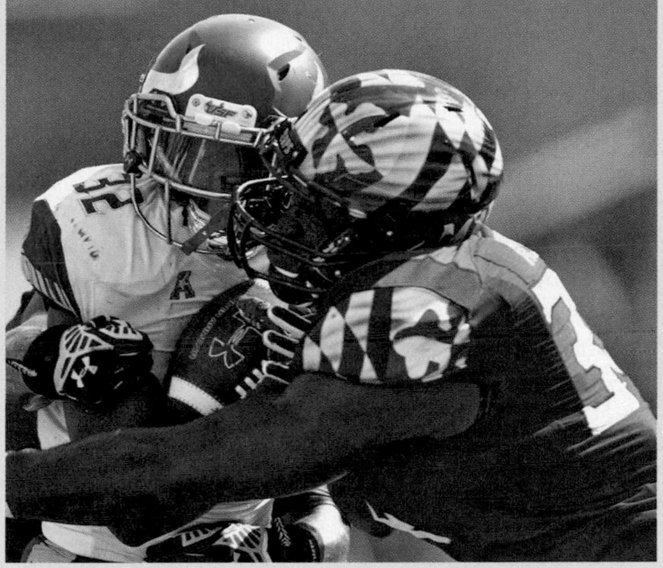

By Aspen Photo/Shutterstock.com

Figure 6.24 Both the NFL and the NCAA have implemented strict new rules in an effort to prevent concussions.

Recent Research

A recent study shows that retired professional football players appear to be at a higher risk of death from diseases of the brain, compared to the general US population. In the study, sponsored by the National Institute for Occupational Safety and Health (NIOSH), researchers examined the medical records of 3,439 former NFL players with an average age of 57. At the time of the analysis, only 10 percent of the participants had died, which is about half the death rate of men that age in the general population. The fact that relatively few had died indicates that the study participants were in better-than-average general health.

The medical records showed, however, that an NFL player's risk of death from Alzheimer's disease or amyotrophic lateral sclerosis (ALS), also known as *Lou Gehrig's disease*, was almost four times higher than in the general population. Furthermore, those players in "speed" positions—such as wide receiver, running back, and quarterback—accounted for most of the deaths from Alzheimer's disease and ALS. The researchers emphasized that the data in this type of study do not establish a cause-effect relationship. They hypothesized, however, that the players in "speed" positions likely had experienced more high-speed collisions, and possibly repeated concussions, compared to the "non-speed" players.

NFL Takes Action

The NFL has donated $30 million to help establish the Sports and Health Research Program within the National Institutes of Health (NIH). This initiative provides funding for research on concussions and other common injuries in athletes across all sports, as well as members of the military.

The NFL also has taken steps to help prevent concussions, such as fining players for dangerous hits, notably helmet-to-helmet tackles. Rule changes at both the professional and collegiate levels now prevent players diagnosed with concussions from returning to play until they have been declared free of symptoms by a medical doctor.

Taking It Further

Working with a group of classmates, determine the standard procedure in athletic departments at local high schools and colleges for dealing with concussions. Are medical professionals involved in evaluating the severity of the concussion and determining when the athlete can resume practice and competitive events? What tests are used for the evaluations? Have rules been instituted to help prevent concussions? Report your findings to the class.

Research is being conducted in scientific and clinical settings to achieve a clearer understanding of the biological effects of TBI. One goal of this research is to develop strategies and interventions that limit the brain damage that occurs during the first few days after a head injury. Another goal is to develop more effective therapies for facilitating recovery of function.

Cerebral Palsy

Cerebral palsy (CP) is a group of nervous system disorders caused by damage to the brain before or during birth (congenital defect), or in early infancy. Congenital defects that can cause CP include a brain that has an abnormal shape or structure, or damaged nerve cells and brain tissues. Infections such as rubella in the mother during pregnancy can produce CP. During the first two years, while the brain is still developing, several conditions—including brain infections, head injury, and impaired liver function—can cause CP. Sometimes, however, the cause is unknown.

The most common symptoms involve varying degrees of motor function impairment, but symptoms may also include hearing, seeing, and cognitive impairment. The degree of impairment may be barely noticeable or very severe (**Figure 6.25**). One or both sides of the body may be affected and the arms, legs, or both may be involved.

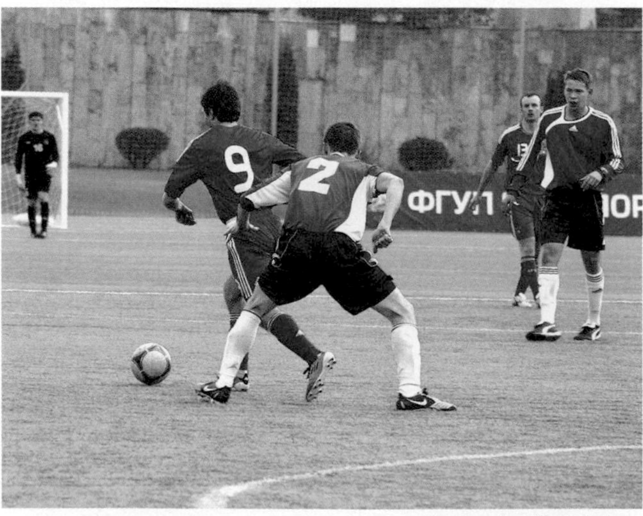

Martynova Anna/Shutterstock.com

Figure 6.25 Russian and British athletes with cerebral palsy play a game of soccer in preparation for the Paralympics.

Several different types of cerebral palsy exist, with some individuals having mixed symptoms. The most common form is spastic CP, with symptoms that include:

- very tight muscles and joints
- muscle weakness
- gait (manner of walking) in which the arms are held close to the body with the elbows in flexion, the knees touch or cross, and the individual walks on tiptoes

In other types of cerebral palsy, motor function degradation may include twisting or jerking movements; tremors; unsteady gait; impaired coordination; and excessive, floppy movements.

Sensory and cognitive symptoms may include learning disabilities or diminished intelligence; problems with speech; problems with hearing or sight; seizures; pain; and problems with swallowing and digestion. Other symptoms may include slowed growth; drooling; breathing irregularities; and incontinence.

No cure for cerebral palsy exists, so the goal of treatment in moderate to severe cases is to promote quality of life and, when possible, independent living. In some cases, surgical intervention can improve gait, alleviate spasticity or pain, or restore joint range of motion.

Spinal Cord Injury

Fractures or displacements of the vertebrae can result in injury to the spinal cord. Such injuries most commonly occur during automobile accidents or participation in high-speed or contact sports. Although injuries to the spinal cord can occur at any level, these injuries most commonly develop in the cervical region because of the flexibility of the neck compared to that of the trunk.

A complete severing of the spinal cord produces permanent paralysis, with a total lack of sensory and motor function below the point of injury. The level of the spine at which the injury occurs is a major factor in determining the extent of injury:

- C_1–C_3—usually fatal
- C_1–C_4—**quadriplegia** (kwah-dri-PLEE-jee-a), characterized by loss of function below the neck

- C_5–C_7—complete paralysis of the lower extremities, partial loss of function in the trunk and upper extremities
- T_1–L_5—**paraplegia** (pair-ah-PLEE-jee-ah), characterized by loss of function in the trunk and legs

Fortunately, most spinal cord injuries do not completely sever the spinal cord. In an *incomplete injury*, the ability of the spinal cord to transmit sensory and motor impulses is not completely lost. This allows some degree of sensory and/or motor function to remain below the point of injury. The prognosis in such cases is typically uncertain; some patients achieve nearly complete recovery, whereas others suffer complete paralysis.

Spinal cord injuries are medical emergencies. Immediate, aggressive treatment and follow-up rehabilitation can help minimize damage and preserve function. Because motion of a fractured or displaced vertebra can cause more damage to the spinal cord after the injury, it is critical that the head, neck, and trunk be immobilized before the victim is moved (**Figure 6.26**). In severe neck injuries of the spinal cord, breathing is affected in about one-third of the cases, and respiratory support is necessary. Surgery is often warranted to remove bone fragments or realign vertebrae to alleviate pressure on the spinal cord.

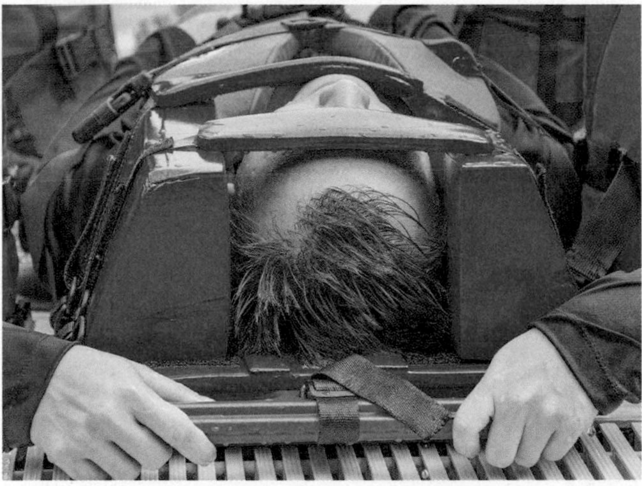

narin phapnam/Shutterstock.com

Figure 6.26 It is critically important that the head, neck, and trunk be immobilized before transporting a patient with a potential spinal cord injury. *What might happen if a patient's head, neck, and trunk are not immobilized after a potential spinal cord injury?*

Ongoing research is aimed at developing techniques for repairing injured spinal cords. Researchers are also working to advance understanding of which rehabilitation approaches are most successful at restoring lost function. Promising new rehabilitation techniques are helping patients with spinal cord injury become more mobile.

Check Your Understanding

1. Identify common causes of traumatic brain injury.
2. List the conditions that can cause cerebral palsy.
3. Explain the usual result of a spinal cord injury that occurs at each of the following levels: C_1–C_3; C_1–C_4; C_5–C_7; and T_1–L_5.

Diseases and Disorders of the CNS

This section explores some of the common diseases and disorders that affect the central nervous system (CNS). The etiology, strategies for prevention, pathology, diagnosis, and common treatments for these diseases and disorders of the CNS are summarized in **Figure 6.27**.

Meningitis

Meningitis (mehn-in-JIGH-tis) is an inflammation of the meninges surrounding the brain and spinal cord. Swelling of these tissues, which is caused by an infection, often produces the signature symptoms of headache, fever, and a stiff neck.

Most infections that cause meningitis are viral, but bacterial and fungal infections can also lead to meningitis. Viral meningitis, the mildest form, may resolve on its own. Bacterial meningitis is much more serious and potentially life threatening. Fortunately, bacterial meningitis can be treated with antibiotics. In either case, a person should seek immediate medical attention if meningitis is suspected.

Diseases and Disorders of the CNS					
	Etiology	**Prevention**	**Pathology**	**Diagnosis**	**Treatment**
Meningitis	infection causes inflammation of the meninges	avoid infection; avoid sick people, wash hands often	swelling of the meninges produces headache, fever, stiff neck	physical exam, MRI, blood tests	antibiotics for bacterial meningitis
Acute flaccid myelitis	cause is unknown; may be viral infection or an immune response	avoid infection; avoid sick people, wash hands often	sudden onset of arm or leg weakness, loss of muscle tone and reflexes; drooping of eyes and face, difficulty swallowing, slurred speech	physical exam, imaging of spinal cord, tests of cerebrospinal fluid	treatment of symptoms
Multiple Sclerosis	immune system attacks the myelin sheath surrounding axons	none	symptoms vary widely, can include impairments in motor, sensory, and autonomic functions	physical exam, tests of nerve function	rest, sound nutrition, avoiding heat and stress; treatment of symptoms
Epilepsy	group of brain disorders caused by disease, injury, or genetics	none	symptoms range from lapses in attention span to uncontrolled seizures	physical exam, brain imaging	medication for seizures, surgery for repairable brain anomalies
Parkinson's disease	unknown; destruction of brain cells that produce dopamine	no known prevention	tremors, difficulty initiating movements, coordination deficits; impaired cognitive and autonomic functions	physical exam, neurological tests	medication to increase dopamine level in the brain
Alzheimer's disease	unknown cause	no known prevention	progressive loss of brain function affecting memory, thinking, and behavior	physical exam, tests for memory and cognition	medications to slow the worsening of symptoms
Spina bifida	spine and spinal cord do not form properly	folic acid supplement before and during pregnancy	varies from no symptoms to myelomeningocele	prenatal blood tests, ultrasound, amniocentesis	pre- or post-natal surgery

Figure 6.27 *Goodheart-Willcox Publisher*

Acute Flaccid Myelitis

Acute flaccid myelitis (AFM) is a rare, but serious neurologic condition that occurs primarily in children. It attacks the gray matter in the spinal cord, affecting the muscles and reflexes. Sudden onset of arm or leg weakness and loss of muscle tone and reflexes are the first signs of AFM. Other symptoms may include drooping eyelids or trouble moving the eyes, facial drooping, difficulty swallowing, and slurred speech. The most severe and life-threatening symptom of AFM is respiratory failure due to weakening of the muscles of respiration.

It is important to see a neurologist as soon as possible if the condition is suspected. Diagnosis is based on a physical exam, imaging of the spinal cord, and tests of the cerebrospinal fluid. The cause of AFM is unknown. However, because most patients had a mild viral infection and symptoms of respiratory illness and fever prior to developing AFM, it may be that viruses play a role. Another possibility is that AFM is caused by an immune response triggered by a virus. To prevent AFM it is prudent to avoid contact with people who are sick, wash the hands frequently, and avoid touching the face with unwashed hands. Vaccination for poliovirus may also be protective.

Multiple Sclerosis

Multiple sclerosis (MS) is an autoimmune disease in which the body's own immune system causes inflammation that destroys the myelin sheath of nerve cell axons. This damage to the myelin sheath, which can occur in any part of the brain or spinal cord, impairs the ability of the affected nerves to transmit impulses. MS can occur at any age, but it is most commonly diagnosed between 20 and 40 years of age and occurs with greater frequency in women. The cause of MS is unknown.

An active attack of MS can last for days, weeks, or months. Periods during which the symptoms vanish or diminish are called *remissions*. Exposure to heat and stress can trigger or worsen attacks.

The symptoms of MS vary widely, depending on location within the CNS and severity of each episode.

- Impairments in motor function may include difficulties with balance, coordination, movement of the arms and legs, tremors, weakness, muscle spasms, and difficulty with speaking or swallowing.
- Sensory impairments may involve numbness, tingling, pain, double vision, uncontrollable eye movements, and loss of vision or hearing.
- Autonomic functions related to urination, defecation, and sexual function may be affected.
- Associated cognitive issues may include decreased attention span, difficulty with reasoning, loss of memory, and depression.

There is no known cure for multiple sclerosis, so treatments are designed to help control symptoms and maintain quality of life. Exercise is often beneficial during the early stages. General recommendations for the MS patient include sufficient rest, sound nutrition, avoidance of hot temperatures, and minimization of stress. Although MS is a chronic condition, life expectancy can be normal. Many individuals with MS continue functioning well in their jobs until retirement.

Epilepsy

Epilepsy (EHP-i-lehp-see) is a group of brain disorders characterized by repeated seizures over time. A seizure is triggered by abnormal electrical activity in the brain that causes widely varying symptoms. Symptoms can range from changes in attention span or behavior to uncontrolled convulsions, depending on the type of epilepsy and area of the brain affected.

Epilepsy may be caused by a disease or injury that affects the brain, although in many cases the cause is unknown, and genetics may play a role. Onset of epilepsy can happen at any age but occurs most frequently in infants and the elderly. Some types of epilepsy completely disappear after childhood.

Epileptic seizures in a given individual are of a relatively consistent nature. Before a seizure, some people have an unusual sensation such as tingling, a strange smell, or an emotional change. This signal is referred to as an *aura*.

Epilepsy can be controlled with medication in most, but not all, people. However, more than 30% of people with epilepsy are not able to control seizure incidence with medications. If epileptic seizures are caused by an observable problem, such as a tumor, abnormal blood vessels, or bleeding in the brain, surgery to address these issues may eliminate further seizures.

Parkinson's Disease

Parkinson's disease (PD) is one of the most common nervous system disorders among the elderly. It is characterized by tremors, difficulty with initiating movements—especially walking—and deficits in coordination. PD most often develops after the age of 50, although a genetic form of the disease may occur in younger adults. Men and women are equally affected.

PD is characterized by slow but progressive destruction of the brain cells responsible for production of the neurotransmitter dopamine, which plays a role in motor function. Without dopamine, the cells in the affected part of the brain cannot initiate nerve impulses, leading to progressive loss of muscle function. The cause of this condition is unknown.

The symptoms of PD tend to begin with a mild tremor or slight stiffness or weakness in one or both of the legs or feet (**Figure 6.28**). As brain cell destruction progresses, symptoms of motor dysfunction affecting one or both sides of the body may include:

- difficulty initiating and continuing movements
- problems with balance and gait
- stiff, painful muscles and tremors
- slowed movement, including blinking
- loss of fine motor control with hand movements
- slowed speech, drooling, and difficulty swallowing
- loss of facial expression
- stooped posture

Autonomic and cognitive functions may also be impaired, as characterized by:

- sweating and fluctuations in body temperature
- fainting and inability to control blood pressure
- constipation
- confusion or dementia
- anxiety or depression

Currently, no cure for PD exists; the goal of treatment is control of symptoms. If untreated, the disorder progresses, resulting in deterioration of all brain functions and early death. The medications prescribed for Parkinson's patients are designed to increase the levels of dopamine in the brain.

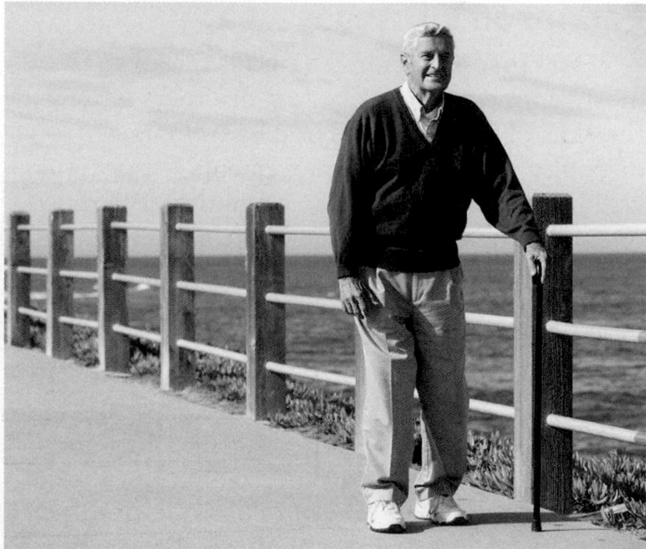

Monkey Business Images/Shutterstock.com

Figure 6.28 Symptoms of Parkinson's disease include weakness and stiffness in the legs and feet, as well as problems with balance and gait.

Dementia and Alzheimer's Disease

Dementia (deh-MEHN-shee-a) is a condition involving loss of function in two or more areas of cognition including memory, thinking, judgment, behavior, perception, and language. Dementia usually occurs after the age of 60, and risk increases with advancing age. Although forgetfulness is often the first sign of dementia, occasional forgetfulness alone does not qualify as dementia.

Dementia can be caused by disruption in the blood supply to the brain, as in stroke or related disorders. However, the single most common cause of dementia is Alzheimer's disease.

Alzheimer's disease (AD), or *senile dementia*, is a progressive loss of brain function with major consequences for memory, thinking, and behavior. In one form of the disease, called *early onset AD*, symptoms appear before 60 years of age. This type of AD tends to worsen quickly and is believed to involve genetic predisposition. The more common form, known as *late onset AD*, occurs after 60 years of age. The risk for developing Alzheimer's disease increases with advancing age. The cause of AD is currently unknown.

Early symptoms of AD may include difficulty with tasks that previously were routine; difficulty learning new ideas, concepts, or tasks; becoming lost in familiar territory; difficulty recalling the names of familiar objects; misplacing objects; a flat mood and loss of interest in activities; and personality changes and loss of social skills.

Worsening symptoms can include difficulty performing activities of daily living; progressive loss of short- and long-term memory; depression and agitation; delusions and aggressive behavior; inability to speak coherently; loss of judgment; and change in sleep patterns.

Advanced symptoms include the inability to understand language and recognize family members. Although no cure currently exists for Alzheimer's disease, medications can help to slow the worsening of symptoms.

Check Your Understanding

1. Describe meningitis.
2. What happens to the body of a person with multiple sclerosis?
3. Describe Parkinson's disease.

LESSON 6.5 Review and Assessment

Mini Glossary

Make sure that you know the meaning of each key term.

acute flaccid myelitis (AFM) a rare, but serious neurologic condition that occurs primarily in children; attacks the gray matter in the spinal cord, affecting the muscles and reflexes

Alzheimer's disease (AD) condition of dementia involving a progressive loss of brain function with major consequences for memory, thinking, and behavior

cerebral palsy (CP) a group of nervous system disorders resulting from brain damage before or during birth, or in early infancy

dementia an organic brain disease involving loss of function in two or more areas of cognition

epilepsy a group of brain disorders characterized by repeated seizures over time

meningitis an infection-induced inflammation of the meninges surrounding the brain and spinal cord

multiple sclerosis a chronic, slowly progressive disease of the central nervous system that destroys the myelin sheath of nerve cell axons

paraplegia disorder characterized by loss of function in the lower trunk and legs

Parkinson's disease (PD) a chronic nervous system disease characterized by a slowly spreading tremor, muscular weakness, and rigidity

quadriplegia disorder characterized by loss of function below the neck

traumatic brain injury (TBI) mild or severe trauma that can result from a violent impact to the head

Know and Understand

1. Describe the body functions that may be affected in a person with cerebral palsy (CP).
2. What is meant by the term "incomplete injury" as it relates to a spinal cord injury?
3. What are the three types of meningitis and which is easiest to treat?
4. Which neurologic condition occurs primarily in children?
5. What is another name for senile dementia?

Analyze and Apply

6. Rheumatoid arthritis is an autoimmune disease described in Chapter 4. How are rheumatoid arthritis and MS similar?
7. Explain what happens in the brain when a person has a seizure.
8. Explain why spinal cord injuries at the C1 to C3 level are usually fatal.
9. Explain why a person should not be moved after an injury if a head or neck injury is suspected. What should be done before the person is moved?
10. In the past, some patients who developed Parkinson's disease were initially misdiagnosed as having Alzheimer's disease. Why might this confusion have occurred?

IN THE LAB

11. Conduct research to find brain images of people with epilepsy and people with Alzheimer's. Explain how the images are alike and how they are different.
12. With a partner, design a medication to treat a disorder associated with neurotransmission. Include the form of the medication, how the medication will be administered (orally, intravenously, etc.), and the desired effects. Also describe any potential side effects and cautions that should be noted before taking the medication.
13. Research has shown that certain activities, begun earlier in life, can reduce the severity of Alzheimer's in people who develop late onset AD. In addition, certain activities undertaken after AD has been diagnosed are thought to slow the progress of the disease. Conduct research to find out what these activities are and how they are thought to help. Collect and create a display of examples of such activities.
14. Guillain-Barré syndrome is a neurological disorder that causes weakness, tingling sensations, and eventually paralysis. Conduct research to find out more about the three types of Guillain-Barré and their symptoms. Write a report of your findings, being sure to cite your sources.

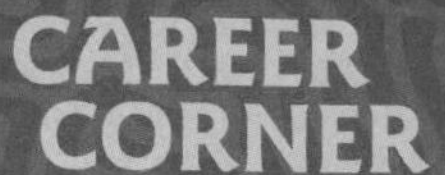

Anatomy & Physiology at Work

The nervous system is a complex organ system that plays an important role in the body's responses to numerous stimuli, both internal and external. That is quite a wide-ranging, significant role! Several careers are dedicated to the study of the nervous system, as well as to the diagnosis and treatment of neural disorders. Two of these careers are described here.

Neurologist

A neurologist (noo-RAHL-oh-jist) is a physician trained in the specialty field of neurology. Neurology involves the diagnosis and treatment of neurological injuries and diseases. A patient is typically referred to a neurologist by another physician who suspects that specialized treatment is needed.

Evaluation of a patient by a neurologist typically begins with a related medical history, followed by a physical examination that focuses on the nervous system. Components of the neurological examination may include assessment of the patient's cognitive function, muscular strength, sensation, reflexes, coordination, and gait. The neurologist may order diagnostic imaging studies when warranted (**Figure 6.29**).

Conditions commonly treated by neurologists include all of those discussed in this chapter. Treatment options vary by condition, and may include prescription of medications, referral for physical or occupational therapy, or referral to a surgeon.

Training to become a neurologist begins with four years of medical school, followed by a residency program or fellowship in pediatric or general neurology. The residency, which is usually four years, involves specific training. After residency, doctors may choose to pursue board certification through the American Board of Psychiatry and Neurology. Some neurologists voluntarily participate in additional training in a fellowship program to gain experience in a subspecialty area.

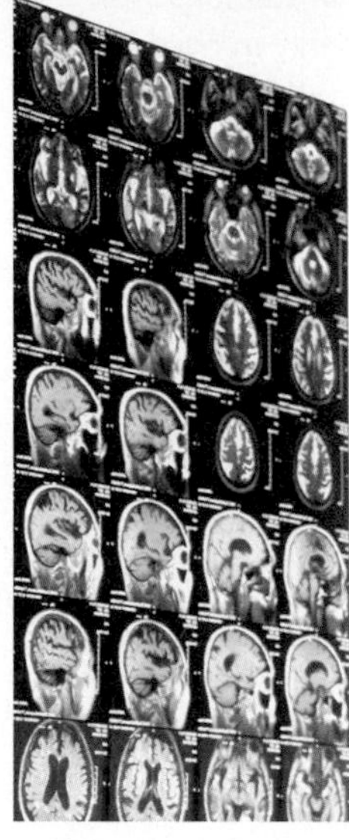
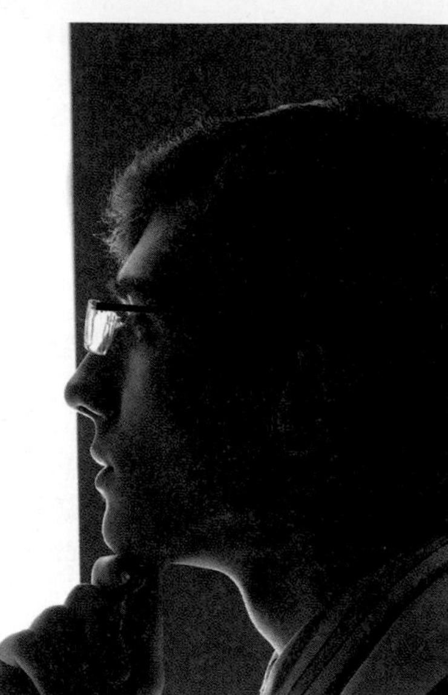

Sergey Nivens/Shutterstock.com

Figure 6.29 A neurologist interprets X-rays and brain scans to diagnose brain disorders and to check the progress of treatments.

Neurosurgery is a different specialty that involves surgical treatment of neurological conditions. Training to be a neurosurgeon requires completion of four years of medical school followed by residency training under the supervision of neurosurgeons for an additional seven to eight years.

Neuroscientist

A scientist who specializes in research of the nervous system is called a neuroscientist. Neuroscientists usually work in a controlled laboratory environment. They conduct experiments to further their understanding of how the nervous system works. They also study the causes, treatment, and prevention of neurological diseases and disorders.

Some neuroscientists study topics such as the characteristics of the normal, aging nervous system and the characteristics of exceptionally well-functioning nervous systems, such as those of elite athletes. The graph in **Figure 6.30**

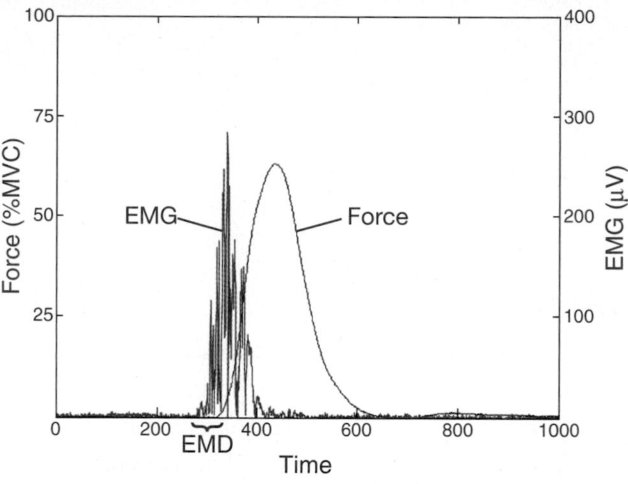

Courtesy of Dr. Chris Knight, University of Delaware

Figure 6.30 This graph shows electrical activity (EMG) in a quadriceps muscle during tension development and the corresponding force output from the leg. Notice that the onset of electrical activity clearly precedes the onset of force production, demonstrating electromechanical delay (EMD). EMD has been found to be longer in elderly individuals and shorter in athletes, particularly those who specialize in speed and power events.

provides an example of the kind of information these scientists gather and study. The graph shows the delay between the electrical stimulation of a muscle and the initiation of tension development in that muscle. This delay increases with aging, but is very short in both speed- and power-trained athletes. Neuroscientists and neurologists often collaborate on research projects—each bringing a different, specialized perspective to the work.

Becoming a neuroscientist requires a four-year bachelor's degree in an area of science, followed by a PhD in neuroscience. It typically takes four to six years to complete the PhD program. This education is often followed by an optional postdoctoral fellowship that lasts two to four years. A neuroscientist is typically employed as a university professor or research scientist. Neuroscientists working as researchers are often employed by a hospital or private company.

Planning for a Health-Related Career

Do some research on the career of a neurologist or neuroscientist. Note that both neurologists and neuroscientists may have dual careers. A neurologist, for example, may practice medicine and teach at a college or university. Likewise, a neuroscientist may teach in addition to performing research.

Alternatively, select a profession from the list of related career options. Using the Internet or resources at your local library, find answers to the following questions:

1. What are the main tasks and responsibilities of a neurologist or neuroscientist?
2. What is the outlook for this career? Are workers in demand, or are jobs dwindling? For complete information, consult the current edition of the *Occupational Outlook Handbook*, published by the US Department of Labor. This handbook is available online or at your local library.
3. What special skills or talents are required? For example, do you enjoy research? Do you need to be good at problem-solving—a skill that would be useful when developing a complicated diagnosis?
4. What personality traits do you think are necessary for success in the career you have chosen to research? For instance, neurologists must work closely with their patients. Do you enjoy working with others?
5. Does the work involve a great deal of routine, or are the day-to-day responsibilities varied?
6. Does the career require long hours, or is it a standard, "9-to-5" job?
7. What is the salary range for this job?
8. What do you think you would like about this career? Is there anything about it that you might dislike?

Related Career Options

- Neuroanatomist
- Neurochemist
- Neuroscience nurse
- Neurosurgeon
- Pathologist

CHAPTER 6

Review

LESSON 6.1

Overview of the Nervous System

Key Points

- The structures within the nervous system are divided into two major divisions: the central nervous system and the peripheral nervous system.
- The two types of tissue within the nervous system are neuroglia and neurons.

Key Terms

afferent nerves
astrocytes
autonomic nervous system
central nervous system (CNS)
dendrites
efferent nerves
ependymal cells
interneurons
microglia
myelin sheath
neuroglia
neurotransmitters
oligodendrocytes
peripheral nervous system (PNS)
satellite cells
somatic nervous system
Schwann cells
synapse

LESSON 6.2

Transmission of Nerve Impulses

Key Points

- Stimuli bring about depolarization, which creates a nerve impulse, or action potential.
- Two major factors influence the speed at which a nerve impulse travels: the presence or absence of a myelin sheath and the diameter of the axon.

Key Terms

action potential
autonomic reflexes
conductivity
depolarized
polarized
reflexes
refractory period
repolarization
saltatory conduction
sodium-potassium pump
somatic reflexes

LESSON 6.3

Functional Anatomy of the Central Nervous System

Key Points

- The brain consists of four major anatomical regions: the cerebrum, diencephalon, brainstem, and cerebellum.
- The spinal cord serves as a major pathway for relaying sensory and motor impulses.

Key Terms

cerebellum
cerebrospinal fluid (CSF)
cerebrum
corpus callosum
diencephalon
epithalamus
fissures
frontal lobes
hypothalamus
lobes
medulla oblongata
meninges
midbrain
occipital lobes
parietal lobes
pons
primary motor cortex
primary somatic sensory cortex
spinal cord
temporal lobes
thalamus

› LESSON 6.4

Functional Anatomy of the Peripheral Nervous System

Key Points

- Nerves are protected by a series of sheaths that surround them.
- The PNS includes spinal nerves and cranial nerves.
- The autonomic nervous system has two branches: the sympathetic branch and the parasympathetic branch.

Key Terms

cranial nerves
craniosacral branch
dorsal ramus
endoneurium
epineurium
ganglion
norepinephrine
paravertebral ganglia
perineurium
plexuses
postganglionic neuron
preganglionic neuron
spinal nerves
thoracolumbar branch
ventral ramus

› LESSON 6.5

Injuries and Disorders of the Nervous System

Key Points

- The brain and spinal cord are well protected, but injuries do occur, and they can have serious consequences.
- Common disorders and diseases of the CNS include meningitis, multiple sclerosis, epilepsy, Parkinson's disease, cerebral palsy, dementia, and Alzheimer's disease.

Key Terms

acute flaccid myelitis (AFM)
Alzheimer's disease (AD)
cerebral palsy (CP)
dementia
epilepsy
meningitis
multiple sclerosis (MS)
paraplegia
Parkinson's disease (PD)
quadriplegia
traumatic brain injury (TBI)

Assessment

› LESSON 6.1

Overview of the Nervous System

Learning Key Terms and Concepts

1. The central nervous system (CNS) includes the spinal cord and the _____.
2. The peripheral nervous system (PNS) is made up of the _____, or sensory, nerves and the efferent, or motor, nerves.
3. The two subdivisions of the efferent nerves are the somatic nervous system and the _____ nervous system.
4. The parts of a neuron that collect stimuli and transport them to the cell body are the _____.
   A. dendrites
   B. cell bodies
   C. glial cells
   D. axons
5. The fatty _____ that wraps around some axons provides an insulating shield that increases the rate of transmission.

6. Nerve fibers that do not have myelin sheaths are known as _____ matter.
   A. yellow
   B. white
   C. gray
   D. black
7. The three types of neurons, when classified by function, are sensory neurons, motor neurons, and _____ (association neurons).
8. The four types of _____, or glial cells, in the CNS are astrocytes, microglia, ependymal cells, and oligodendrocytes.

Thinking Critically

9. Create a flowchart that shows the main components or structures of the nervous system and each of its subdivisions. List the functions and processes that each component controls.
10. Compare and contrast neuroglia and neurons.
11. Briefly describe how the autonomic nervous system keeps a person alive.

›LESSON 6.2

Transmission of Nerve Impulses

Learning Key Terms and Concepts

12. The two behavioral properties of a neuron are irritability and _____.
    A. excitability
    B. conductivity
    C. sustainability
    D. automaticity
13. Because of the difference in electrical charge between the inside and outside of a resting cell, the cell membrane is said to be _____.
    A. depolarized
    B. electrified
    C. polarized
    D. maximized
14. *True or false?* Body temperature can influence the speed of a nerve impulse.
15. Communication between neurons is an electrochemical event that occurs in an area known as a(n) _____.
16. A rapid, involuntary, programmed response to a stimulus is known as a(n) _____.
17. _____ reflexes send involuntary stimuli to the cardiac muscle of the heart and the smooth muscle of internal organs.
    A. Systemic
    B. Autonomic
    C. Somatic
    D. Saltatory

Thinking Critically

18. Recalling what you have learned about nerve impulses, how do you think each of the following substances affects conduction speeds: caffeine, sedatives, and energy drinks?
19. If a person has extremely low blood calcium levels, will that affect the transmission of electrical signals from one cell to another? Explain your answer.
20. How would hypothermia affect a person's nerve impulse transmission?
21. How would a very low sodium level in a person's blood affect action potential and nerve impulse transmission?

›LESSON 6.3

Functional Anatomy of the Central Nervous System

Learning Key Terms and Concepts

22. *True or False?* Recent evidence suggests that the size of a person's brain is related to intelligence.
23. The four major anatomic regions of the brain are the brainstem, cerebellum, cerebrum, and _____.
    A. epithalamus
    B. hypothalamus
    C. pons
    D. diencephalon
24. Each curved, raised area of the brain is called a _____.
    A. gyrus
    B. sulcus
    C. synapse
    D. lobe
25. Each of the grooves between the gyri in the brain is called a(n) _____.
    A. synapse
    B. sulcus
    C. fissure
    D. cortex

26. The four lobes of the brain are the frontal, parietal, temporal, and _____ lobes.
27. The parietal lobes of the brain are located immediately posterior to the _____ lobes.
28. The most inferior lobes of the brain are the _____ lobes.
29. The diencephalon is also called the _____.
    A. hypothalamus
    B. pituitary
    C. brainstem
    D. interbrain
30. The three protective membranes that surround the brain are called the _____.

Thinking Critically

31. If one component or structure in the brain gets damaged, do you think the other structures can compensate enough for the person to function fairly normally? Explain your answer.
32. Examine the importance of the blood-brain barrier. Explain what might happen if this protective measure were no longer in place.
33. Why do you think the brain has gyri and sulci? What would happen if it did not have these areas and was smooth instead?
34. If a person is experiencing jet lag, which part of the diencephalon is being affected? Explain your answer.

LESSON 6.4

Functional Anatomy of the Peripheral Nervous System

Learning Key Terms and Concepts

35. In a nerve, each axon fiber is covered by a fine sheath called the _____.
    A. endometrium
    B. perineurium
    C. endoneurium
    D. epineurium
36. Groups of sheathed axon fibers are bundled into fascicles surrounded by the _____.
37. Groups of fascicles and blood vessels are surrounded by the _____.
38. The body has how many pairs of cranial nerves?
    A. 6
    B. 12
    C. 15
    D. 31
39. _____ nerves are nerves that carry both afferent and efferent impulses.
40. The body has how many pairs of spinal nerves?
    A. 6
    B. 12
    C. 15
    D. 31
41. Spinal nerves are divided into a(n) _____ ramus and a ventral ramus.
    A. inferior
    B. superior
    C. dorsal
    D. caudal
42. The _____ branch of the autonomic nervous system controls all of the automatic functions of the circulatory, respiratory, and digestive systems.

Thinking Critically

43. Explain what happens physiologically when the fight-or-flight response is activated in the body.
44. Explain how the protective membranes covering each part of a nerve help it to resist injury.
45. Why is it important to know from which part of the spine the spinal nerve impulses originate, and from which area of the brain cranial nerve impulses originate?

LESSON 6.5

Injuries and Disorders of the Nervous System

Learning Key Terms and Concepts

46. Symptoms of mild _____ include headache, confusion, dizziness, disturbed vision, ringing in the ears, bad taste in the mouth, fatigue, abnormal sleep patterns, behavioral changes, and trouble with intellectual functions.
    A. multiple sclerosis
    B. acute flaccid myelitis
    C. traumatic brain injury
    D. Parkinson's disease

47. *True or False?* Cerebral palsy can be caused by several disorders or conditions.
48. Some of the first signs of _____ are a sudden onset of loss of muscle tone and reflexes in the arms and legs.
    A. acute flaccid myelitis
    B. epilepsy
    C. dementia
    D. meningitis
49. *True or False?* Multiple sclerosis (MS) is considered an autoimmune disease.
50. Parkinson's disease is the result of low levels of _____ in the brain.
    A. epinephrine
    B. dopamine
    C. sodium
    D. norepinephrine

Thinking Critically

51. Evaluate the cause and effect of cerebral palsy on the structure and function of cells, tissues, organs, and systems.
52. Explain the range of problems that can result from injuries to different parts of the spinal column.
53. Evaluate the cause and effect of TBI on the structure and function of cells, tissues, organs, and systems.
54. Explain how concussion may be related to dementia and Alzheimer's disease.

Building Skills and Connecting Concepts

Analyzing and Evaluating Data

Instructions: The bar graph in **Figure 6.31** shows approximate transmission speeds for several different types of nerve impulses. Use the graph to answer the following questions.

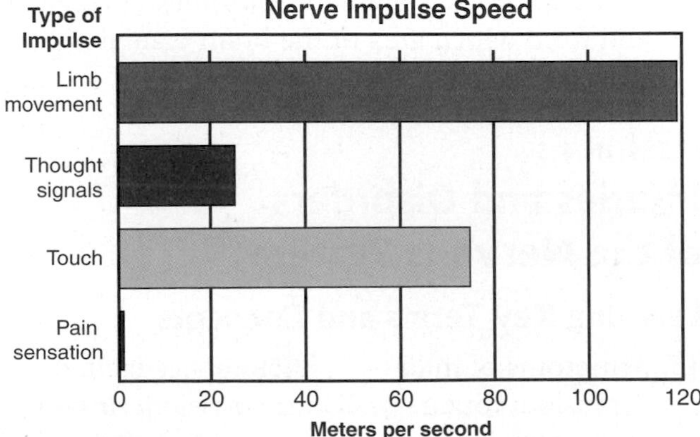

Figure 6.31

55. About how much faster do you *think* than *feel* pain?
56. Do nerve impulses signaling the sense of touch travel at approximately two, three, or four times the speed of thought impulses?
57. Assume that rising temperatures increase all the nerve impulse speeds by 5%. If the limb movement speed shown is 119 meters per second (m/s), what will it be at the higher temperature? Round your answer to the nearest whole meter.
58. Give approximate fps (feet per second) speeds for each type of nerve transmission shown in the graph. Use the conversion chart in the appendices if necessary. Round your answers to the nearest whole foot.
59. If nerve impulse speed increases by 15% when a person has a fever, by how much will the person's pain impulses increase? State your answer in meters per second.

Communicating about Anatomy & Physiology

60. **Writing** *Information technology* is the use of electronic devices such as computers to store, retrieve, transmit, and manipulate information. Write a persuasive essay comparing the use of information technology to the tasks performed by the human brain. Answer this question: Is increasing reliance on information technology decreasing or increasing the capacity of the human brain to think and reason? Provide reasons for your point of view.
61. **Reading** With a partner, make flash cards of the chapter terms for which phonetic spellings have been provided. On the front of the card, write the term. On the back, write the phonetic spelling as written in the text. (You may also choose to use a medical dictionary or multimedia resources such as a reputable online dictionary that allows you to listen to pronunciations.) Practice reading aloud the terms, clarifying pronunciations where needed.
62. **Speaking** Pick 5–10 of the key terms that you practiced pronouncing. Write a brief scene in which those 5–10 terms are used as you imagine them being used by medical professionals in a real-life context. Then rewrite the dialogue using simpler sentences and transitions, as though an adult were describing the same scene to elementary or middle-school students. Read both scenes to the class and ask for feedback on whether the two scenes were appropriate for their different audiences.
63. **Speaking and Writing** Interview your school nurse and several of your school's coaches (for different sports). Prepare for the interview by researching accepted interviewing techniques, and prepare a list of questions in advance. In your interviews, find out what your school district's policies and procedures are for dealing with students who have concussions. Write a report detailing your findings, as well as the people you interviewed. Include quotations from at least two interviewees. Also, identify one area that you think should be changed or improved upon.

Lab Investigations

64. Within a small group, use the following general procedures to create a model of the brain and its protective covers.

    Materials: large Styrofoam™ ball, scalpel or knife, markers, poster board, shower cap.

    Procedure:

    A. Using the scalpel or knife, gently cut grooves in the Styrofoam™ ball and shape it to look like a brain.
    B. Using different colored markers, color each area of the brain: the four lobes (frontal, temporal, parietal, and occipital), the brainstem, cerebellum, and diencephalon.
    C. On a small piece of poster board, using the same colors to correspond to the different colored areas of the model brain, list the bodily functions that each lobe or area controls (some will overlap).
    D. Use the shower cap to illustrate meninges and how they protect and encase the delicate brain.
65. Terms related to the human nervous system are often referred to using abbreviations or acronyms. With a partner, create a chart listing as many abbreviations and acronyms associated with the human nervous system as you can find. Conduct research to find abbreviations and acronyms that are not included in this chapter. Your chart should have three columns: Abbreviation or Acronym, Meaning, and Example of Use. In the Example of Use column, write a sentence using the abbreviation or acronym as it might be used in a healthcare employee's notes. Practice reading your examples to your partner to become more familiar with the use of this terminology.

Building Your Portfolio

66. Take digital photographs of the models and projects you created as you worked through this chapter. Create a folder called "The Nervous System" and insert the photographs, along with written descriptions of what the models show and your reasons for creating them using the materials and forms you chose. Also insert copies of any reports and lab investigations you have performed. Add this folder to your personal portfolio.

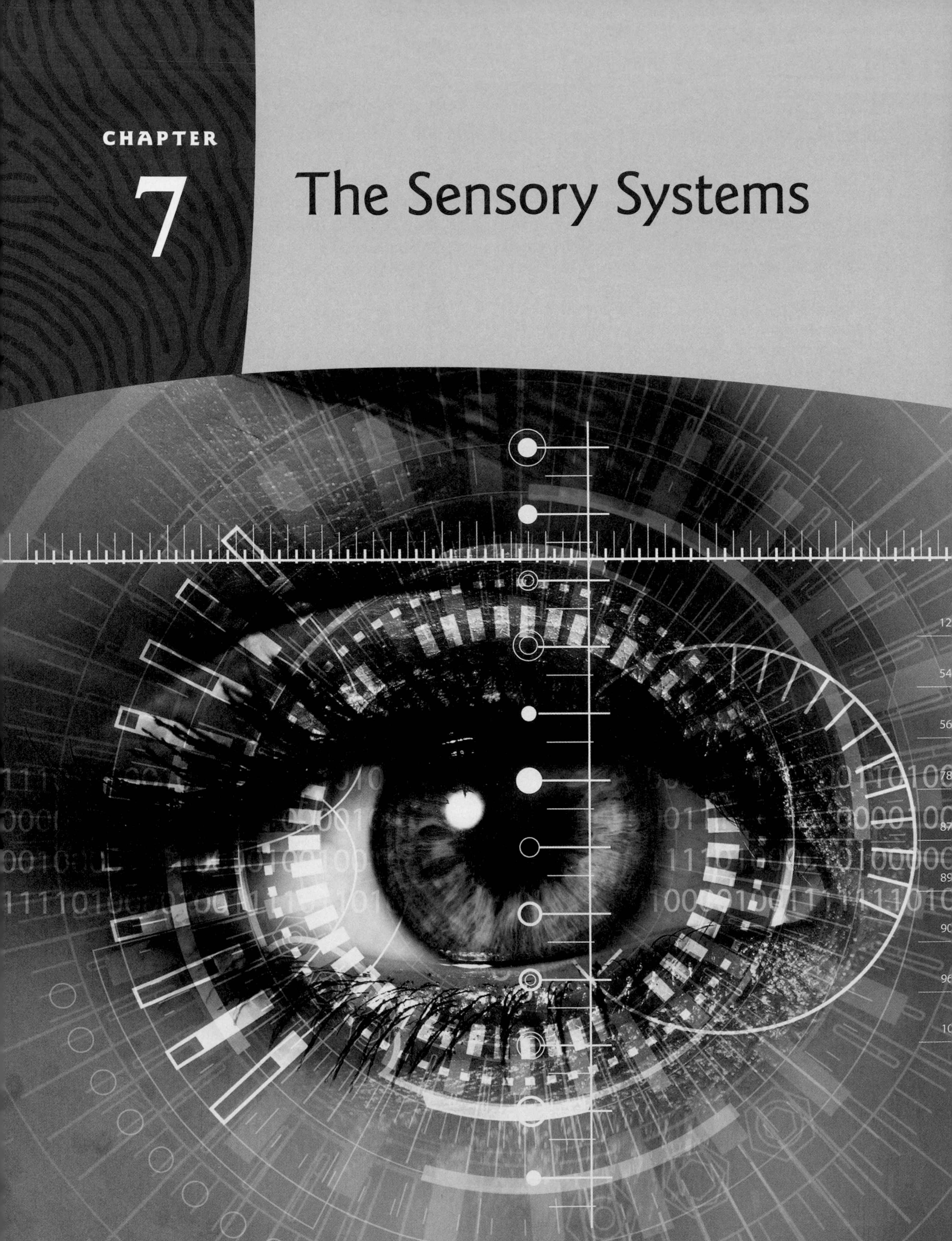

CHAPTER 7 The Sensory Systems

What do the eyes tell you?

Want to capture a picture or video? Use a camera, smartphone, or iPad™. Want to hear music from your portable music player? Use earphones.

The human eyes, ears, nose, and mouth far exceed the ability of today's mechanical devices to capture and transmit sensory information to the brain. The senses, including vision, hearing, smell, and taste, involve extraordinarily well-designed sensory pathways in the nervous system. For each of these senses, highly specialized receptor cells communicate with neurons to begin the virtually instantaneous process of sending sensory messages to the brain. Once in the brain, the input from all the sensory systems is rapidly integrated and interpreted.

This chapter takes a look at the anatomical structures and capabilities of the different components of the sensory systems. In addition, it discusses some of the common injuries and disorders of these systems, along with their symptoms and current treatments.

Chapter 7 Outline

- **Lesson 7.1 The Eye**
  - Anatomy of the Eye
  - Vision
  - Injuries, Diseases, and Disorders of the Eye
- **Lesson 7.2 The Ear**
  - Anatomy of the Ear
  - Functions of the Ear
  - Disorders and Infections of the Ear
- **Lesson 7.3 Smell and Taste**
  - Olfactory Sense
  - Gustatory Sense

Click on the activity icon or visit www.g-wlearning.com/healthsciences/0202 to access online vocabulary activities using key terms from the chapter.

◂ Sergey Nivens/Shutterstock.com

LESSON **7.1**

The Eye

Before You Read

Try to answer the following questions before you read this lesson.

- What enables humans to see colors?
- What causes near- and farsightedness?

Lesson Objectives

- Describe the external and internal anatomical structures of the human eye.
- Explain how the anatomical structures associated with the retina work together to produce vision.
- Discuss common injuries, disorders, and diseases of the eye.

Key Terms

aqueous humor	optic chiasma
choroid	optic nerve
ciliary body	optic tracts
ciliary glands	pupil
cones	retina
conjunctiva	rods
cornea	sclera
extrinsic muscles	suspensory ligaments
iris	tarsal glands
lacrimal glands	vitreous humor
lens	

According to an old English proverb, "The eyes are the windows to the soul." Whether or not this is true, some people do indeed have expressive eyes that help to convey their emotional states. Eyes "twinkling with amusement" or "flashing with anger" are familiar descriptive phrases. A person can also be described as bright-eyed, dark-eyed, shifty-eyed, or eagle-eyed, all of which suggest distinctive images or characteristics.

The eyes obviously are important parts of the human anatomy, because vision is an extremely useful sense. This lesson describes the anatomical components of the eye and explains how they function together to produce the remarkable ability to see.

Anatomy of the Eye

The adult eye, sometimes referred to as the "eyeball," is about 1 inch (2.5 cm) in diameter and has a roughly spherical shape. A variety of external structures serve to protect the eye, and specialized internal structures send sensory signals to the brain, enabling vision.

External Structures

The eye is a delicate structure and, fortunately, is well protected. The eye is encased in the bony, orbital socket of the skull and covered by an eyelid. The eyebrows also function as shields—for example, by helping to protect the eyes from dripping sweat on a hot day. The eyelashes provide considerable protection from circulating dust particles.

Several structures work together to lubricate the eyes (**Figure 7.1**). **Tarsal** (TAR-sal) **glands** in the eyelids produce an oily secretion, and modified sweat glands, called **ciliary** (SIL-ee-air-ee) **glands**, are located between the eyelashes. The **conjunctiva** (kon-junk-TIGH-vuh), a delicate external membrane that covers the exposed eyeball and lines the eyelid, also secretes a lubricating mucus.

The **lacrimal** (LAK-ri-mal) **glands** above the lateral end of each eye continually release the familiar, salty solution known as tears through excretory ducts. Because tears contain antibodies and an enzyme called *lysozyme* that attacks bacteria, they not only lubricate the surface of the eye but also keep it clean.

Tears are flushed into tiny canals called *lacrimal canaliculi* in the medial corner of each eye. These canaliculi then drain into the nasolacrimal (nay-zoh-LAK-ri-mal) duct, which empties into the nasal cavity.

Irritation to the eye produces extra tearing, which helps to wash away foreign substances. Under stressful conditions, tears may be produced at such a high rate that they cannot be drained away fast enough and spill over onto the cheeks.

Six **extrinsic muscles** attach to the outer surface of the eye and are responsible for moving

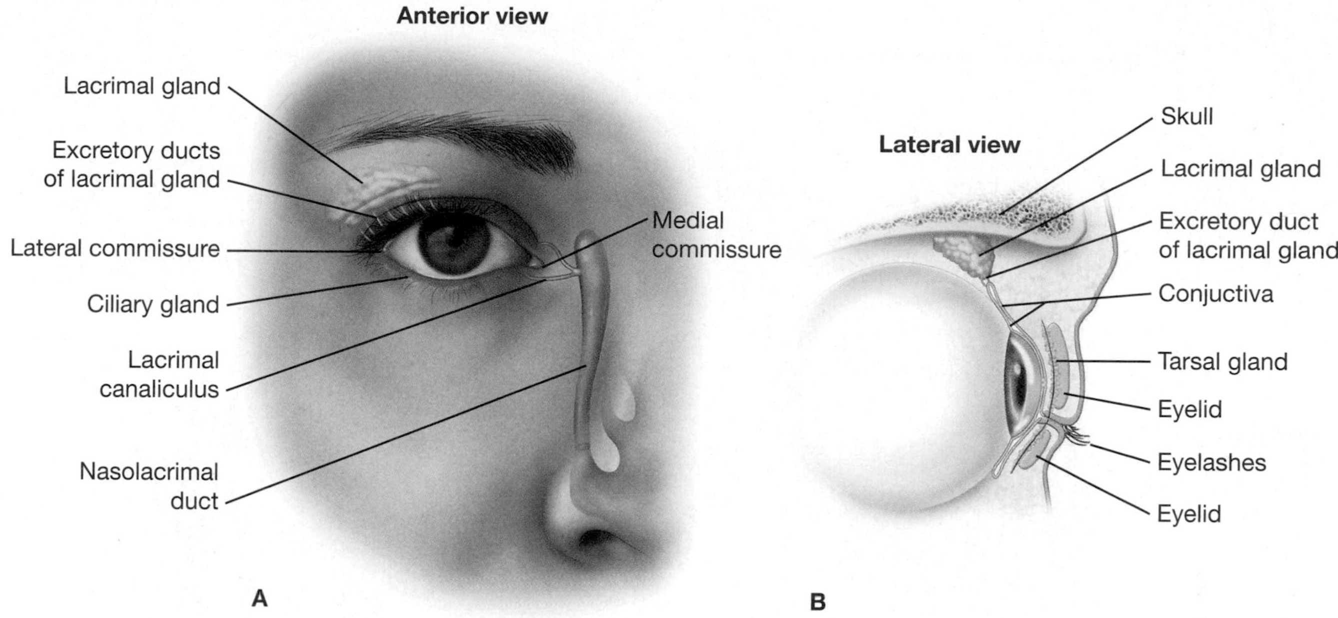

Figure 7.1 Lubricating structures of the eye. A—Anterior view. B—Lateral view. *Some of the structures identified in these drawings serve a function other than lubrication. What are these structures and what is their primary purpose?*

the eye within the orbital socket (**Figure 7.2**). The specific functions of these muscles are listed in the table in **Figure 7.3**.

Internal Structures

The eyeball is a hollow chamber, mostly spherical but somewhat oblong in shape. Three layers of tissue form the walls of the eyeball. The tough, fibrous **sclera** makes up the outer layer of the eye (**Figure 7.4**). The sclera includes the "white of the eye" as well as the transparent **cornea** over the anterior center of the eye. The cornea is called the "window of the eye" because light passes through it. The cornea has no blood supply and is therefore the one body tissue that can be transplanted from one person to another with no concern for rejection.

The middle layer of the eye, called the **choroid** (KOR-oyd), contains a rich supply of blood vessels that provide nourishment to the eye. These blood vessels contribute to a crimson-purple pigmentation that darkens the interior of the eye, preventing light reflections. Anteriorly, the choroid also includes the **iris**, which gives the eye its color. The iris can widen or narrow to control the size of the **pupil**, the opening through which light passes into the interior of the eye.

Superior oblique muscle
Superior rectus muscle
Lateral rectus muscle
Medial rectus muscle
Inferior rectus muscle
Inferior oblique muscle
© Body Scientific International

Figure 7.2 Lateral view of the extrinsic muscles of the eye.

The Extrinsic Eye Muscles	
Muscle	**Action**
superior rectus	upward eye motion
inferior rectus	downward eye motion
lateral rectus	lateral eye motion
medial rectus	medial eye motion
superior oblique	downward and lateral eye motion
inferior oblique	upward and lateral eye motion

Figure 7.3 Goodheart-Willcox Publisher

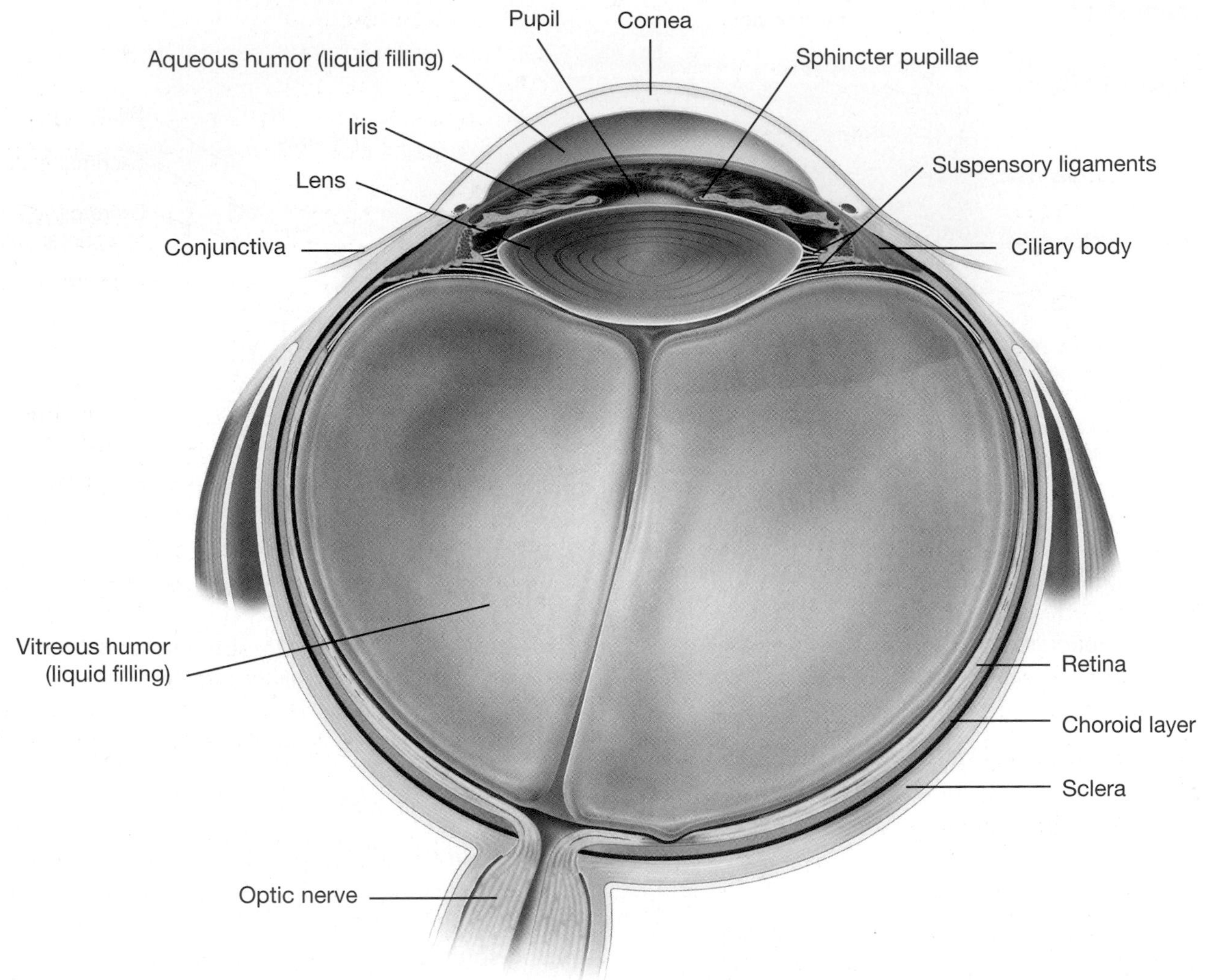

Figure 7.4 Internal structures of the eye. *How would your vision be affected if the iris lacked sphincter pupillae and dilator pupillae muscles to control the amount of light admitted to the eye?*

Two sets of muscles within the iris work to control the amount of light admitted to the eye. The *sphincter pupillae* contracts in the presence of bright light or when the eye focuses on an object within close range, causing the pupil to become smaller. In the presence of dim light or when the eye focuses on a distant object, the *dilator pupillae* muscle contracts, causing dilation (enlargement) of the pupil.

The innermost layer of the eye, the **retina**, is located only around the posterior portion of the eye, anterior to the choroid. The retina is composed of two layers. The outer, or pigmented, layer includes pigmented cells that absorb light, store vitamin A, and serve as phagocytes to remove any damaged receptor cells on the inner layer. The inner, or neural, layer of the retina is dense in specialized, light-sensitive nerve endings. These nerve endings send impulses through the optic nerve to the occipital lobe of the brain, where visual images are interpreted.

The sensory cells in the retina are called **rods** and **cones** (**Figure 7.5**). The rods are activated in dim light and are most densely distributed around the periphery of the retina. They provide peripheral vision and enable perception of shades of gray in dim light. The cones are sensitive to bright light and also provide color vision. They are most densely distributed in the center of the retina, with decreasing distribution moving toward the periphery. Nerve ganglions (GAYNG-glee-ahnz) and bipolar neurons (discussed in Chapter 6) provide connections between the retina and the rods and cones.

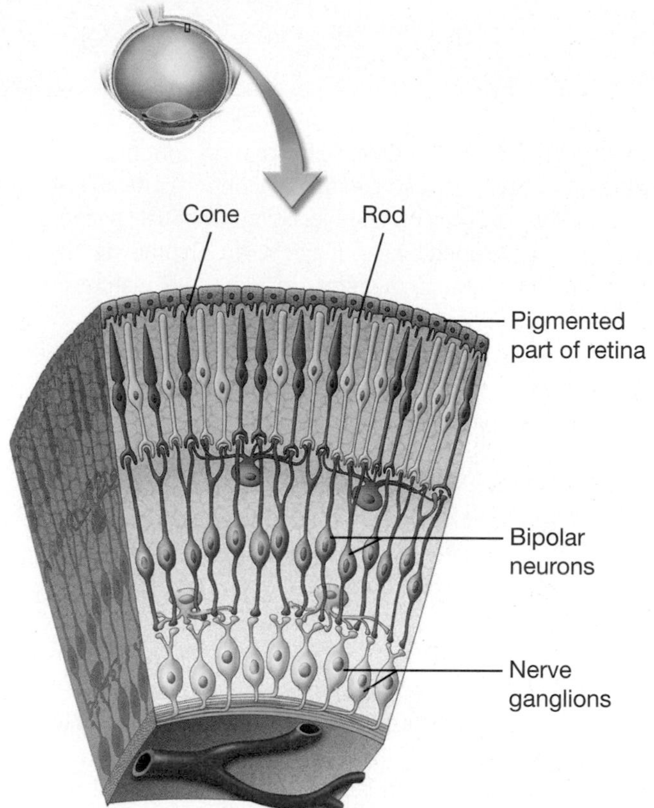

Figure 7.5 Rods and cones in the retina. *Which types of cells—cones or rods—are activated in dim light?*

You may have heard of the "blind spot" on the retina. The physiological blind spot on each retina is called the *optic disc*. The optic disc is the junction between the optic nerve and the eye. Because there are no rods and cones in the optic disc, this tiny area is unable to transmit visual information—hence the term *blind spot*.

Under normal circumstances, you do not perceive the blind spot because the brain fills in the visual information from the other eye. Because of the separation between the two eyes, the blind spots are missing different pieces of the combined visual field.

The **lens** of the eye is located behind the iris. It is a transparent, flexible, crystal-like structure curved outward on both sides. The lens is held in place by tiny **suspensory ligaments** that surround it. These ligaments attach to the **ciliary body**, which merges with the choroid layer.

The lens separates the anterior and posterior chambers of the eye. The anterior chamber is filled with the clear, watery **aqueous** (AY-kwee-us) **humor**. Continually secreted by the choroid, the aqueous humor provides nutrients for the avascular (without blood vessels) lens and cornea, and also helps maintain normal intraocular pressure (pressure inside the eye). The posterior chamber of the eye is filled with the gel-like **vitreous** (VIT-ree-us) **humor**, which also contributes to intraocular pressure.

When at rest, the eye is focused for distance vision. For the eye to clearly view objects closer than about 20 feet, the muscles of the ciliary body contract to change the shape of the lens. This process of contraction, known as *accommodation*, makes the lens thicker, enabling it to focus incoming light rays on the surface of the retina.

After about 40 years of age, the ability of the ciliary body muscles to appropriately contract diminishes. In the absence of other visual corrections, this causes people in the post-40 age group to need reading glasses for up-close vision.

Check Your Understanding

1. What do tarsal glands produce?
2. Describe two different ways by which tears clean the eyes.
3. Name the three layers of the eye.
4. Explain the purpose of aqueous and vitreous humors.

Vision

You see an object when the light that is reflected from that object passes through your cornea, pupil, and lens to your retina. The rods and cones in the retina are stimulated and pass impulses to the **optic nerve**, which transmits sensory signals to the brain.

The optic nerves from the eyes cross at the **optic chiasma** (kigh-AZ-ma). The nerve fibers exiting the optic chiasma are called **optic tracts**. The optic tracts carry visual stimuli to the occipital lobe of the brain.

Check Your Understanding

1. Which nerve is responsible for transmitting sensory signals to the brain?
2. Which part of the brain processes sensory signals from the eyes?

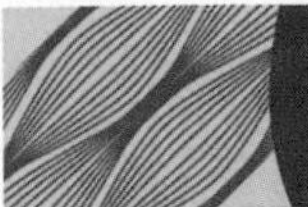

LIFE SPAN DEVELOPMENT: *The Eyes and Vision*

The eyes begin to develop in the embryo during the 17th day after conception through a complex series of events. Optic vesicles form in the neural area and within five days create a cup-shaped beginning of the wall of the eyeball. This allows the retina and lens to begin formation.

Over the next 2 to 3 weeks, the lens, iris, and cornea grow to completion. At four weeks, the orbits and extrinsic muscles begin to develop. During the sixth week, the lacrimal glands begin forming. The lacrimal glands, however, produce no tears until the third month after birth, which is why there are no tears when new infants cry. The sclera develops at seven weeks, followed by the formation of blood vessels. At eight weeks, the eyelids start to form. The maturing cornea becomes transparent when the eye becomes functional in the seventh month. Not until the eight month of pregnancy does the pupil develop the ability to constrict in response to light.

During all this time the retina is evolving, with cells differentiating into rods and cones. Axons from the retinal ganglion cells group to form the optic nerve. The development of the retina occurs between 24 weeks gestation and 3 to 4 months after birth, when the optic nerve becomes fully myelinated. At birth, the rod cells allow newborns to see dark, light, and shades of gray. The ability to see colors does not occur until the cones mature at approximately 3 months of age.

At birth, the infant's eye is only about 65% of its full size. Changes during the first year include growth of the orbit, changes to the lens, and pigmentation of the iris. Eye movements are somewhat uncoordinated and corneal curvature is changing. Full color vision occurs between 5 and 7 months. Visual acuity and stereoscopic vision continue improving through about 15 to 18 months of age.

Focus, tracking, and depth perception continue to develop through early and middle childhood. The ability of both eyes to focus on an object simultaneously becomes more fully developed by about age seven. Depending on eye growth after birth, the orbits may not fully mature until adolescence.

Numerous characteristic changes occur to the lens of the eye as a person ages. The lens becomes stiffer, which causes most people in their 40s to acquire *presbyopia*, making it difficult to see objects closer than two feet without corrective lenses. Because the lens becomes less transparent, it is also more difficult to see well in dim light. The lens also tends to yellow, so colors appear differently.

Other changes due to aging include slowed reaction of the pupil to changes in light level and a decrease in the number of cells transmitting visual information to the brain. These changes result in increased sensitivity to glare, difficulty in discerning fine details and shades of color, and difficulty with depth perception. A decrease in the number of cells producing lubricant to the eyes may cause dryness of the eyes. The eyes also become more susceptible to certain diseases and disorders, as described in the next section.

Lifespan Review

1. Why do infants not produce tears when they cry?
2. What functions of the eyes are still developing at birth?
3. How do changes associated with aging affect vision in healthy elderly individuals?

Injuries, Diseases, and Disorders of the Eye

The eyes are so essential to daily life that any kind of injury or disease can have a major impact on a person's life and well-being. This section describes some common injuries, disorders, and diseases that can affect the ways in which the eye functions. The etiology (cause), strategies for prevention, pathology (clinical characteristics), diagnosis (keys for identifying the condition), and common treatments for these disorders are summarized in **Figure 7.6**.

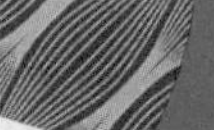

CLINICAL CASE STUDY

Jane is concerned about her dad. When he comes home in the evening, he no longer watches the evening news on TV because he says that his eyes are aching. And the last time she rode in a car with him driving, she had to warn him a couple of times about something on the periphery of his vision that he apparently did not see. As you read this section, try to determine which of the following conditions Jane's dad most likely has.

A. Myopia
B. Cataracts
C. Glaucoma
D. Macular degeneration

Common Vision Disorders					
	Etiology	**Prevention**	**Pathology**	**Diagnosis**	**Treatment**
Myopia	elongated eyeball	none	nearsightedness	vision tests	corrective lenses, laser surgery
Hyperopia	shortened (flattened) eyeball	none	farsightedness	vision tests	corrective lenses, laser surgery
Presbyopia	stiffness of lens	none	age-related farsightedness	vision tests	corrective lenses, laser surgery
Astigmatism	irregular curvature of cornea or lens	none	blurred vision	vision tests	corrective lenses, laser surgery
Amblyopia	abnormal dominance of one eye	none	lazy eye	vision tests	placing a patch over the strong eye for several weeks or months
Diplopia	abnormal alignment of the eyes	none	double vision	vision tests	eye exercises, corrective lenses, surgery
Strabismus	muscles in one eye do not coordinate with those in the other eye	none	one or both eyes turn inward, outward, upward, or downward	vision tests	eye exercises, corrective lenses, surgery
Colorblindness	genetic disorder of cone cells in retina	none	inability to distinguish colors	vision tests	corrective lenses may help
Nyctalopia	disorder of rod cells in retina	none	difficulty seeing at night	vision tests	corrective lenses or surgery

Figure 7.6

Goodheart-Willcox Publisher

Eye Injuries

The structure of the face and eyes helps protect the eyes from injury. The bony socket in which the eyeball is encased, the eyelid, the eyebrows, and the eyelashes all provide a barrier to foreign objects. In fact, these features are so effective in protecting the eye that many eye injuries do not affect the eyeball itself, but rather the surrounding tissues and structures. Still, certain injuries can damage the eyeball, causing impairment or loss of vision.

Usually, minor irritants are flushed from the eye through tear production. Irritating chemicals, however, should be flushed with large quantities of water. Fragments of glass or other solid particles that become lodged in the eye should be removed only by a medical professional.

The cornea is well supplied with pain and touch receptors. Consequently, corneal injuries (abrasions or tears) are extremely painful. Fortunately, however, the cornea has an astonishing ability to self-repair; most injuries resolve themselves within 24 hours.

Trauma to the eye can cause a *detached retina*, in which the retina separates from the underlying support tissue. The detachment may be partial in the beginning, but without treatment it can rapidly progress to complete detachment. The associated vision loss can progress from minor to severe and even to blindness within a few hours or days.

Surgical techniques using lasers, air bubbles, or a freezing probe can be used to reattach the retina. In most cases, surgery can restore good vision. If unrepaired, a detached retina can cause loss of peripheral vision and, subsequently, loss of central vision.

Vision Disorders

A variety of common, but relatively minor, eye defects can impair vision. Many of these defects can be completely corrected with prescription lenses (**Figure 7.7**). These defects, known collectively as *ametropia*, are shown in **Figure 7.8**. For comparison, normal vision is shown in **Figure 7.8A**.

Myopia

Commonly known as *nearsightedness*, *myopia* (migh-OH-pee-uh) results from an elongated eyeball shape, which causes the lens to focus objects in front of the retina rather than directly upon it (**Figure 7.8B**). Nearby objects can be seen clearly, but distant objects appear blurry.

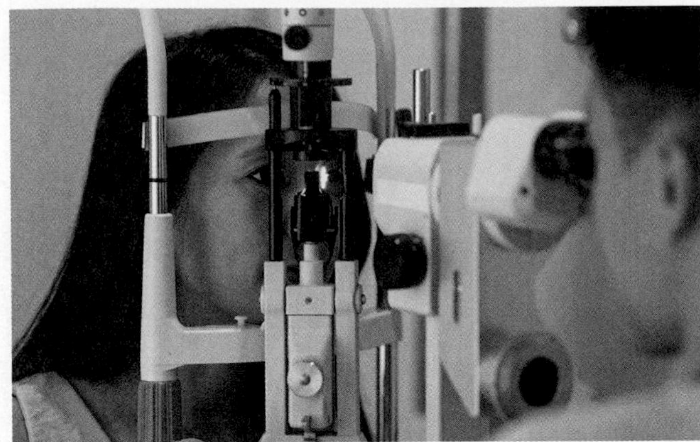

leungchopan/Shutterstock.com

Figure 7.7 Have your eyes examined on a regular basis and as soon as possible if you experience any of the problems discussed in this lesson. Note that several problems can be remedied if treated early but can be very damaging if left untreated.

The classic Snellen chart is used to diagnose myopia. This familiar chart includes rows of letters, with each successive row smaller than the one above. The Snellen chart and other charts similar to it are used only as a first step in diagnosing myopia. Medical eye specialists perform a number of tests before they prescribe corrective lenses for visual defects. Laser surgery techniques also can be performed to correct myopia.

Hyperopia

The opposite condition is *hyperopia* (high-per-OH-pee-uh), also known as *farsightedness*. In hyperopia, the distance from the lens to the retina is shortened because the shape of the eyeball is more flattened (**Figure 7.8C**). Light rays focus behind the retina instead of directly upon it. As a result, objects at a distance can be seen clearly, but objects close up appear blurry. Prescription lenses can correct this condition.

Presbyopia

Presbyopia (prez-bee-OH-pee-uh) is an age-related version of farsightedness. Onset of presbyopia commonly occurs between 40 and 45 years of age because of changes that stiffen and discolor the lens of the eye. Presbyopia causes blurring of up-close vision that impedes the ability to read printed material or text on a computer screen. Like hyperopia, it can be corrected with prescription lenses.

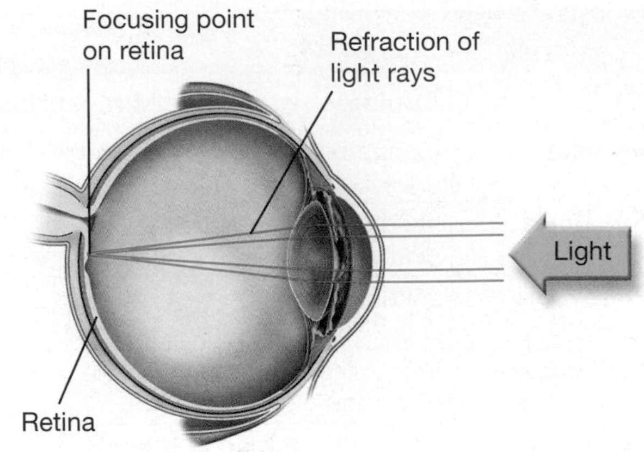

**A Normal vision:
light rays focus on the retina**

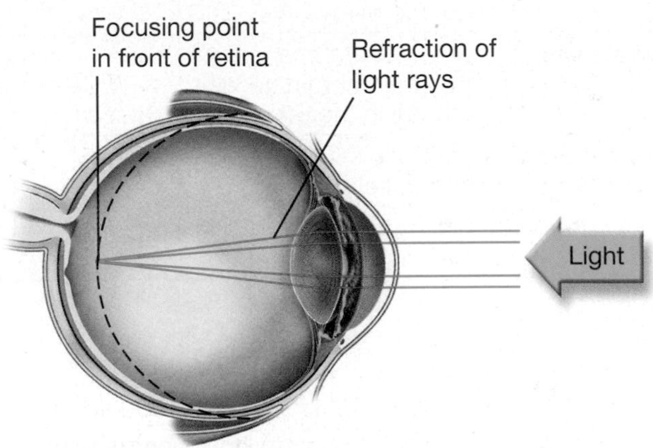

**B Myopia (nearsightedness):
light rays focus in front of the retina**

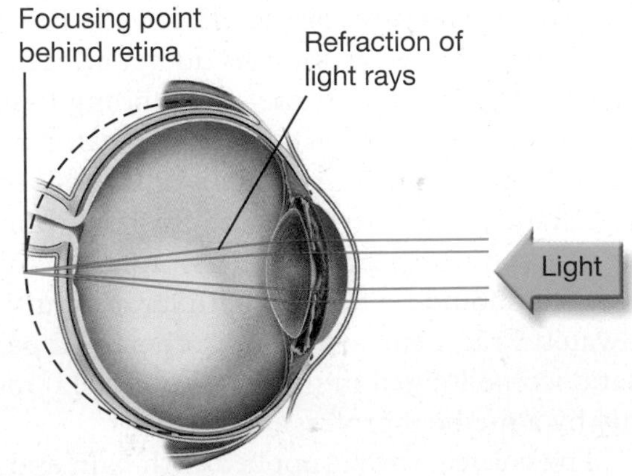

**C Hyperopia (farsightedness):
light rays focus beyond the retina**

© Body Scientific International

Figure 7.8 Common vision disorders compared to normal vision. A—Normal vision. B—Myopia. C—Hyperopia. *If light rays focus on a point in front of your retina, do you have trouble seeing objects close to you or far away?*

MEMORY TIP

You may have heard middle-aged individuals joke that they are "getting old" because they need reading glasses. The word *presbyopia* comes from *presby/o*, a combining form meaning "old," and *-opia*, a suffix that means "the condition of having a visual defect." The term was adopted in the late eighteenth century, when people in their forties were considered old!

The suffix *-opia* is used in conjunction with other combining forms to describe various eye disorders—*myopia, hyperopia*, and *amblyopia*, for example.

Astigmatism

Irregular curvature of the cornea or lens causes *astigmatism* (ah-STIG-ma-tizm), another common eye disorder. The result is blurred vision. Depending on the nature and extent of the curvature, vision may be proportionally affected. Corrective lenses can partially or completely correct astigmatism.

Amblyopia

Amblyopia (am-blee-OH-pee-uh), or *lazy eye*, usually appears during childhood when one eye is extremely dominant and the other eye—the lazy eye—develops poor vision. If uncorrected, the lazy eye can become blind. Treatment generally consists of covering the "good" eye, requiring the extrinsic muscles of the lazy eye to function.

Diplopia

Diplopia (di-PLOH-pee-uh), or double vision, results when one eye is misaligned, causing two images of the object to be perceived simultaneously. Treatment may involve wearing a temporary patch over the affected eye, corrective lenses, or surgery.

Strabismus

In a person with *strabismus* (strah-BIZ-mus), one or both eyes drift in different directions due to malfunctioning of the extrinsic muscles of that eye. The condition is treated with eye exercises, corrective lenses, or surgery.

Colorblindness

Colorblindness affects the cone cells on the retina, impairing an individual's ability to distinguish colors. Red-green colorblindness, the inability to distinguish red from green, is a common form of this disorder.

Colorblindness is an inherited condition. For a son to be colorblind, he needs to inherit the gene for colorblindness only from his mother. By contrast, for a daughter to be colorblind, she must inherit the gene from both parents. This explains why men have a higher incidence of colorblindness compared to women.

Nyctalopia

In nyctalopia (nik-tahl-OH-pee-uh), or *night blindness*, the rods in the retina do not function optimally, making it difficult for a person to see well at night. Nyctalopia is associated with aging, but several other disorders may also affect night vision.

Eye Diseases

This section briefly describes eye diseases that commonly require professional care. The etiology, strategies for prevention, pathology, diagnosis, and common treatments for these common eye diseases and disorders are summarized in **Figure 7.9**.

Conjunctivitis

Commonly known as "pinkeye," *conjunctivitis* (kuhn-junk-ti-VIGH-tis) is a highly contagious inflammation of the conjunctiva. Symptoms include redness, pain, swelling, and mucus discharge. Although it is usually caused by a viral infection, conjunctivitis can be treated with antibiotics if caused by a bacterial infection.

Cataracts

A *cataract* (KAT-uh-rakt) is the development of a progressive clouding of the transparent lens of the eye, causing obstruction of light. The result is blurred vision, poor night vision, yellowing of colors, and "halos" around lights. Cataracts are associated with aging and frequently occur in people older than 70 years of age. Exposure to bright sunlight can speed the development of cataracts. Cataracts are treated with laser surgery.

Common Eye Diseases and Disorders					
	Etiology	**Prevention**	**Pathology**	**Diagnosis**	**Treatment**
Conjunctivitis	infection, causing inflammation of the conjunctiva	avoid contact with infected people	redness, pain, swelling, mucous discharge of the eyes	physical exam, questions regarding symptoms	wet compresses, artificial tears; antibiotics if caused by bacteria
Cataracts	progressive clouding of the lens of the eye	avoid bright sunlight	blurred vision, poor night vision, yellowing of colors, seeing halos around lights	vision tests	surgery to replace the lens with an artificial lens
Glaucoma	increased pressure within the eyeball due to buildup of aqueous humor	none	aching eyes, poor vision in dim light progressing to blurred vision, seeing halos around lights	specialized tests	prescription eyedrops, oral medications, laser treatment, surgery
Dry and wet macular degeneration	dry: progressive thinning of the retina wet: leakage of capillaries within the eye	none	progressive loss of central vision	specialized tests	dry: none wet: medications to hinder growth of new blood vessels
Diabetic retinopathy	long term diabetes causes swelling and leaking of the vessels that supply blood to the retina	health habits to prevent type 2 diabetes	bleeding within the eye causes seeing red spots	eye examination	varies, depending on type and severity of condition
Vitreous floaters	bits of vitreous humor break off and float in the aqueous humor in the center of the eyeball	none	drifting specks in visual field; if combined with flashes of light on lateral periphery may indicate retinal injury	eye examination	none; laser surgery to correct retinal injury if warranted

Figure 7.9

Goodheart-Willcox Publisher

Glaucoma

Glaucoma (glaw-KOH-ma) is a condition of increased pressure within the eyeball caused either by overproduction of aqueous humor or blockage of normal aqueous humor drainage. The onset of symptoms is gradual and includes aching eyes, poor vision in dim light progressing to blurred vision, and the appearance of halos around lights.

As the condition progresses, tunnel vision—or loss of peripheral vision—occurs, and blindness eventually follows. Untreated glaucoma is a common cause of blindness. Glaucoma occurs in about 20 percent of adults older than 40 years of age. Early detection is a must! Glaucoma can be readily treated with medication or surgery.

Macular Degeneration

The hallmark symptom of *macular* (MAK-yoo-lar) *degeneration* is a progressive loss of central vision. This disorder occurs in about 10 percent of elderly people. Peripheral vision, however, remains unaffected. There are two types of macular degeneration: dry and wet.

Dry macular degeneration is caused by progressive thinning of the retina. Although no treatment currently exists, most individuals with this condition do not completely lose their eyesight and are able to function with vision aids. *Wet macular degeneration* involves leakage of small blood vessels within the eye. Some individuals with this condition respond favorably to medication or laser surgery (**Figure 7.10**).

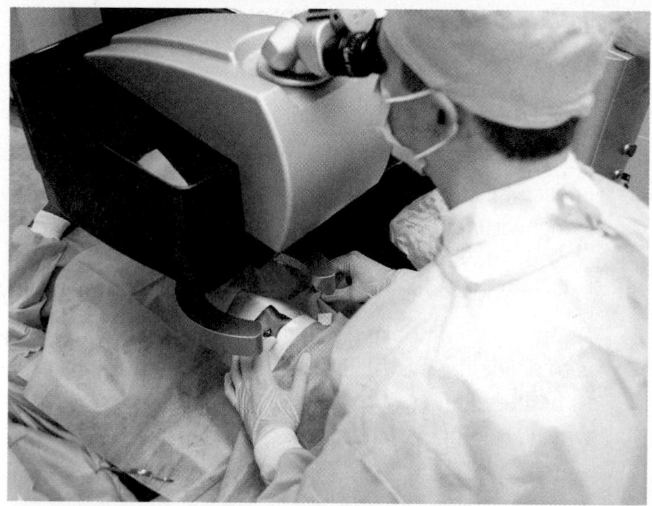

Romaset/Shutterstock.com

Figure 7.10 Eye disorders and diseases, such as detached retinas, myopia, cataracts, and macular degeneration, can often be treated successfully with laser surgery.

Diabetic Retinopathy

Damage to the retina caused by long-term diabetes is called *diabetic retinopathy* (reht-i-NAHP-a-thee). This condition is becoming increasingly prevalent and is currently the leading cause of blindness in American adults. Diabetic retinopathy involves swelling and leaking of the vessels that supply blood to the retina.

When diabetic retinopathy is sufficiently advanced, bleeding occurs, causing the individual to see red spots. Laser surgery typically is effective in treating the condition when it is caught early enough.

Vitreous Floaters

Vitreous floaters are small, irregularly shaped specks that drift around within your field of vision. Floaters form when tiny chunks of the gel-like vitreous humor break off and float in the aqueous humor in the center of the eyeball.

Although sometimes distracting, ordinary eye floaters are common and normally not a cause for alarm. However, the sudden appearance of multiple floaters accompanied by what appear to be flashes of light on the lateral periphery of the eye can be symptoms of a retinal tear or retinal detachment. In such cases, immediate medical attention is required.

Check Your Understanding

1. What is another name for nearsightedness?
2. Presbyopia usually affects people in what age group? Explain.
3. Which disease of the eye is highly contagious?
4. What are the signs and symptoms of cataracts?
5. Distinguish between dry macular degeneration and wet macular degeneration.

LESSON 7.1 Review and Assessment

Mini Glossary

Make sure that you know the meaning of each key term.

aqueous humor the clear, watery fluid that fills the anterior chamber of the eye; provides nutrients for the lens and cornea and helps maintain intraocular pressure

choroid the middle layer of the wall of the eye

ciliary body the structure between the choroid and the iris that anchors the lens in place

ciliary glands modified sweat glands located between the eyelashes

cones sensory cells in the retina that are sensitive to bright light and provide color vision

conjunctiva a delicate external membrane that covers the exposed eyeball and lines the eyelid

cornea a transparent tissue over the anterior center of the eye

extrinsic muscles muscles attached to the outer surface of the eye that are responsible for changing the direction of viewing

iris the anterior portion of the choroid, which gives the eye its color

lacrimal glands tear secretors; located above the lateral end of each eye

lens a transparent, flexible structure that is curved outward on both sides

optic chiasma the point at which the optic nerves cross

optic nerve transmitter of visual sensory signals to the occipital lobe of the brain

optic tracts the continuation of the optic nerve fibers beyond the optic chiasma

pupil the opening through which light rays enter the eye

retina the innermost layer of the eye, containing light-sensitive nerve endings that send impulses through the optic nerves to the brain

rods sensory cells in the retina that are activated in dim light

sclera the tough, fibrous outer layer of the eye

suspensory ligaments tiny structures that attach the lens of the eye to the ciliary body

tarsal glands secretors of an oily substance; located in the eyelids

vitreous humor gel-like substance that fills the posterior chamber of the eye; contributes to intraocular pressure

Know and Understand

1. List the anatomical features that protect the eye from injury.
2. Which glands produce the salty solution known as *tears*?
3. Where are the extrinsic muscles and what is their purpose?
4. What part of the eye is called the "window of the eye?"
5. Rods and cones are located in which layer of the eye?
6. Describe the pathway of vision.
7. What part of the eye has many pain receptors and is able to repair itself quickly?

Analyze and Apply

8. Compare and contrast myopia, hyperopia, and presbyopia.
9. Derrick has had to do a lot of reading in college. He never had a problem with his vision in the past, but lately he has had trouble reading the print in his textbook. When he noticed that he was holding his book farther and farther away from his eyes, he decided to see an ophthalmologist. What do you think the doctor told Derrick? Which injury, disorder, or disease that you read about in this chapter was the diagnosis? What treatment do you think the doctor prescribed?
10. Predict the outcome of a student's ability to do schoolwork without access to medical care for each of the following vision disorders: astigmatism, amblyopia, diplopia, strabismus, and hyperopia.
11. Research the different types of colorblindness and the impact it can have on the following activities of daily living: getting dressed, buying fruits and vegetables, cooking, driving, and spending a day at the beach. Present your findings to the class.
12. Another way of looking at the anatomy of the eye is to divide the eyeball into tunics. Conduct research to find the names of the three tunics of the eye and which structures each tunic includes.

IN THE LAB

13. Make a KWL chart like the one in **Figure 7.11**. Fill in the chart, listing what you know about accommodation, what you want to know, and, after doing the demonstration below, what you learned.

K	W	L
What I Know	What I Want to Know	What I Learned

Figure 7.11 Goodheart-Willcox Publisher

Demonstration: Close one eye and stare at a point about 20 feet away. The point at which you are staring should be in focus. While concentrating on the point, raise one of your fingers into your line of sight just below the point. Your finger should be a bit blurred. Now, change focus—look at the tip of your finger instead of the point 20 feet away. Your finger will come into focus, but the distant point will be blurred.

14. With a partner, obtain a Snellen chart and instructions for using it to assess visual acuity. Also obtain two index cards or other thin, opaque material to be used to cover the eyes. One student acts as the eye examiner and records the other student's responses. Then switch roles so that each student has an opportunity to use the Snellen chart. Record your results.

LESSON 7.2 The Ear

Before You Read

Try to answer the following questions before you read this lesson.

- What is the purpose of earwax?
- How does yawning wide while descending from a height help to equalize pressure in the ears?

Lesson Objectives

- Describe the major anatomical structures of the outer, middle, and inner ear.
- Explain the two major functions of the ear.
- List common diseases and disorders of the ear.

Key Terms

auditory canal	organ of Corti
auricle	ossicles
bony labyrinth	oval window
ceruminous glands	perilymph
cochlea	semicircular canals
cochlear duct	stapes
endolymph	tympanic cavity
Eustachian tube	tympanic membrane
incus	vestibule
malleus	vestibulocochlear nerve
membranous labyrinth	

Just as vision is a highly useful sense, so is the sense of hearing. The ears are remarkable in their ability to capture, amplify, and transmit sounds of varying loudness and pitch (high versus low tones) to the brain. The ears also serve another important function, however. They play a central role in the ability to maintain physical balance and even to recognize which direction is up. This lesson examines the anatomy and inner workings of the ear to learn how the functions of hearing and balance are carried out.

Anatomy of the Ear

The ear includes three anatomical regions—the external (outer) ear, the middle ear (tympanic cavity), and the internal (inner) ear. The external and middle ear contribute to the ability to hear. The internal ear plays roles in both hearing and equilibrium (balance).

External Ear

The irregularly shaped, outer portion of the ear is called the **auricle** (AW-ri-kuhl), or *pinna*. In many animal species, the outer ear serves to channel sound waves into the ear, but in the human species this function is minimal. As **Figure 7.11** shows, the auricle connects with the **auditory canal**, also known as the *external acoustic meatus*.

The auditory canal is a short, tubelike structure about 1 inch long and 1/4 inch in diameter. The walls of this canal are lined with skin that contains **ceruminous** (seh-ROO-mi-nus) **glands**. The ceruminous glands secrete cerumen, also known as *earwax*. Earwax helps to clean, lubricate, and protect the ear.

At the end of the auditory canal is the **tympanic** (tim-PAN-ik) **membrane**, commonly known as the *eardrum*. Sound waves entering the ear cause the tympanic membrane to vibrate. The eardrum also separates the outer ear from the middle ear.

Middle Ear

The middle ear, or **tympanic cavity**, is a small, open chamber in the temporal lobe of the skull (**Figure 7.12**). The tympanic membrane is on the lateral side of the cavity. On the medial side is bone with a membrane-covered opening known as the **oval window**. Beneath the oval window is a *round window*.

Inside the tympanic cavity lie the three smallest bones in the body, known as **ossicles** (AHS-i-kuhls). The ossicles are named for their shapes—the **malleus**, or hammer; the **incus**,

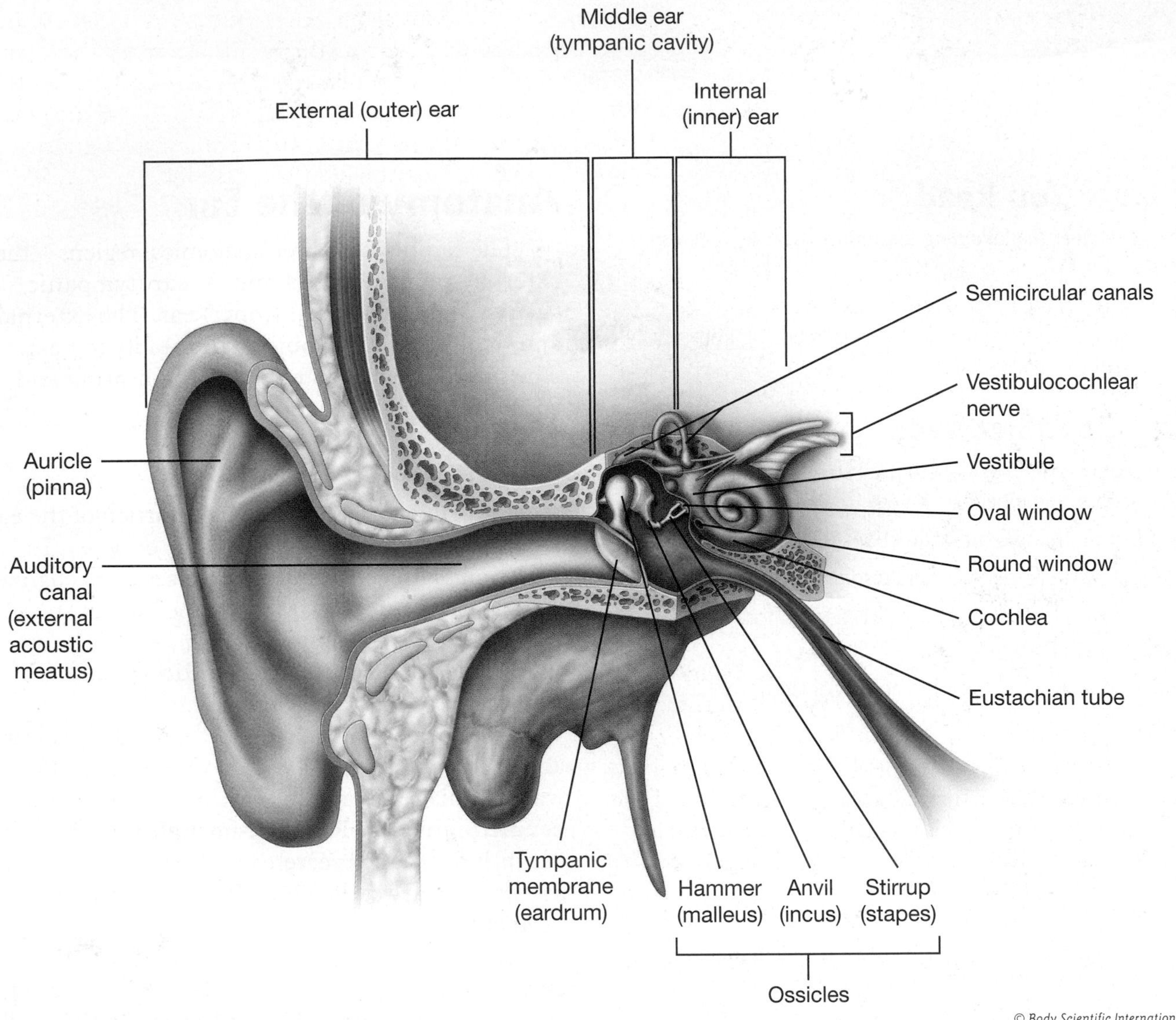

Figure 7.12 Anatomy of the ear. *Which structure separates the outer ear from the middle ear?*

or anvil; and the **stapes**, or stirrup. Together, these bones connect the tympanic membrane to the membrane of the oval window. The hammer attaches to the tympanic membrane, the anvil attaches to the hammer, and the stirrup attaches to the anvil on one side and to the oval window on the other. Because of their mechanical arrangement, the ossicles not only transmit, but also amplify, sound waves.

The **Eustachian** (yoo-STAY-shuhn) **tube** connects the middle ear to the pharynx. The pharynx is the part of the throat that connects the mouth and nasal cavity to the esophagus (the digestive tube between the throat and stomach). The Eustachian tube equalizes the pressure on either side of the tympanic membrane. Yawning widely is a way to help bring pressure in the pharynx, Eustachian tube, and middle ear to the same level as pressure outside the ear. This is a good strategy to use when air (barometric) pressure changes rapidly, such as during an airplane descent or while driving down a mountain road.

Internal Ear

The oval window connects the middle ear with the inner ear. The inner ear structures reside in a hollow tunnel that winds and twists like a bowl of interconnected spaghetti noodles. **Figure 7.13** shows a representation of these winding tunnels, known as the **bony labyrinth**. The three components of the inner ear are the **cochlea** (KAHK-lee-uh), **vestibule** (VEHS-ti-byool), and **semicircular** (sehm-ee-SIR-kyoo-lar) **canals**.

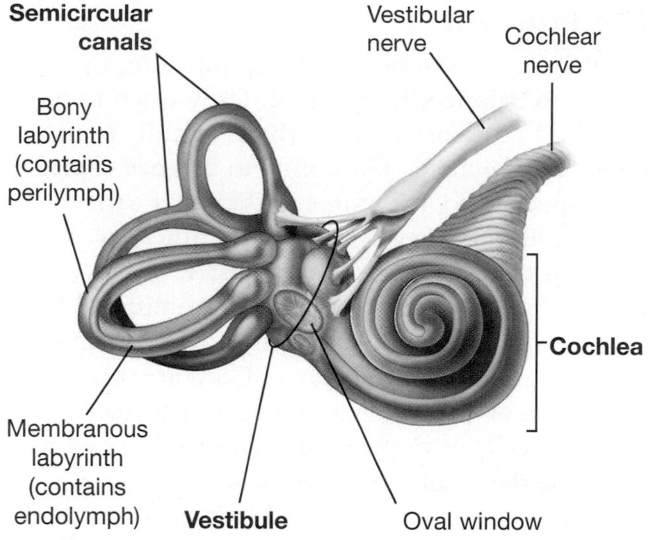

Figure 7.13 Structures of the inner ear. *What role, if any, do you think the inner ear plays in the development of a phobia such as a fear of heights?*

The cochlear nerve and vestibular (vehs-TIB-yoo-lar) nerve transmit sensory information from the cochlea and vestibule, respectively. The cochlear nerve carries information about hearing, and the vestibular nerve carries information about balance. These two nerves join to form a single cranial nerve, the **vestibulocochlear** (vehs-tib-yoo-loh-KAHK-lee-ar) **nerve**.

The bony labyrinth is filled with a clear fluid called **perilymph** (PER-i-limf). Inside the bony labyrinth are membrane-covered tubes called the **membranous labyrinth**, which follow the course of the bony labyrinth. Inside the membranous labyrinth is a thicker fluid called **endolymph** (EHN-doh-limf).

Check Your Understanding

1. What is the purpose of the Eustachian tube?
2. What two types of information are carried by the vestibulocochlear nerve?

Functions of the Ear

You know that the primary function of your ears is to detect sounds in your environment. But did you know that your ears also help your body to maintain its balance, or equilibrium? This section discusses these two important functions of the ear.

Hearing

When sound waves enter the ear, they are transmitted through the auditory canal, causing the tympanic membrane to vibrate. This motion stimulates the malleus, incus, and stapes to amplify and transmit these vibrations to the

LIFE SPAN DEVELOPMENT: *The Ears and Hearing*

The inner ear begins its development with a small area of thickening in the epithelium of the embryo's head during week 4. This area folds inward and pinches off from the surface to form a fluid-filled vesicle called the *otocyst*. The otocyst epithelium evolves to form the primitive membranous labyrinth. The labyrinth then divides into the cochlea and semicircular canals.

Externally, the auricle and external auditory canal begin to form during the fourth and fifth weeks of pregnancy. They are both fully formed at birth but continue to grow into the size and shape of adult ears through about age nine. Ceruminous glands begin development at about five months gestation. They are anatomically complete at birth but do not fully function until puberty.

At what point is the developing baby able to hear? The fetus begins to hear sounds at about four and a half months into the pregnancy. Sensitivity to sound increases and between the sixth and seventh months, fetuses have been observed to respond to voices and other noises.

Young children are able to hear an extremely large range of sound frequencies, from low- to high-pitched. As people age, damage due to loud noise progressively accumulates. At advanced age, there are characteristic age-associated deficits in hearing, as described in the next section. Importantly, however, most of these changes in hearing ability may be as much due to repeated exposure to loud noise as to aging.

Life Span Review

1. What portions of the ear continue to develop after birth?
2. How early is a developing baby in the womb able to hear?
3. Is age-related hearing loss inevitable?

membrane of the oval window. This process of amplification and transmission sets in motion the fluids of the inner ear.

Your ability to hear resides within the snail-shaped cochlea of the inner ear. The portion of the membranous labyrinth inside the cochlea is called the **cochlear duct**. Within the cochlear duct is the spiral **organ of Corti**, which contains hearing receptors called *hair cells* (**Figure 7.14**). The short, stiff hair cells are stimulated by high-pitched sounds; the longer, more flexible hair cells are stimulated by low-pitched sounds.

Motion of the endolymph in the cochlear duct causes the *tectorial membrane* to move. Movement of the tectorial membrane stimulates the hair cells, which in turn stimulate the cochlear branch of the vestibulocochlear nerve. The cochlear nerve then transmits electrical impulses to the auditory region in the temporal lobe of the brain.

Equilibrium

People tend to take their equilibrium, or ability to balance, for granted. Only when they are dizzy or disoriented do they typically even appreciate balance. The ability to balance comes from specialized structures in the inner ear.

Recall that the vestibule of the inner ear contains three semicircular canals. The hair cells in the semicircular canals are stimulated by movement of the endolymph in the canals, much like the hair cells in the organ of Corti are stimulated by motion of the endolymph to produce hearing. The hair cells in the semicircular canals, however, stimulate the vestibular nerve, which communicates with the cerebellum to provide information about the orientation and motion of the head. The semicircular canals play an important role in balance whether a person is stationary or moving.

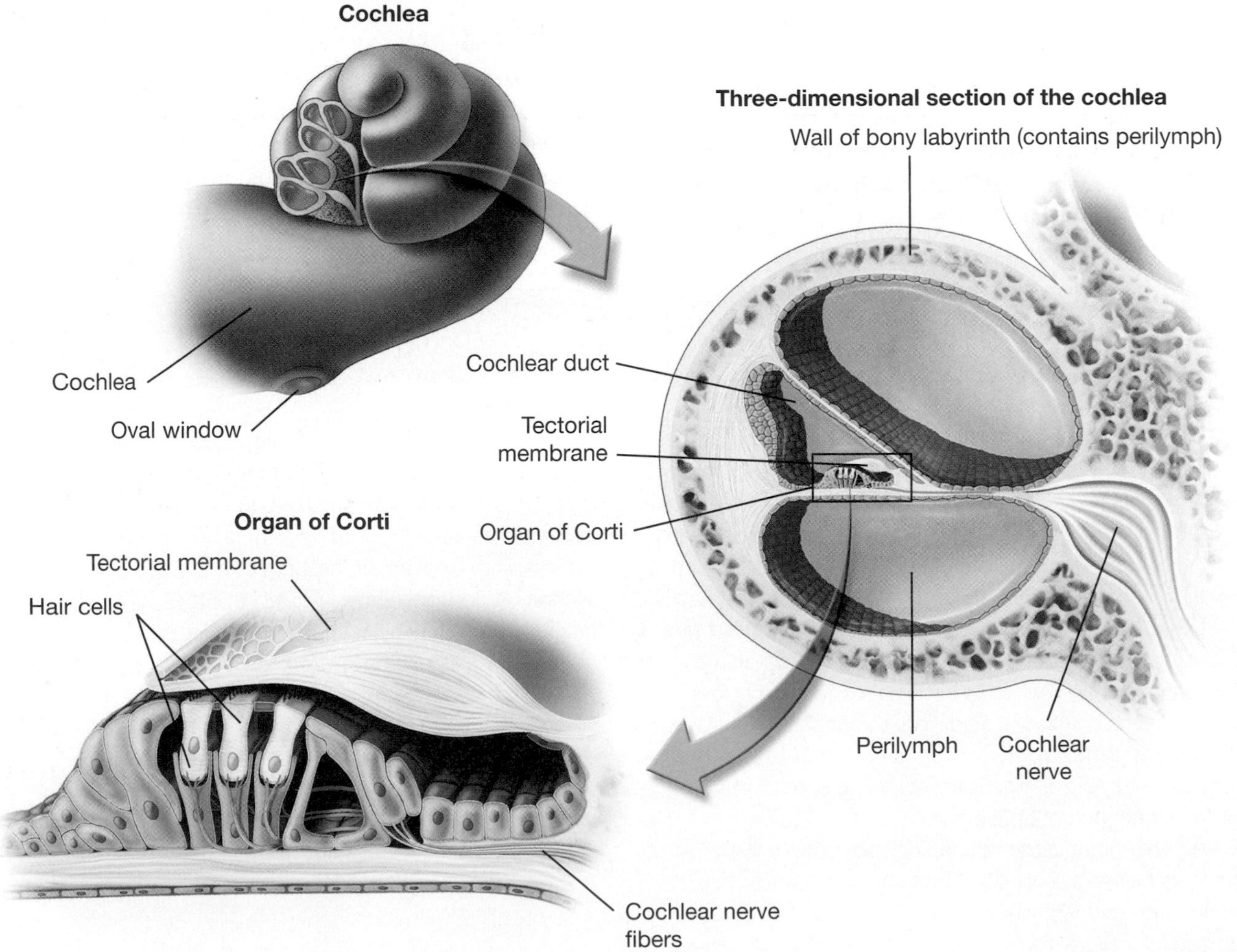

Figure 7.14 Anatomy of the cochlea. *What role do different kinds of hair cells play in relaying sound messages to the brain?*

Check Your Understanding

1. What are the two functions of the ear?
2. What is the function of cerumen?
3. List the ossicles and tell why they are important.
4. Which structure in the inner ear controls equilibrium?

Disorders and Infections of the Ear

A variety of conditions can affect hearing or balance. This section addresses some of the most common disorders and infections of the ear. The etiology (cause), strategies for prevention, pathology (clinical characteristics), diagnosis (keys for identifying the condition), and common treatments for these disorders and infections of the ear are summarized in **Figure 7.15**.

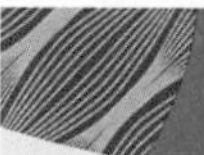

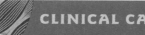

CLINICAL CASE STUDY

George and his friends have been swimming in a nearby lake on weekends during the summer. They enjoy swinging from a rope tied to a tree on the bank of the lake and plunging into deep, cold water. On the day after one of these swimming excursions, George finds that he has a definite pain coming from inside one of his ears. He has no other symptoms. As you read this section, try to determine which of the following conditions George most likely has.

A. Tinnitus
B. External Otitis
C. Otitis media
D. Labyrinthitis

Disorders and Infections of the Ear

	Etiology	Prevention	Pathology	Diagnosis	Treatment
Deafness	injury to middle or inner ear, chronic exposure to loud noise, excessive earwax, scarring of tympanic membrane, damage to auditory nerve or auditory region of brain	avoid exposure to loud noise, keep ears free of excess earwax	partial or complete loss of hearing	physical exam, hearing tests	remove wax blockage, surgical procedures, hearing aid, cochlear implant
Tinnitus	damage to hair cells in organ of Corti, causing them to move randomly	avoid exposure to loud sound; avoid overuse of certain medications, such as NSAIDs	ringing sound in the ears	physical exam, hearing test, imaging test	treat underlying health problem, noise suppression, medications
External otitis (swimmer's ear)	bacterial or fungal infection of the auditory canal	avoid ear immersion in water; irrigate ear with mild alcohol solution after swimming	itching, pain, fever, temporary hearing loss	physical exam, ear exam	cleaning of the ear canal, eardrops for infection, oral medication for pain
Otitis media (middle ear infection)	bacterial or viral infection of middle ear; can result from cold or allergy that causes congestion and swelling of the nasal passages, throat, and Eustachian tubes	keep ears clean and dry; use precautions to avoid colds and allergic reactions	pain, swelling, production of fluid or pus from ear	physical exam, ear exam	antibiotics and pain medication, as indicated
Labyrinthitis (inner ear infection)	inflammation of a vestibular nerve to the inner ear; can result from infections of the ear or systemic infections	maintain healthy lifestyle; avoid stress	dizziness, nausea, loss of hearing, vertigo, loss of balance, tinnitus	physical exam; tests of hearing and blood, imaging tests	antihistamines, medications to reduce dizziness and nausea, sedatives, corticosteroids

Figure 7.15

Goodheart-Willcox Publisher

Deafness

Deafness is the term applied to any loss of hearing, ranging from a slight to a complete inability to hear. Injuries that affect the structures of the middle or inner ear can cause deafness. Regular exposure to extremely loud sounds such as construction noise or loud music can damage the hair receptor cells in the organ of Corti, leading to hearing loss. Other causes of deafness include excessive earwax, scarring of the tympanic membrane following inflammation, and damage to the auditory nerve or auditory region of the brain.

There are two distinct types of deafness: conductive and sensorineural. In *conductive hearing loss*, the transfer of sound waves from the outer ear through the tympanic membrane to the middle ear is disrupted. The source of the disruption may be fluid or an abnormal growth of tissue or bone. *Sensorineural hearing loss* occurs when the cochlea fails to send a signal to the brain.

Presbycusis (prehz-bih-KYOO-sis) is the term for age-related hearing loss. High-pitched sounds, in particular, become harder to hear as people age. This can make words harder to understand, because consonants, such as b, d, p, and t, tend to be high-pitched during normal speech. When these sounds drop out it can make speech difficult to follow. To speak to someone with presbycusis, it is best to articulate words very clearly rather than to just speak loudly. Presbycusis usually can be improved through the use of hearing aids.

Hearing aids amplify and change sounds so that the wearer can better hear the sounds. Some hearing aids amplify all sounds; others specifically boost low- or high-frequency sounds. For elderly individuals with hearing deficits, use of a hearing aid not only improves hearing, but also improves the ability to balance. Scientists are studying this recently discovered phenomenon to try to understand the mechanism by which it works.

Hearing aids are available in a variety of styles and sizes (**Figure 7.16**), and price varies considerably. This is why you would want to carefully analyze all information (from healthcare workers and promotional materials) before making inferences about the best products and services for you or the person you are helping with the purchase.

"In-the-canal" hearing aids are custom-molded to fit inside the auditory canal. This type of hearing aid is recommended for mild to moderate hearing loss.

"Half-shell" hearing aids are custom-fit to sit inside the small, inner bowl-shaped area of the outer ear. These hearing aids are recommended for mild to moderately severe hearing loss. Somewhat larger hearing aids, called "in-the-ear" aids, are custom-designed to fill most of the bowl of the outer ear. This type of hearing aid is recommended for mild to severe hearing loss.

Finally, "behind-the-ear" hearing aids, designed to "ride" behind the ear, are capable of greater amplification than the other types of hearing aids. This model, which transmits amplified sound to a molded piece inside the auditory canal, is appropriate for most types of hearing loss.

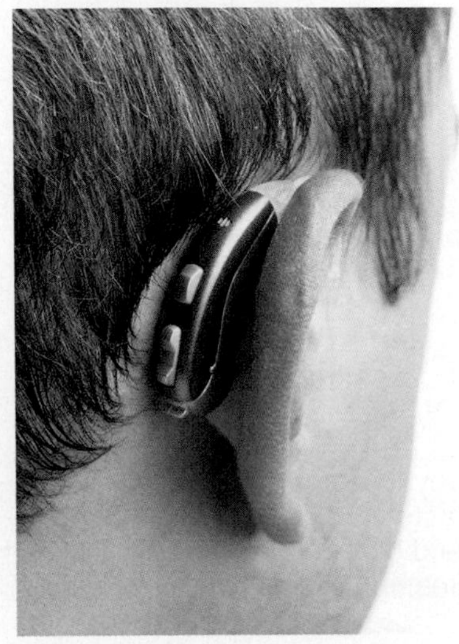
A

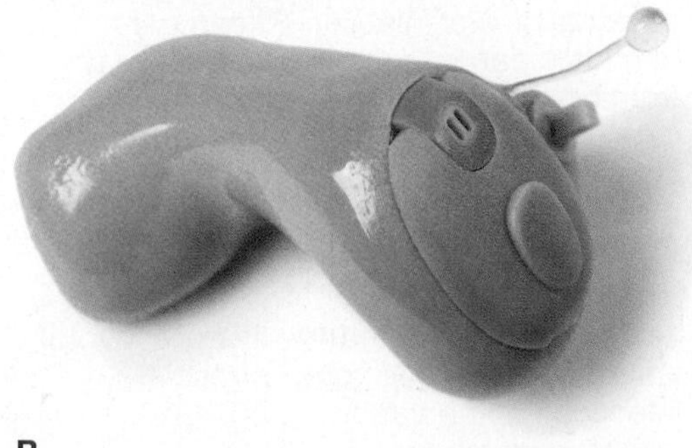
B

Oksix/Shutterstock.com, Jiri Hera/Shutterstock.com

Figure 7.16 Hearing aid models. A—"Behind-the-ear" model. B—"In-the-canal" model.

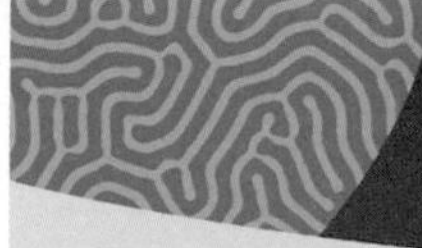

What Research Tells Us

...about Tone-Deafness

You may have noticed that some people have difficulty singing in key with music. It is typically said of such people that they cannot "carry a tune."

A person who sings off-key has *amusia* (uh-MYOO-zee-uh). Amusia is characterized by the inability to distinguish differences in pitch (that is, how high or low a tone is) as well as the inability to remember melodies. Amusia is present in about 3% of people from birth, but it can also result from a brain injury.

Researchers studying this condition have tried to train amusic children to develop the ability to better hear and reproduce musical tones. One method used by the researchers consists of having the children repeatedly listen to popular music for one month. This training, however, has had no apparent effect. Studies of brain activity in amusic individuals indicate that this difficulty in processing musical tones is caused by poor neural connections between the auditory center in the brain and the other related areas of the brain.

Taking It Further

1. Can you carry a tune? Sing a favorite song to friends or relatives, then listen to them as they sing. Compare the results.
2. Do some research on the causes of and treatments for amusia. Share your findings with the class.

Tinnitus

Tinnitus (TIN-i-tus) is a condition that causes a sound like ringing to be heard in the ear. Tinnitus occurs when the hair cells in the organ of Corti that stimulate the auditory nerve are damaged. Normal movement of the hair cells is triggered by sound waves. When the hair cells have been damaged, however, they sometimes move randomly, generating the ringing sound.

What damages these hair cells? The most common culprit is repeated exposure to loud noise, such as loud music. Other causes include overuse or long-term use of certain medications, including nonsteroidal anti-inflammatory drugs (NSAIDs). Tinnitus is a common and growing problem. According to the American Tinnitus Association, some 50 million people in the United States suffer from the disorder.

Otitis Externa

Have you ever gone swimming in a lake and then later developed an earache? You might have had swimmer's ear, formally known as *otitis* (oh-TIGH-tis) *externa*. This bacterial or fungal infection of the auditory canal is caused by immersion in contaminated water. Symptoms may include itching, pain, fever, and, in extreme cases, temporary hearing loss.

Otitis externa can be prevented by thoroughly cleaning and drying the ear canal with a mild alcohol-based solution after swimming, or by avoiding immersion of the ears.

Otitis Media

Otitis media is an infection of the middle ear caused by bacteria or a virus. It is usually associated with an upper respiratory tract infection. Otitis media is relatively common in infants and toddlers because their Eustachian tubes are not yet fully developed. Symptoms of otitis media include pain, swelling, and the production of fluid or pus.

Viral infections do not respond to antibiotics but often improve with time. Mild to moderate middle ear infections caused by bacteria are treated with antibiotics. More serious bacterial infections that do not respond well to antibiotics are frequently treated by a surgical procedure. During the surgery, tiny tubes are inserted into the tympanic membrane. These tubes alleviate the elevated pressure in the inner ear.

Labyrinthitis

Labyrinthitis (lab-uh-rin-THIGH-tis) is an infection of the inner ear that produces inflammation (swelling). It can be caused by inflammation of a vestibular nerve or can result from an infection of the ear or a systemic infection. This condition can disrupt the normal function of the semicircular canals. Symptoms may include severe dizziness, nausea and vomiting, loss of hearing, loss of balance, tinnitus, and vertigo. Individuals with vertigo are unable to stand because their sense of orientation is severely compromised. Labyrinthitis is treated with antihistamines, medications to reduce dizziness and nausea, sedatives, and corticosteroids.

Chronic inflammation of the semicircular canals of the inner ear is called *Ménière's* (men-EERZ) *disease*. This disease causes periodic but severe vertigo, as well as progressive hearing loss.

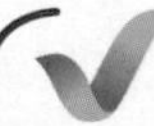

Check Your Understanding

1. List the causes of deafness.
2. Define presbycusis.
3. Name the condition that causes ringing in the ears.
4. Why are infants and toddlers prone to otitis media?

LESSON 7.2 Review and Assessment

Mini Glossary

Make sure that you know the meaning of each key term.

auditory canal a short, tubelike structure that connects the outer ear to the eardrum

auricle the irregularly shaped outer portion of the ear

bony labyrinth winding tunnels located in the inner ear

ceruminous glands secretors of cerumen, or earwax; located in the auditory canal

cochlea a snail-shaped structure in the inner ear that enables hearing

cochlear duct the portion of the membranous labyrinth inside the cochlea

endolymph a thick fluid inside the membranous labyrinth

Eustachian tube a channel that connects the middle ear to the pharynx and serves to equalize pressure on either side of the tympanic membrane

incus one of the three ossicles; tiny bone in the middle ear that attaches to the malleus and transmits sound from the malleus to the stapes

malleus one of the three ossicles; tiny bone in the middle ear that transmits sound from the tympanic membrane to the incus

membranous labyrinth membrane-covered tubes inside the bony labyrinth

organ of Corti a spiral-shaped ridge of epithelium in the cochlear duct lined with hair cells that serve as hearing receptors

ossicles the body's three smallest bones—the malleus, incus, and stapes; found in the middle ear

oval window a membrane-covered opening that connects the middle ear to the inner ear

perilymph a clear fluid that fills the bony labyrinth

semicircular canals inner ear channels containing receptor hair cells that play an important role in balance

stapes one of the three ossicles; tiny bone in the middle ear that attaches to the incus on one side and the oval window on the other

tympanic cavity the middle ear

tympanic membrane a sheet of tissue at the end of the auditory canal; also known as the *eardrum*

vestibule a chamber in the inner ear that contains the three semicircular canals

vestibulocochlear nerve a cranial nerve that rises from the cochlear and vestibular nerves

Know and Understand

1. What are the three anatomical regions of the ear?
2. Name the two terms used to describe the outer portion of the ear.
3. Where are the ceruminous glands located?
4. The Eustachian tube connects the middle ear to the _____.
5. Compare and contrast the function of the short, stiff hairs in the organ of Corti with that of its long, flexible hairs.
6. Describe the pathway of hearing.
7. Which part of the brain controls equilibrium?
8. What is the main function of the semicircular canals?
9. What is labyrinthitis?

Analyze and Apply

10. Explain the relationship between hearing and the brain.
11. Using a T-chart similar to the one in **Figure 7.17**, list the differences between otitis externa, otitis media, and labyrinthitis.

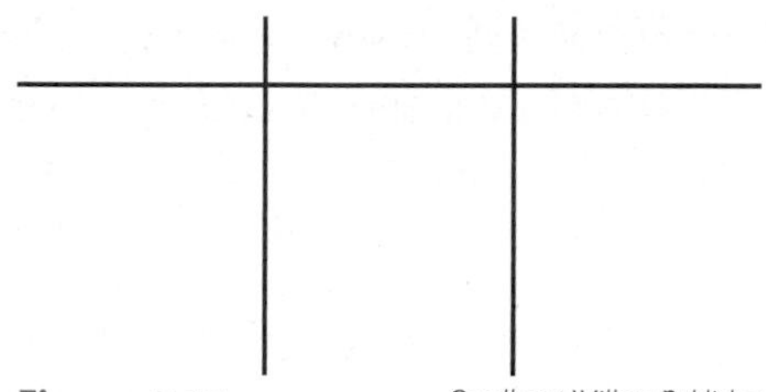

Figure 7.17 *Goodheart-Willcox Publisher*

12. What kind of surgery is sometimes necessary for infants and toddlers who have otitis media, and why does this help?
13. Use the internet to research the three main types of hearing aids: BTE, RIC, and ITE hearing aids. Explain how each type functions.
14. Using a Venn diagram, compare and contrast the advantages and disadvantages of wireless versus non-wireless hearing aids. Discuss your findings and how each would be beneficial to the following groups of individuals with hearing loss: young children, elderly, individuals without health insurance, and individuals of low socioeconomic status in developing countries.
15. Consider the effect of chronic exposure to loud noises on human hearing. What effect would this have on a musician who plays electric guitar in live rock concerts over a 20-year career? How could the musician lower the risk of negative effects?
16. Research the average decibel level of each of the sounds listed below. Create a chart to show the decibel level of each and the effect it would have on hearing over time.
    - whisper
    - commercial plane taking off or landing nearby
    - hair dryer on high setting
    - fireworks
    - normal conversation

IN THE LAB

17. Today's portable electronic devices make it easy to listen to music, podcasts, videos, and movies wherever you may be. This generally includes attaching earphones or earbuds to the device so that you can listen without disturbing others. However, research has shown that using earphones or earbuds can be hazardous if they are not used properly. Conduct research to find out more about using earphones safely. What factors should be considered? Create a brochure recommending safe earphone practices. Use your imagination to illustrate the brochure and make it interesting and eye-catching so that middle school and high school students will be more likely to read the brochure.
18. Research the products and services available for either deafness or otitis media. Collect promotional materials for a variety of products and services from product manufacturers and medical clinics. Analyze the data in these materials based on the knowledge gained from this lesson. Make inferences about the products and services and create an electronic presentation to recommend the best ones to the class.
19. Design an experiment to test the hearing of gerbils. Document the procedure you would use. Identify how you would use controls (some of the gerbils) to make sure that your test is valid. Identify both dependent and independent variables in your experiment. If possible, carry out your experiment, being careful not to harm the animals in any way. Record your results in a formal lab report. Be sure to include enough information that other people can repeat your experiment and verify your results.
20. One hearing screening test that is commonly used in physician offices is the Rinne hearing test. In this test, a tuning fork is used to test a person's hearing in one ear using both bone conduction and air conduction of sound. Conduct research to find out more about how this test works. Then, working with a partner, conduct a Rinne hearing test using a 512 Hz tuning fork and a watch with a second hand.

    Procedure:
    1. Decide who will be the patient and who will be the examiner.
    2. The patient sits in a chair in a quiet environment and covers one ear with his or her hand.
    3. The examiner strikes the tuning fork against the leg or palm to make it start vibrating.
    4. The examiner places the tuning fork against the patient's mastoid process and notes the exact time.
    5. The patient reports when the sound can no longer be heard; the examiner notes the number of seconds that have passed and moves the tuning fork over the ear canal, without touching it.
    6. The patient reports when the sound can no longer be heard; the examiner notes this time as well.
    7. The examiner records both times on a lab sheet.
    8. Repeat steps 3 through 7 for the patient's other ear.
    9. Switch places so that the patient becomes the examiner and the examiner becomes the patient.
    10. Repeat steps 2 through 8.
    11. Organize your results and write a lab report documenting the purpose of a Rinne test, your method, your data, and your results and conclusions.

LESSON 7.3 Smell and Taste

Before You Read

Try to answer the following questions before you read this lesson.

- How can a particular smell trigger an emotion?
- How does the sense of smell influence taste?

Lesson Objectives

- Describe the anatomy of the olfactory region and explain how it functions.
- Discuss the major anatomical structures of the gustatory sense and explain their functions.

Key Terms

antihistamines	olfactory region
gustatory sense	olfactory sense
histamines	papillae
limbic system	septum
olfactory bulb	tastants
olfactory hairs	taste buds
olfactory nerve	taste pores

Have you ever smelled your favorite food cooking and noticed that your mouth was watering? The sense of smell can stimulate your mouth to secrete saliva. Alternatively, imagine a perfectly cooked, scrumptious meal without the ability to smell or taste it.

The senses of smell and taste enable you to enjoy what you eat and drink. These senses can also alert you when food or drink has gone bad, as in the case of sour milk. In addition, your sense of smell can alert you to environmental dangers. For example, you would immediately leave an area in which you smelled toxic fumes or another undesirable or potentially harmful scent.

How are you able to so rapidly interpret what you smell and taste? This lesson explores the anatomy and physiology of the sensory pathways of smell and taste.

Olfactory Sense

Your **olfactory sense** is your sense of smell. Have you ever noticed that when you have a cold, your ability to smell is considerably lessened? The sensors responsible for smell are located in a dime-sized area called the **olfactory** (ohl-FAK-toh-ree) **region**, on the top side of each nasal cavity (**Figure 7.18**). These sensors are called *olfactory receptor cells*. When your nasal cavity becomes congested with mucus from a cold, the olfactory receptors are covered and partially blocked. As a result, odor molecules from foods that normally would trigger your sense of smell do not reach the olfactory receptor cells.

Anatomy and Physiology of the Olfactory Sense

The olfactory receptor cells are neurons. (For a definition of *neuron*, see Chapter 6.) Tiny **olfactory hairs** extend from these neurons into the nasal cavity, where they are covered by a thin, protective layer of mucus. Whenever you inhale an odor, the chemicals that caused the odor dissolve in the mucous layer surrounding the olfactory hairs. This dissolving action stimulates the olfactory receptor cells, which send impulses through the filaments that make up the **olfactory nerve**. The olfactory filaments feed impulses to the **olfactory bulb**, the thickened end of the olfactory nerve. The olfactory nerve sends impulses to the olfactory cortex of the brain.

The nerve pathway between the nose and the brain travels through the **limbic system**, the part of the brain responsible for emotions. A smell may trigger a positive or negative emotion because you have associated a particular experience with that scent. For instance, the scent of cookies baking in an oven may remind you of your family, bringing about a positive emotion. By contrast, the smell of an antiseptic ointment may remind you of an injury that you have experienced—one that you would rather not remember because it triggers a negative emotion.

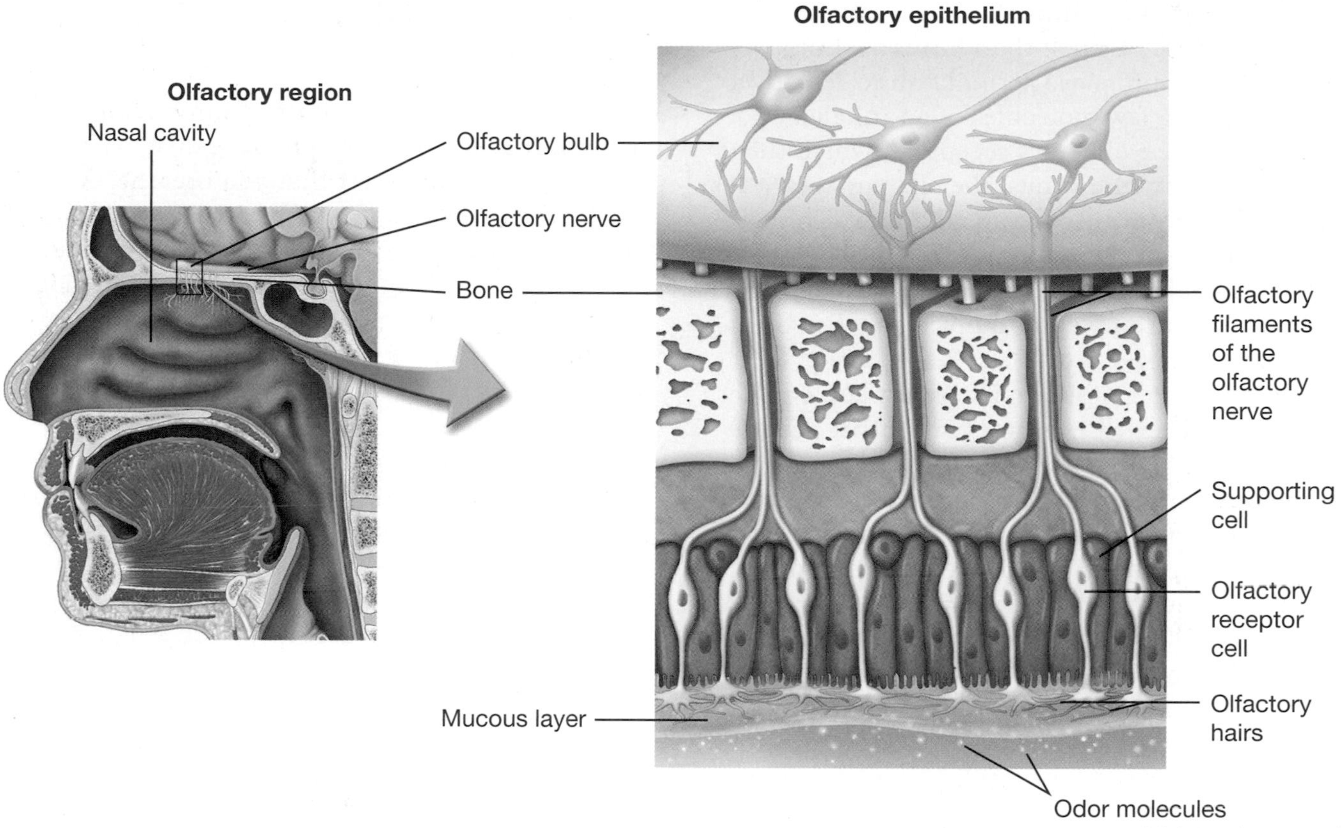

Olfactory region
Nasal cavity
Olfactory bulb
Olfactory nerve
Bone

Olfactory epithelium
Olfactory filaments of the olfactory nerve
Supporting cell
Olfactory receptor cell
Olfactory hairs
Mucous layer
Odor molecules

© Body Scientific International

Figure 7.18 The olfactory region. *Which labeled part of drawing B is covered with mucus when you have a cold? Why does this affect your sense of taste?*

LIFE SPAN DEVELOPMENT: *The Nose and Sense of Smell*

The development of the nose and nasal cavities is most active between the fourth and seventh weeks of pregnancy. The nostrils appear a few weeks later. By 10 weeks, the olfactory receptor cells have formed, and the developing fetus can now become familiar with the scent of the mother's amniotic fluid.

Newborn infants have a highly sensitive sense of smell. They form strong associations between specific scents and related experiences. They also use scents to identify people—especially those who are familiar, such as parents or other caretakers. During the first year babies also rely heavily on odors to identify foods they like and dislike. The ability to differentiate odors continues to develop through about age eight.

The nose and nasal passages are fully formed at birth but continue to grow in proportion to skeletal growth. Sagittal plane growth and anterior projection of the nose continue to increase in females until age 12 to 16 and to increase in males until age 18 and sometimes beyond. During the growth period, the angular shapes and positional relationships of the nose, lips and chin remain relatively constant in both genders. Generally, males have larger noses than females.

The nose continues to grow and change during life, with increasing nasal volume and nostril area. By the age of approximately 30, nose growth has slowed. Between 50 and 60 years of age, nasal volume in men increases by about another 29 percent and by about another 18 percent in women. With advancing age, the cartilage and skin of the nose lose strength, resulting in sagging of the nose. After age 60, loss of olfactory receptor cells may contribute to a diminished sense of smell, resulting in the inability to detect odors in low concentrations.

Life Span Review

1. At what point is the developing fetus able to smell?
2. At what age is the sense of smell fully developed?
3. What changes are characteristic of the nose and sense of smell with advanced age?

Although most animals have a much stronger sense of smell than humans, human olfactory receptors are actually quite sensitive. It takes only a few molecules of an inhaled odor to stimulate the olfactory receptors, which then fire a nerve impulse. Thus, the olfactory receptors can easily become used to an odor to which they are repeatedly exposed. This explains why people who habitually wear a certain perfume or cologne, for example, tend not to smell it on themselves.

Why do you suppose different people prefer or dislike different perfumes and other scents? On a biological level, the answer has to do with individual differences in olfactory receptors. A given smell activates different olfactory receptors in different people. When scientists compared olfactory receptors across people, they found that any two individuals are likely to be approximately 30% different. This may seem surprising, but there are about 400 genes, with 900,000 variations, coding the olfactory receptors. Differences in an individual's sense of smell is therefore not unexpected.

How many different basic odors do you suppose there are? Although many smells are derived from a combination of basic odors, scientists have isolated 10 different basic odor qualities from analysis of olfactory perception data. These have been identified as sweet, fragrant, woody/resinous, fruity (non-citrus), chemical, minty/peppermint, popcorn, lemon, decaying, and pungent.

Injuries and Disorders of the Nose

Your nose is important to your overall health. It acts as a filter to remove dust, irritants, and germs from the air that you breathe. A variety of problems, from the common cold to a deviated septum, can make breathing difficult. The etiology, strategies for prevention, pathology, diagnosis, and common treatments for injuries and disorders of the nose are summarized in **Figure 7.19**.

Rhinitis

Rhinitis (righ-NIGH-tis) is an inflammation of the mucous membranes that line the nasal passage. The most frequent cause of rhinitis is the common cold. However, the condition can be caused by anything that irritates these membranes. Possibilities include infections, allergies, strong chemical odors, and certain drugs.

Irritation of the nasal membranes causes the release of **histamines** (HIS-ta-meenz), molecules that trigger a reaction that produces nasal congestion and drainage. Treatment of rhinitis requires removing or minimizing the original irritant and taking medications that contain **antihistamines** (an-tee-HIS-ta-meenz), which curb the activity of histamines.

Septum Problems

The **septum** of the nose is the structure made of cartilage that divides the left and right air passages in the nose. It is normal for the septum not to be

Disorders and Infections of the Nose

	Etiology	Prevention	Pathology	Diagnosis	Treatment
Rhinitis	inflammation of mucous membranes of nasal passage due to infections, allergies, strong chemical odors, or certain recreational drugs	avoid exposure to infections and nasal irritants	release of histamines causes nasal congestion and drainage	physical exam	rest, antihistamines
Deviated septum	injury or genetics	none	symptoms vary with circumstances	physical exam	treat symptoms; surgical repair when warranted
Perforated septum	injury, ulcer, long-term exposure to toxic fumes, drug abuse	avoid toxic fumes and drug abuse	symptoms vary with circumstances	physical exam	surgical repair when warranted

Figure 7.19 Goodheart-Willcox Publisher

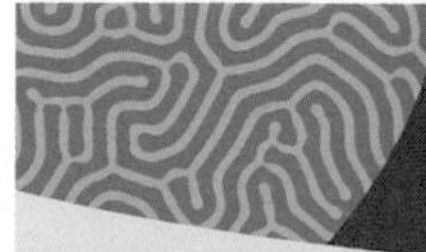

What Research Tells Us

...about Sense of Smell in Animals

How does the human olfactory sense compare to that of animals and fish? The human sense of smell is sufficiently powerful that it can detect the presence of a skunk with only 0.000,000,000,000,071 of an ounce of scent present. Because the sense of smell among many species of animals and fish may be related to survival, however, a larger portion of their brains is devoted to receiving and interpreting scents.

Dogs, for example, have about 125 to 220 million olfactory receptor cells. This is roughly 20 times the number of receptors that humans have. Dogs bred for hunting may have even more olfactory receptors; the bloodhound, for instance, has nearly 300 million. In fact, the percentage of a dog's brain that is responsible for smell is 40 times greater than the corresponding percentage of the human brain.

The wetness of a dog's nose assists with scent detection by capturing odor particles. With all of these advantages, it has been estimated that a dog's sense of smell is 100 thousand to 1 million times more sensitive than that of a human. By comparison, the bloodhound's olfactory sense may be up to 100 million times more sensitive. This is why the bloodhound, sometimes jokingly referred to as "a nose with a dog attached," is often used in law enforcement to track down missing persons and criminals.

A horse's olfactory sense is not as sharp as that of a dog, but it is still stronger than the human sense of smell. Horses use their olfactory sense to identify other horses, people, predators, pastures, feeds, and water sources. A mare's sense of smell is so discriminating that it enables her to pick out her own foal from a group of foals.

Fish such as salmon also have an extremely well-developed sense of smell. Salmon are born in small, freshwater streams. They then swim to the ocean, where they spend one to three years. After this period, they generally return to the same stream where they were born to lay eggs.

How does each salmon locate the exact same stream in which it was born? One hypothesis is that the newborn salmon brain is imprinted with the distinctive odor of the water from the stream of its birth. Researchers tested this hypothesis by tagging a large number of young salmon and recording the location of their births. They then plugged the nostrils of 50 percent of these salmon to block their ability to smell. When the salmon returned to fresh water to lay their eggs, the researchers discovered that the salmon with plugged nostrils did not return to the same stream where they were born. By contrast, most of the salmon with unplugged nostrils returned to the site of their births. Although other factors may influence the salmon's remarkable ability to return to its birth stream, its sense of smell clearly plays a key role.

Taking It Further

1. Do some research to find out how "sniffer" dogs are trained to detect drugs or bombs with their noses. Share your findings with the class.
2. How strong is your own sense of smell? Open an alcohol swab packet near your belly button. Breathe in. Can you detect the odor from the swab? Begin moving it closer to your nose and continue trying to smell it. If you can detect the odor from a distance of 8 to 12 inches from your nose (around chest level), then your sense of smell is normal. If you find that you are having a hard time distinguishing the scent at 4 inches away from your nose, then you may have a loss of the sense of smell.

perfectly centered; a slight deviation to one side is common. However, a large shift in the position of the septum away from the center is called a *deviated septum*. Injury is usually, but not always, the cause of a deviated septum. When warranted, a deviated septum can be surgically repaired.

The septum may also develop one or more holes caused by injury, an ulcer, long-term exposure to toxic fumes, or illegal drug abuse. This condition is known as a *perforated septum*. A perforated septum can be surgically treated to close the open sores.

Check Your Understanding

1. Where are sensors for smell located?
2. Explain the connection between smell and emotions.
3. What is the most common cause of rhinitis?
4. What might cause a perforated septum?

Gustatory Sense

The sense of taste is referred to as the **gustatory** (GUS-ta-toh-ree) **sense**. The human mouth contains approximately 10,000 sensory receptors for the sense of taste. These **taste buds**, or *gustatory receptors*, are scattered throughout the interior of the mouth, including the lips and the sides, top, and back of the mouth. Most of the taste buds, however, reside on the familiar tiny bumps on the tongue known as **papillae** (pa-PIL-ee). Within each taste bud, tiny gustatory hairs run up through the **taste pores**, very small openings in the top of the taste buds (**Figure 7.20**).

When you eat food, the food is mixed in your mouth with saliva, which is produced by the salivary glands in the mouth. Chemical molecules from food dissolve in the saliva to produce compounds called **tastants** (TAYS-tehnts). The tastants stimulate the gustatory hairs to send nerve impulses to the brain. Three of the cranial nerves—the facial nerve, the glossopharyngeal (glahs-oh-feh-RIN-jee-al) nerve, and the vagus (VAY-gus) nerve—are responsible for transmitting taste sensations to the brain. Refer to Chapter 6 for more information about these nerves.

Types of Flavors

Although people enjoy many foods and beverages because of the complexity of the taste sensations they generate, the gustatory sense comprises only five basic tastes. These are *sweet*, *salty*, *sour*, *bitter*, and *umami*. Umami is the taste of beef as well as the taste of monosodium glutamate, a seasoning commonly added to processed foods to enhance their taste. Some scientists have also proposed fat, termed *oleogustus*, as a sixth basic taste. Although a single gustatory cell responds to only one taste sensation, individual taste buds contain 50 to 100 gustatory cells, which typically include all of the taste sensations.

The flavors that you detect in food and beverages are influenced by sensations from your taste buds, but they are also strongly influenced by your sense of smell. An estimated 75% to 90% of what you may attribute to taste is actually due to what you smell. In the absence of smell, you would be able to distinguish only the five basic tastes—sweet, salty, sour, bitter, and umami. But the average person is able to distinguish approximately 10,000 different flavors. The human mouth contains no taste receptors for the distinctly recognizable tastes of peach, tomato, lime, or chocolate, for example. Each of these flavors is produced by a combination of taste and smell. The brain receives sensory information from the receptors for both taste and smell, and then translates this information into the flavors that you recognize (**Figure 7.21**).

Flavor is actually a combination of taste, smell, texture or consistency, and temperature. Many people have aversions to food and beverages whose consistency they simply do not find appealing. A hot food or drink gives off odors that strongly activate the neural pathways for smell, whereas the same food or beverage, when cold, gives off a much weaker odor, making it less appealing.

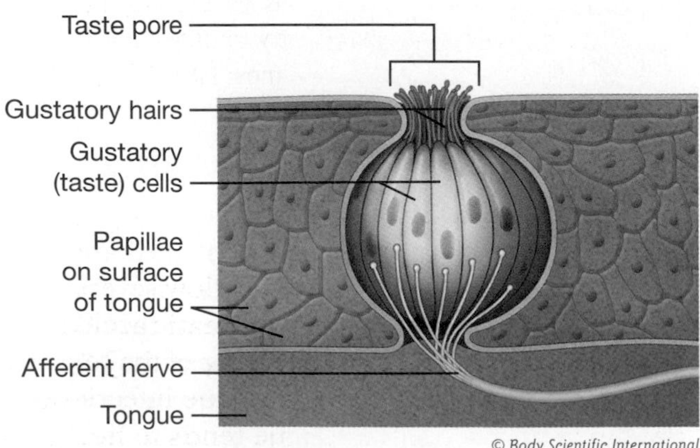

© Body Scientific International

Figure 7.20 Anatomy of a taste bud.

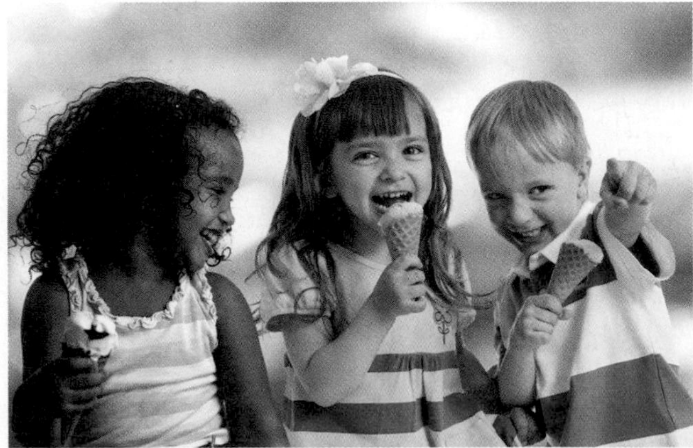

Andrey_Kuzmin/Shutterstock.com

Figure 7.21 These children seem to be enjoying their ice cream cones. *What factors contribute to the tastes and flavors they are experiencing?*

LIFE SPAN DEVELOPMENT: *The Tongue and Sense of Taste*

Specialized taste cells form in the developing fetus around the 7th to 8th week of gestation. By 13 to 15 weeks, these have evolved into fully formed taste buds. Newborn infants are fully responsive to taste. Since both amniotic fluid and breast milk contain molecules from the mother's diet, sampling flavors in foods begins in the womb and continues in early infancy. Mothers who consume a variety of healthful foods during pregnancy and lactation therefore give their babies early exposure to these flavors. Nevertheless, infants are born preferring sweet tastes and avoiding bitter tastes (**Figure 7.22**).

The number of taste receptors remains approximately constant from birth through middle age. By about the age of 50, however, the number of taste buds begins to dramatically decline, making food taste blander. Health issues, including nasal and sinus problems, certain medications, dental problems, cigarette smoking, Alzheimer's disease, and Parkinson's disease, can also diminish the sense of taste.

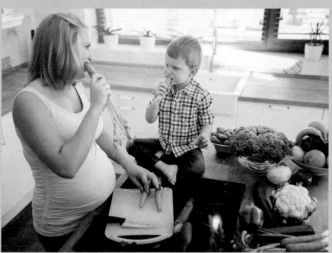

nd3000/Shutterstock.com

Figure 7.22 Mothers who consume a variety of healthful foods during pregnancy and lactation therefore give their babies early exposure to these flavors. Nevertheless, infants are born preferring sweet tastes and avoiding bitter tastes.

Life Span Review

1. Why are developing fetuses able to taste what the mother eats?
2. How well developed is a newborn infant's sense of taste?
3. Why does the ability to discriminate tastes decline with advanced age?

Spicy foods stimulate not only gustatory cells but also pain receptors in the mouth. Because everyone perceives pain differently, some people enjoy the sensation of spicy foods and others do not.

Disorders of the Tongue

The powerful muscles of your tongue enable you to speak and to chew and swallow food. As discussed above, taste buds on the surface of your tongue allow you to experience different taste sensations. A variety of disorders, including infections, injuries, and abnormal tissue growth, can affect the appearance and function of the tongue. Some tongue disorders are short-lived and can be remedied with antibiotics. Other disorders require ongoing treatment for an underlying physical condition. The etiology, strategies for prevention, pathology, diagnosis, and common treatments for injuries and disorders of the tongue are summarized in **Figure 7.23**.

CLINICAL CASE STUDY

Sarah has always practiced good oral hygiene, brushing her teeth and tongue at least twice a day. Two days ago, she had her tongue pierced. Now her tongue is painful and swollen and she feels like she might have a fever. As you read this section, try to determine which of the following conditions Sarah most likely has.

A. Tongue infection
B. Hairy tongue
C. Burning mouth syndrome

Infection of the tongue may follow severe biting of the tongue during a traumatic accident, or it may be associated with piercing of the tongue. Antibiotics are used to treat a tongue infection. Fortunately, the human tongue tends to heal quickly. In fact, it heals more quickly than any other part of the body.

Disorders and Infections of the Tongue					
	Etiology	**Prevention**	**Pathology**	**Diagnosis**	**Treatment**
Tongue infection	bacterial infection following severe biting of the tongue, piercing, or other injury	use measures to keep injury site clean and promote healing	pain, swelling, fever	physical exam	antibiotics
Hairy tongue	inadequate oral hygiene, use of certain medications, excessive drinking of coffee or tea, frequent tobacco use, radiation treatments	good oral hygiene, including brushing the tongue and teeth	unnatural growth of the gustatory hairs of the tongue	physical exam	restoration of good oral hygiene
Burning mouth syndrome	damage to sensory receptors in mouth, persistent dry mouth, nutritional deficiencies, hormonal changes, acid reflux, mouth infection	avoid causal factors when possible	moderate to severe burning in the mouth, may include tingling, numbness, or dryness of the mouth and a bitter or metallic taste	physical exam; blood or other tests related to symptoms	address causal factors and symptoms

Figure 7.23

Goodheart-Willcox Publisher

Certain conditions can promote unnatural growth of the gustatory hairs of the tongue, causing the look and feel of a *hairy tongue.* The most common cause is inadequate oral hygiene, but other causes include use of certain medications, excessive drinking of coffee or tea, frequent tobacco use, or radiation treatments to the head or neck region. Good oral hygiene, including brushing the tongue as well as the teeth, is both a prevention and a cure for hairy tongue (**Figure 7.24**).

Burning mouth syndrome, as the name suggests, involves a sensation of moderate to severe burning in the mouth that may continue for months or even years. When the pain persists, anxiety and depression may develop. Related symptoms may include tingling, numbness, or dryness of the mouth and a bitter or metallic taste. The condition can arise from a variety of causes, including damage to the taste and pain receptors in the mouth, chronically dry mouth, nutritional deficiencies, hormonal changes, acid reflux, and infection in the mouth.

Treatment of burning mouth syndrome is based on the cause, so it may involve addressing an underlying disorder with nutritional supplements, hormone therapy, antibiotics, or other remedies. When no underlying cause is apparent, treatment is designed to reduce the pain associated with burning mouth syndrome.

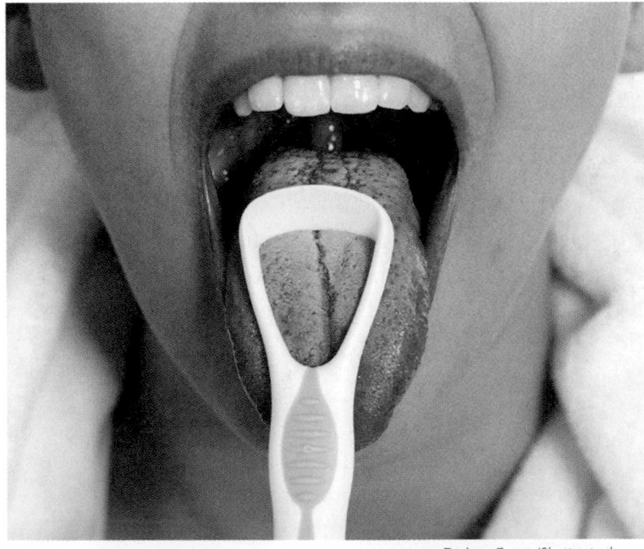

Andrey_Popov/Shutterstock.com

Figure 7.24 This person is using a tongue cleaner to help cure a mild case of hairy tongue. A toothbrush and toothpaste can also be used both to prevent and to cure this disorder.

Check Your Understanding

1. What are papillae?
2. List three nerves responsible for sending taste sensory signals to the brain.

LESSON 7.3 Review and Assessment

Mini Glossary

Make sure that you know the meaning of each key term.

antihistamines medications that work to curb the activity of histamines

gustatory sense the sense of taste

histamines molecules that trigger a reaction to irritation of the nasal membranes, which produces nasal congestion and drainage

limbic system the part of the brain that is responsible for emotions

olfactory bulb the thickened end of the olfactory nerve that sends sensory impulses to the olfactory region of the brain

olfactory hairs threads that extend from the olfactory receptor cells into the nasal cavity

olfactory nerve a cranial nerve that sends impulses to the olfactory cortex of the brain

olfactory region a dime-sized area at the top of each nasal cavity that houses sensors responsible for smell

olfactory sense the sense of smell

papillae tiny bumps on the tongue that house taste buds

septum the structure made of cartilage that divides the left and right air passages in the nose

tastants compounds that stimulate the gustatory hairs to send nerve impulses to the brain

taste buds sensory receptors for taste

taste pores very small openings in the top of the taste buds through which gustatory hairs project

Know and Understand

1. Which part of the brain is responsible for emotions related to scent?
2. Define histamines and state the importance of antihistamines.
3. What is the name of the structure that separates the right and left air passages of the nose?
4. The sense of taste is affected by the sense of _____.
5. Which mouth-related disorder causes a bitter or metallic taste in the mouth?

Analyze and Apply

6. Describe in detail how you are able to taste food.
7. List the five basic tastes and give examples of each.
8. Natural gas has no smell. Explain why utility companies put an unpleasant smell in natural gas.
9. Predict the outcome of an elderly individual without family who lives alone and has experienced a reduction in the number of taste buds due to illness and aging.

IN THE LAB

10. What is the difference between taste and flavor?

    While holding your nose, begin chewing a jelly bean. Can you identify the flavor of the jelly bean? Can you describe what you taste? You might say that you detect a sweet taste, which is due to the sugar in the jelly bean.

    Now, while continuing to chew, let go of your nose. What happens? Did you get a sudden rush of flavor? Can you better identify the flavor of the jelly bean?

    What did you learn from this experiment? Write a brief description of your findings.
11. Aromatherapy is a thriving business throughout the United States. Although scientists agree that aromatherapy is a valid form of therapy, consumers must use caution when purchasing and using aromatherapy-related products. Gather promotional brochures and information about various aromatherapy products. Analyze them and conduct research to determine whether the claims made on the promotional materials are valid. What can you infer about each product? Present your findings to the class.

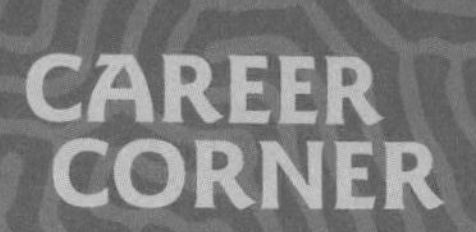

CAREER CORNER

Anatomy & Physiology at Work

A variety of career paths are available that involve working with and treating conditions of the sensory organs. A few of these options are discussed below.

Ophthalmologist

An ophthalmologist (ahp-thal-MAHL-oh-jist) is a medical doctor who specializes in treating injuries, disorders, and diseases of the eye through both medicine and surgery. Training for ophthalmologists in the United States includes a college degree, medical school, and a residency in ophthalmology.

Four years of residency training after medical school is required. The first year of residency training usually consists of a supervised internship in surgery, internal medicine, or pediatrics. During the following three years, residents receive specialized training in ophthalmology. Most residency programs are accredited by the Accreditation Council for Graduate Medical Education (ACGME) and are board-certified by the American Board of Ophthalmology.

Optometrist

Although optometrists (ahp-TAHM-eh-trists) are not doctors of medicine with the MD or OD credential, they are licensed medical professionals trained to prescribe and fit corrective lenses for improving vision (**Figure 7.25**). Optometrists can also diagnose and treat diseases of the eye and can prescribe needed medications. In some states in the United States, optometrists can also perform certain types of laser surgery.

Training for optometrists begins with a four-year college degree that includes successful completion of required courses in math, chemistry, physics, physiology, anatomy, microbiology, and psychology. Students applying for admission to an optometry doctoral program must score well on the standardized Optometry Admission Test. Admission to optometry school is highly competitive, with many more candidates applying than can be accepted.

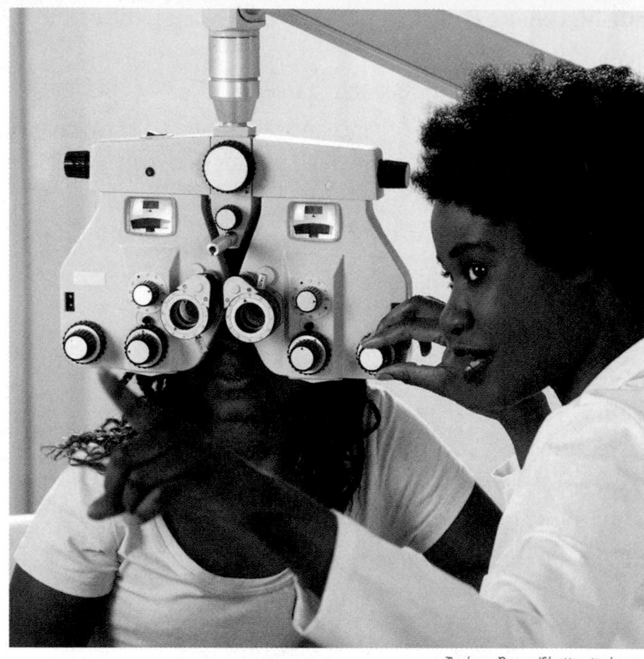

Andrey_Popov/Shutterstock.com

Figure 7.25 An optometrist tests a patient's vision.

The four-year doctoral program in optometry involves specialized classroom and clinical training in all aspects of the anatomy and physiology of the eye, treatment of disorders and diseases of the eye, and procedures for screening and correcting vision deficits. In addition, students receive general training in anatomy, physiology, and systemic diseases of the entire human body. Upon completion of a four-year, accredited optometry program, the optometry degree (OD) is awarded.

To be certified to practice, optometrists must pass a national examination administered by the National Board of Examiners in Optometry (NBEO). This exam encompasses basic science, clinical science, and patient care. Some optometrists elect to complete one- to two-year residencies with training focused on pediatric or geriatric eye care, specialty contact lens prescription, or diseases of the eye.

Audiologist

An audiologist (aw-dee-AHL-oh-jist) is a healthcare professional who specializes in diagnosing and treating disorders of the ear, including problems with both hearing and balance. Audiologists perform screening programs for hearing and prescribe hearing aids (**Figure 7.26**). They can also provide custom-fitted earplugs and other hearing protection devices for individuals who work in noisy environments. Another job of the audiologist is counseling families to help them cope with the diagnosis of a hearing deficit in an infant, and counseling seniors to help them adapt to hearing loss, even after a hearing aid has been prescribed.

Training for audiologists currently requires a four-year college degree followed by a Doctor of Audiology (AuD) degree. Requirements for the AuD degree involve a minimum of 75 semester hours of postbaccalaureate study that includes anatomy and physiology (both general and specific to the ear) as well as diagnosis of hearing deficits and disorders of both hearing and balance. Training in counseling and sign language is required. In addition, the AuD degree requires completion of a 12-month, full-time, supervised practicum; 12 months of full-time, supervised experience with a professional practice; and successful completion of a national exam. To practice, audiologists must receive state licensure or registration.

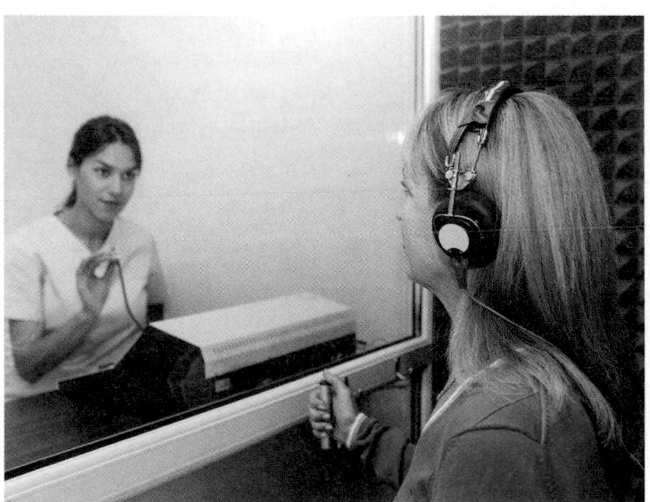

Erica Smit/Shutterstock.com

Figure 7.26 Audiologists have highly sensitive equipment that can detect minute changes in hearing. Typically, a patient is placed in a sound booth wearing headphones and holding a "clicker" to indicate when sounds are heard.

Planning for a Health-Related Career

Do some research on the career of an ophthalmologist or audiologist. Alternatively, select a profession from the list of related career options. Using the internet or resources at your local library, find answers to the following questions:

1. What are the main tasks and responsibilities of this job?
2. What is the outlook for this career? Are workers in demand, or are jobs dwindling? For complete information, consult the current edition of the *Occupational Outlook Handbook*, published by the US Department of Labor. This handbook is available online or at your local library.
3. What special skills or talents are required? For example, do you need to be good at biology or chemistry? Do you need to enjoy interacting with other people?
4. What personality traits do you think are needed to be successful in this job?
5. Does this career involve a great deal of routine, or are the day-to-day responsibilities varied?
6. Does the work require long hours, or is it a standard, "9-to-5" job?
7. What is the salary range for this job?
8. What do you think you would like about this career? Is there anything about it that you might dislike?

Related Career Options

- Biological technician
- Health educator
- Occupational therapist
- Ophthalmic assistant
- Ophthalmic technician
- Optical technician
- Optometrist

CHAPTER 7

Review

LESSON 7.1

The Eye

Key Points

- Exterior structures of the eye include the bony orbital socket and other protective structures, as well as several types of glands that produce secretions to lubricate and protect the eye. Internal structures include the sclera, cornea, pupil, lens, retina, and aqueous and vitreous humor.
- Accommodation is a change in the shape of the lens to allow for near and distant vision.
- Problems commonly associated with the eye include myopia, hyperopia, presbyopia, conjunctivitis, and glaucoma.

Key Terms

aqueous humor
choroid
ciliary body
ciliary glands
cones
conjunctiva
cornea
extrinsic muscles
iris
lacrimal glands
lens
optic chiasma
optic nerve
optic tracts
pupil
retina
rods
sclera
suspensory ligaments
tarsal glands
vitreous humor

LESSON 7.2

The Ear

Key Points

- The ear is divided into three parts—the external ear, middle ear, and internal ear.
- The two main functions of the ear are hearing and maintaining equilibrium.
- Disorders and infections of the ear include deafness, tinnitus, otitis externa, otitis media, and labyrinthitis.

Key Terms

auditory canal
auricle
bony labyrinth
ceruminous glands
cochlea
cochlear duct
endolymph
Eustachian tube
incus
malleus
membranous labyrinth
organ of Corti
ossicles
oval window
perilymph
semicircular canals
stapes
tympanic cavity
tympanic membrane
vestibule
vestibulocochlear nerve

LESSON 7.3

Smell and Taste

Key Points

- In the olfactory sense, or sense of smell, the olfactory receptor cells send impulses to the olfactory nerve, which then sends the stimuli to the olfactory cortex of the brain for interpretation.
- In the gustatory sense, or sense of taste, taste buds collect information and send it to the brain to be interpreted together with information from other senses, including the olfactory sense.

Key Terms

antihistamines
gustatory sense
histamines
limbic system
olfactory bulb
olfactory hairs
olfactory nerve
olfactory region
olfactory sense
papillae
septum
tastants
taste buds
taste pores

Assessment

➤ LESSON 7.1

The Eye

Learning Key Terms and Concepts

1. The _____ is a membrane that lines the eyelid.
2. The muscles responsible for moving the eye within its socket are the _____ muscles.
3. The white of the eye and the cornea make up the _____ of the eye.
4. The eyeball has three layers: the sclera, the choroid, and the _____.
5. The junction between the optic nerve and the eye is the location of the _____, or physiological blind spot on the retina.
6. *True or false?* The muscles of the ciliary body must contract to focus on items more than 20 feet away.
7. Maria wears contact lenses to see the whiteboard at her high school. She probably has an eye disorder called _____.
8. In the eye condition known as _____, malfunctioning extrinsic muscles cause the eyes to drift in different directions.
9. Overproduction of aqueous humor within the eye can result in a condition of high pressure known as _____.

Thinking Critically

10. Compare the anatomy and functions of the iris and the pupil.
11. What would happen if a person's lacrimal glands were clogged?
12. What would be the result of the vitreous humor leaking out of the eyeball?

➤ LESSON 7.2

The Ear

Learning Key Terms and Concepts

13. Another name for the pinna is _____.
14. Cerumen is produced by glands in the _____ canal of the ear.
15. Another name for the eardrum is the _____.
16. In the pathway of hearing, sound waves travel from the tympanic membrane through the _____ to the oval window.
17. The purpose of the _____ is to equalize pressure in the middle ear.
18. The organ of Corti is located in the _____ duct of the ear.
19. The _____ in the ear carries sound impulses to the brain.
20. Damage to the hair cells in the organ of Corti that causes them to move randomly can result in a condition called _____.
21. Chronic inflammation of the semicircular canals of the inner ear causes periodic but severe vertigo, as well as progressive hearing loss; this condition is classified as _____.

Instructions: Identify the letter in **Figure 7.27** that corresponds to the name of each part of the ear.

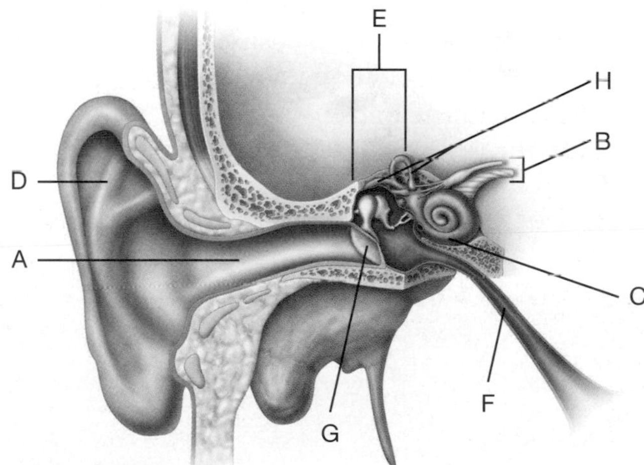

Figure 7.27 © Body Scientific International

22. Auditory canal _____
23. Middle ear _____
24. Semicircular canals _____
25. Auricle _____
26. Vestibulocochlear nerve _____
27. Tympanic membrane _____
28. Cochlea _____
29. Eustachian tube _____

Thinking Critically

30. Mrs. Omar took her baby to the pediatrician because the baby had cried throughout the night and kept holding the left side of his head. Mrs. Omar told the doctor that her baby had suffered a cold for about a week. After examining the baby's ear, the doctor reported that the baby had a bulging, red eardrum. The doctor thought the cause was a middle ear infection. What is the correct name for this condition, and what treatment do you think the doctor prescribed? Explain your reasoning.

› LESSON 7.3

Smell and Taste

Learning Key Terms and Concepts

31. The thickened end of the olfactory nerve, which sends impulses on to the brain, is the olfactory _____.
32. *True or false?* Humans have a better sense of smell than most animals.
33. The common cold is the most frequent cause of inflammation of the mucous membranes in the nasal passages, a condition known as _____.
34. A hole that develops in the nasal septum due to ulcer or long-term exposure to toxic fumes results in the condition known as _____ septum.
35. Where are taste buds *not* found?
    A. in the nose
    B. on the tongue
    C. on the lips
    D. on the roof of the mouth
36. A person has burned his tongue and has trouble tasting food. He has damaged the _____ on his tongue.
37. The flavors of beef and MSG make up the basic taste sensation known as _____.
38. Approximately 75% to 90% of taste is actually supplied by your sense of _____.
39. The gustatory sense comprises only five basic tastes: umami, sweet, bitter, sour, and _____.
40. Maintaining good oral hygiene is the best way to avoid _____ tongue disorder.

Thinking Critically

41. Describe at least three functions of your nose and sense of smell.
42. Explain why a particular smell might trigger a memory. Use the anatomy and physiology you learned in this lesson and previous lessons to support your hypothesis.
43. With a group of friends, taste various foods. Discuss and compare your sensitivity to the five basic tastes with your friends' sensitivity to these tastes. How would you describe your sense of taste compared with their sense of taste?
44. Humans can detect approximately 10,000 different smells. Using the internet, conduct research to discover the name of the general disease state that causes the partial or total loss of a person's sense of smell. Describe its impact on an individual's activity of daily living.

Building Skills and Connecting Concepts

Analyzing and Evaluating Data

Instructions: The chart in **Figure 7.28** shows the age ranges at which people begin to experience hearing loss. For each age range, percentages of the total population are given for both males and females. Use the chart to answer the following questions.

45. In which age range does the highest percentage of people (male and female combined) experience their first hearing loss?
46. Which group—male or female—tends to lose the ability to hear at an earlier age?
47. If you are a female, what are the approximate odds that you will retain your full hearing until you reach 65 years of age? if you are a male?
    A. 1 in 4
    B. 1 in 6
    C. 1 in 3
    D. 1 in 5

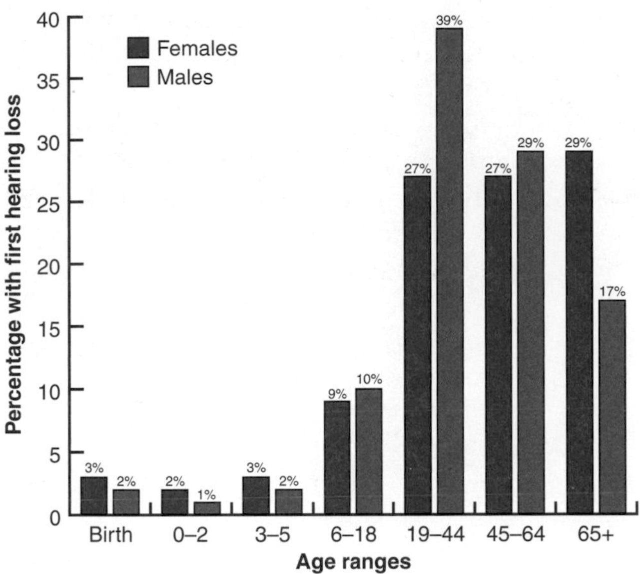

Figure 7.28

Communicating about Anatomy & Physiology

48. **Writing** Write a list of detailed instructions that you would give to a new mother regarding prevention and treatment of ear infections. After each instruction, explain why that particular instruction is important. In preparing your list, be sure to use the new vocabulary that you have learned in this chapter.
49. **Speaking and Listening** With two classmates, role-play a situation in which you are a physician's assistant counseling a young mother and father regarding ear infections. As a basic guide for your counseling, use the list that you developed for the writing activity in #43. Adjust your vocabulary as necessary while responding to their questions and clarifying information. Then switch roles.

Lab Investigations

50. Survey friends and family to identify as many cases as possible of eye and ear disorders. Document each person's disorder, gender, and age at the time of onset. As a class, compile your data and develop a summary chart or graph. What conclusions can you draw?
51. Create a flyer highlighting strategies for preventing blindness. Target the flyer to senior citizens' groups. What key points would you include? How would you design the flyer to attract the attention of your intended audience? Share your flyer and the reasons for your content and design decisions with the class.
52. Perform an experiment to investigate how the human senses distinguish potent smells.

    Note: Do not perform this activity if you have allergies to strong odors.

    Instructions: The instructor will set up four smelling stations around the classroom, one for each essential oil, labeling the stations only by number: 1, 2, 3, and 4. Use a data gathering form similar to the one shown in **Figure 7.29** to record your observations about each smell. After completing all of the stations, answer these questions: Were you able to correctly identify each essential oil? Which of the essential oils did you find appealing to your senses? Research the medicinal values of each of these essential oils and note their value on your data sheet.

Building Your Portfolio

53. Make digital copies of the reports you created and the research studies you performed as you worked through this chapter. Create a document or folder called "The Sensory Systems" and insert the documents. Add this document or folder to your personal portfolio.

Essential Oils				
Data Gathering Form				
Essential Oil #	**Your best guess of its identity**	**Potency on a scale of 1 to 10** *(10 = most potent)*	**Actual identity**	**Medicinal value, if any**
1				
2				
3				
4				

Figure 7.29

Goodheart-Willcox Publisher

CHAPTER

8 The Endocrine System

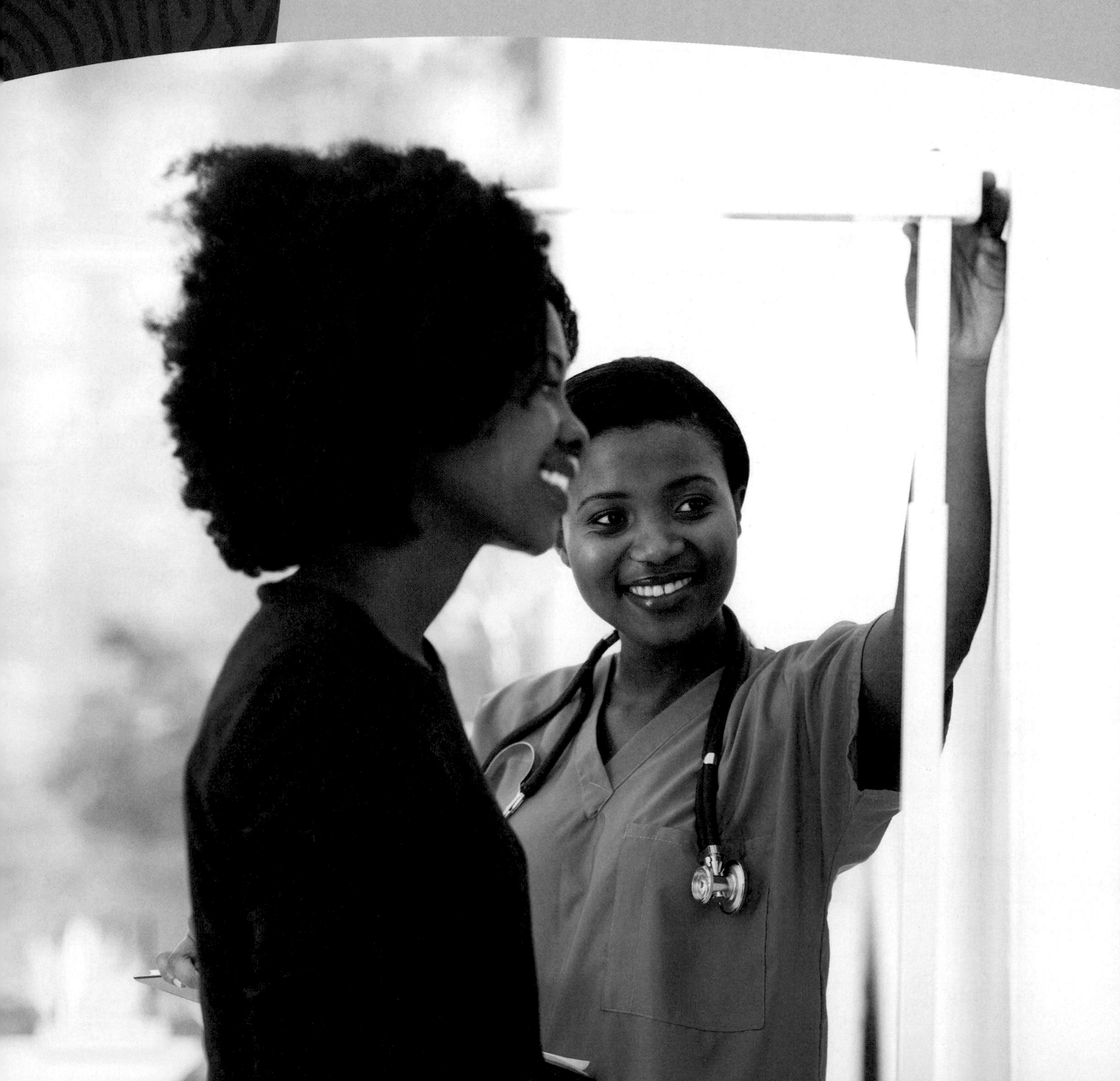

Would you want to become the tallest person on Earth?

In 2010, the *Guinness Book of World Records* named Sultan Kosen, a 29-year-old man from Turkey, the world's tallest man, measuring 8 feet, 3 inches. Kosen also achieved the records for the largest hands (28.5 centimeters, or 11.22 inches) and largest feet (36.5 centimeters, or 14.4 inches). His records still remain today. If you are a basketball player, you are probably thinking, "*Awesome!*"

A tumor caused Kosen's pituitary gland to secrete excessive amounts of growth hormone, resulting in gigantism, a condition in which a person grows to an exceptionally large size. The only way to treat this condition is to stop the excretion of growth hormone.

In 2010, doctors at the University of Virginia's Medical Center put Kosen on drugs to balance his hormone levels. Then they used a gamma knife, which emits focused beams of radiation, to target the tumor. The surgery was a success, and Sultan stopped growing.

Sultan's story highlights the overwhelming effects that the small but powerful endocrine glands and organs can have on the body. This chapter describes these glands and organs and some diseases and disorders that can occur when the endocrine system does not function properly.

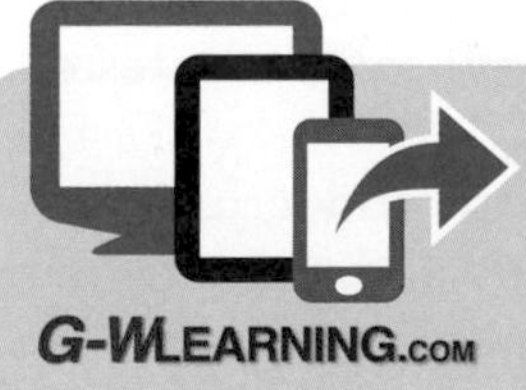

Click on the activity icon or visit www.g-wlearning.com/healthsciences/0202 to access online vocabulary activities using key terms from the chapter.

Chapter 8 Outline

◂ michaeljung/Shutterstock.com

LESSON 8.1

Functions and Control of the Endocrine System

Before You Read

Try to answer the following questions before you read this lesson.

- What roles do the nervous and endocrine systems play in the fight-or-flight response?
- What are hormones?

Lesson Objectives

- Explain how the endocrine and nervous systems work together to regulate bodily functions.
- Describe the functions of hormones, and explain how hormones move through the body.
- Explain how hormones help maintain homeostasis.

Key Terms

downregulated
epinephrine
hormonal control
hormones
humoral control
hypothalamic nonreleasing hormones
hypothalamic releasing hormones
insulin
neural control
non-steroid hormones
steroid hormones
upregulated

Like the nervous system, the endocrine system controls and monitors organs, glands, and processes in the body. The endocrine system does this job using hormones that first collect information and then stimulate organs, glands, and tissues.

The nervous and endocrine systems work together to regulate bodily functions, but they act in very different ways. The nervous system works quickly through electrical impulses, and its effects are short-lived. The endocrine system secretes hormones that are slower to act but whose effects are longer lasting.

It is likely that your body has initiated the fight-or-flight response at some point in your life. Perhaps you have encountered a dangerous situation, such as almost being hit by a car or being startled by something unexpected. The body jumps into action to move out of the way of a speeding vehicle or other impending dangers—that is the nervous system at work. After the danger has passed, a racing heartbeat, an increased respiratory rate, and a thin layer of sweat on your skin may persist for a time. This slower, longer-lasting response is the work of the endocrine system.

Anatomy of the Endocrine System

The endocrine system is a collection of organs and small glands that directly or indirectly influence all the functions of the body. Some of the endocrine glands, such as the hypothalamus (high-poh-THAL-a-mus), pituitary (pi-TOO-i-tair-ee), adrenal, and pineal (PI-nee-al) glands, are also part of the nervous system. This overlap allows the two systems to integrate their responses.

For instance, when the body temperature drops below normal, the sympathetic nervous system (SNS) springs into action by stimulating the secretion of hypothalamic releasing hormones from the hypothalamus. These hormones cause the pituitary gland to secrete hormones that ultimately trigger the thyroid gland to release hormones that increase metabolic rate and generate heat. This process is discussed later in this lesson.

Endocrine Glands

The endocrine system is made up of ductless glands called *endocrine glands*. Endocrine glands are glands of internal secretion; they secrete **hormones**, or chemical messengers, directly into the bloodstream. The endocrine glands include the hypothalamus, pancreas, pituitary gland, adrenal gland, thyroid gland, pineal gland, testes (male), and ovaries (female).

The organs and glands of the endocrine system are spread throughout the body and regulate many functions. **Figure 8.1** illustrates the location of the endocrine glands.

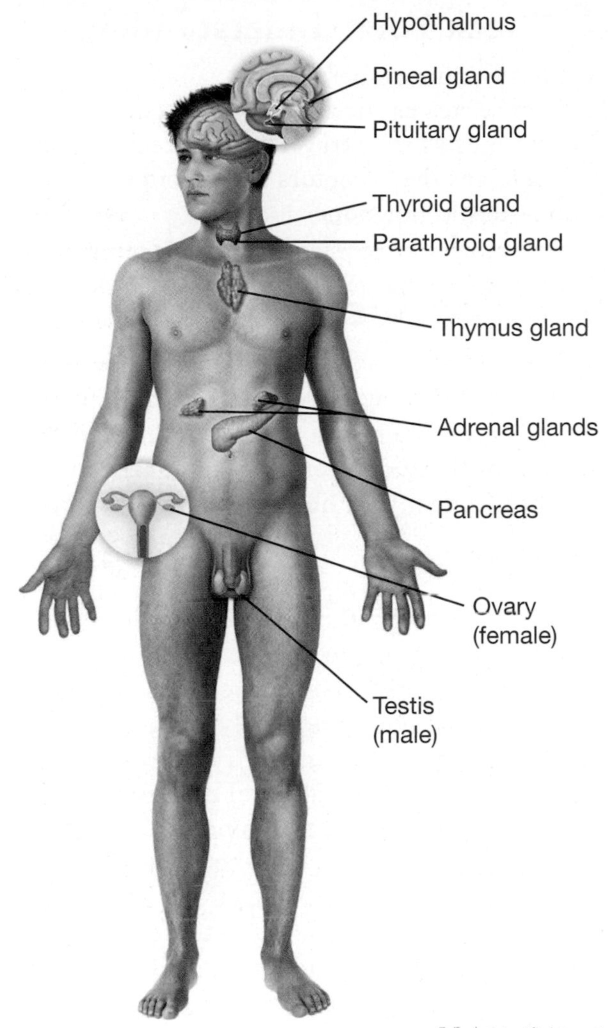

Figure 8.1 The glands and organs of the endocrine system are located throughout the body. *What substances are produced by the glands of the endocrine system?*

Exocrine Glands

Exocrine glands, which are glands of external secretion, are the counterpart to the endocrine glands. Unlike endocrine glands, which secrete hormones directly into the bloodstream, exocrine glands have a duct through which secretions are carried to the body's surface or to other organs. Examples of exocrine glands and their secretions include:

- sweat glands (sweat)
- salivary glands (saliva)
- mammary glands (breast milk)
- lacrimal glands (tears)
- pancreas glands (digestive enzymes)

The pancreas is unique because it functions as both an exocrine gland and an endocrine gland. The pancreas releases hormones that regulate blood glucose levels in the body. It also secretes digestive enzymes through a duct into the small intestine.

Check Your Understanding

1. Name three examples of endocrine glands.
2. What is the difference between an endocrine gland and an exocrine gland?

Hormones

The glands of the endocrine system secrete many different hormones into the bloodstream. As stated earlier, hormones are chemical messengers that influence the activities of other tissues and organs.

Have you ever wondered what stimulates your thirst and hunger? The hypothalamus gland is responsible. Do you feel energized, refreshed, and happier after getting a good night's sleep? You can thank the pineal gland for secreting melatonin, a hormone that induces sleep. Some days, you may be filled with energy; other days, you may feel sluggish and tired. Your thyroid gland secretes several hormones that affect your energy level.

Generally, hormones regulate carbohydrate, fat, and protein metabolism; water and electrolyte balance; reproductive activity; growth and development; and energy balance. Hormones also aid in the body's response to infection and stress. These are just a few of the ways that the endocrine system affects everyday functions, emotions, and behaviors.

The two basic categories of hormones are lipid (fat-based) hormones called **steroid hormones**, and **non-steroid hormones** composed of protein or peptides and amino acid-derived hormones. Hormones are transported throughout the body by the blood, which comes into contact with all the body's tissues and organs. However, hormones affect only the tissues and organs that have receptors specific to those particular hormones. As explained in Chapter 1, a receptor is a transmitter cell that senses and responds to certain stimuli. When a hormone binds with its receptor, the hormone can influence the activity of the cell. It does so by changing the cell membrane's permeability, increasing or decreasing enzyme activity, increasing protein synthesis, or stimulating secretory activity.

Location of Hormone Receptors

The receptors for steroid hormones are found inside the cell nucleus. By contrast, the receptors for the non-steroid hormones are found on the membrane, or surface, of the cell. When a non-steroid hormone binds with the cell surface receptor, it stimulates a second messenger. This second messenger works inside the cell to produce a cascade of responses. There are many secondary messengers, and they vary from cell to cell.

When a steroid hormone binds to the receptor inside a cell nucleus, the interaction between the hormone and receptor alters the cell's DNA and activates mRNA (messenger RNA). mRNA then travels to the cytoplasm and stimulates protein synthesis.

Some hormones, such as **epinephrine** (eh-pi-NEH-frin), have receptors at many different sites, making their effects widespread. Other hormones have fewer target sites, limiting their effects.

Upregulating and Downregulating Hormone Receptors

The activity of hormone receptors can be **upregulated** (increased) or **downregulated** (decreased), making them more or less sensitive to the hormone. Exercise, for example, upregulates insulin receptors, making them more sensitive to **insulin** (a hormone that promotes the uptake of glucose in body tissues). Because exercise upregulates insulin receptors, less insulin is needed to promote glucose uptake in people who are physically active. However, obesity downregulates insulin receptors, so more insulin must be present to promote glucose uptake by cells. These two glucose-uptake scenarios have important implications for diabetics, particularly those who are overweight.

Check Your Understanding

1. What is a hormone?
2. What serves as the transport system for hormones as they travel to their receptor sites?
3. Where are the receptors for steroid and non-steroid hormones located?

Hormone Secretion Control

Now that you know what a hormone is and does, you can discover what prompts a gland to secrete or inhibit a hormone. Endocrine glands are regulated in three different ways: neural control, hormonal control, and humoral control.

Neural Control

In **neural control**, nerve fibers stimulate the endocrine organs to release hormones. Recall that the fight-or-flight response helps people act quickly in potentially dangerous situations. During the fight-or-flight response, the SNS stimulates the adrenal medulla to release epinephrine and norepinephrine, hormones that prime the body to fight or flee from a stressful situation. The effects of these hormones include increased heart rate, blood pressure, respiration, and blood flow to muscles; decreased blood flow to organs; and dilation of the pupils.

The fight-or-flight response is just one example of neural control. Other situations in which the nervous system acts on the hypothalamus include influencing hormone release in other organs and glands of the endocrine system.

Hormonal Control

Hormonal control of the endocrine glands and organs is achieved by a hierarchy, or chain of command, of the endocrine organs. In hormonal control, endocrine organs are stimulated by hormones from other endocrine organs, starting with the hypothalamus. This chain reaction requires a response from the targeted tissue or organ.

Hormonal control can be likened to the hierarchy of a business. Think of the hypothalamus as the president of the company, the pituitary as the vice president, and the other endocrine glands as managers (**Figure 8.2**).

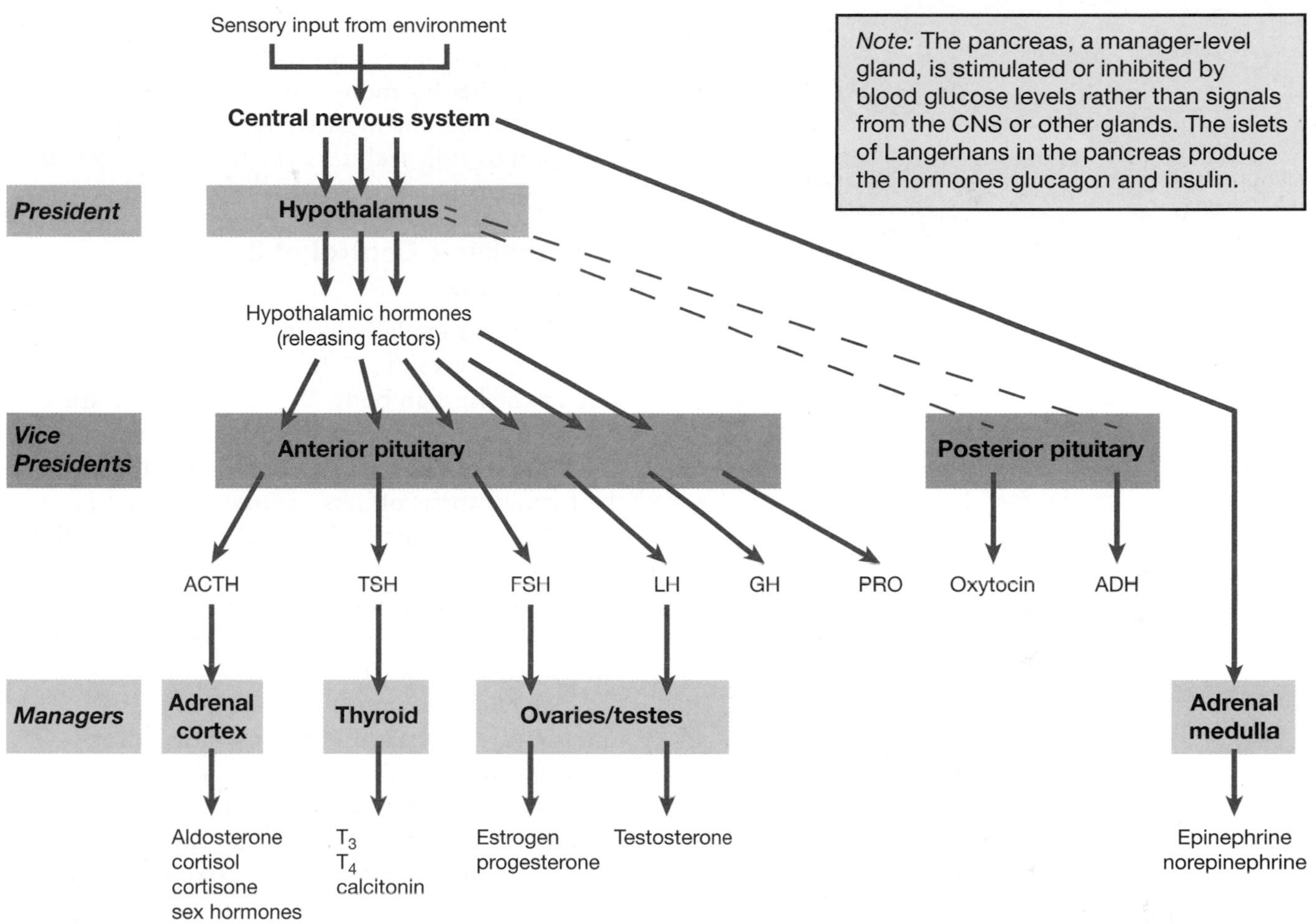

Figure 8.2 Hierarchy of the endocrine system. Each gland in the hierarchy controls the activities of the gland or glands below it. Each gland is controlled by the gland or glands above it. *Why is it appropriate to compare the relationship between endocrine glands to the hierarchy of a business?*

As "president" of the endocrine system, the hypothalamus directs the activities of the pituitary gland (the "vice president"). The hypothalamus does this through the secretion of **hypothalamic releasing hormones**—such as growth hormone releasing hormone (GHRH), thyrotropin releasing hormone, and corticotropic releasing hormone—and **hypothalamic nonreleasing hormones**. The pituitary gland then releases its many hormones to direct the "managers."

When the hormone levels of the "managers" rise in the bloodstream, they have an end goal, such as stimulating target tissues. After the goal has been achieved, the pituitary and hypothalamus receive signals from the "manager" hormones that inhibit, or turn off, the pituitary and hypothalamic hormones, thus ending the chain of hormonal control. Does this process sound familiar? If so, that is because it is a negative feedback loop, a concept discussed in Chapter 1. An example of a negative feedback loop for the endocrine system is shown in **Figure 8.3**.

Humoral Control

Humoral control of the endocrine system is achieved by monitoring the levels of various substances in body fluids, such as the blood. If a homeostatic imbalance is detected, corrective actions are undertaken to help the body regain homeostasis.

For example, when blood glucose levels rise, the pancreas secretes insulin, stimulating the absorption of glucose into body tissues. Greater absorption of glucose into body tissues lowers blood glucose levels. By contrast, when blood glucose levels drop, the pancreas secretes the hormone glucagon (GLOO-kuh-gahn).

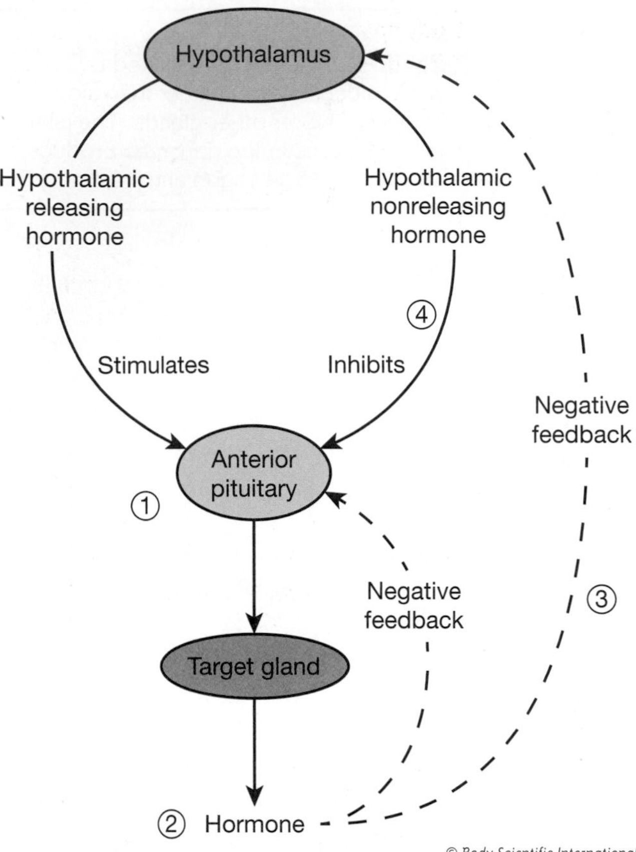

Figure 8.3 Negative feedback loop. 1—The hypothalamus and the pituitary gland direct the target gland to release hormones. 2—The target gland releases hormones to achieve a goal, such as the stimulation of target tissues. 3—After the goal is achieved, the target gland sends signals to the hypothalamus and the pituitary gland. 4—The hypothalamus inhibits the production of additional hypothalamic and anterior pituitary hormones. *What stimulates the hypothalamus to release its hormones?*

Glucagon causes the breakdown of glycogen stored in the liver. The glycogen then enters the bloodstream and increases blood glucose levels.

Hormones and Homeostasis

The body is constantly monitoring all of its systems to ensure that everything is working normally. This functional balance is called *homeostasis*. If the function of any one of the organ systems deviates from the normal range, triggering homeostatic imbalance, the body takes corrective measures to restore homeostasis. Neural, hormonal, or humoral controls trigger the release of hormones during homeostatic imbalance. Increased hormone levels affect the target sites, thereby restoring homeostasis. Homeostatic balance and rising hormone levels inhibit further hormone secretions via a negative feedback loop. The negative feedback loop causes the gland to stop secreting the hormone after the body returns to homeostasis.

Hypothalamic Control of Body Temperature

Chapter 1 explained that the thermostat in a home functions much like the negative feedback loop in the human body. When the temperature falls below the set point, the furnace turns on. When the home reaches the desired temperature, the furnace turns off. As **Figure 8.4** shows, the hypothalamus—the "president" of the endocrine system—functions as a thermostat for the body. The hypothalamus works to maintain the homeostatic set point of the body by keeping its temperature at 98.6°F (37°C).

The hypothalamus monitors body temperature. If your body temperature drops below 98.6°F (37°C), the hypothalamus sets in motion a series of responses. The hypothalamus releases hormones that act on the thyroid gland. The thyroid gland produces thyroxine, a hormone that increases metabolic rate and heat production. The hypothalamus also stimulates the SNS, which initiates shivering and decreases blood flow to the skin. Shivering increases heat production and helps the body maintain core temperature. Once the body temperature has been restored to its hypothalamic set point (homeostasis), the hypothalamus signals the thyroid gland to stop releasing thyroxine. The hypothalamus also signals the SNS to send messages to the body that cause shivering to cease and blood flow to be restored to the skin.

When the body's thermal receptors sense an increase in body temperature above 98.6°F (37°C), the hypothalamus stimulates the SNS. The SNS increases sweat production by stimulating the sweat glands and widening the blood vessels of the skin, increasing blood flow to the area. In addition, the thyroid gland decreases thyroid hormone secretion.

Example: The Endocrine System at Work

When Jordan Romero decided that he wanted to become the youngest person to climb Mount Everest at 13 years of age, he and his dad embarked on a training program to get Romero's

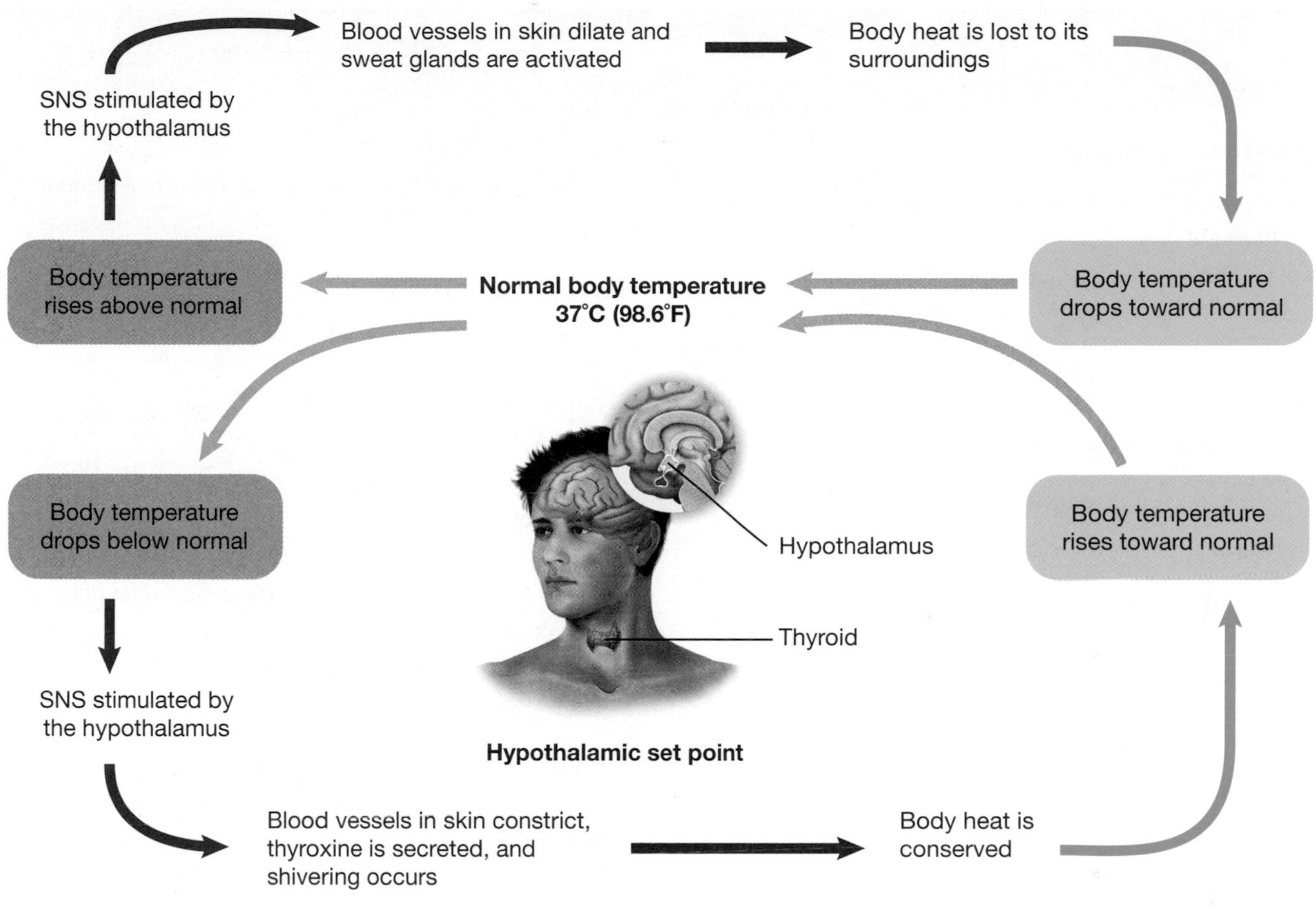

Figure 8.4 The hypothalamus serves as the body's thermostat. *The regulation of body temperature is an example of how the body maintains functional balance. What is this functional balance called?*

body into shape. The 29,029-foot (8,848-meter) climb would challenge Romero's body, particularly because lower oxygen concentration in the air at high altitudes diminishes blood oxygen levels.

While at sea level, Romero spent many hours in an altitude tent, where he was exposed to a hypoxic environment (one with low oxygen content). The hypoxic environment of the altitude tent simulated the environment near the peak of Mount Everest. The low oxygen content of the air that Romero was breathing stimulated his kidneys to secrete the hormone erythropoietin (eh-rith-roh-POY-eh-ten). Erythropoietin stimulates bone marrow stem-cell production of red blood cells (RBCs).

The increased production of RBCs in Romero's blood increased the ability of his blood to carry oxygen. As a result, the effects of the hypoxic environment near the peak of Mount Everest were not as fatiguing and harmful to Romero. Thanks to this hormonal response, Romero achieved his goal of becoming the youngest person to climb Mount Everest.

Check Your Understanding

1. What are the three ways in which hormone secretions are controlled in the endocrine glands?
2. Which two endocrine glands exercise the most control over the others?
3. Which part of the brain maintains the homeostatic set point at 98.6°F (37°C)?
4. How does the secretion of thyroxine by the thyroid gland keep the internal body temperature from falling?

LESSON 8.1 Review and Assessment

Mini Glossary

Make sure that you know the meaning of each key term.

downregulated decreased

epinephrine the chief neurohormone of the adrenal medulla that is used as a heart stimulant, a vasoconstrictor (which narrows the blood vessels), and a bronchodilator (which relaxes the bronchial tubes in the lungs)

hormonal control type of endocrine control in which endocrine organs are stimulated by hormones from other endocrine organs, starting with the hypothalamus

hormones chemical messengers secreted by the endocrine glands

humoral control type of endocrine control in which levels of various substances in body fluids are monitored for homeostatic imbalance

hypothalamic nonreleasing hormones hormones produced in the hypothalamus and carried by a vein to the anterior pituitary, where they stop certain hormones from being released; hypothalamic inhibiting hormones

hypothalamic releasing hormones hormones produced in the hypothalamus and carried by a vein to the anterior pituitary, where they stimulate the release of hormones from the anterior pituitary

insulin a hormone that promotes glucose uptake in body tissues

neural control type of endocrine control in which nerve fibers stimulate the endocrine organs to release hormones

non-steroid hormones hormones composed of protein, or peptide hormones and amino acid-derived hormones

steroid hormones lipid (fat-based) hormones

upregulated increased

Know and Understand

1. What is the purpose of the endocrine system?
2. Which endocrine glands are also part of the nervous system?
3. Which gland has both endocrine and exocrine functions?
4. What are the two basic categories of hormones?
5. Which gland is "president" of the endocrine system? Which is "vice president?"

Analyze and Apply

6. Identify similarities and differences between the nervous and endocrine systems.
7. Describe how the activity of a hormone receptor can be upregulated or downregulated.
8. Explain the role of neural control in a fight-or-flight response.
9. Homeostasis is an equilibrium, or balance, system. List three examples of events that would interrupt this balance.
10. Obesity downregulates insulin receptors to promote glucose uptake by cells. This is a problem for people with diabetes. What other hormones are affected by obesity?

IN THE LAB

11. Following a December snowstorm in Wisconsin, Mark's parents ask him to help shovel the sidewalk in front of their home. After spending some time outside in the cold, Mark begins to shiver. In what other ways is Mark's body responding as his endocrine system works to raise his body temperature?
12. Working with a partner or in a small group, choose one of the following triggers: hunger, thirst, cold temperature, hot temperature, exhaustion, fear. Research how the endocrine system responds to the trigger. Prepare an electronic presentation and share your research with the rest of the class.
13. Generally, hormones regulate the body's electrolyte balance; energy drinks claim to do the same. Select two popular energy drinks and compare them to each other. With what you know about hormones, do you believe these products do what the commercials claim they do? Would you recommend these drinks? Write a short report detailing your investigation, results, and conclusions.

LESSON 8.2

Major Endocrine Organs

Before You Read

Try to answer the following questions before you read this lesson.

- Which hormone makes you sleepy at night?
- Which biological processes are associated with an "adrenaline rush"?

Lesson Objectives

- Identify the functions of the hypothalamus.
- Identify the hormones secreted by the anterior and posterior pituitary gland.
- Describe the location and function of the thyroid gland.
- Explain the function of the parathyroid glands.
- Describe the location and function of the adrenal glands.
- Explain the endocrine and exocrine functions of the pancreas.
- List other hormone-producing organs and tissues.

Key Terms

adrenal cortex
adrenal medulla
adrenocorticotropin (ACTH)
aldosterone
androgens
antidiuretic hormone
calcitonin
catecholamines
cortisol
cortisone
estrogens
follicle-stimulating hormone (FSH)
glucagon
growth hormone (GH)
luteinizing hormone (LH)
melatonin
oxytocin
parathyroid hormone (PTH)
prolactin
thymosin
thyroid-stimulating hormone (TSH)
thyroxine (T_4)
triiodothyronine (T_3)
tropic hormones

As explained in Lesson 8.1, the endocrine system is run by the hypothalamus. The hormones of this tiny gland stimulate the pituitary gland, starting a chain reaction that affects organs and hormones throughout the endocrine system. Each organ plays an important role in ensuring that the endocrine system runs smoothly.

Hypothalamus

The hypothalamus is a very small gland (about 4 grams) buried deep in the brain below the thalamus. The job of the hypothalamus is to collect information from each body system and integrate the responses of the nervous and endocrine systems to maintain homeostatic balance. As explained in Chapter 6, the hypothalamus plays an important role in regulating everyday functions such as metabolism, heart rate, energy level, body temperature, thirst, nutrient intake, blood pressure, and blood composition. It even plays a role in emotions and, to some degree, regulates sleep.

Although the hypothalamus is part of the nervous system, it is also a key part of the endocrine system because it produces hypothalamic releasing hormones and hypothalamic nonreleasing hormones. These hormones stimulate or inhibit the release of hormones from the pituitary gland.

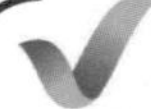

Check Your Understanding

1. Describe the role of the hypothalamus in the endocrine system.
2. List five body functions that are regulated in part by the hypothalamus.

Pituitary Gland

The pea-sized pituitary gland is located in the hypophyseal fossa in the sella turcica of the cranium. It has two lobes: the anterior pituitary (*adenohypophysis*) and the posterior pituitary (*neurohypophysis*). It is located in the depression of the sphenoid bone and is suspended from the underside of the hypothalamus by a short stalk called the *infundibulum* (in-fun-DI-byoo-lum).

Hormones secreted by the pituitary gland function in two ways. They can act directly on target tissue to cause a specific metabolic response, or they can stimulate other endocrine glands (the "manager-level" glands discussed in Lesson 8.1) to release their own hormones (**Figure 8.5**). Pituitary hormones that stimulate other endocrine glands are called **tropic hormones**, or *tropins*.

MEMORY TIP

ACTH, TSH, FSH, and LH are called *tropic* hormones because they are produced by *gonadotropes*, cells in the anterior pituitary. Tropic hormones act on other endocrine glands, *not* body tissue.

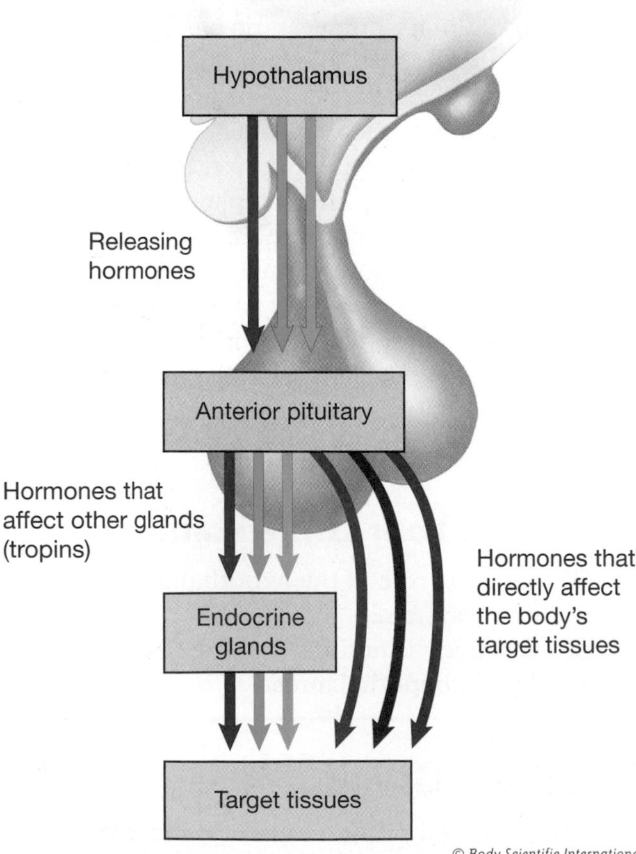

Figure 8.5 Some anterior pituitary hormones act on other glands, and others act directly on the body's tissues. *Which hormones of the anterior pituitary act on other glands? Which hormones act directly on tissues?*

Hormones of the Anterior Pituitary

The anterior pituitary gland secretes six different hormones:

- growth hormone (GH)
- prolactin (PRO)
- adrenocorticotropin (a-dree-noh-kor-ti-koh-TROH-pin) hormone (ACTH)
- thyroid-stimulating hormone (also called *thyrotropin* or TSH)
- follicle-stimulating hormone (FSH)
- luteinizing (LOO-tin-ighz-ing) hormone (LH)

MEMORY TIP

To remember the six hormones secreted by the anterior pituitary gland, try to remember the saying, "**Pro** **A**mateur **G**olfers **T**ake **L**ong **F**lops," with each word representing one of the six hormones:

Pro = prolactin
Amateur = adrenocorticotropic hormone
Golfers = growth hormone
Take = thyroid-stimulating hormone
Long = luteinizing hormone
Flops = follicle-stimulating hormone

Follicle-stimulating hormone and luteinizing hormone are further categorized as gonadotropic (goh-nad-ah-TROP-ik) hormones. **Figure 8.6** shows the hormones produced by the anterior pituitary and their target glands or tissues.

Of the six hormones secreted by the anterior pituitary, four of these are tropic hormones:

- **Adrenocorticotropin (ACTH)** acts on the adrenal cortex to stimulate release of steroid hormones.
- **Thyroid-stimulating hormone (TSH)** acts on the thyroid gland to stimulate release of two thyroid hormones, thyroxine (T_4) (thy-ROK-seen) and triiodothyronine (T_3) (trigh-igh-oh-doh-THIGH-roh-neen).
- **Follicle-stimulating hormone (FSH)** stimulates production of estrogen and eggs in women and production of sperm in men.
- **Luteinizing hormone (LH)** acts on the ovaries to produce progesterone and estrogen in women. It also signals the release of eggs in women. In men, LH stimulates the interstitial cells of the testes to produce testosterone.

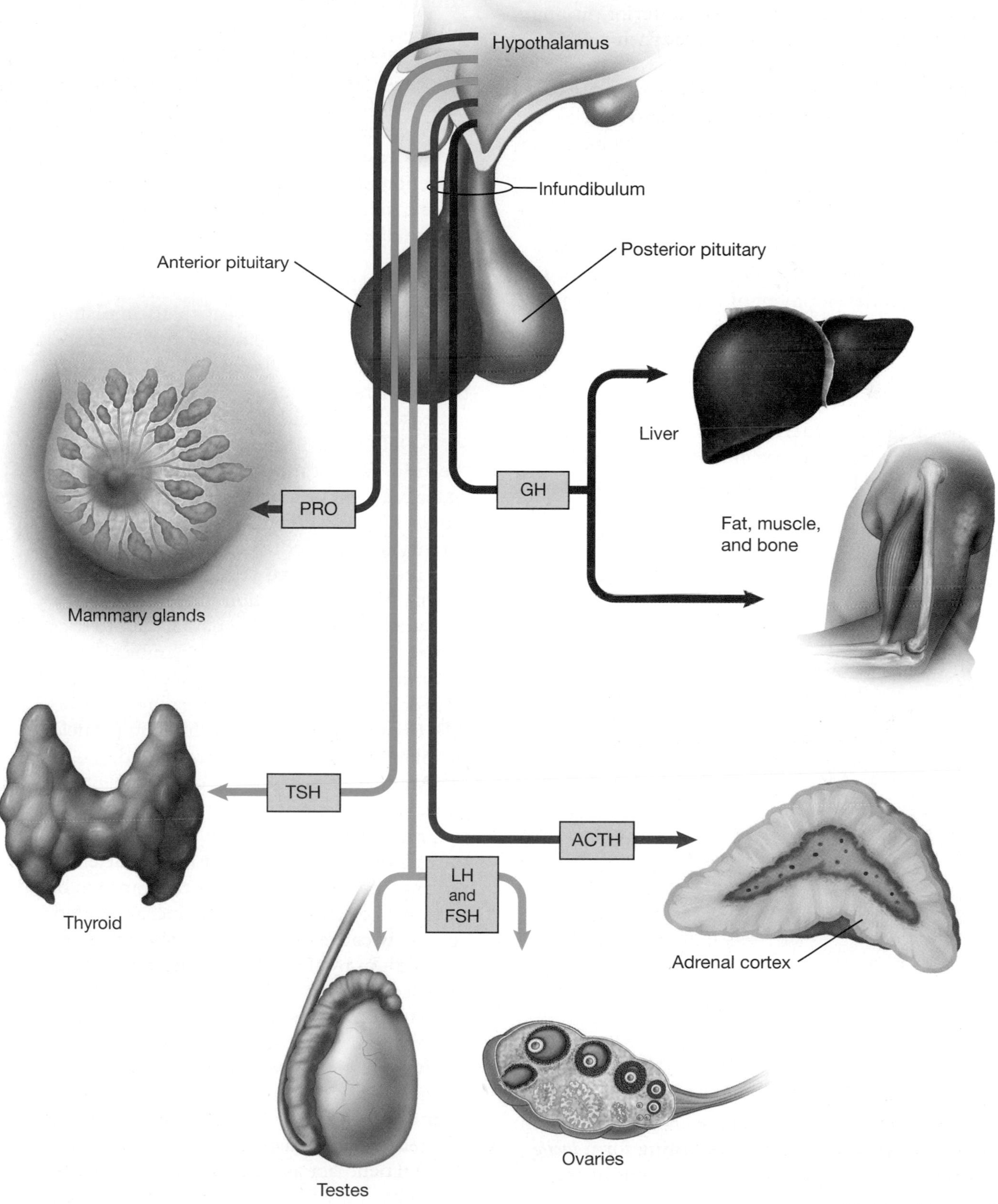

© Body Scientific International

Figure 8.6 Hormones secreted by the anterior pituitary affect many parts of the body. *Of the six hormones shown, which two are not tropic?*

Besides producing these four tropic hormones, the anterior pituitary also stores and releases hormones from the hypothalamus. These hormones are kept in the anterior pituitary until the hypothalamus stimulates their release.

Growth Hormone

Unlike the tropic hormones, **growth hormone (GH)** is an anterior pituitary hormone that acts directly on body tissues. Recall Sultan Kosen, the world's tallest man, from the chapter introduction. Kosen's record-breaking height, hands, and feet are the result of excessive amounts of growth hormone (GH). GH is responsible for the growth and development of the muscles, cartilage, and long bones of the body.

GH also helps break down fats for use as a fuel source by the body. GH is released about 30 to 45 minutes after a person starts to exercise. By using fats as a fuel source, the body can spare the carbohydrates whose glucose is needed for energy by the brain. About 80 minutes into an exercise session, GH stimulates the liver to convert fats (in the form of glycerol) and proteins (in the form of amino acids) into glucose. This process is called *gluconeogenesis* (gloo-koh-nee-oh-JEH-neh-sis). By using fats and proteins as a fuel source, growth hormone plays an important role in a person's ability to maintain prolonged physical activity, such as running a marathon.

MEMORY TIP

Gluconeogenesis, the process by which the liver converts fat and amino acids into glucose, can be easily remembered by examining the combining forms that make up this word. *Gluc/o* refers to "glucose"; *-neo-* means "new"; and *-genesis* means "creation." Put the parts together, and you have the definition of *gluconeogenesis*!

Prolactin

Prolactin stimulates the growth of mammary glands and milk production in a nursing mother. This hormone is named for its function: the prefix *pro-* means "for," and the combining form *lact/o* means "milk." Prolactin is also present in the male body, but its role in males is unclear.

Hormones of the Posterior Pituitary

The posterior pituitary is actually an extension of the hypothalamus. The posterior pituitary does not produce hormones. Rather, it *stores* two hormones—antidiuretic (an-tigh-digh-yoo-REH-tik) hormone (ADH) and oxytocin (ahk-see-TOH-sin)—produced by the hypothalamus.

Because it does not produce its own hormones, the posterior pituitary is not a true endocrine gland. Secretion of hormones from the posterior pituitary is the result of nervous system stimulation of the hypothalamus (**Figure 8.7**).

Antidiuretic Hormone

Diuretics are substances that stimulate urine production to decrease fluid retention in the body. **Antidiuretic hormone (ADH)** does the opposite—it decreases urine output, which increases body fluid volume.

ADH travels in the blood to its target organ, the kidneys. It stimulates the kidneys to increase water reabsorption and return the fluid to the blood. People who engage in regular physical activity have an increased sensitivity to ADH. As a result, they have a higher volume of blood plasma (the liquid portion of blood).

What stimulates the hypothalamus to trigger the release of ADH? ADH, which is subject to humoral control, is secreted when plasma volume decreases from dehydration or profuse sweating during exercise. ADH is also secreted when the solid particles in the blood become more concentrated.

Another important role of ADH is blood pressure regulation. Blood pressure is the tension that blood places on the walls of arteries. ADH raises blood pressure by causing the arteries to narrow, thus increasing their resistance to blood flow. At the same time, ADH increases blood volume because of increased reabsorption of fluid and sodium by the kidneys. The combination of increased blood volume and narrowed arteries leads to higher blood pressure because more blood is flowing through the smaller vessels.

Alcohol inhibits ADH, which leads to increased urination, dehydration, and a dry mouth the morning after a person drinks alcoholic beverages. Caffeine and foods such as asparagus have a similar effect on ADH and act as diuretics.

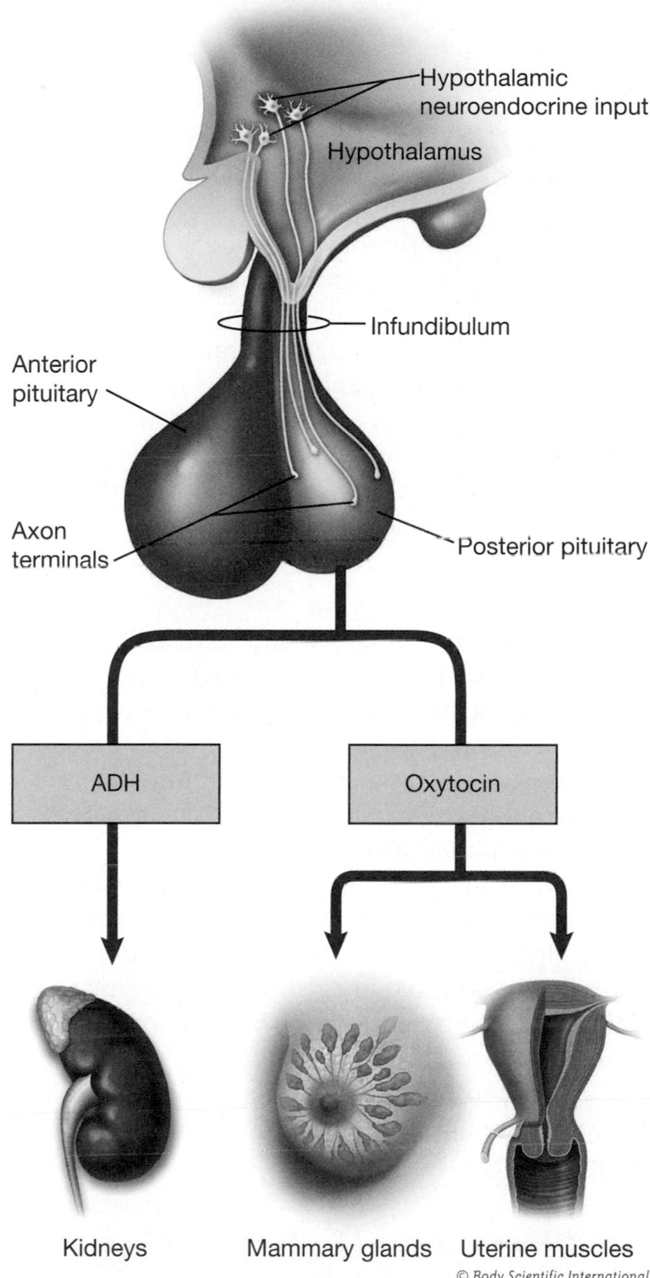

Figure 8.7 The posterior pituitary stores ADH and oxytocin secreted by the hypothalamus. These hormones help maintain the body's fluid balance. In addition, they stimulate uterine contractions in pregnant women and milk production in nursing women.

Oxytocin

Pregnant women produce oxytocin during labor, and the hormone stays in their bodies until they are finished nursing their child. **Oxytocin** facilitates childbirth by stimulating the muscles of the uterus to contract. Oxytocin release is also stimulated by the sucking mechanism of a nursing infant, causing the mammary glands to secrete breast milk from the mammary ducts.

Perhaps you have heard of a pitocin (pi-TOH-sin) drip. A pitocin drip is a synthetic, intravenous form of oxytocin that is administered to induce, or speed up, delivery of a baby.

Check Your Understanding

1. How are the hormones secreted by the pituitary gland classified in relation to their targets?
2. What does FSH stand for, and what is the purpose of this hormone?
3. Which parts of the body does growth hormone help to grow and develop? Name an additional function of GH.
4. Which two hormones does the posterior pituitary store?

Thyroid Gland

The thyroid gland is located inferior to the larynx, or Adam's apple, at the base of the throat. This butterfly-shaped gland is two inches long and lies at the front and sides of the trachea (**Figure 8.8A**). The two lobes of the thyroid gland are divided by a center band of tissue, called the *isthmus* (IS-mus).

The thyroid gland secretes three hormones: two "thyroid hormones" and calcitonin (kal-si-TOH-nin). These hormones drive the body's metabolism. People often blame an underactive thyroid gland for their overweight condition, but the thyroid gland is rarely the reason people become overweight or obese.

T_3 and T_4

The two thyroid hormones are **thyroxine (T_4)** and **triiodothyronine (T_3)**. Both of these hormones are responsible for controlling the rate of energy metabolism and heat production in the body. The follicular cells of the thyroid secrete T_4 and T_3. These hormones are formed from two linked tyrosine (TIGH-roh-seen) amino acids with iodine atoms attached to the amino acids. T_4 has four iodine atoms, and T_3 has three iodine atoms. T_3 is the more powerful of the two hormones

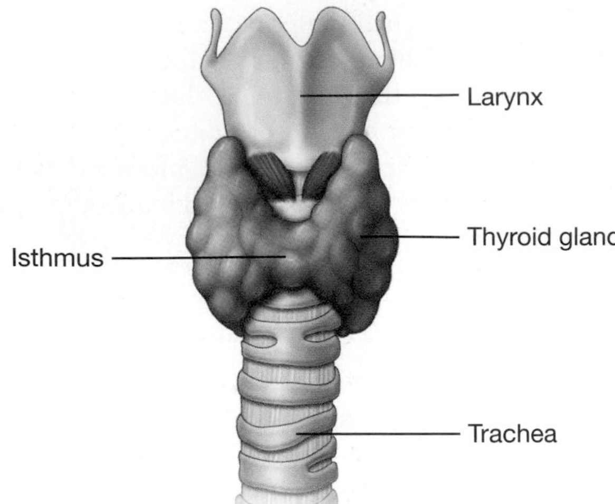

A Location of the thyroid gland

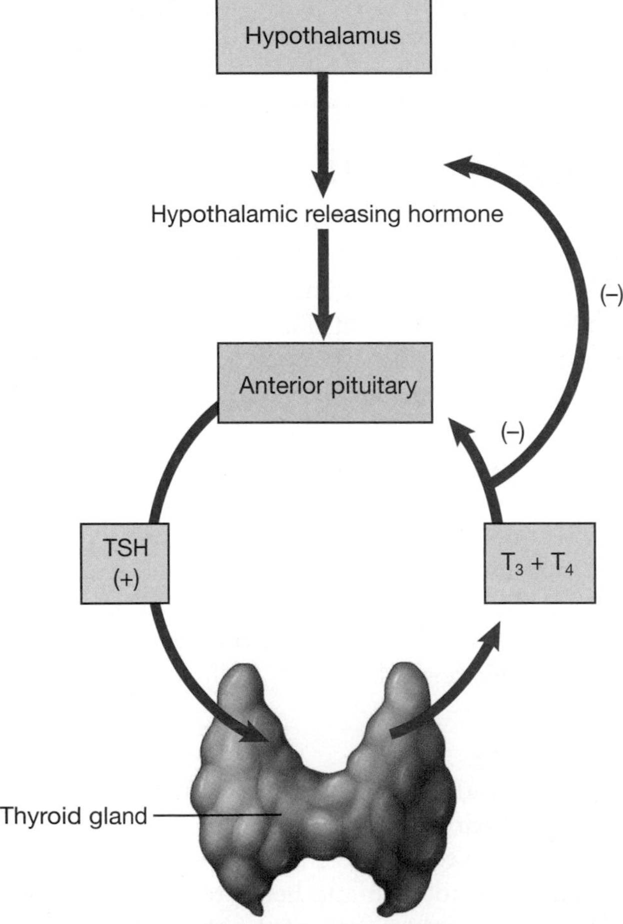

B Regulation of thyroid hormone release

© Body Scientific International

Figure 8.8 The thyroid gland. A—The thyroid gland is located below the larynx and above the trachea. B—The thyroid gland produces the thyroid hormones T_3 and T_4 when signaled by the hypothalamus and anterior pituitary. *Which hormones provide negative feedback to the anterior pituitary and hypothalamus?*

Every cell in the body is affected by T_4 and T_3 because every living cell needs energy to survive. Thyroid hormone also plays a vital role in growth, development, and maturation. The iodine required to make T_4 and T_3 comes from dietary intake, which is why salt is fortified with iodine in many countries. Lesson 8.3 discusses the implications of an iodine deficiency.

The release of thyroid hormone is controlled by the hypothalamus (**Figure 8.8B**). Hypothalamic releasing hormones signal the anterior pituitary to release thyroid-stimulating hormone (TSH). TSH triggers secretion of T_3 and T_4 by the thyroid gland. The increased levels of circulating T_3 and T_4 trigger a negative feedback loop, inhibiting further release of hormones from the hypothalamus (hypothalamic releasing hormone) and pituitary glands.

Calcitonin

Calcitonin is produced and released by the parafollicular cells of the thyroid gland. The parafollicular cells are located between the follicular cells in the connective tissue of the thyroid. Calcium homeostasis is maintained by calcitonin and parathyroid hormone (PTH), which is produced by the parathyroid glands.

When blood calcium levels rise, the thyroid gland releases calcitonin. Calcitonin causes calcium in the blood to be deposited and absorbed into the bone. As a result, blood calcium levels decrease. Calcitonin also reduces the absorption of calcium by the intestines and kidneys.

Once people reach adulthood and their bones are fully developed, very little (if any) calcitonin is released by the thyroid gland.

Check Your Understanding

1. Which three hormones are secreted by the thyroid gland?
2. Which chemical element found in certain foods is necessary for thyroid hormone production?
3. What is the primary function of calcitonin?

Parathyroid Glands

The parathyroid glands are two pairs of glands located on the posterior aspect of the thyroid gland. These four tiny glands (each is the size of a grain of rice) secrete **parathyroid hormone (PTH)** in response to low blood calcium levels. Parathyroid hormone increases blood calcium levels in three ways:

- by stimulating breakdown of bone tissues by osteoclasts, thus moving calcium from the bone into the blood
- by increasing calcium absorption in the intestines with the aid of vitamin D during digestion
- by stimulating kidney resorption of calcium from urine and excreting phosphorus

Figure 8.9 illustrates the regulation of blood calcium levels by both PTH and calcitonin.

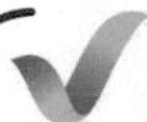

Check Your Understanding

1. Where are the parathyroid glands located?
2. How does parathyroid hormone increase blood calcium levels?

Adrenal Glands

As **Figure 8.10** shows, the adrenal glands are a pair of glands that sit on top of the kidneys. The adrenal glands are actually two organs: the **adrenal cortex** functions as a gland, whereas the **adrenal medulla** is part of the nervous system.

The adrenal cortex makes up the outer layer of each adrenal gland. It comprises three layers that secrete three steroid hormones. The adrenal medulla, which lies beneath the innermost layer of the adrenal cortex, is stimulated by the sympathetic branch of the autonomic nervous system (ANS).

Hormones of the Adrenal Medulla

Lesson 8.1 discussed the fight-or-flight response. This response occurs when the adrenal medulla secretes two hormones—epinephrine (commonly referred to as *adrenaline*) and norepinephrine

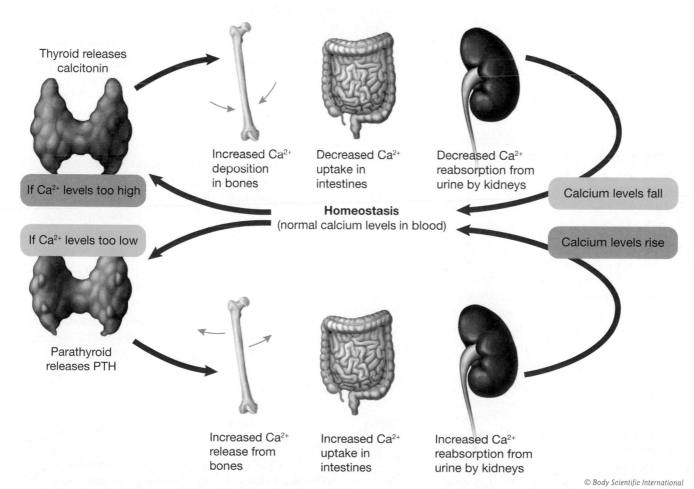

Thyroid releases calcitonin

Increased Ca^{2+} deposition in bones

Decreased Ca^{2+} uptake in intestines

Decreased Ca^{2+} reabsorption from urine by kidneys

If Ca^{2+} levels too high

Calcium levels fall

Homeostasis
(normal calcium levels in blood)

If Ca^{2+} levels too low

Calcium levels rise

Parathyroid releases PTH

Increased Ca^{2+} release from bones

Increased Ca^{2+} uptake in intestines

Increased Ca^{2+} reabsorption from urine by kidneys

Figure 8.9 The thyroid and parathyroid glands act together to maintain healthy blood calcium levels. *Which hormone is responsible for maintaining homeostatic blood calcium levels?*

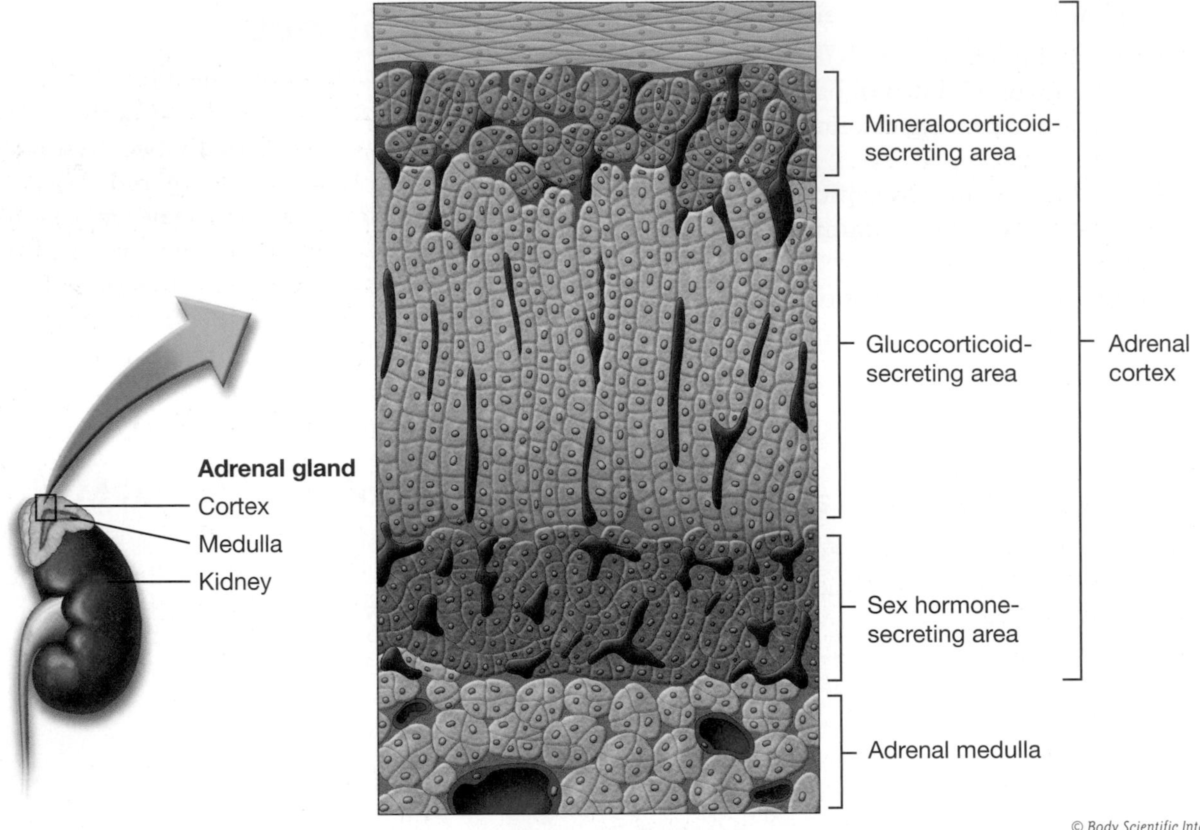

Figure 8.10 The adrenal glands are located on top of each kidney. The adrenal cortex (outer layer) is divided into three layers. The inner layer is the adrenal medulla. *Hormones released by the adrenal medulla are integral in initiating an "adrenaline rush." What is another name for this response?*

(also known as *noradrenalin*). Epinephrine and norepinephrine are both **catecholamines** (kat-eh-KOH-la-meens), hormones released into the blood during times of physical or emotional stress.

The body's response to increased catecholamine levels is called an "adrenaline rush." The telltale signs of an adrenaline rush include increased heart rate, blood pressure, and breathing. In addition, changes that you cannot feel are occurring within the body. For example, blood flow is shunted to the heart, and your muscles prepare you to fight or take flight. Increases in metabolic rate and glucose production by the liver make more energy available for the potential brush with danger.

MEMORY TIP

To remember the hormones secreted by the adrenal medulla, just remember the acronym **AMEN**: **A**drenal **M**edulla secretes **E**pinephrine and **N**orepinephrine.

Hormones of the Adrenal Cortex

The adrenal cortex produces three groups of steroid hormones—mineralocorticoids (min-eh-ra-loh-KORT-i-koids), glucocorticoids (gloo-koh-KORT-i-koids), and sex hormones. Steroid hormones are made from cholesterol and are lipid soluble (that is, they can dissolve in lipids).

The anterior pituitary controls the release of corticoid hormones—hormones of the adrenal cortex. Many of these hormones are vital to survival, so a decrease in their production can be life threatening. These three types of hormones regulate sodium (mineralocorticoids), sugar (glucocorticoids), and sex hormone levels in the body.

MEMORY TIP

The three substances regulated by the hormones of the adrenal cortex all start with an *S*—**S**odium, **S**ugar, and **S**ex hormones.

Mineralocorticoids

The principal mineralocorticoid hormone is **aldosterone** (al-DAHS-ter-ohn). Aldosterone stimulates the kidneys to reabsorb sodium and water from urine and to eliminate potassium. It also plays a major role in blood pressure regulation and plasma levels. When sodium and water are reabsorbed by the kidneys, plasma volume increases, raising blood pressure. Aldosterone also regulates the concentration of blood electrolytes, such as sodium and potassium.

Glucocorticoids

The main glucocorticoid hormones, **cortisone** (KOR-ti-sohn) and **cortisol** (KORT-i-sahl), maintain blood glucose levels by converting fats and amino acids into glucose via gluconeogenesis. This ensures that the brain and nervous system have a constant supply of glucose, their only fuel source.

Sex Hormones

The adrenal cortex produces small amounts of **estrogens** (female sex hormones) and **androgens** (male sex hormones). However, most sex hormones secreted by the adrenal cortex are androgens, primarily testosterone.

The reproductive organs also produce sex hormones. The effects of sex hormones produced by the reproductive organs (discussed in Chapter 15) usually mask the effects of sex hormones produced by the adrenal cortex. This is because the reproductive organs secrete higher volumes of hormones earlier in life. As you age, the reproductive organs secrete smaller quantities of sex hormones. The adrenal cortex, however, continues to produce the same amount of sex hormones; the effects of these hormones can become more noticeable with age. For example, because the adrenal cortex secretes high quantities of androgen, some females develop facial hair and other masculine traits.

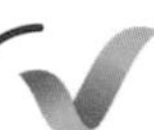

Check Your Understanding

1. Which component of the adrenal gland is actually part of the nervous system?
2. What three groups of steroid hormones are produced by the adrenal cortex?

Pancreas

The pancreas is a long, thin gland located posterior to the stomach in the upper part of the abdominal cavity. It acts as an endocrine gland by secreting hormones that control blood glucose levels. The pancreas is also an exocrine gland that excretes digestive enzymes. The exocrine function of the pancreas is described in Chapter 13.

The hormone-secreting cells of the pancreas are called the *islets* (IGH-lets) *of Langerhans* (LAHNG-er-hahnz), or *pancreatic islets*. The islets of Langerhans are composed of *alpha cells* that secrete **glucagon**, which increases blood glucose levels, and *beta cells* that secrete insulin, which lowers blood glucose levels. Together, the alpha and beta cells work to maintain blood glucose levels between the normal range of 70 and 105 mg/dL.

MEMORY TIP

To remember the hormones secreted by the pancreas, remember the acronym **PIG**: **P**ancreas secretes **I**nsulin and **G**lucagon.

Regulation of blood glucose levels by the pancreas is shown in **Figure 8.11**. When blood glucose level is high (after a meal, for example), the pancreas secretes insulin to lower the blood glucose level.

Insulin targets almost every cell in the body to promote glucose uptake. Once inside a cell, glucose is used for cellular energy. Insulin is essential for providing life-sustaining energy and health because it is the only hormone capable of getting glucose into the body cells. Insulin also stimulates the liver to convert excess glucose as glycogen, or fat.

Glucagon has the opposite effect. When blood glucose level is low, the pancreas secretes glucagon, which increases blood glucose. Glucagon secretion is achieved primarily through gluconeogenesis. Other hormones can raise the blood glucose level, but glucagon is the most effective.

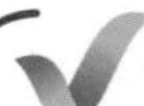

Check Your Understanding

1. What are the islets of Langerhans?
2. What is the difference between the function of an alpha cell and that of a beta cell?

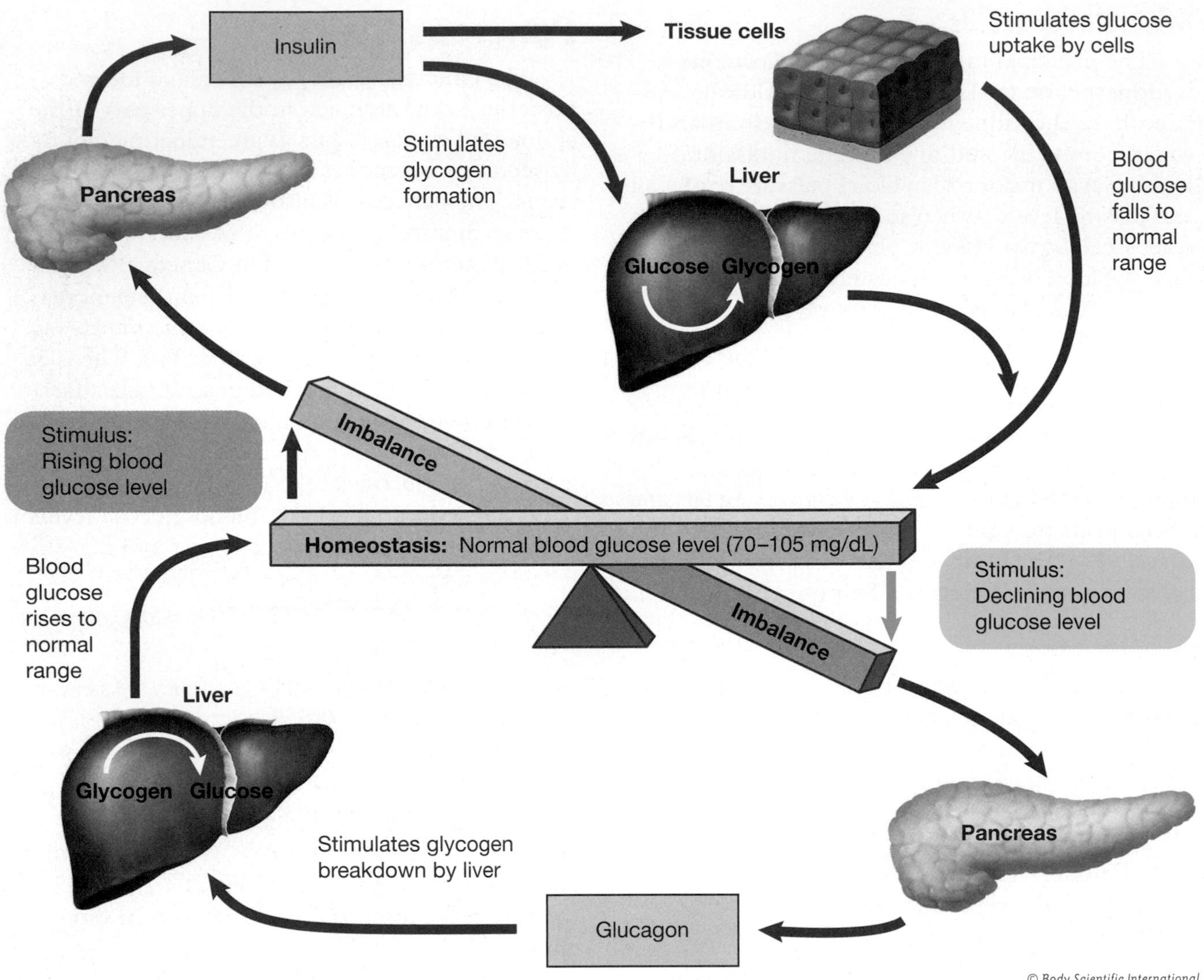

Figure 8.11 Blood glucose levels are maintained through secretion of insulin and glucagon by the pancreas. *What is the normal range for blood glucose levels?*

Other Hormone-Producing Organs and Tissues

Several other organs and tissues produce hormones that help to regulate body systems. These include the thymus, pineal gland, sex glands, and some types of adipose (fatty) tissue.

Thymus

The thymus is both an endocrine gland and a lymphatic organ. It lies under the sternum, anterior to the heart. During childhood, the thymus gland is quite large, but it becomes smaller as we age. At the onset of puberty, the thymus begins to shrink; by adulthood, it is barely visible.

The thymus secretes **thymosin** (THIGH-muh-sin), a hormone essential for the development of white blood cells called T lymphocytes, or T cells. T cells play a key role in the body's immune system.

Pineal Gland

The pineal (PI-nee-al) gland is a pinecone-shaped gland in the brain. Its exact function remains unclear. However, we do know that when the body is exposed to darkness, the pineal gland releases the hormone **melatonin**, causing us to feel sleepy. Melatonin levels are highest at night.

LIFE SPAN DEVELOPMENT: *The Endocrine System*

Although most hormones decrease with age, some remain at the levels found in young adults (post-puberty), and some actually increase. Regardless of whether hormones rise or fall or remain the same, it is generally agreed that endocrine function diminishes with age because the hormone receptors located on target tissues become less sensitive to the circulating hormones, and the rate at which hormones are metabolized is slower. Other factors that affect how the endocrine system functions as people age include chronic diseases, stress, environmental factors, and genetics.

In general, some hormones decrease with age:

- Growth hormone
- Estrogen and prolactin (in women)
- Melatonin
- Testosterone (in men)

Other hormones are unchanged or remain relatively the same with age:

- Cortisol
- Epinephrine
- Insulin
- T_3 and T_4

Still other hormones increase with age:

- Follicle-stimulating hormone
- Luteinizing hormone
- Norepinephrine
- Parathyroid hormone

Effects of the endocrine system during the life span are wide-ranging and are not solely related to levels of hormones. However, some of the more common age-related changes that the body undergoes may be partially explained by decreased levels of growth hormone, sex hormones, and melatonin.

Decreased GH leads to decreased muscle mass and strength. Muscle mass is highly correlated with metabolic rate and thus, as people age they experience a decrease in the number of calories the body burns, which may in part explain age-related weight gain.

Women typically begin menopause in their early 50s as a result of reduced female sex hormones. Decreased estrogen can also lead to increased bone loss. Testosterone declines are evident in men in their 60s and produce several physical changes, such as decreased muscle mass and strength, increased body fat, reduced body hair, and increased fatigue. Both men and women experience sleep disturbances as they age, which could be attributed to decreased melatonin levels.

Although research on hormone replacement to offset aging-related declines is ongoing, most of the current options do not show any noticeable improvements and introduce some negative side effects. For example, studies show that although GH replacement sometimes increases muscle mass, it does not increase strength. However, negative side effects, including carpal tunnel syndrome, were common. In addition, the risks of estrogen replacement therapy outweighs the benefits for many women. For now, exercise, a healthy diet, and maintaining an ideal body weight may be the best way to decrease age-related declines such as muscle loss, increased body fat, weight gain, and lowered bone density.

Gonads

Gonads are sex glands. In men, gonads are called *testes*; in women, they are called *ovaries*.

The paired, oval testes are encased by the scrotum, a sac located outside the body. The testes produce sperm and androgen hormones such as testosterone. Testosterone is responsible for sperm production, development of the male reproductive system, and the emergence of male secondary sex characteristics during puberty. The testes release testosterone when they are stimulated by luteinizing hormone (LH) from the anterior pituitary gland.

The ovaries, which are located inside the female pelvic cavity, produce eggs and the hormones estrogen and progesterone (proh-JES-teh-rohn). Estrogen plays a key role in the development of the female reproductive glands and secondary sex characteristics. Along with progesterone, estrogen also regulates the menstrual cycle.

Other Hormones

Hormones are produced by other tissues in the body, such as adipose tissue and the tissues that line the heart, stomach, and intestines. For example, the kidneys secrete *erythropoietin* (eh-rith-roh-POY-eh-tin), a hormone that stimulates red blood cell production. Fatty tissue secretes *prostaglandins* (prahs-tuh-GLAN-dinz), which act at, or near, the site of production. Prostaglandins regulate the smooth muscle cells that line the blood vessels and respiratory passages, stimulate the muscles of the uterus, and activate the inflammatory response. In addition, adipose cells produce the hormone leptin, which suppresses appetite and increases energy production.

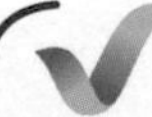

Check Your Understanding

1. Where is the thymus gland located?
2. Which hormone is secreted by the pineal gland?
3. What two hormones are secreted by the ovaries?

LESSON 8.2 Review and Assessment

Mini Glossary

Make sure that you know the meaning of each key term.

adrenal cortex outer layer of the adrenal glands, which itself has three layers that secrete steroid hormones

adrenal medulla the part of the adrenal glands that functions as a part of the nervous system; it secretes the hormones epinephrine and norepinephrine (catecholamines) during the fight-or-flight response

adrenocorticotropin (ACTH) tropic hormone secreted by the anterior pituitary that acts on the adrenal cortex to stimulate release of steroid hormones

aldosterone the principal mineralocorticoid hormone produced by the adrenal cortex; stimulates the kidneys to reabsorb sodium and water from urine and to eliminate potassium

androgens male sex hormones

antidiuretic hormone hormone produced in the hypothalamus and stored in the posterior pituitary; decreases urine output by stimulating the kidneys to increase water reabsorption

calcitonin hormone produced and released by the parafollicular cells of the thyroid gland that helps maintain calcium homeostasis

catecholamines hormones released into the blood during times of physical or emotional stress

cortisol a glucocorticoid hormone produced by the adrenal cortex that works with cortisone to maintain blood glucose levels via gluconeogenesis

cortisone a glucocorticoid hormone produced by the adrenal cortex that works with cortisol to maintain blood glucose levels via gluconeogenesis

estrogens female sex hormones

follicle-stimulating hormone (FSH) tropic hormone secreted by the anterior pituitary that stimulates production of estrogen and eggs in women and production of sperm in men

glucagon hormone secreted by alpha cells in the islets of Langerhans of the pancreas; increases blood glucose levels

growth hormone (GH) nontropic hormone produced by the anterior pituitary that is responsible for growth and development of the muscles, cartilage, and long bones of the body

luteinizing hormone (LH) tropic hormone secreted by the anterior pituitary that stimulates the ovaries to produce progesterone and estrogen and the release of eggs in women; in men, it stimulates the interstitial cells of the testes to produce testosterone

melatonin hormone produced by the pineal gland that causes sleepiness

oxytocin hormone produced in the hypothalamus and stored in the posterior pituitary; facilitates childbirth and causes the mammary glands to secrete breast milk

parathyroid hormone (PTH) hormone produced by the parathyroid glands that works with calcitonin to maintain calcium homeostasis

prolactin hormone secreted by the anterior pituitary that stimulates the growth of mammary glands and milk production in women; it is also present in men, but its purpose is unknown

thymosin hormone produced by the thymus that is essential for the development of white blood cells called T lymphocytes, or T cells

thyroid-stimulating hormone (TSH) tropic hormone secreted by the anterior pituitary that acts on the thyroid gland to stimulate release of two thyroid hormones, thyroxine (T_4) and triiodothyronine (T_3)

thyroxine (T_4) hormone secreted by the thyroid gland that works with T_3 to control the rate of energy metabolism and heat production in the body; called T_4 because it contains four iodine atoms

triiodothyronine (T_3) hormone secreted by the thyroid gland that works with T_4 to control the rate of energy metabolism and heat production in the body; called T_3 because it contains three iodine atoms

tropic hormones pituitary hormones that act on other endocrine glands; tropins

Know and Understand

1. What role does the hypothalamus play in the function of the endocrine system?
2. What is the medical term for the pituitary hormones that stimulate other endocrine glands?
3. Which tropic hormones are secreted by the anterior pituitary gland?
4. Which hormones are secreted when TSH acts on the thyroid gland?
5. What is the purpose of gluconeogenesis?
6. What two functions does prolactin play in a mother nursing an infant?
7. List the two major functions of oxytocin.
8. What general role is played by the hormones secreted by the thyroid?
9. Under what circumstances does the thyroid gland release calcitonin? What effect does this have on the body?
10. List three effects of parathyroid hormone on blood calcium levels.
11. What two organs make up the adrenal glands?
12. What happens when the levels of epinephrine and norepinephrine in the body rise?
13. Name the principal mineralocorticoid hormone in the body and describe its function.
14. Which two hormones regulate the female menstrual cycle?

Analyze and Apply

15. Compare and contrast the adrenal cortex and the adrenal medulla.
16. Explain why the thyroid hormones T_3 and T_4 affect all cells in the body.
17. Discuss the multiple roles ADH plays in the body.
18. Describe the regulation of calcium in the body.
19. Explain how the two types of cells in the islets of Langerhans work together to control blood pressure.
20. In what other body system, besides the endocrine system, does the thymus play a significant role? Explain.
21. Identify the sex hormones produced by the gonads in the female and in the male.

IN THE LAB

22. Lena, a 70-year-old woman, visits her doctor because she is concerned about the slight appearance of facial hair. Explain why it is not unusual for older women to develop masculine traits.
23. Create a mock profile of an endocrine gland for your favorite social media site. Include the following: a brief summary of what it is, where it resides, what type of work it does, and who its friends are. Share your profile with the class.
24. With a partner, create a brochure for the elderly. Your brochure should explain hormonal changes and the effects they have on the body. Use illustrations and perhaps some humor to get your point across. Take into account potential roadblocks that elderly people might have to understanding, such as failing eyesight. Be sure to give credit for any work that you use that is not your own.
25. Choose one of the hormones described in this chapter. Write a short fictional story in which this hormone plays a significant role. You may choose to make the hormone a leading character, or use human characters. You may want to begin by making an outline of your story in order to organize the events. Pay attention to character development and plot development. Share your story with your classmates and ask for feedback. Use the feedback to improve your story. Save the final story in your chapter portfolio.

LESSON **8.3**

Endocrine Disorders and Diseases

Before You Read

Try to answer the following questions before you read this lesson.

- What effect does an overactive thyroid gland have on the body?
- What is the difference between diabetes mellitus and diabetes insipidus?

Lesson Objectives

- Describe the following disorders of the pituitary gland: acromegaly, dwarfism, and diabetes insipidus.
- Discuss the difference between hypothyroidism and hyperthyroidism and name the disorders associated with each.
- Identify disorders and diseases of the parathyroid gland.
- Identify the hormones produced by the adrenal glands and their effects on the body.
- Explain the difference between type 1 and type 2 diabetes mellitus.

Key Terms

acromegaly	hyperglycemia
Addison disease	hyperthyroidism
Cushing syndrome	hypothyroidism
diabetes insipidus	insulin resistance
diabetes mellitus (DM)	ketoacidosis
dwarfism	myxedema
exophthalmos	neonatal hypothyroidism
goiter	peripheral neuropathy
Graves disease	tetany
hypercalcemia	thyroiditis

Because the endocrine system is hierarchical in nature, many of its glands depend on one another, yet also act independently. Therefore, when an endocrine gland is not functioning properly, the effects of its malfunction can be felt throughout the body or at a specific site. This lesson describes some common disorders and diseases of the endocrine system.

CLINICAL CASE STUDY

Madison had always been an active adolescent and adult. As she approached her late fifties, she was frequently tired and felt fatigued much of the time. Although she tried to keep up with her exercise routine, she was gaining weight. Her skin was dry, her hair was thinning, and her normally manicured nails were cracking. Maddie was concerned enough that she made an appointment with her physician. As you read this section, try to determine which of the following conditions Madison most likely has.

A. Hypothyroidism
B. Hyperthyroidism
C. Type 2 diabetes

Pituitary Disorders

The pituitary gland—composed of the anterior and posterior pituitary—releases many important hormones. Thus, a hypofunctioning (underactive) or hyperfunctioning (overactive) pituitary gland can have widespread effects. The etiology (cause), strategies for prevention, pathology (clinical characteristics), diagnosis (keys for identifying the condition), and common treatments for pituitary disorders are summarized in **Figure 8.12**.

Hyperfunction of the Pituitary Gland

Hyperfunction of the pituitary occurs when the gland secretes excessive amounts of a specific hormone. One of the most common disorders caused by hyperfunction of the pituitary is **acromegaly** (ak-roh-MEG-a-lee), or *gigantism*, in which the anterior pituitary secretes too much growth hormone. Acromegaly causes an increase in overall body size, especially in the extremities.

Acromegaly is usually caused by a noncancerous tumor pressing on the pituitary gland. Pressure from the tumor can cause headaches, vision disturbances or loss of vision, seizures, and fatigue. This disorder most often affects middle-aged adults, but it may also affect children. Diagnosis of acromegaly in

Common Pituitary Disorders

	Etiology	Prevention	Pathology	Diagnosis	Treatment
Acromegaly (Gigantism)	anterior pituitary secretes excess growth hormone (GH), usually due to pressure from noncancerous tumor on pituitary gland.	none	headaches, vision disturbances/vision loss, seizures, and fatigue adults: thickened bones, enlarged facial features, hands, and feet children: unusually tall height, large hands and feet	measurement of growth hormone, imaging of pituitary gland	medications to shrink the tumor and decrease GH levels; surgery to remove tumor, if operable
Dwarfism	deficient secretion of GH by anterior pituitary gland; can be congenital or acquired due to brain injury	early diagnosis and treatment with supplemental GH	abnormally short adult stature (approximately 4 feet)	delayed growth markers at well baby checks, GH test, imaging to assess bone development	supplemental GH
Diabetes insipidus	hyposecretion of antidiuretic hormone (ADH) by posterior pituitary	supplemental synthetic ADH	excessive thirst (polydipsia), electrolyte loss, frequent urination	blood tests for ADH; analysis of urine (urinalysis) to determine water levels	supplemental synthetic ADH

Figure 8.12

Goodheart-Willcox Publisher

adults may take years because its effects appear gradually. Measurements of growth hormone and imaging of the pituitary gland are used to help diagnose acromegaly.

Treatment of acromegaly includes medications to shrink the tumor and decrease GH levels. Surgery may be performed to remove the tumor if it is operable. Surgeons may operate on a patient using a radiation beam, or gamma knife, when a tumor is located in a hard-to-reach place. Although medications and surgery can stop excessive growth, the effects of acromegaly cannot be reversed. Unfortunately, the strain that acromegaly places on the body often leads to a shortened life span.

Hypofunction of the Pituitary Gland

Hypofunction of the pituitary gland occurs when the pituitary gland does not secrete enough of its hormones. Hypofunction of the pituitary can cause several disorders, including dwarfism and diabetes insipidus.

Dwarfism

Hyposecretion of GH by the pituitary gland can cause **dwarfism**, a condition in which adult height reaches approximately four feet (**Figure 8.13**). Dwarfism affects only a person's physical size; intellectual ability is normal.

Congenital dwarfism (acquired during development in the uterus) is called *cretinism*. However, it can also be caused by brain injury or a medical condition, such as growth hormone deficiency. When diagnosed at an early age, dwarfism is usually treated with supplemental growth hormone.

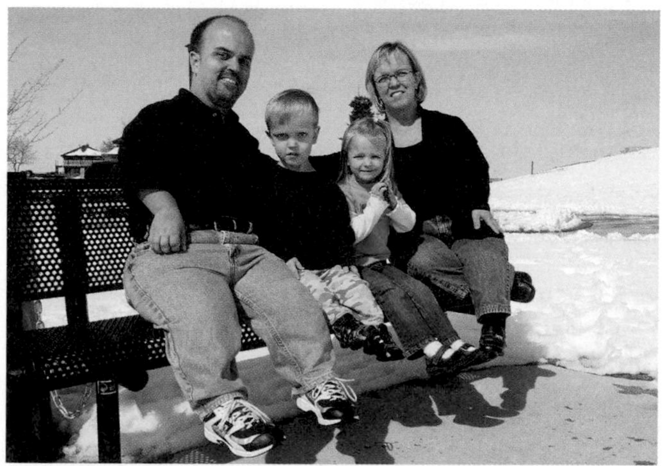

Nolte Lourens/Shutterstock.com

Figure 8.13 Hyposecretion of GH results in dwarfism. *What is the impact of dwarfism on a person's intellectual abilities?*

Diabetes Insipidus.

Hyposecretion of antidiuretic hormone (ADH) from the posterior pituitary causes **diabetes insipidus**. ADH normally targets the kidneys, causing them to reabsorb water from urine. ADH deficiency can cause a large loss of water and electrolytes. People with diabetes insipidus experience excessive thirst, or *polydipsia* (pahl-i-DIP-see-a). Diabetes insipidus is different from diabetes mellitus (MEL-it-uhs), a pancreatic disorder commonly referred to as *diabetes*, which is discussed later in this lesson.

Check Your Understanding

1. Which condition results from hypofunction of the pituitary gland?
2. Which endocrine disorder is caused by an ADH deficiency?

Thyroid Disorders

When inadequate or excessive levels of T_4 and T_3 are secreted, the result is a thyroid disorder. The etiology, strategies for prevention, pathology, diagnosis, and common treatments for thyroid disorders are summarized in **Figure 8.14**.

Hyperthyroidism

Hyperthyroidism, or an overactive thyroid, is characterized by a visibly enlarged thyroid gland in the neck (**Figure 8.15**). An enlarged thyroid is called a **goiter** (GOY-ter). A goiter is caused by insufficient amounts of iodine, a chemical element necessary for the production of thyroid hormones, or by thyroid disorders.

Iodine is not produced by the body, so it is important to eat foods containing iodine. This is one of the reasons that most countries, including the United States, add iodine to salt. An overactive

Thyroid Disorders

	Etiology	Prevention	Pathology	Diagnosis	Treatment
Hyperthyroidism	excess thyroid hormones due to iodine insufficiency, a noncancerous tumor on thyroid gland, or inflamed thyroid	ingestion of a sufficient amount of iodine in the diet.	enlarged thyroid gland (goiter) in the neck, increased metabolism, heart rate, and body temperature, weight loss, diarrhea, difficulty concentrating, anxiety	physical exam, blood tests	medications; radioactive iodine to decrease thyroid hormone production, surgery to reduce some or all thyroid gland activity
Graves disease	form of hyperthyroidism due to autoimmune disorder with a genetic component	none	goiter, bulging eyes (exophthalmos), dry, irritated, red eyes	physical exam, thyroid hormone tests, radioactive iodine uptake test	same as for hyperthyroidism
Hypothyroidism	underactive thyroid, usually caused by inflammation of thyroid gland causing thyroiditis; common in women > 50 years	none	weight gain, fatigue, dry skin, thin hair, brittle fingernails	confirmed by visual observation, testing of thyroid hormone levels	supplemental lifelong thyroid hormone replacement therapy
Myxedema	untreated, severe hypothyroidism	seek treatment for hypothyroidism	swollen, puffy face, low body temperature, dry skin, decreased mental sharpness	physical exam, thyroid blood tests	same as for hypothyroidism
Neonatal hypothyroidism	congenital or shortly after birth due to underdeveloped or absent thyroid gland	early detection and treatment	often symptomless	neonatal screening at birth for thyroid hormones	same as for hypothyroidism

Figure 8.14

Goodheart-Willcox Publisher

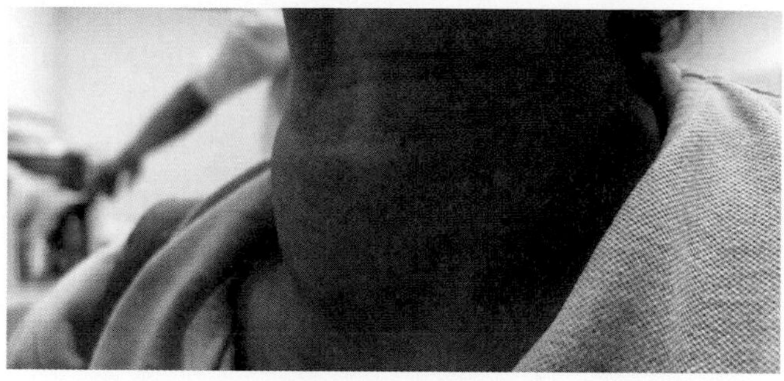

Casa nayafana/Shutterstock.com

Figure 8.15 This woman has a goiter, a result of insufficient iodine levels or thyroid disorders. A goiter may cause difficulty breathing and swallowing, as well as a cough. *How can large goiters be treated?*

thyroid works hard to secrete hormones, but without iodine from the diet, production of thyroid hormones is impaired.

Low levels of the hormones T_3 and T_4 cannot complete the negative feedback loop to "turn off" the hypothalamus and the pituitary glands. As a result, the hypothalamus and pituitary gland continue to produce thyroid-releasing hormone and thyroid-stimulating hormone.

TSH causes the thyroid gland to enlarge. Increased heart rate, elevated body temperature, hyperactivity, weight loss, diarrhea, and difficulty concentrating are other side effects of hyperthyroidism.

Other causes of hyperthyroidism include noncancerous growths on the thyroid or inflammation of the thyroid gland. Treatments for hyperthyroidism include surgery to remove part, or all, of the thyroid gland or tumor, radioactive iodine to destroy thyroid cells, and thyroid drugs to reduce thyroid hormones.

The most common cause of hyperthyroidism is **Graves disease**, an autoimmune disorder that leads to an overactive thyroid gland. A tumor on the thyroid gland causes oversecretion of the thyroid hormones.

Graves disease also causes the eyes to bulge outward, a condition called **exophthalmos** (ek-sof-THAL-muhs). This may make it difficult or impossible to close the eyelid, which can lead to drying and scarring of the cornea. Loss of vision may result from this condition.

Hypothyroidism

Hypothyroidism, or *underactive thyroid*, is usually caused by **thyroiditis**, the result of inflammation that damages thyroid cells. Thyroiditis can be caused by the immune system attacking the thyroid, a cold, a respiratory infection, an inflammation that occurs after pregnancy (postpartum thyroiditis), or prescription drugs.

Hypothyroidism is most common in women and in people over 50 years of age. Symptoms include fatigue, pale and dry skin, thin hair, brittle fingernails, increased sensitivity to cold temperatures, constipation, and weight gain. Treatment involves replacing the T_3 and T_4 hormones through supplemental hormone therapy. Most people with hypothyroidism will need lifelong supplemental hormone therapy to manage their disease.

Myxedema

Adults with hypothyroidism that goes undiagnosed or untreated may develop **myxedema** (miks-eh-DEE-ma). Myxedema is a severe form of hypothyroidism that causes weight gain; a swollen, puffy face; low body temperature; dry skin; and decreased mental acuity, or sharpness. This condition can be treated with an oral form of thyroxine.

Neonatal Hypothyroidism

Newborn children can develop **neonatal hypothyroidism**. This thyroid deficiency may develop congenitally (before birth) or soon after birth. Often, children with neonatal hypothyroidism have a poorly developed thyroid gland or ineffective thyroid hormones.

Untreated neonatal hypothyroidism can lead to mental and physical disability. Dull, dry skin and dry, brittle hair are also common. Early diagnosis is key because the effects of this disorder can be reversed. Like myxedema, neonatal hypothyroidism is treated with oral thyroxine.

Check Your Understanding

1. What is an enlarged thyroid gland called?
2. Which thyroid disorder causes exophthalmos?
3. How is myxedema treated?

Parathyroid Disorders

As explained in Lesson 8.2, the parathyroid glands secrete parathyroid hormone (PTH), and the thyroid gland secretes calcitonin. Calcitonin and PTH work together to regulate blood calcium levels. Abnormal production of PTH can therefore cause calcium-related disorders. The etiology, strategies for prevention, pathology, diagnosis, and common treatments for parathyroid disorders are summarized in **Figure 8.16**.

Hypercalcemia

Hypersecretion of PTH causes too much calcium in the blood, a condition known as **hypercalcemia** (high-per-kal-SEE-mee-a). Hypercalcemia leads to increased calcium absorption by the kidneys. The excess calcium in the kidneys, along with changes in the bones (which develop holes and become brittle), causes kidney stones to form. Hypercalcemia can also affect the nervous and cardiovascular systems, causing depression, decreased heart rate, and fatigue.

Hypocalcemia

Hypocalcemia (high-poh-kal-SEE-mee-a), or low blood calcium, may be due to damage to the parathyroid gland, kidney failure, tumors, or pancreatitis. It has also been linked to vitamin D and magnesium deficiencies, low calcium intake, and medications that can cause calcium loss. Hypocalcemia can cause mild symptoms like muscle cramps or facial twitching, but it can also have serious effects on the body. It can lead to unstable nerve and muscle membranes that continuously fire electrical signals. The result is a condition of sustained muscular contraction known as **tetany** (TET-a-nee). If left untreated, tetany can affect the respiratory muscles, leading to asphyxiation and death. Treatment for hypocalcemia includes PTH replacement therapy, as well as vitamin D, magnesium and calcium supplementation. Blood tests to monitor calcium levels are also helpful in managing this disease.

Check Your Understanding

1. What causes the formation of kidney stones in people with hypercalcemia?
2. What is tetany?

Disorders of the Adrenal Glands

As with other disorders of the endocrine system, disorders of the adrenal glands can result from any number of factors. The etiology, strategies for prevention, pathology, diagnosis, and common treatments for adrenal disorders are summarized in **Figure 8.17**.

Adrenal Medulla

In rare cases, individuals develop a tumor on the adrenal medulla called a *pheochromocytoma* (fee-oh-kroh-moh-sigh-TOH-muh). A pheochromocytoma causes the adrenal medulla to hypersecrete the hormones epinephrine and norepinephrine.

High amounts of epinephrine and norepinephrine in the bloodstream can result in high blood pressure, rapid heart rate, weight loss, nervousness, and sleep disturbances. These symptoms are experienced intermittently (from time to time) and usually resolve within 15 to 20 minutes. However, some episodes may be life threatening if not treated promptly.

Parathyroid Disorders					
	Etiology	**Prevention**	**Pathology**	**Diagnosis**	**Treatment**
Hypercalcemia	hypersecretion of PTH; overuse of calcium supplements	awareness of family history of high calcium levels/kidney stones or brittle bones	painful bones, weakness, stomach upset, kidney stones, increased thirst, decreased heart rate, depression, and fatigue.	blood tests for PTH and blood calcium levels	mild: drinking more water, stopping calcium supplements severe: medications to lower PTH/calcium levels, surgery
Hypocalcemia	hyposecretion of PTH; damage to parathyroid gland, kidney failure, tumor, pancreatitis	awareness of family history of low blood calcium levels, calcium supplements, healthy vitamin D and magnesium levels	mild: muscle cramps, facial twitching severe: tetany, interference with nerve transmissions and normal cell function, asphyxiation, and death	blood tests for PTH, calcium, vitamin D, and magnesium levels; kidney function and pancreatic tests	PTH replacement therapy, vitamin D, magnesium, and calcium supplements

Goodheart-Willcox Publisher

Figure 8.16

Adrenal Gland Disorders					
	Etiology	**Prevention**	**Pathology**	**Diagnosis**	**Treatment**
Pheochromocytoma (adrenal medulla)	tumor on adrenal medulla causes hypersecretion of epinephrine and norepinephrine	none	intermittent high blood pressure, rapid heart rate, weight loss, nervousness, sleep disorders	abdominal CT or MTI scan, blood or urine catecholamine tests, adrenal biopsy	immediate medication to lower blood pressure and heart rate, removal of tumor
Cushing syndrome (adrenal cortex)	hypersecretion of cortisol caused by oversecretion of ACTH by the pituitary gland; tumor on adrenal gland; prolonged use of steroid drugs	limit use of steroid drugs	rounded, moon-shaped face; weight gain; high blood glucose; hypertension; osteoporosis; reddish-purple abdominal stretch marks; facial hair in women; difficulty concentrating	morning salivary cortisol levels and 24-hour urinary cortisol measurements	tumor removal from the adrenal gland if tumor is present; careful weaning from steroid drugs
Addison disease (adrenal cortex)	hyposecretion of ACTH	none	bronze skin tone, muscle atrophy, low blood pressure, kidney damage, high blood potassium, hypoglycemia, fatigue, excessive loss of fluids and electrolytes (especially sodium)	physical exam; blood tests for sodium, potassium, cortisol, and ACTH; CT and MRI imaging	hormone replacement therapy

Figure 8.17 *Goodheart-Willcox Publisher*

Disorders of the Adrenal Cortex

Tumorous growths on the adrenal gland can cause an adrenal cortex disorder. Another cause of adrenal cortex disorders is irregular secretion of hormones from other glands that act on the adrenal cortex. The hyposecretion or hypersecretion of adrenal cortex hormones can also cause a disorder in the body. Common disorders of the adrenal cortex include Cushing syndrome and Addison disease.

Cushing Syndrome

Cushing syndrome is a disorder of the adrenal cortex caused by hypersecretion of cortisol. Cortisol hypersecretion can be caused by:

- oversecretion of adrenocorticotropin hormone (ACTH) by the pituitary gland, which stimulates hypersecretion of cortisol by the adrenal cortex.
- a tumor on the adrenal gland that stimulates hypersecretion of cortisol.
- prolonged use of steroid drugs, such as those prescribed to treat arthritis and other autoimmune disorders. Steroid drugs can suppress the release of ACTH, thus preventing the production of cortisol.

Overproduction of cortisol causes many symptoms, including a rounded, moon-shaped face; weight gain (especially in the upper body); high blood glucose levels; hypertension; osteoporosis; reddish-purple abdominal stretch marks; difficulty concentrating; and facial hair in women (**Figure 8.18**).

It is important to exercise caution when taking steroid drugs. Prolonged use of a steroid drug, whether for illness or to enhance athletic

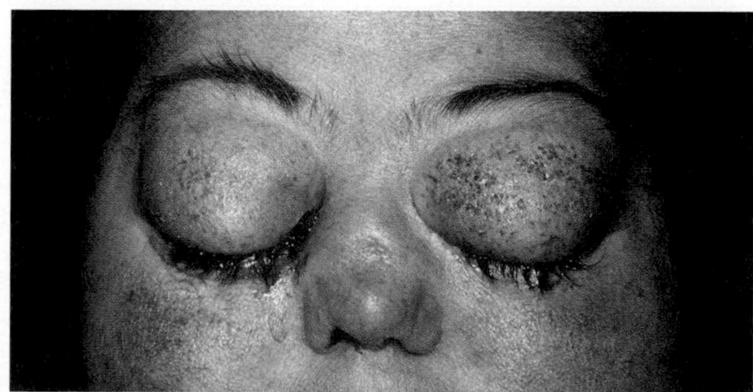

Biophoto Associates/Science Source

Figure 8.18 Cushing syndrome is characterized by a rounded face, bulging eyes, and a reddish complexion. *Which hormone is hypersecreted in a person who develops Cushing syndrome?*

performance, can inhibit the release of ACTH by the anterior pituitary, leading to a lack of cortisol. This puts a person at risk for developing Cushing syndrome. Therefore, it is very important that patients be slowly weaned from steroid drugs, giving the anterior pituitary time to begin producing ACTH again.

Athletes who use anabolic steroids often suffer numerous and long-lasting effects, including decreased heart function, elevated blood pressure, liver damage, premature bone plate closures, aggression, and depression. In males, it can cause impotence or decreased sperm, and in females, it can cause menstrual cycle abnormalities.

Addison Disease

Hyposecretion of adrenal corticoid hormones can cause **Addison disease**, which may result in muscle atrophy, a bronze skin tone, low blood pressure, and kidney damage. Other symptoms include excessive levels of potassium in the blood; hypoglycemia (high-poh-glih-SEE-mee-a); severe loss of fluids and electrolytes (especially sodium); and a general feeling of weakness. Addison disease is life threatening because it can lead to low blood volume, electrolyte disturbances, or shock.

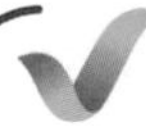

Check Your Understanding

1. What is the cause of Cushing syndrome?
2. What are the possible consequences of prolonged anabolic steroid use?

The Pancreas and Diabetes Mellitus

As you may recall, the pancreas secretes two hormones that regulate blood glucose levels: insulin and glucagon. **Diabetes mellitus (DM)** results when the body cannot produce sufficient amounts of insulin to regulate blood glucose levels. There are two types of diabetes—type 1 and type 2. The etiology, strategies for prevention, pathology, diagnosis, and common treatments for diabetes mellitus are summarized in **Figure 8.19**.

In the United States, 90% to 95% of diabetes cases are type 2; the remaining 5% to 10% are type 1. This disease is so common that almost everyone knows someone with diabetes. According to a recent CDC National Diabetes Statistic report, diabetes is present in 30.3 million Americans of all ages, or 9.4% of the total population. Diabetes is more predominant in older individuals and minority populations, but is on the rise in younger people. Diabetes is the seventh leading cause of death in the United States. It is also the leading cause of kidney failure, nontraumatic lower limb amputation, and new cases of blindness. Diabetes is also a major contributor to heart disease and stroke.

Symptoms and Diagnosis of Diabetes Mellitus

Diabetes mellitus is diagnosed through a fasting blood glucose test, a glucose tolerance test,

Diabetes Mellitus					
	Etiology	**Prevention**	**Pathology**	**Diagnosis**	**Treatment**
Type 1	autoimmune disorder kills insulin-secreting beta cells of pancreas, decreasing or stopping insulin production; genetics may also be a factor	none	dangerously high blood glucose level (> 500 mg/dL); excessive thirst, excessive urination, increased hunger, weight loss, irritability, mood changes, blurred vision, fatigue	measurement of fasting blood glucose levels, glucose tolerance test, HbA1c test	monitoring blood glucose levels, self-administered insulin based on glucose levels; insulin pump to continuously monitor glucose levels and deliver appropriate insulin dosages
Type 2	pancreas secretes insulin but the body's cells are insulin-resistant and do not take up glucose	maintain healthy body weight, exercise regularly, eat a healthy diet, awareness of family history of type 2 diabetes	hyperglycemia, weight gain, especially in the abdominal area	measurement of fasting blood glucose levels, glucose tolerance test, HbA1c test	losing 5-10% of body weight, moderate aerobic exercise on most days, eating a healthy diet; oral hypoglycemic agents or insulin

Goodheart-Willcox Publisher

Figure 8.19

and the HbA1c test, or glycosylated (gligh-KOH-sih-lay-tehd) hemoglobin test.

- Blood glucose test—a blood glucose level of 126 mg/dL or higher after an eight-hour fast is considered positive for diabetes.
- Glucose tolerance test—in this oral glucose tolerance test, a person's blood glucose level is measured at intervals after drinking a liquid that contains 75 grams of glucose, or sugar. A blood glucose level of 200 mg/dL or greater is in the diabetic range.
- HbA1c test—this test measures average blood glucose levels over a three-month period. A glucose level of 5.6% or less is normal, 5.7%–6.4% is prediabetic, and 6.5% or greater indicates diabetes.

Generally, a family history of diabetes mellitus or symptom onset prompts people to be tested for this disorder. The primary symptoms of diabetes include:

- *polyuria* (pahl-ee-YOOR-ee-a)—excessive urination to eliminate glucose
- *polydipsia*—excessive thirst to replenish water lost due to polyuria
- *polyphagia* (pahl-ee-FAY-jee-a)—increased hunger to replace fats and proteins used by the body as fuel sources

Other symptoms of diabetes may include unexplained weight loss or gain, irritability/mood changes, blurred vision, fatigue, nausea, and slow-healing wounds.

Type 1 Diabetes Mellitus

Type 1 diabetes mellitus is an autoimmune disorder in which the immune system attacks and kills the insulin-secreting beta cells of the pancreas. Destruction of these cells causes insulin production to decrease or stop altogether. As a result, blood glucose levels rise from their normal circulating levels of 70–105 mg/dL to dangerously high levels exceeding 500 mg/dL.

Type 1 diabetics receive insulin through several injections over the course of a day. Insulin dosage levels are based on self-administered blood glucose checks. If blood glucose levels are high, a higher insulin dose is administered; if blood glucose levels are low, less insulin is taken (**Figure 8.20**). Type 1 diabetics may regulate their blood glucose levels through an externally worn insulin pump that continuously monitors glucose and delivers appropriate dosages of insulin.

It is unclear what causes the immune system to attack the insulin-secreting beta cells of the pancreas. However, researchers do know that type 1 diabetes mellitus is a hereditary condition. People with this disorder are usually diagnosed at a young age.

Type 2 Diabetes Mellitus

In people with type 2 diabetes, the pancreas secretes insulin, but the body's insulin receptors are downregulated—a condition called **insulin resistance**. Insulin-resistant receptors cannot take up glucose even when insulin is present, so blood glucose levels become elevated, a condition known as **hyperglycemia**. When hyperglycemia is present, the beta cells of the pancreas compensate by producing more insulin. Eventually, even the increased release of insulin fails to have an adequate effect and hyperglycemia occurs. When glucose builds up in the blood, it is absorbed by the kidneys and excreted in the urine.

It is unclear exactly what causes the body's cells to become insulin-resistant but insulin resistance is associated with obesity, physical inactivity, family history of diabetes, and old age. In fact, the NIH estimates that 80% of type 2 diabetics are overweight or obese.

Although large amounts of glucose are available in the body for energy production, diabetics are unable to use this glucose because insulin is unavailable or the body's cells are insulin-resistant. When the body's cells are unable to use glucose as a fuel source, fats and proteins must be used instead.

Using fats for fuel produces ketone bodies that decrease the pH of the blood, making it dangerously acidic. This condition is called **ketoacidosis** (keet-oh-as-i-DOH-sis). If left untreated, ketoacidosis can lead to diabetic coma and death. People with

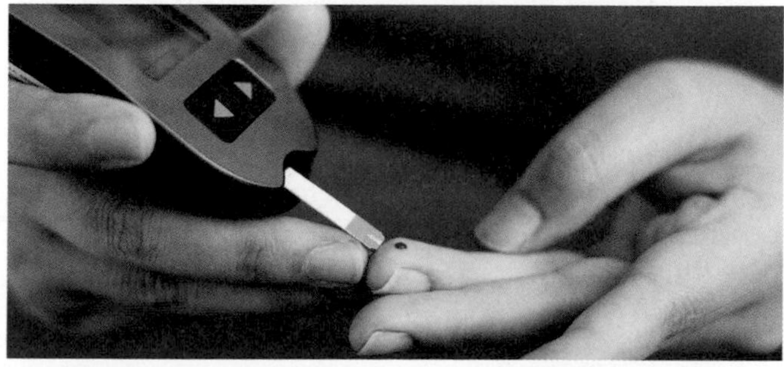

Kwangmoozaa/Shutterstock.com

Figure 8.20 Diabetics use a glucometer to monitor fluctuations in their blood glucose levels. *If a glucometer shows a high blood glucose level, what action should a diabetic take?*

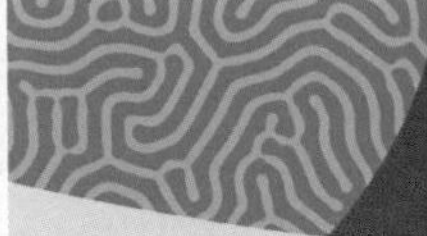

What Research Tells Us

...about Managing Diabetes with Diet and Exercise

Diabetes mellitus has reached epidemic proportions in the United States, largely because of the increased rate of obesity and lack of physical activity. The NIH estimates that there are about 57 million prediabetic cases among people 20 years of age and older in the United States.

Recently, a study of 3,000 diabetic and prediabetic people investigated the effect of a low-fat diet and 30 minutes of moderately intense exercise five days a week (**Figure 8.21**). Most of the study participants chose walking as their exercise activity, and the results were dramatic. On average, participants lost 5% to 7% of their body weight. These two simple but effective lifestyle changes reduced the incidence of type 2 diabetes in the sample group by nearly 60%.

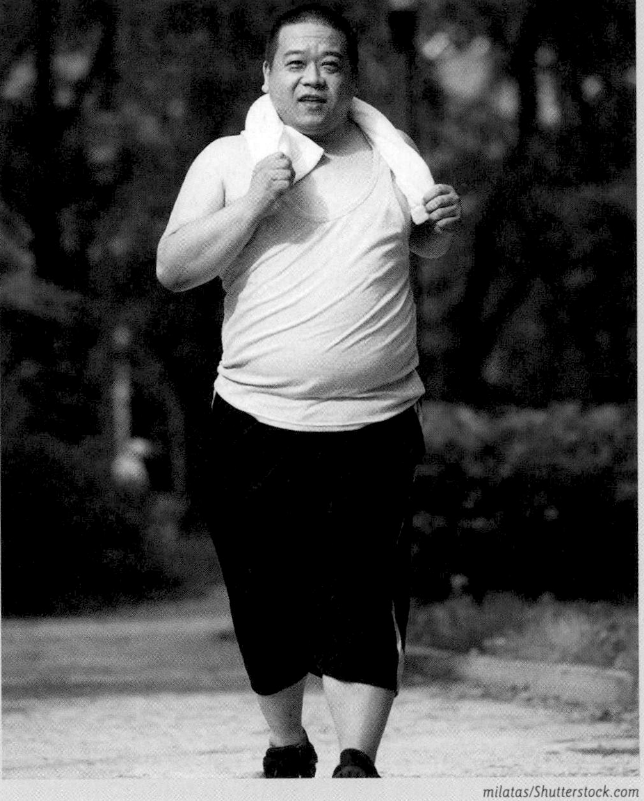

milatas/Shutterstock.com

Figure 8.21 Regular exercise can decrease a person's risk of developing diabetes mellitus.

Taking It Further

1. With a partner, discuss other health benefits of a diet low in fat and calories and a regular exercise routine. How might a healthful diet and regular exercise benefit people with diseases that you have learned about in other chapters of this textbook?
2. Why do you think obesity has reached epidemic proportions in the United States? Brainstorm ways in which society can combat this problem.

ketosis—high levels of ketones in the body—also have fruity-smelling breath because of the presence of acetone.

Recommendations for treating type 2 diabetics include a diet that is lower in calories and refined carbohydrates like sweets, performing aerobic exercise at a moderate intensity for 30–60 minutes most days of the week and reducing body weight by 5–10 percent. If adopting a healthful diet, getting adequate exercise, and reducing body weight are not sufficient for managing type 2 diabetes mellitus, oral hypoglycemic agents or injectable insulin may be required.

Living with Diabetes Mellitus

Patient education is very important for diabetic care. People with diabetes who develop **peripheral neuropathy** (noo-RAHP-a-thee), which causes loss of feeling in the extremities, must take particularly good care of their feet. As a result, diabetics may be unaware when they get a cut or wound on their foot. Unnoticed cuts or wounds can become infected. Severely infected wounds often result in amputation of the affected limb.

There is no known cure for diabetes mellitus. Since there is no cure, the goal for patients is to learn how to successfully manage this disorder. The cornerstones of managing diabetes mellitus are a healthful diet, physical activity to increase insulin sensitivity of the body's cells, weight loss, and taking medications as prescribed.

Check Your Understanding

1. What is the cause of type 1 diabetes mellitus?
2. Why does insulin resistance cause hyperglycemia?

LESSON 8.3 Review and Assessment

Mini Glossary

Make sure that you know the meaning of each key term.

acromegaly a rare condition in which the anterior pituitary hypersecretes growth hormone, causing an increase in overall body size; gigantism

Addison disease a condition caused by hyposecretion of adrenal corticoid hormones that causes muscle atrophy, a bronze skin tone, low blood pressure, kidney damage, hypoglycemia, severe loss of fluids and electrolytes, and a general feeling of weakness

Cushing syndrome a disorder of the adrenal cortex caused by hypersecretion of cortisol; symptoms include weight gain, high blood glucose levels, hypertension, and osteoporosis

diabetes insipidus a disorder resulting from hyposecretion of antidiuretic hormone (ADH) by the posterior pituitary

diabetes mellitus (DM) a disease that results from the body's inability to produce sufficient amounts of insulin to regulate blood glucose levels

dwarfism a condition in which the pituitary gland hyposecretes growth hormone, resulting in an adult height of less than four feet

exophthalmos condition in which the eyes bulge outward

goiter an enlarged thyroid gland caused by insufficient amounts of iodine or a thyroid disorder

Graves disease an autoimmune disorder that causes an overactive thyroid gland and outward bulging of the eyes

hypercalcemia a condition caused by the hypersecretion of parathyroid hormone (PTH), leading to increased blood calcium levels and increased calcium absorption by the kidneys

hyperglycemia a condition in which blood glucose levels become elevated

hyperthyroidism a condition characterized by a visibly enlarged thyroid gland in the neck; *overactive thyroid gland*

hypothyroidism a condition caused by an underactive thyroid gland

insulin resistance a condition common in type 2 diabetes in which the pancreas secretes insulin, but the body's insulin receptors are downregulated, causing elevated blood glucose levels

ketoacidosis condition in which the pH of the blood is decreased, making the blood dangerously acidic; results from using fats for fuel, which produces ketone bodies in the blood

myxedema a condition in adults with hyperthyroidism that causes weight gain; a swollen, puffy face; low body temperature; dry skin; and decreased mental acuity

neonatal hypothyroidism hypothyroidism that occurs in infants and children

peripheral neuropathy a disease or degenerative state of the peripheral nerves often associated with diabetes mellitus; marked by muscle weakness and atrophy, pain, and numbness

tetany a condition of sustained muscular contraction

thyroiditis inflammation of the thyroid gland

Know and Understand

1. What causes diabetes insipidus?
2. Why are goiters uncommon in the United States today?
3. What are the symptoms of hypothyroidism?
4. Which disease is caused by the hyposecretion of adrenal corticoid hormones?
5. Which tests are used to diagnose diabetes mellitus?

Analyze and Apply

6. Compare and contrast type 1 and type 2 diabetes mellitus.
7. Why does hypercalcemia cause brittle bones?
8. Make a list of the symptoms of acromegaly. Why might someone with this condition have a shorter life span?
9. Review the table in Figure 8.14. How might a physician diagnose hypothyroidism?
10. Diabetes is the seventh leading cause of death in the United States. What factors do you think contribute to this statistic?

IN THE LAB

11. Dominick, a 37-year-old male, has developed type 2 diabetes mellitus. Dominick is 5 feet, 8 inches tall and weighs 300 pounds. Make a list of questions that you would ask Dominick if you were counseling him about beneficial lifestyle changes. Also, make a list of guidelines that could help Dominick manage his disease.
12. Create a time line for a day in the life of a high school student with type 1 diabetes mellitus. Use text and images to describe the day's events. Pay special attention to how often the student checks her glucose levels, and determine how she receives insulin.
13. Choose a partner. One of you will be a reporter and the other will be a patient. The patient will choose a disease discussed in this chapter and learn a few more details about it. The reporter will make a list of ten questions about lifestyles, diet, medications, and other factors and will use the list to interview the patient.

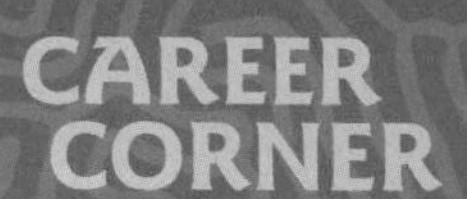

CAREER CORNER Anatomy & Physiology at Work

The organs and hormones of the endocrine system have wide-ranging effects on the body. Many careers require highly specific or general knowledge of this complex body system. Two occupations involving work with patients who have endocrine system disorders and diseases are endocrinologist and physician assistant.

Endocrinologists use their advanced knowledge of the endocrine system to diagnose and treat hormonal imbalances and diseases. Physician assistants treat patients in a variety of settings and circumstances; thus, they need a broad understanding of the body.

Endocrinologist

Endocrinologists (ehn-doh-kri-NAHL-uh-jists) are medical doctors who specialize in the treatment of hormone imbalances with the goal of restoring hormonal activity to normal, homeostatic levels (**Figure 8.22**). Disorders commonly treated by endocrinologists include diabetes mellitus, obesity, osteoporosis, thyroid disorders, infertility, and other endocrine system disorders. Many of these disorders can affect other body systems, so a comprehensive understanding of human biology and anatomy and physiology is a must for endocrinologists.

Extensive education, beyond a four-year bachelor's degree in biology or a related field, is required to become an endocrinologist. After four years of medical school, future endocrinologists spend three to four years at an internship, or residency in internal medicine. The internship culminates with a two- to three-year fellowship spent focusing on hormone conditions and diseases.

Endocrinologists typically work in hospitals, private practices, or medical research facilities. They work closely with patients to diagnose and establish treatment plans for endocrine system diseases.

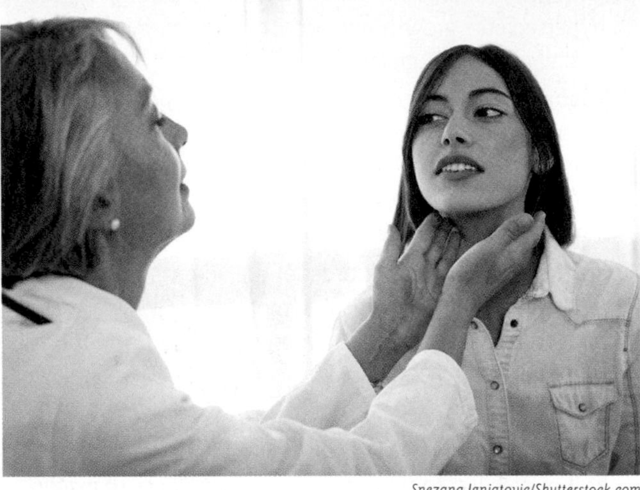

Snezana Ignjatovic/Shutterstock.com

Figure 8.22 Endocrinologists work to diagnose and treat hormonal disorders.

Physician Assistant

Physician assistants (PAs) practice medicine under the direction and observation of physicians and surgeons. Although they are formally trained to examine and treat patients, physician assistants do not attend medical school. Physician assistants diagnose and treat injuries and illnesses, take patients' medical histories, order and interpret test results, and give vaccinations. In some states they are allowed to write prescriptions. One example of the difference between a physician assistant and a doctor is that a physician assistant may perform the "prep" work on a patient right before surgery (making the opening incision), but a doctor performs the surgery.

To become a physician assistant, candidates must earn a bachelor's degree that includes coursework in biology, chemistry, anatomy and physiology, and other science-based courses. PAs must also complete an accredited two- to three-year physician assistant master's program and pass a national licensing exam.

PAs work in hospitals, clinics, emergency rooms, surgery centers, private physicians' offices, and schools. PAs may treat patients when a doctor is unavailable—for example, during house calls, nursing home visits, or rural or inner-city clinics that a doctor might not visit daily (**Figure. 8.23**). In these circumstances, PAs communicate with the supervising physician on staff or other medical personnel as necessary, or as required by law.

Planning for a Health-Related Career

Do some research on the career of a physician assistant or an endocrinologist. Keep in mind that many practice specialties are available to endocrinologists. Some endocrinologists may focus on researching and treating one disease in particular—for example, diabetes mellitus or thyroid disorders. If you are a person with good problem-solving skills, these two career options require a person with good analytical skills.

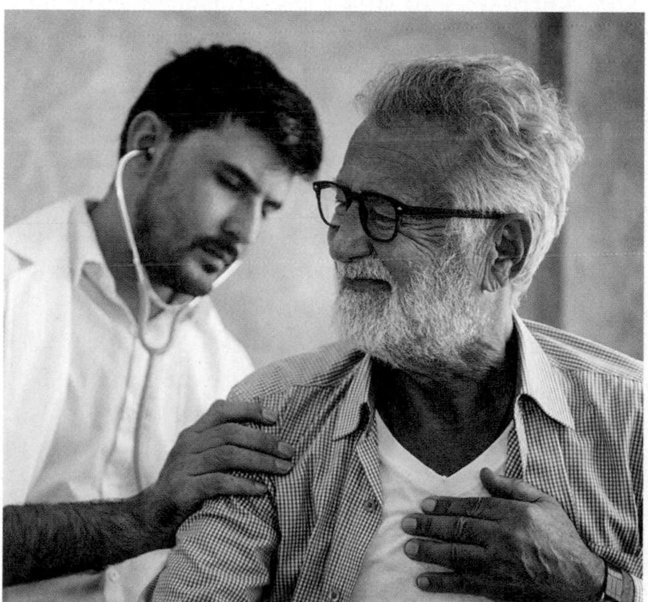

K.D.P./Shutterstock.com

Figure 8.23 Many physician assistants work in senior clinics and other walk-in clinics.

You may choose instead to research a profession from the list of related career options. Using the Internet or resources at your local library, find answers to the following questions:

1. What are the main tasks and responsibilities of this job?
2. What is the outlook for this career? Are workers in demand, or are jobs dwindling? For complete information, consult the current edition of the *Occupational Outlook Handbook*, published by the US Department of Labor. This handbook is available online or at your local library.
3. What special skills or talents are required? For example, do you need to be good at biology and chemistry? Do you need to enjoy interacting with other people?
4. What personality traits do you think are needed to be successful in this job? For example, a career as a physician assistant requires collaboration with other people, particularly a supervising doctor. Do you enjoy teamwork?
5. Does this career involve a great deal of routine, or are the day-to-day responsibilities varied?
6. Does the work require long hours, or is it a standard, "9-to-5" job?
7. What is the salary range for this job?
8. What do you think you would like about the career? Is there anything about it that you might dislike?

Related Career Options

- Gynecologist
- Nurse practitioner
- Occupational therapist
- Occupational therapy aide
- Paramedic
- Pediatrician
- Pharmacist
- Physician
- Registered nurse
- Surgeon

CHAPTER 8

Review

LESSON 8.1

Functions and Control of the Endocrine System

Key Points

- The endocrine system is a collection of organs and small glands that secrete hormones that directly or indirectly influence all the functions of the body.
- The two basic categories of hormones are steroid hormones and non-steroid hormones.
- When a hormone binds with a receptor in or on a cell, the hormone can influence the activity of the cell in various ways.
- Hormone secretion is controlled in three different ways: neural control, hormonal control, and humoral control.

Key Terms

downregulated
epinephrine
hormonal control
hormones
humoral control
hypothalamic nonreleasing hormones
hypothalamic releasing hormones
insulin
neural control
non-steroid hormones
steroid hormones
upregulated

LESSON 8.2

Major Endocrine Organs

Key Points

- The hypothalamus collects information from every body system and integrates the responses of the nervous and endocrine systems to maintain homeostatic balance.
- The anterior pituitary secretes six different types of hormones; the posterior pituitary gland stores ADH and oxytocin.
- The thyroid gland secretes three hormones: thyroxine, triiodothyronine, and calcitonin.
- The parathyroid glands are located behind the thyroid gland and secrete parathyroid hormone.
- The adrenal medulla is part of the nervous system; the cortex secretes three steroid hormones, which regulate sodium, sugar, or sex hormone levels.
- The pancreas secretes hormones that regulate blood glucose levels.
- Other hormone-producing organs include the thymus, the pineal gland, and the male and female gonads.

Key Terms

adrenal cortex
adrenal medulla
adrenocorticotropin (ACTH)
aldosterone
androgens
antidiuretic hormone
calcitonin
catecholamines
cortisol
cortisone
estrogens
follicle-stimulating hormone (FSH)
glucagon
growth hormone (GH)
luteinizing hormone (LH)
melatonin
oxytocin
parathyroid hormone (PTH)
prolactin
thymosin
thyroid-stimulating hormone (TSH)
thyroxine (T_4)
triiodothyronine (T_3)
tropic hormones

➤ **LESSON 8.3**

Endocrine Disorders and Diseases

Key Points

- Major disorders of the pituitary gland include acromegaly, dwarfism, and diabetes insipidus.
- Major disorders of the thyroid gland are hyperthyroidism (goiter and Graves disease, for example), and hypothyroidism.
- Parathyroid gland disorders affect calcium levels in the blood.
- A tumor on the adrenal medulla can cause life-threatening hypersecretion of the hormones epinephrine and norepinephrine; abnormal levels of hormones from the adrenal cortex are responsible for Cushing syndrome and Addison disease.
- Diabetes mellitus results from the inability of the pancreas to produce sufficient amounts of insulin to regulate blood glucose levels.

Key Terms

acromegaly
Addison disease
Cushing syndrome
diabetes insipidus
diabetes mellitus (DM)
dwarfism
exophthalmos
goiter
Graves disease
hypercalcemia
hyperglycemia
hyperthyroidism
hypothyroidism
insulin resistance
ketoacidosis
myxedema
neonatal hypothyroidism
peripheral neuropathy
tetany
thyroiditis

Assessment

➤ **LESSON 8.1**

Functions and Control of the Endocrine System

Learning Key Terms and Concepts

1. The chemical messengers secreted by the endocrine glands are _____.
   A. electrolytes
   B. enzymes
   C. hormones
   D. lacrimals
2. Which of the following is *not* an example of an exocrine gland?
   A. salivary glands
   B. sweat glands
   C. mammary glands
   D. adrenal glands
3. _____ glands are glands that have ducts through which hormones are transported to other organs or to the surface of the body.
   A. Exocrine
   B. Humoral
   C. Neural
   D. Endocrine
4. What are lipid-based hormones called?
   A. steroid hormones
   B. hypothalamic hormones
   C. non-steroid hormones
   D. glucagon
5. Receptors for _____ hormones are found on the surfaces of cells.
   A. lipid
   B. steroid
   C. carbohydrate
   D. non-steroid

6. The hormone epinephrine is under _____ control.
   A. hormonal
   B. neural
   C. electrical
   D. humoral
7. Which endocrine gland maintains the body's homeostatic set point at 98.6°F (37°C)?
   A. hypothalamus
   B. pituitary gland
   C. adrenal glands
   D. pancreas

Thinking Critically

8. The body's fight-or-flight response can be triggered in situations that pose no real physical threat or danger. For example, think about the last time you were very anxious in a social situation. What physical sensations did you feel? Relate your sensations to the description of the fight-or-flight response in the chapter.
9. Compare and contrast the three control systems (neural, hormonal, and humoral) of the endocrine system.
10. How do hormones help maintain homeostasis?
11. What does the hypothalamus do to help maintain homeostasis when the body becomes too cold? What are the physical signs that it is doing its job?

› LESSON 8.2

Major Endocrine Organs

Learning Key Terms and Concepts

12. The hypothalamus is located _____.
    A. just below and to the right of the liver
    B behind the sternum, above the diaphragm
    C. deep inside the brain
    D. inside the thyroid gland
13. The hormone prolactin, which stimulates milk production in a nursing mother, is produced by the _____.
    A. adrenal cortex
    B. adrenal medulla
    C. anterior pituitary
    D. posterior pituitary
14. Of the six hormones secreted by the anterior pituitary gland, the two that are *not* tropic are GH and _____.
    A. ACTH
    B. prolactin
    C. follicle-stimulating hormone
    D. luteinizing hormone
15. Which two hormones are stored in the posterior pituitary?
    A. ADH and oxytocin
    B. ADH and LH
    C. TSH and oxytocin
    D. LH and oxytocin
16. Which of the following statements about the posterior pituitary gland is *true*?
    A. It is not a true endocrine gland.
    B. It stores the hormones prolactin and ADH.
    C. It is an extension of the brainstem.
    D. It produces the hormones oxytocin and FSH.
17. Antidiuretic hormone is responsible for which of the following effects?
    A. increasing urine output
    B. decreasing body fluid volume
    C. decreasing urine output
    D. decreasing water absorption
18. Which endocrine gland is located in front of the trachea?
    A. adrenal gland
    B. thymus gland
    C. pituitary gland
    D. thyroid gland
19. TSH is secreted by the pituitary gland and acts on the _____ gland.
    A. thymus
    B. thyroid
    C. adrenal
    D. parathyroid
20. Parathyroid hormone raises concentrations of _____ in the blood.
    A. oxygen
    B. potassium
    C. sodium
    D. calcium

21. Which organ is a part of the nervous system?
    A. adrenal medulla
    B. adrenal cortex
    C. anterior pituitary
    D. posterior pituitary
22. Another name for the hormone epinephrine is _____.
    A. aldosterone
    B. renin
    C. adrenaline
    D. cortisone
23. The hormones produced by the adrenal cortex that regulate sodium levels are known as _____.
    A. mineralocorticoids
    B. natriocorticoids
    C. glucocorticoids
    D. carbocorticoids
24. Which gland plays a key role in maintaining proper glucose levels in the blood?
    A. adrenal gland
    B. thymus
    C. pancreas
    D. thyroid gland
25. The purpose of the islets of Langerhans in the pancreas is to secrete _____.
    A. insulin and cortisone
    B. glucagon and insulin
    C. cortisone and aldosterone
    D. aldosterone and glucagon
26. Which gland secretes the hormone melatonin?
    A. pancreas
    B. parathyroid
    C. anterior pituitary
    D. pineal
27. _____ is the hormone responsible for sperm production and the development of the male reproductive system.
    A. Estrogen
    B. Epinephrine
    C. Progesterone
    D. Testosterone

Thinking Critically

28. Both antidiuretic hormone and aldosterone play major roles in blood pressure regulation. Explain the role of each hormone.
29. Explain the relationship between insulin and glucagon with regard to blood glucose levels.
30. Describe the process of gluconeogenesis and give examples of circumstances that may stimulate it.
31. What triggers the hypothalamus to release ADH? What "artificial" methods can be used to provide the same effect as ADH?

LESSON 8.3

Endocrine Disorders and Diseases

Learning Key Terms and Concepts

32. Unusually tall height, along with enlargement of the hands, feet, and facial features, are common symptoms of _____.
    A. goiter
    B. Graves disease
    C. acromegaly
    D. myxedema
33. When diagnosed at a young age, dwarfism is treated by administering supplemental _____.
    A. GH
    B. FSH
    C. ACTH
    D. LH
34. Which of the following disorders is *not* associated with growth hormone imbalance?
    A. acromegaly
    B. diabetes
    C. dwarfism
    D. gigantism
35. A goiter is caused by a lack of _____ in the diet.
    A. calcium
    B. phosphate
    C. sodium
    D. potassium
36. A person suffering from _____ would most likely have a goiter.
    A. myxedema
    B. diabetes insipidus
    C. hyperthyroidism
    D. hypocalcemia

37. Hypocalcemia can cause _____.
    A. diabetes
    B. leukemia
    C. elevated blood sugar levels
    D. tetany
38. Which of the following is *not* a common symptom of Cushing syndrome?
    A. weight gain
    B. moon-shaped face
    C. enlarged thyroid
    D. hypertension
39. Normal blood glucose levels fall in the range of 70 to _____ mg/dL.
    A. 500
    B. 105
    C. 80
    D. 135

Thinking Critically

40. A young woman is brought into a medical clinic by her husband. She complains of hyperactivity and weight loss. She also appears to be mentally sluggish and has difficulty concentrating when questioned by a nurse. There is a slight swelling in the anterior of her neck. Which condition do you suspect? What are some possible causes and treatment options?
41. Selik is experiencing extreme thirst, unexplained weight changes, mood changes, and fatigue. He also notices that minor cuts and injuries are taking longer than normal to heal. What disease might you suspect, given these symptoms? How could you confirm your suspicion?
42. What practice, common to the United States and several other countries, has reduced the incidence of goiters?

Building Skills and Connecting Concepts

Analyzing and Evaluating Data

Instructions: Use the bar graph from the Centers for Disease Control and Prevention (**Figure 8.24**) to answer the following questions.

43. How many new cases of type 1 diabetes mellitus occurred per 100,000 children under ten years of age? How many cases of type 2 occurred? What conclusion can you make from this data?
44. Which ethnic group experienced the highest number of new cases of type 1 diabetes? Which group experienced the fewest number of cases?
45. The number of new cases of type 2 diabetes increases dramatically in the 10 to 19 age group, as compared to the under 10 age group. Based on your reading of this chapter and any research you might need to do, develop reasons why new cases of type 2 diabetes mellitus are more prevalent in the older age group.

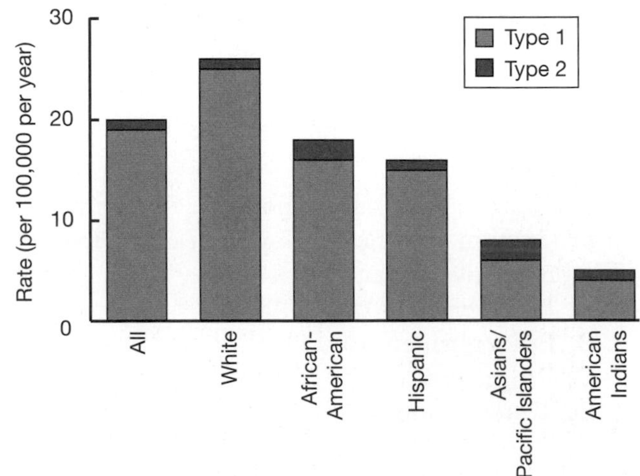

Figure 8.24 *Centers for Disease Control and Prevention (CDC)*

46. According to the CDC's Diabetes Fast Facts, 9.4% of the US population, or 30.3 million people, currently have diabetes. Of these, only 23.1 million people have been diagnosed. Use this information to create a bar graph showing the number of people who have diabetes, and the number and percentage of those people who are diagnosed and undiagnosed. Compare your graph with the text information in this question. Which method do you think would have more of an impact on people reading the facts? Explain your answer.

Communicating about Anatomy & Physiology

47. **Writing** In the competitive world of professional sports, athletes are sometimes tempted to take performance-enhancing drugs. One such drug is human growth hormone, a manufactured version of growth hormone. Research the use of human growth hormone by professional athletes. Identify an athlete who has tested positive for human growth hormone. How did this revelation affect his or her career? Excessive amounts of growth hormone can lead to acromegaly. Does human growth hormone also cause this disease? What other negative side effects does this drug have on the body? Create a presentation and share your findings with the class.
48. **Listening and Speaking** Listen closely as your classmates present their findings on human growth hormone. Take notes on anything you find particularly interesting, or write down any questions you think of during their presentations. Once they are finished presenting, share with the class one thought or question you had regarding their research.
49. **Speaking** Assume that you are the new CEO of a foundation to raise awareness about juvenile diabetes. Create a public service announcement that would make young people pay attention to the risks. Be creative—get their attention! Give your announcement to the class, being sure to vary the pitch and volume of your voice as appropriate to generate interest. To take it to the next level, see if your school will allow you to read it over the PA system.

Lab Investigations

50. Visit the Centers for Disease Control (CDC) website and research the prevalence of obesity and diagnosed diabetes among US adults. Working with another student or in a small group, prepare a report on the steady rise in obesity and diabetes in the United States. Start by making a list of states by region. Then study the most recent CDC maps. What trends do you notice about the link between obesity and diabetes throughout the United States? Share your findings with the class.
51. Research information on becoming a physician assistant. Create a flyer that will stimulate other students' interest in exploring this career. Include information on salary, schooling, and duties. Be creative; you may use clip art photos or graphics, but remember to comply with copyright laws. Talk to a school counselor to find out information about high school courses that could help a student prepare for a career as a physician assistant. Include a list of your references on the back of the flyer.
52. Using a commercial lab kit, perform a simulation of a blood glucose test. Follow the instructions in the kit. Then evaluate the lab experience. Was it realistic? What did you learn?

Building Your Portfolio

53. Gather the reports and presentations you created as you worked through this chapter. Place them in a document or folder called "The Endocrine System" and add this document to your personal portfolio.

CHAPTER

9 The Respiratory System

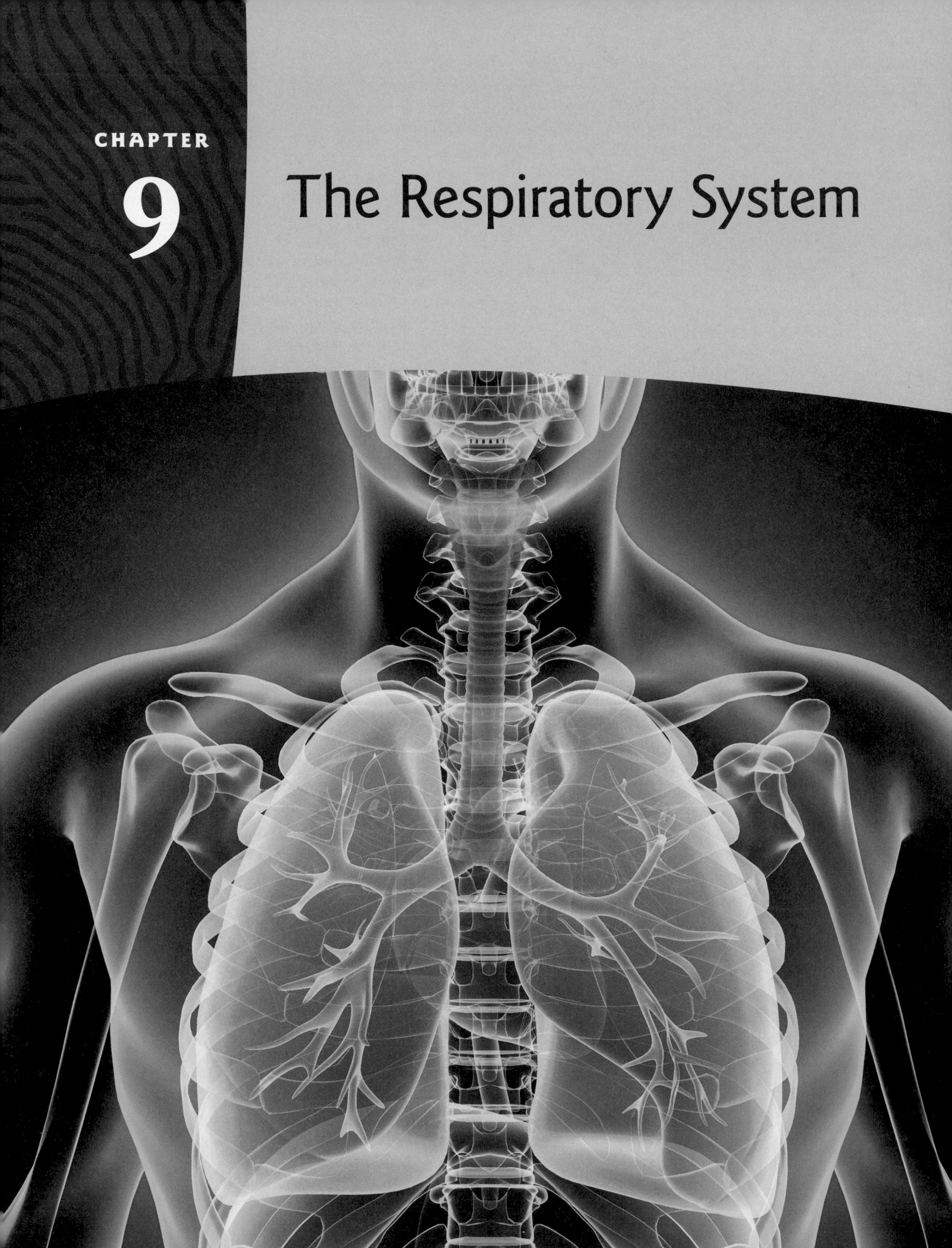

Can a larger lung volume contribute to athletic success?

Every breath you take puts your respiratory system in direct contact with the environment. Have you ever stopped to think about what your lungs are exposed to on a daily basis? Do you walk to school along a busy street and breathe in exhaust fumes from cars? Does a friend or relative expose you to secondhand smoke?

The respiratory system has a big job to do; appropriately, it is one of the largest organ systems in the body. The lungs contain about 1,500 miles of airways and almost 1,000 miles of capillaries. If you were to spread out the 300 million air sacs found in the lungs, they would nearly cover the surface of an entire tennis court. In fact, the surface area of your lungs is about 80 times greater than the surface area of your skin.

Because the body cannot go without oxygen for long, the respiratory system is vital to survival. Working with the cardiovascular system, the respiratory system ensures that a supply of fresh oxygen is always available, while removing harmful carbon dioxide from the body. This chapter explores the anatomy of the respiratory system and describes how it carries out the life-sustaining process of respiration.

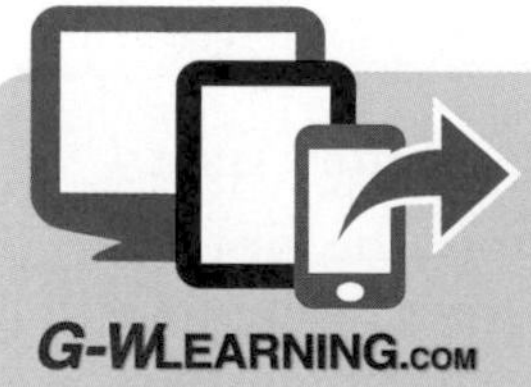

Click on the activity icon or visit www.g-wlearning.com/healthsciences/0202 to access online vocabulary activities using key terms from the chapter.

Chapter 9 Outline

◂ MDGRPHCS/Shutterstock.com

LESSON **9.1**

Anatomy of the Respiratory System

Before You Read

Try to answer the following questions before you read this lesson.

- Which organs and structures are part of the respiratory system?
- Where within the lungs does gas exchange take place, and why does it happen so effortlessly?

Lesson Objectives

- Name the structures of the upper respiratory tract.
- Understand the anatomy of the lower respiratory tract.

Key Terms

alveolar capillary membrane	pharynx
alveoli	pleural sac
bronchioles	pores of Kohn
epiglottis	primary bronchi
larynx	sinuses
mediastinum	surfactant
nares	thyroid cartilage
nasal conchae	tonsils
palate	trachea

Humans can survive for weeks without food and days without water, but only minutes without oxygen. In most cases, the brain will cease to function, and death will occur, after the brain has been deprived of oxygen for 5 to 6 minutes. However, there have been incidents in which individuals have survived for longer durations with effective CPR and emergency medical treatments.

The main purpose of the respiratory system is to provide body cells with a constant supply of oxygen, while at the same time eliminating carbon dioxide, a waste product, from the body. This process is called *gas exchange*.

The respiratory system (sometimes called the *pulmonary system*) works cooperatively with the cardiovascular system to conduct gas exchange. These two systems are often collectively referred to as the *cardiopulmonary system*.

The blood, which is pumped through the body by the cardiovascular system, acts as the transport vehicle for oxygen and carbon dioxide. Fresh oxygen from the lungs is delivered to all cells of the body. The body's cells discharge carbon dioxide into the bloodstream, which then carries the carbon dioxide to the lungs for elimination.

Most people understand why we need sufficient amounts of oxygen, but they do not realize that removal of carbon dioxide from the body is equally important. Excessive levels of carbon dioxide can be toxic to the body, causing damage to cells and organs and even resulting in death.

The Upper Respiratory Tract

The major organs of the respiratory system include the nose, pharynx, larynx, trachea, bronchi, bronchioles, and lungs (**Figure 9.1**). The respiratory system is divided into two parts: the upper respiratory tract and the lower respiratory tract. The upper respiratory tract includes the nose, mouth, nasal cavity, pharynx, and larynx.

The structures of the upper respiratory tract not only serve as a passageway for air moving in and out of the lungs, but also perform other vital functions:

- filter and remove foreign particles from inspired (inhaled) air
- humidify and control the temperature of the inspired air
- produce sound (voice)
- provide a sense of smell (olfactory sense)
- aid in immune defense
- conduct air to the lower respiratory tract

As a result of these functions, the air that reaches the structures of the lower respiratory tract is warm, moist, and filtered—important qualities for the health of the lungs.

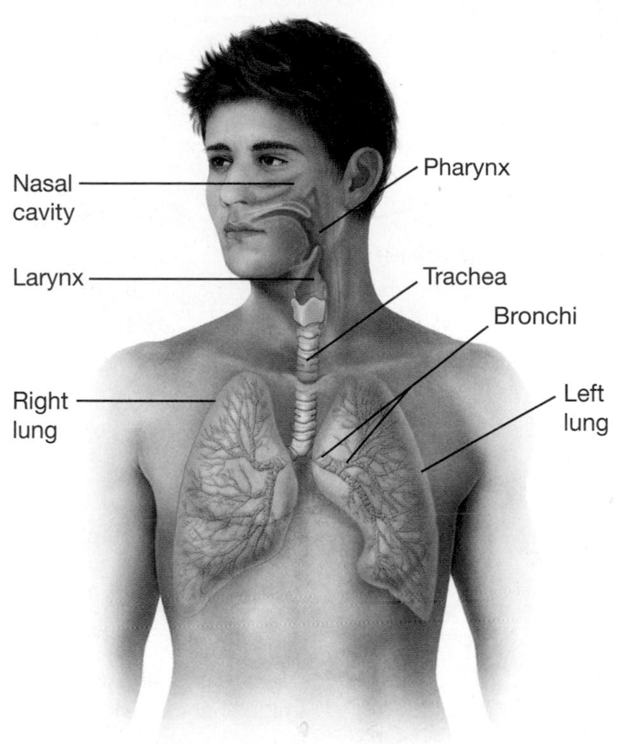

© Body Scientific International

Figure 9.1 Simplified overview of the major respiratory structures. *What is another name for the respiratory system?*

The Nose

The nose is the only part of the respiratory system that is external to the body. During inspiration (inhalation, or breathing in), air enters the nose through two openings called **nares**, or *nostrils*. As you read about the anatomy of the nose and its internal structures, refer to **Figure 9.2**.

The nose comes in many shapes and sizes. The nose's prominent location makes rhinoplasty (surgical modification of the nose) one of the most commonly performed plastic surgeries. Reconstructive rhinoplasty is performed to correct breathing issues associated with birth defects or trauma to the nose. Cosmetic rhinoplasty is performed to change the shape or appearance of the nose.

The Nasal Cavity

As you may recall from Chapter 1, the nasal cavity occupies the space behind the nose. It is divided into right and left chambers by the nasal septum.

The nasal cavity is lined with mucous membranes that filter and purify inspired air. At the front of the nasal cavity, just inside each naris (the singular form of *nares*), is the *vestibular* (vehs-TIB-yoo-lar) *region*. This region contains oily, coated nasal hairs called *cilia*, which trap and prevent particles from entering the nose.

Along the mucous membrane that lines the roof of the nasal cavity is an area called the *olfactory region*. Olfactory receptors located in this region provide your sense of smell. Your sense of smell is closely tied to your sense of taste. The next time you have a stuffy nose and your sense of taste seems "off," an accumulation of mucus on your olfactory receptors may be the culprit. Refer to Chapter 7 for more information about how the gustatory and olfactory senses work together.

The rest of the nasal cavity is called the *respiratory cavity*, despite the fact that no respiration occurs there. The respiratory region is lined with a mucosal membrane occupied by a dense network of thinly walled veins. This mucosal membrane warms the air that you breathe, but the thin walls of these veins and their location can cause nosebleeds.

Conchae

Three uneven, scroll-like **nasal conchae** (KAHN-kee) bones extend down through the nasal cavity. The conchae are categorized based on their location in the nasal cavity: superior, middle, and inferior conchae. These bones create three passageways that greatly increase the surface area available for filtering inspired air.

The conchae also increase the turbulence of the airflow in the nasal passage. This movement of air allows more particles to be trapped in the mucous membranes that line the nasal cavity and the conchae. If you have ever flown in an airplane, there is a good chance that you have experienced turbulence. When a plane is subjected to turbulent airflow, the ride is bumpy. The erratic movement of the plane is similar to the turbulent movement of inspired air when it enters the conchae.

The Palate

The **palate** (PAL-at) is the roof of the mouth, which separates the mouth from the nasal cavity. The anterior part of the palate is supported by bone; for this reason, it is called the *hard palate*.

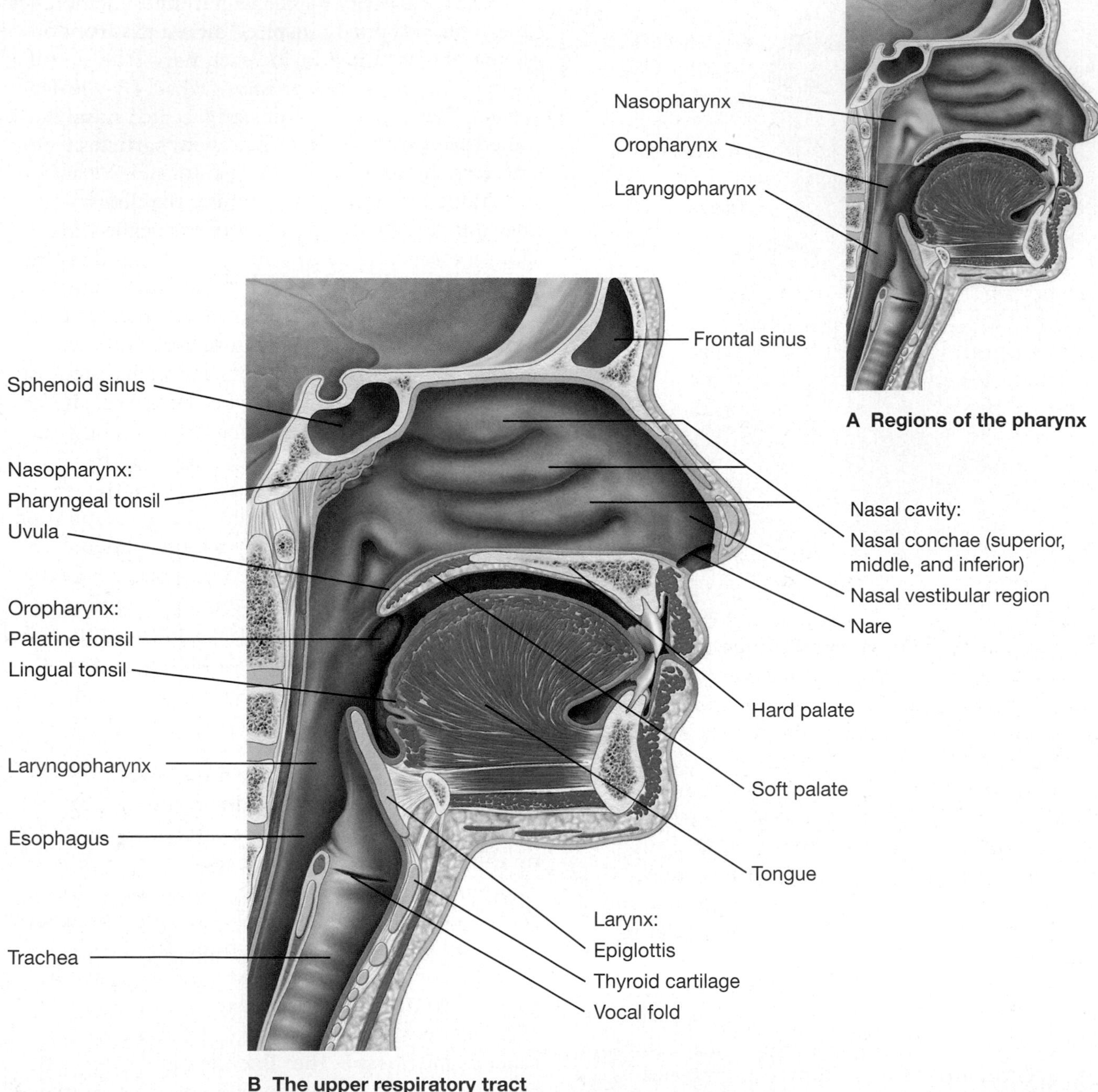

Figure 9.2 Detailed overview of the major structures of the upper respiratory tract. A—Regions of the pharynx. B—The upper respiratory tract. *What normally passes through the pharynx? How might you describe the air that reaches the lower respiratory tract as a result of the work done by the upper respiratory tract?*

The posterior palate is called the *soft palate* because it is composed of soft muscle and tissue and is unsupported by bone.

Hanging from the end of the soft palate is the uvula, a small, conical mass of connective tissue and muscle fibers. The uvula is believed to play a small role in speech, but it also helps prevent food from entering the nasal cavity.

When the parts of the palate do not completely fuse together during fetal development, a *cleft palate* is the result. The upper lip can also be cleft, or separated. A cleft palate or lip leaves an opening in the roof of the mouth or a gap between the lip and nose. This condition occurs in 1 out of every 700 babies. Surgery to close and repair the cleft palate or lip typically fixes this problem.

The Sinuses

The **sinuses** are air-filled cavities that surround the nose. They are lined with mucous membranes and are connected to the nasal cavities by ducts that drain into the nose.

There are four sinuses. Each is named for the bone on which it lies: the *frontal sinus*, *ethmoidal sinus*, *sphenoidal sinus*, and *maxillary sinus* (**Figure 9.3**).

The sinuses lighten the weight of the head, warm and moisten inspired air, and amplify, or strengthen, the tone of the voice. Have you ever noticed how "nasal" a person's voice becomes during a sinus infection? That is because an infection causes the sinuses to become swollen and filled with fluid and bacteria. This prevents the voice from projecting in its normal tone.

The Pharynx

The **pharynx** (FAIR-ingks) is a muscular passageway that transports air, food, and liquids from the nasal and oral cavities to the trachea and esophagus. Thus, it is part of both the respiratory system and the digestive system. The pharynx, commonly called the *throat*, is approximately 12.7 centimeters (5 inches) long. The pharynx is composed of an upper section called the *nasopharynx* (nay-zoh-FAIR-ingks), a middle section called the *oropharynx* (ohr-oh-FAIR-ingks), and a lower region called the *laryngopharynx* (la-ring-goh-FAIR-ingks).

The nasopharynx is located behind the nasal cavity, superior and posterior to the soft palate. The Eustachian tubes of the middle ear drain into the nasopharynx. Because of this connection, an inner ear infection can cause an upper respiratory infection, or vice versa. Whereas air is the only thing that passes through the nasopharynx, the oropharynx and laryngopharynx are passageways for air, food, and liquid.

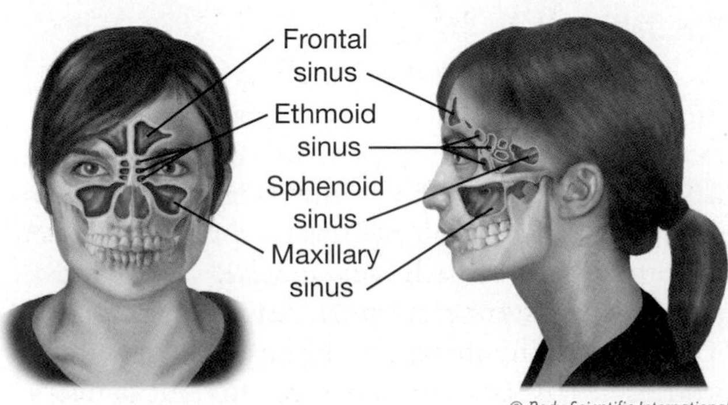

Figure 9.3 Front and side views of the sinuses. *Where do the names of the sinuses come from?*

The Tonsils

The **tonsils** are clusters of lymphatic tissue in the pharynx. The pharyngeal tonsil is located in the upper part of the nasopharynx; the palatine and lingual tonsils lie in the upper portion of the oropharynx.

The tonsils are a first line of defense against infection. When bacteria and other pathogens enter the throat, they become trapped in the tonsils. This is why the tonsils themselves can become infected and inflamed, causing a condition called *tonsillitis*.

The Larynx

The **larynx** (LAIR-ingks), or voice box, routes air and food to the proper passageways and houses the structures that produce speech. It is a triangular-shaped space located inferior to the pharynx. The larynx is composed of eight cartilaginous plates. The largest plate, the **thyroid cartilage**, is commonly called the *Adam's apple*. Below the thyroid cartilage is a ring of cartilage known as the *cricoid cartilage*.

At the top of the larynx is a flap of cartilaginous tissue called the **epiglottis** (ehp-i-GLAHT-is), which lies between the root of the tongue and the larynx. The epiglottis acts as a "gatekeeper" by controlling the destination of ingested food and liquid and inspired air. As food or liquid is swallowed, the epiglottis covers the opening of the larynx, preventing the substance from entering the trachea. If food or liquid does enter the trachea, a cough is triggered to expel the substance so that it does not enter the lungs. When you are not swallowing food or liquid, the epiglottis allows air to flow freely into the lower respiratory tract.

The structures that produce the distinctive sound of your voice are located in the larynx. The larynx is lined with a mucous membrane that forms a pair of folds called the *vocal cords*. Between the vocal cords is a space called the *glottis*, which gives the vocal cords room to vibrate. When air enters the vocal cords, they vibrate, producing sound. The ventricular folds are similar to the true vocal cords, but do not play a role in voice production, so they are also known as *false vocal cords*.

Check Your Understanding

1. List the structures that make up the respiratory system.
2. Besides serving as a passageway for air, what functions do the structures of the upper respiratory tract perform?
3. Which two structures does the palate separate?
4. The pharynx is a part of which two body systems?
5. What are the two major functions of the larynx?

The Lower Respiratory Tract

The lower respiratory tract consists of the trachea, bronchi, bronchioles, and lungs. The lungs contain alveoli (al-VEE-oh-ligh), air sacs in which the important gas-exchange function occurs.

The Trachea

The **trachea** (TRAY-kee-uh), also called the *windpipe*, extends about 10 centimeters (4 inches) from the end of the larynx to the fifth thoracic vertebra (mid-chest). The walls of the trachea are lined with a mucous membrane that contains ciliated epithelium, a covering with tiny, hair-like structures. The ciliated epithelium continuously sweeps foreign matter (such as dust) upward toward the larynx and pharynx, where it can be swallowed or coughed up.

The walls of the trachea are reinforced by a series of cartilaginous, C-shaped rings (**Figure 9.4**). The rings are made of rigid cartilage that provides support for the anterior side of the trachea and prevents the airway from collapsing. However, the rings are open on the posterior side of the trachea. This provides a flexible area that allows the trachea to expand. The C-shaped rings serve two functions. The cartilage provides support and prevents the airway from collapsing, and the opening posterior to the rings allows the trachea to expand. This flexibility is helpful when large food particles pass through the esophagus, the structure that lies behind the trachea.

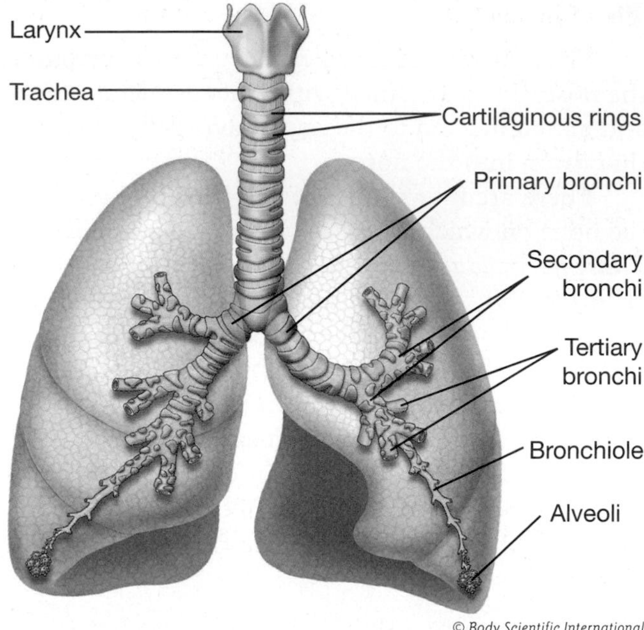

Figure 9.4 The larynx, trachea, and bronchial tree. The cartilaginous rings of the trachea continue throughout the passageways, ending at the bronchioles.

The Bronchi

At its bottom end, the trachea divides into right and left **primary bronchi** (BRAHNG-kigh). The primary bronchi lead to the right and left lungs. The wider, shorter bronchus (singular form of *bronchi*) on the right also hangs more vertically than the left bronchus. Because of these structural differences, inhaled substances are more likely to become lodged in the right bronchus. This understanding of the shape of the bronchi has helped doctors quickly locate and remove inhaled objects, preventing many choking deaths.

The bronchi subdivide into Y-shaped, smaller branches called the *secondary* and *tertiary bronchi*, until they end in the smallest air-conducting passageway—the **bronchioles** (BRAHNG-kee-ohls). The walls of the bronchial branches—but not the walls of the bronchioles—are reinforced by cartilaginous rings. The increasingly smaller branches of the bronchi are often compared to the branches of a tree. This is why the lungs are sometimes referred to as the *respiratory tree*.

The Alveoli

The bronchi and bronchioles are collectively known as the *conducting zone* because they are passageways that conduct air to and from the lungs. The terminal bronchioles lead into the *respiratory zone*. The respiratory zone contains the respiratory bronchioles, *alveolar ducts*, and grape-like clusters of **alveoli**. A limited amount of gas exchange occurs in the respiratory bronchioles, which are connected to the clusters of alveoli by the alveolar ducts.

The alveoli, or air-filled sacs, are the main sites of gas exchange in the lungs. Millions of alveoli clusters make up the bulk of the lung tissue. The alveoli walls are composed of a very thin layer of squamous epithelial cells. The interior of these walls is coated with **surfactant**, a phospholipid. Surfactant reduces the surface tension in the alveoli and prevents them from collapsing.

The internal environment of the alveoli is kept clean and healthy by bacteria-ingesting cells called *macrophages*. Gases and macrophages travel between alveoli via the **pores of Kohn**, small openings in the alveolar wall.

The Alveolar Capillary Membrane

The alveoli and the capillaries that surround them make up the **alveolar** (al-VEE-oh-lar) **capillary membrane** (**Figure 9.5**). The alveolar capillary membrane is built for gas exchange. Oxygen easily diffuses across the membrane of the alveolar sacs into the capillaries, and carbon dioxide passes from the blood into the alveolar sac.

Gas exchange occurs rapidly for a few reasons. First, the surface area of the lungs is immense. If we were to lay the alveolar sacs side by side on the ground, they would cover almost the whole length of a tennis court. The millions of alveolar sacs provide an almost unlimited number of sites for gas exchange between the blood and alveolar sacs.

Second, the oxygen and carbon dioxide molecules only have to travel from the red blood cell, through the capillary wall and its membrane, and then through the alveolar wall and its membrane. These membranes are razor thin—thinner than even a sheet of tissue paper. This razor-thin quality makes it easy for oxygen and carbon dioxide to move freely between the alveoli and the bloodstream.

The third reason that gas exchange occurs rapidly is that gases always diffuse from areas of high concentration to areas of low concentration. Carbon dioxide has a high concentration in the capillary blood, but its concentration in the lungs is low. As a result, carbon dioxide diffuses rapidly from the blood into the alveolar sacs.

By contrast, there is a high concentration of oxygen in the alveolar sacs of the lungs, and a low concentration in the capillary blood. Thus, oxygen readily diffuses into the blood, where it binds with hemoglobin molecules in the red blood cells.

So just how fast does gas exchange occur in the lungs? Faster than you might think. Your blood becomes 98% oxygenated in 0.75 second—in about the blink of an eye!

The Lungs

The lungs are large organs that occupy almost the entire thoracic (chest) cavity (**Figure 9.6**). The **mediastinum** (mee-dee-uh-STIGH-num),

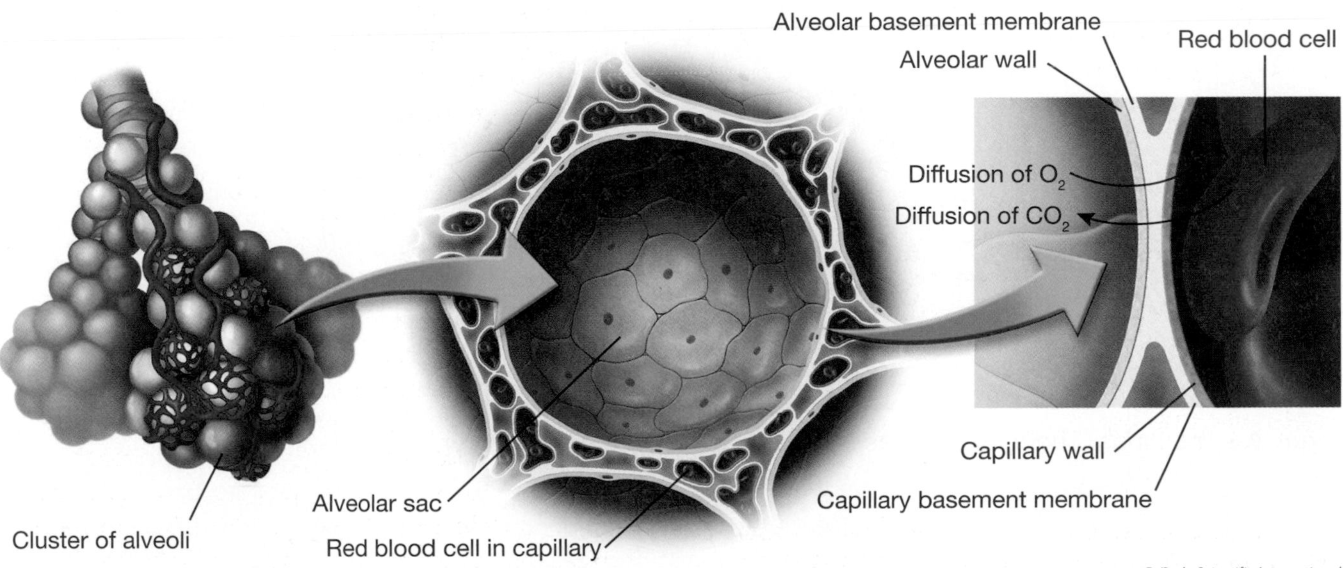

Figure 9.5 Lung tissue is made up of millions of alveoli clusters. Pulmonary gas exchange occurs rapidly because the capillary walls of the alveolar sacs are much thinner than even a sheet of tissue paper. *What are other reasons that gas exchange occurs very rapidly?*

the central area of the thoracic cavity, lies between the lungs. It houses the heart, great blood vessels, trachea, esophagus, thoracic duct, thymus gland, and other structures. The mediastinum creates a deep, concave (rounded inward) indentation along the border of the left lung.

The upper part of the lung, called the *apex*, is located just below the clavicle, or collarbone. The broad base of the lung rests on the diaphragm. The lungs are divided into lobes by fissures. The right lung has three lobes: the superior, middle, and inferior lobes. The left lung has only two lobes: the superior left lobe and inferior left lobe.

Most of the tissue in the lungs is filled with air. In fact, the lungs weigh only 2.5 pounds and would float if placed in water.

The lungs are surrounded by a thin, double-walled **pleural sac**. The pleural sac is composed of two slippery, serous membranes. One membrane, the *parietal pleura*, lines the thoracic wall and diaphragm. The other membrane, the *visceral pleura*, covers the lungs and dips into the fissures. Both pleural membranes secrete a serous, or watery, fluid that allows the two linings to slide smoothly against each other as the lungs expand and contract during respiration. The serous fluid also acts like glue, keeping the two linings from pulling apart. The area between the two membranes is known as the *pleural space*, or *pleural cavity*.

Check Your Understanding

1. Which structures are included in the lower respiratory tract?
2. What is the purpose of surfactant in the alveoli?
3. Name the two layers of the pleural sac.

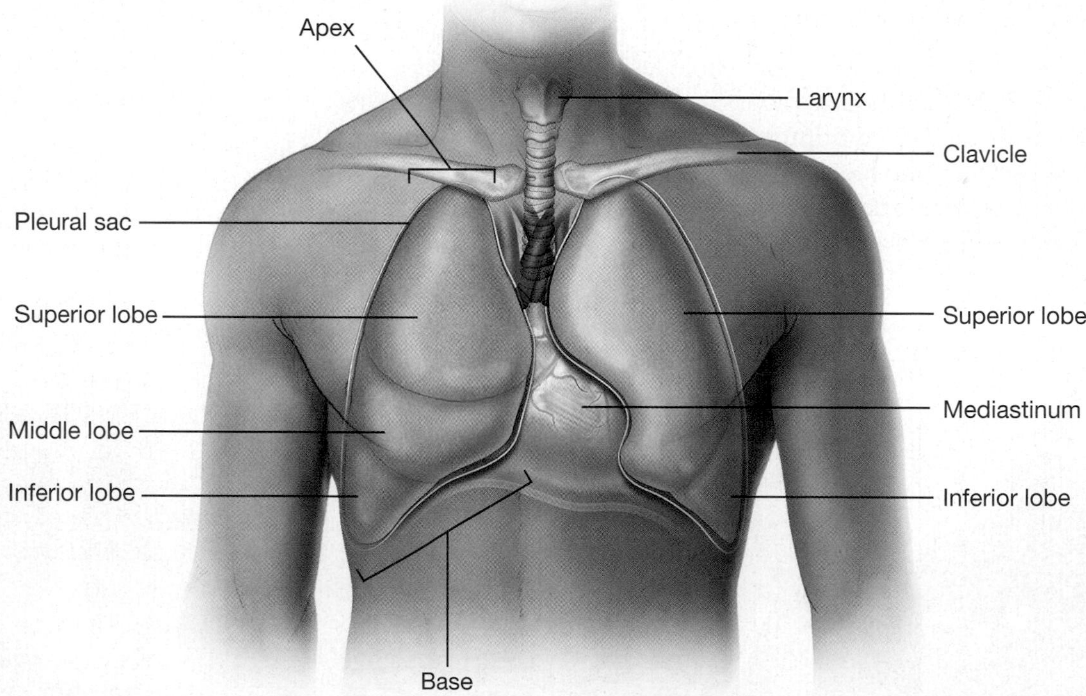

Figure 9.6 The lungs. The right lung has three lobes, but the left lung has only two lobes.

LESSON 9.1 Review and Assessment

Mini Glossary

Make sure that you know the meaning of each key term.

alveolar capillary membrane gas-exchange structure that contains the alveoli and the capillaries surrounding the alveoli

alveoli air sacs in the lungs from which gas is exchanged with the capillaries

bronchioles the thin-walled branches of the bronchi; the smallest air-conducting passageways of the bronchi. The terminal bronchioles conduct a small amount of gas exchange in the respiratory zone.

epiglottis a flap of cartilaginous tissue that covers the opening to the trachea; diverts food and liquids to the esophagus during swallowing

larynx a triangular-shaped space inferior to the pharynx that is responsible for voice production; the *voice box*

mediastinum the area of the thoracic cavity between the lungs; houses the heart, great blood vessels, trachea, esophagus, thoracic duct, thymus gland, and other structures

nares the two openings in the nose through which air enters; nostrils

nasal conchae three uneven, scroll-like nasal bones that extend down through the nasal cavity

palate the structure consisting of hard and soft components that separates the oral and nasal cavities; the *roof of the mouth*

pharynx the muscular passageway that extends from the nasal cavity to the mouth and connects to the esophagus; *the throat*

pleural sac the thin, double-walled serous membrane that surrounds the lungs

pores of Kohn small openings in the alveolar walls that allow gases and macrophages to travel between the alveoli

primary bronchi the two passageways that branch off the trachea and lead to the right and left lungs

sinuses the air-filled cavities that surround the nose

surfactant a phospholipid that reduces the surface tension in the alveoli and prevents them from collapsing

thyroid cartilage the largest cartilaginous plate in the larynx; the *Adam's apple*

tonsils clusters of lymphatic tissue in the pharynx that function as the first line of defense against infection

trachea the air tube that extends from the larynx into the thorax, where it splits into the right and left bronchi; the *windpipe*

Know and Understand

1. What is the main purpose of the respiratory system?
2. What is the job of the cilia in the nasal cavity?
3. Describe the two parts of the palate.
4. Which structures are housed in the larynx?
5. Which structures provide rigid support for the trachea and prevent it from collapsing?
6. Why are the bronchi and bronchioles together called the *conducting zone*?
7. How many lobes does each lung have?

Analyze and Apply

8. Explain why a person's sense of taste is diminished when he or she has a stuffy nose.
9. Imagine that you are a physician and one of your patients recently gave birth to an infant with a cleft palate and lip. How would you explain this condition and the treatment required?
10. In what way does the epiglottis function as a gatekeeper?
11. Consider all of the functions of the sinuses. Which one function do you consider most important? Why?

IN THE LAB

12. Working in a group of three or four students, create a clay model of the respiratory system. Use different colored clay for each organ. Once you have created individual pieces for each major structure, connect all the clay organs to form the respiratory system. Then create a label for each organ. Share your model with other groups in your class.
13. Children are born every day with cleft palates, and repair can take up to 3 years. Press your tongue against your hard palate, on the roof of your mouth. If the palate were not there, where would your tongue go? Make a list of the problems you think a baby with a cleft palate would have. Use your imagination and design a piece of equipment to fix one of those problems. Sketch out your design and explain it in writing to a new parent.

LESSON 9.2 Respiration: Mechanics and Control

Before You Read

Try to answer the following questions before you read this lesson.

- Which muscles are used for breathing?
- How do oxygen and carbon dioxide levels regulate your breathing?

Lesson Objectives

- Understand the mechanics of respiration.
- Explain how breathing is affected by neural, chemical, and emotional factors as well as conscious control.
- Identify different methods of measuring lung volume and how each method works.

Key Terms

central chemoreceptors
expiration
expiratory reserve volume (ERV)
external respiration
forced expiratory volume in one second (FEV_1)
forced expiratory volume in one second/forced vital capacity (FEV_1/FVC)
functional residual capacity (FRC)
Hering-Breuer reflex
inspiration
inspiratory reserve volume (IRV)
internal respiration
mechanoreceptors
peripheral chemoreceptors
pulmonary ventilation
residual volume (RV)
respiration
respiratory gas transport
tidal volume (TV)
total lung capacity (TLC)
vital capacity (VC)

Every minute of every day, your respiratory system works hard to deliver oxygen and dispose of carbon dioxide. Breathing may seem like a subconscious action—something you are not even aware that you are doing—but there are actually many factors that control respiratory activity. This lesson explores the mechanics of breathing and the mechanisms by which it is controlled.

Respiration

As explained in Lesson 9.1, the main function of the respiratory system is gas exchange. Gas exchange is done through a process called **respiration**, or breathing.

The cardiovascular system and the respiratory system work together to accomplish respiration. This process involves four key tasks:

- **pulmonary ventilation**: air is continuously moved into and out of the lungs
- **external respiration**: fresh oxygen from outside (external to) the body fills the lungs and alveoli, allowing gas exchange between the alveoli and pulmonary blood capillaries
- **respiratory gas transport**: the oxygen and carbon dioxide gases in the blood are transported between the lungs and body tissues
- **internal respiration**: gas exchange occurs inside the body between the tissues and capillaries

This chapter describes the first two processes: pulmonary ventilation and external respiration. Respiratory gas transport and internal respiration are discussed in Chapters 10 and 11.

Boyle's Law

The mechanics of breathing can be explained by Boyle's law. Boyle's law states that the volume of a gas is inversely proportional to its pressure. In simpler terms, as the volume of a gas increases, the pressure of the gas decreases.

Boyle's law affects breathing because of differences between atmospheric (outside) air pressure and intrapulmonary (lung) air pressure. At rest, both atmospheric and intrapulmonary air pressures are 760 millimeters of mercury (mmHg). When these pressures are the same, lung volume, or the amount of air in the lungs, does not change. At this point, there is no airflow (**Figure 9.7**).

For the lungs to be able to take in air, the intrapulmonary pressure must be *less than* the atmospheric pressure. When the direction of airflow is reversed to expel air from the lungs, the intrapulmonary pressure must be *greater than* atmospheric pressure.

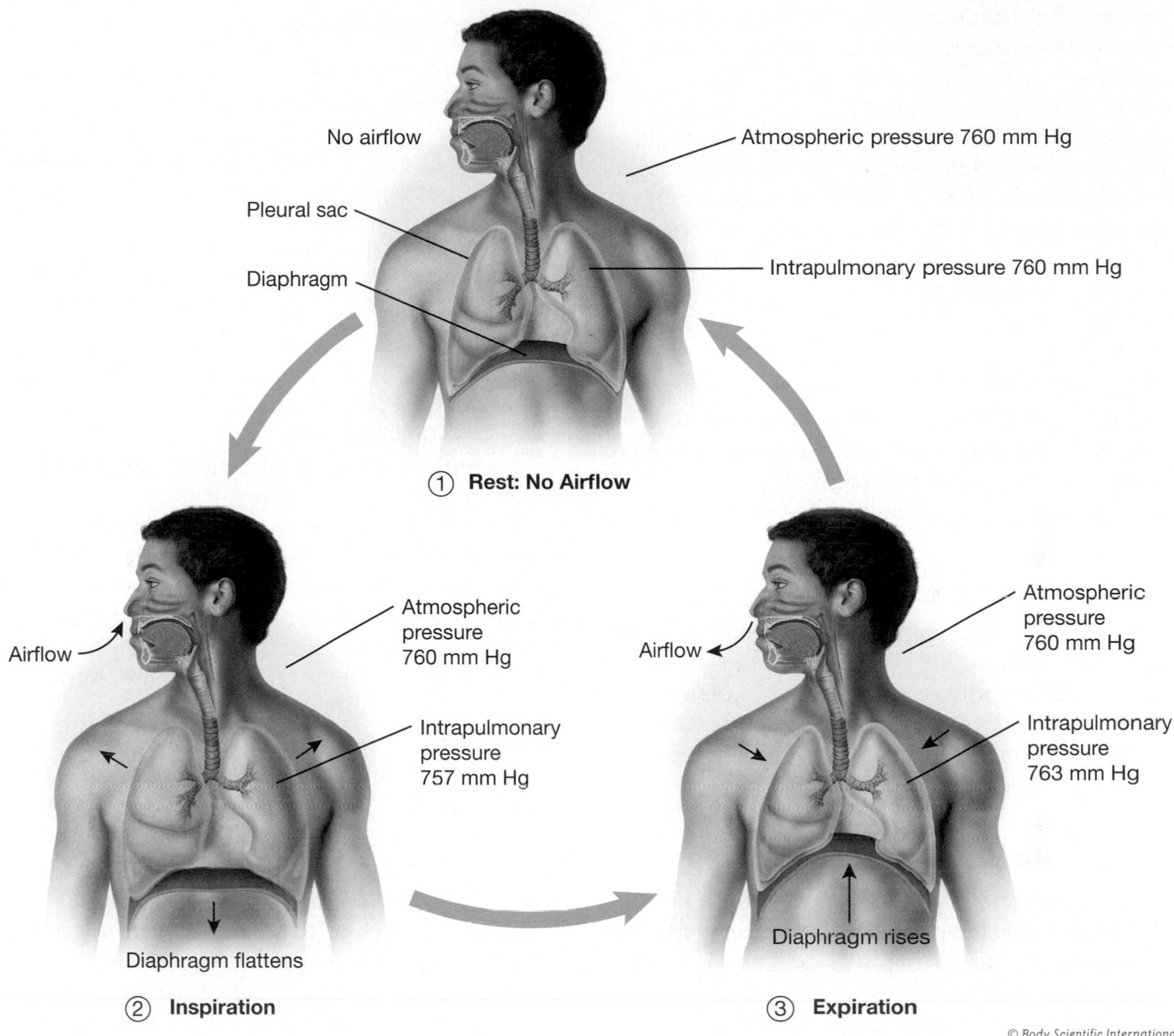

Figure 9.7 Changes in intrapulmonary and atmospheric pressure allow air to flow into and out of the lungs. *Explain the processes that cause intrapulmonary pressure to rise and fall.*

Inspiration

Inspiration is the process by which air flows into the lungs; it is also called *inhalation*. Inspiration begins when the external intercostal muscles contract, lifting the ribs upward and outward. At the same time, the dome-like diaphragm muscle contracts downward and flattens. Both of these maneuvers expand the thoracic cavity, decreasing its internal pressure. As the thoracic cavity expands, it pulls the lungs with it, and the lungs also expand.

As the lungs expand, the intrapulmonary pressure falls below the atmospheric pressure. When the intrapulmonary pressure is lower than the atmospheric pressure, a vacuum is created. The vacuum sucks air into the lungs until the pressure inside the lungs is equal to the atmospheric pressure.

Expiration

The process by which air is expelled from the lungs is called **expiration**, or *exhalation*. Expiration begins when the external intercostal muscles and the diaphragm relax, decreasing the space in the thoracic cavity and increasing the intrapulmonary pressure to 763 mmHg. When the intrapulmonary pressure exceeds the atmospheric pressure (760 mmHg), air is forced out of the lungs.

It is important to note that expiration does not require muscle contraction. This is because normal expiration is a *passive* process. When asthma or mucus accumulation narrows the respiratory passageways, or when your respiration rate increases during exercise, expiration becomes an *active* process. Active expiration requires the internal intercostal muscles to forcibly depress the rib cage to expel air from the lungs. At the same time, the abdominal muscles contract to push air out of the lungs.

Nonrespiratory Air Maneuvers

Did you know that a sneeze can travel up to 40 miles per hour? A sneeze is a nonrespiratory air maneuver. Besides breathing, there are other ways in which air moves into and out of the lungs.

You are familiar with coughing, sneezing, hiccupping, and yawning, but have you ever wondered why they happen? These nonrespiratory maneuvers often occur as a reaction, or reflexive response, to a stimulus, such as dust or debris, entering the respiratory passages. **Figure 9.8** explains how and why these nonrespiratory air maneuvers occur.

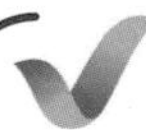

Check Your Understanding

1. What does Boyle's law state?
2. For inspiration to occur, must the intrapulmonary pressure be higher or lower than atmospheric pressure?
3. Which process—inspiration or expiration—normally requires muscle contractions?

Control of Breathing

Breathing is controlled mainly by neural and chemical factors, although emotions and conscious control play a small role. The average respiratory rate for adults at rest is 12 to 15 breaths per minute. The average respiratory rate varies based on biological and physical factors.

One biological factor that affects the way you breathe is gender. In general, women have higher respiratory rates because they have a smaller lung capacity than men. Age is another important biological factor. Infants take between 40 and 60 breaths each minute because they have a very small lung capacity.

A physical factor that influences respiratory rate is postural position (whether you are sitting or standing). When you move from a reclined position to a standing position, your breathing rate almost doubles. During maximal exercise, your respiratory rate can increase dramatically—by about 50 breaths per minute. However, respiration does not usually limit the exercise ability of people with healthy lungs.

Neural Factors

Rate and depth of breathing are controlled by inspiratory and expiratory breathing centers in the brain (**Figure 9.9**). These centers are located in the medulla oblongata and the pons, which are part of the brainstem.

The medulla oblongata and pons work as a team to make breathing a smooth, rhythmic process. The medulla is like the quarterback of the team, setting the normal breathing pace. By contrast, the pons is more of a utility player, fine-tuning respiratory rate and depth while also coordinating the transition between inspiration and expiration.

Nonrespiratory Air Maneuvers		
Air Maneuver	**Cause**	**Result**
cough	a need to clear dust or other debris from the lower respiratory tract	a deep breath closes the epiglottis, and then a forceful exhalation is performed
sneeze	a need to clear the upper respiratory passageways of dust or other debris	stimulation of nerve endings in the nasal passages trigger a reflex in the brain, causing the forceful expulsion of air through the nose and mouth
hiccup	an irritation of the phrenic nerves that causes the diaphragm muscle to spasm	sudden inspirations against the vocal cords of a closed glottis cause the hiccupping sound
yawn	thought to be caused by a need for increased oxygen in the lungs	prolonged, deep inspirations (taken with the jaws widely open) saturate the alveoli with fresh air

Figure 9.8 Goodheart-Willcox Publisher

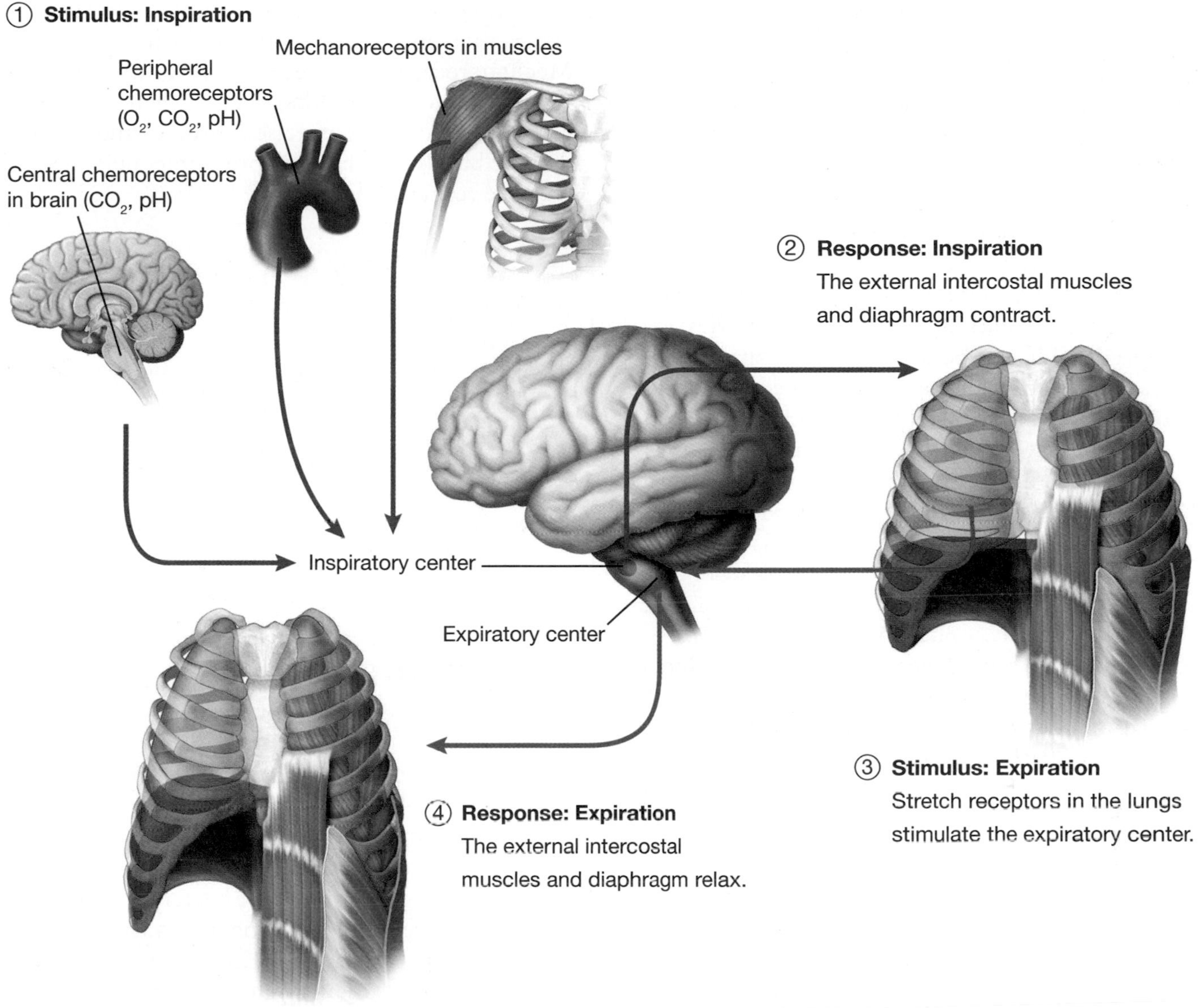

Figure 9.9 Regulation of breathing. The inspiratory and expiratory breathing centers, located in the medulla oblongata and pons, control the rate and depth of breathing. These centers are stimulated by sensory triggers (central chemoreceptors, peripheral chemoreceptors, and mechanoreceptors) and neural triggers (stretch receptors).

The medulla and pons work together to create a normal, rhythmic breathing pattern. The medullary inspiratory center stimulates the diaphragm and the external intercostals. This stimulation is achieved by afferent nerve impulses sent through the phrenic and intercostal nerves. As the lungs fill with air, stretch receptors in the bronchioles and alveoli trigger the **Hering-Breuer reflex** to prevent overinflation of the alveolar sacs. Once activated, the stretch receptors send nerve impulses to the medulla via the vagus nerve. These impulses alert the medulla to stop inspiration and start exhalation. The pons works to achieve smooth transitions between inspiration and expiration.

Chemical Factors

Most people don't think of oxygen and carbon dioxide as chemicals, but when it comes to respiration, that is how they are classified. Oxygen (O_2) and carbon dioxide (CO_2) are chemicals that influence the inspiratory and expiratory centers of the brain. Because oxygen is essential for maintaining life, you might think it exerts greater control over the rate and depth of breathing than carbon dioxide. However, as **Figure 9.9** shows, several chemical factors regulate breathing.

Central Chemoreceptors

Within the respiratory centers of the brain are sensory cells called **central chemoreceptors** (KEE-moh-ree-sehp-torz). Central chemoreceptors constantly monitor changes in the pH (acidity or alkalinity) of cerebrospinal fluid (CSF). A decrease in CSF pH indicates a high amount of carbon dioxide in the body.

When metabolism increases, oxygen consumption accelerates and the body produces more carbon dioxide. In excessive quantities, carbon dioxide can be dangerous because it can cross the blood-brain barrier, a protective border between brain tissues and circulating blood.

A high level of carbon dioxide increases the number of hydrogen ions in the body. These hydrogen ions cause the pH of the CSF to decrease. When the central chemoreceptors sense a decrease in pH, they stimulate the brain's inspiratory center by sending impulses to the inspiratory center via the vagus and glossopharyngeal nerves. When the inspiratory center receives this information, it stimulates an increase in the rate and depth of breathing. The result is a fresh supply of oxygen and a lower carbon dioxide level. As you can see, carbon dioxide is the chemical driving force behind respiration.

Peripheral Chemoreceptors

Located in the aorta and carotid arteries, **peripheral chemoreceptors** are sensitive to changes in blood oxygen level. Peripheral chemoreceptors are also mildly sensitive to carbon dioxide and pH, but less so than they are to oxygen. Like the central chemoreceptors, peripheral chemoreceptors stimulate respiration by sending sensory information to the brain via the vagus and glossopharyngeal nerves.

MEMORY TIP

Central chemoreceptors are sensitive to **C**arbon dioxide. Both of these terms start with C. **P**eripheral chemoreceptors are most sensitive to **O**xygen. P and O are close together in the alphabet.

Mechanoreceptors

Yet another type of sensory cells that play a role in regulating respiration are the **mechanoreceptors** (MEHK-a-noh-ree-sehp-torz). Located in muscles and joints, mechanoreceptors detect muscle contraction and force generation during exercise. Mechanoreceptors are responsible for the quick increase in ventilation that occurs when you first begin to exercise. As exercise continues and carbon dioxide builds up, the chemoreceptors help to regulate respiration.

Check Your Understanding

1. By which two types of factors is breathing mainly controlled?
2. What is the average breathing rate for adults?
3. How many breaths per minute does an infant take?
4. Where are the inspiratory and expiratory control centers located?
5. What processes do the inspiratory and expiratory centers control?

Lung Volume

Lung volume measurements are used to assess whether or not a person's lung capacity is normal. The total volume for a pair of healthy adult lungs is about six liters of air.

Do you think lung volume plays a major role in an athlete's success? Does the swimmer with the largest lung volume have a better chance of winning an event than the one with a smaller lung capacity? Before answering these questions, it is important to understand how to measure and interpret lung volume.

Lung volume varies according to age, height, weight, gender, and race. Therefore, it is important that an appropriate set of normative values be used as a reference source. There are two types of lung volume: static and dynamic. *Static lung volume* measures only volume at a fixed point in time; *dynamic lung volume* measures volume over a specific period of time. For instance, a dynamic lung volume measurement might assess the ability of the lungs to forcibly expire air in one second.

Static lung volume is measured by a *spirometer* (spigh-RAHM-eh-ter). Dynamic lung volume is measured using a *flow volume meter.*

Static Lung Volume

Measures of static lung volume are important because they can be used to determine whether a lung deficiency or disorder exists. In static lung volume measurement, a person performs a series of breathing maneuvers. First, the person is instructed to breathe normally for at least six breaths so that a measurement of **tidal volume (TV)** can be obtained. Tidal volume is the amount of air inhaled during a normal breath. Then, the person inspires maximally (breathes in as deeply as possible), followed by a maximal expiration. This last breathing maneuver helps identify the person's **vital capacity (VC)**, or the total amount of air that can be forcibly expired after a maximal inspiration.

The volume of air that never leaves the lungs, even after the most forceful expiration, is called the **residual volume (RV)**. Residual volume is important because it allows gas exchange to occur continuously between inspiration and expiration. Residual volume cannot be measured by a spirometer; it requires advanced measurement techniques.

Static lung volume can be measured in other ways:

- **functional residual capacity (FRC)**: the amount of air that remains in the lungs after a normal expiration; ERV + RV
- **inspiratory reserve volume (IRV)**: the amount of air that can be inhaled immediately after a normal inspiration
- **expiratory reserve volume (ERV)**: the amount of air that can be exhaled, or forced from the lungs, immediately after a normal expiration
- **total lung capacity (TLC)**: a combination of the vital capacity plus the residual volume; IRV + TV + ERV + RV (which usually measures about 6L of air)

Each of these forms of static lung volume measurement can be obtained with a spirometer except for the FRC, which requires more sophisticated equipment. See **Figure 9.10** for an example of spirometer test results of static lung volume. Test results are usually compared to normal values matched to the patient's age, height, weight, gender, and ethnicity.

Generally, lung volume does not predict the average athlete's performance. During maximal exercise, you use only about 65% of your lungs' vital capacity. Because high-intensity exercise does not require 100% of the lungs' vital capacity, lung volume is not a limiting factor for healthy individuals.

Dynamic Lung Volume

Dynamic lung volume is a measurement of flow rate during a forced vital capacity maneuver.

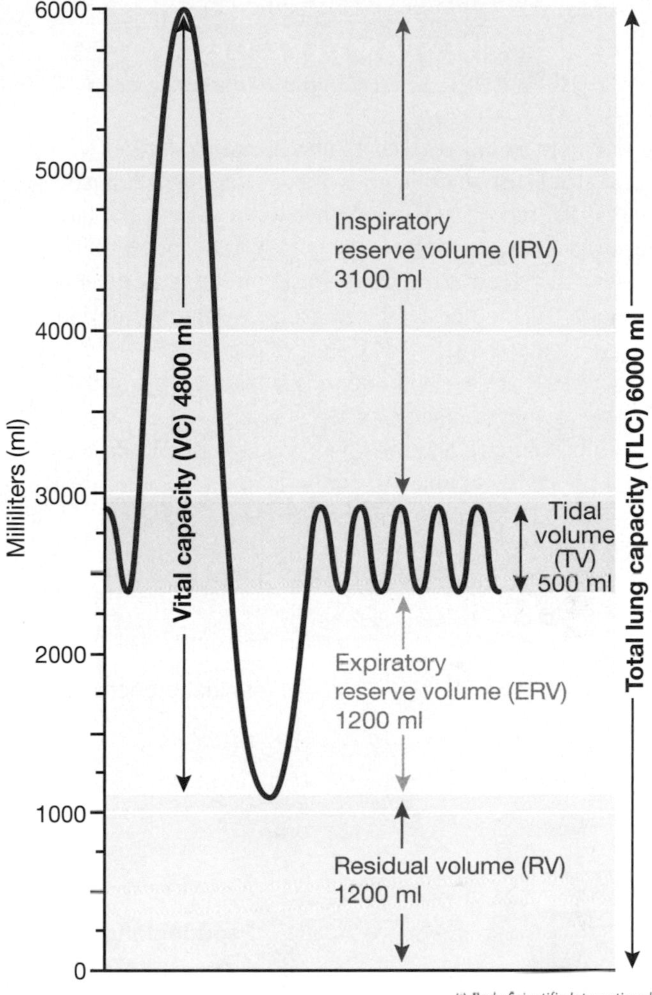

Figure 9.10 Lung volume chart. This lung volume tracing was obtained by a test using a spirometer. *How might a lung volume chart be used?*

Pulmonary function testing by a computerized flow-volume meter is used to measure dynamic lung volume. The pulmonary function test is very important because it can determine whether a person has asthma, obstructive lung disease, or restrictive lung disease. Like those for static lung volume measurements, normal values for dynamic lung volume measurements vary based on age, height, weight, gender, and race.

During a test of dynamic lung volume, a person is instructed to breathe normally into a mouthpiece connected to a flow volume machine. After several tidal (normal) respirations, the person is instructed to inspire maximally and then expire as long, hard, and fast as possible. The goal is for the person to breathe out for at least six seconds. This may not sound very hard, but most people cannot expire for six seconds on their first attempt. The most

LIFE SPAN DEVELOPMENT: *The Respiratory System*

Before an infant takes its first breath of air, the respiratory system undergoes dramatic and amazing changes within the mother's uterus. While in the uterus, the fetus receives all oxygen and nutrients from the mother's blood, and carbon dioxide and other waste products are removed through the mother's umbilical blood. Fetal lungs develop in five stages (**Figure 9.11**). An explanation of the lung structures that develop in utero is shown in **Figure 9.12**. Following these dramatic changes, alveoli will increase in size and blood supply, and the lungs will continue to develop until the chest wall finishes growing in size at adulthood.

Generally speaking, lung capacity peaks in the mid-twenties, then gradually declines until approximately age 55 to 60 years, when the lung tissue becomes less elastic, the respiratory muscles weaken, and the chest wall becomes stiffer. All of these factors decrease lung capacity and the ability to ventilate the lung. In fact, by the age of 70, lung capacity is reduced by approximately 30 percent. These physical changes, combined decreased ciliary activity, a weakened immune system, and diminished gas exchange, make older individuals more susceptible to respiratory tract illnesses, pneumonia, influenza, and lung diseases.

Life Span Review

1. How are waste products removed from a developing fetus?
2. Why are older people more susceptible to respiratory tract illness than younger people?

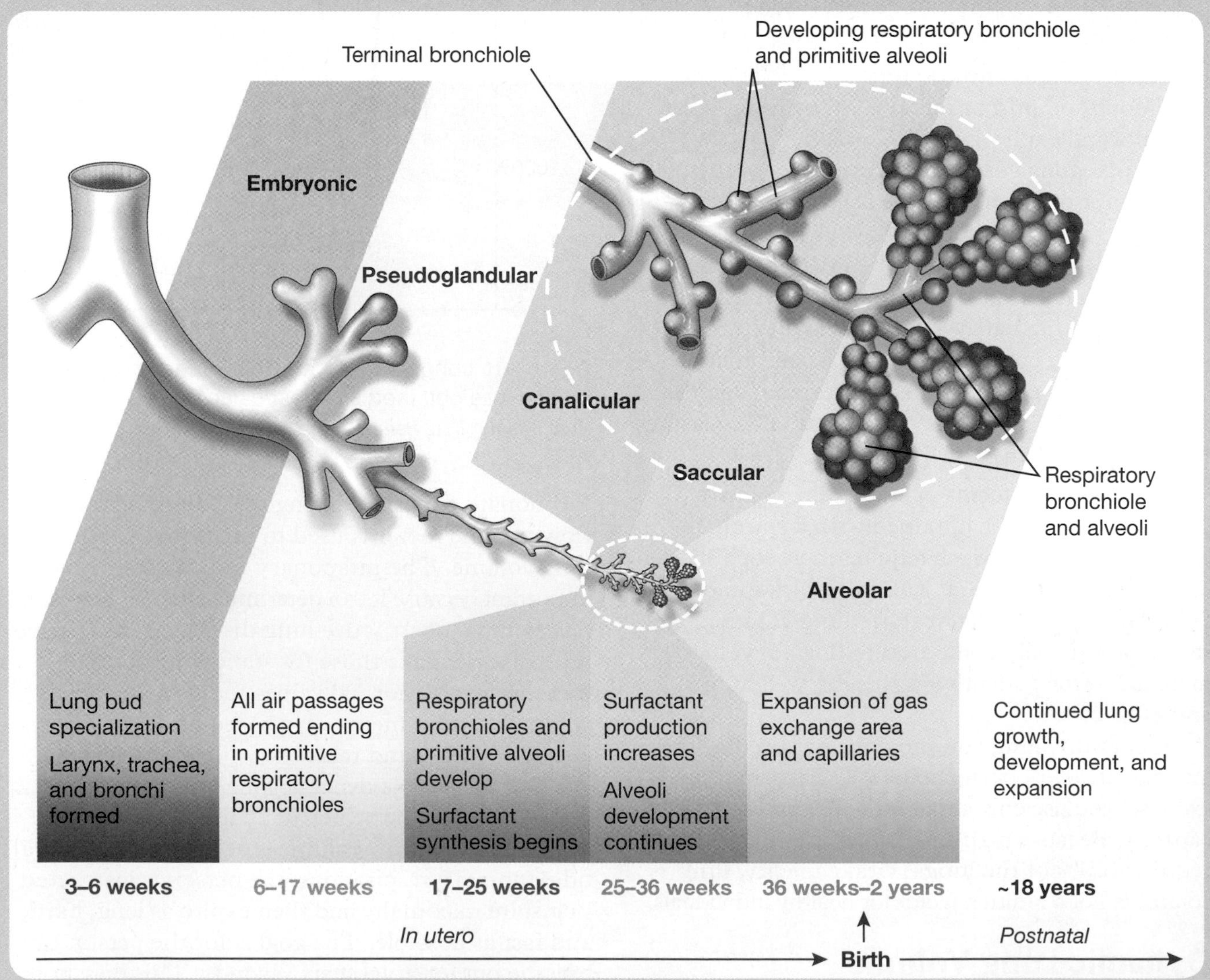

Figure 9.11 The stages of fetal lung development.

(continued)

Lung Development in Utero		
Stage	**Duration**	**Description**
Embryonic	3–6 weeks	Two small buds branch off to form right and left lungs; larynx and trachea are formed. Buds of the two main bronchi develop; these will eventually form the bronchi and all other lower respiratory structures.
Pseudoglandular	6–17 weeks	Further branching of lung buds into smaller and more numerous units. All air passages are formed and terminate in the primitive respiratory bronchioles. Cilia and cartilage begin to form, and amniotic fluid production begins.
Canalicular	17–25 weeks	Respiratory bronchioles, alveolar ducts, and primitive alveoli develop. Basic structure of the gas-exchange portions of lungs are formed and vascularized; air-blood barrier is formed, allowing oxygen to enter the respiratory capillaries and remove carbon dioxide. Surfactant production begins in small quantities.
Saccular	25–36 weeks	Surfactant production increases. This crucial step allows amniotic fluid to drain from the lungs and allows the lungs to fill with air during delivery. Surfactant is composed of fatty molecules produced by cells in the alveoli that reduce the attraction between water molecules within the alveoli. It keeps the alveoli open, allowing them to fill with air during inspiration. Premature babies born at 28 weeks usually can breathe on their own.
Alveolar	36 weeks through birth and early childhood (2 years)	Surfactant production continues to increase, more bronchioles and alveolar sacs develop, leading to greater gas exchange and lung expansion as a newborn and as a growing child. Mature alveoli are not present until 5 weeks after birth. The 20 million primitive alveoli present at birth develop into 300 million alveoli by age 2 years.

Figure 9.12 Goodheart-Willcox Publisher

important measurements obtained from this test include the following:

- **forced expiratory volume in one second (FEV_1)**: the maximum amount of air that a person can expire in one second. This test measures the ability of the lungs to expel air
- **forced expiratory volume in one second/forced vital capacity (FEV_1/FVC)**: the overall expiratory power of the lungs

People with asthma or a chronic obstructive pulmonary disease (COPD) such as emphysema or chronic bronchitis often have increased airway resistance because of an obstruction. As a result, their FEV_1 and FEV_1/FVC values are less than 80% of those for healthy individuals.

People with restrictive lung disease such as cystic fibrosis or pneumonia have an increased stiffness in the lungs, which prevents the lungs from expanding normally. Lung stiffness causes static and dynamic lung volume values to be much lower than normal. Lung volumes indicative of some pulmonary disorders will be discussed in greater length in Lesson 9.3.

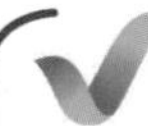

Check Your Understanding

1. What does vital capacity (VC) measure?
2. Explain the difference between inspiratory reserve volume and expiratory reserve volume.
3. What can a pulmonary function test determine?

LESSON 9.2 Review and Assessment

Mini Glossary

Make sure that you know the meaning of each key term.

central chemoreceptors chemical receptor cells that monitor changes in the pH of the cerebrospinal fluid in an effort to regulate carbon dioxide levels and respiration

expiration the process by which air is expelled from the lungs; exhalation

expiratory reserve volume (ERV) the additional amount of air that can be exhaled, or forced from the lungs, immediately after a normal exhalation

external respiration the process by which gas exchange occurs between the alveoli in the lungs and the pulmonary blood

forced expiratory volume in one second (FEV_1) the amount of air that a person can expire in one second

forced expiratory volume in one second/forced vital capacity (FEV_1/FVC) the overall expiratory power of the lungs

functional residual capacity (FRC) the amount of air that remains in the lungs after a normal expiration; ERV + RV

Hering-Breuer reflex an involuntary impulse triggered by stretch receptors in the bronchioles and alveoli that halts inspiration and initiates exhalation

inspiration the process by which air flows into the lungs; inhalation

inspiratory reserve volume (IRV) the amount of air that can be inhaled immediately after a normal inhalation

internal respiration the process of gas exchange between the tissues and arterial blood

mechanoreceptors chemical receptor cells that detect muscle contraction and force generation during exercise; they quickly increase respiration rates when exercise begins

peripheral chemoreceptors sensory receptor cells located in the aortic arch and carotid arteries that are sensitive to changes in blood oxygen level

pulmonary ventilation the process of continuously moving air in and out of the lungs

residual volume (RV) the volume of air that never leaves the lungs, even after the most forceful expiration

respiration the process by which the lungs provide oxygen to body tissues and dispose of carbon dioxide; breathing

respiratory gas transport the process by which oxygen and carbon dioxide are transported to and from the lungs and tissues

tidal volume (TV) the amount of air inhaled in a normal breath

total lung capacity (TLC) a combination of the vital capacity plus the residual volume; IRV + TV + ERV + RV

vital capacity (VC) the total amount of air that can be forcibly expired from the lungs after a maximum inspiration

Know and Understand

1. What are the four key tasks the cardiopulmonary system works to accomplish?
2. Describe the mechanics of a cough.
3. How does posture affect your breathing rate?
4. Where are the neural centers for breathing located?
5. What instruments are used to measure static and dynamic lung volume?

Analyze and Apply

6. What are stretch receptors, and what role do they play in the Hering-Breuer reflex?
7. Explain Boyle's law and how it relates to breathing.
8. Imagine that you are a pediatrician. A frantic mother visits you in your office with her newborn son. The mother expresses concern that her baby's breathing rate is too high. She tells you that the baby takes many more breaths each minute than his older brother. After testing the baby's respiratory rate, you discover that it falls in the normal range for newborns. How do you explain this to the mother?
9. Using the information shown in Figure 9.11, when do you think the baby will take its first breath of air?
10. Consider the anatomical structures of the chest. Why do you think the right lung has three lobes, but the left lung only has two?

IN THE LAB

11. You can determine lung capacity with a balloon, ruler, pencil, and graph paper.

    Take several deep breaths and then exhale as much air as possible into the balloon. Measure and record the diameter of the balloon, labeling it *vital capacity*. Repeat three times, and then calculate your average vital capacity.

    Exhale normally. Before inhaling again, quickly put the balloon to your lips and exhale into the balloon. Measure the diameter of the balloon as before, and record this measurement as the *expiratory reserve*. Repeat three times and calculate your average expiratory reserve.

    Take a normal breath, and as you exhale normally, put the balloon to your lips. Measure the diameter of the balloon as before, recording the measurement as *tidal volume*. Repeat three more times, then calculate your average tidal volume.

    Make a bar graph that compares your three average lung volume measurements. Compare your results with those of your classmates.
12. Compare respiratory rates as related to lung age. Begin with a partner in the classroom and practice counting each other's respiration for a full minute. Remember, one respiration equals one inhalation and one exhalation. Then, outside the classroom, obtain permission to count the respirations of an infant, toddler, middle school student, adult, and senior citizen. Graph your results. When you return to class, compare your graph to that of other students.

LESSON 9.3 Respiratory Disorders and Diseases

Before You Read

Try to answer the following questions before you read this lesson.

- How common is the "common cold"?
- What is the leading cause of chronic obstructive pulmonary disease?

Lesson Objectives

- Identify common illnesses of the upper respiratory tract.
- Differentiate among lower respiratory tract illnesses.
- Identify the most common forms of chronic obstructive pulmonary disease and describe strategies for symptom management.
- Describe potential causes for asthma attacks and how to avoid asthma triggers.
- Understand the causes, symptoms, and treatments associated with other common respiratory disorders and diseases.

Key Terms

acute bronchitis
asthma
bronchospasms
chronic bronchitis
chronic obstructive pulmonary disease (COPD)
emphysema
hyperventilation
hypoxia
influenza
laryngitis
nasopharyngitis
pharyngitis
pneumonia
sinusitis
tonsillitis
tuberculosis (TB)

CLINICAL CASE STUDY

Demetrius was a straight-A student, and he was determined to keep it that way because had had his sights set on career as a physical therapist. On Wednesday, he felt a little fatigued but otherwise fine, so he was surprised when he woke up Thursday feeling horrible. He had a fever, chills, headache, was coughing a lot and his whole body ached. Despite wanting to attend school to maintain his grades, Demetrius knew he had to stay home. As you read this section, try to determine which of the following conditions Demetrius most likely has.

A. Nasopharyngitis
B. Laryngitis
C. Sinusitis
D. Influenza

It is likely that you have had a "common cold" several times in your life—after all, it is called the *common* cold for a reason! In fact, you have probably had the flu, have a friend with asthma, or know someone whose tonsils have been removed. But do you know how to prevent the cold or flu? Do you know what causes your friend's asthma attacks?

This lesson discusses the causes and symptoms of several respiratory disorders, along with treatment options. You may be surprised to learn that some of these disorders cannot be cured, yet others can be prevented by behavior as simple as washing your hands.

Upper Respiratory Tract Illnesses

Upper respiratory tract illnesses, or URIs, are the most common acute respiratory illnesses. As explained in Lesson 9.1, the upper respiratory tract includes the nose, nasal cavity, sinuses, pharynx, and larynx. Infection and inflammation of the upper respiratory tract can lead to a variety of illnesses, including:

- **nasopharyngitis** (nay-zoh-fair-in-JIGH-tis): the common cold
- **pharyngitis** (fair-in-JIGH-tis): inflammation of the pharynx, or throat
- **sinusitis** (sigh-nyoos-IGH-tis): inflammation of the sinuses
- **laryngitis** (lair-in-JIGH-tis): inflammation of the larynx, or *voice box*
- **tonsillitis** (tahn-si-LIGH-tis): inflammation of the tonsils

Figure 9.13 lists the causes and symptoms of upper respiratory tract illnesses. The chart also provides recommended treatments for these illnesses.

Avoiding URIs

Most people get between two and four colds (nasopharyngitis) each year. Typical symptoms of a cold come on gradually and include a runny or stuffy nose with a sore throat. Sometimes you may feel little fatigued or have a slight cough, but rarely does a common cold develop into a more serious health problem. Treatment is just rest, drinking plenty of fluids and, if needed, taking over-the-counter medication to relieve nasal congestion or discharge and a sore throat. According to the Cleveland Clinic, there are 12 million medical visits for pharyngitis and 20 billion cases of bacterial sinusitis each year.

Upper Respiratory Tract Illnesses					
	Etiology	**Prevention**	**Pathology**	**Diagnosis**	**Treatment**
Pharyngitis	infection from common cold or flu virus; bacterium such as group A streptococcus (strep throat)	wash hands with soap and hot water often; use alcohol-based hand sanitizer if you cannot wash your hands; cover your mouth and nose with a tissue when sneezing, or sneeze into your sleeve	sore, scratchy throat; fever; headache; swollen lymph nodes	self-diagnosis, physical exam, throat swab to test for strep, if suspected	gargle with saline solution; drink warm fluids; suck on freezer pops or throat lozenges; over-the-counter pain relievers and antibiotics if strep is diagnosed
Sinusitis	caused by bacteria, viruses, or fungi	same as pharyngitis	sinus pain; nasal stuffiness and discharge; headache; fever; sore throat; postnasal drip; fatigue	self-diagnosis; if serious, nasal/sinus cultures, imaging, nasal endoscopy, allergy testing	drink fluids; apply warm, moist cloth to face; use humidifier, nasal saline spray; see a doctor about severe/chronic symptoms
Laryngitis	viral infections such as common cold of flu, bacterial infections, allergies, or inhaled irritants	same as pharyngitis	sore throat; hoarseness; loss of voice; fever, dry cough, swollen glands	self-diagnosis; see physician if it persists more than 2 weeks, or if you cough up blood, have a temperature over 103°F, or have trouble breathing	rest your voice; use a humidifier, decongestants, or pain relievers as necessary
Tonsillitis	viral or bacterial infection; streptococcus A is the most common bacterial infection	same as pharyngitis	red, swollen tonsils; white/yellow patches on tonsils; difficult, painful swallowing; bad breath; swollen neck glands	physical exam; throat swab for strep; rarely, blood test	gargle with saline solution; drink warm fluids such as tea with honey; over-the-counter pain medications (no aspirin for those under 21 years of age); antibiotic, if strep is diagnosed; surgery
Influenza (both upper and lower respiratory infection)	viral infection	proper hand washing, annual flu shot, avoid smoking; strengthen immune system through diet, exercise, and adequate sleep	quick onset of fever, headache, nasal congestion, alternating chills/sweats, dry cough, fatigue, aching muscles	medical exam; rapid influenza diagnostic test	antiviral medication, bed rest, plenty of fluids, over-the-counter pain relievers

Figure 9.13 Goodheart-Willcox Publisher

Transmission of upper respiratory illnesses such as nasopharyngitis and other URIs occurs by direct hand-to-hand contact, handling a contaminated object, or inhaling airborne droplets produced by unprotected sneezing or coughing. Proper respiratory etiquette and hand hygiene are the most effective ways to prevent URIs (**Figure 9.14** and **Figure 9.15**):

- Cover your nose and mouth with a tissue when you cough or sneeze. If a tissue is unavailable, sneeze or cough into your sleeve to avoid contaminating your hands.
- Wash your hands often with soap and hot water. Use an alcohol-based hand sanitizer if soap and water are not available.
- Avoid touching your hands to your eyes, nose, or mouth to decrease the spread of germs.

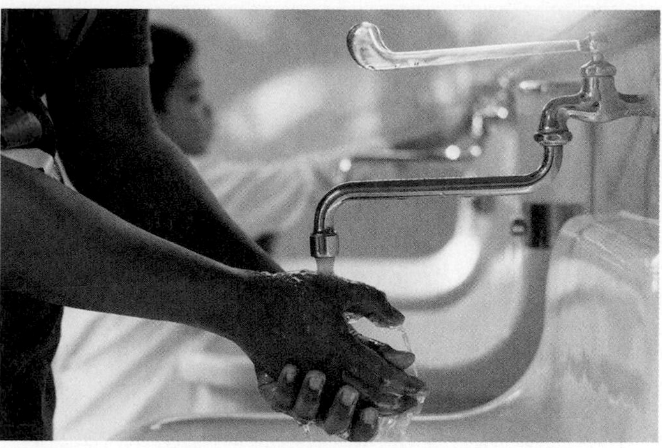

CC7/Shutterstock.com

Figure 9.15 Wash your hands with hot, soapy water for 20 seconds, about the length of time it takes to sing "Happy Birthday" twice.

Influenza

Influenza, or the flu, is a viral infection that affects the respiratory system. Unlike a cold, whose symptoms come on slowly, the flu strikes quickly. Symptoms include a fever above 100°F (38°C), headache, nasal congestion, alternating chills and sweats, dry cough, fatigue, and aching muscles, especially in the back, arms, and legs.

From November through March, the flu strikes the Northern Hemisphere in epidemic proportions. According to the Centers for Disease Control (CDC), 5% to 20% of the US population is infected with the flu each year, and more than 200,000 people are hospitalized because of flu-related complications. The CDC also reports that influenza-related deaths average about 25,000 annually in the United States, although this number can vary greatly from year to year. The CDC also estimates that school-aged children (5 to 17 years of age) in the United States miss 38 million days of school each year because of the flu. The single best way to protect against seasonal flu is to get the seasonal influenza vaccine each year.

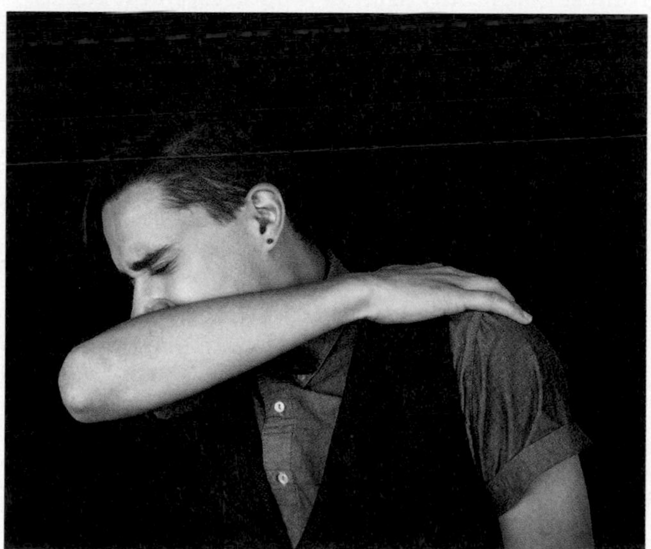

Brenda Carson/Shutterstock.com

Figure 9.14 Sneezing into your sleeve decreases the transmission of germs. *What other ways can you avoid spreading germs?*

Check Your Understanding

1. How many colds does the average person contract each year?
2. What is the scientific name for the common cold?
3. Which URI is characterized by red, swollen tonsils and swollen neck glands?

Lower Respiratory Tract Illnesses

Like the upper respiratory tract, parts of the lower respiratory tract are susceptible to certain ailments. Bronchitis, pneumonia, and tuberculosis are among the most common. **Figure 9.16** summarizes common lower respiratory tract illnesses.

Lower Respiratory Tract Illnesses					
	Etiology	**Prevention**	**Pathology**	**Diagnosis**	**Treatment**
Acute bronchitis	inflammation of mucous membranes of the trachea and bronchial passages; develops as a result of ongoing viral infection such as flu	proper hand washing; annual flu shot; no smoking; strengthen immune system through diet, exercise, and enough sleep	cough with or without mucus production	physical exam	non-steroidal anti-inflammatory drugs (NSAIDS), decongestants, and expectorants
Pneumonia	infection of the lungs caused usually by a virus or bacterium. Can also be caused by fungus or parasite	same as acute bronchitis; pneumonia shot for people over age 60	cough, fever, chills, fatigue, shortness of breath, nausea, vomiting, diarrhea	medical history, physical exam including auscultation of lungs; blood tests, chest X-ray, pulse oximetry, sputum test	antibiotics, cough medicine, fever reducer/ over-the-counter pain medication
Tuberculosis	infection caused by mycobacterium tuberculosis	avoid contact with TB-infected individual; same as for acute bronchitis	fever, fatigue, unintended weight loss, excessive sweating	medical history, physical exam, TB skin test, blood test, imaging, sputum tests	long-term use of antibiotics; confinement to room at home or in hospital for 2-4 weeks to prevent spreading

Figure 9.16

Goodheart-Willcox Publisher

Acute Bronchitis

Bronchitis is classified as either acute or chronic. **Acute bronchitis** is an inflammation of the mucous membranes that line the trachea and bronchial passageways. Chronic bronchitis is discussed later in this lesson.

Acute bronchitis is characterized by a cough that may or may not produce mucus. This illness usually develops as a result of an ongoing viral infection such as influenza or a cold. Treatment for acute bronchitis varies based on the patient's symptoms. It often includes the use of nonsteroidal anti-inflammatory drugs (NSAIDs), decongestants, and expectorants (medications that expel mucus).

Pneumonia

Pneumonia (noo-MOH-nee-ah) is an infection of the lungs. It is usually caused by a virus or bacterium, but some pneumonia infections are caused by a fungus or parasites.

The immune response to the invading virus or bacterium damages and sometimes kills the cells of the lungs. Fluid also builds up in the lungs, making gas exchange difficult. Symptoms of pneumonia include cough, fever, chills, fatigue, shortness of breath, nausea, vomiting, and diarrhea. Diagnosis is made by examining chest X-rays and cell cultures. Treatment of pneumonia includes antibiotics and supplemental oxygen, as necessary.

Tuberculosis

Tuberculosis (TB) is a highly contagious infection caused by *Mycobacterium tuberculosis*. It most commonly attacks the lungs, but it can spread to other organs such as those in the digestive, nervous, or lymphatic systems. TB is contracted by breathing in air droplets from the cough or sneeze of an infected person.

Symptoms of TB include fever, fatigue, unintentional weight loss, and excessive sweating, especially at night. People with TB also develop a cough that may produce mucus or blood.

Most forms of TB can be treated with antibiotics, but some new forms are drug resistant. Individuals with TB must be confined to their home or the hospital for two to four weeks to avoid spreading this contagious disease to others.

Check Your Understanding

1. What are the two general classifications of bronchitis?
2. List common symptoms of pneumonia.
3. How is tuberculosis contracted?

Chronic Obstructive Pulmonary Diseases

Chronic obstructive pulmonary disease (COPD) is any lung disorder characterized by a long-term airway obstruction, making it difficult to breathe. Two of the most common forms of COPD are **emphysema** (ehm-fi-SEE-ma) and **chronic bronchitis**. Bronchitis is classified as *chronic* when a person has a cough that has lasted from three months to two years. **Figure 9.17** summarizes these and other common chronic obstructive pulmonary diseases.

The CDC reports that COPD is the third leading cause of death in the United States and is a major cause of long-term disability. According to the World Health Organization, COPD accounts for 5% of all deaths worldwide.

Causes of COPD

The primary cause of COPD is cigarette, cigar, or pipe smoking. The longer a person smokes, the more susceptible he or she becomes to COPD. The risk of developing COPD is also increased by long-term, regular exposure to secondhand smoke or occupational exposure to chemical fumes, dust, or pollution.

People with COPD are more likely to have frequent respiratory infections such as cold and flu viruses, pneumonia, or a cough that produces mucus. They also experience dyspnea (difficulty breathing), which progressively worsens. Breathing—something that many people take for granted—is an exhausting experience for COPD patients. Difficulty breathing leaves many COPD patients unable to participate in everyday activities. The challenges associated with managing COPD can also cause patients to develop depression.

Chronic Obstructive Pulmonary Diseases and Other Lung Disorders

	Etiology	Prevention	Pathology	Diagnosis	Treatment
Emphysema	ruptured alveolar sacs that prevent proper gas exchange	stop smoking; avoid second-hand smoke, air pollution, chemical fumes, and dust	shortness of breath, difficulty breathing, frequent respiratory infections, depression	medical exam, pulmonary function tests, chest X-rays, bronchoscopies, arterial blood gases for oxygen and carbon dioxide	smoking cessation, pulmonary rehabilitation, purse-lipped breathing, respiratory muscle training, supplemental oxygen
Chronic Bronchitis	obstructed airway due to ongoing inflammation of the bronchi and excessive mucus production	same as for emphysema, hand washing to prevent infection, drinking plenty of fluids, healthy lifestyle	cough, mucus production, wheezing, and shortness of breath that last for more than 3 months	same as for emphysema	stop smoking; bronchodilators, inhaled corticosteroids, antibiotics, chest physical therapy, oxygen therapy
Asthma	inflammation and narrowing of airways accompanied by mucus production	same as for emphysema; for exercise–induced asthma, warm up for 20 minutes at low-intensity, and use bronchodilator 30 minutes before exercise	wheezing, shortness of breath, coughing, chest tightness	medical exam; family history of allergies, symptoms triggered by allergens, exercise, emotional stress; pulmonary function testing, exercise challenge test	limit exposure to allergens, exercise, stress; bronchodilators, anti-inflammatory drugs, inhaled corticosteroids
Obstructive Sleep Apnea	muscles in the back of throat relax and occlude upper airway, causing hypoxia (lack of oxygen)	maintain healthy weight, sleep on side, avoid alcohol, sedatives and opioid usage; stop smoking	loud snoring, intermittent bouts of stopping breathing during sleep; obesity, male gender, minority status, smoking, use of narcotics or alcohol, older age	medical exam; history of obesity, daytime drowsiness, and fatigue and other risk factors for OSA; sleep study	wearing a CPAP device or other appliance or surgery to keep airways open while sleeping, weight loss, side sleeping

Figure 9.17 *Goodheart-Willcox Publisher*

Living with COPD

There is no cure for COPD. The main goals of treatment are to help the patient manage symptoms, improve the quality of life, slow the progression of the disease, and treat infections. The key factor in achieving these goals is smoking cessation. A person with COPD *must* stop smoking and avoid exposure to substances that may irritate the lungs.

Smoking causes 1 in 5 deaths annually, or 480,000 deaths each year with more than 41,000 of these deaths attributed to exposure to second-hand smoke. The CDC estimates that 25 million people alive today will die prematurely from the harmful effects of smoking. This includes 5 million people under 18 years of age.

The nicotine in tobacco is more addictive than cocaine, so a person may experience several failed attempts at quitting the smoking habit before success is achieved. The use of nicotine gum or patches increases the likelihood of smoking cessation; however, these can also be addictive.

COPD symptoms can be alleviated through a variety of methods. One technique, purse-lipped breathing, helps maximize breathing and ease shortness of breath. Patients using this technique are advised to inhale through their nose and then slowly release the air through pursed, or puckered, lips. Respiratory muscle training, pulmonary rehabilitation, and supplemental oxygen can also help reduce COPD symptoms. Pharmacological therapies such as bronchodilators, anti-inflammatory medications, and inhaled steroids can help expand airways and are often prescribed for COPD patients. However, none of these methods slows the progression of COPD more effectively than smoking cessation. Pulmonary function tests, X-rays, bronchoscopies (brahng-KAHS-koh-pees), and monitoring of gas levels in arterial blood are used in both the diagnosis and management of COPD.

Figure 9.18 illustrates the results of a pulmonary function test for normal individuals and for those with emphysema, chronic bronchitis, and restrictive disease (any chest disease that reduces lung volumes). Note the concave-shaped expiration pattern for individuals with emphysema and chronic bronchitis. This is due to trapped air in the lungs. Additionally, when you examine the curve for restrictive disease, you will see how limited inspiration and expiration are, compared to the curve for normal individuals. This is because the lungs are unable to expand due to stiffness.

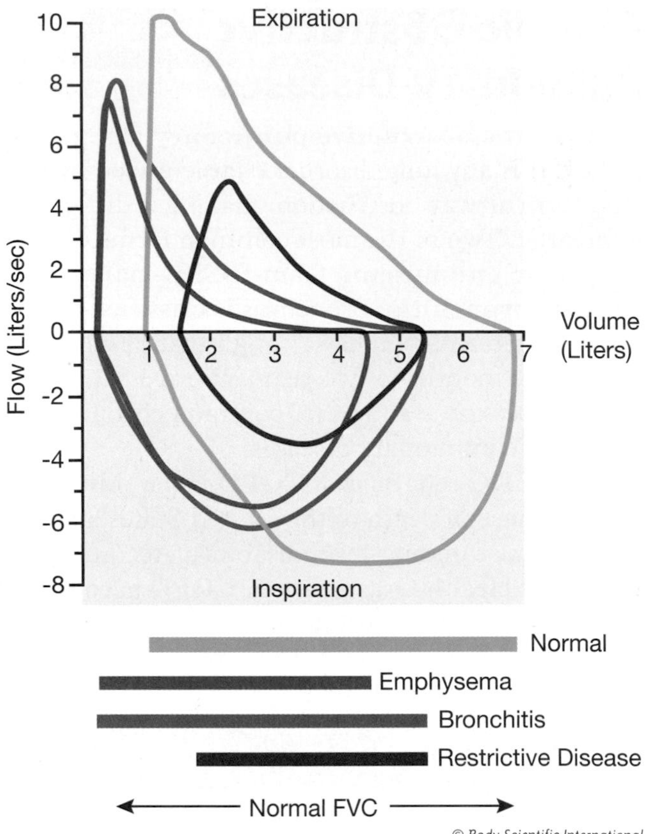

Figure 9.18 Results of a pulmonary function test for healthy individuals, and for people diagnosed with emphysema, chronic bronchitis, and restrictive disease. *Can you explain the concave-shaped expiration pattern for individuals with emphysema and chronic bronchitis?*

Emphysema

Commonly caused by tobacco smoke, emphysema is a form of COPD that leads to chronic inflammation in the lungs. This inflammation damages the air passages distal to the terminal bronchioles, namely the alveolar ducts and the alveolar sacs (**Figure 9.19**). The pulmonary capillary bed is also damaged. This damage decreases the surface area of the lungs, limiting the number of sites available for gas exchange. As emphysema progresses, the alveolar sacs rupture, leading to poor gas exchange and buildup of carbon dioxide in the lungs.

To compensate for the poor gas exchange, the body triggers **hyperventilation**, or an abnormally high respiratory rate. Hyperventilation brings in oxygen while allowing the lungs to dispose of accumulated carbon dioxide.

People with emphysema work so hard to breathe that they often lose weight. This exertion also causes emphysema patients to develop a pink

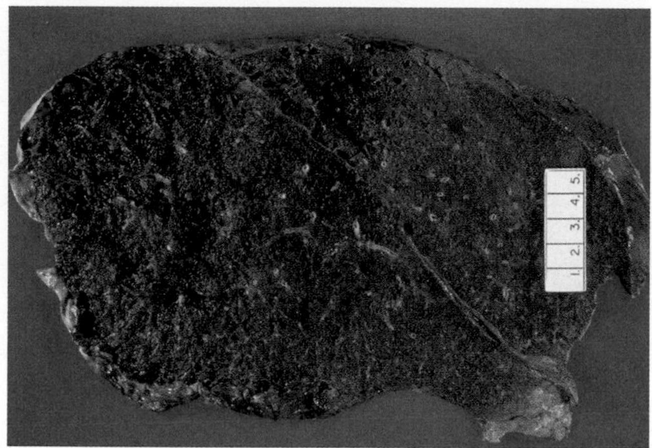

Dr. E. Walker/Science Source

Figure 9.19 Lung of a smoker with emphysema. The accumulation of inhaled irritants from smoking blackened the lung. *What other diseases are associated with smoking?*

appearance to the face. The characteristic pink cheeks and labored breathing of the COPD patient have led to the descriptive term "pink puffers" among people in clinical circles.

Chronic Bronchitis

People with chronic bronchitis have an obstructed airway due to inflammation of the bronchi and excessive mucus production that lasts for more than 3 months. The excessive mucus limits respiration and gas exchange. It also increases the risk of infection because bacteria can become trapped and breed in the warm, moist environment of the lungs. The body responds to the mucus accumulation by decreasing the respiratory rate and increasing cardiac output. Unlike emphysema, chronic bronchitis does not damage the pulmonary capillary bed.

The face and lips of a person with chronic bronchitis develop a blue color due to *hypoxemia*, or lowered arterial blood oxygen content. Residual volume also increases, causing a bloated appearance. These two side effects have led to the description of chronic bronchitis patients as "blue bloaters."

Check Your Understanding

1. What is the difference between acute and chronic bronchitis?
2. What is the primary cause of COPD?
3. Which respiratory disease is associated with the term "pink puffer"?

Asthma

Asthma (AZ-ma) is a respiratory disease in which the airways of the lungs become narrow or inflamed during episodes called *asthma attacks*. During an asthma attack, the airways are temporarily constricted by **bronchospasms** (BRAHN-koh-spazmz), contractions of the smooth bronchial muscles. Also, the lining of the inflamed airways produces mucus that causes further narrowing. Bronchospasms, inflammation, and mucus production result in symptoms such as wheezing, breathlessness, coughing, and tightness in the chest.

People with a family history of allergies are at an increased risk of developing asthma because many of the stimuli that trigger allergies also cause asthma attacks. A variety of substances can trigger an asthma attack. Asthma triggers include cigarette smoke, mold, air pollution, pet hair and dander, cold air, exercise, dust, pollen, and emotional stress.

If you lose your breath easily, feel very tired or weak when exercising, wheeze and cough after exercise, or experience a frequent cough (especially at night), these may be early symptoms of asthma. A school nurse or other healthcare professional can use a peak flow meter to measure the airflow from your lungs (**Figure 9.20**).

Your doctor may use a more detailed pulmonary function test to diagnose asthma. Proper diagnosis is important because it leads to treatment options that enable an asthmatic person to lead a healthy, productive life; participate in physical activities; and limit the frequency and severity of asthma attacks.

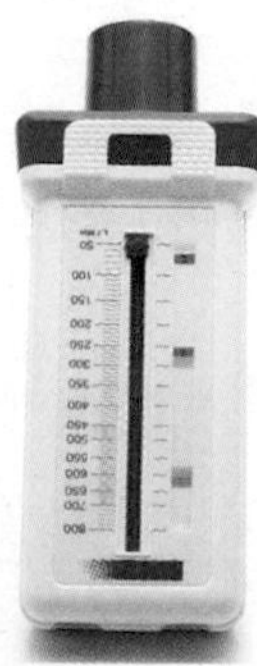

mayer kleinostheim/Shutterstock.com

Figure 9.20 A peak flow meter is used to measure airflow from the lungs. Blowing forcefully into the end of the device causes the marker to move up the numbered scale.

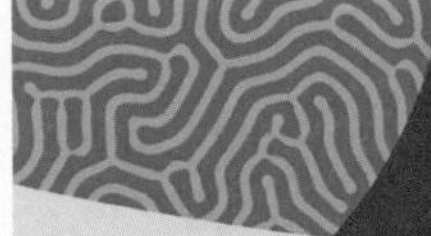

What Research Tells Us

...about Exercise-Induced Asthma

Asthma attacks triggered by exercise are called *exercise-induced bronchospasms (EIBs)*, or *exercise-induced asthma*. Exercise-induced asthma is not uncommon. Many people who exercise regularly have asthma, even professional athletes. Hundreds of athletes successfully compete at the Olympic Games despite having asthma.

Researchers investigated the incidence of EIBs among members of the US Olympic Winter Sports teams. The athletes tested for EIBs included members of seven different teams: biathlon, cross-country skiing, figure skating, ice hockey, Nordic combined events, long-track speed skating, and short-track speed skating.

All the athletes in the study were tested for EIBs during actual or simulated competition. The overall incidence of EIBs was 23%. This percentage included nearly half of the cross-country skiing team as well as winners of gold, silver, and bronze medals. This study demonstrated that athletes can compete at the international level—even winning an Olympic gold medal—despite having exercise-induced asthma.

Taking It Further

1. Research the career of a famous athlete with asthma. What challenges did asthma cause for the athlete? How did he or she cope with the disease? Present your findings in an oral report to the class.
2. If you were a coach and a member of your team showed symptoms of exercise-induced asthma, what advice would you give him or her for managing this disease?

Treatments for asthma include limiting exposure to irritants that can trigger an asthma attack and using prescription medications such as bronchodilators, anti-inflammatory drugs, and inhaled steroids (**Figure 9.21**). These medications work by relaxing the muscles of the bronchi and expanding the airways.

Currently more than 25 million people in the United States have asthma, with an incidence of about 8% of all adults and children. According to the CDC's 2016 prevalence data, African-Americans and Puerto Ricans have the highest rates among minority populations, with rates of 11.6 and 14.3 percent respectively. This respiratory disease can be fatal; it kills more than 3,500 people each year. In the United States, the costs associated with asthma treatments and lost productivity in the workplace amount to roughly $56 billion each year.

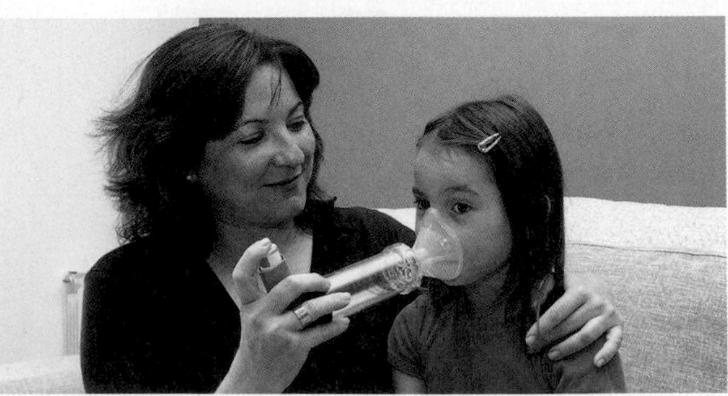

xavier gallego morel/Shutterstock.com

Figure 9.21 A mother helps her child use an asthma inhaler with a spacer. The spacer allows more of the medicine to get into the child's lungs.

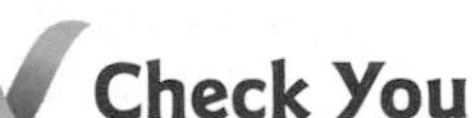

Check Your Understanding

1. What percentage of people in the United States has asthma?
2. What are some treatments for asthma?

Obstructive Sleep Apnea

Sleep apnea affects more than 12 million Americans, and many of them go undiagnosed because the primary symptom happens during sleep. There are many forms of sleep apnea. This discussion relates to the most common form: obstructive sleep apnea. OSA is usually characterized by loud snoring with intermittent partial or complete obstruction of the upper airway. It occurs when an individual's tongue falls against the soft palate and the soft palate and the uvula fall back against the throat, obstructing the airway, which results in **hypoxia** (too little oxygen).

Sleep apnea is diagnosed when an individual stops breathing for 10 seconds or longer for a minimum of five times per hour while sleeping. Many individuals experience moderate to severe OSA, having 20 or more episodes per hour. These people are at a significantly greater risk for detrimental side effects, some of which are life threatening. Side effects of OSA-induced hypoxia include abnormal heartbeat (dysrhythmias), increased risk of sudden cardiac death, high blood pressure, stroke, diabetes and glaucoma. A recent study showed that pregnant women with sleep apnea had a higher chance of developing high blood pressure and giving birth prematurely. Other side effects include diminished work performance, drowsy driving, and increased risk of accidents due to sleeplessness.

While OSA affects people of all ages, races, and genders, it is more prevalent in African American males, Native Americans, Hispanics, and Asians than in Caucasians. Risk factors for OSA include excessive weight, male gender, large neck circumference, older age, smoking, nasal congestion, and use of alcohol, sedatives, tranquilizers or opioids. Excessive weight is a primary risk factor because excess fat can cause thickening of the airway walls and narrowing of the trachea, making occlusion more likely.

People are usually diagnosed with OSA by a medical history that identifies loud snoring, periods during which breathing stops while sleeping, daytime sleepiness, fatigue, and chest pain during sleep. A sleep study is performed at home or at an overnight medical facility where breathing is monitored during a night's sleep and the number of times a person partially or fully stops breathing is recorded, along with the duration of the lack of breathing.

Treatment for OSA includes weight loss, sleeping on your side, exercising throat muscles, use of a device that delivers a continuous positive air pressure to keep the airway open (CPAP), appliances to open the nose and mouth during sleeping, or surgery to widen the breathing passages (**Figure 9.22**).

Check Your Understanding

1. What is hypoxia?
2. Why might sleeping on your side help ease OSA?

Other Respiratory System Diseases

The respiratory system is also the target of other diseases and disorders. Two such diseases are lung cancer and cystic fibrosis, as explained in **Figure 9.23**.

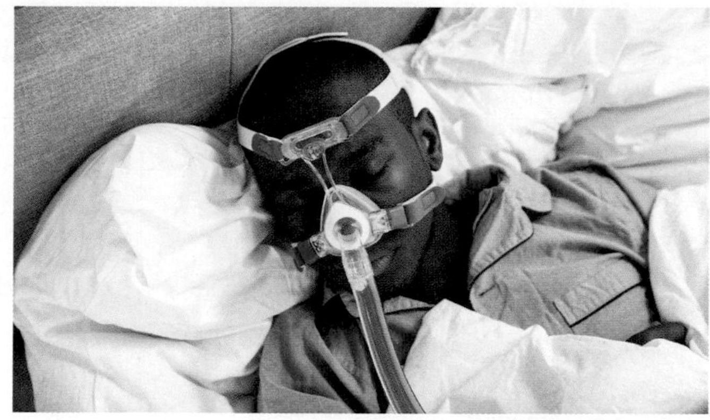

Andrey_Popov/Shutterstock.com

Figure 9.22 A CPAP machine provides a constant air pressure that helps people who have obstructive sleep apnea breathe more easily while they are sleeping.

Lung Cancer

More people in the United States die from lung cancer than any other form of cancer. This statistic is particularly tragic because lung cancer is highly preventable. In about 90% of cases, smoking is the main cause of lung cancer. Exposure to secondhand smoke, radon, asbestos, and other toxins are other risk factors for lung cancer.

The majority of people with lung cancer die within a year because the cancer was not diagnosed at a treatable stage. Lung cancer metastasizes (spreads) quickly to lymph nodes and other organs, such as the brain and the breasts.

Lung cancer is usually classified as non-small cell or small cell lung cancer. Non-small cell lung cancer is the more common of the two forms and is prevalent in smokers. Non-small cell lung cancer spreads more slowly than small cell lung cancer. Small cell lung cancer develops and spreads quickly in the early stage of the disease, often before a detectable tumor forms on one of the lungs. Because a tumor is usually the identifying element of lung cancer, small cell cancer has ample time to spread before it is detected.

Treatment options for both non-small cell and small cell lung cancer include radiation therapy and chemotherapy. In some cases, surgery is performed to remove the cancerous growth. However, surgery is usually not an option because the cancer typically is too advanced when it is diagnosed. Unfortunately, radiation therapy and chemotherapy are often not very effective because lung cancer tends to spread quickly throughout the body. Alternate treatment options have been developed, including an inhalable, dry chemotherapy drug. One promising treatment

Other Respiratory System Diseases					
	Etiology	**Prevention**	**Pathology**	**Diagnosis**	**Treatment**
Lung Cancer	non-small and small cancer cells develop in the lungs due to smoking, radon, second-hand smoke, occupational exposure to carcinogens like asbestos	never smoke, limit exposure to second-hand smoke and other carcinogens	coughing, coughing up blood, wheezing, shortness of breath; weight loss, fever, clubbing of fingernails; chest pain, bone pain, difficulty swallowing, pneumonia	medical exam, chest X-rays, imaging, low-dose CT scan, Positron emission tomography (PET) scan, lung biopsy, bronchoscopy, blood tests	radiation, chemotherapy, surgery, counseling targeted therapies such as immuno-therapy, clinical trials
Cystic Fibrosis	inherited autosomal recessive disease that affects multiple organs, especially the lungs and pancreas	none	bronchiectasis, lung infections, coughing up blood, shortness of breath, wheezing, nasal congestion, pneumothorax, respiratory failure; digestive compli-cations, including nutritional deficiencies, poor growth, blocked bile duct, inability to digest food properly, painful bowel movements, and intestinal blockage	medical exam, measurement of electrolytes in sweat, genetic testing	mucus-thinning drugs, chest clapping, antibiotics, nutritional modifications, psychosocial support networks; possibly gene therapy in the future

Figure 9.23

Goodheart-Willcox Publisher

option involves tailoring chemotherapy drugs based on a patient's unique biological response to treatment methods.

Cystic Fibrosis

Cystic fibrosis (CF) is an inherited lung disorder that can cause severe damage to the lungs, digestive system and other body organs. It is an autosomal recessive disease, which means that children need to inherit one copy of the mutated gene from each parent. If they only inherit one copy, they will only be carriers of the gene with the potential to pass it to their own children. It is the most commonly inherited respiratory disease, afflicting 1 in every 2,500 newborns. The average life expectancy for those with CF is mid- to late 30s, but some people live into their 40s and 50s. CF is caused by a mutation in the cystic fibrosis transmembrane conductance regulator gene (CFTR), which regulates salt flow into and out of cells. There are more than 1,500 variations of the CFTR gene, and the type of CFTR gene mutation inherited determines the severity of the disease.

A defective CFTR gene affects the cells that produce mucus, sweat, and digestive juices. This causes the secretions to thicken, clogging passage-ways, ducts, and tubes, particularly in the lungs and pancreas. Thickening of mucus in the airways and in the pancreatic duct make individuals with CF more susceptible to fatal lung infections. They may also be unable to digest food properly due to a lack of pancreatic enzymes and bile in the small intestine. Their sweat also has an increased salt content.

Individuals with CF may present with the following lung symptoms and conditions: damaged lungs (bronchiectasis), chronic lung infections, wheezing, nasal congestion, coughing up blood, shortness of breath, pneumothorax, and respiratory failure. Digestive complications include nutritional deficiencies, a blocked bile duct, diabetes, intestinal obstruction, poor weight gain, poor growth, foul-smelling stools, intestinal blockage, especially in newborns, and painful constipation.

Measurement of electrolyte levels in sweat is the optimal diagnostic tool for diagnosing CF. People with CF will present with elevated sodium and chloride levels.

Treatment for CF includes early detection, mucus thinning drugs, chest clapping, antibiotics to treat infections, nutritional modifications, and psychosocial support networks. Investigations into gene therapy for CF are ongoing.

Check Your Understanding

1. What causes nearly 90% of all lung cancers?
2. Why is lung cancer difficult to treat?

LESSON 9.3 Review and Assessment

Mini Glossary

Make sure that you know the meaning of each key term.

acute bronchitis a temporary inflammation of the mucous membranes that line the trachea and bronchial passageways; causes a cough that may produce mucus

asthma disease of the lungs characterized by recurring episodes of airway inflammation causing bronchospasms and increased mucus production

bronchospasms spasmodic contractions of the bronchial muscles that constrict the airways in the lungs during an asthma attack

chronic bronchitis a long-lasting respiratory condition in which the airways of the lungs become obstructed due to inflammation of the bronchi and excessive mucus production

chronic obstructive pulmonary disease (COPD) any lung disorder characterized by a long-term airway obstruction, making it difficult to breathe

emphysema chronic inflammation of the lungs characterized by an abnormal increase in the air spaces near the bronchioles; causes an accumulation of carbon dioxide in the lungs

hyperventilation excessive ventilation that leads to abnormal expulsion of carbon dioxide

hypoxia condition of not having enough oxygen

influenza a viral infection that affects the respiratory system; the flu

laryngitis inflammation of the larynx, or voice box

nasopharyngitis inflammation of the nasal passages and pharynx; the common cold

pharyngitis inflammation of the pharynx, or throat

pneumonia an infection of the lungs that causes inflammation; caused by a virus, bacterium, fungus, or—in rare cases—parasites

sinusitis inflammation of the sinuses

tonsillitis inflammation of the tonsils

tuberculosis (TB) a highly contagious bacterial infection caused by *Mycobacterium tuberculosis*

Know and Understand

1. List five common upper respiratory tract infections.
2. List some ways in which upper respiratory tract illnesses can be prevented.
3. Which symptoms indicate influenza?
4. Name three lower respiratory tract illnesses.
5. What is COPD?
6. In which respiratory disorder do the airways of the lungs become narrow and inflamed, constricting air flow?
7. Describe obstructive sleep apnea from a physiological point of view.
8. What are the two basic forms of lung cancer?

Analyze & Apply

9. Montee has not been feeling well for a few weeks. He has been coughing frequently. His cough regularly produces mucus, but sometimes it also contains blood. Montee has been very tired and feverish, often waking in the middle of the night because he is warm and sweating profusely. After considering his symptoms, what disease do you think Montee has?
10. Explain how the results of a pulmonary function test differ between a person with healthy lungs and someone with emphysema or chronic bronchitis.
11. Why are people with a family history of allergies at a higher risk for having asthma?
12. Why is purse-lipped breathing recommended for people with COPD?
13. Both cigarette smoking and inhaling second-hand smoke are major contributors to respiratory disorders and diseases. In your opinion, would vaping have the same effects? Explain your answer.

IN THE LAB

14. Create an informational pamphlet on the respiratory disorder of your choice. Research the causes of the disorder, symptoms, age groups affected, tests or scans used to diagnose the disorder, treatments, and prognosis. Include images in your pamphlet. Present your pamphlet to the class.
15. Create a poster to educate young children in correct respiratory hygiene. Remember to take your audience into account. You may need to rely more heavily on pictures than on words, and keep your words simple enough for young children to understand. The CDC recommends that children cough and sneeze using the "vampire method." Be creative.
16. Conduct research to find out more about sudden infant death syndrome (SIDS). What are its possible causes? Create an informational brochure for new parents explaining steps they can take to reduce the chance that their newborn will be affected by SIDS.

CAREER CORNER

Anatomy & Physiology at Work

The respiratory system is a vital body system that delivers life-sustaining oxygen to body tissues and removes harmful carbon dioxide.

A number of careers are dedicated to the study of the respiratory system, the health and maintenance of its components, and the diagnosis and treatment of respiratory disorders and diseases. Two of these careers are respiratory therapist and pharmacy technician.

Respiratory Therapist

A respiratory therapist (RT) is a healthcare professional who, under the supervision of a physician, cares for people with respiratory disorders. RTs also provide emergency care for people who have breathing problems resulting from heart attack, stroke, near-drowning, or other circumstances (**Figure 9.24**).

RTs perform diagnostic tests on patients, including pulmonary function tests, static lung volume measurements, cardiopulmonary exercise testing, and arterial blood gas tests. RTs also treat patients with poor pulmonary health. They control patients' supplemental oxygen levels and provide respiratory muscle training. In addition, RTs educate patients about effective ways to minimize symptoms and manage their pulmonary disease.

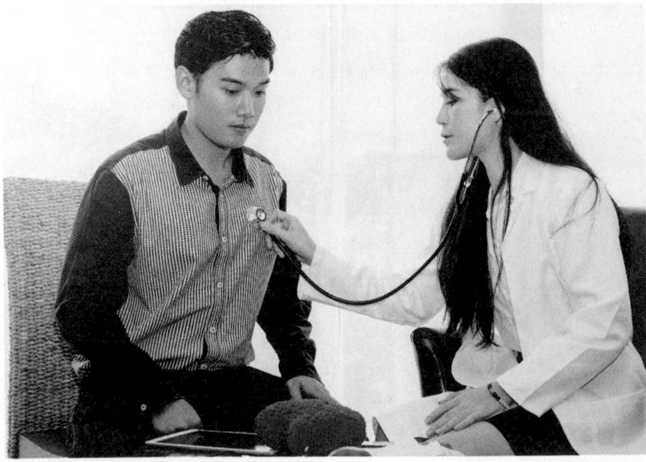

Akira Kaelyn/Shutterstock.com

Figure 9.24 A respiratory therapist assists her patient with a breathing exercise.

RTs administer drug treatments to patients, including nebulizer therapy treatments. A nebulizer is a machine that turns liquid medication into a mist, which is breathed directly into the lungs.

To become a respiratory therapist, you need an associate's degree or a bachelor's degree in respiratory therapy from an accredited institution. You must also pass a national certification exam and meet the licensing requirements of your state. Most hospitals hire registered respiratory therapists (RRTs) who have passed the Registered Respiratory Therapist exam.

The demand for respiratory therapists is expected to increase by more than 25% in the next 10 years. Much of the growth in this field, and in other healthcare-related careers, is due to the aging of a large segment of the population called *baby boomers*. Baby boomers are people who were born in the decades after World War II, when the birth rate in the United States increased dramatically. The baby boomers are now moving into old age, a time when many people develop health problems, including respiratory system disorders.

Pharmacy Technician

A pharmacy technician assists licensed pharmacists in dispensing prescription medications. They work in hospitals and in retail pharmacies (**Figure 9.25**).

Because pharmacy technicians interact frequently with patients or customers, they must have excellent interpersonal, or "people," skills. After receiving a prescription from a customer, the pharmacy technician may need to request additional information from the customer or a physician in order to provide the correct medication. Prescriptions also come into the pharmacy electronically from physician offices, so pharmacy technicians must have a working knowledge of computers and electronic document handling.

Pharmacy technicians must be very attentive to detail. Dispensing the wrong medication or the wrong dosage (amount) to a customer or patient

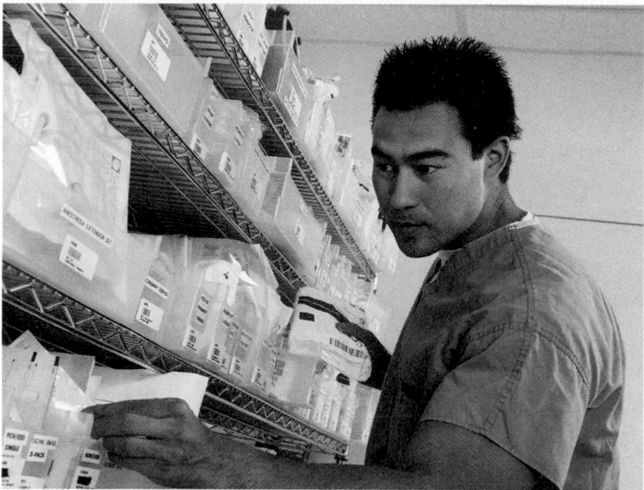

sirtravelalot/Shutterstock.com

Figure 9.25 A pharmacy technician works under the direct supervision of a licensed pharmacist.

can cause illness or even death. After reading a prescription, the pharmacy technician retrieves the correct medication from the shelves. Under the supervision of a pharmacist, the pharmacy technician counts out the correct number of tablets or capsules, measures the prescribed amount of a liquid, or mixes substances to produce the drug. Pharmacy technicians who work in healthcare facilities may also dispense intravenous (IV) medications.

After prescriptions have been packaged and labeled, a pharmacist checks them. The pharmacy technician then dispenses the medications to customers and takes payment. Pharmacy technicians may also create and maintain medical profiles of their customers or patients, prepare and submit health insurance forms, and manage the pharmacy inventory.

Pharmacy technicians must possess a high school diploma or its equivalent. Some pharmacy technicians receive on-the-job training; others attend a certificate program at a vocational school or community college. Certification for pharmacy technicians is offered by the National Pharmacy Technician Certification Board and the National Healthcare Association. To find out the certification requirements for your state, check the website of your state pharmacy board.

The job outlook for pharmacy technicians is promising. As people age, they often need more prescription medications. A shortage in the number of licensed pharmacists has also created a demand for pharmacy technicians.

Planning for a Health-Related Career

Do some research on the career of a respiratory therapist or a pharmacy technician. You may choose instead to research a profession from the list of related career options. Using the internet or resources at your local library, find answers to the following questions:

1. What are the main tasks and responsibilities of a person employed in the career that you chose to research?
2. What is the outlook for this career? Are workers in demand, or are jobs dwindling? For complete information, consult the current edition of the *Occupational Outlook Handbook,* published by the US Department of Labor. This handbook is available online or at your local library.
3. What special skills or talents are required? For example, do you enjoy research? Do you enjoy communicating with other people?
4. What personality traits do you think are necessary for success in the career that you have chosen to research? For example, are you meticulous and accurate? Pharmacy technicians must have these traits.
5. Does the work involve a great deal of routine, or are the day-to-day responsibilities varied?
6. Does the career require long hours, or is it a standard, "9-to-5" job?
7. What is the salary range for this job?
8. What do you think you would like about this career? Is there anything about it that you might dislike?

Related Career Options

- Athletic trainer
- Medical assistant
- Medical records and health information specialist
- Occupational therapist
- Pharmacist
- Physical therapist
- Registered nurse

CHAPTER 9

Review

› LESSON 9.1

Functions and Anatomy of the Respiratory System

Key Points

- The major organs of the respiratory system include the nose, pharynx, larynx, trachea, bronchi, bronchioles, and lungs
- The lower respiratory tract consists of the trachea, bronchi, bronchioles, and lungs.

Key Terms

alveolar capillary membrane
alveoli
bronchioles
epiglottis
larynx
mediastinum
nares
nasal conchae
palate
pharynx
pleural sac
pores of Kohn
primary bronchi
sinuses
surfactant
thyroid cartilage
tonsils
trachea

› LESSON 9.2

Respiration: Mechanics and Control

Key Points

- One respiration, or breath, consists of an inspiration and an expiration. Inspiration and expiration occur according to Boyle's law.
- Neural, chemical, and mechanical factors play key roles in breathing control.
- Lung volume varies based on age, height, weight, gender, and race.

Key Terms

central chemoreceptors
expiration
expiratory reserve volume (ERV)
external respiration
forced expiratory volume in one second (FEV_1)
forced expiratory volume in one second/forced vital capacity (FEV_1/FVC)
functional residual capacity (FRC)
Hering-Breuer reflex
inspiration
inspiratory reserve volume (IRV)
internal respiration
mechanoreceptors
peripheral chemoreceptors
pulmonary ventilation
residual volume (RV)
respiration
respiratory gas transport
tidal volume (TV)
total lung capacity (TLC)
vital capacity (VC)

➤ **LESSON 9.3**

Respiratory Disorders and Diseases

Key Points

- Upper respiratory tract illnesses are transmitted by hand-to hand contact, handling of a contaminated object, or airborne droplets from an infected person's cough or sneeze. Thorough hand washing is one of the most effective ways to prevent their transmission.
- Bronchitis, pneumonia, and tuberculosis are among the most common lower respiratory tract illnesses.
- Chronic obstructive pulmonary diseases (COPD) include lung disorders that cause long-term airway obstruction and difficulty breathing.
- The prevalence of asthma in the United States has risen dramatically in recent years.
- Obstructive sleep apnea involves intermittent partial or complete obstruction of the upper airway.
- Other major respiratory diseases include lung cancer and cystic fibrosis.

Key Terms

acute bronchitis
asthma
bronchospasms
chronic bronchitis
chronic obstructive pulmonary disease (COPD)
emphysema
hyperventilation
hypoxia
influenza
laryngitis
nasopharyngitis
pharyngitis
pneumonia
sinusitis
tonsillitis
tuberculosis (TB)

Assessment

➤ **LESSON 9.1**

Functions and Anatomy of the Respiratory System

Learning Key Terms and Concepts

1. The main purpose of the respiratory system is to provide a constant supply of oxygen while eliminating _____.
2. Which of the following is *not* part of the respiratory system?
   A. nose
   B. lungs
   C. duodenum
   D. trachea
3. The nasal cavity contains oily, coated hairs called _____ that trap and prevent particles from entering the nose.
4. *True or False?* The roof of the mouth is known as the *palate*.
5. _____ are air-filled cavities that surround the nose.
6. *True or False?* The pharynx is part of both the respiratory and digestive systems.
7. The anatomical term for the voice box is the _____.

8. The flap of cartilage that covers the opening of the larynx during swallowing to prevent food or liquids from entering the trachea is called the _____.
   A. uvula
   B. tonsils
   C. epiglottis
   D. pharynx
9. *True or False*? *Trachea* is the anatomical term for the *windpipe*.
10. The trachea divides into right and left _____.
11. The air-filled sacs in the lungs where gas exchange occurs are called _____.
12. The central area of the thoracic cavity is the _____.

Thinking Critically

13. Explain in your own words how the nasal conchae filter inspired air. Why do you think this filtering method is so effective?
14. The anterior part of the trachea is supported by cartilaginous C-shaped rings that prevent it from collapsing. On the posterior side, the C-shaped rings are open and contain no cartilage. Why is this beneficial?
15. Which passageway in the human body is used for air, food, and water? Why do you not drown or choke when using this passageway?

LESSON 9.2

Respiration: Mechanics and Control

Learning Key Terms and Concepts

16. Another name for breathing is _____.
17. _____ is the respiratory process by which air is continuously moved into and out of the lungs.
   A. Pulmonary ventilation
   B. External respiration
   C. Respiratory gas transport
   D. Internal respiration
18. _____, also called *inhalation*, is the process by which air flows into the lungs.
19. *True or False*? Normal expiration is an active process.
20. *True or False*? Breathing rate cannot be consciously controlled.
21. *True or False*? Your postural position affects your breathing rate.
22. _____ monitor cerebrospinal fluid pH to detect excess carbon dioxide levels in the body.
   A. Stretch receptors
   B. Central chemoreceptors
   C. Peripheral chemoreceptors
   D. Mechanoreceptors
23. Lung volume varies according to all of the following factors *except* _____.
   A. temperature
   B. weight
   C. height
   D. race
24. During maximal exercise, humans use only about _____ of their lungs' vital capacity.
   A. 30%
   B. 50%
   C. 65%
   D. 85%
25. *True or False*? Lung volume generally does not predict the average athlete's performance.

Thinking Critically

26. Explain in your own words the difference between each of the following pairs of lung capacity measurements.
   A. tidal volume and inspiratory reserve volume
   B. expiratory volume and vital capacity
   C. FEV_1 and ERV
27. Explain the following formula:
   IRV + TV + ERV + RV = TLC.
   What does each abbreviation mean? Why do these four elements equal TLC?
28. Recalling what you have learned about neural and chemical factors that control breathing rate, why is it not possible to hold your breath for long periods of time?
29. Compare and contrast the effects of central chemoreceptors and peripheral chemoreceptors.
30. Explain the Hering-Breuer reflex.

LESSON 9.3

Respiratory Disorders and Diseases

Learning Key Terms and Concepts

31. Respiratory infections occur most commonly in the _____.
    A. upper respiratory tract
    B. lower respiratory tract
32. Inflammation of the throat is called _____.
    A. laryngitis
    B. pharyngitis
    C. tonsillitis
    D. sinusitis
33. Laryngitis is an inflammation of the _____, or voice box.
    A. palatine tonsil
    B. pharynx
    C. vomer
    D. larynx
34. *True or False*? Sinusitis can be caused by fungi.
35. *True or False*? Influenza causes white or yellow patches to form on the tonsils.
36. Acute bronchitis usually develops in response to an ongoing _____ infection.
    A. viral
    B. bacterial
    C. fungal
    D. helminthic
37. *True or False*? People with tuberculosis must be confined to their home or the hospital for two to four years to avoid spreading this highly contagious disease.
38. The two most common forms of COPD are emphysema and _____.
    A. tuberculosis
    B. chronic bronchitis
    C. pneumonia
    D. respiratory distress syndrome
39. Bronchitis is considered chronic when a person has a cough that has lasted _____.
    A. two to three weeks
    B. five or six days
    C. three months to two years
    D. ten years or longer
40. The primary cause of COPD is _____.
41. *True or False*? Emotional stress can trigger an asthma attack.
42. About _____ of adults and children in the United States have asthma.
    A. 3%
    B. 10%
    C. 8%
    D. 14%
43. Sleep apnea is diagnosed when a person stops breathing for a period of _____ seconds or longer for a minimum of five times per hour while sleeping.
    A. 3
    B. 10
    C. 18
    D. 20
44. Surgery, radiation therapy, and _____ are treatment options for lung cancer.

Thinking Critically

45. Imagine that you are a doctor, and a female patient visits your office with a complaint of headache, fatigue, sinus pain and stuffiness, body aches, and chills. You take her temperature and discover that she has a fever of 102°F (38.9°C). She tells you that she felt fine the night before but woke up that morning feeling terrible. Based on the patient's symptoms, what do you think her diagnosis might be? Why?
46. Identify the respiratory diseases associated with the terms "pink puffers" and "blue bloaters." Why are these terms appropriate for each disease?
47. Given that many forms of lung cancer can be prevented, why do you think the incidence of lung cancer is so high?
48. Suppose one of your best friends contracts a contagious lung disease. What could you do to protect yourself while visiting your friend?
49. Respiratory syncytial virus (RSV) is a common virus that causes an infection in the lungs and respiratory tract. In many cases, it causes symptoms similar to those of the common cold, and it goes away on its own. In some people, however, the infection can be severe and can lead to more dangerous illnesses. What factors or characteristics may cause RSV to be a severe threat to a person? Why?

Building Skills and Connecting Concepts

Analyzing and Evaluating Data

Imagine that you are a doctor and one of your patients is an active, 15-year-old boy named Toua. Toua complains of tightness in his chest, wheezing, and breathlessness. Using a computerized flow-volume meter, you test Toua's dynamic lung volumes. His test results are shown in **Figure 9.26**. Review Toua's test results and then answer the questions that follow.

Test	Predicted	Toua's Value
FVC	3.86 L	2.81 L
FEV_1	3.20 L	2.20 L
FEV_1/FVC	83%	78%

Figure 9.26 *Goodheart-Willcox Publisher*

49. In your own words, what does the forced expiratory volume in 1 second (FEV_1) represent?
50. What does the ratio of FEV_1/FVC measurement mean about a person's ability to breathe?
51. What percentage of the predicted values are Toua's FEV_1 and FEV_1/FVC measurements?
52. Do these measurements show that Toua has asthma? Explain your answer.

Communicating about Anatomy & Physiology

53. **Speaking and Writing** Working in a group of three or four students, recall the last time that you had a cold or the flu. Discuss common symptoms. Write down the five most common symptoms. Do research to find out why these symptoms occurred. For example, a sore throat is caused by mucus dripping into your pharynx (throat), producing irritation and inflammation. Share your findings with the class.
54. **Reading and Writing** In this chapter, you learned that the respiratory and cardiovascular systems work together to conduct gas exchange. Think about the body systems that you have studied so far and skim ahead looking for similar relationships between the structures and functions of systems. Write a detailed report that describes and analyzes one or more of these relationships.
55. Speaking Form two teams for a debate. The topic for the debate is: If you know you are a carrier for a severe lung disease such as cystic fibrosis would you choose to have children? Debate this question as a class, using the following Health Occupations Students of America (HOSA) guidelines:

    Affirmative Constructive Speech (4 minutes).
    The speaker for the affirmative presents their arguments.

    Negative Cross-Examination (2 minutes).
    The speaker(s) for the negative questions the affirmative speaker on the points made in the affirmative constructive speech.

    Negative Constructive Speech (4 minutes).
    The speaker for the negative presents their arguments.

    Affirmative Cross-Examination (2 minutes).
    The speaker(s) for the affirmative questions the negative speaker on the points made in the negative constructive speech.

    Affirmative Rebuttal (3 minutes).
    The affirmative speaker rebuts the points made by the negative speaker.

    Negative Rebuttal (4 minutes).
    The negative speaker rebuts the points made by the affirmative speaker.

    Final Affirmative Rebuttal (1 minute).
    The affirmative speaker again rebuts.

Lab Investigations

56. Work with a partner to determine breathing recovery rates after exercise.

    Important: *If you have asthma, do not attempt this lab activity.*

    Take turns measuring your resting breathing rate. Count the number of breaths in one minute. (Refer to the "Measuring Vital Signs" section in Chapter 11 for instructions on counting respirations.) Do this three times, find the average, and then record your resting breathing rate.

    Next, do 25 jumping jacks. Immediately afterward, have your partner count the number of breaths that you take in one minute. Record this number. Continue to record the number of breaths that you take each minute after that. Then count the number of minutes that it takes you to return to your resting breathing rate. Record this number.

    Finally, run in place for two minutes. Immediately afterward, have your partner count the number of breaths that you take during the first minute. Record this number. Then record the number of breaths that you take each minute until you have returned to your resting breathing rate. Record these numbers.

    A. Compare your average resting rate, your respiratory rate one minute after doing the jumping jacks, and your respiratory rate after running in place. Is there a great difference between these numbers? Explain your results.
    B. Examine the number of minutes that it took to return to your resting rate after doing 25 jumping jacks and after running in place. Are these numbers higher or lower than you expected?
    C. The faster that your respiratory rate returns to its resting value, the more physically fit you are. Based on your results, what do you think your level of physical fitness is? If your physical fitness is lower than you'd like, what are some strategies that you can undertake to improve it?

57. Conduct an experiment to simulate different levels of respiratory distress. To do this, design an experiment to measure the impact of a respiratory disorder on respiratory rate and pulse. You will need at least one volunteer "subject" on which to perform the experiment. Measure the subject's respiratory rate and pulse at rest and after a period of activity. Ask the subject to breathe through straws of various sizes to simulate breathing restrictions.

    Important: *Do not accept any volunteers who have asthma or are sick or have recently been sick. If any subject shows signs of distress or feels dizzy, stop the experiment immediately.*

    Prepare a full lab report describing the materials and the procedure you used. Create a graph or chart to present your experimental data. Include a discussion of your results and form a conclusion about the impact of a respiratory disorder on respiratory rate and pulse.

Building Your Portfolio

58. Take digital photographs of the models and projects you created as you worked through this chapter. Create a document or folder called "The Respiratory System" and insert the photographs, along with written descriptions of what the models show and your reasons for creating them using the materials and forms you chose. Add the reports from your laboratory experiments and add this document to your personal portfolio.

CHAPTER

10 The Blood

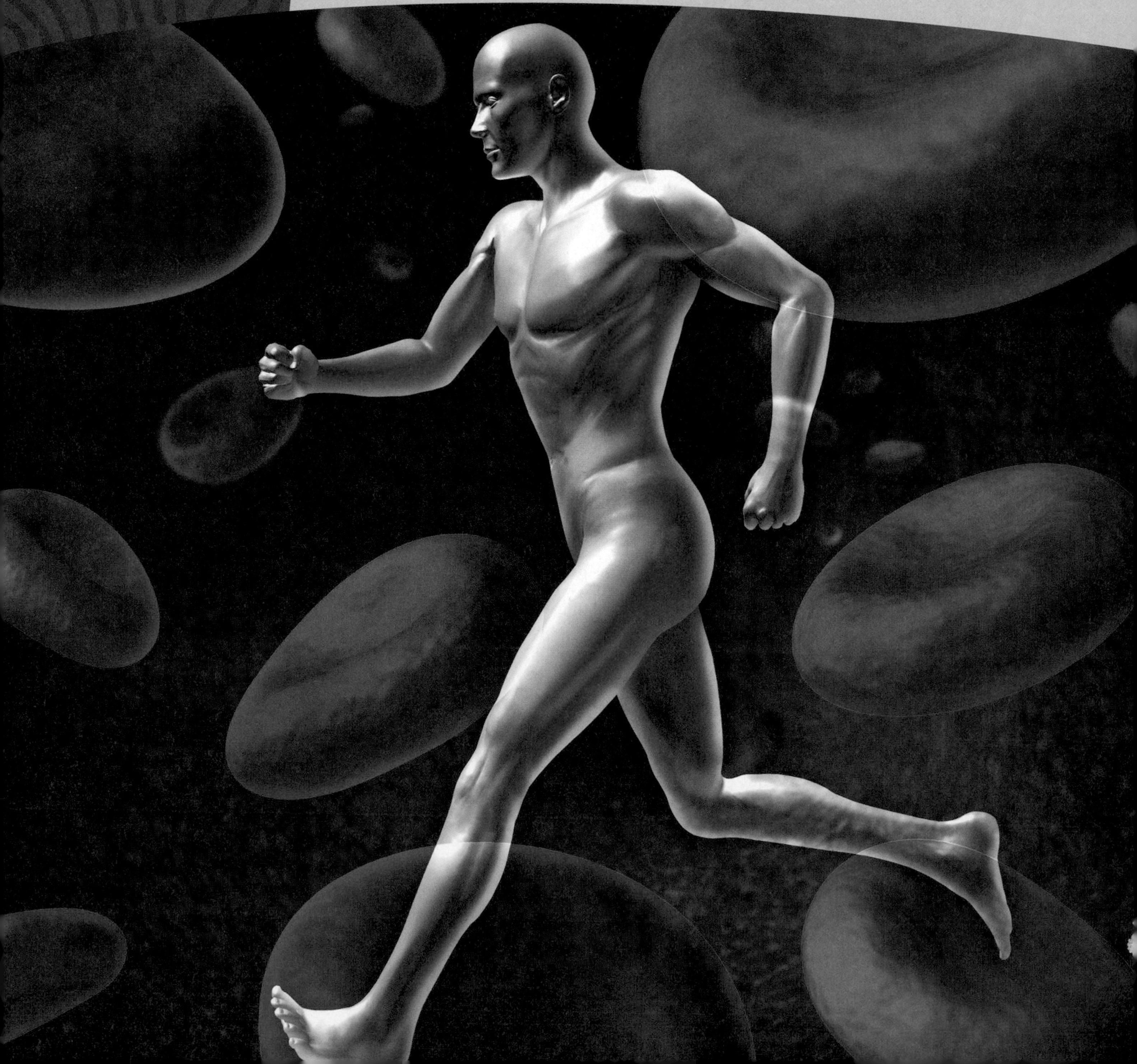

Why is it important to know your blood type?

The life-giving functions of blood has not always been clear. As early as Greek times, physicians thought that draining blood from the body, a procedure known as *bloodletting*, would cure the sick and restore health to the body. This practice continued into the late 1800s.

As you might suspect, some individuals did not fare well from bloodletting. Bloodletting contributed to the death of President George Washington. During a brief illness that began with a sore throat and fever, Washington's physicians bled him. Over the course of 16 hours, physicians drained 5 to 7 pints of Washington's blood. That's equivalent to 40% to 60% of the body's supply of blood! Not surprisingly, President Washington died shortly thereafter.

Today the important role that blood plays in maintaining a person's health and sustaining life is better understood. For this reason, many people donate their blood to organizations such as the American Red Cross, which maintains blood banks. When you donate blood, you really are giving the gift of life: one pint can feed, protect, clean, and heal up to three people. This chapter explains the functions and composition of blood, blood types, and common blood disorders and diseases.

Click on the activity icon or visit www.g-wlearning.com/healthsciences/0202 to access online vocabulary activities using key terms from the chapter.

Chapter 10 Outline

◂ Lightspring/Shutterstock.com

LESSON **10.1**

The Function and Composition of Blood

Before You Read

Try to answer the following questions before you read this lesson.

- What substances does blood transport?
- How does blood protect the body from infection?

Lesson Objectives

- Identify the functions of blood in the human body.
- Describe the physical properties of blood.
- Explain the components of blood and their functions, including red blood cells, white blood cells, and platelets.

Key Terms

buffy coat
carbaminohemoglobin
coagulation
diapedesis
erythrocytes
erythropoiesis
erythropoietin
fibrin
formed elements
hematocrit
hematopoiesis
hemoglobin
hemolysis
hemostasis
leukocytes
oxyhemoglobin
plasma
platelet plug
platelets

Every day, your body undergoes so many changes that it would be hard to quantify them. Even with all of these changes, however, the body maintains homeostasis through many dynamic regulatory systems. Blood is one of the body's regulatory and transport systems. Blood plays a vital role in gas exchange; body temperature maintenance; and acid-base, fluid, and electrolyte balance.

The Functions of Blood

The blood is responsible for providing transportation, regulation, and protection throughout the body. It plays a key role in gas exchange, which, as explained in Chapter 9, involves supplying oxygen and other nutrients to cells, while also removing carbon dioxide and other waste products. The blood carries waste to the kidneys and carbon dioxide to the lungs, where both the waste and carbon dioxide are eliminated from the body.

Blood also protects the body against infection and regulates body temperature by directing heat toward the skin and lungs. In addition, buffers and amino acids transported in the blood help maintain the body's pH at healthy levels between 7.35 and 7.45. **Figure 10.1** summarizes the roles that blood plays in maintaining homeostasis.

Check Your Understanding

1. The functions of blood can be divided into what three major categories? Give two specific examples for each category.
2. What is a healthy pH for the human body?

Physical Properties of Blood

Blood is a sticky, thick fluid that makes up roughly 8% of total body weight. Both men and women have, on average, between 4 and 5 liters of blood in their bodies. However, blood volume

Functions of the Blood	
Transports	oxygen and carbon dioxide
	waste products of metabolism (urea and lactic acid)
	hormones
	enzymes
	nutrients (glucose, fats, amino acids, vitamins, and minerals)
	blood cells (white and red)
	plasma proteins (fibrinogen, albumin, globulin)
Regulates	body temperature
	acid-base balance (pH)
	fluid and electrolyte balance
Protects	white blood cells protect against infection
	antibodies detect foreign material
	clotting factors prevent excessive bleeding

Figure 10.1 *Goodheart-Willcox Publisher*

depends on body size, muscle mass, and physical fitness. Athletes, for example, have higher blood volumes than nonathletes.

Blood is slightly salty, with a sodium chloride concentration of 0.9%. It has a pH between 7.35 and 7.45 and an average temperature of 100.4°F (38°C). The color of blood varies based on the oxygen level in the bloodstream. Oxygen-rich blood in the arteries is a brighter red than the oxygen-poor blood in the veins.

The old saying that "blood is thicker than water" is literally true. At 100.4°F (38°C), the viscosity (thickness) of blood is about five times thicker than that of water. This is because blood contains solid components such as the formed elements and plasma proteins. Blood viscosity contributes to blood flow resistance. In general, the thicker the blood, the harder the heart has to work to maintain blood flow. Factors that increase blood viscosity are decreased blood temperature, prolonged exposure to a high altitude, and an elevated number of red blood cells.

Check Your Understanding

1. What are the two basic components of blood?
2. Typically, what percentage of the blood is made up of plasma?
3. Which physical property of blood is affected by differences in the blood oxygen level?

Composition of Blood

Blood has two basic components: the liquid component, called **plasma**, and the solid components, collectively referred to as the **formed elements** (**Figure 10.2**). The formed elements consist of **erythrocytes** (red blood cells), **leukocytes** (white blood cells), and **platelets** (thrombocytes). Red blood cells carry oxygen to tissue, white blood cells protect the body, and platelets play a vital role in blood clotting. The formed elements make up about 45% of the blood's content, and plasma comprises the remaining 55%.

Components of blood are readily identified when a blood sample is taken and spun down in a centrifuge. A *centrifuge* is a machine that spins rapidly, generating a centrifugal force that separates elements in the blood. The blood separates into three layers: liquid plasma rises to the top of the tube, red blood cells settle at the bottom of the tube, and a thin layer called the **buffy coat** settles between the red blood cells and plasma. The buffy coat contains white blood cells and platelets (**Figure 10.3**).

Separating the blood elements allows a common blood measurement called **hematocrit** (hee-MAT-oh-krit). Hematocrit is the proportion of the total blood volume that is composed of red blood cells. This proportion of red blood cells is expressed as a percentage of total blood volume.

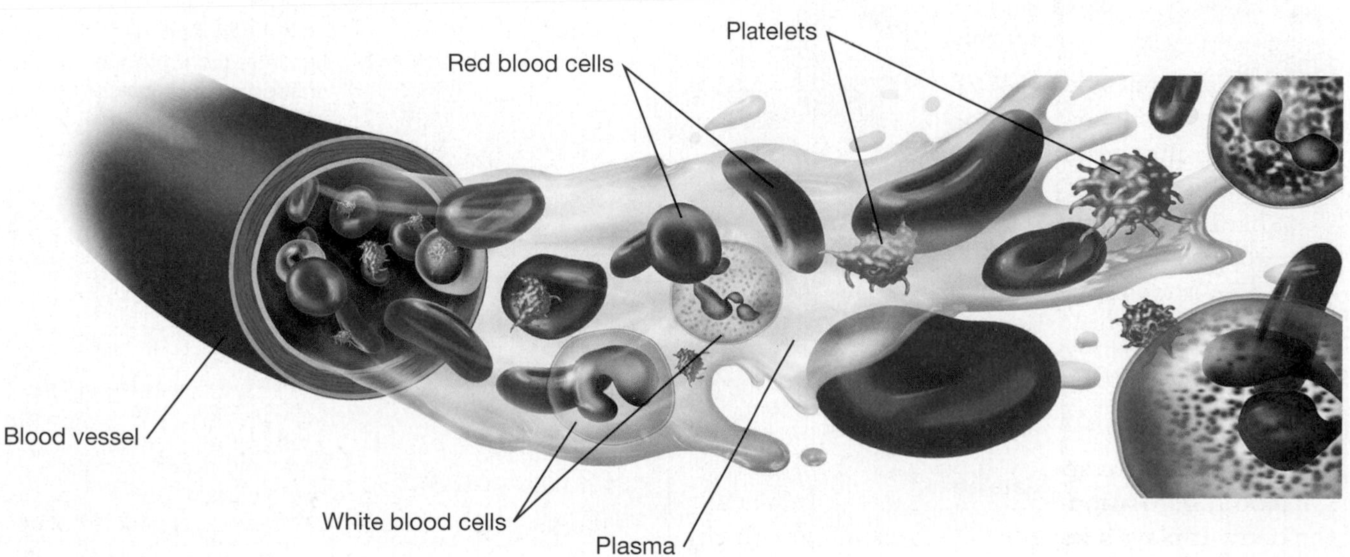

Figure 10.2 Blood is made up of both liquid (plasma) and solid components (the formed elements). *What three substances comprise the formed elements?*

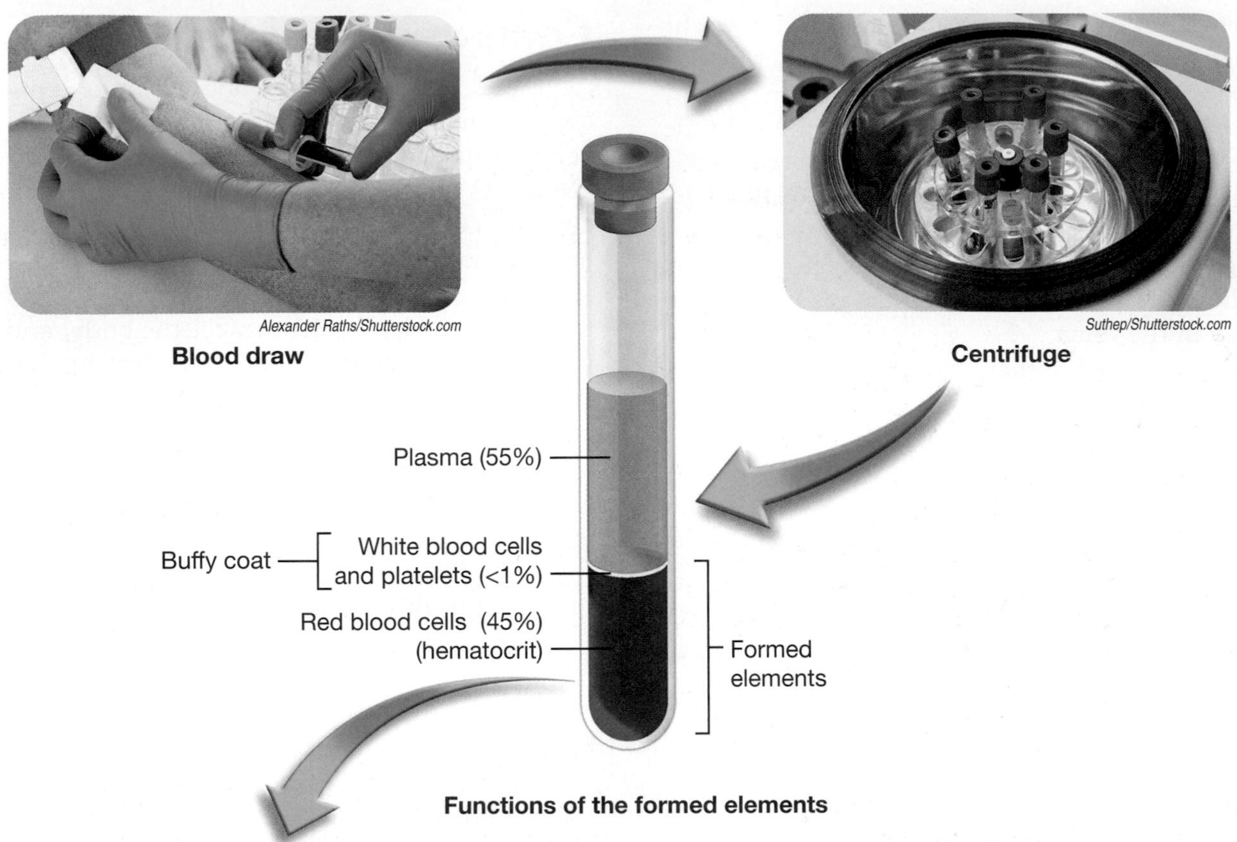

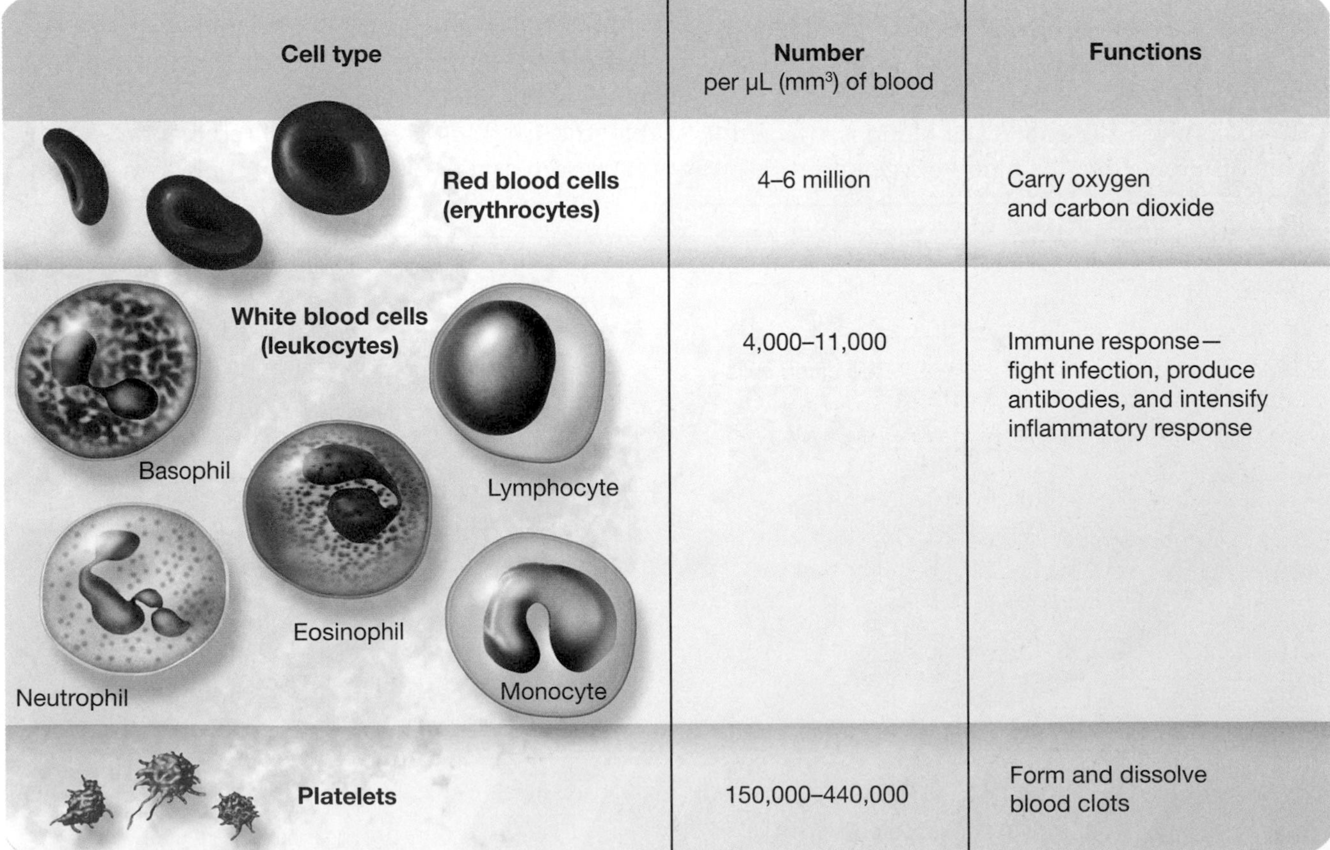

Cell type	Number per µL (mm³) of blood	Functions
Red blood cells (erythrocytes)	4–6 million	Carry oxygen and carbon dioxide
White blood cells (leukocytes) Basophil, Lymphocyte, Eosinophil, Neutrophil, Monocyte	4,000–11,000	Immune response—fight infection, produce antibodies, and intensify inflammatory response
Platelets	150,000–440,000	Form and dissolve blood clots

Figure 10.3 Drawn blood is spun through a centrifuge to separate the plasma and formed elements. *What property of blood does hematocrit measure?*

Hematocrit averages 45% of total blood volume in men and 40% of total blood volume in women. Hematocrit is fairly constant, but dehydration can cause it to increase due to loss of blood plasma or decreased blood volume. However, if you live at a high altitude, your hematocrit may increase to 60% or 65% of your total blood volume because altitude exposure increases red blood cell production.

Plasma

The formed elements are transported in the plasma, or liquid part of the blood. Plasma is a pale yellow fluid composed mostly of water. Although the levels vary slightly, plasma consists of approximately 90% water and 8% plasma proteins; the remaining 2% is a mixture of electrolytes, nutrients, ions, respiratory gases, hormones, and waste products.

Blood plasma contains three types of proteins: fibrinogen, albumin, and globulin (**Figure 10.4**). These proteins perform a variety of functions, including transporting lipids (fats) and fat-soluble vitamins, regulating blood pressure and volume, and assisting in blood clot formation.

Besides water and plasma proteins, blood plasma contains a mixture of electrolytes and buffers. The electrolytes include sodium, potassium, chloride, magnesium, and calcium, all of which help maintain fluid and electrolyte balance. Buffers such as bicarbonate, phosphate, and sulfate regulate blood pH.

As blood travels through the body, it collects and removes carbon dioxide, a waste product. Plasma contains a bicarbonate that provides the primary means for carbon dioxide transport. Because of gas exchange and different substances being added to or removed from plasma, its composition varies from minute to minute. However, homeostatic mechanisms monitor and maintain relatively constant plasma composition. In short, blood plasma transports elements throughout the body to maintain homeostasis.

Maintaining homeostasis requires constant effort. Think about all the changes that take place in the body during a 30-minute run, for example. Blood glucose levels decline, blood pH becomes more acidic, and blood temperature increases. The body's feedback systems sense these changes and respond accordingly. To maintain homeostasis in this situation, gluconeogenesis begins, respiration increases to buffer (balance) the acidic pH of the blood, the sweat glands are activated, and blood flow is shifted closer to the surface of the skin to cool the body. Plasma plays an important role in each of these responses. It would be impossible to maintain homeostasis without it.

Erythrocytes

You will often hear erythrocytes, or red blood cells, referred to as *RBCs*. RBCs perform one of the most important functions in the body—gas exchange. They carry oxygen to every living cell in the body and carry carbon dioxide away. RBCs are the most abundant cells in the blood, numbering between 4 and 6 million per cubic millimeter. To put this number into perspective, a cubic millimeter is so small that it is almost invisible to the naked eye. Imagine 4 to 6 million cells in a tiny, nearly invisible speck!

Shape and Size

Mature RBCs are disk-shaped cells that look like a doughnut without the hole in the center. Anatomically, this shape is called a

Plasma Proteins

Protein	Percent of Plasma Composition	Origin	Function
albumin	58%	liver	regulates osmotic pressure of blood and blood volume; transports lipids, hormones, and other solutes
globulin	38%		aids in blood clot formation;
alpha		liver	transports lipids and fat-soluble vitamins
beta		liver	transports lipids and fat-soluble vitamins
gamma		plasma cells	helps fight infection
fibrinogen	4%	liver	aids in blood clot formation

Figure 10.4

Goodheart-Willcox Publisher

biconcave disk. They are small, measuring only 7 or 8 micrometers in diameter. To put this measurement into perspective, 1 millimeter is equal to 1,000 micrometers.

As RBCs develop, the nucleus is forced out of the cell, causing the center of the cell to collapse. This mechanism of development serves three important functions:

- It increases the surface area of the cell, providing a larger binding area for oxygen and carbon dioxide.
- It increases the flexibility of the cell, allowing it to change shape so it can fit into capillary openings that are half the size of the cell.
- It limits the cell's life span to 120 days; without a nucleus, the cell is unable to replicate.

Hemoglobin

The **hemoglobin** (HEE-moh-gloh-bin) molecule is the "workhorse" of the red blood cell because it carries out the important job of gas exchange. Oxygen and carbon dioxide attach to the hemoglobin molecules of the RBC; thus, hemoglobin is known as the *binding site*.

Hemoglobin is actually composed of two molecules: a large protein called *globin* (GLOH-bin) and an iron molecule called *heme* (heem). Each hemoglobin molecule has four heme binding sites for oxygen (**Figure 10.5**). Before you donate blood, your hemoglobin level is measured, because removing blood from your body lowers the iron level. Iron is necessary for maintaining your energy and strength.

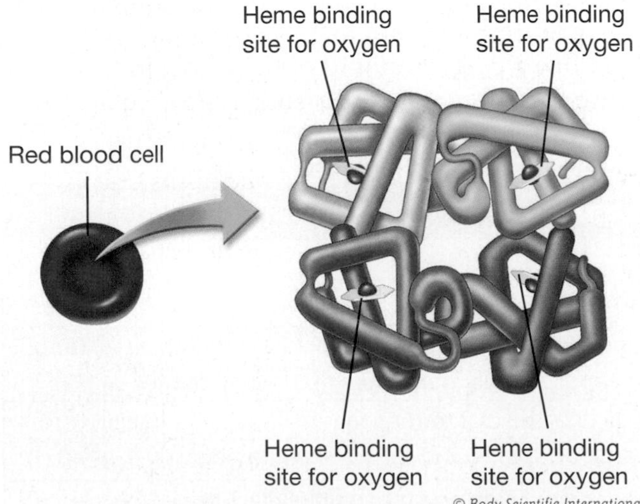

Figure 10.5 During gas exchange, oxygen binds to hemoglobin at each of the four heme binding sites.

One RBC contains approximately 250 million hemoglobin molecules. This means that one RBC carries almost 1 billion oxygen molecules. Hemoglobin levels differ between men and women. In men, they range from 12 to 16 grams per deciliter (g/dL); in women, hemoglobin levels range from 13 to 18 grams per deciliter.

Oxygen binds to hemoglobin, forming an **oxyhemoglobin** (ahk-see-HEE-moh-gloh-bin) molecule in the capillaries of the lung. The oxygen-rich RBCs then travel to tissue capillaries. There the oxygen is unloaded from the hemoglobin, diffusing from the blood into the oxygen-deprived tissues.

The globin protein serves as the binding site for carbon dioxide. Once carbon dioxide has attached to the hemoglobin molecule, a **carbaminohemoglobin** (kar-bahm-i-noh-HEE-moh-gloh-bin) molecule is formed. The carbaminohemoglobin molecule transports carbon dioxide back to the lungs to be expelled from the body. Keep in mind, however, that the bicarbonate ion in plasma is the chief means by which carbon dioxide is transported.

Erythropoiesis

The kidneys regulate red blood cell production through a process called **erythropoiesis** (eh-rith-roh-poy-EE-sis). When blood oxygen content decreases—as it does where the altitude is above 5,000 feet—the kidneys secrete a hormone called **erythropoietin** (eh-rith-roh-POY-eh-tin), or EPO. Erythropoietin stimulates stem cell production of RBCs in the red bone marrow (**Figure 10.6**).

When additional RBCs are produced and blood oxygen levels rise, erythropoietin levels diminish, slowing RBC production. Thus, any condition or factor that lowers blood oxygen levels (such as emphysema or high altitude exposure) causes the kidneys to release erythropoietin and stimulate RBC production. If too many RBCs are produced, polycythemia (pahl-ee-sigh-THEE-mee-ah) can develop. Polycythemia is discussed in more depth in Lesson 10.3.

Iron, folic acid, vitamin B_{12}, and protein are needed for RBC production, as well as for red bone marrow. People who are anemic, and potentially those with an iron-deficient diet, lack enough iron to properly form the heme component of hemoglobin. The result is iron-deficient anemia, a blood disorder that you'll learn more about later in this chapter.

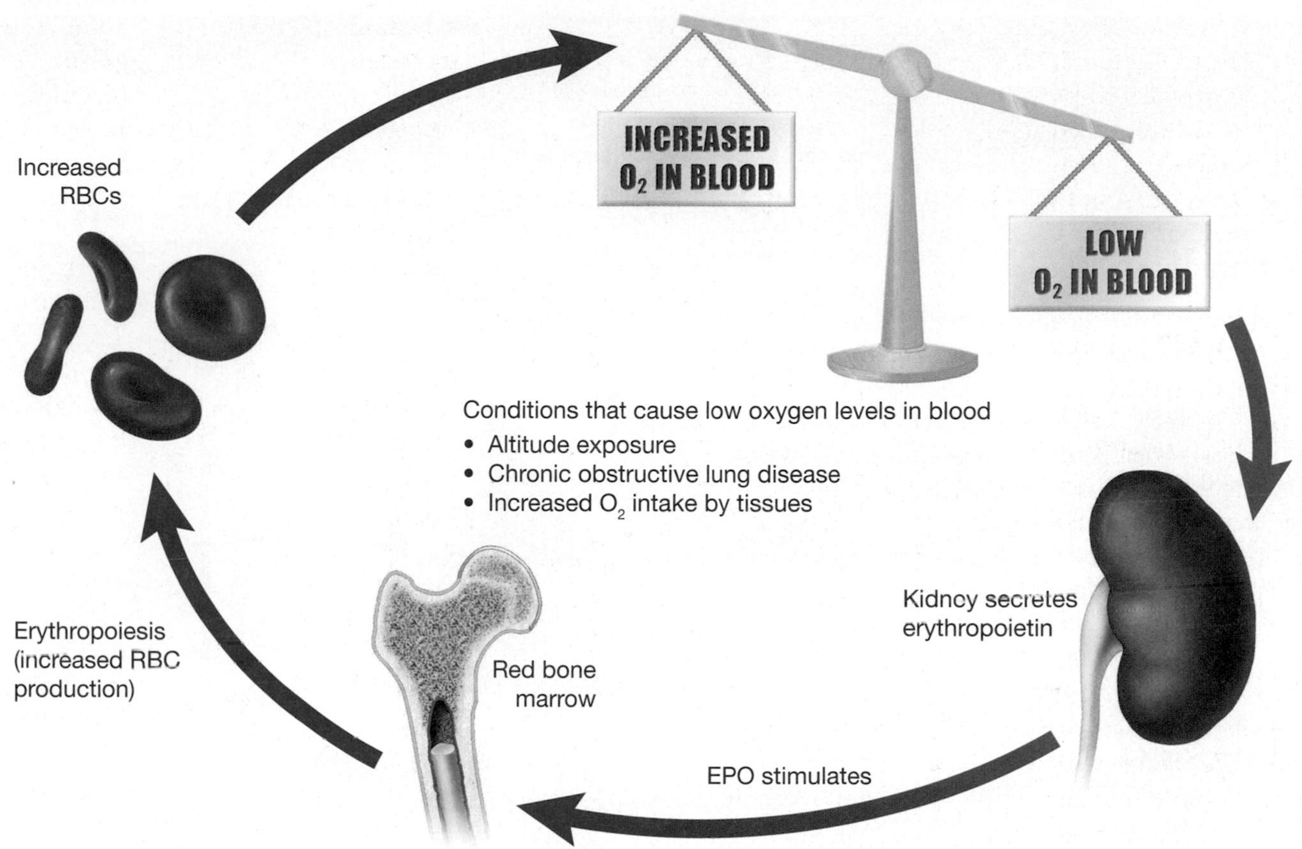

Figure 10.6 The endocrine system works with the blood to release the hormone erythropoietin, which stimulates red blood cell production.

Your Body Goes Green: Recycling Red Blood Cells

Red blood cells have the remarkable ability to bend, twist, and turn, allowing them to fit into capillaries half their size. All these contortions take their toll on the RBC, causing its membrane to quickly become ragged. The ragged membrane, coupled with the lack of a nucleus, seals the fate of the RBC—death by phagocytosis.

Phagocytosis (fayg-oh-sigh-TOH-sis) is the process by which macrophages (MAK-roh-fayj-ez) in the liver and spleen eat and recycle old RBCs, as well as other types of cells. Macrophages are cells that play a major role in immune system function. Macrophages, phagocytes, and phagocytosis are described in Chapter 12.

Hemolysis (hee-MAHL-i-sis) is the rupture of RBCs. It occurs when RBCs approach the end of their 120-day life span. Hemolysis can also result from diseases of the RBCs caused by antibodies, infections, or blood transfusion complications.

With the exception of the hemoglobin molecules, the RBC breaks down quite easily. For a hemoglobin molecule to be recycled, it must first be separated into its two parts—globin and heme. The globin protein is further broken down into amino acids that are later used to make new proteins. The heme is broken down into iron and bilirubin (BIL-i-roo-bin), a waste product.

The iron is stored in the liver until the bone marrow needs it to manufacture new RBCs. The bilirubin is excreted into bile. The bile is transported to the gallbladder and then travels through the intestines, before finally being excreted in the feces.

Leukocytes

Leukocytes, or white blood cells (WBCs), serve as the body's infection fighters and therefore play an important role in immune response. At any given time, blood contains about 4,300 to 10,800 WBCs per cubic millimeter. For every 1 white blood cell in your blood, there are approximately 700 red blood cells.

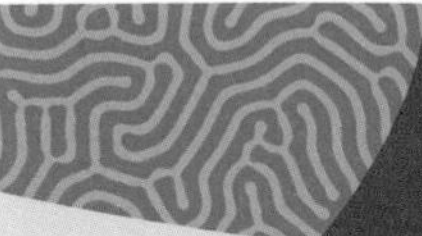

What Research Tells Us

...about Bioengineering Red Blood Cells to Create an Unlimited Supply

Since Roman times, scientists have been looking for viable (usable) substitutes for blood. Doctors and scientists have experimented with animal blood and animal milk. Even wine has been suggested as a possible alternative to blood.

Researchers at the Université Pierre et Marie Curie in Paris, France, have been studying the possibility of manufacturing red blood cells from stem cells. The researchers at this university were able to generate billions of RBCs from a single stem cell. The RBCs were then injected into the stem cell donor. The stem cells were treated with several different growth factors to stimulate them to develop into mature RBCs.

After 5 days, the survival rate of the human-engineered RBCs was 94% to 100%. Of this number, 41% to 63% were still alive after 26 days. This is similar to the survival rate of a normal RBC. This research is critical, especially when you consider how these engineered RBCs might be used.

Each year, the American Red Cross alone distributes about six million units of RBCs (**Figure 10.7**). According to the World Health Organization (WHO), each year more than 90 million blood donations are made at hospitals, clinics, blood banks, and donation centers around the world. However, some of these donations come from paid donors. In addition, the majority of blood donations are made in high-income countries.

Successful engineering of RBCs would limit dependence on paid donors, especially in low-income nations where voluntary donation is less common. Research continues, but this first successful attempt holds promise for a new way to achieve an unlimited blood supply.

plenoy m/Shutterstock.com

Figure 10.7 Every day, many units of blood are needed for transfusions and surgeries around the world.

Taking It Further

According to WHO, most blood transfusions in low-income countries are given to children with severe anemia and to women during childbirth. By contrast, the main reasons for blood transfusion in high-income countries are physical trauma (such as from a car accident), blood loss during organ-transplant surgeries, and blood disorders that require transfusion therapy. With your classmates, brainstorm possible reasons that donated blood is used for different purposes in low-income and high-income countries.

Although RBCs far outnumber WBCs, the ratio of 1 WBC for every 700 RBCs is a bit misleading. That's because WBCs can leave the blood, but RBCs cannot. Through a process called **diapedesis** (digh-a-peh-DEE-sis), WBCs slip through spaces in the capillary walls as they move from the blood to infection sites in body tissues. Therefore, the ratio of 1:700 does not really tell the complete story.

When a foreign microorganism, such as a virus or bacterium, is detected, the body dramatically increases WBC production. Within a matter of hours, the number of WBCs doubles. The WBCs then race to battle the infection.

WBCs have an arsenal of weapons that they use to fight infection. Some WBCs engulf and digest bacteria and other antigens in a process called *phagocytosis* (**Figure 10.8**). Other WBCs produce antibodies, intensify the inflammatory response (which increases swelling and draws more white blood cells to the site of an injury or infection), play a role in allergic reactions, or destroy parasitic worms.

The five types of white blood cells are neutrophils, eosinophils, basophils, lymphocytes, and monocytes. Each type varies by size, appearance, and function.

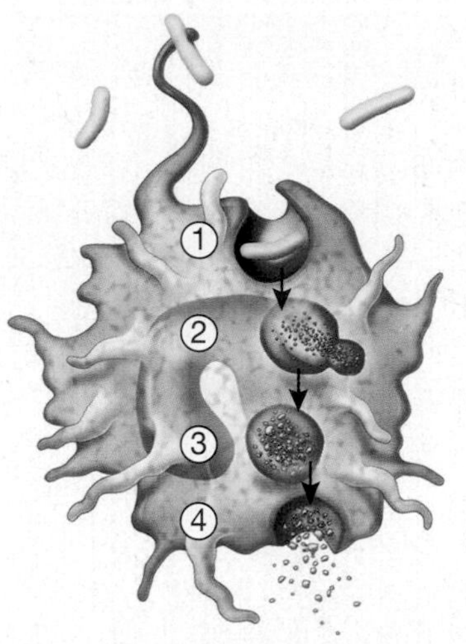
① White blood cell engulfs enemy cell (bacteria, dead cells)
② Enzymes start to destroy enemy cell
③ Enemy cell breaks down into small fragments
④ Indigestible fragments are discharged
© Body Scientific International

Figure 10.8 White blood cells engulf foreign antigens, such as bacteria, in an effort to fight infection and keep the body healthy.

Neutrophils, eosinophils, and basophils are classified as *granulocytes* (GRAN-yoo-loh-sights). Granulocytes have granules in their cytoplasm. Lymphocytes and monocytes are classified as *agranulocytes* (AY-gran-yoo-loh-sights) because their cytoplasm lacks granules.

Unlike RBCs, WBCs have a nucleus. The nucleus of a WBC is visible under a microscope when exposed to Wright's stain, a staining solution that scientists use to differentiate blood cell types. The size of a WBC, the shape and color of its nucleus, and the color of any granules after staining help scientists classify WBCs (**Figure 10.9**).

Neutrophils

Neutrophils are the most abundant type of white blood cells and are the most important component of the body's immune system because they are the "first responders." Neutrophils are active phagocytes, cells that engulf and kill foreign invaders such as bacteria, viruses, and fungi. Neutrophils are vital to fighting infection; therefore, a neutrophil deficiency is a life-threatening condition.

Eosinophils

Eosinophils make up only a small portion of the white blood cell count—about 1% to 3%. Eosinophils participate in many inflammatory processes, especially allergic reactions, and are capable of phagocytosis. They are particularly active in the presence of parasites and worms.

Basophils

Basophils are the least abundant white blood cells in the body. They produce histamine, which induces an inflammatory response and summons more infection-fighting WBCs to a site of injury or infection. Basophils also produce heparin, an anticoagulant that prevents blood clotting. Basophils are often associated with allergic reactions and asthma. They also play an important role in T cell adaptive immune responses.

Lymphocytes

Lymphocytes are the second most abundant white blood cells in the body. There are two types of lymphocytes: T cells and B cells. More than 80% of lymphocytes are T cells. Lymphocytes play an important role in the immune response by forming antibodies to fight antigens. Lymphocytes are also essential in fighting cancer cells.

Monocytes

Monocytes, the largest white blood cells in the body, are produced in red bone marrow and then move to the blood, where they remain for one to three days before migrating into body tissues. Once they have arrived in the tissues, monocytes develop into macrophages that devour microorganisms.

Platelets

Platelets (also called *thrombocytes*) are small, irregularly shaped cell fragments. As cell fragments, platelets do not have a nucleus. Old platelets are removed from the body by phagocytosis in the spleen and liver.

Platelets are derived from multinucleated megakaryocytes (mehg-a-KAIR-ee-oh-sights), which are specialized bone marrow cells. Like red and white blood cells, megakaryocytes develop from a hematopoietic stem cell. The hormone *thrombopoietin* (thrahm-boh-POY-eh-tin) regulates platelet production from megakaryocytes. Thrombopoietin is produced by the liver and kidneys.

Platelets play an important role in **hemostasis** (hee-moh-STAY-sis), the sequence of events that causes blood clots to form and bleeding to stop (**Figure 10.10**). Hemostasis involves four key steps.

Characteristics of White Blood Cells				
Type	**Microscopic appearance**	**Percentage of WBCs**	**Diameter**	**Function**
Granulocytes				
neutrophil	pale pink stain with fine granules in the cytoplasm; multilobed, deep purple nucleus	55%–77%	10–12 micrometers	performs phagocytosis; kills bacteria and fungi
eosinophil	rose-colored stain with coarse granules in the cytoplasm; two blue-red, irregularly shaped nuclei	1%–3%	10–12 micrometers	destroys parasitic worms; controls allergic responses
basophil	dark blue stain with large purple granules in the cytoplasm; nucleus with 2–3 lobes	<1%	8–10 micrometers	releases histamine, intensifying the inflammatory process; liberates the anticoagulant heparin; active in allergic reactions
Agranulocytes				
lymphocyte	light blue-stained cytoplasm and dark blue, disk-shaped nucleus	25%–33%	7–8 micrometers	B cells produce antibodies; T cells and natural killer cells fight cancerous tumors and viruses
monocyte	grayish-blue cytoplasm; blue-purple stained, kidney-shaped nucleus	2%–10%	7.5–10 micrometers	performs phagocytosis; lives longer than neutrophil; morphs into macrophage that removes dead cell debris and attacks microorganisms

Figure 10.9

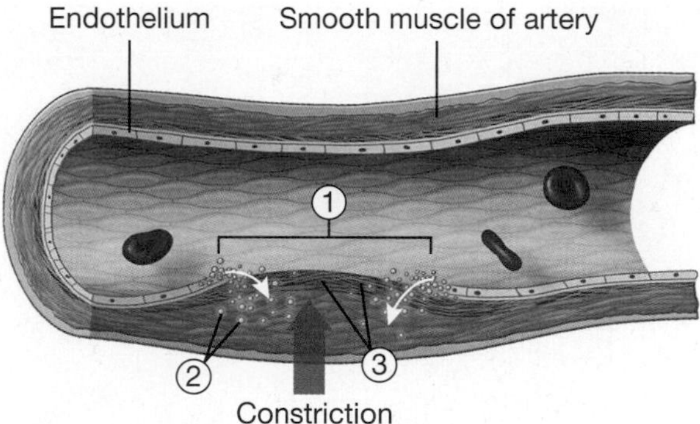

1 Vessel wall injury and constriction

1. Site of injury
2. Endothelin release causes constriction
3. Collagen fibers exposed

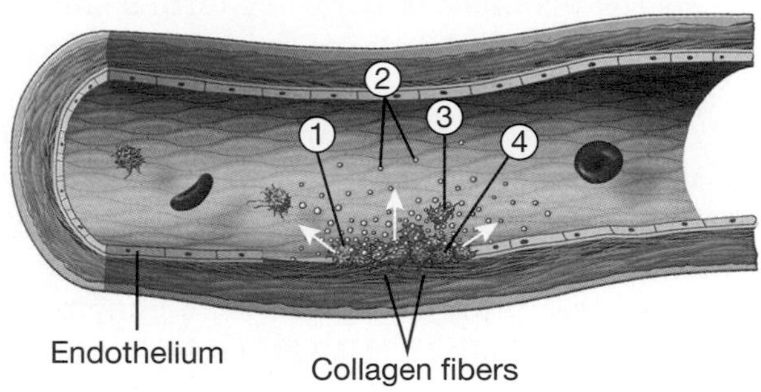

2 Platelet aggregation

1. Platelet adhesion
2. Chemicals released by platelets
3. Platelets gather
4. Platelets cluster to repair wall

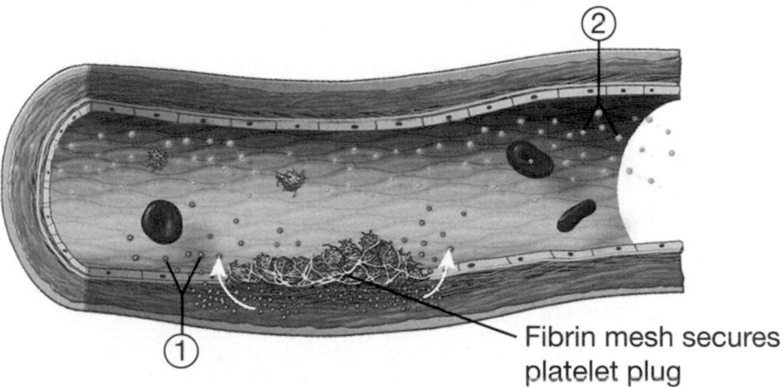

3 Platelet plug formation and coagulation

1. Tissue factor released
2. Clotting factors released

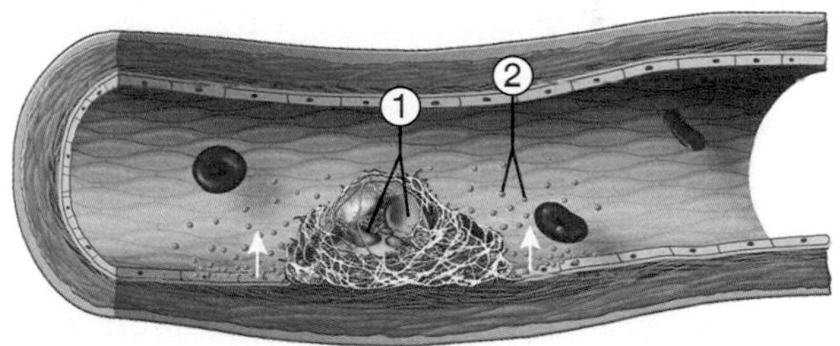

4 Blood clot formation

1. Red and white blood cells are trapped in mesh
2. Release of coagulation inhibitors and other chemicals

Figure 10.10 Injured vessel walls are repaired during a process called *hemostasis*. *When a blood vessel wall is injured, what hormone is released to constrict the vessel wall?*

1. **Vessel wall injury and constriction.** When the endothelium, or inner lining of a blood vessel, is injured, it releases endothelin (en-doh-THEE-lin). Endothelin is a hormone that causes the blood vessel to constrict and spasm for several minutes. This constriction helps reduce blood loss at the site of the injury. Under normal circumstances, platelets do not adhere to the blood vessel wall because the wall is coated with a platelet repellent called *prostacyclin* (prahs-ta-SIGH-klin). When the blood vessel wall is injured, the prostacyclin is breached, exposing the collagen fibers along the wall.
2. **Platelet aggregation.** Platelets stick to the collagen fibers and to the rough edges of the blood vessel wall (*platelet adhesion*). The platelets act like a spackling compound to repair the hole or tear. In addition, the platelets release chemicals that maintain constriction of the blood vessel and attract more platelets to the damaged wall.

3. **Platelet plug formation and coagulation.** As the platelets gather, they form a small, loose mass at the site of the injury called a **platelet plug**. To initiate **coagulation** (koh-ag-yoo-LAY-shun), the injured blood vessel releases a chemical called *tissue factor*. Tissue factor activates 11 different clotting factors in the blood. These clotting factors, which are proteins, combine an enzyme called *thrombin* (THRAHM-bin) with the protein *fibrinogen* (figh-BRIN-oh-jehn). The combination of thrombin and fibrinogen produces **fibrin**, a long, thread-like fiber. The fibrin strands weave in and around the platelet plug, forming a strong, tightly woven fibrin mesh. The process can be compared to throwing a fishing net around the platelet plug.
4. **Blood clot formation and retraction.** Red and white blood cells get trapped in the fibrin mesh, giving the blood clot a red color (**Figure 10.12**). When coagulation is complete—usually somewhere between 2 and 15 minutes—the blood clot has formed. Shortly after the fibrin mesh is in place, the blood clot begins to retract, or shrink in size. This process normally takes 30 to 60 minutes.

As the blood clot retracts, platelets pull the fibrin threads together. This, in turn, draws the edges of the ruptured vessel together. Meanwhile, the factors that started the hemostasis sequence are rapidly inactivated to prevent excessive clotting. In addition, coagulation inhibitors are released to prevent further clot formation. Eventually, other chemicals cut the fibrin strands and dissolve the blood clot completely.

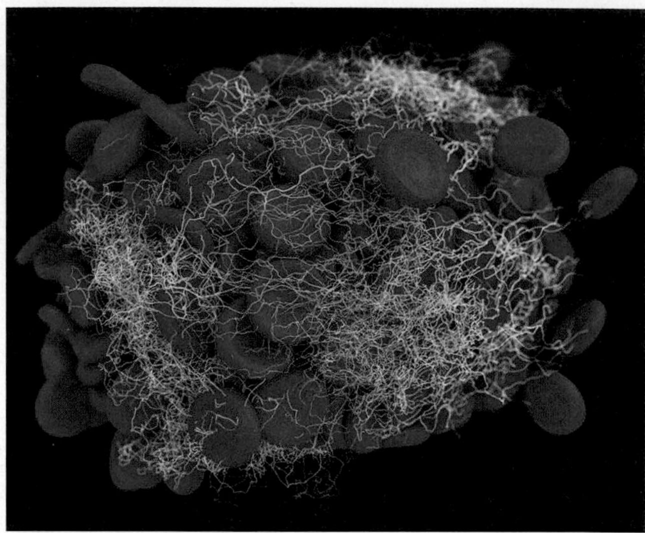

somersault18:24/iStock.com

Figure 10.12 Red and white blood cells are trapped in a fibrin mesh to form a blood clot.

Check Your Understanding

1. Which three proteins are found in plasma?
2. Which blood cells are most abundant in the blood?
3. Which two molecules make up hemoglobin?
4. Which organs regulate red blood cell production through the process of erythropoiesis?
5. List the five different types of white blood cells.
6. What are the four steps of hemostasis?

LIFE SPAN DEVELOPMENT: *The Blood*

Blood formation begins well before birth. At weeks 3–8 of fetal development, **hematopoiesis**, or the formation and development of blood cells, occurs in collections of blood cells called *blood islands* in the yolk sac. Large, nucleated erythrocytes are produced and a small number of monocytes/macrophages and megakaryocytes (precursors of platelet cells) are formed.

At approximately week 12, the site of blood cell formation shifts from the blood islands to the liver primarily, with some formation occurring in the spleen and lymph nodes. At this stage, erythrocytes become adult-type cells, without a nucleus. During the fifth month of fetal development, bone marrow develops from the mesoderm layer of the embryo and becomes the main site of hematopoiesis.

(continued)

After birth and during early childhood, the majority of hematopoiesis occurs in the red bone marrow of long bones. As people age, it becomes limited to the pelvis, vertebrae, ribs, sternum, skull and the proximal heads of the femur and the humerus.

In the human adult, red bone marrow produces all RBCs and platelets and approximately 60%–70% of WBCs. The remaining 20%–30% of WBCs are produced in the lymphatic tissues (lymph nodes, liver, and spleen). All blood cells start with a self-renewing, multipotent, hematopoietic stem cell that differentiates into either a lymphoid or myeloid stem cell. Depending on a variety of factors that influence gene expression, the lymphoid or myeloid stem cells undergo irreversible changes that determine whether they form lymphocytes or all of the other types of blood cells (RBCs, platelets, or other types of WBCs). **Figure 10.11** shows this process. Once the blood cells have matured, they are carried into the circulatory system by blood as it passes through the bone marrow.

The "river of life" called blood is constantly renewing its cellular blood components and nutrients while simultaneously disposing of older, damaged blood cells and waste products. It is hard to believe that 3 million new red blood cells enter the bloodstream every second and a comparable number of old, ruptured cells are cleared by the liver and spleen, because this dynamic process goes unnoticed unless a problem, such as anemia, develops. Blood's other cellular components undergo similar changes. A more in-depth explanation is included in Chapter 10.

Life Span Review

1. Into what two types of stem cells do the hematopoietic stem cells differentiate?
2. Where in the adult body are leukocytes produced?

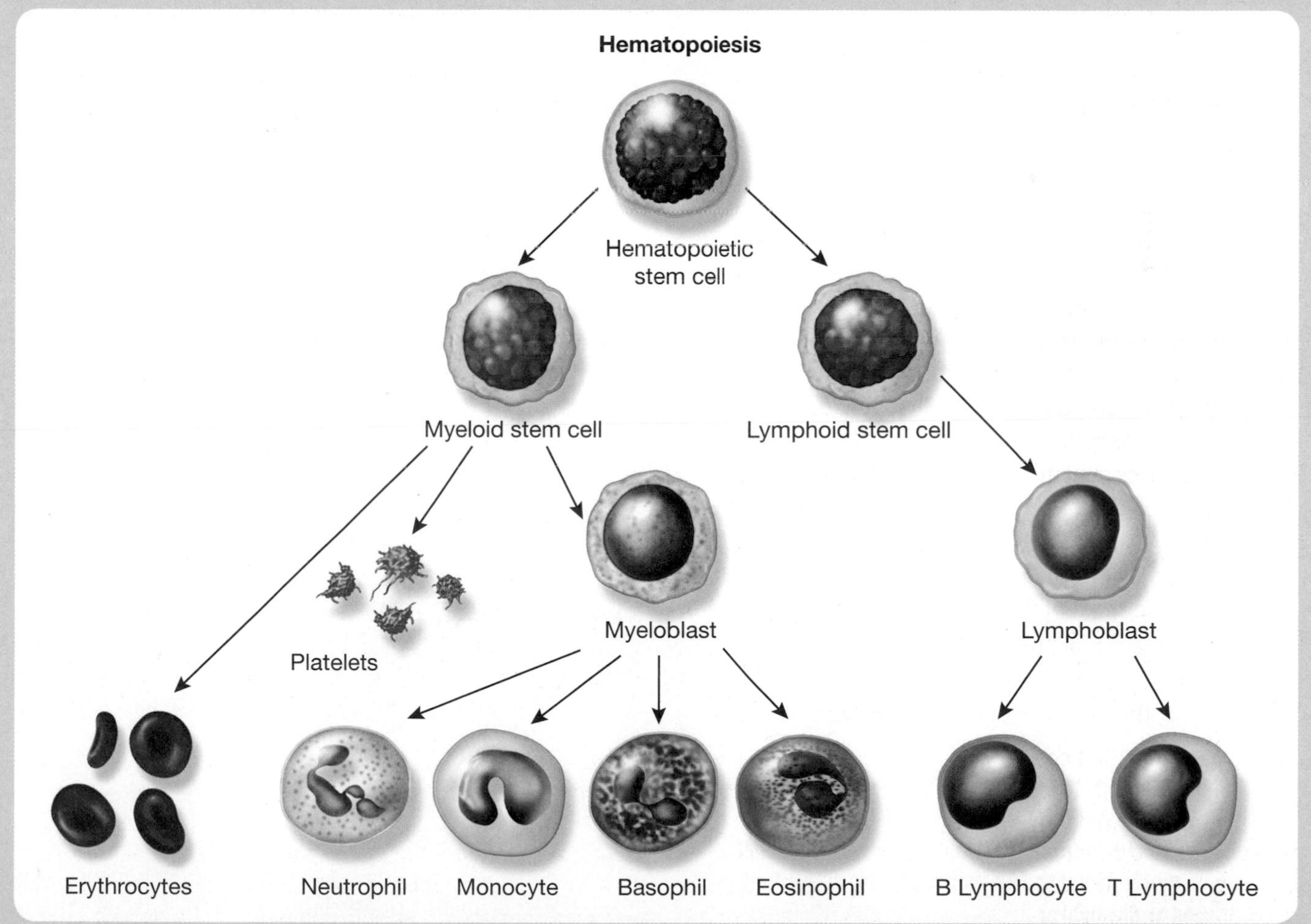

Figure 10.11 Hematopoiesis is the formation of the cellular components of blood from hematopoietic stem cells.

LESSON 10.1 Review and Assessment

Mini Glossary

Make sure that you know the meaning of each key term.

buffy coat a thin layer of white blood cells and platelets that lies between the red blood cells and plasma in a blood sample that has gone through a centrifuge

carbaminohemoglobin hemoglobin molecule with carbon dioxide molecules attached; transports carbon dioxide to the lungs where it can be expelled from the body

coagulation the process by which the enzyme thrombin and the protein fibrinogen combine to form fibrin, a fiber that weaves around the platelet plug to form a blood clot; takes between 2 and 15 minutes to complete

diapedesis the passage of blood, or any of its formed elements, through the blood vessel walls into body tissues

erythrocytes red blood cells; contain hemoglobin, a protein responsible for oxygen and carbon dioxide exchange

erythropoiesis the process by which red blood cells are produced

erythropoietin a hormone secreted by the kidneys that stimulates the production of red blood cells

fibrin a long, thread-like fiber created by the combination of thrombin and fibrinogen; weaves around the platelet plug to form a blood clot

formed elements the solid components of blood; red blood cells, white blood cells, and platelets

hematocrit the percentage of total blood volume that is composed of red blood cells

hematopoiesis the formation and development of red blood cells

hemoglobin an essential molecule of the red blood cell that serves as the binding site for oxygen and carbon dioxide; composed of two molecules: globin and heme

hemolysis the rupture of red blood cells as a result of disease or old age

hemostasis the sequence of events that causes a blood clot to form and bleeding to stop

leukocytes white blood cells; fight infection and protect the body through various mechanisms

oxyhemoglobin hemoglobin molecule with attached oxygen molecules; transports oxygen from the lungs to the body tissues

plasma the liquid component of blood

platelet plug gathering of platelets that forms a small mass at the site of an injury

platelets part of the formed elements of the blood; play a vital role in blood clotting

Know and Understand

1. List at least six functions of blood, two in each of the three major categories described in this lesson.
2. Name at least four physical properties of blood.
3. A centrifuge is used to separate the elements of blood into three layers. Describe the components of each layer.
4. List the components that make up plasma.
5. What is the average life span of an erythrocyte?
6. During hemolysis, hemoglobin is broken into heme and globin. Into what two components is heme broken?
7. Which WBCs are considered granulocytes? Which are considered agranulocytes? What is the difference?
8. What is blood coagulation?

Analyze and Apply

9. Explain why having a critically low platelet count could be life-threatening.
10. Explain how kidney disease could affect erythropoiesis and the production of thrombocytes.
11. One reason a potential blood donor's hemoglobin level is checked before he or she donates blood is to ensure that the donor will have enough iron-carrying capacity after the donation. Suggest another possible reason for checking the donor's hemoglobin.

IN THE LAB

12. Draw and color an example of each of the five types of white blood cells. Identify the function of each next to its image.
13. Write a song, rap, poem, or story about the formed elements of blood. Include these things:
    - the function of erythrocytes
    - the five types of leukocytes and their functions
    - the function of platelets

LESSON **10.2** **Blood Types**

Before You Read

Try to answer the following questions before you read this lesson.

- Why can't someone with type A blood receive blood from a person with type B blood?
- What role does the Rh factor play in pregnant women?

Lesson Objectives

- Identify the four blood types and the role of antigens and antibodies in differentiating blood types.
- Explain the Rh classification system and why it is important.

Key Terms

agglutination	Rh factor
antibody	RhoGAM
antigen	universal donor
erythroblastosis fetalis	universal recipient

Lesson 10.1 explained that everyone's blood contains some similar elements—red blood cells, white blood cells, and platelets. But when blood from different people is viewed under a microscope, there are distinct differences. This is because there are four blood types: A, B, AB, and O.

Do you know your blood type? Have you ever wondered what determines your blood type? Like your eye or hair color, your blood type is inherited. The table in **Figure 10.13** provides a list of possible blood types a person may have based on the blood types of his or her parents.

ABO Blood Types

Blood typing was made possible by the groundbreaking work of Karl Landsteiner, an Austrian scientist who won the Nobel Prize for his discovery. In 1901, Landsteiner classified blood according to the microscopic differences he found on the surface of the red blood cell. His system is commonly known as the *ABO blood typing system.*

The presence of molecule A on the red blood cell indicates type A blood, molecule B indicates type B blood, and the presence of both A and B molecules indicates type AB blood. Some people have neither A nor B molecules on their red blood cells. These people have type O blood.

Of the four blood types, type O is the most common in the United States, and type AB is the rarest. Blood types tend to vary among ethnic groups and regions of the world (**Figure 10.14**).

Antigens and Antibodies

The molecules on the surface of the red blood cells are called **antigens**. Antigens are large, complex molecules, such as proteins and glycolipids, that identify cells as "self" or "nonself." In this way, antigens make it possible for the body to tell the difference between its own cells and any nonself, or foreign, cells. The presence of foreign antigens causes the immune system to produce **antibodies** that mark the foreign cells for destruction. The antibodies circulate in plasma and mark any cells with antigens different from those found in the host's blood (or blood recipient's blood during a

Inherited Blood Type											
	Parent 1	AB	AB	AB	AB	B	A	A	O	O	O
	Parent 2	AB	B	A	O	B	B	A	B	A	O
Possible blood type of child	**O**					X	X	X	X	X	X
	A	X	X	X	X		X	X		X	
	B	X	X	X	X	X	X		X		
	AB	X	X	X			X				

Figure 10.13 *Goodheart-Willcox Publisher*

Blood Type Prevalence by Ethnicity					
Prevalence (% of US Population)					
Blood Group	Caucasian	African-American	Hispanic	Asian	Native American
AB	3	4	2	5	1
B	9	20	10	27	4
A	41	27	31	28	16
O	47	49	57	40	79

Figure 10.14

Goodheart-Willcox Publisher

transfusion). The role of antigens and antibodies in the immune system is discussed in greater detail in Chapter 12.

Figure 10.15 shows the antigens and antibodies associated with each blood type. People with AB blood have antigens A and B on their red blood cells, but neither A nor B antibodies in their plasma, making them a **universal recipient**. A universal recipient can safely receive blood of any type due to the lack of attacking antibodies. People with type O blood have neither antigen A nor antigen B on their red blood cells, but both A and B antibodies in their plasma. Because type O blood has no antigens that can be attacked by the host's blood, anyone can receive type O blood. Thus, people with type O blood are considered **universal donors**.

Blood Transfusions

Understanding blood types is critical for blood transfusions and surgery. If you look at the history of blood transfusions, you will see that the earliest outcomes of this technology were grim. In the fledgling days of medicine, physicians did not know about the different blood types. Some transfusions were successful due in large part to luck, but others resulted in serious complications or death.

The ABO Blood Group System				
Blood Type	Erythrocyte (Red Blood Cell) Antigens	RBC Antigens	Antibodies	Blood That Can Be Received
AB	A and B	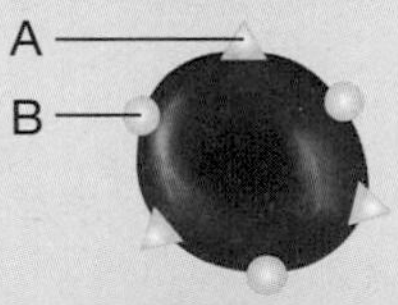 A B	Neither anti-A nor anti-B antibodies	A, B, AB, O (Universal recipient)
B	B	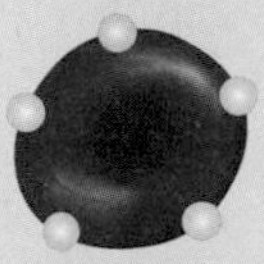	Anti-A	B, O
A	A	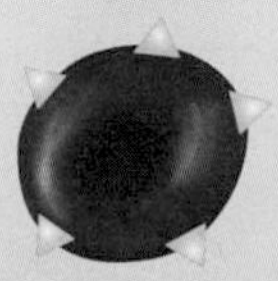	Anti-B	A, O
O	Neither A nor B	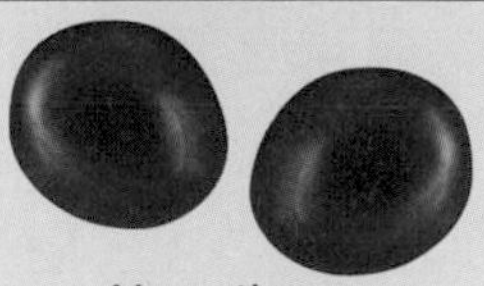 No antigens	Anti-A and Anti-B	O (Universal donor)

Figure 10.15

© Body Scientific International, Goodheart-Willcox Publisher

When a person with type A blood is transfused with blood from a type B blood donor, the recipient's B antibodies attack the donor's red blood cells. This causes the donated red blood cells to clump together in a process called **agglutination** (ah-gloo-ti-NAY-shun). Agglutination creates blockages in smaller blood vessels and is potentially fatal.

Agglutination also causes hemolysis, or destruction, of the donated red blood cells. Hemolysis releases hemoglobin into the bloodstream. Hemoglobin can accumulate in the kidneys, causing kidney damage and failure, or even death. Usually, however, blood transfusion reactions are milder, with symptoms ranging from fever and chills to vomiting. Regardless, it is *extremely important* that blood types be classified and matched *before* transfusion.

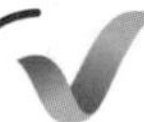

Check Your Understanding

1. What determines a person's blood type?
2. What molecules are found on the surface of red blood cells?
3. Which blood type classifies someone as a universal recipient? A universal donor?

The Rh Classification System

Besides the antigen that determines blood type, there is another antigen on the surface of the red blood cells. This second antigen is called the **Rh factor**. The Rh factor is named after the rhesus monkey in which it was first discovered.

Not everyone possesses the Rh factor. Those who have the Rh factor on the surface of their red blood cells are classified as *Rh-positive*; those who lack it are classified as *Rh-negative*. The majority of people (approximately 85%) are Rh-positive.

When writing out a blood type, you drop the "Rh" and simply add a plus or minus superscript to the blood type's letter. For example, a person who has the Rh factor and type AB blood would say that she or he is AB^{+}.

Rh Factor Complications

Plasma does not naturally contain an antibody for the Rh factor. However, antibodies to the Rh factor can develop if a person with Rh^{-} blood is transfused with Rh^{+} blood. After exposure to the Rh^{+} blood, antibodies begin to form against the Rh factor. If the person is exposed to Rh^{+} blood again, the antibodies will cause agglutination and hemolysis.

Females can become sensitized to the Rh factor during pregnancy. If a mother who is Rh^{-} has a baby who is Rh^{+}, her first pregnancy will not cause a problem because the mother's blood has not yet developed antibodies to the Rh^{+} blood. However, some of the baby's Rh^{+} blood may come in contact with the mother's Rh^{-} blood through the placenta, the organ that transports nutrients from the mother to her child. Once the mother's blood has been exposed to the Rh^{+} blood, she develops anti-Rh^{+} antibodies.

If the mother becomes pregnant with another child who is Rh^{+}, the mother's Rh^{+} antibodies will attack the red blood cells of the fetus, causing agglutination and hemolysis. This depletes the number of mature RBCs in the fetus. As a result, erythroblasts (immature RBCs) leave the bone marrow of the fetus before they are mature. If left untreated, the baby will develop **erythroblastosis fetalis** (eh-rith-roh-blas-TOH-sis fee-TAL-is), or *hemolytic disease of the newborn (HDN)*. Erythroblastosis fetalis can be fatal.

Preventing Complications

Fortunately, erythroblastosis fetalis is becoming increasingly less common due to the development of the immune serum **RhoGAM**. RhoGAM is administered to the Rh^{-} mother shortly after she has given birth to her first child. The addition of RhoGAM prevents the mother's blood from becoming sensitized to the child's antibodies.

Any woman considering pregnancy should know her blood type and get early prenatal healthcare. It is essential for the health of the mother and her baby.

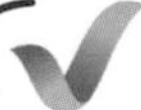

Check Your Understanding

1. How would you indicate a person's blood type if the person has A antigens and the Rh factor on their red blood cells?
2. Besides blood transfusions, what other condition can sensitize the body to the Rh factor?

LESSON 10.2 Review and Assessment

Mini Glossary

Make sure that you know the meaning of each key term.

agglutination the process by which red blood cells clump together, usually in response to an antibody; can block small blood vessels and cause hemolysis

antibody a cell that circulates in plasma and attacks red blood cells with foreign antigens, or antigens that are different from those of the host

antigen a protein on the surface of RBCs that is used to identify blood type; a molecule on the surface of cells that identifies cells as either "self" or "nonself" (foreign) cells

erythroblastosis fetalis a severe hemolytic disease of a fetus or newborn caused by the production of maternal antibodies against the fetal red blood cell antigens, usually involving Rh incompatibility between the mother and fetus

Rh factor the antigen of the Rh blood group that is found on the surface of red blood cells; people with the Rh factor are Rh^+ and those lacking it are Rh^-

RhoGAM an immune serum that prevents a mother's blood from becoming sensitized to foreign antibodies from her fetus

universal donor a person with type O blood; type O blood has no antigens that can be attacked by the host's blood, so it can be donated to anyone

universal recipient a person with type AB blood; type AB blood has neither A nor B antibodies, so a universal recipient can safely receive a transfusion of any blood type

Know and Understand

1. If a person's parents both have type B blood, what blood types might that person have?
2. What are the four blood types?
3. What is an antigen?
4. Describe agglutination.
5. Besides the antigen that determines blood type, what other antigen is sometimes found on the surface of red blood cells?
6. If you have type B blood, what kind of antibodies do you have?

Analyze and Apply

7. What is the difference between an antigen and an antibody?
8. Explain why a person with type AB blood is a universal recipient.
9. Explain why a person with type O blood is a universal donor.
10. In terms of antigens and antibodies, explain why it is critical that a patient be transfused with a blood type that is compatible with his or her own.

IN THE LAB

11. Using the information that you learned in this lesson, copy and complete the chart shown in **Figure 10.16**. Identify whether the recipient (column A) can safely receive a blood donation from each potential donor (column B).

Blood Donation		
Recipient Blood Type	**Potential Donor Blood Type**	**Safe to Receive Blood from Donor?**
B^-	A	
AB	O	
AB	B	
O	AB	
O	O	
A^-	B^+	
B^-	O^-	

Figure 10.16 Goodheart-Willcox Publisher

12. With a partner, make a large blood type chart on poster board. Glue cut-out pictures of RBCs onto the poster board to show how the RBC looks in each blood type. Include the Rh factor. Glue cut-out letters for the antigens along the outside of the RBC cutouts. Use more cut-out letters to show the different antibodies. Glue these to the top of the chart. Your chart should contain four columns:
    - Antigens on RBC Surface
    - Antibodies in the plasma
    - Can Receive Blood From
    - Can Donate Blood To

    To complete your chart, use a permanent marker and fill out each column for each of the eight blood types (A^+, A^-, O^+, O^-, B^+, B^-, AB^+, AB^-).

LESSON 10.3 Blood Disorders and Diseases

Before You Read

Try to answer the following questions before you read this lesson.

- What does it mean to be anemic?
- Which blood disorder causes yellowing of the whites of the eyes and skin?

Lesson Objectives

- Identify the purpose of a complete blood count.
- Describe the differences between acquired and inherited anemias.
- Identify common blood disorders and diseases.

Key Terms

acute lymphocytic leukemia (ALL)
acute myeloid leukemia (AML)
anemia
aplastic anemia
chelation therapy
chronic lymphocytic leukemia (CLL)
chronic myeloid leukemia (CML)
hemophilia
iron-deficient anemia
jaundice
leukemia
multiple myeloma
pernicious anemia
phlebotomy
polycythemia
sickle cell anemia
thalassemia

Blood disorders and diseases can be diagnosed in a variety of ways, including a complete blood count test. But what causes a disorder or disease of the blood? Many health problems affecting the blood are inherited, but some are caused by environmental factors, poor diet, or even old age. This lesson describes the complete blood count diagnostic test and then explores some of the most common disorders and diseases of the blood and their causes, symptoms, and treatments or management strategies.

CLINICAL CASE STUDY

Sam was diagnosed with type 1 diabetes mellitus when he was six years old. Although the constant blood monitoring of his glucose levels and limiting his intake of refined sugars was restrictive at first, he and his family ultimately embraced his condition as a means of eating a healthy diet. Now, in high school, Sam has decided to compete in cross-country running. He is committed to excelling in his sport and has made some dietary adjustments. He has decided a plant-based, vegan diet would help him lose those last 10 pounds and best fuel his workouts and competitive races. Sam's training and diet strategy worked well his first season and he won several races. Over the summer, Sam continued to train and became very strict about his commitment to being vegan, cutting out all animal-based foods.

Since the start of the second season, he has been feeling unusually fatigued and short of breath, and he has had bouts of diarrhea. His resting heart rate, which he checks regularly, has consistently been 10–15 beats higher than normal and his tongue is sore, red, and swollen. Sam mentions his symptoms to his mother and she promptly makes an appointment with their family physician. As you read this section, try to determine which of the following conditions Sam most likely has.

A. Aplastic anemia
B. Iron-deficient anemia
C. Pernicious anemia

Complete Blood Count

A complete blood count (CBC) helps detect blood disorders or diseases such as anemia, abnormal blood cell counts, clotting problems, immune system disorders, and cancers of the blood. The test measures the number of RBCs, WBCs, and platelets in a person's blood.

A low RBC count may indicate anemia, bleeding, or dehydration. In addition, the number of each of the five different types of WBCs is measured for signs of infection, blood cancer, or immune disorder. A reduced platelet count may indicate bleeding or a thrombotic (clotting) disorder. Hemoglobin and hematocrit levels are also measured for signs of anemia. **Figure 10.17** shows the results of a complete blood count test. Values that are higher or lower than the normal range appear in red.

Check Your Understanding

1. What basic tests are performed in a CBC?
2. What might a low platelet count indicate?

Anemia

Anemia is a condition characterized by a decrease in the number of RBCs or an insufficient amount of hemoglobin in the RBCs. In both cases, the oxygen-carrying capacity of the RBCs is reduced.

Anemia can be acquired or inherited. The three main causes of anemia are excessive blood loss, decreased RBC production, or a high rate of RBC destruction. Symptoms of anemia include headache, dizziness, weakness, fatigue, and difficulty breathing or shortness of breath.

There are several types of anemia. Some forms are mild and easily treated by adopting a healthful diet; others can be severe, debilitating, and even life-threatening if they remain undiagnosed or untreated. A healthful diet provides the building blocks for RBC production: iron, folic acid, and vitamin B.

Acquired Anemias

Acquired anemias include iron-deficient anemia, aplastic anemia, pernicious anemia, and anemia related to chronic disease. Anemia can be caused by a dietary deficiency or exposure to parasitic worms. It can also be a symptom of another disease. The table in **Figure 10.18** describes the etiology, prevention, pathology, diagnosis, and treatment of acquired anemias.

Iron-Deficient Anemia

The most common type of anemia, **iron-deficient anemia**, accounts for nearly 50% of all anemias worldwide. Iron-deficient anemia results from an insufficient dietary intake of iron or loss of iron from intestinal bleeding.

Low red blood count, hemoglobin, and hematocrit signal anemia.

Elevated white blood count may signal disease or infection.

Complete Blood Count Example Test Results

Test	Results	Low/High	Units	Normal Ranges
CBC with Differential				
Red Blood Count		3.5 (L)	× 10–6/µl	4.1–5.1 (F) / 4.70–6.10 (M)
Hemoglobin		10.8 (L)	g/dL	12.0–16.0 (F) / 14.0–18.0 (M)
Hematocrit		31.1 (L)	%	37.0–48.0 (F) / 42.0–52.0 (M)
Platelets	302		× 10–3/µl	140–415
White Blood Count	7.2		× 10–3/µl	4.5–11
Lymphocytes		48 (H)	%	17–44
Monocytes	7.0		%	3–10
Neutrophils		43 (L)	%	45–76
Eosinophils	2.0		%	0–4
Basophils	0		%	0–2

M = Male
F = Female

Goodheart-Willcox Publisher

Figure 10.17 The results of a complete blood count can be used to determine the presence of a disease or disorder. The Low/High column shows counts lower (L) or higher (H) than normal. *What are some diseases that can be identified by examining the results of a complete blood count?*

Acquired Anemias					
	Etiology	**Prevention**	**Pathology**	**Diagnosis**	**Treatment**
Iron-deficient anemia	insufficient iron intake, blood loss, alcohol abuse, anti-coagulant or antiplatelet medications, trauma, inability to absorb iron, pregnancy, parasites, colorectal cancer	eat an iron-rich diet, if vegan, take in enough iron and vitamin B_{12}; eat foods rich in vitamin C, take supplements	shortness of breath, extreme fatigue, headache, dizziness, rapid heart rate, pale skin, unusual craving for nutrient-lacking substances (dirt, starch, ice), rectal bleeding/blood in stool/urine	physical exam, CBC, imaging, rectal bleeding, blood in stool	iron-rich diet, iron supplements, correct internal bleeding problem
Aplastic anemia	damage to stem cells in bone marrow due to exposure to toxins, cancer treatment, viral infections	avoid exposure to toxins such as insecticides, herbicides, paint removers, or organic solvents	fatigue, shortness of breath, rapid heart rate, pale skin, unexplained bruising, prolonged bleeding from cuts, nosebleeds, bleeding gums, frequent or prolonged infections	physical exam, CBC, bone marrow biopsy	toxin removal, stop radiation/chemotherapy, blood transfusions, or immunosuppressant drugs; in severe cases, bone marrow stem-cell transplants
Pernicious anemia	inability of intestine to absorb vitamin B_{12}, diet lacking in vitamin B_{12}, type 1 diabetes, Addison disease, chronic thyroiditis	diet rich in vitamin B_{12}; B_{12}-fortified foods	fatigue; shortness of breath; red, sore, swollen tongue; dizziness; headache, diarrhea, constipation, cold hands/feet, rapid or irregular heartbeat	physical exam, CBC, serum folate, iron, and iron-binding blood tests, bone marrow test	vitamin B_{12} pills/injections, or nasal spray; treat underlying cause
Anemia caused by chronic diseases	autoimmune diseases, cancer, HIV/AIDS, diabetes, inflammatory bowel diseases, heart failure	none	shortness of breath, extreme fatigue, headache, dizziness, rapid heart rate	CBC, blood tests to measure iron content in blood and body	treat underlying condition, blood transfusions, erythropoiesis-stimulating agents, eat iron-rich diet

Figure 10.18 *Goodheart-Willcox Publisher*

Parasitic worms that result in intestinal bleeding are the main cause of iron-deficient anemia worldwide. Parasitic worms are most commonly found in developing or low-income countries.

Pregnant women may also suffer from iron-deficient anemia. This happens because their bodies supply the fetus with hemoglobin, which depletes the mother's iron levels. (Recall from Lesson 10.1 that the heme molecule in hemoglobin is composed of iron.)

If iron-deficient anemia is caused by a poor diet, an iron supplement can be prescribed. Foods rich in iron (such as lean beef, poultry, fortified cereals, and leafy, green vegetables) are also recommended (**Figure 10.19**).

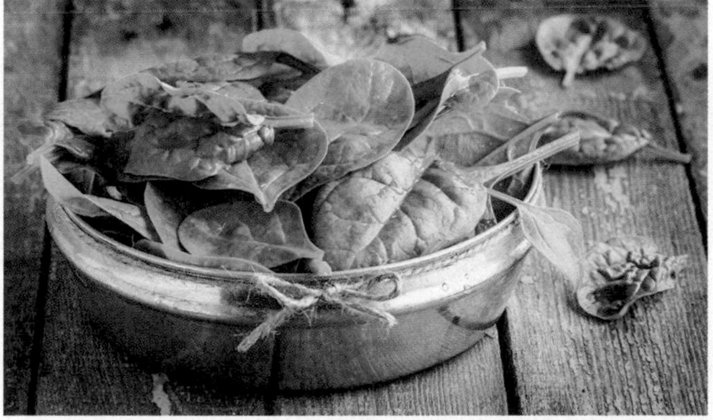

Nikola Bilic/Shutterstock.com

Figure 10.19 Spinach is an iron-rich food. Adopting a diet rich in leafy, green vegetables such as spinach is one way to help fight iron-deficient anemia. *What other foods are high in iron?*

Aplastic Anemia

A rare but serious condition, **aplastic anemia** is caused by damage to the stem cells in the bone marrow. When bone marrow stem cells are damaged, they cannot produce a sufficient number of RBCs, WBCs, and platelets. The blood cells manufactured in the bone marrow have problems developing into mature blood cells, resulting in aplastic anemia. Causes of aplastic anemia include:

- toxins (such as those found in pesticides)
- radiation therapy or chemotherapy
- infectious diseases such as hepatitis, Epstein-Barr virus (which may also cause mononucleosis), and human immunodeficiency virus (HIV)
- autoimmune disorders such as rheumatoid arthritis and lupus
- heredity

Treatments for aplastic anemia include toxin removal, discontinuing radiation or chemotherapy, and blood transfusions. In severe cases, bone marrow stem cell transplants may be performed.

Pernicious Anemia

When the intestines are unable to absorb B_{12}, a vitamin essential for RBC production, the result is **pernicious anemia**. This condition develops when the stomach stops producing intrinsic factor, a key protein in vitamin B_{12} absorption. A weakened stomach lining or an autoimmune disorder may cause the body to attack intrinsic factor.

Pernicious anemia usually develops later in life; on average, diagnosis occurs in patients around 60 years of age. Certain diseases, such as type 1 diabetes mellitus, Addison disease, and chronic thyroiditis, can increase the risk of developing pernicious anemia.

Signs and symptoms common among people with pernicious anemia include a red, swollen tongue; pale skin; fatigue; and shortness of breath. Diarrhea or constipation are other symptoms. Treatment usually consists of vitamin B_{12} supplements.

Anemias Caused by Chronic Disease

Chronic illnesses such as rheumatoid arthritis or kidney disease can cause anemia. For example, kidney disease may lower production of the hormone erythropoietin, which regulates RBC production. Inflammatory conditions associated with diseases such as rheumatoid arthritis can affect the bone marrow's response to erythropoietin. As a result, RBC production may decrease. Diseases characterized by chronic infections, such as HIV, tuberculosis, cirrhosis of the liver, and certain cancers, also can cause anemia.

Treatment of anemia caused by chronic disease involves diagnosing and resolving the underlying disease. In the short term, blood transfusions may be used as part of the treatment plan for managing anemia.

Inherited Anemias

Inherited anemias are determined by genetic makeup. A child must receive an anemia gene from both parents to experience symptoms of an inherited anemia. If an anemia gene is received from only one parent, the child will be a carrier but will not experience symptoms. Two commonly inherited anemias are sickle cell anemia and thalassemia. The table in **Figure 10.20** describes the etiology, prevention, pathology, diagnosis, and treatment of inherited anemias.

Sickle Cell Anemia

Recall from Lesson 10.1 that normal RBCs are disk-shaped. However, the RBCs of a person with **sickle cell anemia** are shaped like a crescent or sickle, which is a large cutting instrument with a curved metal blade. This is because the hemoglobin molecules in the RBCs of a patient with sickle cell anemia are misshaped, causing the RBCs to take on the abnormal shape.

Sickle-shaped hemoglobin molecules carry less oxygen than normal hemoglobin molecules. Because of their shape and sticky texture, sickle-shaped RBCs easily get stuck in small blood vessels, disrupting normal blood flow. **Figure 10.21** illustrates how the sickle-shaped RBCs become lodged in blood vessels.

Symptoms of sickle cell anemia include excruciatingly painful episodes called *crises*. Crises can last anywhere from a few hours to several days, and require hospitalization. The pain usually occurs in the back and around long bones, such as the femur, where tissues can be damaged from oxygen deprivation. Other symptoms include bacterial infection, fatigue, shortness of breath, rapid heart rate, and a yellowing of the skin and eyes. Strokes may also occur if RBCs become lodged in the small vessels of the brain.

Inherited Anemias					
	Etiology	**Prevention**	**Pathology**	**Diagnosis**	**Treatment**
Sickle cell anemia	gene mutation causes crescent- or sickle-shaped RBCs, which carry less oxygen and become stuck in small blood vessels; more common in African-Americans and people of Mediterranean descent	awareness of family history of sickle cell anemia	extremely painful episodes called *crises*, back pain, pain in the long bones, O_2 deprivation, fatigue, shortness of breath, bacterial infection, rapid heart rate, jaundice, stroke	physical exam, CBC, hemoglobin electrophoresis test	daily antibiotics, folic acid supplements, blood transfusions, pain medications, fluids, gene therapy in the future
Thalassemia (Cooley's anemia)	gene mutation causes RBCs with underdeveloped hemoglobin and low RBC count, decreasing O_2 carrying capacity	awareness of family history of thalassemia	bone deformities (especially facial), dark urine, delayed growth and development, excessive fatigue, yellow or pale skin, swollen stomach, shortened life span	physical exam, CBC, hemoglobin electrophoresis test, heart and liver function tests	frequent blood transfusions, iron chelation therapy, daily folic acid, bone marrow transplant

Figure 10.20

Goodheart-Willcox Publisher

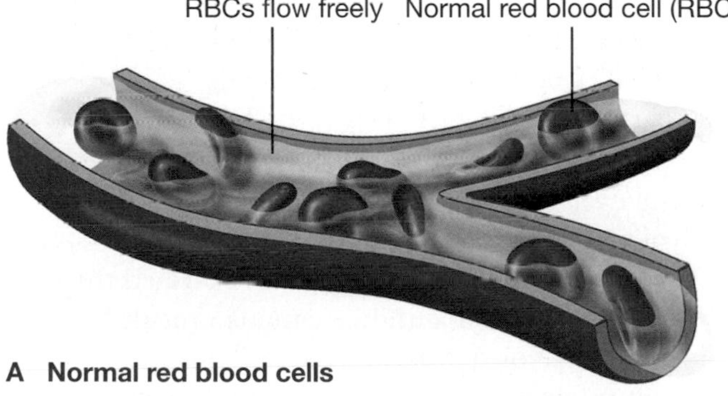

A Normal red blood cells

Cross section of RBC

Normal hemoglobin

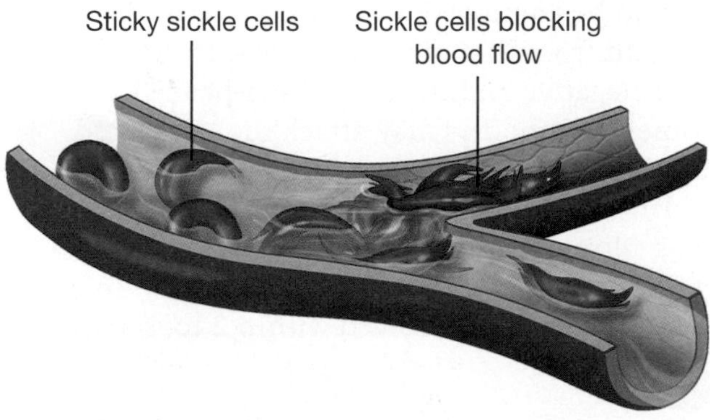

B Abnormal red blood cells (sickle cells)

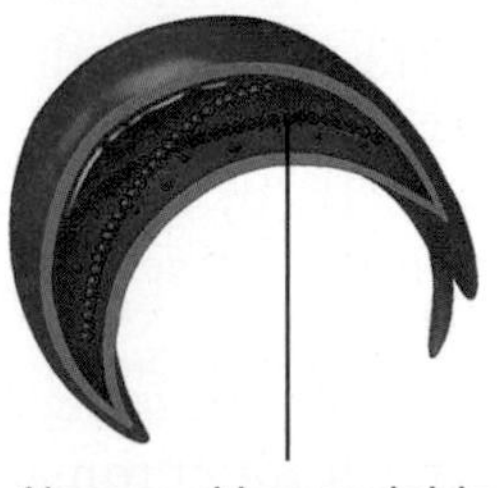
Cross section of sickle cell
Abnormal hemoglobin forms strands, causing the sickle, or crescent shape

© Body Scientific International

Figure 10.21 Sickle-shaped red blood cells get stuck more easily in smaller blood vessels, causing painful episodes called *crises*. *Why does sickle cell anemia increase the risk of stroke?*

Treatment of sickle cell anemia may require daily doses of antibiotics to prevent bacterial infection, especially in small children. Folic acid supplements are also recommended. In the event of a crisis, the patient is given blood transfusions, pain medications, and fluids. In addition, blood transfusions are given frequently to increase the patient's RBC count.

Individuals who inherit the sickle cell gene from only one parent have the sickle cell trait, which means they are a carrier but will not develop any of the symptoms of the disease. Sickle cell anemia is most common in African-Americans and individuals of Mediterranean descent.

In the past, sickle cell anemia resulted in death at an early age, but medical advances are helping people with this disease live into their fifties and beyond.

Thalassemia

Thalassemia (thal-a-SEE-mee-a), also called *Cooley's anemia*, is a type of anemia that affects hemoglobin proteins. Thalassemia limits the body's ability to produce fully developed hemoglobin and the proper number of RBCs. As a result, the blood's oxygen-carrying capability is reduced.

People with thalassemia require frequent blood transfusions to increase their RBC counts. However, these transfusions can be dangerous because they can increase the iron in the blood to toxic levels. Excessive amounts of iron are especially harmful to the heart, liver, and endocrine organs. Iron accumulation leads to heart attack and death in 50% of people with thalassemia before they reach 35 years of age.

Chelation therapy is a special procedure that removes excess metals, such as iron, from the blood. Chelation therapy is essential for preventing organ damage and failure in thalassemia patients. During this therapy, the chelating drug is pumped into the body either intravenously (through an IV) or subcutaneously (by injection). It then binds with whatever metal is present in excess amounts.

In the case of iron poisoning, the chelating drug binds with the iron and prepares it for elimination from the body through the urine. The drug is usually administered at night and is infused slowly over an 8-hour period, 4 to 6 nights a week.

Check Your Understanding

1. What are the three main causes of anemia?
2. Which type of anemia is the most common worldwide?
3. Which anemia is caused by the inability of the intestines to absorb vitamin B_{12}?
4. Why might a person with rheumatoid arthritis be more likely to develop anemia than someone without rheumatoid arthritis?
5. Why does a sickle-shaped red blood cell take on its abnormal structure?

Other Diseases and Disorders of the Blood

Anemia is not the only disorder associated with the blood. Other conditions and diseases include jaundice, hemophilia, polycythemia, leukemia, and multiple myeloma. The table in **Figure 10.22** describes the etiology, prevention, pathology, diagnosis, and treatment of these disorders.

Jaundice

Jaundice is a blood disorder characterized by yellow-tinted skin and yellowing of the whites of the eyes. It can be caused by an excess of bilirubin—a by-product of RBC breakdown—in the bloodstream. Bilirubin is typically excreted through bile in the liver, so jaundice can also result from liver damage or disease.

Jaundice is common in newborns, usually as the result of an immature liver. A newborn is more likely to be jaundiced when his or her Rh factor is different from that of the mother's. If the mother is Rh-negative and the baby is Rh-positive, the mother's antibodies may attack the baby's red blood cells.

Infant jaundice is treated with phototherapy using ultraviolet light, which lowers the bilirubin levels in the baby's blood (**Figure 10.23**). Infant jaundice is usually resolved within 2 to 4 weeks of birth.

Hemophilia

Hemophilia (hee-moh-FIL-ee-a) is a disorder in which the blood does not clot properly because one of the clotting factors responsible for coagulation is missing. There are 13 clotting

Other Blood Disorders					
	Etiology	**Prevention**	**Pathology**	**Diagnosis**	**Treatment**
Jaundice	yellowing of the skin or whites of the eyes due to excess bilirubin, caused by inflamed liver or bile duct, blocked bile duct, or an immature liver in newborns	eat a healthy diet; limit or abstain from alcohol; avoid use of non-steroidal anti-inflammatory drugs (NSAIDs) and other medications affecting liver function	yellow pigmentation of skin and whites of eyes, itchiness, dark urine, pale stools, fatigue, abdominal pain, fever, vomiting	physical exam; CBC; liver function, bilirubin, and hepatitis blood tests, imaging, biopsy	avoid toxins (alcohol and medications) known to cause liver damage; ultraviolet phototherapy, especially for infants
Hemophilia	genetic disorder resulting in the absence of clotting factors in the blood, which can cause abnormal bleeding and hemorrhage; may be acquired due to autoimmune disorder, cancer, pregnancy, or multiple sclerosis	awareness of family history	symptoms vary based on severity of missing clotting factor; unexplained and/or excessive bleeding from cuts/injuries, surgeries, or dental work or vaccinations; large bruises, blood in urine/stool, painful, swollen joints; internal bleeding, including brain bleeds	physical exam with positive history of hemophilia; clotting-factor deficiency blood tests	regular replacement of missing clotting factor, hormones to increase clotting factors, drugs to promote clotting, first aid for cuts, physical therapy for damaged joints
Polycythemia	slow-developing blood cancer that causes bone marrow to produce too many RBCs; results in blood thickening and increased likelihood of organ damage, clot formation (thrombosis), and/or heart attack	awareness of family history	symptomless in many; itchiness, headache/dizziness, fatigue, excessive sweating, shortness of breath, numbness/tingling in hands, feet, arms, legs; blurred vision, fever, unexplained weight loss	physical exam, CBC, blood tests for hormone and erythropoietin levels, bone marrow biopsy, gene mutation testing	regular blood donations to reduce RBC count, low-dose aspirin, medications to suppress RBC production by the bone marrow, therapy to reduce itchiness if present
Leukemia	acute: cancer of the blood characterized by bone marrow's overproduction of immature WBCs that lack infection-fighting properties chronic: over- or underproduction of WBCs	avoid exposure to high doses of radiation, benzene, or other carcinogens, avoid tobacco use; knowledge of family history of leukemia; refrain from alcohol during pregnancy	may be symptomless for years if chronic, symptoms include fatigue, fever, unexplained weight loss, easy bleeding/bruising, bone and joint pain, stomach swelling, pain from enlarged liver or spleen, enlarged lymph nodes (acute lymphocytic leukemia)	physical exam, CBC and other blood tests, imaging tests, bone marrow biopsy, lymph node biopsy	chemotherapy and/or radiation therapy, targeted therapy, biological therapy that helps the immune system attack leukemia cells, lymph node biopsy, stem cell transplant, imaging, support system
Multiple myeloma	cancer of plasma cells in bone marrow, causing cancerous plasma cells called myelomas; leads to bone and kidney damage	none	may be symptomless; bone pain, especially in spine/chest; fatigue, frequent infections, loss of appetite, nausea, constipation, weight loss, mental confusion, excessive thirst	CBC, blood and urine tests for M proteins and beta$_2$-microglobulin produced by myeloma cells, urinalysis for M proteins, bone marrow biopsy, kidney function test, imaging tests	targeted therapies, immunotherapy, chemotherapy and/or radiation therapy, corticosteroid medications, treatments to relieve pain and complications like bone pain, anemia, kidney damage, infections, if present

Figure 10.22 *Goodheart-Willcox Publisher*

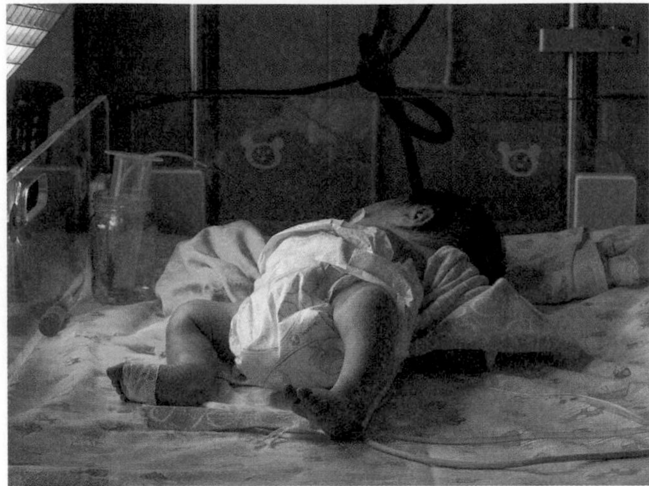

mindfullness/Shutterstock.com

Figure 10.23 Phototherapy helps break down excess bilirubin so that it can be excreted in the urine and feces.

factors involved in the coagulation process. Recall from Lesson 10.1 that platelets and clotting factors form a blood clot to stop an injured blood vessel from bleeding. People with hemophilia typically lack either clotting factor VII or IX.

Hemophilia is usually inherited, but in very rare cases may be acquired if the body forms antibodies that fight one of the clotting factors. This disease is more common in males, and occurs in one out of every 5,000 births each year.

Polycythemia

Polycythemia (pahl-ee-sigh-THEE-mee-a), also known as *polycythemia primary* or *polycythemia vera*, is a rare, slow-developing blood cancer that increases bone marrow production of red blood cells. It leads to an increased hematocrit that causes the blood to thicken, which can increase the likelihood of organ damage, blood clot formation, and/or heart attack.

Polycythemia can also be caused by exposure to atmospheric air with a low concentration of oxygen, which is common at high elevations. Living at a high altitude contributes to polycythemia because long-term exposure to high altitude causes the kidneys to produce more erythropoietin. Erythropoietin stimulates stem cell production in the bone marrow, leading to increased RBC production. However, people who live at a high

What Research Tells Us

...about Extending Life Expectancy of Patients with Sickle Cell Anemia

People with sickle cell anemia are prone to life-threatening infections, fatigue, and painful episodes called *crises*. Historically, this has meant that people with sickle cell anemia have a shortened life span.

In the 1960s, 15% of children born with sickle cell anemia died before two years of age; many more died as teenagers. Since that time, research funded by the National Heart, Lung, and Blood Institute (NHLBI) has shown that infants given daily doses of penicillin have an 84% reduction in infections, thus greatly improving their life expectancy.

Because sickle-shaped RBCs can become lodged in the blood vessels of the brain, people with sickle cell anemia are prone to stroke. NHLBI-funded research led to the development of the Transcranial Doppler (TCD) screening test, which can identify whether a patient with sickle cell anemia is at risk for stroke. Frequent blood transfusions have proven to lower the risk of stroke and increase life expectancy.

In another effort to increase the life expectancy of patients with sickle cell anemia, NHLBI researchers performed a partial stem cell transplant on 10 individuals with severe sickle cell disease; nine of them were cured.

Research continues with the goal of finding a permanent cure for sickle cell anemia. Meanwhile, a disease that was once associated with an early death is now a manageable condition, with life expectancies ranging from 40 to 50 years of age and beyond.

Taking It Further

1. Research treatment options for sickle cell anemia that are not discussed in this chapter. Are any advanced technologies available? Write a report on your findings and present it to the class.
2. Denzel and Maya are considering having a baby. Denzel has the sickle cell trait. Do you think the couple should seek genetic counseling? Why or why not? Do research to support your case. Share your argument with the class.

altitude do not develop polycythemia unless they also have a rare genetic mutation that increases bone marrow sensitivity to erythropoietin, causing even more RBCs to be produced.

Polycythemia is diagnosed by testing hemoglobin or hematocrit levels. Unusually high levels of hemoglobin or hematocrit indicate excessive RBC production.

Phlebotomy (fleh-BAHT-oh-mee), or drawing blood from the body, is the standard treatment for polycythemia. Phlebotomy reduces the number of RBCs circulating in the body. This helps correct hematocrit levels. Aspirin has also been used to thin the blood, but aspirin therapy is not advised for anyone with a history of spontaneous bleeding or stroke.

Intravascular Clotting

Normally, blood clots do not form in an undamaged blood vessel. However, sometimes they do form, usually in a vein. This intravascular clot is called a *thrombus*. If it does not dissolve on its own, it may cause a blockage in the vessel. If the clot breaks away from the vessel wall and enters the bloodstream, it is known as an *embolus*. Both thrombi and emboli can be dangerous. A thrombus that forms in a coronary artery may cause a heart attack. An embolus that travels to and becomes lodged in a coronary artery may also cause a heart attack. If it travels to the brain, it may cause a stroke.

Leukemia

Leukemia is a cancer of the blood. It is caused by the production of an extremely high number of immature white blood cells in the bone marrow. These immature, cancerous WBCs grow larger and faster than normal WBCs, but they lack the infection-fighting ability of normal WBCs. The cancerous WBCs live longer than healthy WBCs, crowding the healthy blood cells and making it hard for them to do their job. Cancerous WBCs can spread to lymph nodes (resulting in lymphocytic leukemia) and to other organs and tissues, causing swelling and pain.

Leukemia is classified as either acute or chronic. Acute leukemia worsens quickly, while chronic leukemia progresses more slowly. Children with leukemia usually have acute leukemia. Adults may contract either acute or chronic leukemia. Of the four types of leukemia, two are acute and two are chronic.

- **Acute lymphocytic leukemia (ALL)**: Most common in adults over 70 years of age, ALL is characterized by an overproduction of lymphocytes.
- **Acute myeloid leukemia (AML)**: AML is the most common form of leukemia in adults. It develops when the bone marrow produces too many myeloblasts, cells that fight bacterial infections. Myeloblasts are blast cells that later develop into RBCs, platelets, and some WBCs.
- **Chronic lymphocytic leukemia (CLL)**: Like acute lymphocytic leukemia, CLL is characterized by extremely high levels of lymphocytes. CLL is rare in children and most often affects middle-aged adults (**Figure 10.24**).
- **Chronic myeloid leukemia (CML)**: CML is a type of leukemia in which the bone marrow manufactures too many granulocytes (neutrophils, eosinophils, and basophils).

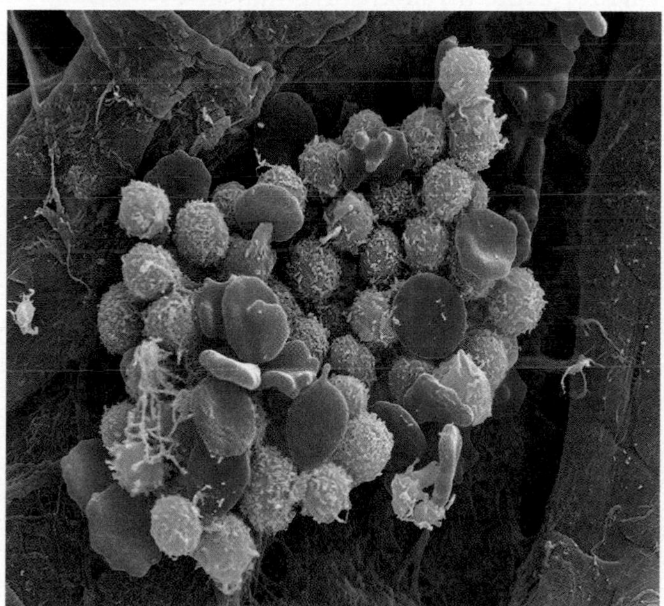

SPL/Science Source

Figure 10.24 This micrograph shows a blood sample from a person with chronic lymphocytic leukemia (CLL). Notice the disproportionate number of WBCs (lymphocytes, which are purple in this micrograph) to RBCs. In a healthy person, RBCs far outnumber WBCs. CLL results from the creation of a high number of lymphocytes, which causes a reduction in the number of RBCs.

People with chronic leukemia may not experience any symptoms, sometimes even for years after they develop the disease. By comparison, people with acute leukemia often seek medical care because they feel sick. Symptoms of both chronic and acute leukemia include weakness, fever, bone and joint pain, and stomach swelling and pain from an enlarged spleen or liver. People with leukemia also have frequent infections because cancerous WBCs are unable to aid in the immune response.

A complete blood count is often used to help diagnose leukemia. This disease increases the number of WBCs and decreases platelet and hemoglobin counts. A physical examination is done to check for swelling in the lymph nodes, spleen, or liver. In addition, physicians may perform a biopsy (removal and examination of body tissues) and other tests to look for cancerous cells.

Treatment options for leukemia vary, but often include chemotherapy, radiation therapy, and stem cell transplants. The five-year survival rate for acute myeloid leukemia varies with age. Those *under* 50 years of age at the time of diagnosis have a survival rate of 25% over a five-year period, while those *over* 50 years have a survival rate of 50% over a five-year period. New drug treatments for chronic myeloid leukemia have led to a promising 90% survival rate over the course of five years.

Multiple Myeloma

Multiple myeloma (migh-eh-LOH-ma) is a cancer of the plasma cells in bone marrow. The plasma cells of a person with this disease divide many times, creating even more cancerous plasma cells, called *myelomas*.

Myeloma cells deposit in the bone marrow, forming tumors that can damage the bone. As a result, people with multiple myeloma are prone to bone fractures and bone pain, particularly in the back and ribs. Other symptoms of this disease include excess blood calcium levels, kidney damage, and frequent infections.

Multiple myeloma is a treatable but incurable condition. It is treated with steroid drugs, chemotherapy, and stem cell transplants (**Figure 10.25**).

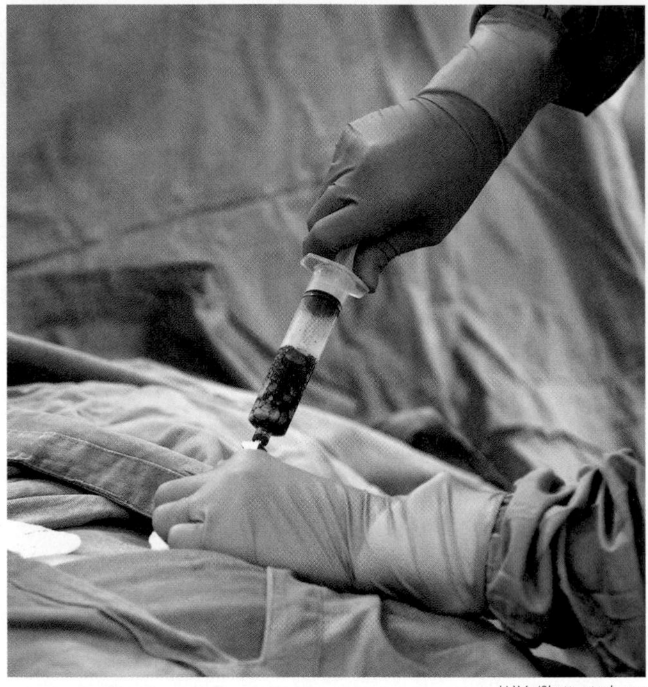

Li Wa/Shutterstock.com

Figure 10.25 Bone marrow is harvested (removed) from a healthy individual in preparation for a stem cell transplant. Transplanted bone marrow replaces the diseased bone marrow of a person with leukemia or multiple myeloma and produces healthy WBCs, RBCs, and platelets.

Multiple myeloma is the second most common blood cancer in the United States, accounting for 15% of all blood cancer cases. Each year, this disease affects between 1 and 4 of every 100,000 people. African-Americans are twice as likely as Caucasians to develop multiple myeloma. Survival rates continue to improve as a result of new drug therapies and stem cell transplant techniques.

Check Your Understanding

1. What type of drug therapy is used to remove excess metals, such as iron, from the blood?
2. What distinct changes in a person's physical appearance indicate jaundice?
3. What is the difference between acute and chronic leukemia?
4. Which cancer affects the plasma cells in bone marrow?

LESSON 10.3 Review and Assessment

Mini Glossary

Make sure that you know the meaning of each key term.

acute lymphocytic leukemia (ALL) the most common form of leukemia in adults over 70 years of age; characterized by overproduction of lymphocytes

acute myeloid leukemia (AML) the most common form of leukemia in adults; develops when the bone marrow produces too many myeloblasts

anemia a condition characterized by a decrease in the number of red blood cells or an insufficient amount of hemoglobin in the red blood cells

aplastic anemia a rare but serious condition in which the bone marrow is incapable of making new red blood cells

chelation therapy a procedure in which excess metals, such as iron, are removed from the blood

chronic lymphocytic leukemia (CLL) a form of leukemia characterized by extremely high levels of lymphocytes; most often found in middle-aged adults

chronic myeloid leukemia (CML) a form of leukemia characterized by overproduction of granulocytes

hemophilia a condition in which blood does not clot properly due to the absence of a clotting factor

iron-deficient anemia the most common anemia; caused by an insufficient dietary intake of iron, loss of iron from intestinal bleeding, or iron-level depletion during pregnancy

jaundice a blood disorder characterized by yellow-colored skin and whites of the eyes

leukemia a cancer caused by the production of an extremely high number of immature white blood cells in the bone marrow

multiple myeloma a cancer of the plasma cells in bone marrow

pernicious anemia a severe anemia caused by the inability of the intestines to absorb vitamin B_{12}, which is essential for the formation of red blood cells; usually develops in older adults

phlebotomy the drawing of blood; a standard treatment for polycythemia

polycythemia a condition in which the bone marrow manufactures too many red blood cells; caused by prolonged altitude exposure and a genetic mutation

sickle cell anemia a disease in which the red blood cells are shaped like a sickle, or crescent, rather than a disk; caused by irregularly shaped hemoglobin molecules in the red blood cells

thalassemia a condition that affects the body's ability to produce fully developed hemoglobin and red blood cells; Cooley's anemia

Know and Understand

1. What does a complete blood count detect?
2. What type of food and what mineral supplements are recommended for a person with iron-deficient anemia?
3. What condition results from damage to bone marrow stem cells, making them unable to produce mature blood cells?
4. Diseases such as type I diabetes mellitus, Addison disease, or chronic thyroiditis increase the risk of developing which type of anemia?
5. What are the major treatments for sickle cell anemia?
6. What is another name for Cooley's anemia?
7. What factor might increase the likelihood that a newborn will develop jaundice?
8. What disease would cause people to be more concerned than normal about skin punctures and cuts?
9. What is the most common form of leukemia in adults?

Analyze and Apply

10. How does long-term exposure to high altitude contribute to polycythemia?
11. Explain the cause of leukemia.
12. Using what you have learned about stem cells, explain why a stem cell transplant would help a person with multiple myeloma.
13. Explain why someone with sickle cell anemia is at greater risk for stroke than someone with a different type of anemia.
14. Explain why an elderly patient with liver disease will likely have jaundice.

IN THE LAB

15. Using library resources or the Internet, research multiple myeloma. Focus on any developing therapies and stem cell transplant techniques. What do these new treatment options involve? How do they work? Create a poster to illustrate your findings and present it to the class.
16. Assume that you are a physician whose patient has iron-deficient anemia. You need to develop a treatment plan for your patient that focuses on nutrition. Research foods that are good sources of iron to include in your treatment plan. Develop a sample meal plan for one week, including breakfast, lunch, and dinner. Present your plan to the class.

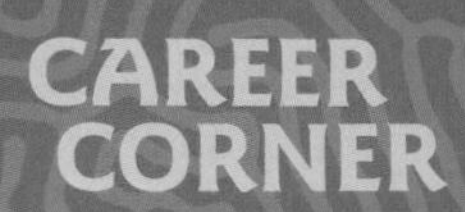

Anatomy & Physiology at Work

The blood touches every cell and tissue in the body. Therefore, blood samples, or specimens, can be used to diagnose many disorders and diseases.

Phlebotomists are people who collect blood specimens. These specimens are frequently analyzed and evaluated by medical technologists.

Phlebotomist

Phlebotomists are trained in blood collection techniques and in the handling and storage of blood. Phlebotomists collect blood for diagnostic tests, blood banks, transfusions, and clinical research.

Phlebotomists can collect blood in different ways. For example, they might simply stick a finger using a sterile lancet to draw a small amount of blood. To take more blood they would draw it from a vein, usually in the arm (**Figure 10.26**). It is critical that phlebotomists follow proper procedures and safety precautions for collecting blood. They must also ensure that their equipment is sterile and safe for use.

opard wattanasakul/Shutterstock.com

Figure 10.26 Phlebotomists collect and store blood specimens for use in laboratory testing.

Phlebotomists work in a variety of settings, including hospitals, medical clinics, and private practices. Some physicians do not have phlebotomists on staff, so they send their patients to laboratories that employ phlebotomists. These laboratories specialize in collecting and analyzing blood specimens for physician offices and blood banks.

Students interested in a career as a phlebotomist must possess a high school diploma or its equivalent. They must also complete a brief certification program. Each state has different program and licensure requirements. States that do require a license to be a phlebotomist may require successful completion of an exam administered by an accrediting agency such as the American Society for Clinical Pathology.

Most licensing exams have questions about specimen collection, clinical laboratory procedures, proper handling of blood samples, and safety protocols. Some employers prefer to hire phlebotomists who are not only state licensed but also nationally certified.

Medical Technologist

Medical technologists analyze human blood and tissue specimens. They perform a full range of laboratory tests on these specimens. For example, they match blood types before transfusions or surgery. They also check blood specimens for signs of disease, parasites, drugs, chemicals, and other elements. Medical technologists are responsible for confirming the accuracy of their test results and reporting laboratory findings to physicians and pathologists.

The medical technology laboratory has a wide array of instruments, including microscopes and complex computerized equipment. Therefore, medical technologists must be comfortable operating such machines.

Medical technologists must be precise, thorough, and able to handle high levels of stress. Physicians often need lab results quickly, so medical technologists must be comfortable working in a fast-paced, sometimes stressful environment. Medical technologists are employed in hospitals, clinics, independent laboratories, and public health facilities (**Figure 10.27**).

Students interested in pursuing a career as a medical technologist should establish a strong science foundation in high school by taking courses such as biology, chemistry, math, and computer science. A bachelor of science degree in medical technology from a program recognized by the national accrediting agency for clinical laboratory sciences is also required. Aspiring medical technologists must also pass a national certification exam administered by the American Society for Clinical Pathology.

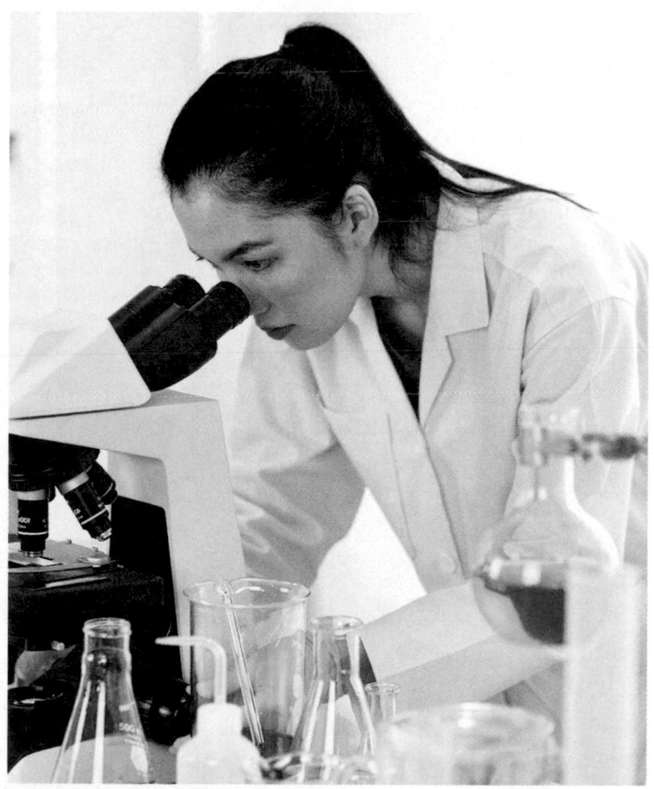

Jarun Ontakrai/Shutterstock.com

Figure 10.27 Medical technologists analyze blood, urine, saliva, and tissue specimens.

Planning for a Health-Related Career

Do some research on the career of a phlebotomist or a medical technologist. You may choose instead to research a profession from the list of related career options. Using the Internet or resources at your local library, find answers to the following questions:

1. What are the main tasks and responsibilities of a person employed in the career that you chose to research?
2. What is the outlook for this career? Are workers in demand, or are jobs dwindling? For complete information, consult the current edition of the *Occupational Outlook Handbook*, published by the US Department of Labor. This handbook is available online or at your local library. More specific information for your state or local area may also be available.
3. What special skills or talents are required? Does the idea of working with blood make you feel queasy?
4. What personality traits do you think are necessary for success in the career that you have chosen to research? Some people are afraid of sharp instruments such as needles. Would you be able to calm a person's fear of needles and make them feel comfortable as you obtain a blood specimen?
5. Does the work involve a great deal of routine, or are the day-to-day responsibilities varied?
6. Does the career require long hours, or is it a standard, "9-to-5" job?
7. What is the salary range for this job? Is this salary range in line with your expectations?
8. What do you think you would like about this career? Is there anything about it that you might dislike?

Related Career Options

- Biological technician
- Chemical technician
- Emergency medical technician (EMT)
- Epidemiologist
- Medical assistant
- Medical transcriptionist
- Occupational health and safety technician

CHAPTER 10

Review

LESSON 10.1

The Functions and Composition of Blood

Key Points

- Blood is responsible for providing transportation, regulation, and protection throughout the body.
- Blood is slightly salty, with a sodium chloride concentration of 0.9%. It has a pH between 7.35 and 7.45 and an average temperature of 100.4°F (38°C).
- Erythrocytes carry oxygen and other essential nutrients to every cell of the body. Leukocytes protect against infection. Platelets promote blood clotting.

Key Terms

buffy coat
carbaminohemoglobin
coagulation
diapedesis
erythrocytes
erythropoiesis
erythropoietin
fibrin
formed elements
hematocrit
hematopoiesis
hemoglobin
hemolysis
hemostasis
leukocytes
oxyhemoglobin
plasma
platelet plug
platelets

LESSON 10.2

Blood Types

Key Points

- The four blood types in the ABO blood typing system are A, B, AB, and O. These types are based on antigens on the surface of the red blood cells and antibodies the body produces against them.
- The Rh factor is an antigen on the surface of red blood cells. People with the Rh factor are Rh-positive (Rh^+). People without it are Rh-negative (Rh^-).

Key Terms

agglutination
antibody
antigen
erythroblastosis fetalis
Rh factor
RhoGAM
universal donor
universal recipient

LESSON 10.3

Blood Disorders and Diseases

Key Points

- A complete blood count is a test that measures the number of red blood cells, white blood cells, and platelets. It is often used to diagnose blood disorders and diseases.
- Anemia is characterized by a decreased number of red blood cells or an insufficient amount of hemoglobin in red blood cells. Acquired anemias are the result of dietary deficiency or internal bleeding, whereas inherited anemias are determined by genetic makeup.
- Other diseases and disorders of the blood include jaundice, hemophilia, polycythemia, leukemia, and multiple myeloma.

Key Terms

acute lymphocytic leukemia (ALL)
acute myeloid leukemia (AML)
anemia
aplastic anemia
chelation therapy
chronic lymphocytic leukemia (CLL)
chronic myeloid leukemia (CML)
hemophilia
iron-deficient anemia
jaundice
leukemia
multiple myeloma
pernicious anemia
phlebotomy
polycythemia
sickle cell anemia
thalassemia

Assessment

LESSON 10.1

The Functions and Composition of Blood

Learning Key Terms and Concepts

1. *True or False*? Blood is considered a regulatory system.
2. Blood makes up approximately _____% of total body weight.
3. The two basic components of blood are the formed elements and _____.
4. What percentage of blood is composed of plasma?
5. Which of the following is *not* a protein in blood plasma?
   A. fibrinogen
   B. albumin
   C. erythropoietin
   D. globulin
6. *True or False*? Red blood cells have an unlimited life span.
7. The kidneys regulate red blood cell production through a process called _____.
8. In adults, RBCs, platelets, and the majority of WBCs are produced in the _____.
9. _____ are the most abundant type of white blood cells in the body.
10. Basophils are leukocytes that _____.
    A. attack invading microorganisms
    B. produce histamine
    C. give red blood cells their disk shape
    D. give blood its color

Thinking Critically

11. A healthy blood vessel normally repels platelets to prevent unnecessary clotting. Explain hemostasis when a blood vessel wall has been injured.
12. Explain why checking a patient's hemoglobin and hematocrit levels is necessary before the patient undergoes surgery.
13. Explain the process of phagocytosis and how old RBCs are recycled. Name the organs involved in recycling RBCs.
14. Explain the process by which WBCs fight infection.

LESSON 10.2

Blood Types

Learning Key Terms and Concepts

15. *True or False*? There are three major blood types in the ABO system of blood typing.
16. _____ are molecules on the surface of cells that help the body distinguish between "self" and "nonself" cells.
17. In the ABO system, a universal recipient has blood type _____.
18. In the ABO system, a universal blood donor has blood type _____.
19. The potentially fatal process that causes blood of different types to clump and create blockages is called _____.
20. Agglutination can cause _____, or destruction of donated red blood cells.
21. *True or False*? The term *Rh factor* was inspired by the rhesus monkey.
22. RhoGAM, when administered to an Rh^- woman shortly after the birth of an Rh^+ child, can help prevent _____.

Thinking Critically

23. Explain the characteristics used to identify the different blood types. Why is it dangerous to mix certain blood types for blood transfusions?
24. Identify the characteristic that makes blood types either positive (+) or negative (–). Explain the significance of these classifications.
25. Why is it important for a woman to know her blood type before she has a baby?

LESSON 10.3

Blood Disorders and Diseases

Learning Key Terms and Concepts

26. Which of the following *cannot* be detected by a CBC?
    A. abnormal kidney function
    B. blood clotting problems
    C. cancers of the blood
    D. immune system disorders
27. *True or False*? It is possible to inherit an anemic condition.

28. The three main causes of anemia are a high rate of RBC destruction, decreased RBC production, and _____.
    A. increased production of leukocytes
    B. platelet destruction
    C. polycythemia vera
    D. excessive blood loss
29. *True or False*? Iron-deficient anemia accounts for almost 50% of all anemias around the world.
30. Aplastic anemia is caused by damage to the _____ in the bone marrow.
31. _____ anemia is caused by the inability of the intestines to absorb vitamin B_{12}.
32. To develop sickle cell anemia, you must inherit the sickle cell gene from _____.
    A. your mother
    B. your father
    C. both parents
    D. a grandfather
33. _____ is a disease that affects proteins in hemoglobin and prevents the body from producing fully developed hemoglobin.
34. The type of therapy used to remove excess iron from the blood is called _____ therapy.
35. An immature liver is a common cause of _____ in newborns.
36. People who have _____ are typically missing clotting factor VII or IX.
37. The type of leukemia in which the bone marrow produces too many granulocytes is _____ leukemia.
38. *True or false*? Multiple myeloma is a curable form of cancer.

Thinking Critically

39. Why is a complete blood count a beneficial test to run? What kinds of things can it tell the physician about a patient?
40. Kelsey is a fifteen-year-old girl whose parents moved to Chicago from their native Sicily five years before she was born. When Kelsey was a baby, she was diagnosed with a blood disorder. As a result of this disorder, Kelsey experiences back and leg pain. She is often short of breath and tired. Which blood disorder do you think Kelsey is living with? What can she do to manage her disease?
41. Rachael is a young mother with Rh-negative blood. Her first child, Hazel, was born two years ago and has Rh-positive blood. Rachael is now pregnant with her second child. What complications might arise if her second baby also has Rh-positive blood? What could Rachael's doctor have done to avoid these complications?
42. Some of the symptoms of anemia are headache, dizziness, fatigue, and shortness of breath. What is the underlying reason for these symptoms?
43. Explain the role a healthy diet plays in preventing or treating anemia.
44. Explain chelation therapy. Why might a person with thalassemia need this type of therapy?

Building Skills and Connecting Concepts

Analyzing and Evaluating Data

Instructions: The chart in **Figure 10.28** shows survival rates for leukemia and multiple myeloma patients from 1960–2007. Use this chart to answer the following questions.

45. By what percentage did survival rates for multiple myeloma cases improve between the 1960s and 2007?

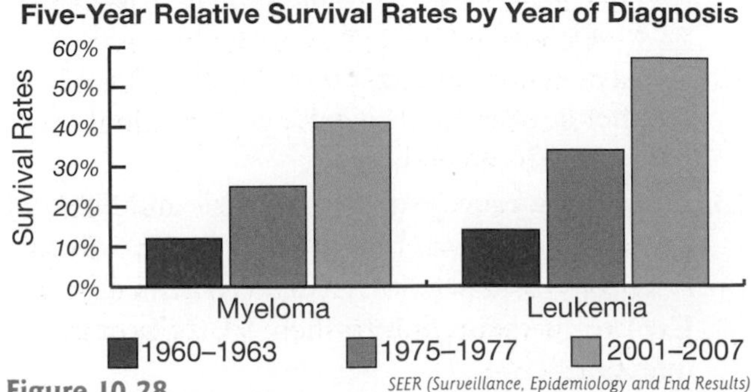

Figure 10.28

46. If a person was diagnosed with leukemia in 1976, what survival rate could they expect?
47. If a person was diagnosed with multiple myeloma in 2003, what survival rate could they expect?
48. Survival rates for both multiple myeloma and leukemia have consistently risen since the 1960s. Why do you think this is?
49. What are the current five-year survival rates for multiple myeloma and leukemia? Research the statistics online and determine the survival-rate percentage for both diseases. Then, recreate the chart shown here on a sheet of paper. Add a new bar to represent the current survival rates.
50. By what percentage did survival rates increase for leukemia between the 1960s and 2007?
51. What is the difference in percentage of survival rates in the 1970s for someone diagnosed with multiple myeloma compared to someone diagnosed with leukemia?

Communicating about Anatomy & Physiology

52. **Reading and Writing** In 1985, the United States established mandatory screenings of donated blood for bloodborne diseases such as HIV. Research the blood donation process. For what other diseases is donated blood screened to prevent transmission of diseases? Besides screening for bloodborne diseases, what steps must be taken to ensure that donors are healthy candidates for donation? Can people with tattoos donate blood? What about someone with a cold virus? Write a report highlighting the precautions that are taken to ensure that donated blood is healthy and free of disease.
53. **Writing** One of the most well-known carriers for hemophilia was Queen Victoria of England. Research the history of hemophilia in Queen Victoria's family. Did this disease affect royal families in other nations? If so, why? Also, look into which members of her family were carriers and which suffered from the disease. Create a family tree that incorporates your findings and present it to the class.
54. **Speaking** Research the history of sickle cell anemia and why it is more prevalent in African Americans and people of Mediterranean descent. Create a presentation to share your findings with your class.

Lab Investigations

55. Working in a small group, research the history of blood transfusions from the 1600s to the present. Why did some early transfusion efforts fail? What technological developments improved transfusion success rates? Create a time line highlighting the major successes and failures. Present your time line to the class.
56. Working with a partner, create clay models of red blood cells, platelets, and each type of white blood cell. Pay special attention to the presence of granules in the white blood cells, as well as their stain color. Use the illustrations in this chapter to help you create your models.

    Once you have finished constructing the models, label each model with its name and a brief description of the purpose it serves in the body. Share your models with the class. Do your models resemble those of other groups? If not, what is different and why?
57. Perform a bloodless transfusion. First cut out red circles to represent RBCs. Draw different shapes on the red circles to represent the different antigens. For example, a triangle might represent antigen A, and a circle might represent antigen B. Then cut out corresponding shapes to represent the antibodies. Make RBCs and antibodies for all of the different blood types.

    Place one RBC for a particular blood type on the desk with the appropriate antibodies around it. Place another RBC, for another blood type, on the desk with the appropriate antibodies around it. Perform the transfusion by placing one donor RBC on top of one recipient RBC. See if the antibody shapes match the shapes on the donor RBC. Document whether this transfusion was successful or harmful.

Building Your Portfolio

58. Take digital photographs of the models and posters you created as you worked through this chapter. Create a document or folder called "The Blood" and insert these items, along with written descriptions of what the models show and your reasons for creating them using the materials and forms you chose. Also make copies of your research and other documents. Add these items to your personal portfolio.

CHAPTER

11 The Cardiovascular System

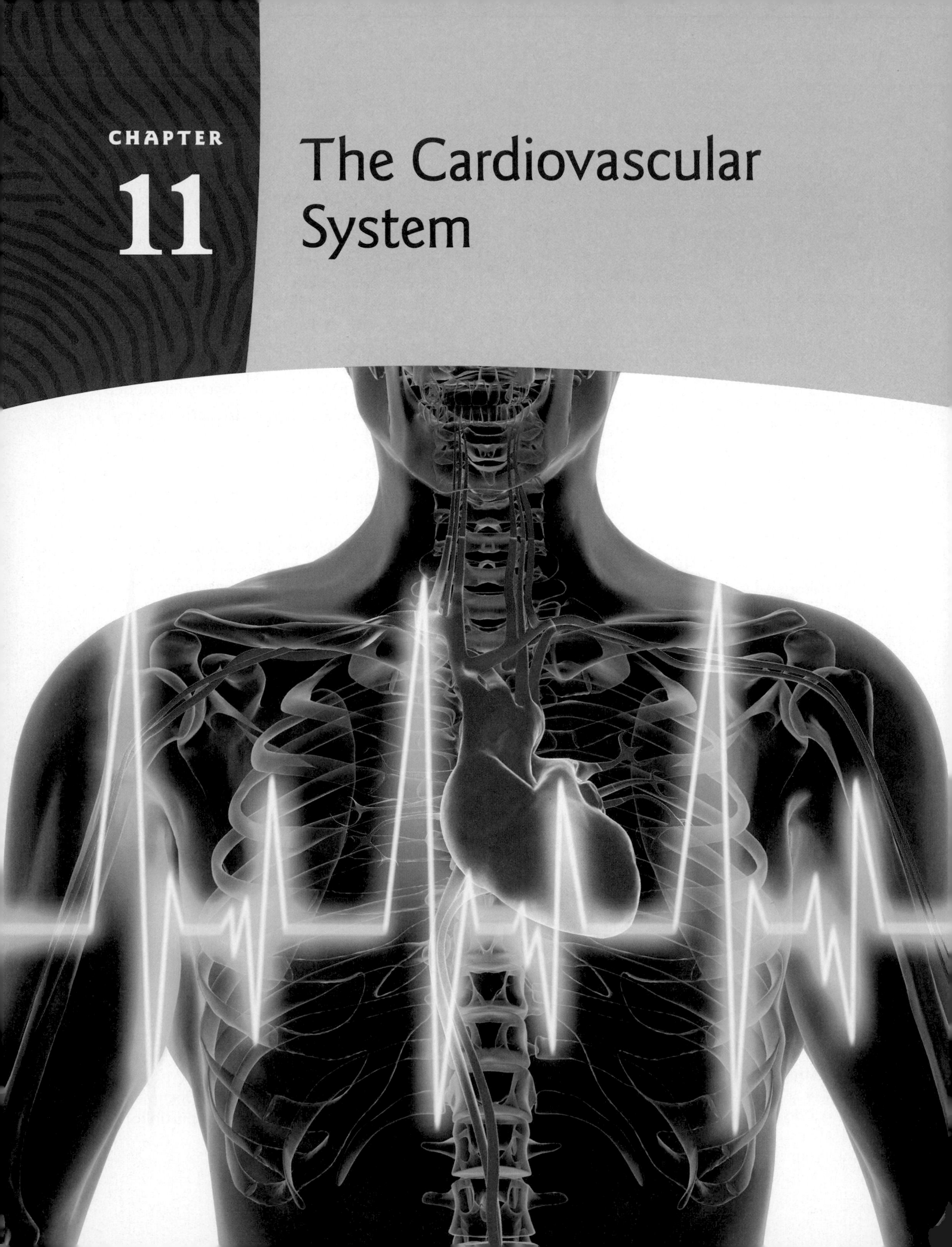

What important role does electricity play in regulating the heart?

"You gotta have *heart*!"
"Follow your *heart*."
"Know it by *heart*."
"Let's get to the *heart* of the matter!"

Is there an organ in the human body that is referenced in everyday language more often than the heart? What does this say about the function and importance of the heart?

The beating heart is just one part of the complex cardiovascular system. This system—comprising the heart, blood, and blood vessels—has a major impact on every living cell in the body.

Your heart beats 24 hours a day, 7 days a week. It pumps approximately 1.3 gallons (5 liters) of blood per minute, or approximately 2,000 gallons (7,571 liters) of blood each day. By comparison, a typical oil well pumps about 94 gallons of oil a day. The amount of blood pumped through your heart can fill 45 oil barrels a day and 2 oil super tankers in your lifetime. Isn't that an extraordinary feat for a muscle that is the size of a fist and weighs less than one pound? The heart is an amazing pump! This chapter explains how blood is pumped through thousands of miles of passageways in the body to nourish every cell.

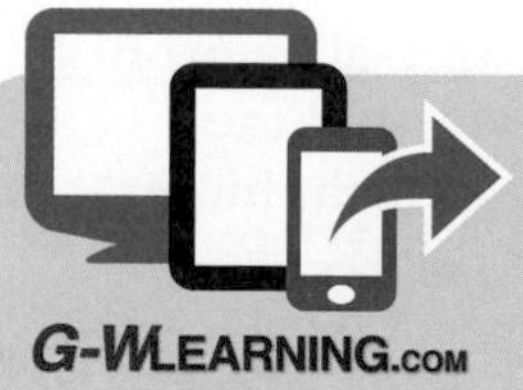

Click on the activity icon or visit www.g-wlearning.com/healthsciences/0202 to access online vocabulary activities using key terms from the chapter.

Chapter 11 Outline

◂ ancroft/Shutterstock.com

LESSON 11.1 Heart Anatomy and Physiology

Before You Read

Try to answer the following questions before you read this lesson.

- Besides serving as a transportation system throughout the body, what are the functions of the cardiovascular system?
- Why does blood flow in only one direction in the heart?

Lesson Objectives

- Describe the location, size, and structures of the heart.
- Outline the flow of blood through the heart and describe the cardiac cycle.

Key Terms

aorta	mean arterial pressure (MAP)
aortic valve	mitral valve
atrioventricular (AV) valves	myocardium
cardiac cycle	papillary muscles
cardiac output (CO)	pulmonary valve
diastole	semilunar valves
endocardium	stroke volume
epicardium	superior vena cava
Frank-Starling law	systole
inferior vena cava	tricuspid valve
interatrial septum	vasoconstriction
interventricular septum	vasodilation

The cardiovascular system, also called the *circulatory system*, consists of a strong, muscular pump (the heart), an extensive network of pipes (blood vessels), and fluid (blood). The system transports oxygen, hormones, and other nutrients to cells and rids the body of carbon dioxide and other metabolic waste products. Additionally, the cardiovascular system helps to regulate body temperature by **vasodilation** (va-soh-digh-LAY-shun) and **vasoconstriction** (va-soh-kun-STRIK-shun) of blood vessels. Vasodilation expands the diameter of blood vessels, which increases blood flow. Vasoconstriction decreases the diameter of blood vessels, which decreases blood flow.

The cardiovascular system has many functions:

- transportation of oxygen and other nutrients
- removal of carbon dioxide and other waste products
- regulation of body temperature
- maintenance of the body's acid-base balance
- transportation of hormones
- assistance with immune function

Anatomy of the Heart

The heart is the hardest-working organ in the human body. The normal rate of an adult heart is 72 to 82 beats per minute (bpm), or approximately 3 billion times in a person's lifetime. This fatigue-resistant organ is about the size of a clenched fist. It weighs a little less than the combined weight of two baseballs, or about 8 to 10 ounces in women and 10 to 12 ounces in men.

Location and Size of the Heart

The heart is located in the thoracic cavity under the sternum, or breastbone. It is centered in the chest and tilted slightly to the left. The heart is flanked on either side by the lungs and sits on top of the diaphragm. The broad *base* of the heart is positioned closer to the neck, at the second rib. The pointed *apex*, or bottom of the heart, lies at approximately the fifth rib and points down toward the left hip (**Figure 11.1**).

The Four Chambers of the Heart

The heart has an atrium and a ventricle on its right side and an atrium and a ventricle on its left side. The two atria (plural for *atrium*) act as low-pressure collecting chambers, and the two ventricles act as powerful pumps.

An **interatrial** (in-ter-AY-tree-al) **septum** separates the right and left atria, and the two ventricles are divided by a much thicker **interventricular** (in-ter-ven-TRIK-yoo-lar) **septum**. The septal walls prevent oxygen-rich blood from mixing with oxygen-poor blood.

The right atrium receives deoxygenated blood from the venous system (system of veins) via the

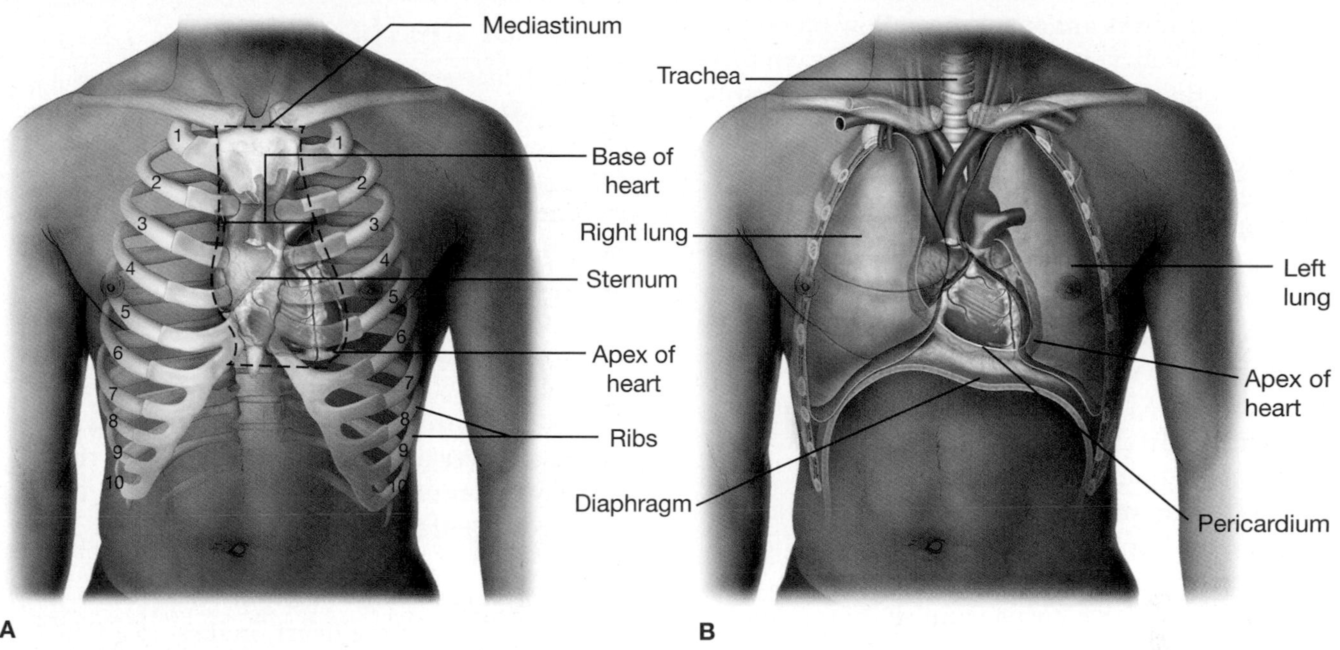

Figure 11.1 Position of the heart. A—Position of the heart in the thoracic cavity. B—Position of the heart in relation to the lungs and diaphragm. *Write one sentence describing the position of the heart in relation to a structure(s) in the thoracic cage (see Chapter 4 if necessary) and one sentence describing the location of the apex of the heart in relation to the lungs.*

inferior vena cava and the **superior vena cava** after the blood has made its trip around the body. The right ventricle then pumps the blood to the lungs. The left atrium receives the oxygenated blood from the lungs, and the left ventricle pumps the blood through the **aorta** (ay-OR-ta) to the body. The two ventricles contract almost simultaneously—as the right ventricle pumps blood to the lungs, the left ventricle pumps blood to the body.

The Heart Valves

The heart is outfitted with four valves, which permit blood to flow in only one direction. **Figure 11.2** shows the heart valves in open and closed states.

The AV Valves

The **atrioventricular** (ay-tree-oh-vehn-TRIK-yoo-lar) **valves**, or AV valves, are the two valves located between the atria and the ventricles.

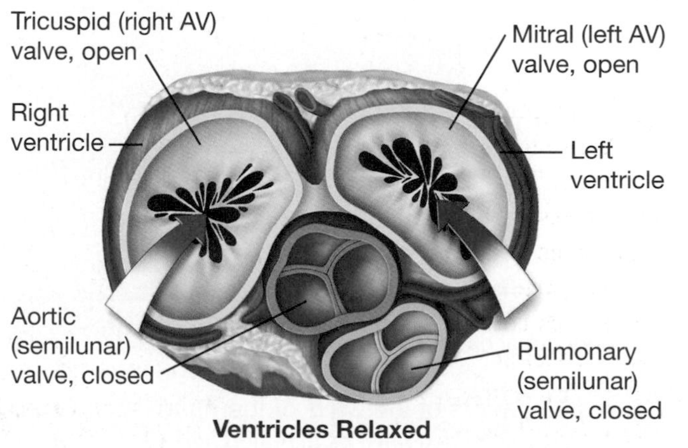

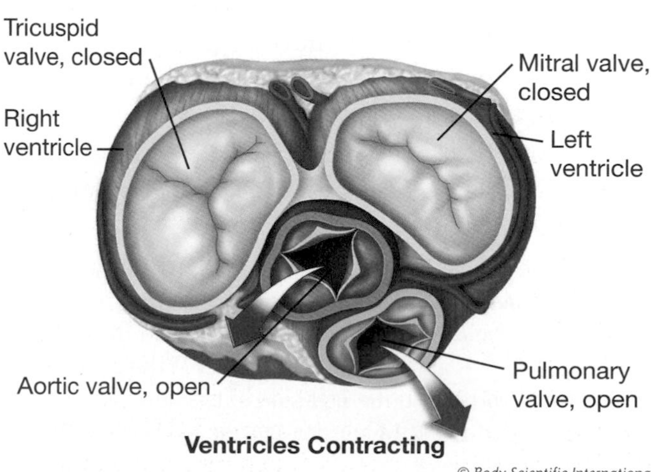

Figure 11.2 Anterior superior view of the heart valves. The red arrows indicate the flow of oxygenated blood. The blue arrows indicate the flow of deoxygenated blood. *When the ventricles are relaxed, are the AV valves open or closed? When the ventricles contract, are the semilunar valves open or closed?*

When these valves are open, they allow blood to flow from the atria into the ventricles. When they are closed, the AV valves prevent blood from flowing from the ventricles backward into the atria as the ventricles contract.

The AV valve on the right side of the heart is called the **tricuspid** (trigh-KUS-pid) **valve** because it has three cusps, or flaps. The AV valve on the left side of the heart is called the *bicuspid* (bigh-KUS-pid) *valve*, or the **mitral** (migh-tral) **valve**, because it has two cusps.

Attached to these cusps are *chordae tendineae* (KOR-dee TEHN-di-nee), which are thin, fibrous cords that are connected to the **papillary** (PAP-i-lair-ee) **muscles**. When the ventricles contract, the papillary muscles contract. These contractions pull on the chordae tendineae, preventing the valve cusps from swinging into the atria. If the valves were not secured by the chordae tendineae and the papillary muscles, the AV valve cusps would be pushed upward into the atria, allowing blood to flow backward into the atria. This backward blood flow is what happens when you have a heart murmur.

The Semilunar Valves

The next set of valves, the **semilunar** (sehm-ee-LOO-nar) **valves**, allows blood to flow from the ventricles to the lungs and the rest of the body. The **pulmonary** (PUL-muh-nair-ee) **valve** and **aortic** (ay-OR-tik) **valve** each have three semilunar (half-moon) cusps that do not need to be anchored. When they close, the cusps are strong enough to brace each other, similar to the three legs of a stool.

The pulmonary valve is located at the opening of the pulmonary artery on the right side of the heart. The aortic valve is located at the opening of the aorta on the left side of the heart.

MEMORY TIP

These tips should help you remember the locations of the different heart valves. You can remember that the **T**ricuspid valve is on the **R**ight side of the heart by noting that the letters **R** and **T** are close together in the alphabet. The **M**itral valve is on the **L**eft side of the heart, so remember that **L** and **M** are side by side in the alphabet.

Layers of the Heart

The heart is a hollow organ enclosed in a fluid-filled, double-walled sac called the *pericardium* (per-i-KAHR-dee-um). The fibrous outer wall of the sac anchors the heart to surrounding structures such as the sternum, diaphragm, and lungs. The inner wall of the sac is divided into two layers, which are separated by a fluid-filled cavity, called the *pericardial cavity*, that allows the heart to beat in a frictionless environment.

The heart wall has three layers of tissue. The **epicardium** (ehp-i-KAHR-dee-um) is the outermost layer of the heart, and it is also the innermost layer of the pericardium (**Figure 11.3**). The coronary arteries lie on the epicardial surface.

The **myocardium** (migh-oh-KAHR-dee-um), the middle layer of the heart, makes up about two-thirds of the heart muscle. It is the workhorse of the heart, contracting with enough force to pump blood through roughly 60,000 miles of vessels and back to the heart.

The innermost layer, the **endocardium** (ehn-doh-KAHR-dee-um), lines the interior of the heart chambers and covers the valves of the heart. The endocardium helps the blood to flow smoothly through the heart.

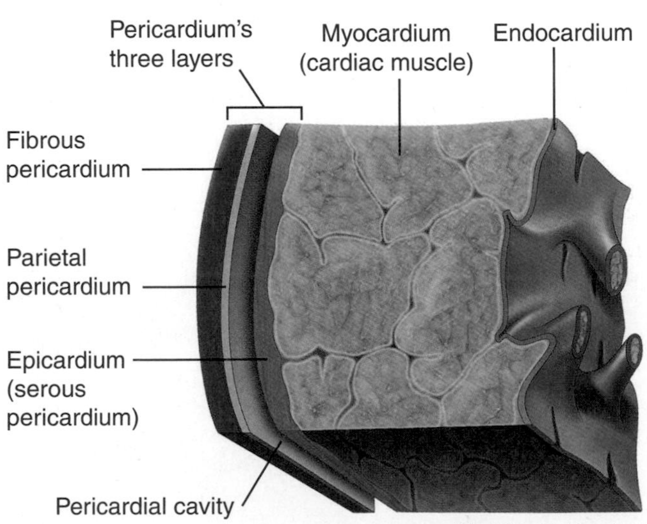

Figure 11.3 Layers of the walls of the heart. *Which layer of the heart can be described as the "workhorse"?*

Check Your Understanding

1. Is the blood leaving the left ventricle oxygenated or deoxygenated?
2. Which valve does blood move through as it goes from the right atrium to the right ventricle?
3. When the pulmonary valve opens, blood is forced into which artery and which main respiratory organ?
4. What is the name of the sac that encases the heart?
5. Name the three layers of the heart.

Physiology of the Heart

The anatomical structures of the heart are well suited to the heart's role as manager of blood flow throughout the body. This section explains the route blood takes through the heart, as well as the cycle of events that cause the blood to flow.

Blood Flow through the Heart

The following steps describe blood flow through the heart. Notice that the steps are also numbered and shown in **Figure 11.4**.

1. Deoxygenated blood enters the right atrium from both the inferior vena cava and the superior vena cava. The blood collects in the right atrium.

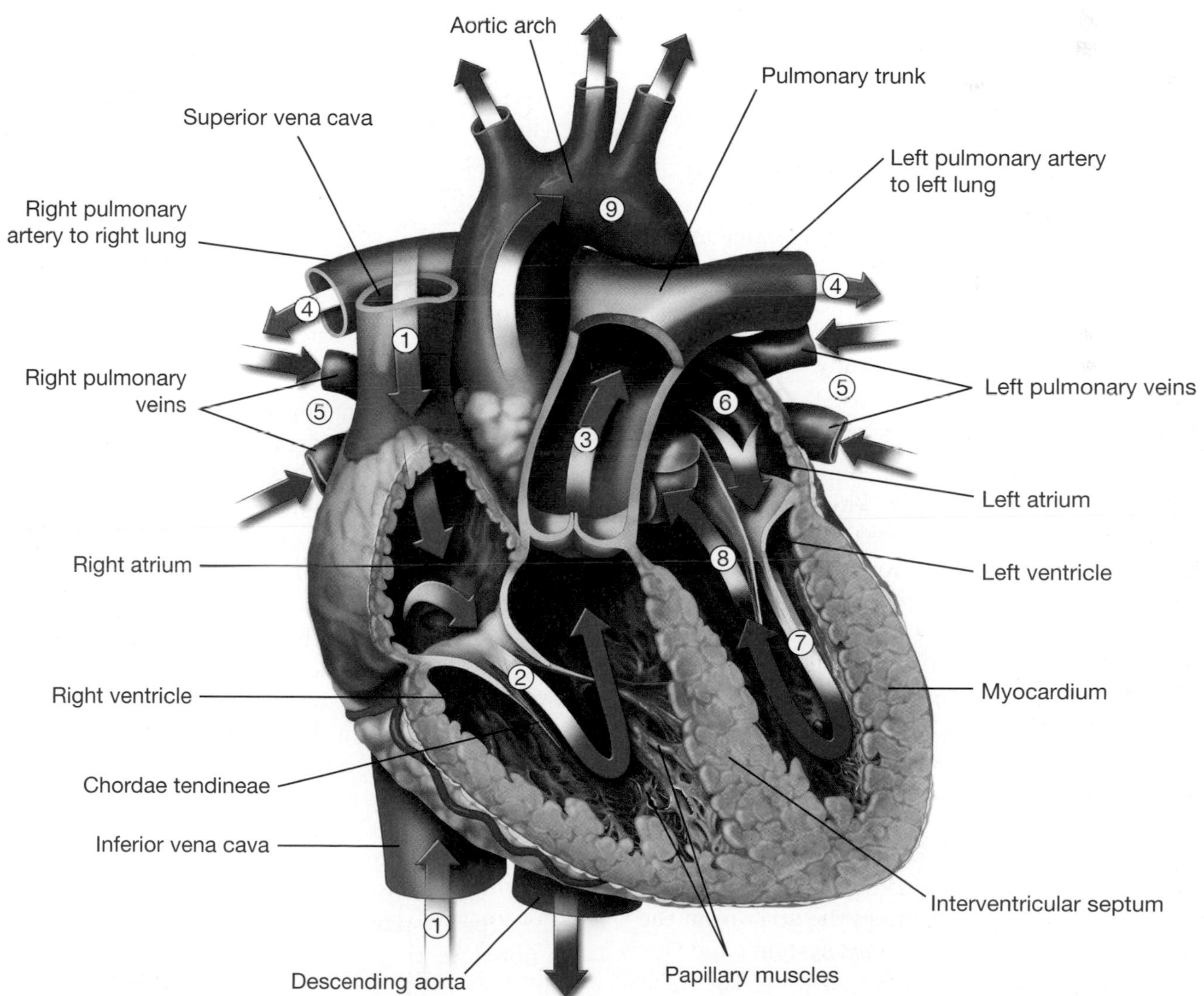

© Body Scientific International

Figure 11.4 Heart chambers, great vessels, and blood flow through the heart. The arrows indicate the direction of blood flow. The blue arrows indicate deoxygenated blood. The red arrows indicate oxygenated blood. *Has the blood that is shown in the left ventricle already been through the lungs, or is it on its way to the lungs?*

2. The collecting blood increases the pressure against the tricuspid valve, causing the valve to open. At this stage, with the tricuspid valve open, the right ventricle fills passively. Then, the right atrium contracts, forcing the remaining blood from the atrium into the ventricle.
3. The right ventricle contracts, and pressure increases in the chamber. This causes the tricuspid valve to close and the pulmonary valve to open, forcing blood into the pulmonary artery.
4. The pulmonary artery carries the blood to the lungs, where it becomes oxygenated in the capillary network of the lungs.
5. Oxygenated blood returns to the left atrium via the pulmonary veins.
6. Blood collects in the left atrium, causing pressure to increase in the chamber, thereby forcing the mitral valve to open. At this stage, the left ventricle is filling passively.
7. Atrial contraction forces the remaining blood into the left ventricle.
8. The ventricle contracts, and the pressure increases in the chamber. The increased pressure in the chamber causes the mitral valve to close and the aortic valve to open. The blood is forced into the aorta.
9. Oxygenated blood begins its journey to supply oxygen to all parts of the body.

Cardiac Cycle

The events included in a single heartbeat are known as the **cardiac cycle**. This cycle consists of two phases: contraction and relaxation. During one complete cardiac cycle, the four chambers of the heart undergo a period of relaxation called **diastole** (digh-AS-toh-lee), when the chambers are filling with blood. Each cycle also includes a period of contraction called **systole** (SIS-toh-lee), when the chambers are pumping blood out of the heart.

The cardiac cycle can be further divided into early and late ventricular diastole, atrial systole, and ventricular systole. During late ventricular diastole, both the atria and the ventricles are completely relaxed and the pressure inside the chambers is low. At this point, blood enters the atria from the pulmonary and systemic venous systems and flows passively into the right and left ventricles. About 80% of the blood entering the ventricles does so passively. During this time, the AV valves (tricuspid and mitral) are open and the semilunar valves (pulmonary and aortic) are closed.

During atrial systole, the atria contract and pump the remaining 20% of blood into the ventricles. As the pressure in the ventricles increases, the AV valves are forced closed. Ventricular pressure then rises rapidly.

When the ventricular pressure exceeds the pressure in the pulmonary trunk and aorta, the semilunar valves open and blood is ejected from the ventricles into the pulmonary and systemic circulatory systems. This phase is called *ventricular systole*. During this stage, the atria are relaxed and filling with blood. At the end of ventricular systole, the semilunar valves close and the pressure in the ventricles begins to drop. At this point the AV valves are also closed, so the ventricles are completely relaxed and the pressure continues to decrease. This is called *early diastole*. When the pressure in the ventricles is lower than that of the atria, the AV valves are forced open and the ventricles begin to fill with blood again, starting a new cardiac cycle.

One cardiac cycle is approximately 0.81 seconds in duration. In general, for an individual who has a resting heart rate of 72 to 82 bpm, approximately two-thirds of the cardiac cycle is spent in diastole, and one-third is spent in systole. This ratio is the basis for the formula for **mean arterial pressure (MAP)**:

$$\text{MAP} = \frac{\text{2/3 diastolic}}{\text{blood pressure}} + \frac{\text{1/3 systolic}}{\text{blood pressure}}$$

The mean arterial pressure measures the overall pressure within the cardiovascular system, which determines blood flow to various organs. If this pressure falls below 60 millimeters of mercury (mmHG), the organs of the body will become damaged from lack of oxygen. A lower blood pressure also means that the body will not receive the nutrient-rich blood flow that it needs.

At your next physical examination, your physician may use a stethoscope to listen to your heart. During the cardiac cycle, the AV valves and the semilunar valves make sounds when they close. The sounds are referred to as "lub-dub" sounds. The "lub" sound is produced when the AV valves (tricuspid and mitral) close, and the "dub" sound is produced when the semilunar valves (pulmonary and aortic) close. If the valves do not close properly, there may be an additional sound, called a *heart murmur*. Many children have a heart murmur. Most of these murmurs are harmless and are not caused by a heart abnormality, but rather by a rapid growth spurt.

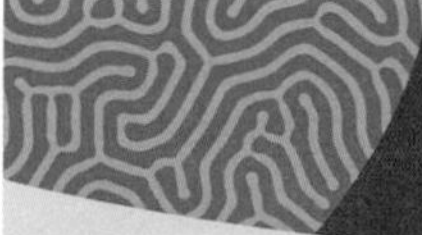

What Research Tells Us

...about How the Hearts of Athletes Adapt to Exercise

An *echocardiogram* (ehk-oh-KAHR-dee-oh-gram) is an ultrasound test that looks at the structures of the heart to determine whether the heart valves are opening and closing properly (**Figure 11.5**). This test can also measure the pumping capacity of the heart.

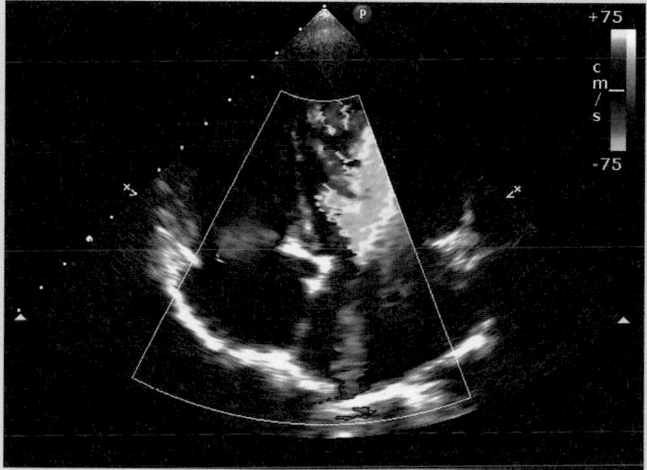

kalewa/Shutterstock.com

Figure 11.5 Modern Doppler echocardiographs use color to provide information about heart health.

Echocardiogram studies have shown that athletes who train aerobically (by running, cycling, or swimming, for example) have increases in both the size of their left ventricular chamber and in the thickness of the left ventricular wall. However, athletes who train using resistive exercise (weight lifting) have an increase in the left ventricular wall thickness but not in the size of the ventricular chamber.

Athletes also have an increase in their parasympathetic tone, causing their resting heart rate to decrease to 30 to 40 beats per minute. These adaptations are one of the reasons why stroke volume among athletes is almost twice that of untrained individuals.

Taking It Further

1. Working with a partner, research the impact of regular exercise on the hearts of individuals who ordinarily do not exercise. What types of exercise bestow the greatest benefit? Develop a report for the class on the benefits of exercise and on exercise recommendations for different age groups.
2. Investigate the different types of echocardiogram tests and what each test reveals. Report your findings to the class.

Cardiac Output

Cardiac output (CO) is the amount of blood pumped from the ventricles in 1 minute. The average cardiac output for men is approximately 5 L/min (5,000 mL). Cardiac output from the left ventricle is important because it is a measure of the pumping capacity of the heart, which determines the effectiveness of the heart to deliver blood and oxygen to the entire body. If cardiac output is lowered due to cardiovascular disease, the delivery of oxygen to the peripheral tissues and organs is diminished and negative side effects occur.

The two factors that determine cardiac output are heart rate and stroke volume. Heart rate is the number of times the heart beats in 1 minute (beats per minute or bpm) and is normally about 72 bpm. **Stroke volume** is the amount of blood pumped from the heart per beat (mL/beat) and is usually about 60–80 mL/beat. Cardiac output is adjusted to meet the oxygen needs of the body by changing heart rate and/or stroke volume.

Cardiac output is the product of heart rate and stroke volume:

$$\text{CO (L/min)} = \frac{\text{heart rate (bpm)} \times \text{stroke volume (mL/beat)}}{1{,}000 \text{ mL/L}}$$

For example, if heart rate is 75 bpm and stroke volume is 80 mL/beats/min, the cardiac output would be:

$$\text{CO} = \frac{75 \text{ bpm} \times 80 \text{ mL/beat}}{1{,}000 \text{ mL/L}} = 6 \text{ L/minute}$$

Several factors may influence heart rate and stroke volume, and consequently, cardiac output. At rest, heart rate can be influenced by the size of the heart or a person's fitness level. Generally, the larger the heart, the lower the heart rate. Why does this occur? A larger heart has a larger left ventricular chamber, which means it can hold more blood. As a result, when the heart contracts, there is a higher stroke volume.

At rest, there is an inverse relationship between heart rate and stroke volume. If stroke volume is higher, then heart rate is lower because the system tries to maintain a cardiac output of about 5 L/minute. Conversely, if the heart is smaller and stroke volume is lower, then heart rate has to be higher to maintain a cardiac output of 5 L/minute. This is the why a baby's heart rate is much higher than that of an adult and also why females tend to have higher resting heart rates than men.

Generally, people who are more fit have a lower resting heart rate, which increases the amount of time that the ventricle can fill with blood. A trained athlete's resting heart rate is usually well under 60 beats/minute. Thus when the heart contracts, there is an increased

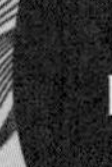

LIFE SPAN DEVELOPMENT: *The Cardiovascular System*

One of the most exciting moments in an expectant parent's life is to hear the baby's heartbeat for the first time. This miracle occurs at around day 21 when the primitive heart starts to pump blood in the developing fetus. The heart is the first organ to form, due to its vital role in providing oxygen and nutrients to the developing fetus.

Fetal Development

The heart's development actually starts from embryonic tissue around day 18 in a region called the *cardiogenic* (*cardi/o* = heart; *-genic* = creation) *area*. During the following week, the primitive heart undergoes five developmental changes so that by the fourth week, the atria and the ventricles are oriented as they are in an adult, with the atria lying superior to the ventricles. At about four weeks after fertilization, partitioning of the chambers begins and the primitive interatrial septum begins to fuse with structures called *endocardial cushions*.

When the fusion of the interatrial septum and the endocardial cushions is complete, an opening in the septum called the *foramen ovale* is formed. The foramen ovale allows blood entering the right atrium to flow into the left atrium until birth, when it normally closes. The interventricular septum that partitions the ventricles into the right and left ventricles also forms during this time. The partitioning of the chambers is complete by the fifth week. The atrioventricular and semilunar valves are formed during weeks 5–9.

Blood cells begin to develop from blood islands beginning at week 3, or 15 days after fertilization. Blood vessels begin to form about two days later. Blood islands contain angioblasts that form endothelial cells, which line the inside of every blood vessel. In this early stage of fetal development, *vasculogenesis* is the main process for blood vessel development. As fetal development continues, vessels are developed through the process of *angiogenesis*, the formation of blood vessels from preexisting vessels. Angiogenesis continues after the baby is born and continues through old age.

Effects of Aging

Cardiovascular function declines by about 10% every decade after age thirty. As people get older, there is a decrease in cardiac muscle size and cardiac muscle strength, a reduced cardiac output, a decreased maximal heart rate, an increased systolic blood pressure, and a stiffening of walls of the aorta.

Increased stiffness occurs in all of the other arteries and vessels in the cardiovascular system. Vascular stiffness is greatly affected by the accumulation of plaque in the arteries, or atherosclerosis. What does this mean in practical terms? These changes increase the likelihood of hypertension, coronary artery disease, myocardial infarctions, and other cardiovascular disorders. The good news is you can delay the onset of aging-related changes by following the healthy lifestyle recommendations on exercise, diet, weight maintenance, and stress management outlined in this chapter!

Life Span Review

1. What is the difference between vasculogenesis and angiogenesis?
2. How can you minimize age-related changes to the cardiovascular system?

stroke volume. In fact, a well-trained athlete may have a resting stroke volume of more than 100 mL/beat.

During exercise, heart rate increases because of the effects of increased sympathetic nervous system stimulation and certain hormones on the heart, which increases cardiac output. Other factors that can increase or decrease heart rate include:

- certain cardiovascular diseases
- fever
- ingested substances (such as caffeine)
- illegal drugs (such as cocaine)
- medications (such as antihistamines and decongestants)
- emotions

In addition to the size of the left ventricular chamber and the amount of blood in the left ventricle, there are two other factors that influence stroke volume. When there is more blood in the left ventricle, the myocardial muscle fibers are stretched to a greater degree. The more the myocardial muscle fibers are stretched, the greater the strength of the contraction, which increases stroke volume. This principle is known as the **Frank-Starling law**. You can liken this to stretching a rubber band and releasing it. If you stretch it a little, the rubber band will not go far, but if you stretch it a lot, the rubber band may shoot across the room.

The last factor that can increase stroke volume is the amount of sympathetic nervous system stimulation. When there is an increase in sympathetic nervous system stimulation, the cardiac muscle fibers contract more forcibly, causing an increase in stroke volume.

The changes in cardiac output due to changes in heart rate or stroke volume or both, and the change in cardiac output can be quite dramatic. For example, at rest, cardiac output is normally 5 L/minute, but during maximal exercise for the average person it may increase 4- to 5-fold to a level of 20 to 25 L/minute. In elite athletes during maximal exercise, cardiac output may even increase 8-fold to as high as 40 L/minute!

Check Your Understanding

1. What events are included in a single cardiac cycle?
2. What produces the "dub" sound heard through a stethoscope?
3. What is the formula for cardiac output?

LESSON 11.1 Review and Assessment

Mini Glossary

Make sure that you know the meaning of each key term.

aorta a large arterial trunk that arises from the base of the left ventricle and channels blood from the heart into other arteries throughout the body

aortic valve the semilunar valve between the left ventricle and the aorta that prevents blood from flowing back into the left ventricle

atrioventricular (AV) valves the two valves (tricuspid and mitral) situated between the atria and the ventricles

cardiac cycle the events that occur during a single heartbeat

cardiac output (CO) the amount of blood pumped from the heart per minute

diastole the period of relaxation in the heart when the chambers are filling with blood

endocardium the innermost layer of the heart, which lines the interior of the heart chambers and covers the valves of the heart

epicardium the outermost layer of the heart and the innermost layer of the pericardial sac

Frank-Starling law an increase in blood volume in the ventricles of the heart causes an increase in stroke volume

inferior vena cava largest vein in the human body that returns deoxygenated blood to the right atrium of the heart from body regions below the diaphragm

interatrial septum the wall that separates the right and left atria in the heart

interventricular septum thick wall that divides the two ventricles in the heart

mean arterial pressure (MAP) measure of the overall pressure within the cardiovascular system, which determines blood flow to various organs

mitral valve the valve that closes the orifice between the left atrium and left ventricle of the heart; bicuspid valve

myocardium the middle layer of the heart, which makes up about 2/3 of the heart muscle

papillary muscles small, muscular bundles attached at one end to the chordae tendineae and at the other to the innermost or endocardial wall of the ventricles; maintain tension on the chordae tendineae as the ventricles contract

pulmonary valve semilunar valve located between the right ventricle and the pulmonary artery

semilunar valves valves situated at the opening between the heart and the aorta and at the opening between the heart and the pulmonary artery; they prevent backflow of blood into the ventricles

stroke volume the volume of blood pumped from the heart per beat

superior vena cava second largest vein in the body that returns deoxygenated blood to the right atrium of the heart from the upper half of the body

systole a period of contraction when the chambers are pumping blood out of the heart

tricuspid valve the valve that closes the orifice between the right atrium and right ventricle of the heart; composed of three cusps

vasoconstriction narrowing of the blood vessels, which decreases blood flow

vasodilation widening of the blood vessels, which increases blood flow

Know and Understand

1. What are the names of the large blood vessels that bring blood back to the heart and empty it into the right atrium?
2. Which muscles control the AV valves?
3. Which layer of the heart is responsible for contractions?
4. What kind of vessels carry blood to the lungs?
5. In which phase of the cardiac cycle do the semilunar valves open, ejecting blood from the ventricles into the pulmonary and systemic circulatory systems?
6. What is the difference between cardiac output and stroke volume?

Analyze and Apply

7. What is the main difference between the function of the AV valves and that of the semilunar valves?
8. What does the name *chordae tendineae* tell you about the characteristics of these structures?
9. What have echocardiogram studies revealed about the different effects of exercise on the hearts of aerobic athletes (runners, for example) and anaerobic athletes (weight lifters)?
10. Calculate cardiac output for a person with a heart rate of 40 beats/min and a stroke volume of 93 mL/beat.
11. In your own words, explain why a baby has a higher heart rate than an adult.

IN THE LAB

12. Create a hemisectional diagram of the heart (imagine cutting from top of right atrium to bottom of left ventricle). Label the three layers and the following structures: chambers, valves, septums, major blood vessels, and pericardium.
13. Starting with the inferior and superior venae cavae, trace the pathway of the blood through the heart diagram.
14. With a partner, make flash cards of important terminology from this lesson. After the cards are made, have flash card races with your classmates to see who can match up the cards in the fastest time. Use these terms for your flash cards: vasodilation, vasoconstriction, interatrial septum, interventricular septum, tricuspid valve, mitral valve, pulmonary valve, aortic valve, pericardium, epicardium, myocardium, endocardium, diastole, systole.

LESSON 11.2 Regulation of the Heart

Before You Read

Try to answer the following questions before you read this lesson.

- What is the internal (intrinsic) mechanism that allows the heart to beat on its own?
- What are the two external (extrinsic) systems that regulate the heart?

Lesson Objectives

- Describe the mechanisms that regulate the heart.
- Identify the components of the conduction system of the heart.

Key Terms

atrioventricular (AV) node	Purkinje fibers
baroreceptors	repolarize
bundle of His	right bundle branch
depolarize	sinoatrial (SA) node
left bundle branch	

Several mechanisms combine to cause the heart to beat and to control its function. An entire system—the conduction system—ensures that the heart cells contract in the right sequence.

Internal and External Control of the Heart

The heart is regulated by three different mechanisms. One is inside the heart; the other two are outside of the heart.

Internal Control

When a heart is transplanted from one individual to another, it will still beat on its own. How is this possible? The heart continues to beat on its own because of a very important internal control mechanism called a *pacemaker*. The heart's primary pacemaker is the **sinoatrial** (sigh-noh-AY-tree-al) **node**, or SA node. The SA node is located at the top of the right atrium, slightly lateral and inferior to the opening of the superior vena cava (**Figure 11.6** and **Figure 11.7**). The SA node sends out an electrical impulse that tells the heart to beat at a rate between 60 and 100 bpm.

External Control

The heart is also regulated by two external mechanisms. One is the cardiac center located in the medulla oblongata of the brain. The other is the endocrine system.

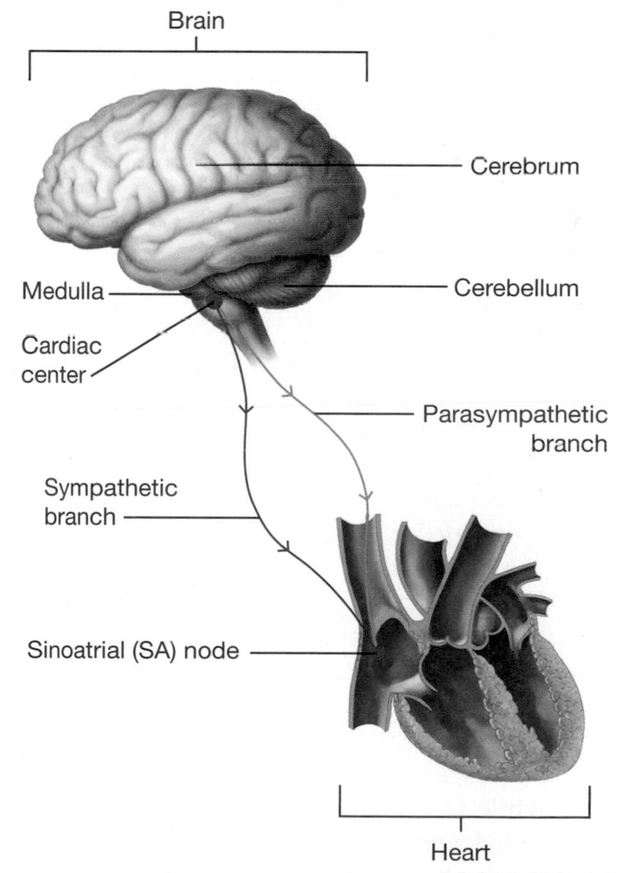

Figure 11.6 Location of the cardiac center in the medulla of the brain. *What type of stimulation—sympathetic or parasympathetic—causes the heart rate to increase?*

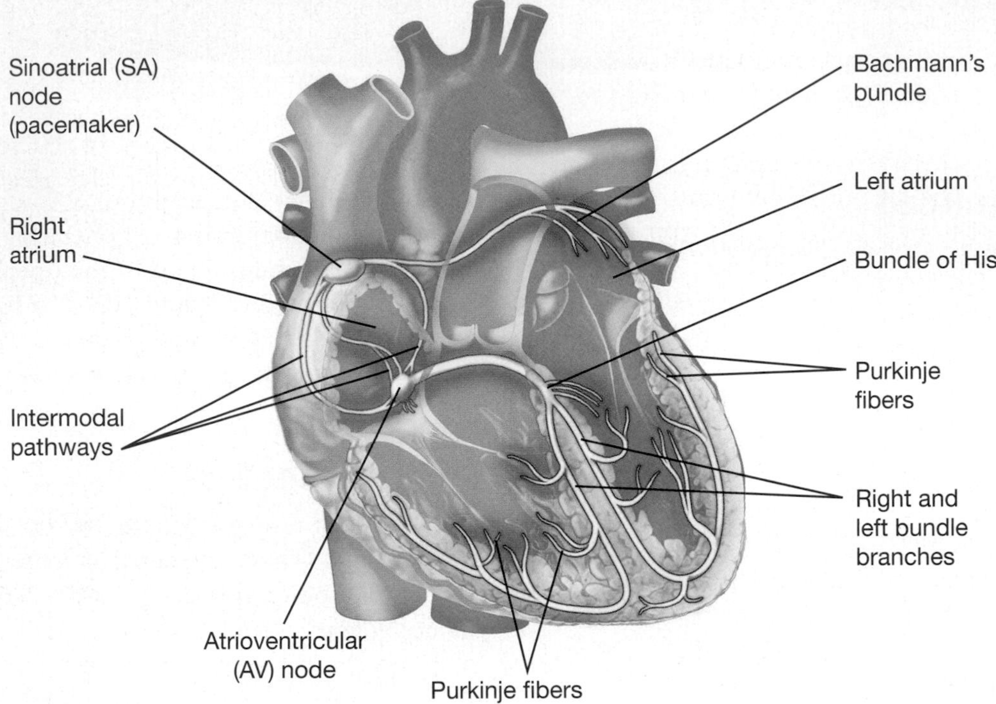

Figure 11.7 Conduction system of the heart. *Describe the pathway of an electrical impulse generated by the SA node.*

The Cardiac Center

The cardiac center has sympathetic and parasympathetic branches, which are collectively referred to as the *autonomic nervous system*. (For a discussion of the autonomic nervous system, see Chapter 6.) The cardiac center continuously makes adjustments in heart rate, contraction strength, and stroke volume. It gives the heart a "green light" (sympathetic stimulation) when it wants the heart rate to increase, or a "red light" (parasympathetic stimulation) when the heart rate needs to slow down.

Baroreceptors (BAIR-oh-ree-sep-terz) that are sensitive to pressure are located in the atrium of the heart, aortic arch, and carotid arteries. The baroreceptors constantly monitor blood pressure and send sensory information back to the cardiac center, stimulating either the parasympathetic or the sympathetic branch.

The parasympathetic branch is the dominant branch while you are at rest, which is why your heart rate is lower at rest than when you are active. As necessary, the parasympathetic branch releases acetylcholine, which decreases heart rate.

The cardiac center is also affected by emotions and physical activity. The sympathetic branch takes over during exercise and when you are emotionally stressed.

MEMORY TIP

Barometers measure the atmospheric pressure. Baroreceptors measure blood pressure.

Chapters 6 and 8 described the characteristics of the fight-or-flight response. When faced with a dangerous situation, the body has to prepare itself to fight or run from the danger at hand. In such a situation, a set of brain structures called the *limbic system* stimulates the sympathetic branch in the cardiac center. The sympathetic nerve fibers stimulate the SA node to fire faster, which causes the heart rate to increase.

The Endocrine System

The endocrine system is composed of glands that secrete hormones, which can cause many changes within the body. The adrenal medulla and the thyroid glands, for example, can affect the cardiovascular system. When the adrenal medulla secretes epinephrine (ehp-i-NEHF-rin) and norepinephrine (nor-ehp-i-NEHF-rin), heart rate increases. Similarly, when the thyroid gland releases thyroxine (thigh-RAHK-seen), heart rate increases.

Check Your Understanding

1. What three mechanisms regulate the heart?
2. Which structure is the primary pacemaker of the heart?
3. Which part of the nervous system signals the heart to increase the number of beats per minute?
4. Name three hormones released by the endocrine system that affect heart rate.

The Conduction System

Conduction is the process of conveying or transmitting types of energy, such as electrical impulses. The conduction system in the heart transmits signals that control both heart rate and contraction strength of the muscle tissues.

The conduction system of the heart includes two areas of nodal tissue and a network of conduction fibers. These structures allow the electrical impulses formed by the SA node to travel to the ventricles, telling the ventricles to contract (**Figure 11.7**).

Once the SA node fires, the electrical impulse is carried to the left atrium via Bachmann's bundle. The impulse also goes to the **atrioventricular node**, or AV node, via three internodal pathways. The AV node is a very dense network of fibers, which causes the electrical impulse to get "tied up," or delayed there, for approximately a tenth of a second.

Once the electrical impulse leaves the AV node, it is carried through conducting fibers called the **bundle of His**, or the atrioventricular bundle, in the ventricular septum. The bundle of His then divides, and the electrical impulse travels down the **left bundle branch** and the **right bundle branch** to millions of **Purkinje fibers** in both ventricles. When the Purkinje fibers receive the impulse, they stimulate the ventricles to contract.

The *electrocardiogram* (ee-lehk-troh-KAHR-dee-oh-gram), known as an *ECG* or *EKG*, is a recording of the electrical activity of the heart (**Figure 11.8** and **Figure 11.9**). In a sense, an ECG speaks the language of the heart. It illustrates what is happening electrically in the conduction system and mechanically in the atria and ventricles when they **depolarize** (contract) and **repolarize** (relax).

Check Your Understanding

1. What role does the AV node play in the conduction system of the heart?
2. Which structures carry electrical impulses from the common bundle to the individual Purkinje fibers, causing the ventricles to contract?
3. What does ECG stand for, and what is it used for?

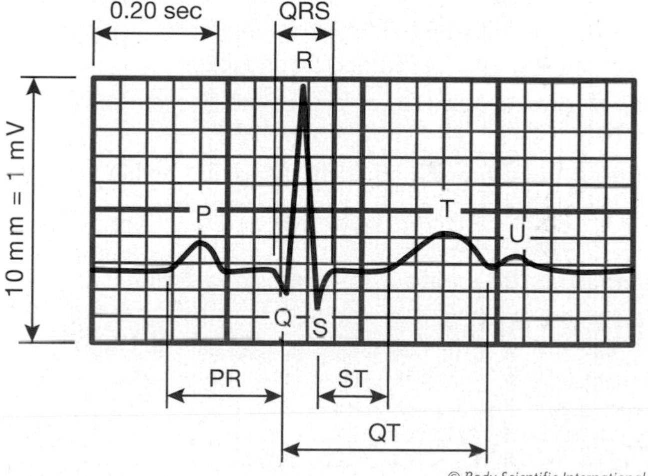

© Body Scientific International

Figure 11.8 An ECG is a piece of graph paper containing a record of the electrical events in the heart. The placement of the electrodes on the body surface affects the size and shape of the waves recorded. This example shows a normal ECG.

Electrical and Mechanical Events on an ECG Tracing

ECG Recording	Electrical Event	Mechanical Event
P wave	SA node fires and depolarization occurs	atrial contraction
QRS complex	impulse travels to Purkinje fibers and ventricular depolarization occurs	ventricular contraction
T wave	ventricular repolarization occurs	ventricular relaxation
U wave (not always seen)	repolarization of the bundle of His and Purkinje fibers	relaxation of the bundle of His and Purkinje fibers

Figure 11.9

Goodheart-Willcox Publisher

LESSON 11.2 Review and Assessment

Mini Glossary

Make sure that you know the meaning of each key term.

atrioventricular (AV) node a small mass of tissue that transmits impulses received from the sinoatrial node to the ventricles via the bundle of His

baroreceptors pressure-sensitive nerve endings in the atrium, aortic arch, and carotid arteries

bundle of His a slender bundle of modified cardiac muscle that conducts electrical impulses from the AV node to the left and right bundle branches to Purkinje fibers in the ventricle

depolarize to contract; the atria and ventricles depolarize as the heart beats

left bundle branch the left branch arising from the bundle of His, through which electrical impulses are transmitted through the left ventricle

Purkinje fibers part of the impulse-conducting network of the heart that rapidly transmits impulses throughout the ventricles, causing ventricular contraction

repolarize to relax; the atria and ventricles repolarize as the heart beats

right bundle branch the right branch arising from the bundle of His, through which electrical impulses are transmitted through the right ventricle

sinoatrial (SA) node a small mass of specialized tissue located in the right atrium that normally acts as the pacemaker of the heart, causing it to beat at a rate between 60 and 100 bpm

Know and Understand

1. What do baroreceptors monitor and where do they send messages?
2. Which two components of the endocrine system release hormones that affect heart rate?
3. Where are the Purkinje fibers located?
4. List in order the structures through which an electrical impulse travels on its way to the muscle fibers of the heart's ventricles.

Analyze and Apply

5. How does the nervous system help to regulate heart rate?
6. What happens to an electrical impulse when it reaches the AV node in the conduction system of a normally functioning heart?
7. At what point in the conduction of an electrical impulse through the heart do the atria contract?

IN THE LAB

8. While sitting at your desk, take your heart rate at your carotid artery/pulse and record it. (You may want to refer to the information on taking a pulse later in this chapter.) Now run in place for 45 to 60 seconds. Take and record your heart rate again. Sit down and wait two minutes before taking and recording your heart rate again. Did your resting heart rate qualify as bradycardia? Did your exercising heart rate qualify as tachycardia? What happened to your heart rate after you sat down for two minutes? Explain the role of the sympathetic and parasympathetic nervous systems during this experiment. Share your answers with your lab group.

   Using the data that you and your lab partners collected, your own experimental testing, your observations, and logical reasoning, analyze and evaluate the explanations given by your partners. Identify potential sources of bias in your own and your partners' explanations. If you find any sources of bias, discuss as a group how your conclusions could be restated to avoid bias.
9. Make a poster depicting the development of the heart starting right after conception. Be specific about how and when the heart starts to form and how it changes structurally and functionally during its development up until birth. Include pictures on your poster to illustrate the changes.
10. Create a flowchart showing the normal electrical pathway through the heart.

LESSON 11.3 Blood Vessels and Circulation

Before You Read

Try to answer the following questions before you read this lesson.

- What are the three types of blood vessels and the most important function of each?
- Why are capillaries well suited for gas exchange?

Lesson Objectives

- Identify the differences among the three types of blood vessels.
- Outline the flow of blood through the cardiopulmonary system.
- Demonstrate how to measure a person's vital signs.
- Explain how keeping track of your weight, blood pressure, and cholesterol levels can help you stay healthy.

Key Terms

aortic arch
arteries
arterioles
brachial artery
capillaries
capillary beds
cardiac circulation
carotid artery
coronary sinus
ductus arteriosus
fetal circulation
foramen ovale
hepatic portal circulation
precapillary sphincter
pulmonary circulation
radial artery
systemic circulation
tunica externa
tunica intima
tunica media
veins
venules
vital signs

The purpose of the cardiovascular system is to move blood throughout the body to deliver nutrients and pick up wastes for removal from the body. Although the heart is the primary organ in the cardiovascular system, other components are necessary to transport the blood. This lesson describes the network of blood vessels that carry blood throughout the body.

Blood Vessels: The Transport Network

Three types of blood vessels form a closed loop of tubes that carry blood from the heart to the rest of the body and back to the heart. These vessels are the **arteries**, **capillaries**, and **veins**. Two other important subdivisions of vessels are the **arterioles** (ar-TEER-ee-ohlz), or smaller arteries, and **venules** (VEN-yoolz), or smaller veins. **Figure 11.10** summarizes the structure and function of each of these types of blood vessels.

Blood Vessel Layers

All blood vessels, with the exception of capillaries, are composed of three layers that surround the blood-filled opening called the *lumen* (LOO-mehn). The **tunica intima** (TOO-ni-ka IN-ti-ma), the innermost layer, is composed of a single layer of squamous (flattened) epithelial cells over a sheet of connective tissue. The tunica intima provides a smooth, frictionless surface that allows blood to flow smoothly through the vessel (**Figure 11.11**).

Tunica media, the middle layer, is a thicker layer containing smooth muscle cells, elastic fibers, and collagen. The smooth muscle cells in this layer are directed by the sympathetic nervous system to *vasodilate* (increase the opening of the lumen) and *vasoconstrict* (decrease its opening). This process allows blood flow to be increased to certain tissues and decreased to other tissues as needed.

Vasodilation and vasoconstriction of the vessels also play a major role in regulating and determining blood pressure. When a vessel dilates, blood pressure becomes lower; when the vessel constricts, blood pressure increases.

The **tunica externa**, the outermost layer of a blood vessel, is composed mostly of fibrous connective tissue. The purpose of the tunica externa is to support and protect the blood vessel.

Structure and Function of Vessels		
Vessel Type	**Structure**	**Function**
Artery*	three-layered vessel (intima, media, adventitia), thick, elastic, muscular walls	transports oxygen-rich blood away from heart to arterioles; influenced by the sympathetic nervous system (contraction/dilation)
Arteriole	thinner, three-walled vessel, mostly smooth muscle cells	transports blood from arteries to capillaries; greater impact by the sympathetic nervous system; acts to direct blood flow in the body
Capillary	single layer of epithelial cells	gas/nutrient and waste-product exchange between blood and tissues
Venule	thin-walled vessels bundled together to form a vein	transports blood from capillary to vein
Vein	three-layered (intima, media externa), thin-walled vessel with one-way valves	transports oxygen-poor blood back to the heart

*Exception: Pulmonary arteries carry deoxygenated blood.

Figure 11.10

Goodheart-Willcox Publisher

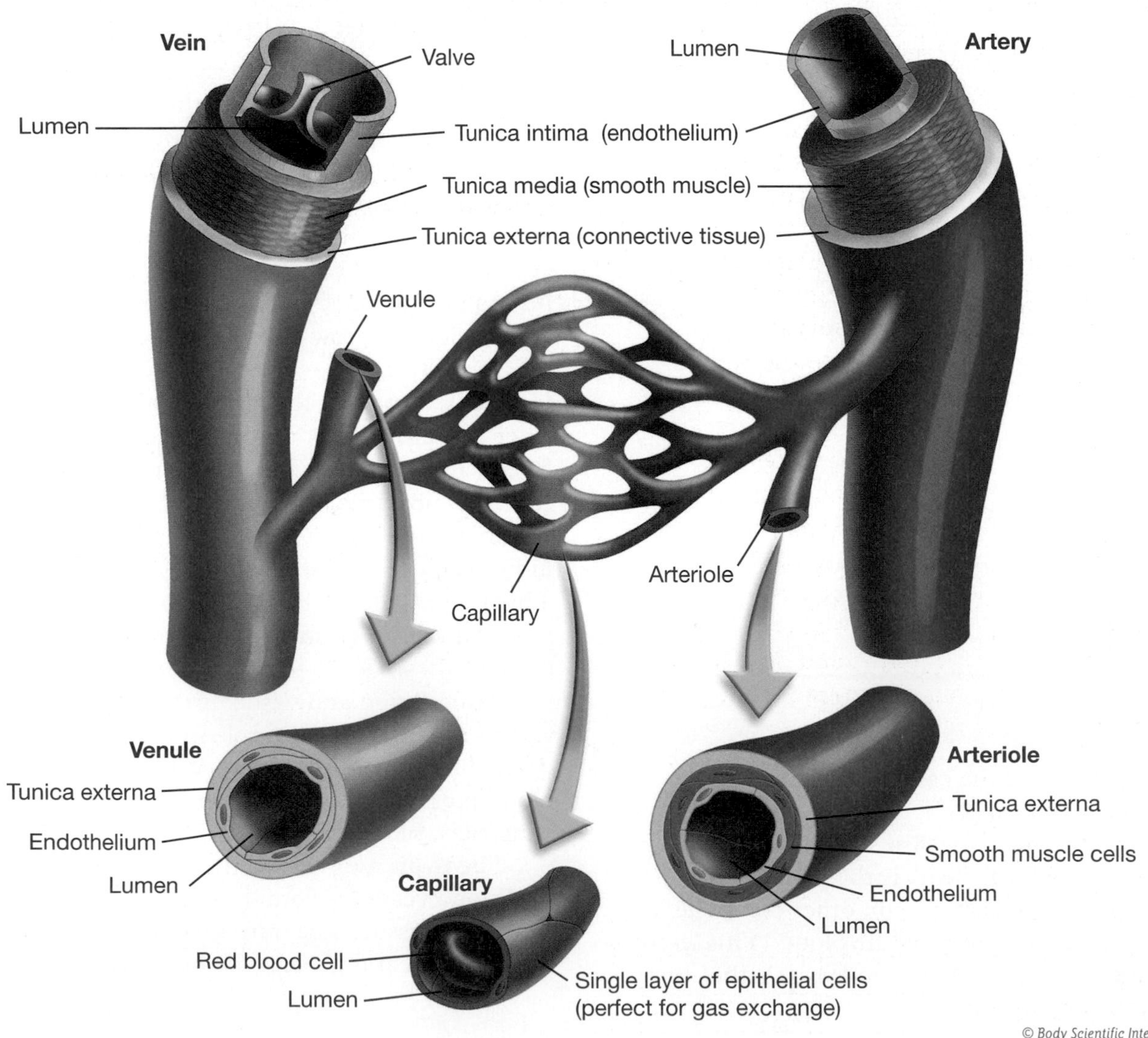

© Body Scientific International

Figure 11.11 Sizes and layers of different types of blood vessels. *What size differences do you notice between the arteries and veins?*

Differences between Arteries and Veins

Although arteries and veins both have three layers, the relative thickness and composition of the layers differ, as does the size of the lumen. These differences exist because the two vessels have very different functions in the cardiovascular system.

Figure 11.12 details the structural difference between arteries and veins. The arterial vessels carry blood away from the heart, so they must withstand large increases in pressure when the heart contracts. The aorta, the largest artery, leaves the heart and branches into progressively smaller arteries that eventually become arterioles (**Figure 11.13**). Arteries have the thickest, strongest, most elastic walls of all the blood vessels.

The venous system (system of veins) carries blood back to the heart. Unlike arteries, veins do not have to deal with large increases in pressure. Thus, the walls of the veins are thinner and less elastic than those of the arteries. In addition to carrying blood from the body cells back to the heart, the venous system acts as a reservoir, housing 65% of the blood in the body.

The blood enters the venules from the capillaries. The venules merge together to form progressively larger veins until they reach the largest veins, the inferior and superior venae cavae. These two veins empty into the right atrium of the heart.

The venous system can pump blood back to the heart because it has one-way valves that allow blood to flow only toward the heart. In addition, when the muscles that surround the veins contract, they "milk" the blood toward the heart (**Figure 11.14**). Venous return of blood is also assisted by the pump-like action of the respiratory system. Changes in abdominal and thoracic pressure that occur with breathing help to pump blood back to the heart.

Differences between Arteries and Veins		
Structures	**Arteries**	**Veins**
walls	strong, thick, elastic	thin, less elastic
pressure	high	low
lumen	small	large
valves	no	yes

Figure 11.12 Goodheart-Willcox Publisher

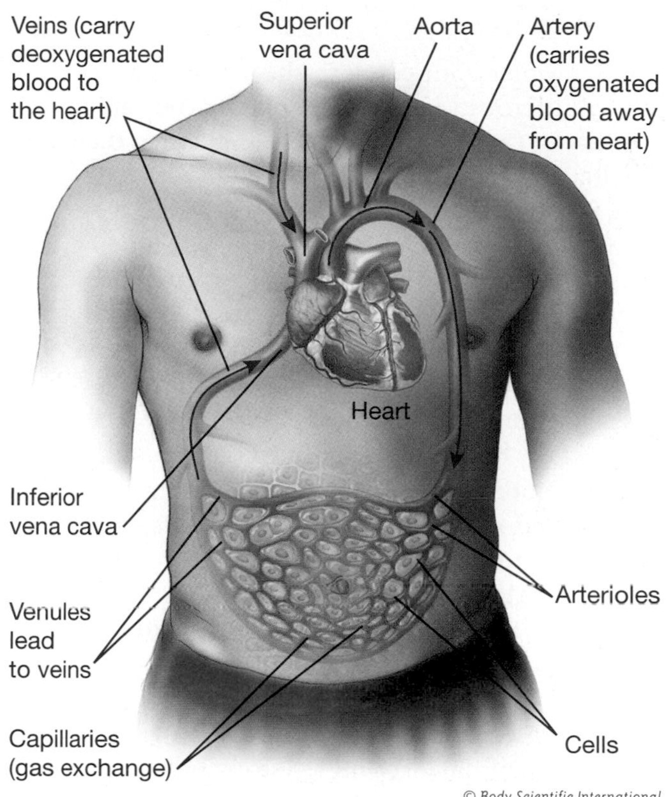

Figure 11.13 Network of blood vessels in the cardiovascular system.

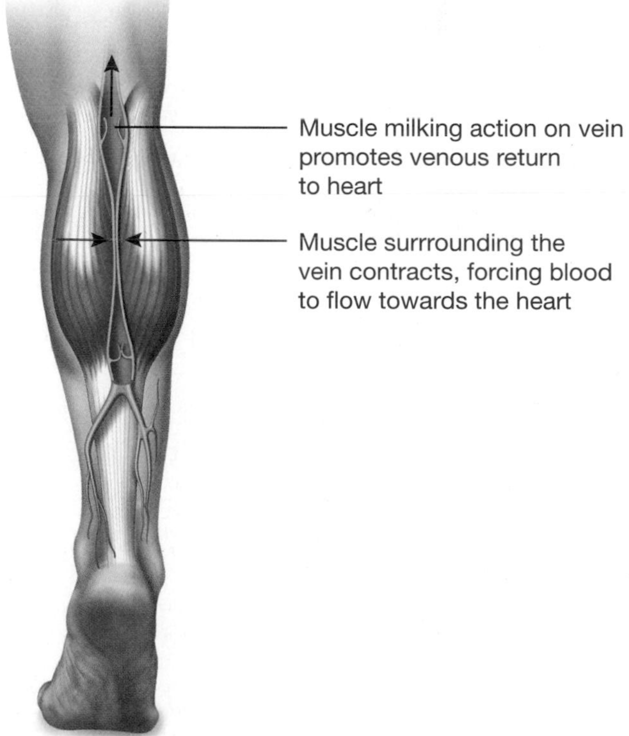

Figure 11.14 Muscle milking action. *Where is the muscle in relation to the vein on which it performs its milking action?*

Capillaries

Arterioles connect with the smallest and most numerous vessels in the body—the capillaries. Capillaries range in size from 0.0025 cm to 0.25 cm. Capillaries are so narrow that red blood cells must pass through them in a single line, one at a time.

Capillaries are called *exchange vessels* because oxygen and carbon dioxide gas exchange occurs between the capillaries and the tissues. Capillaries in the kidneys, liver, small intestines, and endocrine glands also have microscopic pores that allow the passage of small molecules. For instance, these pores allow hormones to pass into the bloodstream when the pores come in contact with endocrine glands, and they allow white blood cells to pass into tissue to kill harmful bacteria.

Blood flow through the capillaries is controlled by a **precapillary sphincter** (pree-KAP-i-lair-ee SFINGK-ter), a band of smooth muscle fibers that encircles the capillaries at the arteriole-capillary junctions. Contraction of the precapillary sphincter stops blood flow to the capillary; relaxation increases blood flow. Contraction or relaxation of the precapillary sphincter is based on the local conditions (pH, oxygen, carbon dioxide, temperature) in the tissue. For instance, approximately 15% of blood flow goes to your muscles at rest. During exercise, however, when the metabolic needs of the muscles dramatically increase, approximately 85% of blood flow goes to the working muscles.

Capillaries do not operate separately; they form an expansive network of intertwined vessels called **capillary beds**. Blood begins its journey back to the heart when the capillaries merge with venules. The venules then merge with larger, thicker-walled veins that eventually lead back to the heart.

Check Your Understanding

1. All blood vessels, with the exception of capillaries, consist of what three layers?
2. What type of vessel connects arteries with capillaries?
3. What types of vessels carry blood back to the heart?
4. Why are capillaries called *exchange vessels*?

Circulation: Moving Blood around the Body

The circulatory system is an extensive network of blood vessels that stretches 60,000 miles within the body. To gain a better understanding of this vast network, this section breaks it down into manageable parts.

Pulmonary Circulation

As explained earlier in the chapter, the right side of the heart pumps oxygen-poor blood to the lungs (**pulmonary circulation**), and the left side of the heart pumps oxygen-rich blood to the rest of the body (**systemic circulation**) (**Figure 11.15**). This section first explores the pulmonary system. Note that this information builds on information provided earlier in the chapter.

1. Deoxygenated blood enters the right atrium from the inferior and superior venae cavae.
2. Deoxygenated blood flows through the tricuspid valve into the right ventricle.
3. The right ventricle contracts, and deoxygenated blood is ejected through the pulmonary valve into the pulmonary artery.
4. The pulmonary artery splits into smaller arteries, which carry the deoxygenated blood to the lungs.
5. The two smaller pulmonary arteries branch into arterioles that merge with the capillary network in the lungs.
6. The blood becomes oxygenated in the lungs and then flows through the venules, which merge with the four pulmonary veins that carry the oxygenated blood back to the heart.
7. The pulmonary veins empty oxygenated blood into the left atrium.

Systemic Circulation

The systemic circulatory system refers to the closed-loop network of arteries, arterioles, capillaries, venules, and veins that circulate oxygen, hormones, water, and other nutrients to tissues and then carries carbon dioxide and waste products back to the heart. This section traces the journey of a red blood cell through systemic circulation. Keep in mind that it has 60,000 miles to go!

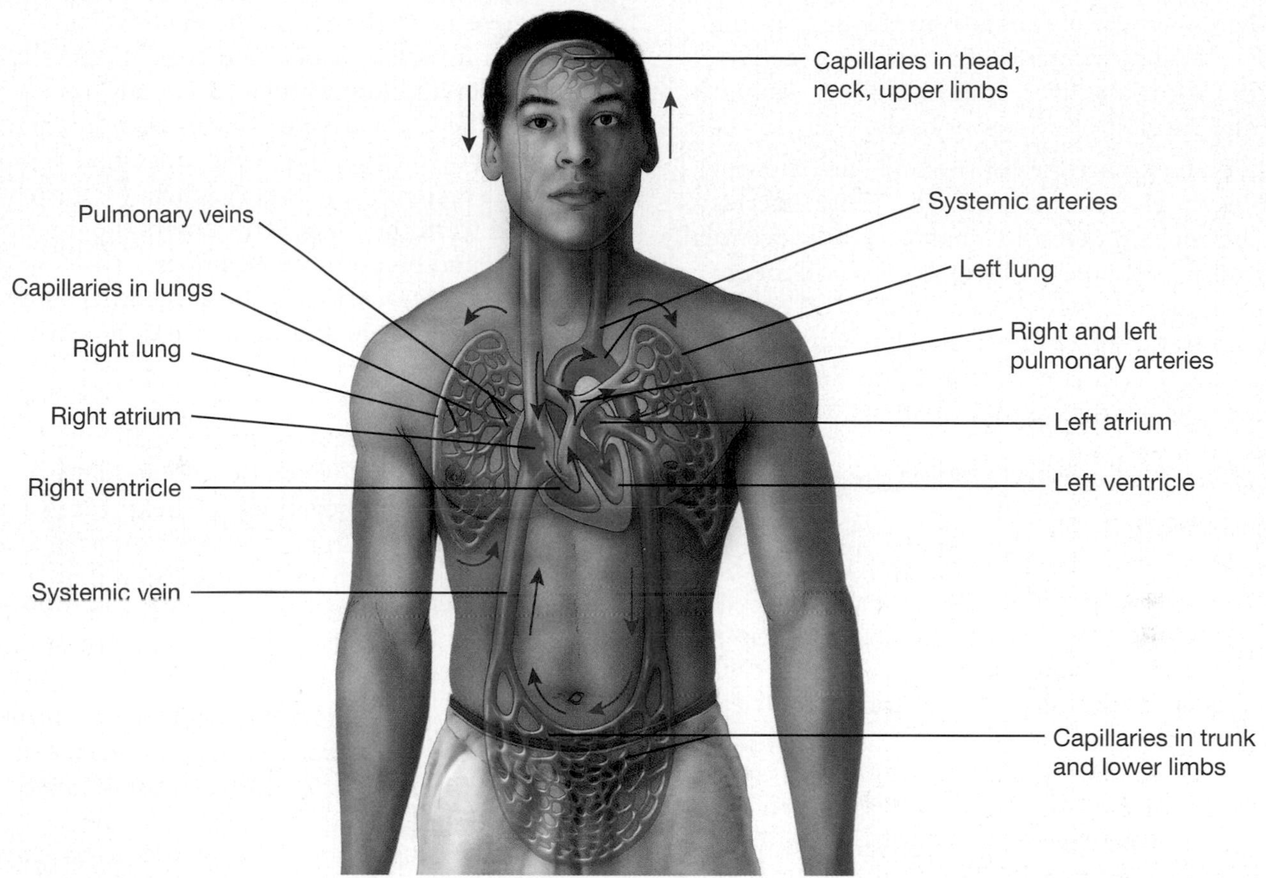

Figure 11.15 The heart pumps blood through two major circuits: the pulmonary circuit and the systemic circuit. The right side of the heart pumps blood to the lungs (pulmonary circulation), and the left side of the heart pumps blood throughout the body (systemic circulation). *Is the blood entering the lungs in the pulmonary circuit oxygen rich or oxygen poor? Is the blood pumped from the left side of the heart to the rest of the body in the systemic circuit oxygen rich or oxygen poor?*

The journey begins when the left ventricle pumps blood through the aorta, the largest artery in the body. The ascending branch of the aorta rises up from the heart, arches to the left (thus the term **aortic arch**), and then proceeds downward through the descending aorta into the thorax along the spine, through the diaphragm, and into the abdomen. Once this vessel reaches the abdomen, it is called the *abdominal aorta*.

Many other arteries arise from the aorta:

- The right and left coronary arteries branch from the ascending aorta and supply the heart with blood.
- The brachiocephalic (bray-kee-oh-seh-FAL-ik), left common carotid, and left subclavian (sub-KLAY-vee-an) arteries branch from the aortic arch to supply the head, neck, and arms with blood. These arteries subdivide into many more arteries. **Figure 11.16** illustrates the arteries that arise from the aorta.

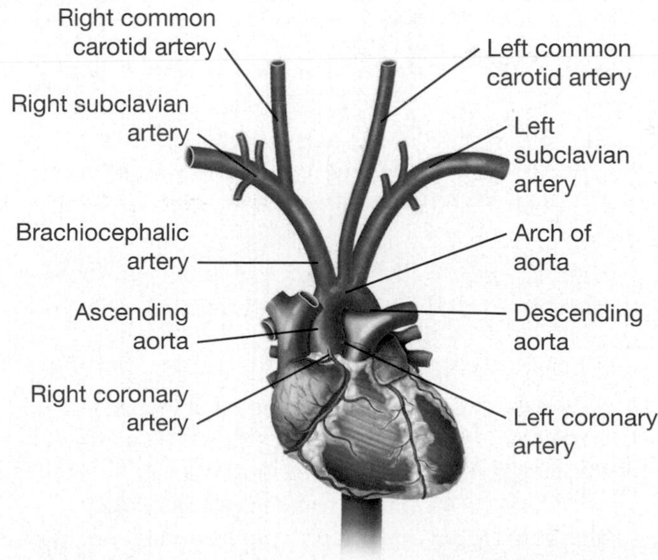

Figure 11.16 Arteries arising from the aorta. *To which areas of the body will these arteries supply blood? Which of the arteries labeled in this drawing is the major artery supplying blood to the lower limbs?*

- Many arteries branch from the descending aorta, supplying blood to various organs including the liver, spleen, kidneys, stomach, and the rest of the lower body.

The major arteries of the body are shown in **Figure 11.17**. As you can see, these arteries branch into smaller and smaller vessels, eventually becoming arterioles. The arterioles will merge with capillaries, where tissue and blood exchange nutrients and waste materials. The journey back to the heart begins with blood draining into the venules, which merge to form veins.

MEMORY TIP

Keep in mind that the names of the arteries and veins often refer to the organ or location that they supply with blood. For example, the *femoral* artery supplies blood to the femoral region of the leg, and the *lumbar* artery supplies blood to the lumbar area of the back.

Figure 11.18 illustrates the major veins that drain from the head and the trunk, as well as the upper and lower limbs. Generally, the names of the veins are the same as their arterial counterparts (for example, *renal artery* and *renal vein*). The systemic circulatory journey ends when the blood from the lower veins enters the inferior vena cava and blood from the upper veins empties into the superior vena cava. Both the inferior and superior venae cavae drain into the right atrium.

Cardiac Circulation

You have read that oxygen is supplied to the body by the arteries, which carry blood away from the heart. But how does the heart receive its oxygen supply?

Perhaps you thought that the blood that circulates through the chambers of the heart provides the oxygen for the heart, but it does not. The oxygen-rich blood that nourishes the heart is supplied by the right and left coronary arteries that lie on the epicardial (outermost) surface of the heart (**Figure 11.19**). This system is called **cardiac circulation**.

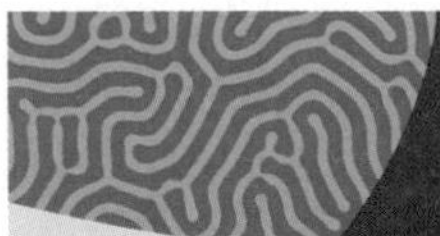

What Research Tells Us

...about Why Records Are Not Broken on Hot, Humid Days

Marathoners will not soon forget the environmental conditions at the 2012 Boston Marathon: direct sunlight, temperatures in the mid-80s, and high humidity. This was a recipe for slow race times and heat-related mishaps! Geoffrey Mutai, the 2011 winner, dropped out with heat-related cramps at mile 18, and the 2012 winner was 10 minutes slower than Mutai's 2011 time. Why do you think this occurred?

Research indicates that exercise in a heated environment causes internal competition in the body for blood supply. As body temperature increases, a greater percentage of blood goes to the skin to cool the body. In addition, increased sweat rates cause blood volume to decrease. The result of these conditions is that less blood goes back to the heart. Less blood to the heart means that the stroke volume must decrease.

How does the heart react to a decrease in stroke volume? For sufficient cardiac output to be maintained, heart rate must increase. This means that the heart has to work harder, causing the body to use fuel more quickly. Over time performance declines.

What can be learned from this research? To minimize performance declines during severe heat conditions, keep hydrated by drinking plenty of plain water or water that contains a mixture of salt and carbohydrates (electrolytes).

Taking It Further

1. Research how the cardiovascular system reroutes blood through the body as body temperature increases. Describe your findings in a report.
2. Besides excessively warm temperatures, what other environmental factors can affect heart rate?
3. Use a heart-rate monitor to measure your heart rate at various times over several days. Note any patterns. For example, is your heart rate higher or lower in the morning than later in the day? Do you notice a relationship between your body temperature and heart rate?

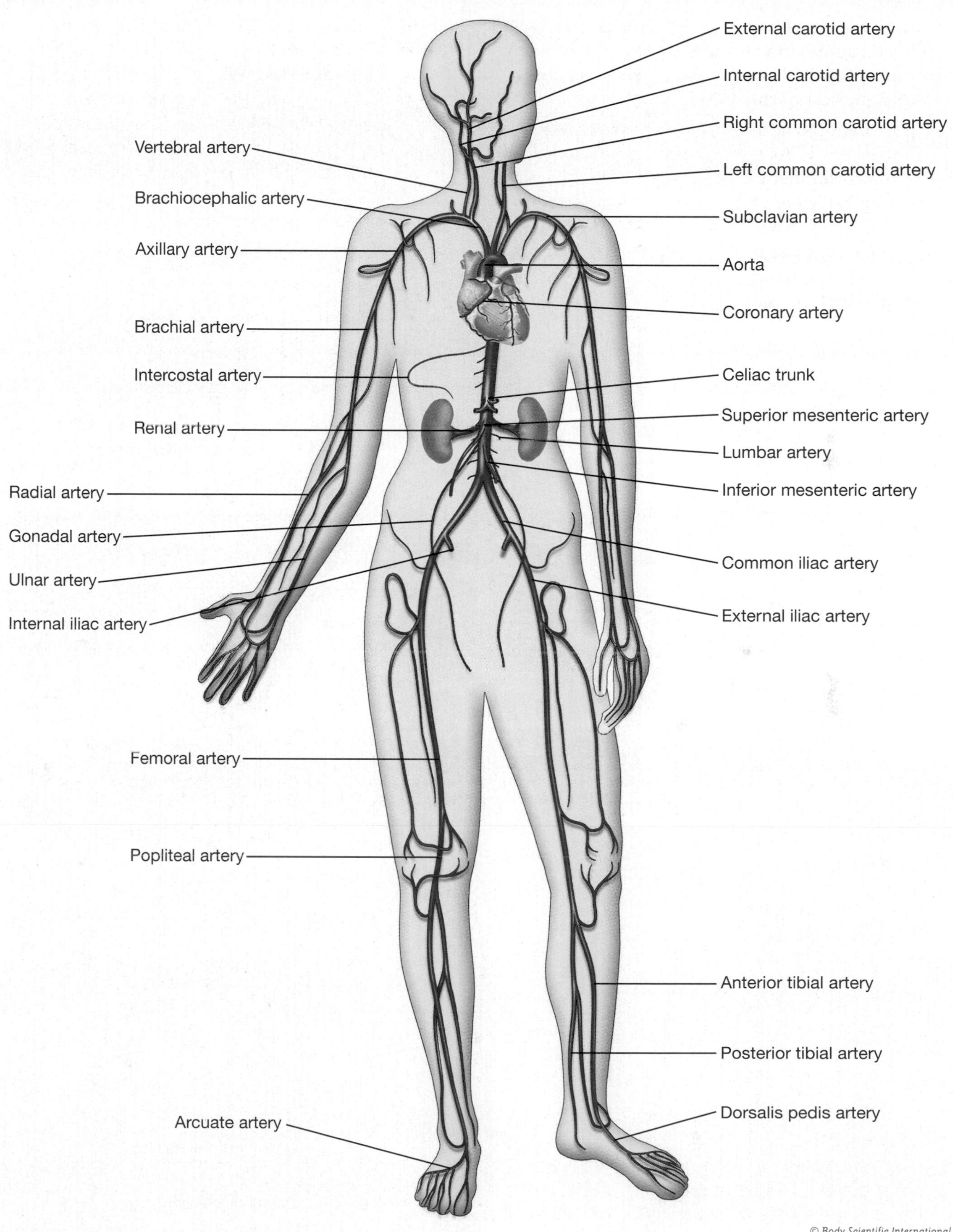
External carotid artery
Internal carotid artery
Right common carotid artery
Vertebral artery
Left common carotid artery
Brachiocephalic artery
Subclavian artery
Axillary artery
Aorta
Coronary artery
Brachial artery
Intercostal artery
Celiac trunk
Superior mesenteric artery
Renal artery
Lumbar artery
Inferior mesenteric artery
Radial artery
Gonadal artery
Common iliac artery
Ulnar artery
Internal iliac artery
External iliac artery
Femoral artery
Popliteal artery
Anterior tibial artery
Posterior tibial artery
Dorsalis pedis artery
Arcuate artery
© Body Scientific International

Figure 11.17 Major arteries of the body.

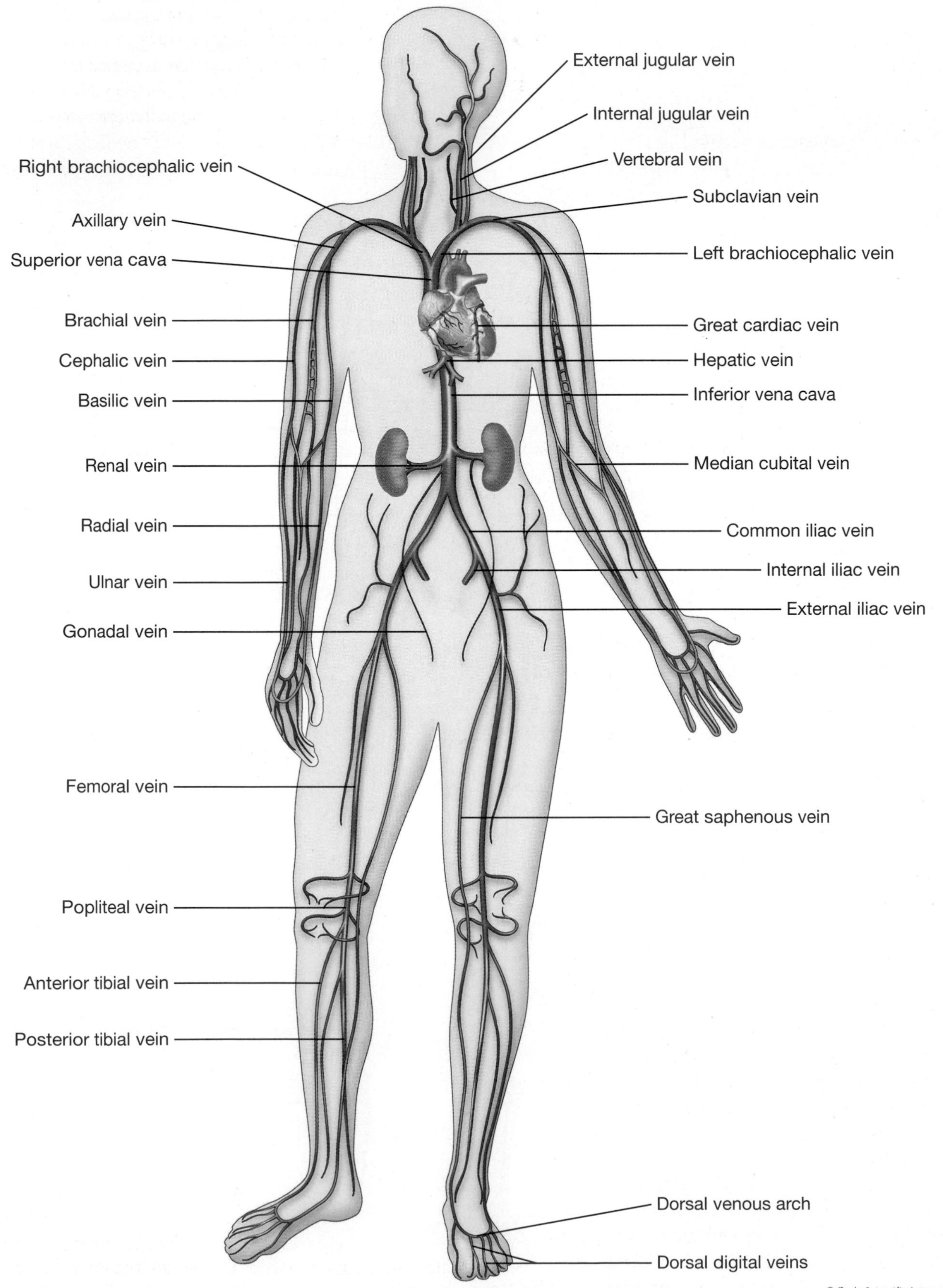

Figure 11.18 Major veins of the body. *Which two veins represent the end of the blood's journey through the body?*

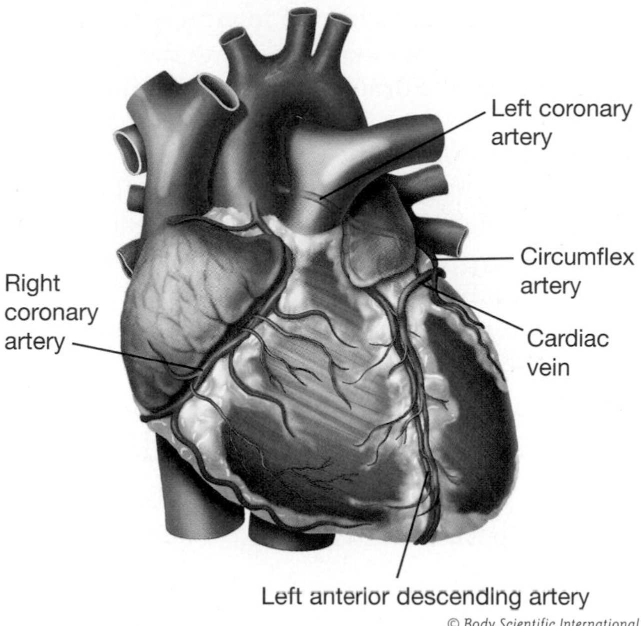

Figure 11.19 Anterior view of the coronary arteries.

The right coronary artery has two main branches, which supply blood to the inferior and posterior walls of the heart. The left main coronary artery divides into two arteries (the left anterior descending artery and the circumflex artery) that supply oxygen-rich blood to the anterior, lateral, and posterior walls of the heart.

The coronary arteries arise from the base of the aorta and fill when the ventricles are relaxed. The coronary arteries are closed when the ventricles contract, so they are protected from the high pressure that is generated during contraction. Blood from the coronary arteries empties into several cardiac veins, which drain into a large vessel called the **coronary sinus**, which is located on the posterior wall of the right atrium.

Hepatic Portal Circulation

In addition to blood, other nutrients, such as carbohydrates, fats, and proteins, are stored in or released into the bloodstream. Storage and circulation of these valuable nutrients is critical if you are to have the energy you need to perform your daily activities.

Hepatic portal circulation plays a vital role in maintaining proper carbohydrate, fat, and protein levels in the blood. The hepatic portal circulation system does something unusual. Whereas the arteries of the cardiovascular system deliver blood to different parts of the body, the veins of the hepatic portal circulation system supply the blood to the liver.

The veins that drain the stomach, spleen, pancreas, small intestine, and colon deliver blood to the liver through the hepatic portal vein (**Figure 11.20**). This blood is rich with nutrient sources from carbohydrates and fats. As the blood percolates through the liver, some of the nutrients are removed, stored, or repackaged for another use.

The best example is the fate of glucose. After a meal, the blood that drains into the liver may be high in glucose. The liver, which plays a role in regulating blood glucose levels, stores glucose as glycogen until a later date, when the body needs the glucose for energy. Suppose that a person is exercising and her blood glucose level starts to drop. As this happens, the liver breaks down its stored glycogen and releases it into the bloodstream as glucose, thereby maintaining blood glucose levels.

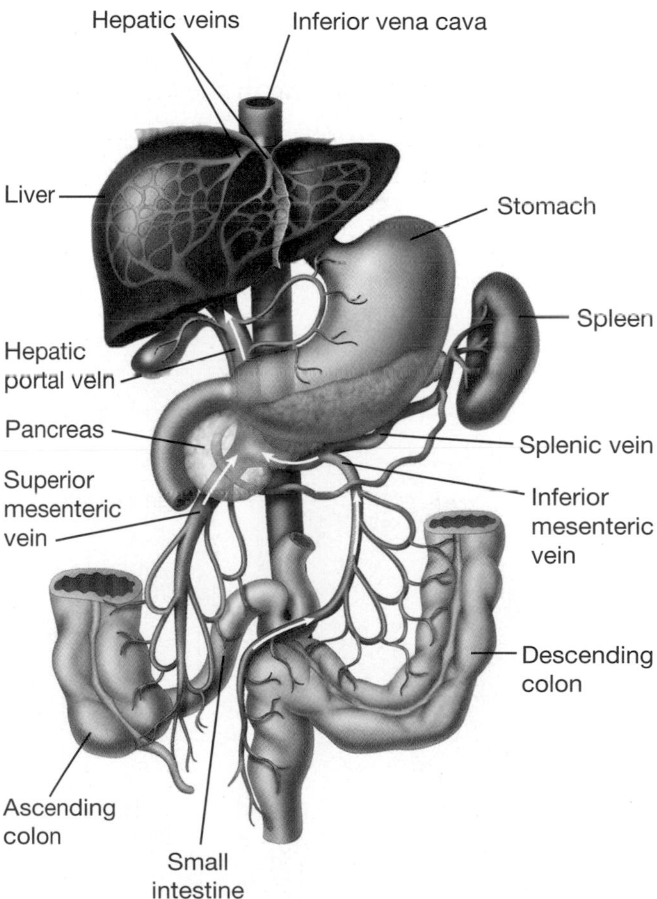

Figure 11.20 Hepatic portal circulation. Veins from the stomach, spleen, pancreas, small intestine, and colon drain into the hepatic portal vein. The liver filters the blood before the blood empties into the inferior vena cava. *What is the vital role of hepatic portal circulation?*

Once blood has been filtered by the liver, it returns to the inferior vena cava through the hepatic veins. Chapter 13 describes this process in greater detail.

Fetal Circulation

Fetal circulation is the process by which an unborn infant receives oxygen and nutrients and disposes of waste products. The infant receives oxygen and nutrients from the mother's blood through one large umbilical vein. The waste products are cleared through the two umbilical arteries in the placenta that pass through the umbilical cord to the fetus (**Figure 11.21**). This process is necessary because the lungs and digestive system of the fetus are underdeveloped and not yet functioning.

Most blood enters the fetus through the fetal ductus venosus vein, bypassing the liver and going directly to the right atrium by way of the inferior vena cava. Blood bypasses the right ventricle and is shunted (diverted) to the left atrium because of an opening in the septal wall, between the atria, called the **foramen ovale**. A small amount of blood does go to the right ventricle, but it is drained through the **ductus arteriosus**, a vessel that connects the pulmonary artery to the aorta.

Once the blood is pumped from the left ventricle, the oxygenated blood flows through the fetus's body. Deoxygenated blood returns to the placenta via the umbilical arteries. Shortly after birth, the ductus arteriosus and ductus venosus close, as does the foramen ovale.

Check Your Understanding

1. Is the blood in the pulmonary veins oxygenated or deoxygenated? Explain your answer.
2. Which arteries arise from the ascending aorta?
3. Where are the coronary arteries located in the heart?
4. What is the role of hepatic portal circulation?
5. Which blood vessel delivers blood to the liver?

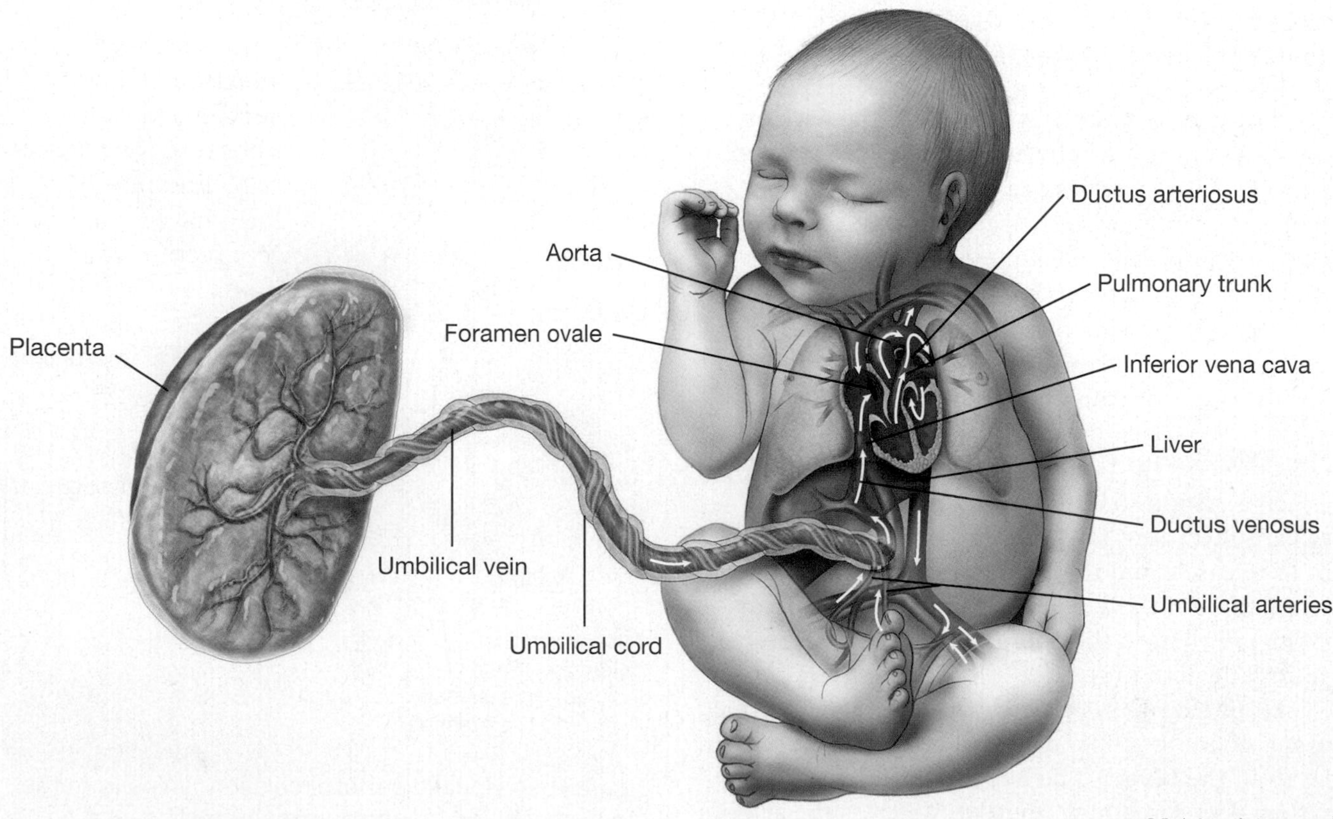

Figure 11.21 Fetal circulation in a full-term fetus (before birth). *Describe how blood flows into and through the fetal heart during the development of the fetus. How does this process change after the baby is born?*

Measuring Vital Signs

For those who are interested in—and proactive about—their health, pulse monitoring and blood pressure measurement are important skills to acquire. These skills are even more important for students who are interested in pursuing a healthcare career.

Have you ever checked your pulse? Pulse monitoring is essential if you want to ensure that you are exercising at an intensity level that will improve your cardiovascular fitness. Blood pressure measurement is another simple procedure that can provide lifesaving information about your physical condition. In certain circumstances, you may also want to monitor your breathing rate (respirations) and temperature. Pulse, blood pressure, respiration, and body temperature measurements are commonly referred to as **vital signs**.

Checking Your Pulse

Pulse is a rhythmic, throbbing sensation that can be felt when the heart contracts and blood is forced through the arteries. To measure your pulse, use your index and third fingertips to apply light pressure to any point where an artery comes close to your skin. Count the number of beats for 15 seconds and multiply that number by 4. The most common anatomic locations for measuring your pulse are as follows:

- **Radial artery:** With your palm facing upward, feel for your pulse on the thumb side of your wrist (**Figure 11.22A**).
- **Carotid artery:** On the side of your neck, feel for your pulse to the right of your trachea, or windpipe (**Figure 11.22B**).
- **Brachial artery:** At the fold of your elbow, feel for your pulse along the inner portion of your arm.

MEMORY TIP

What makes your body healthy?

Your body **MENDS** itself with the right lifestyle!

Make sure that your weight, blood pressure, cholesterol, and glucose are normal.

Exercise most days for 30 minutes at a moderate intensity level.

No smoking or use of tobacco products.

Diet should be rich in fruits and vegetables and low in saturated fat and sodium.

Stress less, laugh more. Recent research shows that laughter may lower disease risk!

Measuring Body Temperature

Normal body temperature ranges from 97.8 to 99°F (36.5 to 37.2°C) for a healthy adult. Today electronic, digital monitors are recommended for use. The American College of Pediatrics does *not* recommend the use of glass mercurial thermometers because they can break, and mercury is poisonous. They are no longer being made, but if you still have a glass thermometer, dispose of it by contacting your

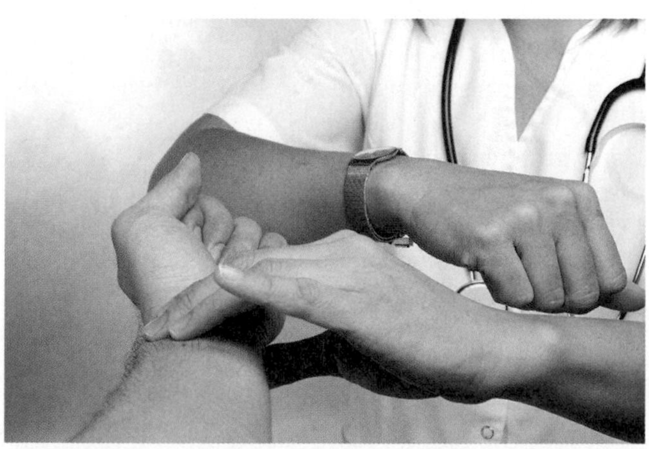

A

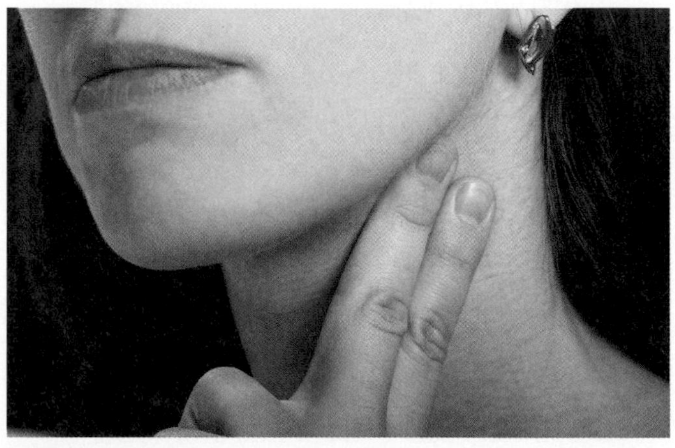

B

otherstock/Shutterstock.com, LeventeGyori/Shutterstock.com

Figure 11.22 Measuring pulse. A—Radial artery. B—Carotid artery. *What are other sites on the body where pulse can be measured?*

local health department, fire department, or waste disposal authority. Listed below are the recommended ways to measure body temperature.

- **Oral:** Insert a digital thermometer probe, covered with a disposable plastic sheath, under the tongue. Close the mouth and breathe through the nose. Leave the probe in the mouth until the device beeps. Read the temperature displayed on the thermometer's screen.
- **Rectal:** This method is typically used for infants and small children. Make sure to clean the probe thoroughly, then insert it in a disposable plastic sheath. Place a small amount of petroleum jelly on the tip of the probe. Place the child face down on a flat surface or on your lap. Spread the buttocks and insert the probe about 0.5 to 1 inch (1 to 2.5 cm) into the anal canal. *Do not insert the probe any farther than this.* Also try to prevent the child from struggling, because struggling can push the probe in farther. Remove the probe when the device beeps and read the display. A rectal temperature is 0.5°F (0.3°C) to 1°F (0.6°C) higher than an oral temperature.
- **Aural (through the ear):** Use a clean, disposable probe tip each time, and follow the manufacturer's instructions carefully. Gently tug on the ear, pulling it up and back to straighten the ear canal (**Figure 11.23**). Gently insert the thermometer until the ear canal is fully sealed off. Remove the thermometer and read the temperature when the probe beeps. An ear temperature is 0.5°F (0.3°C) to 1°F (0.6°C) higher than an oral temperature.
- **Axillary (in the armpit):** Place digital probe under the arm and press the arm against the body until the probe beeps. Research indicates that the axillary temp plus 1°C is a good indication of rectal temperature in infants older than one month. Read the temperature display. An axillary temperature is usually 0.5°F (0.3°C) to 1°F (0.6°C) lower than an oral temperature.

Measuring Respiration

Respiratory rate is the number of times a person inhales and exhales in one minute. Normal respiratory rates for healthy adults range from 12 to 20 breaths per minute at rest. The procedure for measuring respiratory rate is to count the number of times the chest rises in one minute with the person at rest. If the person's breathing rate seems regular, you can count the number of times the upper part of the chest rises in 30 seconds and multiply by 2. Other aspects of breathing to note are the rhythm (does inspiratory time equal expiratory time?), ease of breathing (labored or difficult) and strength of breathing (shallow vs. normal).

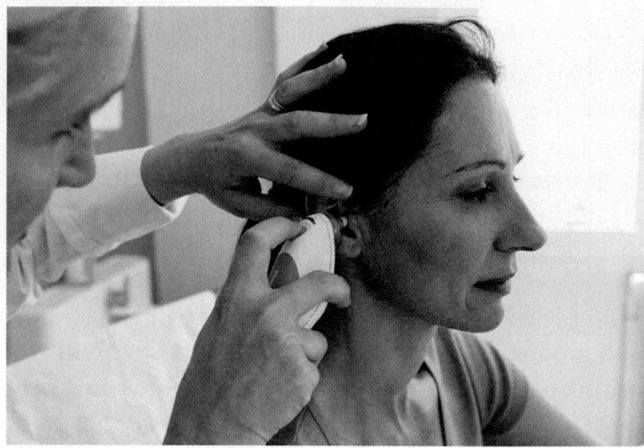

Image Point Fr/Shutterstock.com

Figure 11.23 In adults, pull the ear up and back to straighten the ear canal before inserting the ear probe. Always use a probe cover, and discard the cover when you are finished taking the patient's temperature.

Measuring Blood Pressure

Optimal blood pressure for an adult is 110/70 mmHg. Generally, lower blood pressure is not a problem, but it could cause you to become dizzy if you get up too quickly. Adults with blood pressure in excess of 140/90 mmHg should consult their physician.

Blood pressure is measured at the brachial artery using a stethoscope (STETH-oh-skohp) and a sphygmomanometer (sfig-moh-ma-NAHM-eh-ter), or blood pressure cuff. Inflating the cuff causes the brachial artery to collapse. As the cuff is deflated, the brachial artery gradually reopens, and you can hear the pulse, which creates a tapping sound. When the artery is completely open, the tapping sound disappears. Following are the steps for measuring blood pressure (**Figure 11.24**):

- Place the blood pressure cuff around the arm, with the arrow on the cuff pointed toward the brachial artery. Place the cuff approximately the distance of two fingertips above the fold in the elbow.

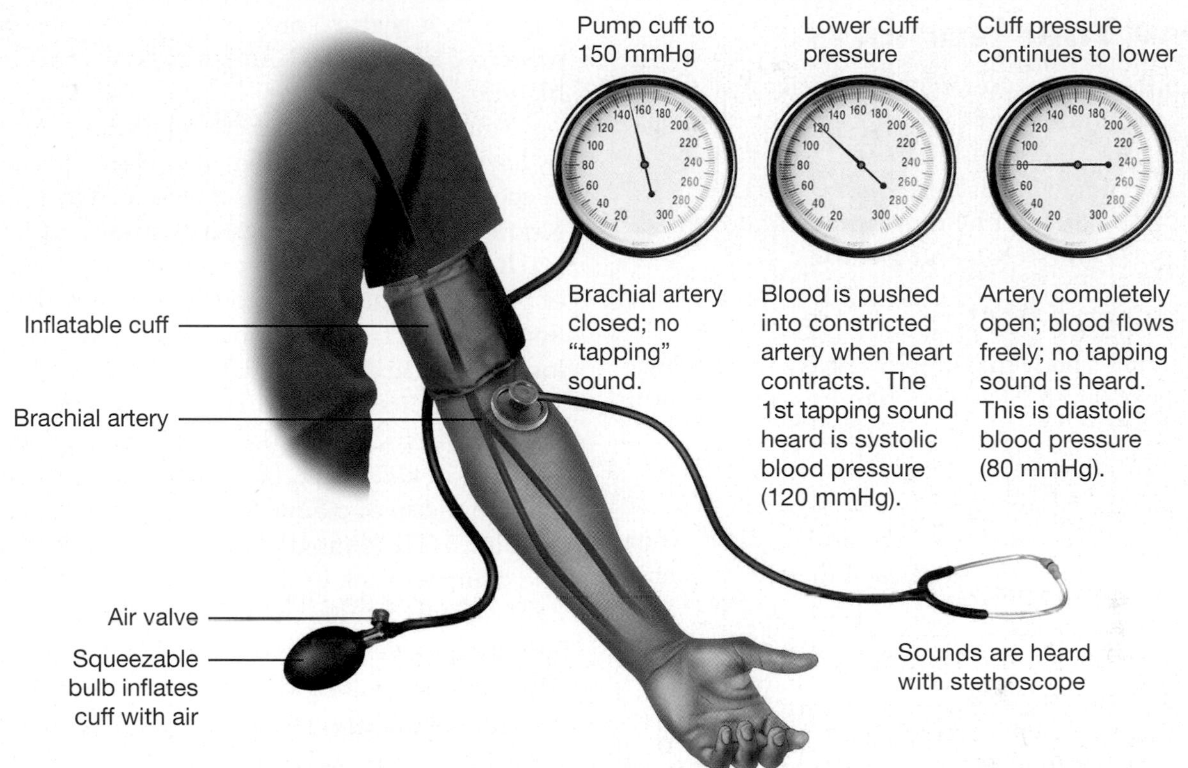
Pump cuff to
150 mmHg
Lower cuff
pressure
Cuff pressure
continues to lower
Brachial artery
closed; no
"tapping"
sound.
Blood is pushed
into constricted
artery when heart
contracts. The
1st tapping sound
heard is systolic
blood pressure
(120 mmHg).
Artery completely
open; blood flows
freely; no tapping
sound is heard.
This is diastolic
blood pressure
(80 mmHg).
Inflatable cuff
Brachial artery
Air valve
Squeezable
bulb inflates
cuff with air
Sounds are heard
with stethoscope

Figure 11.24 Blood pressure measurement. *Explain the difference between systolic and diastolic blood pressure measurements.*

- Insert the stethoscope's earpieces in your ears and make sure that your stethoscope is in the "on" position by gently tapping the diaphragm of the chest piece.
- Place the head of the stethoscope over the brachial artery.
- Squeeze the bulb of the sphygmomanometer repeatedly while listening for a "tapping" sound.
- Continue to pump up the cuff 30 millimeters of mercury (mmHg) more after the "tapping" sound stops. This would be approximately 150 mmHg for someone with a normal blood pressure of 120/80 mmHg (**Figure 11.25**).
- Open the release valve so that the cuff deflates at a rate of about 2 mmHg/second.
- The first "tap" that you hear is the systolic blood pressure. The last muffled sound that you hear is the diastolic blood pressure.

The systolic blood pressure is the pressure in the brachial artery when the left ventricle contracts. The diastolic blood pressure is the pressure in the brachial artery when the left ventricle is relaxed and filling with blood.

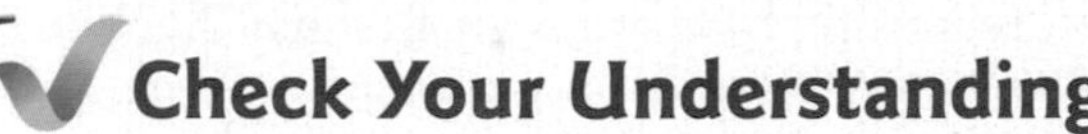

Check Your Understanding

1. What four measurements are often referred to as vital signs?
2. A person's pulse is taken by placing the fingertips over the skin near which type of blood vessel?
3. What is the medical term for a blood pressure cuff?
4. What does systolic blood pressure measure?

Blood Pressure Classification			
Normal	**Pre-Hypertension**	**Stage 1 Hypertension**	**Stage 2 Hypertension**
<120/80 mmHg	systolic: 120–129 mmHg AND diastolic: <80 mmHg	systolic: 130–139 mmHg OR diastolic: 80–89 mmHg	systolic: 140 mmHg or greater OR diastolic: At least 90 mmHg

Figure 11.25

Know Your Numbers

In addition to knowing how to measure vital signs, you should know and monitor some other key numbers. These numbers will give you an indication of how healthy you are compared to the general population. The most important of these are weight, cholesterol, and glucose.

Weight and BMI

An adult's body mass index (BMI) should range between 18.0 and 24.9, which represents a healthy weight. BMIs less than 18 are classified as thin. BMIs equal to or greater than 25 are considered overweight. BMIs greater than 30 are classified as obese.

To calculate your body mass index, divide your weight in kilograms by your height in meters squared.

$$\text{BMI} = \frac{\text{Weight (kg)}}{\text{Height (m}^2\text{)}}$$

If you are an athlete or you have a lot of muscle mass, this BMI calculation method may incorrectly classify you as overweight or obese. This could happen because the formula does not take into account your body composition. The same incorrect result could occur if you use height and weight tables, whether or not you are in the normal range for your age and size.

Body composition is a way of identifying your body's proportion of lean tissue to fat tissue. If you want to know your body composition, you can measure it using a weight scale that has bioelectric impedance technology. These special scales are available in many pharmacies and schools. Another way to measure body composition is to use a caliper to do a skinfold test.

Cholesterol

As explained in Chapter 2, cholesterol is a steroid found in blood. Cholesterol is essential for cell function and for absorption of fat-soluble vitamins. It is also a precursor to the development of steroid hormones. Cholesterol is carried in the blood by lipids.

You can learn the cholesterol level in your blood by having your blood drawn and tested. The amount of cholesterol in the blood is represented by a number. Knowing your total cholesterol number is helpful.

It is more helpful, however, to know how much of your total cholesterol consists of high-density lipoprotein (HDL) and how much consists of low-density lipoprotein (LDL). HDL is the "good type" of cholesterol, and LDL is the "bad type."

LDL carries fat to the arterial walls and deposits it. Over time, these fatty deposits can cause buildup of plaque leading to blockages in the arteries. HDL removes fat from the arterial walls and brings it back to the liver, where it is broken down. Triglycerides are another form of fat that can increase your risk of cardiovascular disease. Desirable levels for each of these substances are:

- Total cholesterol: less than 200 mg/dL
- LDL: less than 100 mg/dL
- HDL: more than 40 mg/dL, preferably more than 60 mg/dL
- Triglycerides: less than 150 mg/dL

MEMORY TIP

To remember the differences between HDL (the good type of cholesterol) and LDL (the bad type), keep in mind the following hint: **H**DL is **H**ealthy, and **L**DL is **L**ousy.

Check Your Understanding

1. What is the normal range for an adult's body mass index?
2. Name two ways to check your body composition.
3. What is the good type of cholesterol and what does it do?

LESSON 11.3 Review and Assessment

Mini Glossary

Make sure that you know the meaning of each key term.

aortic arch the curved portion of the aorta between the ascending and descending parts of the aorta

arteries vessels that carry blood away from the heart

arterioles microscopic arteries that connect with capillaries

brachial artery the artery located at the fold of the elbow where the brachial pulse is detected

capillaries small, thin-walled vessels where oxygen and carbon dioxide gas exchange occurs

capillary beds network of intertwined vessels formed by multiple capillaries

cardiac circulation blood circulation through the coronary arteries, providing the heart with nutrients and removing wastes

carotid artery the artery located on the side of the neck, where the carotid pulse is felt

coronary sinus large venous channel between the left atrium and left ventricle on the posterior side of the heart that empties into the right atrium at the junction of the four chambers

ductus arteriosus a short, broad vessel in the fetus that connects the left pulmonary artery with the descending aorta, allowing most of the blood to bypass the infant's lungs

fetal circulation the process by which an unborn infant receives oxygen and nutrients and disposes of waste products

foramen ovale opening in the septal wall between the atria; normally present only in the fetus

hepatic portal circulation blood circulation through the liver, helping to regulate the levels of nutrients (carbohydrates, proteins, and fats) in the blood

precapillary sphincter a band of smooth muscle fibers that encircles the capillaries at the arteriole-capillary junctions and controls blood flow to the tissues

pulmonary circulation circulation of oxygen-poor blood from the right ventricle, through the lungs, and returning to the left atrium with oxygen-rich blood

radial artery the artery located on the thumb side of the wrist, where the radial pulse is detected

systemic circulation circulation of oxygenated blood through the arteries, capillaries, and veins of the circulatory system, from the left ventricle to the right atrium

tunica externa the outermost layer of a blood vessel, composed mostly of fibrous connective tissue that supports and protects the vessel

tunica intima the innermost layer of a blood vessel, composed of a single layer of squamous epithelial cells over a sheet of connective tissue; its smooth, frictionless surface allows blood to flow smoothly through the vessel

tunica media the thicker middle layer of a blood vessel that contains smooth muscle cells, elastic fibers, and collagen; its muscle cells are directed by the sympathetic nervous system to increase or decrease blood flow to tissues as needed

veins vessels that carry blood to the heart

venules the smallest veins; connect the capillaries with the larger systemic veins

vital signs measurements of pulse and blood pressure

Know and Understand

1. Which layer of a blood vessel is responsible for vasodilation and vasoconstriction?
2. Which structures in the venous system prevent blood from flowing away from the heart? How is this accomplished?
3. How many pulmonary veins take blood back to the heart? Is the blood oxygenated or deoxygenated? Explain your answer.
4. Starting at the heart, list the vessels through which blood travels and returns to the heart during systemic circulation.
5. At which artery in the neck is the heart rate sometimes measured?
6. List four methods of measuring a person's temperature.
7. How is a person's BMI measured?

Analyze and Apply

8. Calculate your BMI. Do you think it is accurate? What fact, which may skew the results, is not taken into account when calculating a person's BMI?
9. Suppose that you are at baseball practice and it is extremely hot and humid. What can you do to ensure that you perform at the top of your game?
10. The carotid pulse is stronger than the radial pulse. Why do you think that is the case?
11. Why do arteries need to be stronger, thicker, and more elastic than veins?

IN THE LAB

12. **Taking Blood Pressure.** Following the steps described in this lesson, take your lab partner's blood pressure at rest. Next, ask your partner to run in place for one minute and repeat the same steps. Analyze the results. Did your partner's blood pressure change? If so, why?
13. Research ways to lower LDL cholesterol and raise HDL cholesterol. Write a treatment plan for a person who has high total cholesterol, low HDL, and high LDL cholesterol levels. Include dietary changes and exercise as part of your treatment plan.
14. Find examples on the internet of normal and abnormal heart sounds. Create a chart listing the normal heart sounds and heart sounds for various heart conditions or disorders. For each condition or disorder, describe in your own words how the sounds differed from normal heart sounds.
15. Investigate how electronic medical records (EMR) are used to record patient vital signs in physician offices and hospitals. Write a comparison, including pros and cons, of using EMR technology versus the traditional method of recording vital signs and other patient information by hand.

LESSON 11.4 Cardiovascular Disease

Before You Read

Try to answer the following questions before you read this lesson.

- Why does your body create plaque?
- What is the window of time, after cardiac symptoms begin, for preventing irreversible tissue damage?

Lesson Objectives

- Describe common cardiac dysrhythmias.
- Explain common valve abnormalities and how they are treated.
- Compare various types of cardiac inflammatory conditions.
- Describe the buildup of plaque in the arteries and the problems that can occur as a result.
- Identify several common types of heart diseases and disorders and their symptoms.

Key Terms

aneurysm
angina pectoris
atherosclerosis
atrial fibrillation
bradycardia
cardiomyopathy
cerebrovascular accident (CVA)
coronary artery disease
dysrhythmia
endocarditis
heart block
heart murmurs
hypertension
ischemia
mitral valve prolapse
myocardial infarction
myocarditis
palpitations
pericarditis
peripheral vascular disease (PVD)
premature atrial contractions (PACs)
premature ventricular contractions (PVCs)
tachycardia
transient ischemic attack (TIA)
valvular stenosis
ventricular fibrillation (VF)
ventricular tachycardia (VT)

CLINICAL CASE STUDY

Mr. Willis is a 78-year-old male who has been hypertensive for almost 15 years. He is on three medications for his hypertension, and it is well controlled. Ten years ago he had a myocardial infarction (heart attack) and had a stent inserted to open his coronary artery. Five years later, he had a second heart attack and had to have a coronary artery bypass graph surgery to repair two of his coronary arteries. During his checkup four months ago, his BMI was 26 kg/m^2 , his blood pressure was 142/90 mmHg, total cholesterol was 220 mg/dL, LDL was 130 mg/dL, and his HDL was 35 mg/dL. Recently, he has been very short of breath and fatigued while performing his normal daily activities, and he has stopped taking his daily walk. In addition, he has noticed that the longer he stands, the tighter his shoes feel on his feet. In fact, he noticed that when he took his shoes off, his ankles were swollen. Mr. Willis has made an appointment with his cardiologist in two weeks.

1. What do Mr. Willis's BMI, blood pressure, and cholesterol numbers tell you about his current cardiovascular disease risk and why?
2. As you read this section, try to determine which of the following conditions Mr. Willis most likely has.
   A. Peripheral vascular disease
   B. Pericarditis
   C. Heart failure

Cardiovascular diseases account for one in six deaths in the United States, or approximately 2,200 deaths per day, according to the American Heart Association. To put this statistic into perspective, someone will have a coronary event—a heart attack or chest pain, for example—approximately every 25 seconds. Also, every minute someone will die from a coronary event. Heart disease is not only epidemic; it is also costly: the direct and indirect costs of heart disease in the United States are estimated at $300 billion annually. This lesson describes some of the more common types of heart disease.

Cardiac Dysrhythmias

Usually the heart follows a sequence of events at regular intervals. In a normal, healthy heart the rhythm is regular, and the rate is between 60 and 100 beats per minute. This is called a *normal sinus rhythm*, or *normal contractility condition*.

Sometimes, however, a beat comes too soon, or the conduction system may not work properly, and an abnormal heartbeat occurs. This irregularity is called a **dysrhythmia** (dis-RITH-mee-uh), or *abnormal contractility condition*. Generally, dysrhythmias that originate in the atria or AV node are not immediately life threatening, but those that originate in the ventricle are more dangerous and can be life-threatening. Ventricular dysrhythmias can affect blood flow to the heart and to the rest of the body, whereas atrial dysrhythmias do not. Dysrhythmias have many causes, including damage to the heart muscle (such as from a heart attack), coronary artery disease, hypertension, smoking, excessive alcohol consumption, excessive caffeine ingestion, electrolyte imbalances, illicit drug use, dietary supplements that contain stimulants, stress, and certain medications.

Types of Dysrhythmias

The ECG is the best tool for detecting abnormal rhythms. Listed below, and shown in **Figure 11.26**, are several types of dysrhythmias. A normal rhythm is shown in **Figure 11.26A**.

B. **Bradycardia** (brad-ee-KAHR-dee-a)—a normal rhythm but with a heart rate below 60 bpm. This condition is common and is considered normal in athletes.

C. **Tachycardia** (tak-i-KAHR-dee-a)—a normal rhythm but with a heart rate above 100 bpm.

D. **Premature atrial contractions (PACs)**—a condition in which an irritable piece of atrial heart tissue fires before the SA node. This causes the contraction to occur too early in the rhythm. Usually PACs are harmless. Caffeine ingestion, other types of stimulants, and stress can increase their likelihood.

E. **Atrial fibrillation**—a condition in which the atrial tissue is very irritated, causing the atria to beat at a rate greater than 350 bpm. The atrial cells do not contract in a coordinated manner; they simply quiver. On an electrocardiogram, the baseline is a wavy line, and the rhythm is irregular. Atrial fibrillation is the most common type of arrhythmia worldwide. In fact, many people with atrial fibrillation go about their daily routine without any symptoms. But if the ventricular rate is too low or too high, pharmacological intervention, cardioversion, or a pacemaker may be needed. *Cardioversion* (KAHR-dee-oh-ver-zhun) is a process in which an electrical shock is administered to stop the heart in the hope that when it restarts, the SA node will be reestablished as the dominant pacemaker of the heart and the new rhythm will be normal sinus rhythm.

F. **Premature ventricular contractions (PVCs)**—a condition in which Purkinje fibers fire before the SA node, causing the ventricles to contract prematurely. Single PVCs are not dangerous. However, frequent PVCs (more than six per minute) or multifocal PVCs (those that occur at multiple sites in the ventricle) can be dangerous and require treatment.

G. **Ventricular tachycardia (VT)**—a life-threatening dysrhythmia in which the ventricles, rather than the SA node, initiate the beat. The heart rate is between 150 and 250 bpm, requiring immediate medical intervention such as intravenous lidocaine (LIGH-doh-kayn) or cardioversion.

H. **Ventricular fibrillation (VF)**—a life-threatening condition in which the ventricles quiver, producing no distinct heartbeats. Essentially, there is no cardiac output in this condition. Immediate steps must be taken to convert the system to a normal, healthy rhythm.

I. **Heart block**—a condition in which the impulses traveling from the SA node to the ventricles are delayed, blocked intermittently, or completely blocked by the AV node. These are commonly called *first-* (impulse-delayed), *second-* (intermittently blocked) and *third-degree* (completely blocked) *heart blocks*. Third-degree heart block is a dangerous dysrhythmia because there is no electrical communication between the atria and the ventricles. The atria fire at the rate of the SA node between 60 and 100 bpm, and the ventricles beat at their own rate, between 15 and 40 bpm. Because the ventricles fire at such a slow rate, cardiac output is too low to adequately supply blood to the rest of the body. A pacemaker is usually inserted into the heart to remedy this condition.

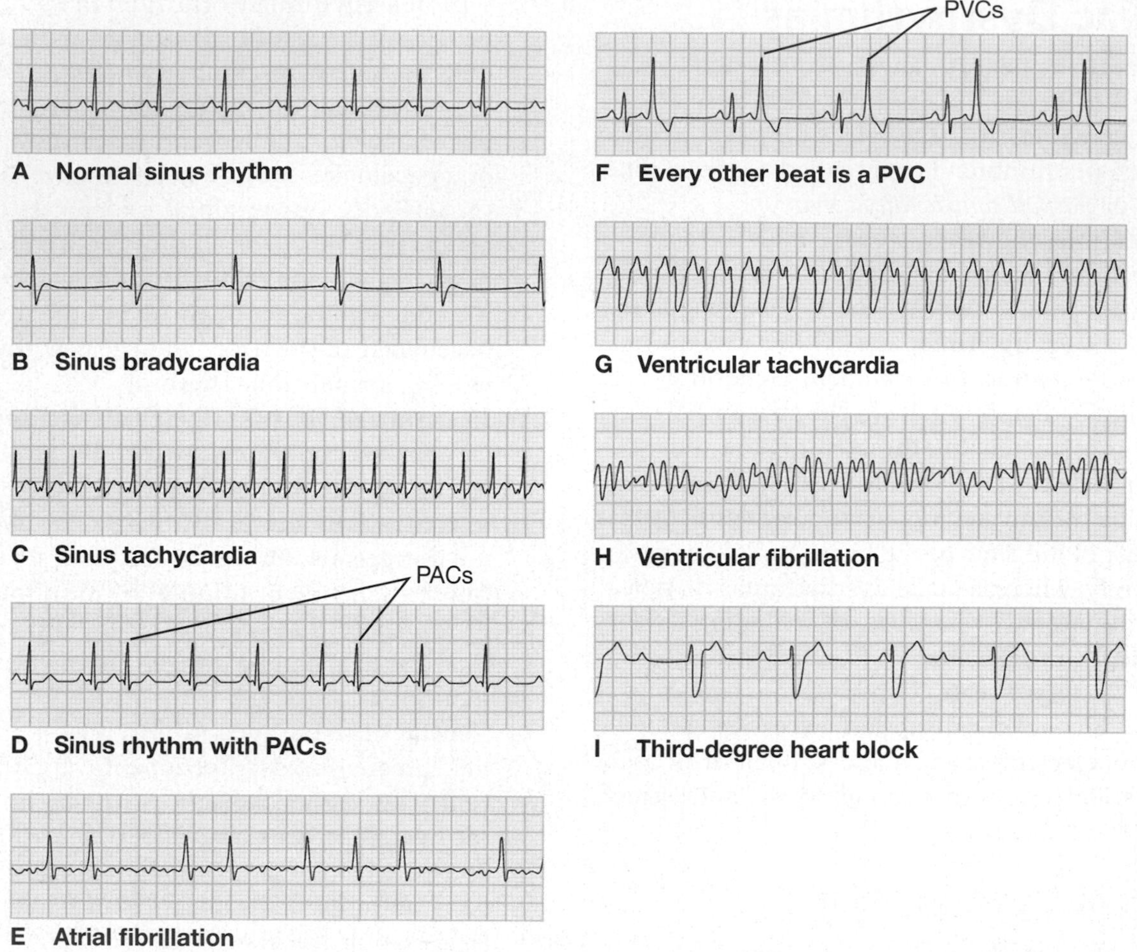

© Body Scientific International

Figure 11.26 A—A normal ECG. B through I—Different types of dysrhythmias.

Defibrillators and Life-Threatening Arrhythmias

A *defibrillator* is a device that can deliver a therapeutic dose of electric current that momentarily stops the heart, allowing its built-in pacemaker, the SA node, to assume control and produce a normal rhythm. Automatic external defibrillators (AEDs) are available in many public gathering places, such as airports, shopping malls, and schools. These devices automatically detect the type of dysrhythmia present and deliver an electrical shock if appropriate, thus allowing people with little to no training to use them (**Figure 11.27**).

The American Heart Association offers a basic cardiopulmonary resuscitation (CPR) course that can train you to perform CPR and to use an automatic external defibrillator. This course is recommended for everyone. If, however, you are involved in a rescue and have not taken such a course, you can still use the AED. With its foolproof, two- to three-step process, it is easy to use.

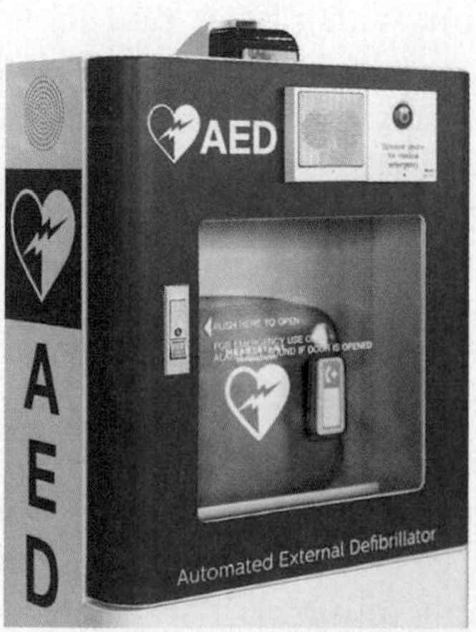

Quality Stock Arts/Shutterstock.com

Figure 11.27 An automated, external defibrillator, or AED.

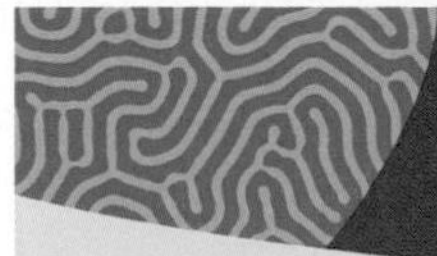

What Research Tells Us

...about How Transplanted Hearts Function

Research on heart transplant patients found that their resting heart rates are higher than normal at approximately 90 bpm. According to exercise stress-test studies, increases in heart rates occur more slowly in transplant patients, and recovery heart rates remain elevated for longer periods of time.

Why are the hearts of transplant patients different in this way? The parasympathetic and sympathetic systems do not regulate heart rate in a transplanted heart. This means that heart rate is higher at rest, and it only begins to rise during exercise from an increase in hormones such as epinephrine and norepinephrine.

Taking It Further

Research the development of the total artificial heart (TAH). How do these hearts function in patients awaiting heart transplantation? Present your findings to the class.

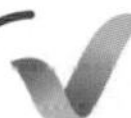

Check Your Understanding

1. What are PACs?
2. Which type of heart block is life-threatening and why?

Valve Abnormalities

In a normal heart, when your healthcare provider listens to your heart, he/she will hear "lub-dub" during a normal cardiac cycle when the valves are opening and closing. Improper functioning of these valves can cause a variety of problems. Three common abnormalities of the heart valves are heart murmurs, valvular stenosis, and mitral valve prolapse (**Figure 11.28**). summarizes the etiology, prevention, pathology, diagnosis, and treatment of these disorders.

Heart murmurs are whooshing or swishing sounds heard upon *auscultation* (aws-kul-TAY-shun)—the act of listening to internal sounds of the body using a stethoscope—that are caused by

Valve Abnormalities					
	Etiology	**Prevention**	**Pathology**	**Diagnosis***	**Treatment**
Heart murmurs	abnormal heart sounds; produced by turbulent blood flow through the heart valves	reduce CAD risk factors	congenital or underlying heart abnormalities	medical exam or well-baby check with auscultation, chest X-ray, echocardiogram, other imaging studies	harmless: no treatment. pathological: medication and/or surgery
Valvular stenosis	narrowing of heart valve due to stiff, calcified, or fused valve cusps	prevent rheumatic fever, reduce CAD risk factors, prevent and treat gum disease and kidney disease	mild: no symptoms Moderate to severe: chest pain, shortness of breath, fatigue, heart palpitations; poor growth in children	medical exam; chest X-ray, echocardiogram, ECG, exercise stress test, cardiac imaging, cardiac catheterization	based on severity; ongoing monitoring, surgery to repair or replace valve
Mitral valve prolapse	incomplete closure of the mitral valve, which may cause regurgitation or blood flow back into left atrium	none	may be without symptoms; light-headedness, shortness of breath, fatigue, irregular heartbeat, chest pain	medical exam with auscultation, echocardiogram, ECG, exercise stress test, coronary angiogram	no treatment for symptomless patients; medications, surgical repair or replacement of valve

*Note: CT scans, MRIs, cardiac catheterizations, echocardiograms, and angiograms are all imaging techniques used to evaluate cardiac abnormalities.

Figure 11.28

Goodheart-Willcox Publisher

one of the heart valves not closing properly. Heart murmurs are common in young children and usually do not require any special treatment. They can also be caused by congenital heart defects, which are present at birth, and by valvular disease as a result of aging, infection, rheumatic fever, or other diseases.

Valvular stenosis is a narrowing of the heart valve due to stiff or fused valve cusps (**Figure 11.29**). Valvular stenosis can occur in one or more of the valves, making the heart work very hard to pump blood through the smaller-than-normal valve opening. People with a mild case of stenosis may be symptom-free. Those with a moderate form, however, may have to restrict their physical activity, and those with a severe case may need surgery to replace the valve.

Mitral valve prolapse occurs when the mitral valve does not close completely. Mitral valve prolapse is fairly common, occurring in up to 10% of the population. It is usually benign and does not require any restrictions. In a small number of cases, mitral regurgitation occurs. This is a disorder in which blood flows backward through the valve into the left atrium when the ventricle contracts. Symptoms may include shortness of breath, **palpitations** (sensation of rapid or pounding heartbeat), fatigue, and chest pain. In some instances the valve has to be repaired or replaced.

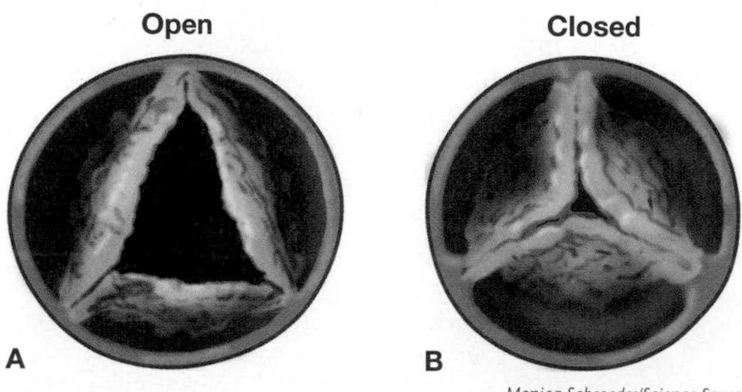

Figure 11.29 Valve abnormalities. A—When a stenotic aortic valve is open, the opening is a little smaller than in a normal valve due to the stiffness and irregularities. The white areas show calcification of the valve leaflets (flaps), which makes them stiff and unable to open properly. B—A stenotic valve is unable to close all the way, so blood can leak through when the valve is closed. *What physical symptoms might be experienced by a person with stenosis of the aortic valve?*

Check Your Understanding

1. What is valvular stenosis?
2. Describe mitral regurgitation and list the symptoms it may cause.

Inflammatory Conditions

The suffix *-itis* means "inflammation." For example, if you have **pericarditis** (per-i-kahr-DIGH-tis), you have an inflammation of the pericardial sac that surrounds your heart, usually due to infection. This condition causes the heart to rub against the pericardial sac as the heart contracts, producing a stabbing pain in the chest. Shortness of breath, fatigue, and rapid pulse may also occur. Drugs are usually prescribed to fight the infection and to decrease inflammation and pain.

Myocarditis (migh-oh-kahr-DIGH-tis) is an inflammation of the myocardium, which is the middle layer of the heart. Myocarditis can cause symptoms similar to those of pericarditis.

Endocarditis (ehn-doh-kahr-DIGH-tis) is an inflammation of the innermost lining of the heart, including the inner surface of the chambers and the valves. It can destroy the heart valves and cause life-threatening complications if left untreated. **Figure 11.30** summarizes the etiology, prevention, pathology, diagnosis, and treatment of these disorders, as well as heart failure, which is discussed in the next section.

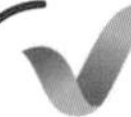

Check Your Understanding

1. What is the name of the condition in which the sac covering the heart is inflamed?
2. Which of the inflammatory conditions described in this chapter is most serious? Why?

Diseases of the Arteries

As explained earlier in this chapter, the arteries transport blood throughout the body. Here are some of the most common problems and diseases that can inhibit or prevent this vital function. **Figure 11.31** summarizes the etiology, prevention, pathology, diagnosis, and treatment of these disorders.

Inflammation/Infection of the Heart Walls and Heart Failure					
	Etiology	**Prevention**	**Pathology**	**Diagnosis***	**Treatment**
Pericarditis	inflammation of the pericardial sac, causing the heart to rub against the sac wall	none	stabbing pain under sternum or in the left side of the chest; fatigue, shortness of breath, rapid pulse	medical exam, chest X-ray, echocardiogram, ECG, other imaging	mild: rest, OTC pain medication, or Colchicine severe: corticosteroids or hospitalization
Myocarditis	inflammation of the cardiac muscle, usually caused by a virus; can lead to heart failure	get all vaccinations; avoid people with viral or flu-like symptoms; wash hands frequently; avoid illegal drug use and other risky behaviors	chest pain, fatigue, shortness of breath and dysrhythmias, swelling in legs, ankles, feet; signs of viral infection: headache, body aches, fever, joint pain, sore throat, diarrhea	medical exam, chest X-ray, echocardiogram, ECG, blood tests, cardiac imaging	mild: rest, antiviral drugs, stop sports severe: hospitalization, IV medications, ventricular assist devices, treatments to decrease heart's workload
Endocarditis	inflammation and infection of the endocardium	good oral hygiene; treat underlying causes; avoid illegal drug use and other risky behaviors	flu-like symptoms, night sweats, shortness of breath, fatigue, swelling in abdomen, feet, or legs; new or changed heart murmur	medical exam; chest X-ray, echocardiogram, ECG, blood tests, cardiac imaging	hospitalization, IV antibiotics, surgery to repair or replace damaged valves
Heart failure	heart loses its ability to pump enough blood to meet oxygen needs of the body, or the heart becomes too stiff and has difficulty filling with blood	heart-healthy lifestyle; avoid excessive alcohol use; have sleep apnea treated	shortness of breath, fatigue, swelling in legs, ankles, and feet; dysrhythmias, inability to exercise, swelling of abdomen, rapid weight gain, persistent cough with phlegm	physical exam, blood tests, chest X-ray, echocardiogram, ECG, imaging tests, coronary angiogram, myocardial biopsy	medication and surgery to treat underlying causes: implantable cardioverter-defibrillators, ventricular assist devices, heart transplant, coronary bypass, heart valve surgery

*Note: CT scans, MRIs, cardiac catheterizations, echocardiograms, and angiograms are all imaging techniques used to evaluate cardiac abnormalities.

Figure 11.30 *Goodheart-Willcox Publisher*

Aneurysms

An **aneurysm** (AN-yoo-rizm) is an abnormal ballooning of a blood vessel—usually an artery—due to a weakness in the wall of the vessel (**Figure 11.32**). Although the causes of an aneurysm are unclear, hypertension, high cholesterol, and smoking increase the risk of developing an aneurysm.

Pain and swelling are common symptoms of an aneurysm, but some individuals have no symptoms. Common locations for aneurysms include the aorta, the brain, the artery behind the knee, and the abdomen. Imaging techniques such as computed tomography (CT), ultrasound, and magnetic resonance angiography (MRA) are used to diagnose an aneurysm.

Aneurysms can rupture, causing sudden death or life-threatening side effects. This condition requires immediate surgical attention to repair the ruptured wall of the artery.

Coronary Artery Disease

Coronary artery disease is caused by a narrowing of one or more of the coronary arteries from a buildup of plaque. This buildup hardens over the course of many years, becoming the disease known as **atherosclerosis** (ath-er-oh-skler-OH-sis), or hardening of the arteries. Atherosclerosis is one form of *arteriosclerosis*, which is a general term for thickening or stiffening of the arteries.

Diseases of the Arteries					
	Etiology	**Prevention**	**Pathology**	**Diagnosis***	**Treatment**
Aneurysm	abnormal ballooning of a blood vessel	healthy lifestyle, quit smoking, avoid excessive alcohol consumption, manage stress	pain/swelling at or near site of aneurysm; if rapid expansion and rupture occur, pain, dizziness, nausea, vomiting, rapid heart rate, shock, low blood pressure	medical exam, CT scan, ultrasound, magnetic resonance angiography (MRA)	depends on risk of rupture; if small, physician monitoring; if high, surgery to reinforce the vessel wall using a stent
Coronary artery disease (CAD)	narrowing of 1 or more of the coronary arteries	awareness of family history of cardiovascular disease; same as for aneurysm	When vessel is narrowed by 50% or more: in men—chest pain, throat dryness, jaw pain, left arm pain, nausea, shortness of breath, perspiration, fainting; in women—fatigue, flu-like symptoms	medical exam, ECG, exercise stress test, stress echocardiogram, nuclear stress test, cardiac catheterization and angiogram, cardiac CT scan	medications to control chest pain, blood pressure, cholesterol, and glucose levels; cardiac rehabilitation
Myocardial infarction	coronary artery becomes completely blocked	awareness of family history; 911 within 5 minutes of onset of symptoms; same as for aneurysms	heart attack and death are first symptom in 33% of cases; other symptoms: same as for CAD	medical exam, ECG, blood tests for cardiac enzymes, chest X-ray, echo-cardiogram, cardiac catheterization and angiogram, CT scan	immediate hospital treatment: drugs to dissolve clot, surgery to insert stent; coronary artery bypass surgery; cardiac rehabilitation

*Note: CT scans, MRIs, cardiac catheterizations, echocardiograms, and angiograms are all imaging techniques used to evaluate cardiac abnormalities.

Figure 11.31 Goodheart-Willcox Publisher

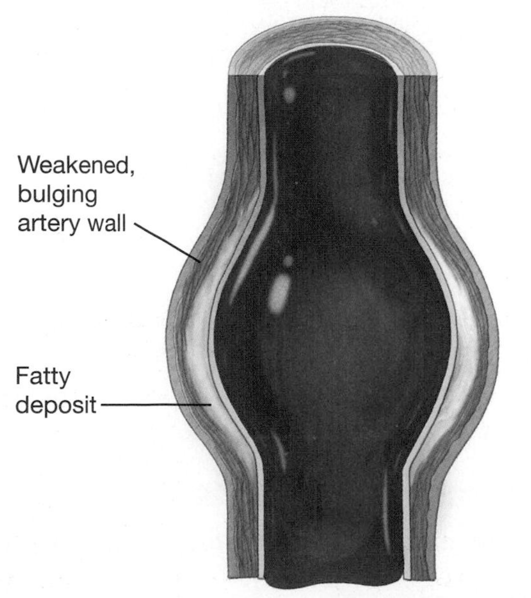

Figure 11.32 Aneurysm.

The buildup of arterial plaque usually starts with an injury to the tunica intima, the innermost lining of the artery. The injury can be caused by high blood pressure, smoking, high blood glucose levels from insulin resistance or diabetes, or high levels of fats and cholesterol in the blood.

Once an injury to an artery occurs, the body tries to repair it by applying its version of a spackling compound, which consists of certain fats and cholesterol, calcium, and other substances in the blood. LDL cholesterol is one of the main culprits in the formation of plaque because it enters the intimal wall and starts to accumulate (**Figure 11.33**). White blood cells digest the LDL particles, become engorged with fat, and create a foamy substance, which is why they are called *foam cells*. In addition, smooth muscle cells migrate from the tunica media of the vessel wall into the intimal lining, where they ingest fats, multiply, and deposit collagen and elastin fibers.

The arterial plaque grows gradually, narrowing the channel through which the blood flows. When the vessel opening is decreased by 50% or more, the heart may not receive a sufficient amount of blood at certain times, such as during exercise or stressful situations. This insufficient blood supply may cause **angina** (an-JIGH-na) **pectoris**, or chest pain. The drug nitroglycerine can be given to dilate (open) the coronary arteries, which helps to alleviate the pain.

Chest pain is the most common symptom arising from lack of oxygen and **ischemia** (is-KEE-mee-a),

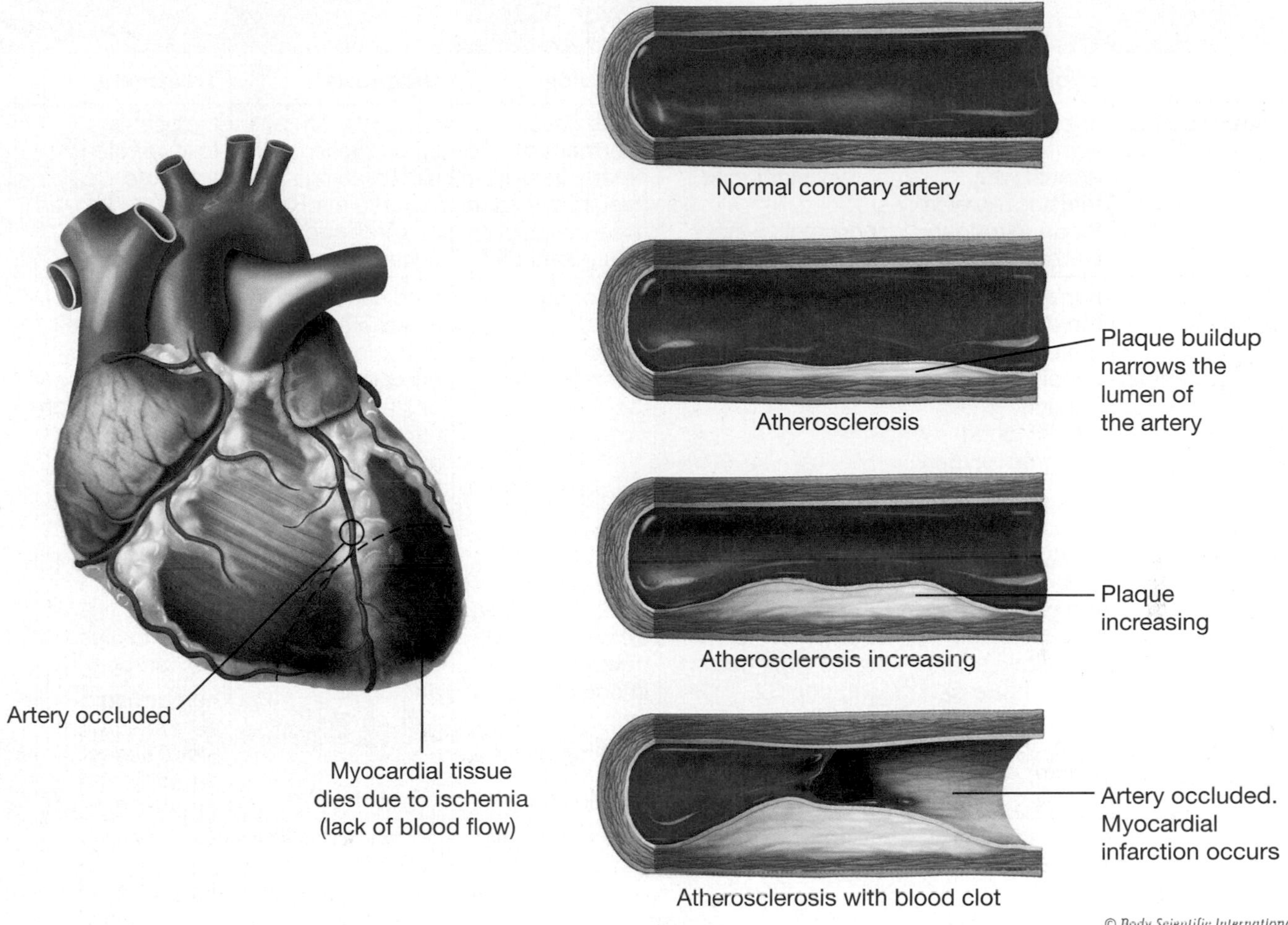

Figure 11.33 Progression of atherosclerosis and development of myocardial infarction. *How does LDL cholesterol cause the formation of plaque in blood vessels?*

lack of blood flow to the heart. Other symptoms include throat dryness, jaw pain, pain going down the left arm, nausea, increased perspiration, shortness of breath, and fainting. These are all "classic" symptoms because they are the symptoms that men typically experience. It was long thought, mistakenly, that heart disease was primarily a problem for men. By contrast, women often do not have any of the classic symptoms. Instead, they may feel unusually fatigued, have flu-like symptoms, or experience no pain at all.

Check Your Understanding

1. Name three factors that can increase the risk of someone developing an aneurysm.
2. What is atherosclerosis?
3. What materials contribute to the buildup of plaque?

Other Cardiovascular Diseases and Disorders

Several other conditions also affect the heart. This section describes a few of them. **Figure 11.34** summarizes the etiology, prevention, pathology, diagnosis, and treatment of these disorders.

Heart Failure

Heart failure is a condition in which the heart cannot adequately pump blood to meet the oxygen needs of the body, sometimes because the heart muscle becomes stiff and has difficulty filling with blood. Heart failure can occur in the right or left ventricle. More commonly, it occurs in both ventricles.

When the heart's pumping ability diminishes, fluid backs up in the lungs, liver, arms, legs, and gastrointestinal tract. Other symptoms include

Other Cardiovascular Abnormalities					
	Etiology	**Prevention**	**Pathology**	**Diagnosis***	**Treatment**
Hypertension	force of blood against the arterial wall remains elevated for an extended period of time	healthy lifestyle, low-salt diet, normal body weight, quit smoking, limit alcohol consumption, have sleep apnea treated	headaches, shortness of breath, light-headedness and nosebleeds; often asymptomatic	medical exam with blood pressure (BP) reading >140/90 mmHg on three separate occasions	medications to lower blood pressure
Peripheral vascular disease (PVD)	narrowing of the arteries in the extremities, usually the legs, resulting in a lack of blood flow and oxygen	limit cardiovascular and diabetes risk factors; quit smoking	pain or burning sensation in calf muscle, and fatigue in the lower extremities	medical exam, ankle-brachial index (compares brachial BP to ankle BP), ultrasound and angiography, blood tests for cholesterol and glucose	medication to lower BP, cholesterol, and glucose levels, prevent clots, and provide symptom relief; surgical interventions and cardiac rehabilitation
Stroke	interruption in blood flow to the brain due to a blockage (ischemic stroke) or a rupture of one of the arteries (hemorrhagic stroke)	limit cardiovascular and diabetes risk factors; awareness of family history of stroke, limit use of birth control	drooping or paralysis of face, arm, or leg, slurred speech, trouble seeing in one or both eyes, trouble walking, headache, confusion	medical exam, ECG, blood tests, CT scan, MRI, carotid imaging, cerebral angiogram, echocardiogram	immediate hospital treatment: ischemic stroke: drugs to dissolve clot, surgery hemorrhagic stroke: surgical blood vessel repair; rehabilitation

*Note: CT scans, MRIs, cardiac catheterizations, echocardiograms, and angiograms are all imaging techniques used to evaluate cardiac abnormalities.

Figure 11.34 Goodheart-Willcox Publisher

shortness of breath, cough, edema (excessive fluid) in the ankles, weight gain, and frequent waking at night to urinate.

Heart failure is not curable, but several different drugs are used to treat it with good outcomes. These include diuretics to prevent water retention, vasodilators, and cardiostimulatory and cardioinhibitory drugs. Cardiostimulatory drugs enhance heart function by increasing heart rate; cardioinhibitory drugs reduce heart rate.

The most common cause of heart failure is coronary artery disease, but heart failure can also be caused by an infection that weakens the heart muscle. This condition is called **cardiomyopathy** (kahr-dee-oh-migh-AHP-uh-thee). Heart failure usually happens gradually, but it can develop quickly after a heart attack has damaged the heart muscle.

Heart transplants are often performed on individuals with end-stage heart failure and, in some rare cases, on children with congenital heart defects. Open-heart surgery is performed, and the patient's diseased heart is replaced with the donor's heart while the patient is hooked up to a heart-lung machine. The first-year survival rate among heart-transplant patients (81%) has greatly improved with the advent of immunosuppressant drugs. Five-year survival rates are 75%, and most individuals are able to return to their normal activities of daily living. However, they need to stay on a lifelong regimen of multiple medications to prevent rejection of the donated heart.

Myocardial Infarction

If an artery becomes completely blocked, a **myocardial infarction**, or heart attack, occurs. This can happen suddenly when a piece of arterial plaque ruptures and occludes (closes) the artery. Many people who have had a heart attack remark that they "felt like an elephant was sitting on [their] chest" or that "the pain was crushing." Morphine and other pain medications are administered to diminish the pain.

You may not think that people who have symptoms such as chest pain or shortness of breath before a heart attack are lucky, but in a way they are. These symptoms are early warnings, giving the person a chance at survival. Others are not so lucky: in approximately one-third of all heart attacks, the first symptom is death.

People with cardiac symptoms should take an aspirin and call 911 within five minutes of onset of the symptoms. Time is of the essence. The first two phases of a heart attack—ischemia and injury to the heart tissue—are reversible with proper intervention. But there is only a 20- to 60-minute window before death of cardiac tissue occurs, which is irreversible.

A goal of the American College of Cardiology (ACC) is to ensure that heart attack patients receive treatment within 90 minutes of their arrival at a hospital. Within 30 minutes of their arrival in the emergency room, patients should receive fibrinolytic (figh-brin-oh-LIT-ik) therapy, the use of special drugs to dissolve the clot. This therapy minimizes the threat of permanent damage to the heart. The ACC also recommends that heart attack patients receive *balloon angioplasty* to open the blocked vessel and that a *stent* (a circular, hollow, wire mesh tube) be inserted within 90 minutes of arrival in the ER (**Figure 11.35**).

Hypertension

Hypertension is another word for high blood pressure. It occurs when the force of blood against the arterial wall remains elevated for an extended period of time. In many cases, doctors are unable to determine what causes hypertension. Individuals with a blood pressure reading greater than 140/90 mmHg on three separate occasions are considered to have high blood pressure.

Many people do not know that they have high blood pressure because there are often no symptoms. This is why hypertension is called the *silent killer.* In fact, the Centers for Disease Control (CDC) estimates that one in five US adults has high blood pressure without knowing it. Approximately one-third of the people in the United States have high blood pressure, and the risk of developing it increases substantially with age. Risk factors for developing hypertension include a family history of hypertension, obesity, smoking, physical inactivity, and sensitivity to salt.

When energy intake exceeds the body's energy needs, the excess energy is stored for future use, in the form of triglycerides or glycogen. Because the body's glycogen storage capacity is limited, chronic energy excess leads to fat formation and obesity. In turn, obesity increases the risk of hypertension, stroke, and coronary artery disease.

Peripheral Vascular Disease (PVD)

Peripheral vascular disease (PVD) is a condition caused by a narrowing of the arteries in the legs. PVD usually results in a lack of blood flow

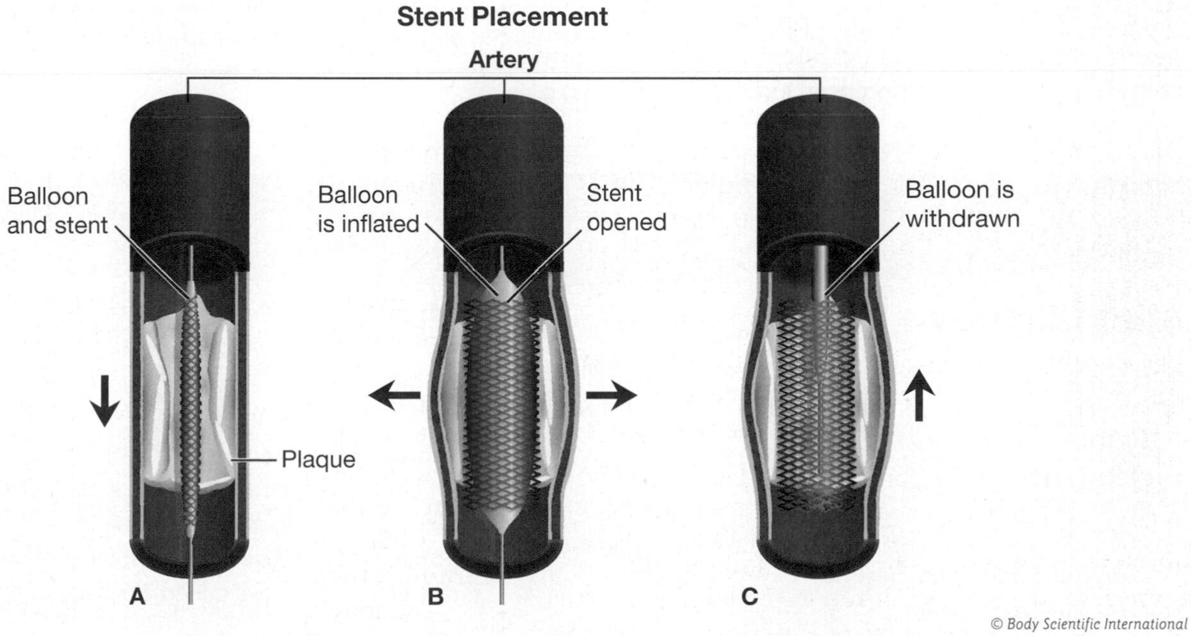

Figure 11.35 Balloon angioplasty and stent placement. A—A hollow wire is threaded through the blood vessel to the blockage. B—A balloon is inflated to press the plaque against the walls of the blood vessel, opening the lumen. C—A stent is placed at the location to hold the vessel open after the balloon is removed.

to the thighs, calf muscles, and feet. Symptoms generally include pain, fatigue in the lower extremities, and a burning sensation in the calf muscle. Initially, these symptoms may be apparent only while walking, but they may also occur at rest as the condition worsens.

The disease strikes both men and women, but African-Americans are at greater risk. Smoking greatly increases a person's risk of developing PVD. Exercise lowers the risk and lessens the symptoms. Medications to dilate the arteries and prevent blood clots help control the disorder. In severe cases, surgery or the placement of a stent to open a narrowed artery may be required.

Cerebrovascular Accident

A stroke, or **cerebrovascular accident (CVA)**, is a medical emergency that occurs when blood flow to the brain stops. There are two different types of strokes. An *ischemic CVA* occurs when one of the arteries of the brain becomes blocked. A *hemorrhagic CVA* occurs when one of the arteries ruptures, causing bleeding in the brain. Within minutes, the brain is deprived of oxygen, causing many complications and possibly death.

According to the CDC, stroke is the fourth leading cause of death in the United States and the leading cause of long-term, severe disability. The CDC estimates that the cost of care for stroke survivors in the United States is approximately $20 billion annually.

Paralysis, loss of speech, problems walking, uncontrolled emotional outbursts, depression, and coma are some of the potential side effects of stroke. These side effects may be temporary if a person experiences a **transient ischemic attack (TIA)**, a temporary lack of blood flow to the brain. In this case, symptoms usually disappear within one to two hours. TIAs are a warning sign that stroke could occur in the future, so steps should be taken to correct the underlying condition and risk factors.

Risk factors for stroke include family history of stroke, high blood pressure, diabetes, high cholesterol, use of birth control pills, and African-American ancestry. Smoking, excessive alcohol consumption, illicit drug use, overweight or obese conditions, and physical inactivity also increase the risk of stroke.

MEMORY TIP

Signs of a stroke are easy to remember if you use the F.A.S.T. tip developed by Methodist Health Systems.

F—Face Is one side drooping?
A—Arms Is one arm weak or numb?
S—Speech Is speech slurred?
T—Time Time is critical. Call 911 or get to the hospital quickly.

Check Your Understanding

1. What is the most common cause of heart failure?
2. What should you do if you think you are experiencing cardiac symptoms?
3. What is the medical term for a stroke?

LESSON 11.4 Review and Assessment

Mini Glossary

Make sure that you know the meaning of each key term.

aneurysm abnormal ballooning of a blood vessel, usually an artery, due to a weakness in the wall of the vessel

angina pectoris condition characterized by severe, constricting pain or sensation of pressure in the chest, often radiating to the left arm; caused by an insufficient supply of blood to the heart

atherosclerosis hardening of the arteries

atrial fibrillation condition in which the atria contract in an uncoordinated, rapid manner (rate above 350 bpm), causing the ventricles to contract irregularly

bradycardia a normal heart rhythm but with a rate below 60 bpm; a condition common among athletes

cardiomyopathy heart failure caused by infection and weakening of the myocardium, or heart muscle

cerebrovascular accident (CVA) a sudden blockage of blood flow, or rupture of an artery in the brain, that causes brain cells to die from lack of oxygen

coronary artery disease a narrowing of one or more of the coronary arteries due to a buildup of plaque; coronary heart disease

dysrhythmia an irregular heartbeat or rhythm

endocarditis inflammation of the innermost lining of the heart, including the inner surface of the chambers and the valves

heart block a condition in which the impulses traveling from the SA node to the ventricles are delayed, intermittently blocked, or completely blocked by the AV node

heart murmurs extra or unusual sounds heard by a stethoscope during a heartbeat; may be harmless or indicative of a problem with one of the heart valves

hypertension condition that occurs when the force of blood against the arterial wall remains elevated for an extended period of time; high blood pressure

ischemia a lack of blood flow, usually due to the narrowing of a blood vessel

mitral valve prolapse an incomplete closing of the mitral valve, causing blood to flow backward into the left atrium when the left ventricle contracts

myocardial infarction tissue death that occurs in a segment of heart muscle from blockage of a coronary artery; heart attack

myocarditis inflammation of the myocardium, the middle layer of the heart (also known as the heart muscle)

palpitations sensation of rapid heartbeat

pericarditis inflammation of the pericardial sac that surrounds the heart

peripheral vascular disease (PVD) condition caused by a narrowing of the arteries in the legs

premature atrial contractions (PACs) condition in which an irritable piece of atrial heart tissue fires before the SA node, causing the atria to contract too soon

premature ventricular contractions (PVCs) condition in which Purkinje fibers fire before the SA node, causing the ventricles to contract prematurely

tachycardia a normal heart rhythm but with a rate above 100 bpm

transient ischemic attack (TIA) a temporary lack of blood flow to the brain

valvular stenosis a narrowing of the heart valve due to stiff or fused valve cusps

ventricular fibrillation (VF) a life-threatening condition in which the heart ventricles quiver without producing a heartbeat

ventricular tachycardia (VT) a life-threatening arrhythmia in which the ventricles, rather than the SA node, initiate the heartbeat; the heart rate is between 150 and 250 bpm, requiring swift medical attention

Know and Understand

1. What are the differences between atrial and ventricular fibrillation?
2. What surgical method can be used to remedy some valve abnormalities?
3. What fluid-related problem results from the heart's inability to pump sufficient blood to meet the body's oxygen needs?
4. What is the cause of myocardial infarction?
5. What is the maximum amount of time that should elapse before a heart attack patient arriving at the hospital receives treatment?
6. What disease is known as the "silent killer"?

Analyze and Apply

7. Further investigate AEDs. What are their therapeutic uses and effects?
8. Using the illustrations in this chapter, explain how you would interpret normal and abnormal contractility conditions.
9. Explain why the body's attempt at repairing an injury to an artery can become a problem.
10. Compare and contrast a CVA and an aneurysm.
11. Explain how the cholesterol level in a person's blood makes the person susceptible to coronary artery disease.
12. Explain why ventricular dysrhythmias are more dangerous, and potentially more life-threatening, than atrial dysrhythmias.
13. Explain the difference between an ischemic stroke, a hemorrhagic stroke, and a transient ischemic attack (TIA).
14. Why does the risk of developing hypertension increase as a person ages?

IN THE LAB

15. Working with a partner, create a new-patient questionnaire for a medical center, focusing on questions to detect high blood pressure. Share and compare your questionnaire with the questionnaires created by other teams. Compile the best questions into one final questionnaire.
16. Working with a small group of students, pick one of the conditions discussed in this lesson that is of particular interest to you and the members of your group. Create a collage that represents the causes, symptoms, anatomy, physiology, and remedies for that condition. Share your collage with the class.
17. Research ways to treat hypertension and/or decrease a person's risk of developing hypertension. Create an informational pamphlet or brochure and include your findings. Include at least five ways to lower your risk of developing hypertension and at least three ways it can be treated if you already have it.

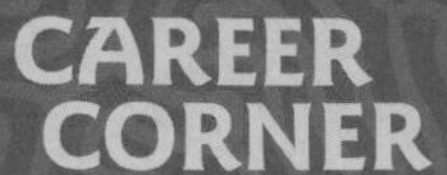

Anatomy & Physiology at Work

The cardiovascular system, which consists of the heart, blood, and blood vessels, influences every living cell in the body. Many people have found challenging and fulfilling careers in the promotion of cardiovascular health and the diagnosis and treatment of cardiovascular diseases. Healthcare providers who manage the health of cardiac patients often deal with patients in life and death situations. Therefore, people who are interested in a career in this area need to be able to relate to patients and their families in a kind, caring, and compassionate way.

Cardiologist

Cardiologists are medical doctors who specialize in the heart and the cardiovascular system. They work with patients, usually on referral from the patient's primary physician, to diagnose and treat various cardiovascular diseases and disorders.

Cardiologists must have extensive training beyond normal medical school training. They need a 4-year degree from a medical school, followed by 3 years of training in internal medicine, and then 3 additional years of specialty training. They must then go through a residency in which they apply their skills in a hands-on setting under the guidance of more experienced cardiologists.

Cardiology Physician Assistant

Some people interested in cardiology choose to become physician assistants (PA) with a specialty in cardiology. Although they are not medical doctors, cardiology PAs can assist the cardiologist and can even perform certain procedures, such as draining fluid from the chest cavity, or inserting chest tubes. They may also care for patients after cardiovascular surgery.

To become a cardiology physician assistant, you must first obtain the normal physician assistant degree—usually a bachelor's or master's degree—from an accredited university. You must also pass a national certification exam, and then become licensed in the state in which you will practice. The outlook for cardiology physician assistants is especially good, as hospitals and medical facilities try to keep rising costs under control while maintaining a high level of patient care.

Clinical Exercise Physiologist

A clinical exercise physiologist performs many tasks, including exercise screening, clinical exercise testing, exercise prescription, and health education. The clinical physiologist does this for individuals with cardiovascular, pulmonary, metabolic, orthopedic, musculoskeletal, and hematologic diseases. These physiologists work in hospitals, physical therapy clinics, rehabilitation programs, corporate health programs, and colleges and universities.

Clinical exercise physiologists monitor heart rate and blood pressure responses to exercise, perform electrocardiogram monitoring, and supervise exercise participation for at-risk and diseased populations (**Figure 11.36**).

Clinical exercise physiology is a relatively new medical career that requires a master's degree in exercise science, exercise physiology, or kinesiology from an accredited institution. Most master's programs are two years but there are a few that offer a one-year intensive program of study. The Registered Clinical Exercise Physiology Certification from the American College of Sports Medicine is recommended. Job prospects are considered to be very good in the near future. This is largely due to the emphasis placed on exercise as a rehabilitative tool.

Cardiovascular Technologist and Technician

Professionals who perform—or assist in performing—diagnostic tests on patients with cardiovascular diseases are referred to as *cardiovascular technologists* and *technicians*. These

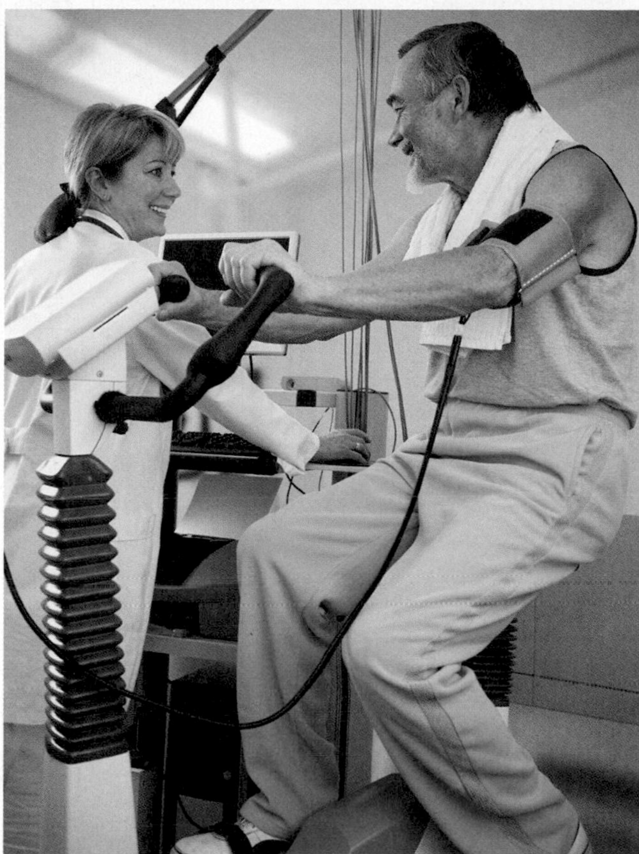
Alexander Raths/Shutterstock.com

Figure 11.36 A clinical exercise physiologist monitors a patient during exercise screening.

tests may include electrocardiograms, cardiac catheterizations, pulmonary function tests, echocardiograms, and graded exercise testing.

Most cardiovascular technologists have a two-year associate's degree from an accredited community college. Some institutions offer a four-year degree in cardiovascular technology. Cardiovascular technicians, also known as EKG technicians, may have a one-year certificate or receive on-the-job training. Certification can be obtained from the American Board of Cardiovascular Perfusion, American Society of Phlebotomy Technicians, or the American Certification Agency for Healthcare Professionals.

Planning for a Health-Related Career

Do some research on the career of a cardiologist, cardiology PA, clinical exercise physiologist, or a cardiovascular technologist/technician. Alternatively, select a profession from the list of related career options. Using the internet or resources at your local library, find answers to the following questions:

1. What are the main tasks and responsibilities of a person employed in the career that you chose to research?
2. What is the outlook for this career? Are workers in demand, or are jobs dwindling? For complete information, consult the current edition of the *Occupational Outlook Handbook*, published by the US Department of Labor. This handbook is available online or at your local library.
3. What special skills or talents are required? For example, do you need to be good at biology and anatomy and physiology? Do you need to enjoy interacting with other people?
4. What personality traits do you think are necessary for success in the career you have chosen to research? For example, a career as an exercise specialist involves educating people about exercise training and lifestyle modifications designed to promote health. Do you enjoy teaching or coaching others?
5. Does the work involve a great deal of routine, or are the day-to-day responsibilities varied?
6. Does the career require long hours, or is it a standard, "9-to-5" job?
7. What is the salary range for this job?
8. What do you think you would like about this career? Is there anything about it that you might dislike?

Related Career Options

- Athletic trainer
- Cardiovascular nurse
- Diagnostic medical sonographer
- Electrocardiographic (ECG) technician
- Fitness trainer
- Kinesiotherapist
- Physical therapist
- Radiologist
- Recreational therapist
- Vascular technologist

CHAPTER

11 Review

›LESSON 11.1

Heart Anatomy and Physiology

Key Points

- The heart is located in the center of the thoracic cavity and is encased in the pericardium. It has four chambers: two atria and two ventricles.
- The "lub-dub" sounds of the heart are the closing of one-way valves between the atria and ventricles and between the ventricles and blood vessels; these valves maintain the correct flow of blood through the heart.

Key Terms

aorta
aortic valve
atrioventricular (AV) valves
cardiac cycle
cardiac output (CO)
diastole
endocardium
epicardium
Frank-Starling law
inferior vena cava
interatrial septum
interventricular septum
mitral valve
myocardium
papillary muscles
pulmonary valve
semilunar valves
stroke volume
superior vena cava
systole
tricuspid valve
vasoconstriction
vasodilation

›LESSON 11.2

Regulation of the Heart

Key Points

- The heart is regulated internally by the sinoatrial node (SA node), and externally by the nervous and endocrine systems.
- The conduction system of the heart consists of the SA node, which sends an impulse through the AV node to the bundle of His and down the left and right bundle branches to the Purkinje fibers.

Key Terms

atrioventricular (AV) node baroreceptors
bundle of His
depolarize
left bundle branches
Purkinje fibers
repolarize
right bundle branches
sinoatrial (SA) node

›LESSON 11.3

Blood Vessels and Circulation

Key Points

- Arteries carry blood away from the heart and have thick, strong, elastic walls. Veins carry blood back toward the heart and have thin, less elastic walls and one-way valves. Capillaries are tiny vessels that perform the actual gas exchange between the blood and the body cells.
- Cardiopulmonary circulation is the process of transporting deoxygenated blood from the right side of the heart to the lungs and then transporting oxygenated blood back to the left side of the heart. Systemic circulation is the process of transporting oxygenated blood from the left side of the heart out to the rest of the body. Systemic circulation also includes cardiac and hepatic portal circulation.
- Vital signs are assessed by measuring a person's blood pressure, pulse, respirations, and temperature.

Key Terms

aortic arch
arteries
arterioles
brachial artery
capillaries
capillary beds
cardiac circulation
carotid artery
coronary sinus
ductus arteriosus
fetal circulation
foramen ovale
hepatic portal circulation
precapillary sphincter
pulmonary circulation
radial artery
systemic circulation
tunica externa
tunica intima
tunica media
veins
venules
vital signs

›LESSON 11.4

Cardiovascular Disease

Key Points

- Cardiac dysrhythmias occur when other irritable cells in the heart fire, taking over or outpacing the rhythm set by the SA node.
- Valve conditions are often not life-threatening, but in some cases they require surgical repair or replacement.
- Inflammatory conditions in the heart can be treated with drugs that decrease inflammation.
- Plaque buildup in the arteries can cause coronary artery disease and other serious heart conditions.
- Other heart conditions include heart failure, myocardial infarction, hypertension, peripheral vascular disease, and cerebrovascular accident.

Key Terms

aneurysm
angina pectoris
atherosclerosis
atrial fibrillation
bradycardia
cardiomyopathy
cerebrovascular accident (CVA)
coronary artery disease
dysrhythmia
endocarditis
heart block
heart murmurs
hypertension
ischemia
mitral valve prolapse
myocardial infarction
myocarditis
palpitations
pericarditis
peripheral vascular disease (PVD)
premature atrial contractions (PACs)
premature ventricular contractions (PVCs)
tachycardia
transient ischemic attack (TIA)
valvular stenosis
ventricular fibrillation (VF)
ventricular tachycardia (VT)

Assessment

> LESSON 11.1

Heart Anatomy and Physiology

Learning Key Terms and Concepts

1. The heart is flanked on either side by the _____.
   A. diaphragm
   B. hips
   C. sternum
   D. lungs
2. The wall that separates the atria from each other is called the _____.
3. The bicuspid valve is located between the _____.
   A. right and left ventricles
   B. left atrium and left ventricle
   C. left and right atria
   D. left ventricle and the aorta
4. Attached to the cusps of heart valves are thin, fibrous cords called chordae tendineae, which are connected to _____ muscles.
5. The fluid-filled, double-walled sac that surrounds the heart is the _____.
   A. pericardium
   B. endocardium
   C. myocardium
   D. epicardium
6. The myocardium is the _____.
   A. sac surrounding the heart
   B. thick, muscular layer of the heart wall
   C. inner lining of the heart
   D. septum between the chambers of the heart
7. The "lub" of the heart's "lub-dub" sound is caused by the closing of the _____ valves.
8. Cardiac output is calculated by multiplying _____.
   A. heart rate and systolic blood pressure
   B. diastolic blood pressure and systolic blood pressure
   C. stroke volume and heart rate
   D. diastolic blood pressure and heart rate

Thinking Critically

9. What would happen if the interventricular septum had a hole in it?
10. It is widely believed that arteries carry only oxygenated blood and veins carry only deoxygenated blood. Is this a correct statement? Explain and defend your answer.
11. In your own words, describe the function of the chordae tendineae. Why are they important to the functioning of the heart?
12. Explain what is happening in the heart during systole and diastole.

> LESSON 11.2

Regulation of the Heart

Learning Key Terms and Concepts

13. The primary pacemaker of the heart is the _____.
   A. mitral valve
   B. atrioventricular node
   C. sinoatrial node
   D. bundle of His
14. The SA node is located _____.
   A. at the top of the right atrium
   B. near the junction of the left atrium and left ventricle
   C. between the bundle of His and the bundle branches
   D. at the distal end of the Purkinje fibers
15. The cardiac center of the brain is made up of the sympathetic and parasympathetic branches of the _____ nervous system.
16. When sympathetic nerve fibers stimulate the SA node, the effect is _____.
   A. an increase in heart rate
   B. a decrease in heart rate
   C. contraction of the ventricles
   D. an irregular heart rhythm
17. The _____, which are sensitive to pressure, are located in the aortic arch and carotid arteries.
18. Which of the following is *not* considered a component of the heart conduction system?
   A. sinoatrial (SA) node
   B. epicardium
   C. Purkinje fibers
   D. atrioventricular (AV) node

Thinking Critically

19. What would happen if the parasympathetic branch of a person's autonomic nervous system did not function?
20. How do the endocrine and limbic systems work together to help a person escape from a dangerous situation?

›LESSON 11.3

Blood Vessels and Circulation

Learning Key Terms and Concepts

21. Which layer of a blood vessel provides a smooth, frictionless surface for the flow of blood?
    A. tunica media
    B. tunica intima
    C. tunica externa
    D. medulla oblongata
22. Which type of blood vessel has the thickest, strongest, and most elastic walls?
    A. artery
    B. capillary
    C. venule
    D. vein
23. The smallest, most numerous blood vessels in the body are the _____.
    A. venules
    B. arterioles
    C. capillaries
    D. veins
24. Blood returning to the heart via the inferior vena cava and the superior vena cava collects in the _____.
    A. left ventricle
    B. right ventricle
    C. left atrium
    D. right atrium
25. Blood is carried to the lungs by the _____.
    A. pulmonary vein
    B. pulmonary artery
    C. aorta
    D. inferior vena cava
26. From which part of the aorta does the brachiocephalic artery arise?
    A. aortic arch
    B. ascending aorta
    C. descending aorta
    D. abdominal aorta
27. The heart receives oxygen and nutrients through _____ circulation, which is part of the systemic circulatory system.
28. Through which blood vessel does a fetus receive oxygen and nutrients?
    A. carotid artery
    B. ductus arteriosus
    C. aorta
    D. umbilical vein
29. The artery located on the side of your neck, where you can clearly feel your pulse, is called the _____ artery.
30. An axillary temperature is measured in the _____.
    A. ear
    B. anus
    C. armpit
    D. mouth
31. Blood pressure measured when the left ventricle contracts is called _____ pressure.
    A. diastolic
    B. stroke
    C. systolic
    D. mean
32. To be considered normal, a person's total cholesterol level should be _____.
    A. less than 200 mg/dL
    B. less than 100 mg/dL
    C. more than 60 mg/dL
    D. more than 150 mg/dL

Thinking Critically

33. Why is blood considered a connective tissue?
34. Drawing on the information you studied in the first three lessons, explain why low blood pressure is considered a potentially dangerous condition.
35. Consider how blood vessel structure relates to its function. Why is it beneficial that capillaries are only a single layer thick?
36. Explain how hepatic portal circulation is different from other circulation in the body.

›LESSON 11.4

Cardiovascular Disease

Learning Key Terms and Concepts

37. The condition in which the atria quiver, rather than contract in a coordinated manner, is known as atrial _____.

38. The condition in which the electrical impulse is completely blocked by the AV node is _____.
    A. first-degree heart block
    B. second-degree heart block
    C. third-degree heart block
    D. fourth-degree heart block
39. The process of listening to heart sounds using a stethoscope is called _____.
40. What is the term for a narrowing of the heart valve due to stiff or fused valve cusps?
    A. valve prolapse
    B. valvular stenosis
    C. palpitations
    D. heart murmurs
41. Inflammation of the middle layer of the heart is called _____.
42. One common location for an aneurysm is the _____.
    A. carotid artery
    B. aorta
    C. jugular vein
    D. brachial artery
43. Atherosclerosis is the medical term for hardening of the _____.
    A. peripheral veins
    B. capillary beds
    C. coronary arteries
    D. pulmonary veins
44. The most common cause of heart failure is _____.
45. A general term for any infection that weakens the heart muscle is _____.
46. Which of the following is *not* considered a risk factor for hypertension?
    A. physical activity
    B. smoking
    C. salt sensitivity
    D. obesity
47. The common abbreviation of the medical term for a narrowing of the arteries in the legs is _____.

Thinking Critically

48. Which of the dysrhythmias described in this chapter do you think is *least* serious? Explain your answer.
49. How is the function of the heart affected by a myocardial infarction?
50. Compare and contrast a TIA and a hemorrhagic stroke.
51. How would having too much LDL cholesterol in your blood vessels increase your risk of having a myocardial infarction?
52. Explain how having valvular stenosis could impact the function of the heart.

Building Skills and Connecting Concepts

Analyzing and Evaluating Data

Instructions: The bar graph in **Figure 11.37** shows the number of deaths from heart disease for selected years. Use the graph to answer the following questions.

53. How many people died from heart disease in 1980?
54. Between which years did the greatest reduction in the number of heart disease-related fatalities occur?

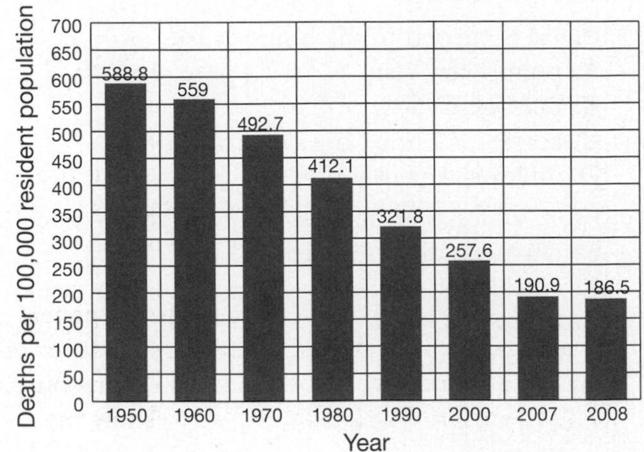

Figure 11.37

Goodheart-Willcox Publisher

55. Between which 10-year periods did the smallest reduction in the number of heart disease-related fatalities occur? How might this be interpreted in a positive way?
56. What is the difference in the number of heart disease-related fatalities between 1950 and 2008?
57. By what percentage did the number of heart disease-related deaths go down from 1950 to 2008? Round to the nearest whole percent.
58. What is the difference in the number of heart disease-related deaths from 1970 to 2000?

Communicating about Anatomy & Physiology

59. **Writing** Create a children's story describing the adventures of a red blood cell as it travels through the human cardiovascular (circulatory) system. Include as many of the terms from the chapter as possible in your story. Devise a creative way to tell your story. For example, you may want to include color illustrations or make a pop-up book.
60. **Speaking** Research the early signs and symptoms of a stroke and what should be done if you suspect that someone is having a stroke. Compile your research into a presentation and present it to your class to educate your classmates on what to look for and what to do.
61. **Listening** Work with two partners, and each of you choose one of the following conditions: pericarditis, myocarditis, and endocarditis. Research your chosen condition, looking for signs and symptoms, treatments/medications used, and prognosis. Each of you should then present your findings to the other two. Listen carefully and take notes on each other's presentations.

Lab Investigations

62. Refer again to **Figure 11.37**. With a small group of classmates, discuss the data in the graph. Then create a list of possible explanations for the dramatic decrease in the number of heart disease-related fatalities. Expand your list into a poster for your classroom.
63. Draw a human form on a large sheet of paper. Then draw and label the following structures of the cardiovascular system. Make the veins blue and the arteries red. Add arrows to show the direction of blood flow. Use your textbook as a guide and do internet research if necessary.
    structures of/circulation through the heart: *right atrium, left atrium, right ventricle, left ventricle, inferior vena cava, superior vena cava, aorta, tricuspid valve, bicuspid valve, pulmonary veins, pulmonary artery, aortic valve, pulmonary circulation, pulmonary valve, myocardium, endocardium, pericardium, apex, interventricular septum*
    structures of/circulation throughout the body: *brachial artery, femoral artery, radial artery, popliteal artery, dorsalis pedis artery, temporal artery, carotid artery, renal artery, hepatic vein, renal vein, jugular vein, portal vein, cerebral circulation, coronary circulation*
    In your drawing, write the name of each of the following conditions on the part of the cardiovascular system in which the condition originates or occurs: *aneurysm, atherosclerosis, hypertension, pericarditis, ischemic stroke, hemorrhagic stroke, myocardial infarction.*
64. Measure your pulse (heart rate) three times for a full minute each time. Record your heart rate for each trial on a piece of paper. Add up the three heart rates and divide that total by 3 to get your average pulse rate. Record your average heart rate on your paper.
    Next, find your cardiac output. To do that, multiply your average heart rate by the stroke volume. For this experiment, you may use 70 mL for the stroke volume. Be sure to state your answer in L/min. Show your calculations.
    Next, record your answers to these questions:
    - What is your cardiac output based on your calculations?
    - If your body contains about 5 L of blood, based on your results, is the entire volume of your blood pumped through your heart in less than a minute or more than a minute?

Building Your Portfolio

65. Take digital photographs of the models and projects you created as you worked through this chapter. Create a document or folder called "The Cardiovascular System" and insert the photographs, along with written descriptions of what the models show and your reasons for creating them using the materials and forms you chose. Add posters and brochures you created and the reports from your laboratory experiments. Add this document or folder to your personal portfolio.

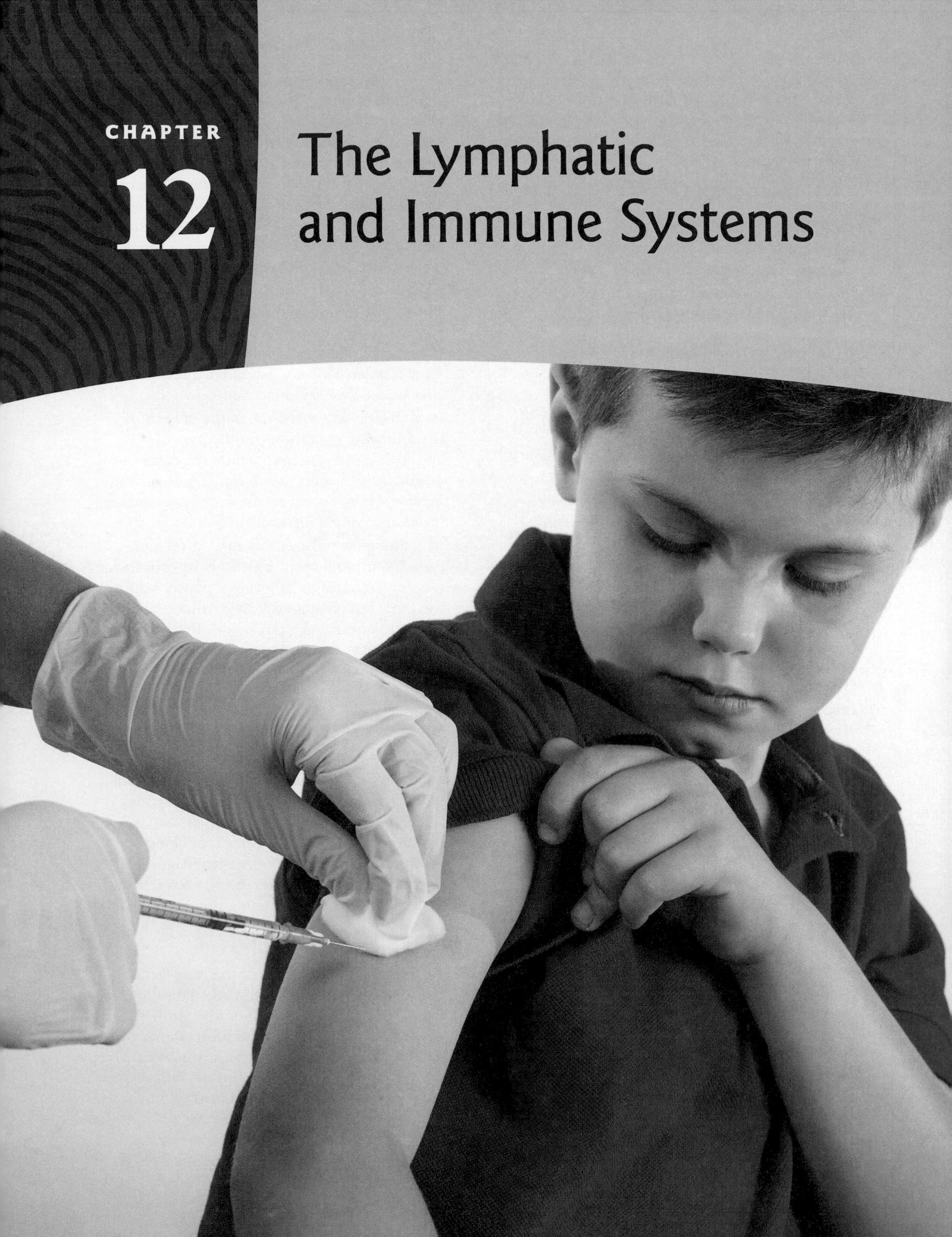

CHAPTER

12 The Lymphatic and Immune Systems

How does the lymphatic system work with the immune system to help keep your body healthy?

The world is a dangerous place—full of bacteria, viruses, fungi, and toxins. Because the human body is an attractive host for these and other infectious agents, your body must defend itself against constant assault by disease-producing microbes. You are usually unaware of this battle, which takes place on a microscopic level. Like a medieval town protected by walls, pots of burning oil, and soldiers, your body is protected by physical and chemical barriers and a cellular defense system.

This chapter explores the lymphatic system and the body's defense systems against infection and disease. First, it discusses the anatomy and basic physiology of the lymphatic system and related lymphatic tissues. Next, it describes the nonspecific defense systems, whose mechanisms work without regard for the specific identity of an infectious agent. Finally, the chapter examines the body's specific defense systems, which generates cells and antibodies that are custom-made for targeting an invading organism.

Click on the activity icon or visit www.g-wlearning.com/healthsciences/0202 to access online vocabulary activities using key terms from the chapter.

Chapter 12 Outline

◂ Luiscar74/Shutterstock.com

LESSON 12.1 The Lymphatic System

Before You Read

Try to answer the following questions before you read this lesson.

- What are the two primary functions of the lymphatic system?
- What would happen to the human body if it did not have a lymphatic system?

Lesson Objectives

- Trace the formation and flow of lymph, including the parts of the body drained by the major lymph vessels.
- Identify and describe the cells, tissues, and organs that make up the lymphatic system.

Key Terms

B lymphocytes (B cells)
cisterna chyli
endothelial cells
interstitial fluid
lingual tonsils
lymph
lymph nodes
lymphatic nodules
lymphatic trunks
lymphatic valves
lymphatic vessels
lymphocytes
macrophages
mucosa-associated lymphatic tissue (MALT)
natural killer (NK) cells
palatine tonsils
pathogens
pharyngeal tonsil
spleen
T lymphocytes (T cells)

The lymphatic system performs two vital functions in the human body: it solves a "plumbing" problem, and it constantly remains on the lookout for foreign invaders that can cause infection and disease.

The plumbing problem is caused by capillaries that naturally leak. As blood travels through the blood capillaries, a small amount of blood plasma leaks out of the capillaries and into the surrounding tissue. The normal leakage rate, across the entire body, is 2 to 3 mL per minute, a tiny amount compared to the 5,000 mL of blood that pass through capillaries each minute. But even this tiny amount would, in less than one day, cause a potentially fatal drop in blood pressure if the excess fluid were not returned to the cardiovascular system.

The lymphatic system also manages the challenge of quickly recognizing and mounting a counter-attack against infectious agents. As the lymphatic system reabsorbs fluid from the leaking capillaries, it removes bacteria and virus-infected cells from body tissues. It also "sounds the alarm" that activates specific immune defenses. The lymphatic system therefore plays a vital role in the body's immune system, which provides protection against disease.

Organization of the Lymphatic System

The lymphatic system includes lymphatic vessels, lymphatic fluid (called *lymph*), and lymphatic organs such as lymph nodes and the spleen (**Figure 12.1**). Many of the cells that fight infection develop within, and travel through, the organs and vessels of the lymphatic system.

The lymphatic system resembles the cardiovascular system in that both extend throughout almost all parts of the body. Both systems also have a network of vessels that vary in size from microscopic capillaries to large vessels. Unlike the circulatory system, however, the lymphatic system is not a closed loop.

Lymph Formation and Flow

Lymph formation begins with fluid that leaks out of blood vessel capillaries, the tiniest blood vessels in the body that connect the smallest arterioles to the smallest venules (**Figure 12.2**). When this fluid is inside the blood vessels, it is called *blood plasma*. When it leaks out and enters the spaces between cells, it is called **interstitial** (in-ter-STISH-al) **fluid**.

The slow but steady trickle of fluid out of the blood vessel capillaries amounts to about 4 liters per day. Because the average adult has only about 3 liters of blood plasma, all of a person's blood plasma would be lost in less than a day, if there were not a way for the fluid to return to the circulatory system.

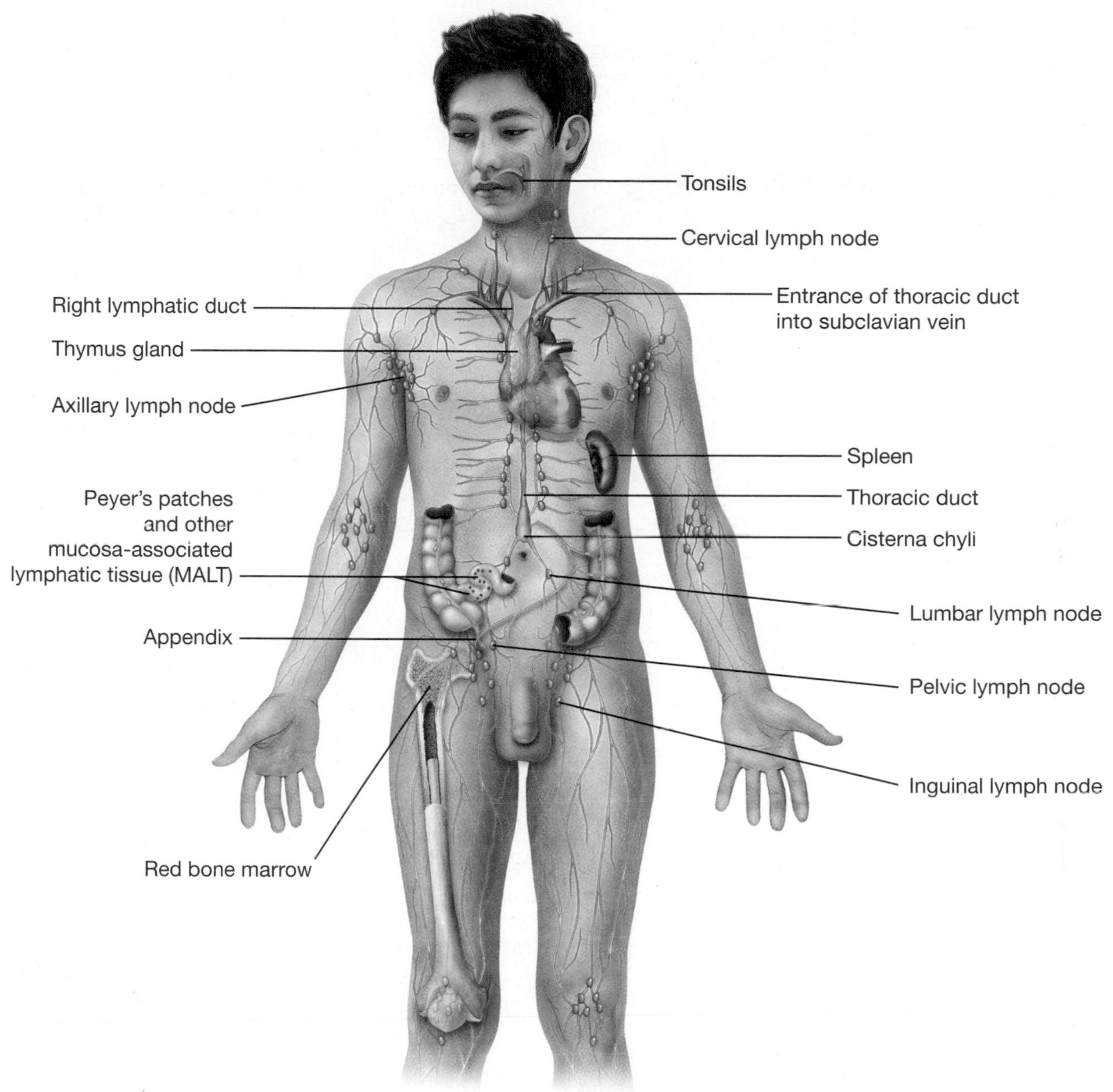

Figure 12.1 The lymphatic system includes lymph, lymphatic vessels, lymphatic cells and tissues, and lymphatic organs. *Is a lymph node an organ?*

MEMORY TIP

The word *lymph* comes from the Latin word *lympha*, which means "water." Most of the time, lymph is a clear fluid that resembles water. However, its composition, produced by a combination of chemical substances, differs throughout the body. When lymph drains from the small intestine, for example, it takes on a milky appearance from the lipids (fats) that it collects as it travels through the small intestine.

As the fluid builds up in the interstitial space, some of it enters the lymphatic capillaries through small gaps between the **endothelial** (ehn-doh-THEE-lee-al) **cells**, which form the walls of the lymphatic capillaries. These endothelial cells overlap and are tethered to one another in a way that makes it easy for fluid to enter the lymphatic capillaries but hard for it to leave. Once the fluid is in the lymphatic capillaries or the larger **lymphatic vessels**, it is called *lymph*.

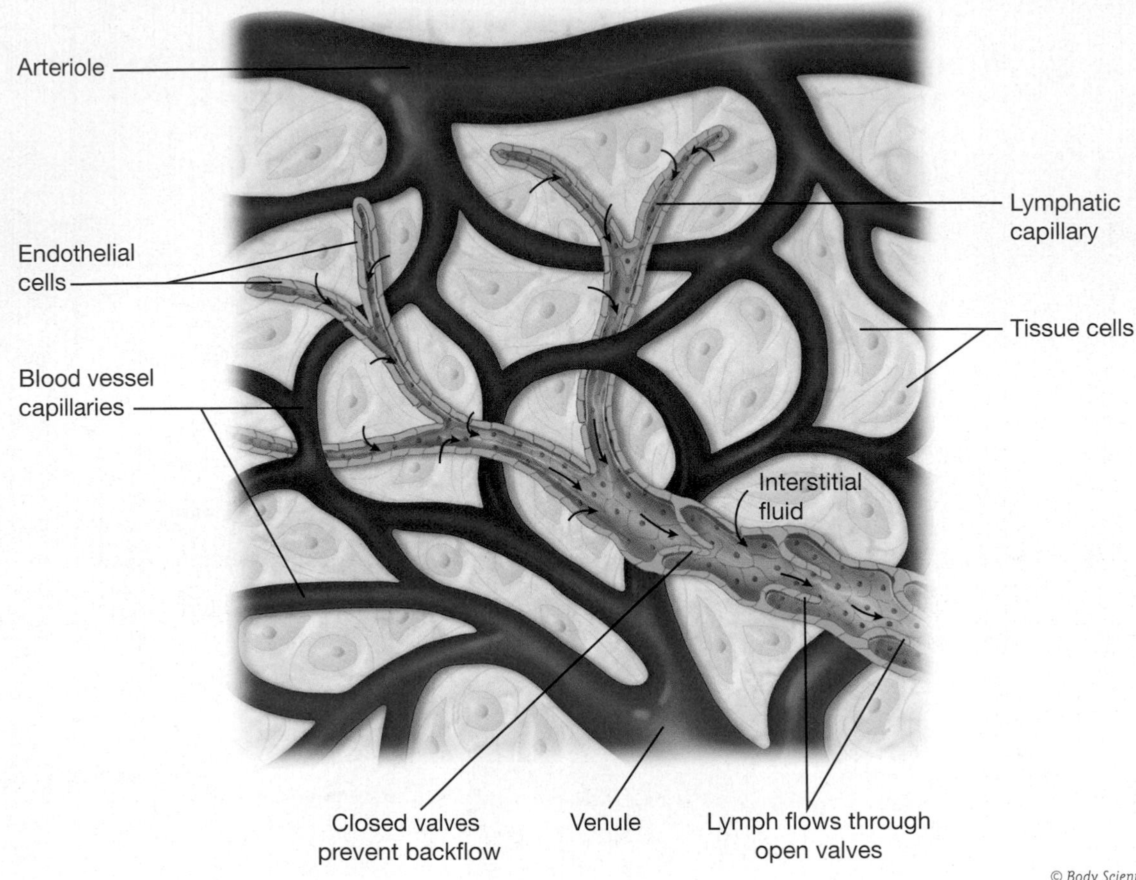

Figure 12.2 Lymph formation and flow. Blood plasma leaks out of blood capillaries and mixes with the interstitial fluid. It then enters lymphatic capillaries. The overlapping endothelial cells of the lymphatic capillaries make it easy for fluid to enter the capillaries but hard to leave. Lymph flows from lymphatic capillaries to progressively larger lymphatic vessels. Lymphatic vessels have internal flaps that act as one-way valves, which prevent lymph from flowing backward to the capillaries.

The lymphatic capillaries join together to form collecting vessels, which in turn link together to form even larger vessels called **lymphatic trunks**. The lymphatic trunks drain lymph from different parts of the body.

The human body does not have a pump similar to the heart to help propel lymph through this network of vessels. However, muscular contractions and movement of organs compress the lymphatic vessels, advancing the lymph along its route. This process is aided by **lymphatic valves**, tissue flaps that act as one-way valves inside the lymphatic vessels. When a lymphatic vessel is compressed by surrounding tissue, the valves allow the lymph to go only in one direction—away from the lymphatic capillaries.

Lymph Drainage

The lymphatic trunks are named for their location and the part of the body they drain. These include the left and right *jugular trunks*, the left and right *subclavian* (sub-KLAY-vee-an) *trunks*, the left and right *bronchomediastinal* (brahn-koh-mee-dee-as-TIGHN-al) *trunks*, the *intestinal trunk*, and the left and right *lumbar trunks*. The two lumbar trunks and the intestinal trunk converge at the **cisterna chyli** (sis-TER-na KIGH-ligh), an enlarged chamber located just in front of the vertebral column, at the diaphragm level (**Figure 12.3A**).

The thoracic duct carries lymph superiorly, or upward, from the cisterna chyli. At its superior end, the thoracic duct receives the left jugular, subclavian, and bronchomediastinal trunks. These trunks drain lymph from the head, left arm, and

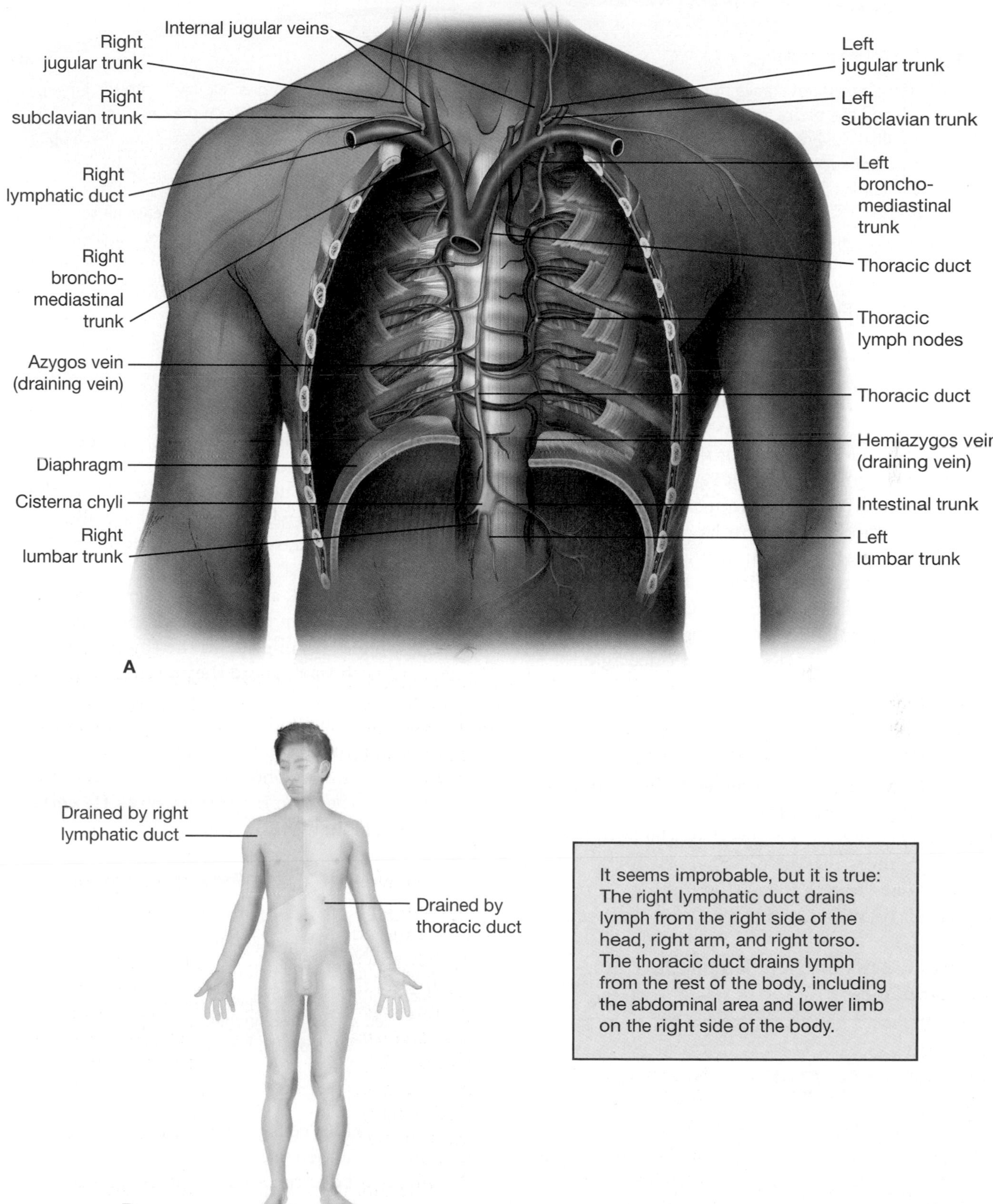

Figure 12.3 A—Locations of the lymphatic ducts and vessels. B—The right lymphatic duct collects lymph from the right jugular, subclavian, and bronchomediastinal trunks and drains into the right subclavian vein. The thoracic duct collects lymph from the left jugular, subclavian, and bronchomediastinal trunks and drains into the left subclavian vein. *How are lymphatic ducts named?*

MEMORY TIP

The term *interstitial* comes from the Latin root word *stat* (stand) and the prefix *inter-* ("between" or "among"). Thus, interstitial fluid occupies the spaces between cells, or the *interstitial space*. Interstitial fluid is also sometimes called *extracellular fluid*, which simply means "fluid outside of cells."

The bronchomediastinal trunks are so named because they receive lymph from the lungs and from the mediastinum, the collection of thoracic organs and tissues between the lungs, including the heart, trachea, esophagus, and thymus. The root word *bronch/o* means "airway" (into the lungs). The word *mediastinum* comes from the Latin word meaning "middle." The organs and tissues that make up the mediastinum lie in the middle of the chest cavity, between the lungs.

The subclavian trunks, veins, and arteries all lie beneath the clavicle, or collarbone. The word *subclavian* comes from the Latin prefix *sub-* ("under") and the Latin word *clavicula* ("little key"). Ancient Roman physicians thought the clavicle resembled a small door key.

left side of the chest and lower neck, respectively (**Figure 12.3B**). Ultimately, the thoracic duct drains into the left subclavian vein.

The right lymphatic duct receives contributions from the right jugular, subclavian, and bronchomediastinal trunks. These trunks drain lymph from the right arm and the right side of the thorax and head (**Figure 12.3B**). The right lymphatic duct drains into the right subclavian vein. Lymph rejoins the blood via the lymphatic duct and the thoracic duct, and it once again becomes blood plasma.

Check Your Understanding

1. What two vital functions does the lymphatic system perform in the body?
2. What other body system does the lymphatic system most resemble? Why?
3. How does lymph formation begin?
4. How is lymph moved throughout the lymphatic vessels?
5. How did the different lymphatic trunks get their names?

Lymphatic Cells, Tissues, and Organs

The lymphatic system is made up of a complex network of cells, tissues, and organs that play a vital role in the body's nonstop battle against invasion by disease-causing agents. This section discusses the structure and function of the lymphatic cells, tissues, and organs.

Lymphatic Cells

Lymphocytes (lymphatic cells) are the distinctive cells of the lymphatic system. Lymphocytes make up about 20% to 30% of the white blood cells in whole blood and are abundant in lymphatic tissues, such as lymph nodes and the spleen.

All lymphocytes, along with other white and red blood cells, begin their lives in bone marrow. Some lymphocytes migrate to the thymus, an organ in the thorax, where they complete their maturation before they move out to the blood and the rest of the body. These lymphocytes are called **T lymphocytes (T cells)**. (The *T* stands for *thymus*.) The lymphocytes that remain in the bone marrow become **B lymphocytes (B cells)** or **natural killer (NK) cells**.

MEMORY TIP

It is helpful to remember that **B** cells mature in **b**one marrow—although their name comes from the fact that they were first discovered in the bursa (a fluid-filled sac involved in joint or muscle movement) of a chicken. Some people like to remember that **B** cells make anti**b**odies.

Natural killer cells play an important role in the nonspecific defense system of the body. They recognize and destroy virus-infected cells and cancer cells. By contrast, B and T cells are the key cells in the specific defense system. For example, B cells provide antibody-mediated immunity. This means that when they are activated, B cells produce antibodies, which are proteins involved in immune function. Antibodies circulate as free proteins in the bloodstream.

T cells include cytotoxic T cells, which provide cell-mediated immunity. They also include helper and suppressor T cells, which regulate the activity of B cells and T cells.

Although they are not lymphocytes, **macrophages** (MAK-roh-fay-jehz) are important cells in lymphatic tissues. They start out as white blood cells called *monocytes*. When a monocyte migrates out of lymphatic circulation into the surrounding tissue, it develops into a macrophage. Macrophages phagocytize (surround and destroy) foreign cells and substances, and they help to activate T lymphocytes.

Lymphatic Tissues

Lymphatic tissue is loose connective tissue that contains many lymphocytes. Lymphatic tissue is present in mucous membranes and certain organs throughout the body. Mucous membranes, which line passageways open to the outside world (including the respiratory, gastrointestinal, urinary, and reproductive tracts), are potential routes of entry for infectious agents. Inside these passageways, **mucosa-associated lymphatic tissue (MALT)** keeps lymphocytes ready and waiting to stop the pathogens (**Figure 12.1**).

The tonsils—small, almond-shaped masses of lymphatic tissue—form a ring of MALT around the pharynx (throat). A single **pharyngeal** (fa-RIN-jee-al) **tonsil** (sometimes called the *adenoid*) lies at the back of the nasopharynx (nay-zoh-FAIR-inks), the part of the throat above the palate, and opens into the nasal cavity. The left and right **palatine** (PAL-uh-tighn) **tonsils** lie at the back of the mouth. The palatine tonsils are the largest and the most commonly infected. The **lingual** (LING-gwal) **tonsils** are located on either side of the base of the tongue.

In some parts of the body, lymphocytes and macrophages form small, localized clusters of dense tissue called **lymphatic nodules**. These nodules develop in areas often exposed to foreign microorganisms and help protect those areas against infection.

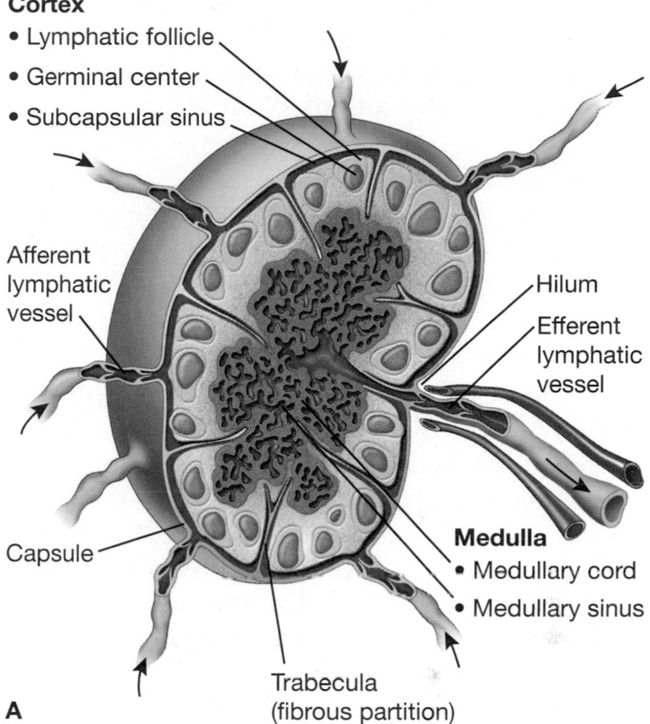

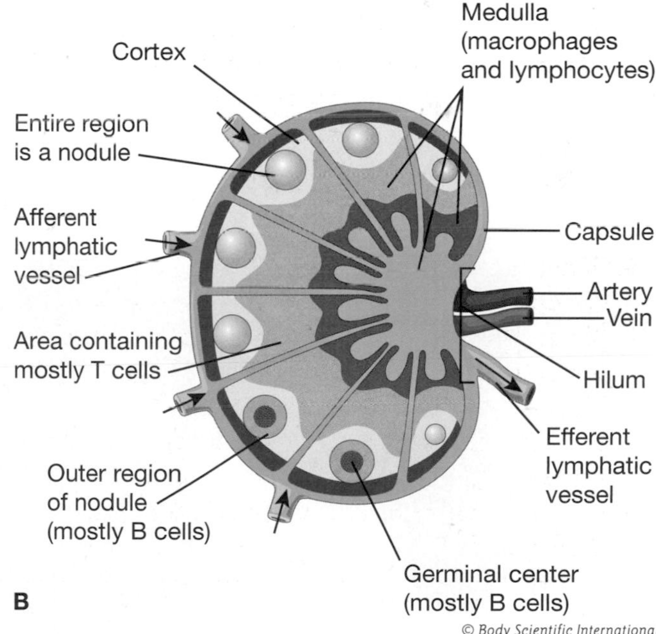

Figure 12.4 Lymph nodes. A—Cross section through a lymph node and associated lymphatic vessels. B—Simplified diagram distinguishing the cortex and medulla of a lymph node. *Do the lymph nodes in your neck become larger or smaller when you have a throat infection? Why?*

Clusters of MALT in the small intestine are called *Peyer's patches*. MALT also protects the appendix, a small, worm-shaped tube at the junction of the large and small intestines.

Lymphatic Organs

The three organs of the lymphatic system are the lymph nodes, spleen, and thymus. This section takes a closer look at each of them.

Lymph Nodes

Small, bean-shaped organs called **lymph nodes** are located along the lymphatic vessels throughout the body (**Figure 12.4**). Lymph nodes serve a dual purpose. They cleanse the lymph by trapping bacteria, viruses, and other harmful substances, which in turn are destroyed by white blood cells. Lymph nodes also store and produce T cells and B cells that help fight infection.

Lymph nodes vary in size from smaller than a pea to the size of a lima bean (0.04 to 1 in., or 1 to 25 mm, in diameter). They have a fibrous capsule and a spongy interior, packed with lymphocytes and macrophages.

Afferent lymphatic vessels carry lymph *into* the lymph nodes. The lymph moves slowly from the cortex, or outer portion of the lymph node, to the deeper medulla.

One or two *efferent lymphatic vessels* emerge from the *hilum* (HIGH-lum), a small indentation on one side of the node, and carry lymph to the next node. Efferent lymphatic vessels carry lymph *away from* the lymph nodes.

Most lymph passes through several lymph nodes on its way from a lymphatic capillary to the subclavian vein. Because lymph flows slowly, foreign particles such as bacteria or viruses are quickly detected. When a foreign particle is detected, it may be "eaten" by a macrophage, or it may activate an immune response.

When an immune response is activated, the lymphocytes quickly multiply, causing the lymph nodes to enlarge. When you have a throat infection, for example, the lymph nodes in your neck may become swollen. If you go to a doctor, she or he will examine your neck for "swollen glands"—a common description for enlarged lymph nodes.

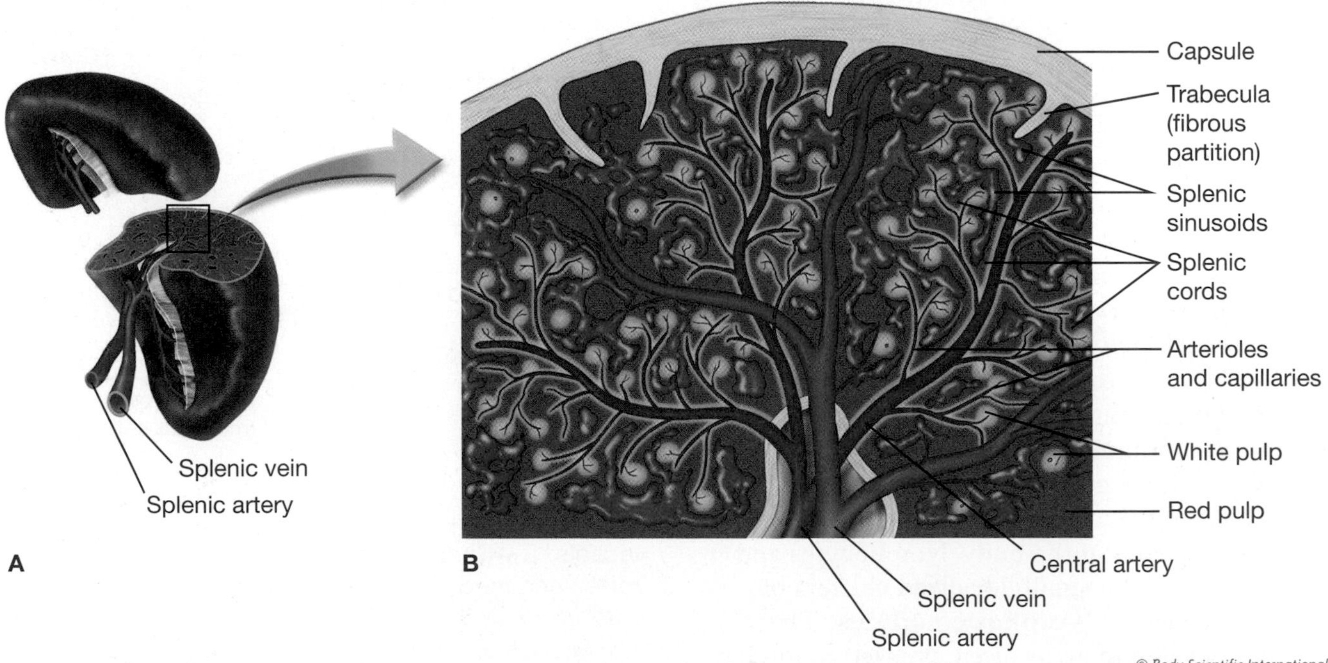

Figure 12.5 A—Diagram of the spleen, anterior view. B—Simplified diagram of the histology (tissue structure) of the spleen. *Explain why you would not want to have your spleen removed even if you knew you could live a normal life without it.*

Spleen

The **spleen**, located in the abdomen below the diaphragm, is the largest lymphatic organ in the human body (**Figure 12.5**). It measures 4 to 5 inches (10 to 12 cm) long and weighs 5 to 7 ounces (150 to 200 g). Its size can vary considerably, even among healthy people. The spleen is located between the stomach and the body wall in the upper left quadrant of the abdomen.

You could say that lymph nodes filter lymph, and the spleen filters blood. There is some truth to this simple statement, although "scan, clean, and, if necessary, activate the immune response" more accurately describes the cleansing process than does the term "filter."

Like a lymph node, the spleen has a thin capsule and a spongy interior. It is dark red due to its large blood supply, which enters and leaves via the splenic artery and vein. The functional tissue inside the spleen contains red pulp and white pulp. The white pulp is rich in lymphocytes, which monitor blood flowing through the spleen for infectious cells and viruses. When cells in the spleen detect an infectious agent, an immune response is activated, and lymphocytes begin to multiply.

Within the red pulp of the spleen, macrophages destroy old, worn-out red blood cells. The macrophages also remove **pathogens**, or disease-causing agents, and old blood platelets from the blood. Like lymph nodes, the spleen often becomes enlarged during an infection.

LIFE SPAN DEVELOPMENT: *The Lymphatic and Immune Systems*

The lymphatic vessels develop from the middle layer, the mesoderm, of the early embryo. Some anatomists in the first half of the 20th century believed that lymphatic vessels developed by budding off of central veins and grew outward toward the periphery. This is known as the *centrifugal hypothesis*. Others argued that many lymphatic vessels first arise in the periphery and grow inward toward the large veins near the heart; this is the *centripetal hypothesis*. More recent studies with newer techniques indicate that both hypotheses about lymphatic vessel development are true.

The thymus is the first lymphoid organ to appear in the embryo, and the first to stop functioning later in life. In childhood, it is the site for the development and maturation of T lymphocytes. The thymus reaches peak size in childhood and starts to atrophy, or shrink, by puberty. By that time, the body has a mature population of T cells that have populated the lymphoid tissues throughout the body. In adults, the thymus is nonfunctional, and the former spaces for lymphoid development have been replaced with a few fat cells.

The specific immune responses of the fetus are suppressed before birth. This is probably beneficial, on the whole, because it reduces the chance of harmful attacks by the infant's immune system on the maternal tissues of the placenta and other structures before birth. This means the newborn immune system's B- and T-cell responses are not fully active. This is one of the reasons why newborns are more susceptible to respiratory and GI infections than older children and healthy adults. The infant immune system is significantly aided by breast-feeding, because breast milk delivers antibodies that help protect the baby.

There is evidence that children in large families, children who live on farms, and children who are exposed to pets and other animals early in life have a reduced risk of developing allergies, asthma, and related immune disorders. This has led to the *hygiene hypothesis*, which states that exposure to a variety of immune stimuli early in life is important for good immune function later in life. This hypothesis is still somewhat controversial and continues to be studied.

Immune function gradually declines as people get older. Older adults are more susceptible to infectious diseases, including pneumonia and influenza, which take a high toll on the elderly. They also do not respond as vigorously as younger adults to vaccination for influenza. Autoimmune disorders are also more common in the elderly. This remains an area of active investigation.

Life Span Review

1. What is the difference between the centrifugal hypothesis and the centripetal hypothesis of lymphatic vessel origin?
2. What is the hygiene hypothesis?

Because the spleen has a thin capsule and a soft interior, it may tear during a traumatic blow to the abdomen. This can happen during contact sports or a motor vehicle accident, for example. It may surprise you to learn that when the spleen has been surgically removed, a person can still lead a normal life, although with increased susceptibility to infection.

MEMORY TIP

A pathogen is a source of disease, such as a virus or bacterium. The word *pathogen* comes from the Greek words *pathos* ("suffering" or "disease") and *genos* ("birth/origin" or "race/kind"). You are perhaps already familiar with many words that share the *path/o* combining form, including *sympathy*, *pathetic*, and *psychopath*. The number of words that share the *gen/o* combining form is practically infinite. Examples include *gene*, *genesis*, *genital*, and *carcinogen*.

What other words containing the *path/o* or *gen/o*-root can you think of?

Thymus

The thymus (THIGH-mus) is a lymphatic organ that extends from the base of the neck downward into the thorax. It lies in front of the heart, trachea, and esophagus (**Figure 12.1**). The thymus is also an endocrine gland. (See Chapter 8.) The thymus is largest during childhood. It slowly but steadily shrinks after puberty.

All lymphocytes first develop in bone marrow from lymphatic stem cells. Some lymphocytes then migrate to the thymus, where they complete their maturation into T cells. Unlike lymph nodes, MALT, and the spleen, the thymus is *not* a site where lymphocytes wait to detect and attack infectious agents. Rather, the thymus functions as a nursery for T cells.

Primary care providers must understand lymphatic organ anatomy in order to do an effective physical examination. A typical physical exam may include palpation (examination by touching) of lymph nodes in the neck, visual examination of the palatine tonsils in the mouth, and palpation of the spleen. Any of these organs may become enlarged and inflamed under certain pathologic conditions.

Check Your Understanding

1. Which two cell type are the "soldiers" of the body's specific defense system?
2. Where are lymphatic tissues found in the body?
3. What two purposes do lymph nodes serve?
4. Where in the body do all lymphocytes first develop?

LESSON 12.1 Review and Assessment

Mini Glossary

Make sure that you know the meaning of each key term.

B lymphocytes (B cells) lymphocytes that mature in the bone marrow before moving out to the blood and the rest of the body; also called *B cells*

cisterna chyli an enlarged lymphatic vessel located just in front of the vertebral column, at the diaphragm level, at which the two lumbar trunks and the intestinal trunk converge

endothelial cells cells that form the walls of lymphatic capillaries; their overlapping structure helps fluid enter the lymphatic capillaries and makes it hard for the fluid to leave

interstitial fluid fluid in the spaces between cells

lingual tonsils two masses of lymphatic tissue that lie on either side of the base of the tongue

lymph clear, transparent, sometimes faintly yellow fluid that is collected from tissues throughout the body and flows in the lymphatic vessels

lymph nodes small, bean-shaped structures found along the lymphatic vessels throughout the body

lymphatic nodules small, localized clusters of dense tissue formed by lymphocytes and macrophages

lymphatic trunks large lymphatic vessels that drain lymph from different parts of the body

lymphatic valves tissue flaps that act as one-way valves inside the lymphatic vessels

lymphatic vessels vessels that carry lymph

lymphocytes white blood cells that are abundant in lymphatic tissue

macrophages cells that phagocytize (surround and destroy) foreign cells, such as bacteria and viruses

mucosa-associated lymphatic tissue (MALT) lymphatic tissue found in mucous membranes that line passageways open to the outside world; these include the respiratory, gastrointestinal, urinary, and reproductive tracts

natural killer (NK) cells lymphocytes that play an important role in the nonspecific defense system of the body by killing virus-infected cells and cancer cells

palatine tonsils two masses of lymphatic tissue that lie in the back of the mouth, on the left and right sides; the largest and most commonly infected tonsils

pathogens disease-causing agents

pharyngeal tonsil lymphatic tissue that lies at the back of the nasopharynx, the part of the throat above the palate, and opens into the nasal cavity; commonly called the *adenoid*

spleen the largest lymphatic organ in the body, located in the abdomen below the diaphragm; filters blood and activates an immune response if necessary

T lymphocytes (T cells) lymphocytes that complete their maturation in the thymus before they move out to the blood and the rest of the body; also called *T cells*

Know and Understand

1. Explain the role the lymphatic system plays in maintaining blood pressure.
2. List the differences among lymphatic fluid, blood plasma, and interstitial fluid.
3. Identify the type of cells that form the walls of the lymphatic capillaries.
4. Identify the point at which blood plasma becomes lymph.
5. List the lymphatic trunks and identify the parts of the body in which they are located.
6. Distinguish between T lymphocytes and B lymphocytes.
7. What are lymphatic nodules?

Analyze and Apply

8. In a sense, the lymphatic system is a plumber and a soldier. Which role do you think is more important? Build a case to support your choice.
9. Explain why lymphatic fluid, which usually has a clear color, takes on a milky appearance when it has drained from the small intestine.
10. Summarize the process by which lymphatic fluid moves through the lymphatic system.

IN THE LAB

11. In some ways, the lymphatic system is similar to the cardiovascular system. Create simple models of both systems that clearly show one or two of the major differences between these two systems.
12. Create your own figure of the human body. Label the lymphatic trunks and identify the organs associated with each trunk:
    A. Left and right jugular trunks
    B. Left and right subclavian trunks
    C. Left and right bronchomediastinal trunks
    D. Intestinal trunk
    E. Left and right lumbar trunks
13. Create a poster to demonstrate your understanding of a pathogen and how it works, as well as how the lymphatic system responds to a pathogen. Do research beyond the text. Be creative and give credit for any borrowed work.

LESSON 12.2 Nonspecific Defenses

Before You Read

Try to answer the following questions before you read this lesson.

- What are phagocytes, and what role do they play in the defense systems of the body?
- Why does inflammation occur in the body? What important purpose does it serve?

Lesson Objectives

- Describe the microbial and other challenges that humans face from disease-causing organisms.
- Describe the physical barriers that help protect humans from disease-causing organisms.
- Explain the components of the cellular and chemical defenses against disease.
- Describe the inflammatory response and explain its purpose.
- Explain what happens during a fever.

Key Terms

alternative pathway
chain of infection
classical pathway
complement proteins
complement system
exocytosis
fever
germ theory of disease
inflammatory response
interferons
mast cells
monocytes
neutrophils
opsonins
phagocytes
phagocytosis
prostaglandins
pyrogens

You have seen how the lymphatic system works to keep fluids in balance and to activate immune responses against foreign substances. This lesson examines the challenges people face and the body's arsenal of defense against diseases that do *not* involve recognition of the precise identity of pathogens. These defensive systems of the body include physical barriers, cellular and chemical defenses, inflammation, and fever.

Microbial and Other Disease-Causing Challenges

Humans share the world with organisms that can cause disease. These include both microorganisms and organisms that may be large enough to see with the naked eye. Microorganisms that can cause disease in humans include bacteria, fungi, and viruses. The **germ theory of disease** is the theory, which is now proven beyond doubt, that microscopic organisms can cause disease in humans.

Bacteria

Bacteria are single-celled *prokaryotic* (proh-kayr-ee-AH-tik) *organisms*, or prokaryotes. Prokaryotes are generally a few microns in size, which makes them smaller than most human cells, but large enough to be seen using a light microscope. Unlike a human cell, a prokaryotic cell does not have a nucleus with a membrane around it, and it does not have mitochondria or endoplasmic reticulum or Golgi apparatus or other membranous structures inside the cell.

There are many ways of classifying bacteria. One way is to see whether a chemical stain called *Gram stain* sticks to them or not. Some bacteria have a single-layered cell membrane, and Gram stain does not stick to them, so they are called *gram-negative* (**Figure 12.6**). Other bacteria have an outer and an inner cell membrane. Gram stain sticks to them, so they are called *gram-positive*. This distinction is clinically important, because some

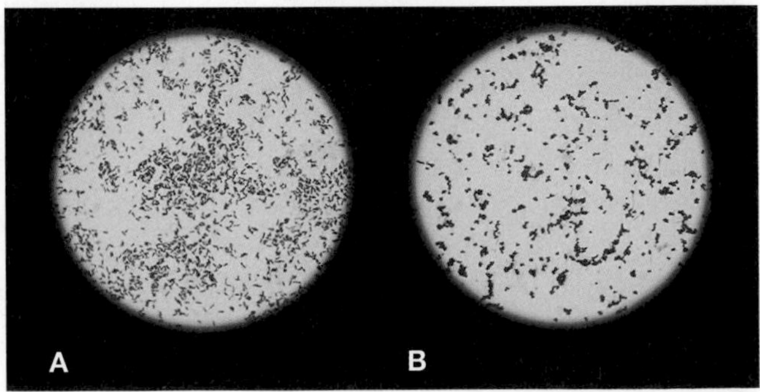

toeytoey/Shutterstock.com

Figure 12.6. A—Gram-negative bacteria. B—Gram-positive bacteria.

antibiotic drugs, including penicillin, work against gram-positive organisms, not against gram-negative organisms. Examples of gram-positive bacteria include the *Streptococcus* and *Staphylococcus* families, which cause "strep" and "staph" infections. Gram-negative bacteria include the *E. coli* and *Salmonella* families. An adult human has more bacterial cells than human cells: 40 trillion versus 30 trillion, according to recent estimates. However, the great majority of bacteria in and on humans live in the colon, and usually do not cause disease.

Drugs that kill bacteria are called *antibiotics*. The profound differences between prokaryotes, including bacteria, and human cells makes it possible to find drugs that kill bacteria without killing human body cells. This does not mean that antibiotics are harmless. Antibiotics can, and often do, kill beneficial bacteria that live inside the human body. This can disrupt gastrointestinal function and cause other problems.

Fungi

Fungi (singular: *fungus*) are a class of *eukaryotic* (yoo-kar-ee-AH-tik) *organisms*. Eukaryotic cells have a nucleus with a membrane. They may have other membrane-bound organelles, such as mitochondria. They are more complex, and almost always larger, than bacteria. Plants, animals, and humans are also eukaryotic organisms.

The fungi of greatest importance in human healthcare are the *Candida* family, which are a kind of yeast. They can cause infections in the gastro-intestinal tract, the reproductive tract, the skin, and elsewhere. Antibiotics, which kill bacteria, generally do not affect fungi. In fact, antibiotics can increase the risk of a yeast infection. When antibiotics kill beneficial bacteria, *Candida* can multiply more easily. Because human cells and fungi are both eukaryotic, many drugs that kill fungi can also harm human cells. This is why there are fewer good antifungal drugs than antibiotics. It is also why most antifungal drugs are applied on the surface of the body, rather than being taken internally as pills.

Viruses

Viruses are very different from bacteria and fungi. They are not cells. They are packages of protein, nucleic acids, and sometimes lipids. They are too small to see using a light microscope. Viruses can only reproduce inside of living cells. A virus enters a host cell and uses the enzymes, nutrient molecules, and energy of the host cell to make copies of itself. The copies of the virus are released by lysing the host cell (which immediately destroys the host cell) or by budding, which allows the host cell to live somewhat longer. The unique biology of viruses means that unique drugs are needed to eliminate them.

Other Threats

Not all human infectious diseases are caused by microorganisms. Multicellular organisms, especially roundworms and tapeworms, are a major source of illness, disability, and death, especially in low-income countries in the tropics. These organisms, collectively referred to as *helminthic parasites*, reproduce in, and cause illness in, humans. They spread through contaminated water and by other means. Drug therapy for infected individuals and improvements in public health, especially in water quality, can reduce the health burden of helminthic diseases.

Chain of Infection

The **chain of infection** is a useful concept for understanding how infectious diseases spread. The chain begins with the infectious organism. The infectious agent lives in a reservoir, which could be a human, another animal, or the environment. The organism leaves the reservoir through an exit portal. A mode of transmission carries the infectious agent from the exit portal to the next entry portal. For example, a mosquito carrying blood from an infected host is the mode of transmission for malaria. Contaminated water is the mode of transmission for many infectious diseases. The organism then uses an entry portal to gain access to a susceptible host. The mouth, or a cut on the skin, could be an entry portal.

The chain of infection concept is the basis for approaches to infection control. Breaking one or more of the links in the chain of infection stops the infection from spreading. *Standard precautions* are steps that healthcare workers should take with all of their patients to help prevent the spread of infections. These precautions include, but are not limited to, good hand hygiene, using personal protective equipment such as gloves and eye protection when appropriate, and disposing of needles and other contaminated equipment safely.

Check Your Understanding

1. What three types of microorganisms can cause disease in humans?
2. In what significant way are viruses different from bacteria and fungi?
3. List in order the links in the chain of infection.
4. What are standard precautions?

Physical Barriers

The defense against infectious agents begins with physical barriers to their entry. The skin is quite effective as a barrier, as long as it is intact (**Figure 12.7**). Its outer layer, the epidermis, is a stratified squamous epithelium. That is, the epithelial, or surface, cells of the skin are flattened (squamous) and arranged in layers (stratified). The protein keratin, a major constituent of hair and nails, fills the flattened keratinocytes (keratinized cells) in the top layer of the epidermis. This keratin layer is flexible, strong, and hard to penetrate, due in part to the desmosomes (DEHZ-moh-sohmz) that bind the deeper epithelial cells together.

Hair on the skin provides additional protection from chafing, sunburn, and insects. The acidic secretions of sweat glands and sebaceous glands (which produce sebum, a fatty lubricating substance) contain toxic chemicals that thwart bacterial growth. When the integrity of your skin is breached—by cuts or punctures, for example—you are at a much greater risk for infection. Burns also compromise—and can destroy—the protective function of the skin. For this reason, patients with serious burns are at a high risk for infection.

As stated in the previous lesson, protective mucous membranes line the respiratory, digestive, urinary, and reproductive tracts. Such protective linings are important because these tracts are open to the outside world and are therefore vulnerable to invasion. The mucus they secrete

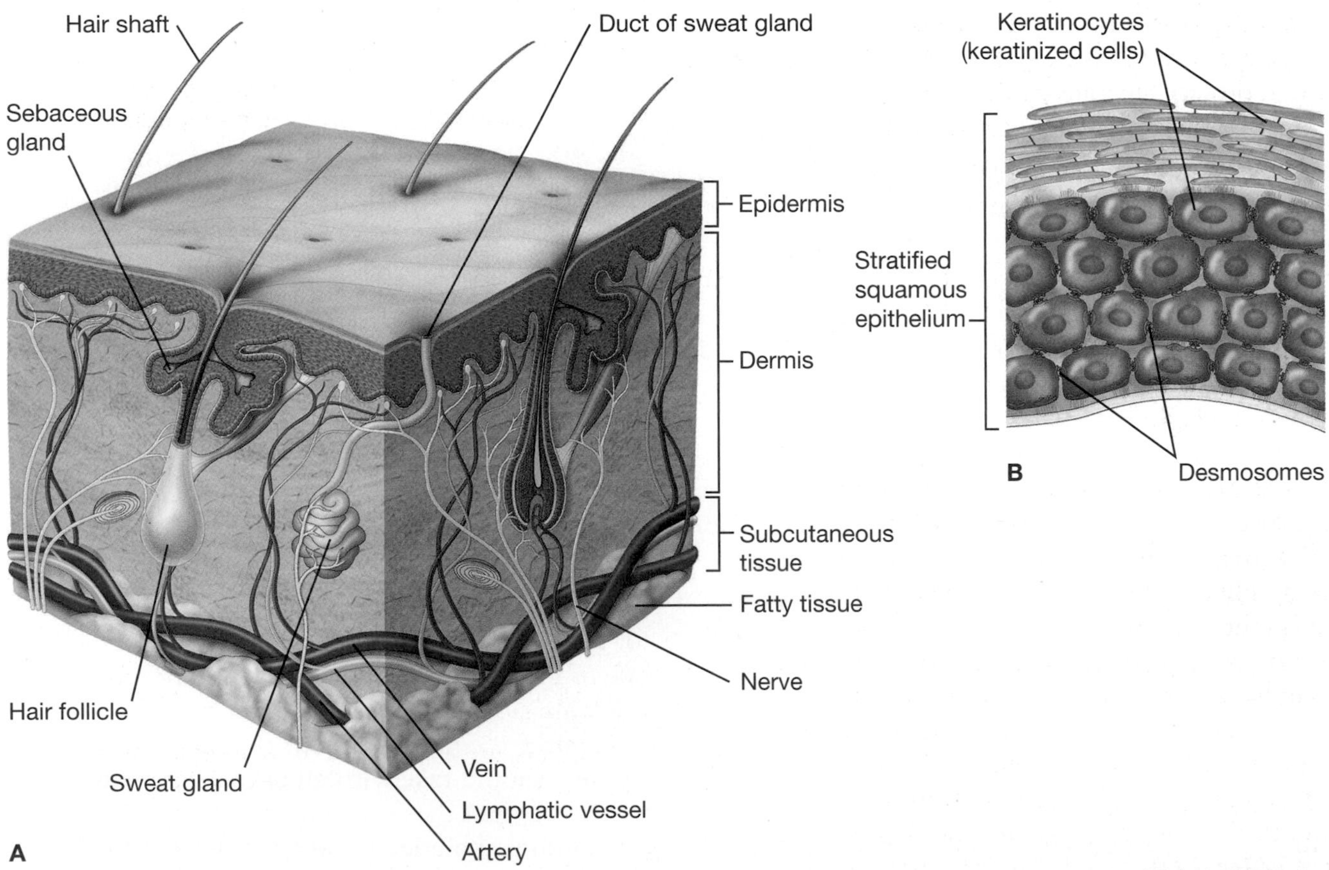

Figure 12.7 A—The skin and its structures help protect the body by serving as physical barriers against infectious agents. B—A layer of flattened cells filled with keratin, and deeper cells connected by desmosomes, make the skin strong and tough. Hair and the secretions of sweat glands and sebaceous glands provide additional protection. *When is the skin not an effective barrier to infectious agents?*

forms a sticky layer that can trap microorganisms. Underlying mucosa-associated lymphatic tissue increases the chances that the microorganisms will be quickly recognized and destroyed.

The cells in the mucous membranes of the respiratory tract contain cilia, tiny hair-like structures that continually sweep the mucus upward to the throat, where it is swallowed. Bacteria caught in the respiratory mucus are then likely to be destroyed in the acidic environment of the stomach.

Check Your Understanding

1. What role do physical defenses play in keeping the body healthy?
2. What protein makes the epidermis flexible, strong, and hard to penetrate?

Cellular and Chemical Defenses

If pathogens penetrate the physical barriers, they face an array of cellular and chemical defenses. Within these defense systems, cells such as **phagocytes** (FAYG-oh-sights) and NK cells work hard to protect the body against foreign invaders. In addition, interferons and antimicrobial complement proteins act as chemical defenders against pathogens.

Each of these defense systems prevents or fights infection in its own way. These systems also interact to produce an inflammatory response. The inflammatory response is important because it speeds up tissue repair and boosts the body's ability to fight infection.

Phagocytosis

The process by which cells engulf and destroy foreign matter and cellular debris is called **phagocytosis** (Figure 12.8). Phagocytosis begins when a phagocyte recognizes its target and binds to it.

For example, **neutrophils** (NOO-troh-filz), the most common type of leukocytes (LOO-koh-sights), or white blood cells, can slip out of capillaries and into surrounding tissue. There they phagocytize (FAY-goh-sigh-tighz) bacteria and cellular debris. Some **monocytes**, another class of leukocytes, develop into macrophages when they leave the bloodstream and enter tissues to phagocytize pathogens.

How does phagocytosis work? The phagocyte wraps its cytoplasm (the membrane surrounding the cell nucleus) around the target and encloses it in a membrane-bound compartment. This compartment protects the cell from damaging itself with the chemicals that it uses to destroy the engulfed material.

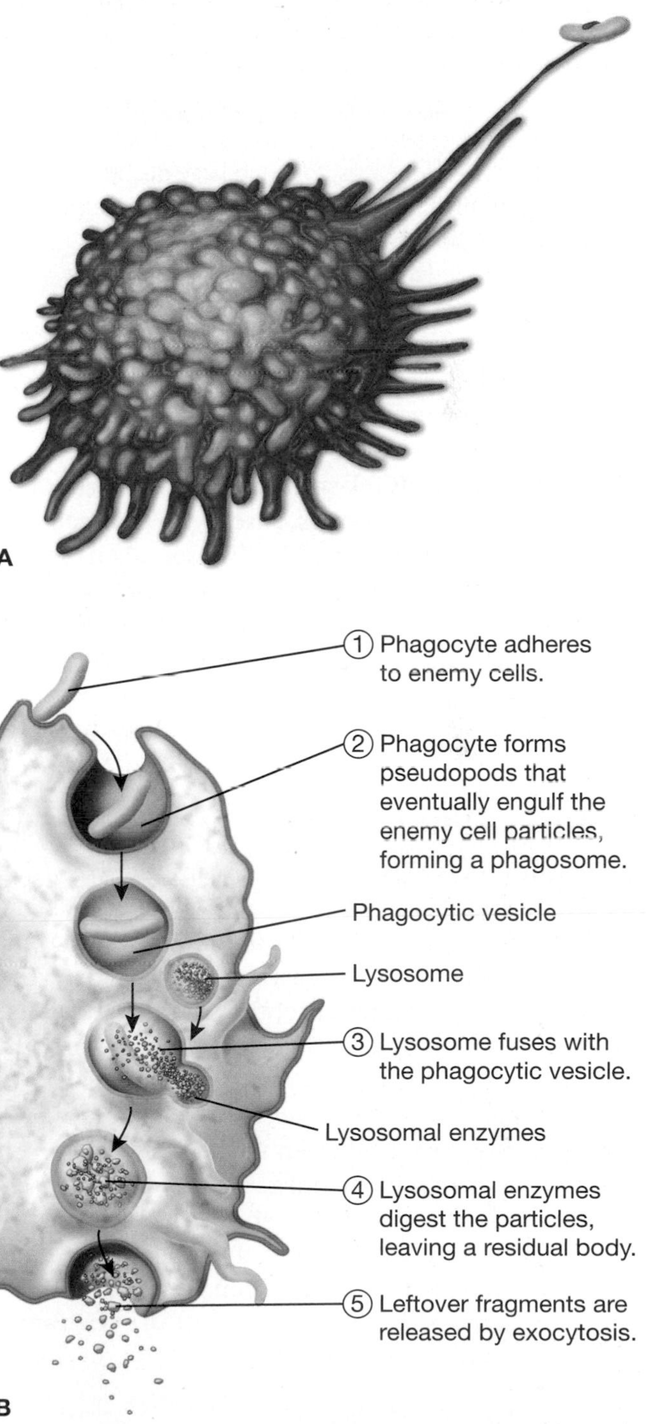
A
B
1 Phagocyte adheres to enemy cells.
2 Phagocyte forms pseudopods that eventually engulf the enemy cell particles, forming a phagosome.
Phagocytic vesicle
Lysosome
3 Lysosome fuses with the phagocytic vesicle.
Lysosomal enzymes
4 Lysosomal enzymes digest the particles, leaving a residual body.
5 Leftover fragments are released by exocytosis.
© Body Scientific International

Figure 12.8 A—Illustration of a phagocyte (purple) extending its cytoplasm to engulf a bacterium (yellow). B—The events of phagocytosis. *In your own words, describe what happens during phagocytosis.*

MEMORY TIP

A leukocyte is any white blood cell in the body. The word *leukocyte* comes from the combining form *leuk/o-* ("white") and the suffix *-cyte* ("cell").

The word *phagocyte* gets its name from the combining form *phag/o-* ("eat" or "swallow") and the suffix *-cyte*. Phagocytes "eat" foreign cells and debris in the body. Thus, the word *macrophage*, made up of the prefix *macro-* ("large") and the combining form *phag/o-*, literally means "big eater." This makes sense when you consider that macrophages, found in large quantities in the spleen, tonsils, and lymph nodes, act as the main phagocytes of the immune system.

The word *inflammation* is a combination of the prefix *in-* ("on" or "in") and the Latin word *flamma* ("flame" or "fire"). So, when you suffer inflammation from an injury or illness, you might feel as though a part of your body is "on fire."

A lysosome (LIGH-soh-zohm), which contains acid and lysosomal enzymes, fuses with the material engulfed by the phagocyte. The lysosomal enzymes and acid usually destroy the target material, and the debris is released from the cell through **exocytosis** (ehk-soh-sigh-TOH-sis). Exocytosis is a process in which the cell membranes fuse together and then push the debris from the cell vesicles to the outside of the cell.

Natural Killer Cells

Natural killer (NK) cells are lymphocytes that recognize and destroy abnormal body cells. Virus-infected cells and cancer cells often display unusual proteins on their surface, or they fail to display the usual proteins. In either case, they attract NK cells.

NK cells bind to cells that appear abnormal. The NK cells then release *perforins* (PER-for-inz)—proteins that destroy target cells—by exocytosis into the narrow space between the cells. The perforins embed themselves in the target cell membrane and self-assemble into doughnut-shaped pores. This process causes perforations in the target cell. The target cell, now full of holes, soon dies. Cytotoxic T cells (discussed in the next lesson) use the same technique to kill their targets.

Complement System

The **complement system** is a set of more than 30 proteins that circulate in the blood plasma through the body and work together to destroy foreign substances. The complement system is so named because it *complements*, or balances out, the effects of antibodies.

The complement system can be activated in two primary ways: via the **classical pathway** or the **alternative pathway**. The route to the classical pathway begins when one of the circulating **complement proteins**, usually inactive, recognizes antibodies bound to a target. The complement protein does not seek any particular antibody; any bound antibody will activate the complement protein. The activated protein kicks off a cascade of complement-protein activation.

The alternative pathway is initiated when another circulating, normally inactive complement protein recognizes foreign materials, such as bacterial cell walls. The classical and alternative pathways converge at complement protein C3. Activation of either pathway causes C3 to split into C3a and C3b (**Figure 12.9**). C3b sticks to target cells and makes them more attractive to phagocytes. Proteins that make cells more attractive to phagocytes are called **opsonins** (AHP-soh-ninz). The process of making cells attractive to phagocytes is called *opsonization*.

Antibodies can also act as opsonins. C3a and another complement protein, C5a, cause **mast cells**, a type of cell found in connective tissue, to release histamine, a compound that activates an inflammatory response. (Mast cells and the inflammatory response will be discussed in more detail in the next section.) Additional proteins in the complement cascade are converted from inactive to active form. Once activated, complement proteins insert themselves into the bacterial cell membrane and form a *membrane attack complex* (*MAC*), which creates a large, lethal hole in the cell membrane. The process by which complement proteins penetrate the cell membrane is similar to the way in which perforin molecules, produced by NK cells, make holes in their targets.

Interferons

A virus, unlike a bacterium, is not a cell. A virus is tiny, even when compared with the smallest bacterium. In short, a virus is a little bundle of nucleic acids with a protein coat. Because a virus cannot reproduce itself, it enters a cell and takes over the intracellular machinery. This process enables the virus to make many copies of itself. When the newly reproduced copies of the virus are released, they invade nearby cells. Thus, an infection is borne and spread.

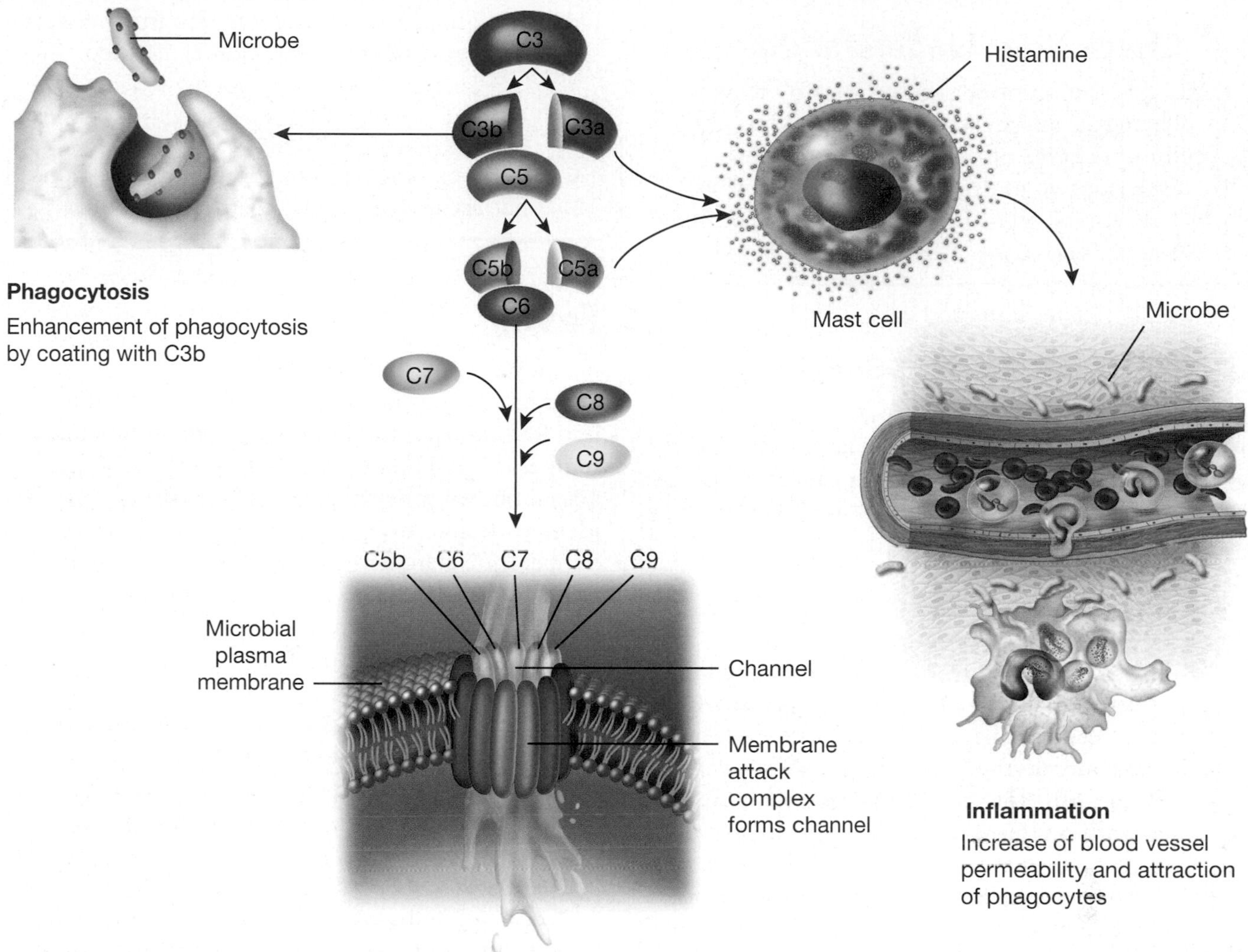

Figure 12.9 The classical and alternative pathways converge at the complement protein identified as C3. Activation of either pathway causes the protein to split. The proteins then attack bacteria or viruses in different ways.

Interferons (in-ter-FEER-ahnz) are proteins released by cells that have been infected with viruses. Interferons are so named because they interfere with viral replication and spreading. They do not help the already-infected cells. They do, however, help neighboring cells to resist viral infection.

There are several classes of interferons, and each class has multiple members. *Alpha interferons* are produced by virus-infected leukocytes. *Beta interferons* are produced by virus-infected fibroblasts (connective tissue cells). Both types of interferons can bind to receptors on neighboring cells, causing those cells to express proteins that slow down protein synthesis and hinder the reproduction of viral particles. *Gamma interferons* are produced by NK cells and T cells that have been activated by detection of foreign materials. Gamma interferons help macrophages resist viral infection and attack virus-infected cells more quickly.

Because interferons help block protein synthesis, they tend to hinder cell growth and division, including the rapid growth and division of cancer cells. When interferons were first discovered, the scientific community held high hopes that these antiviral proteins would be able to halt or cure many types of cancer. Although these hopes have not been fully realized, interferons have turned out to be useful therapeutic agents for treating certain diseases, including hepatitis C, some forms of leukemia (a cancerous disease of the white blood cells), and certain types of lymphoma (cancer that affects lymphatic tissue).

Check Your Understanding

1. What is the name for the process by which cells engulf and destroy foreign matter and cellular debris?
2. Name the two main complement pathways.
3. What do NK cells and MACs have in common?
4. What are the three classes of interferons?

Inflammatory Response

The **inflammatory response**, also called *inflammation*, occurs when tissues have been injured by bacteria, toxins, trauma, or other causes. Although inflammation often is uncomfortable, its purpose is to promote the repair of damaged tissue.

Key steps in the inflammatory response are illustrated in **Figure 12.10**. When cells are damaged, they release proteins and chemicals that are usually stored within the cells. The appearance of these unusual chemicals in the interstitial fluid causes mast cells in the area to *degranulate*. This means that the mast cells release their intracellular stores of histamine granules, **prostaglandins** (PRAHS-ta-glan-dinz), and other chemicals.

Histamine and the other chemicals attract phagocytes and lymphocytes to the injured or diseased area, make the capillaries more permeable, and cause the arterioles to dilate. The phagocytes consume cellular debris and pathogens. Increased permeability causes more capillary fluid leakage, which increases interstitial fluid volume and tissue swelling.

The increased permeability of the capillaries allows clotting proteins to move from the blood into the tissues, where they are activated to form a clot. The stretching of tissue from swelling, and the direct effect of histamine on nerve fibers, causes pain. The dilation of arterioles in the affected region causes more blood to flow to that region, which produces redness and localized warming, or heat. Heat, redness, swelling, and pain are the signs of inflammation.

The chemical processes involved in the inflammatory response cause an increase in local temperature, which boosts the metabolic rate of cells in the area. The accompanying increase in blood flow means that plenty of nutrients will be available for repair processes. You have probably noticed that when you experience swelling and pain from an injury or infection, you instinctively protect the part of your body that is affected.

Check Your Understanding

1. What event causes the inflammatory response?
2. What are the four signs of inflammation?

Fever

Fever is the maintenance of body temperature at a higher-than-normal level. Neurons in the hypothalamus of the brain work to regulate body temperature. The neurons in this area compare actual body temperature to its "set point," the ideal or desired body temperature. If the actual temperature is higher or lower than the set point, the hypothalamic neurons send commands throughout the body to make adjustments that will bring the temperature to the desired level.

If the body is warmer than the desired temperature, sweat glands are activated and blood flow is redirected toward the skin to help dissipate heat. If the body is cooler than the desired temperature, blood flow to the skin and extremities is reduced to minimize heat loss. If the reduction in blood flow does not fix the problem, shivering begins.

Think of temperature control in a building, which works similarly: a thermostat compares the actual temperature to the set-point temperature. If the building is colder than desired, the thermostat turns on the heater. If the building is too warm, the thermostat turns on the air conditioner.

As you probably know, the normal set point for body temperature is about 98.6°F (37°C). But activation of leukocytes and macrophages can cause the cells to release **pyrogens** (PIGH-roh-jehnz), chemicals that raise the set-point temperature of the neurons in the hypothalamus. The hypothalamic neurons then cause reflex adjustments that raise body temperature. The increase in temperature boosts the rate of biochemical reactions in cells by about 10% for every 1.8°F (1°C) rise in temperature.

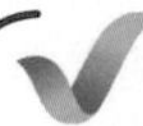

Check Your Understanding

1. In which part of the brain do neurons work to regulate body temperature?
2. What body temperature is considered "normal"?

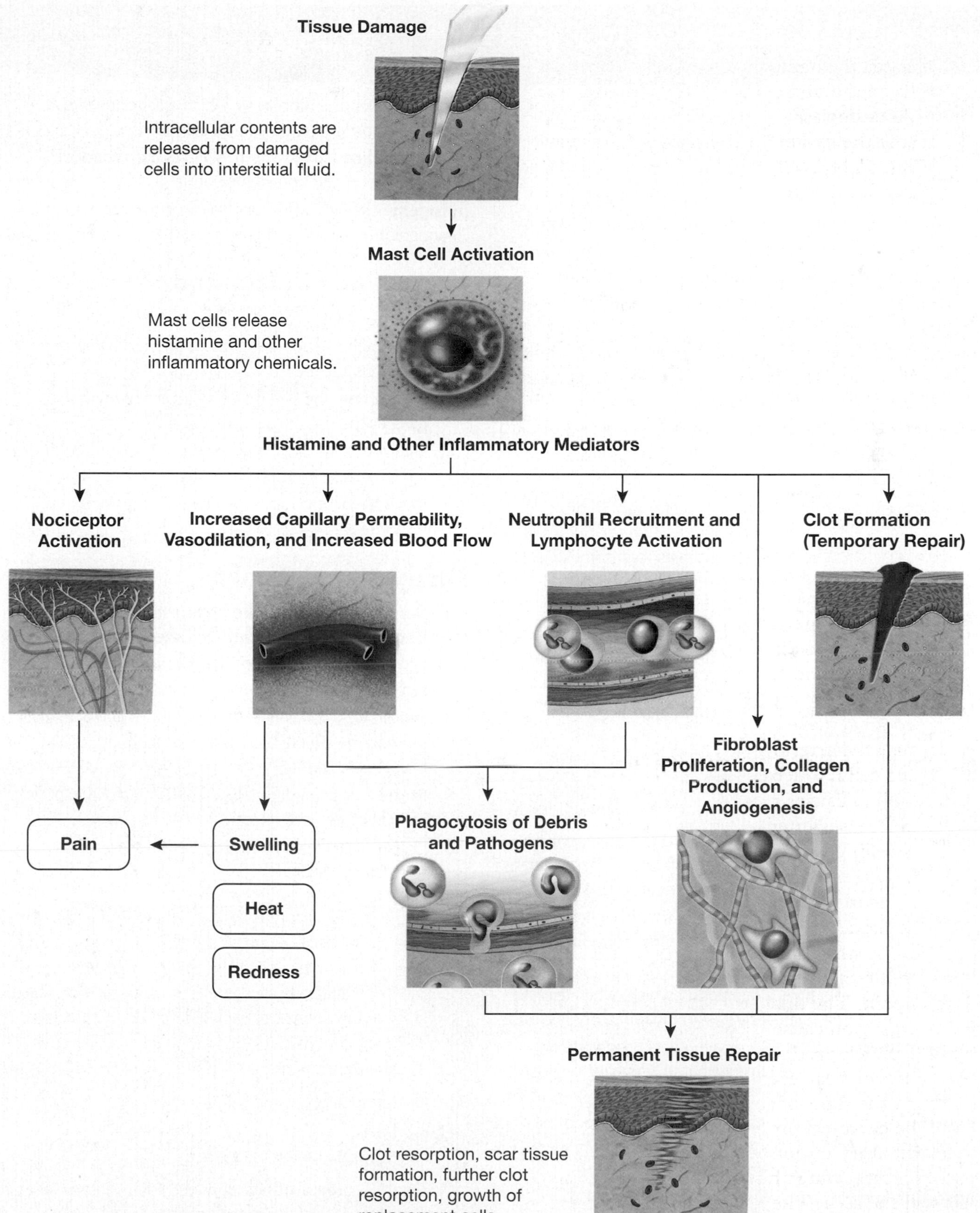

Figure 12.10 The development of inflammation. The hallmarks of inflammation are heat, redness, swelling, and pain. *What important purpose does inflammation serve in the body?*

LESSON 12.2 Review and Assessment

Mini Glossary

Make sure that you know the meaning of each key term.

alternative pathway one of the two primary ways in which the complement system can be activated; this pathway is triggered when the C3b complement protein binds to foreign material

chain of infection the disease process for infections, starting with the causative pathogen and ending with the actual infection

classical pathway a mode of complement system activation in which a circulating complement protein recognizes an antibody bound to foreign material

complement proteins proteins in the blood that work with immune system cells and antibodies to defend the body against infection

complement system a system of more than 30 proteins that circulate in the blood plasma through the body and work together to destroy foreign substances; complements, or balances out, the specific and nonspecific defense systems of the body

exocytosis the process in which cell membranes fuse together and then push debris from the cell vesicles to the outside of the cell

fever the maintenance of body temperature at a higher-than-normal level

germ theory of disease the well-proven theory that microscopic organisms, or "germs," can cause disease in humans

inflammatory response physiological response to tissue injury or infection, also called *inflammation*; the four signs of inflammation are heat, redness, swelling, and pain

interferons proteins released by cells that have been infected with viruses; interfere with virus reproduction

mast cells connective tissue cell with granules (particles) that contain histamine, a compound which, when released into surrounding fluid, activates an inflammatory response

monocytes leukocytes that develop into phagocytizing macrophages when they migrate out of lymphatic circulation into surrounding tissue

neutrophils the most common type of white blood cell; can slip out of capillaries and into surrounding tissue, where they destroy bacteria and cellular debris

opsonins proteins that make cells more attractive to phagocytes

phagocytes cells that engulf and consume bacteria, foreign material, and debris

phagocytosis the process by which a cell engulfs and destroys foreign matter and cellular debris

prostaglandins fatty acids involved in the control of inflammation and body temperature

pyrogens chemicals that tend to cause fever by raising the set-point temperature of the neurons in the hypothalamus

Know and Understand

1. Name two examples of gram-positive bacteria.
2. Describe how the skin acts as a physical barrier against infectious agents.
3. Explain how the skin thwarts bacterial growth and reduces the risk of infection.
4. Summarize the process by which cells engulf and destroy foreign matter and cellular debris.
5. Describe the role of histamine in the inflammatory response.

Analyze and Apply

6. Describe in detail the two primary ways in which the complement system can be activated.
7. Explain how an infection caused by a virus develops and spreads. Be sure to include the characteristics of a virus.
8. Explain why someone with an injury or illness might say that the affected part of his or her body feels as though it is "on fire."
9. Create a diagram depicting the inflammatory response; include causes and effects.
10. Consider the chain of infection. Name at least five ways to break the chain.

IN THE LAB

11. Using any materials available, make a model of each of the following structures associated with the lymphatic system. Be sure to include a detailed description of each structure.
    A. Neutrophil
    B. Monocyte
    C. Lysosome
    D. Natural killer cell
12. Create a cartoon that explains the inflammatory process. Make it obvious who each character is. Your cartoon should be both accurate and creative. Use a large piece of poster board so you can show plenty of detail. Create an appropriate slogan for your cartoon.

LESSON 12.3 Specific Defenses

Before You Read

Try to answer the following questions before you read this lesson.

- Why is the specific immune system also called the adaptive immune system?
- What is an antibody, and what function does it serve?

Lesson Objectives

- Explain the differences between humoral immunity (antibody-mediated immunity) and cellular immunity (cell-mediated immunity).
- Describe the role of antigen-presenting cells (APCs) in immune system function.
- Define the term *antibody* and explain its role in the specific defense system of the body.
- Explain the difference between the primary and secondary immune responses.

Key Terms

active immunity
antigenic determinants
antigen-presenting cells (APCs)
apoptosis
cellular immunity
clonal selection
humoral immunity
immune system
immunoglobulins
interleukins
major histocompatibility complex (MHC) glycoproteins
memory cells
passive immunity
precipitation
primary immune response
secondary immune response
severe combined immune deficiency (SCID)

Of the human body's defenses against disease, its specific defense systems are the most remarkable and complicated. The cells and chemicals that contribute to these specific defenses make up the **immune system**. The *specific immune system* is also called the *adaptive immune system*. These terms are used because the immune system is highly specific in its responses to foreign substances. It is able to recognize new challenges, adapt to those challenges, and "remember" what it has learned. The lymphatic organs and tissues are the physical "home" of the immune system.

As with many body functions, people do not notice or appreciate the immune system as it works. The immune system is constantly finding, targeting, and eliminating bacteria and viruses. It even kills the body's own cells when they show signs of infection or cancerous development.

Patients with a compromised immune system are susceptible to diseases that never trouble people with a normal immune system. For example, babies born with **severe combined immune deficiency (SCID)**, a genetic immune system deficiency, have a tragically poor prognosis unless they receive a successful bone marrow transplant. SCID, also known as the "bubble boy disease," gained global attention in the 1970s with news reports of David Vetter, a boy with SCID who had to live in a sterile, plastic bubble to avoid contact with bacteria and viruses. An infection that is minor for a person with a healthy immune system is potentially fatal for a person with SCID (**Figure 12.11**).

The many cells and chemicals of the immune system interact with one another in complex ways that are still not completely understood. This complexity makes the immune system challenging to study. Scientists do, however, know a great deal about this fascinating system.

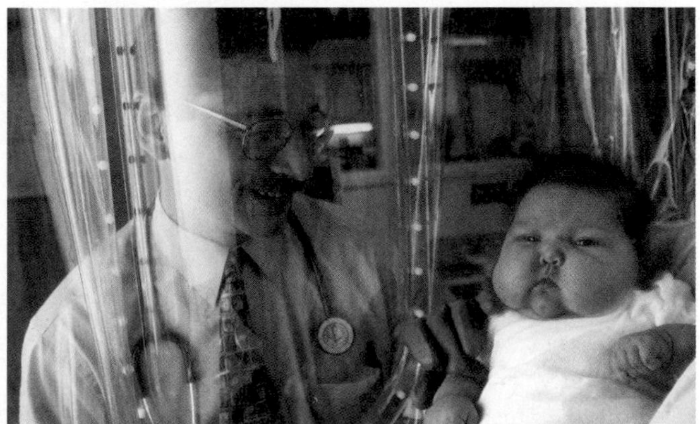

Peter Menzel/Science Source

Figure 12.11 Severe combined immune deficiency (SCID) results in a poor prognosis unless the patient receives a bone marrow transplant that is successful.

Antigens

Antigens, as explained in Chapter 10, are large molecules, such as proteins, polysaccharides, glycolipids, or nucleic acids, on the surface of cells. Antigens identify cells as either "self" or "nonself" cells, thereby making it possible for the body to distinguish between its own cells and any nonself, or foreign, cells. This makes it possible for the immune system to recognize foreign cells and respond, which it does by producing antibodies that bind to and mark the foreign antigens. The foreign antigens may be parts of bacteria, viruses, or abnormal cells, but they are not necessarily pathogens. For example, substances that people are allergic to are foreign antigens, but they are not pathogens.

A single complex antigen molecule can have multiple foreign parts, or **antigenic determinants**. Larger molecules, especially proteins, are more likely to provoke an immune response than small ones because they have more antigenic determinants.

The antigens on the surfaces of the body's own cells (the "self" antigens described above) do *not* provoke an immune response. Why not? Because any immature lymphocytes that *do* respond to "self" molecules are killed off early in the development process.

Check Your Understanding

1. What is an antigen?
2. Why are larger antigen molecules more likely to provoke an immune response than smaller ones?

Immune System Cells

You read earlier that lymphocytes are the signature cells of the immune system. Other cells, such as **antigen-presenting cells (APCs)**, are also essential for proper immune function. Macrophages, dendritic cells (immune system cells in the skin and lymphatic organs), and B cells all can act as APCs (**Figure 12.12**).

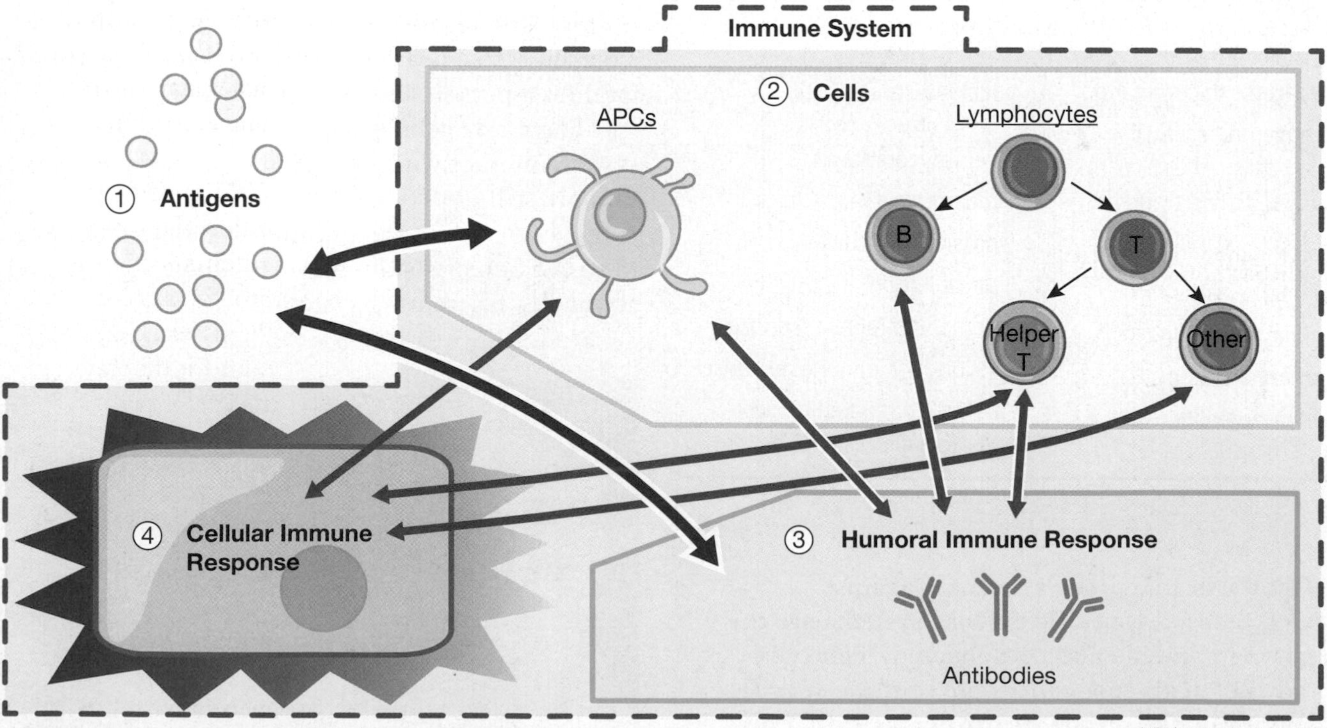

Figure 12.12 Diagram of the immune system. Helper T cells play a significant role in both the humoral and cellular immune responses. Other T cells are associated mainly with the cellular response. B cells are associated with the humoral response. APCs (antigen-presenting cells) are involved in both types of responses. *In general, how do humoral and cellular responses differ from the immunity provided by interferons or inflammation?*

Lymphocytes

Remember from Lesson 12.1 that lymphocytes initially develop from stem cells in red bone marrow. Some travel to the *t*hymus to complete their maturation; these are called *T* (for *thymus*) *lymphocytes*. Some lymphocytes complete their maturation in *b*one marrow; these are called *B lymphocytes*.

All lymphocytes go through a screening process. If, during the screening process, a lymphocyte responds to the body's self-antigens as foreign matter, which it is not supposed to do, it undergoes **apoptosis** (ap-ahp-TOH-sis). Apoptosis, a programmed process of cellular self-destruction, ensures that the surviving lymphocytes do not attack the body's own tissues. This weeding-out process does not always work with 100% success. When it does not work perfectly, autoimmune disease, in which the immune system attacks the body's own tissue, can result. Immune disorders are described in Lesson 12.4.

Each lymphocyte has many antigen receptors in its membrane. All the receptors in a lymphocyte membrane recognize one—and only one—type of antigen. The human body has millions of lymphocytes, and each one recognizes a particular antigen. So, you can see why this lesson is entitled "Specific Defenses."

Once the lymphocytes have matured, they travel throughout the blood to all parts of the body. Some lymphocytes circulate continuously while others "settle down" in lymph nodes, the spleen, or other lymphatic tissues.

Over the course of a lifetime, only a fraction of the lymphocytes will ever encounter the antigen that binds to their particular antigen receptors. Lymphocytes that do not meet their antigen remain *quiescent*, or inactive.

When a lymphocyte does meet its antigen, the binding of the antigen to the antigen receptor stimulates the lymphocyte to *differentiate*, or divide repeatedly, making many copies of itself. Each copy is an exact genetic duplicate, or clone, of the original cell that was stimulated. This process is called **clonal selection**.

Most of the clones produced by lymphocytic differentiation become short-lived effector cells that fight an infectious invader. A few of the clones become **memory cells** that reside in lymphatic tissues, ready to respond if the same antigen reinvades the body.

MHC Proteins

For an immune response to be activated, it is not enough for antigens to be present—the antigens must be presented in a particular way. Antigens are displayed on the surfaces of cells by **major histocompatibility complex (MHC) glycoproteins**, or MHC proteins.

There are two main classes of MHC proteins. Class I MHC proteins are found on the surfaces of *all* cells that contain nuclei. Class II MHC proteins are found only on the surfaces of antigen-presenting cells (APCs) and lymphocytes.

Class I MHC proteins, which are found on cell surfaces, display fragments of the many different proteins found inside the cells. This means that a normal body cell displays normal protein fragments (*self-antigens*) on its surface. When the immune system is working properly, passing lymphocytes ignore these self-antigens.

Just as class I MHC proteins display fragments of normal proteins, they display fragments of abnormal, undesirable proteins that might be inside the cell. So, if a cell is infected or cancerous, it displays parts of the infectious agent, or cancer-related proteins, on its surface.

When a passing cytotoxic T (T_C) cell "sees" a cell that displays an unfamiliar antigen (for example, cancer-related proteins) on a class I MHC protein, it goes into "attack" mode. As **Figure 12.13** shows, an APC internalizes and breaks down a foreign particle, and it displays on its surface the particle fragments of class II MHC proteins.

Check Your Understanding

1. Name at least three types of antigen-presenting cells.
2. What are MHC proteins, and how many classes are there?
3. What has to happen to prevent a lymphocyte from being characterized as *inactive*?

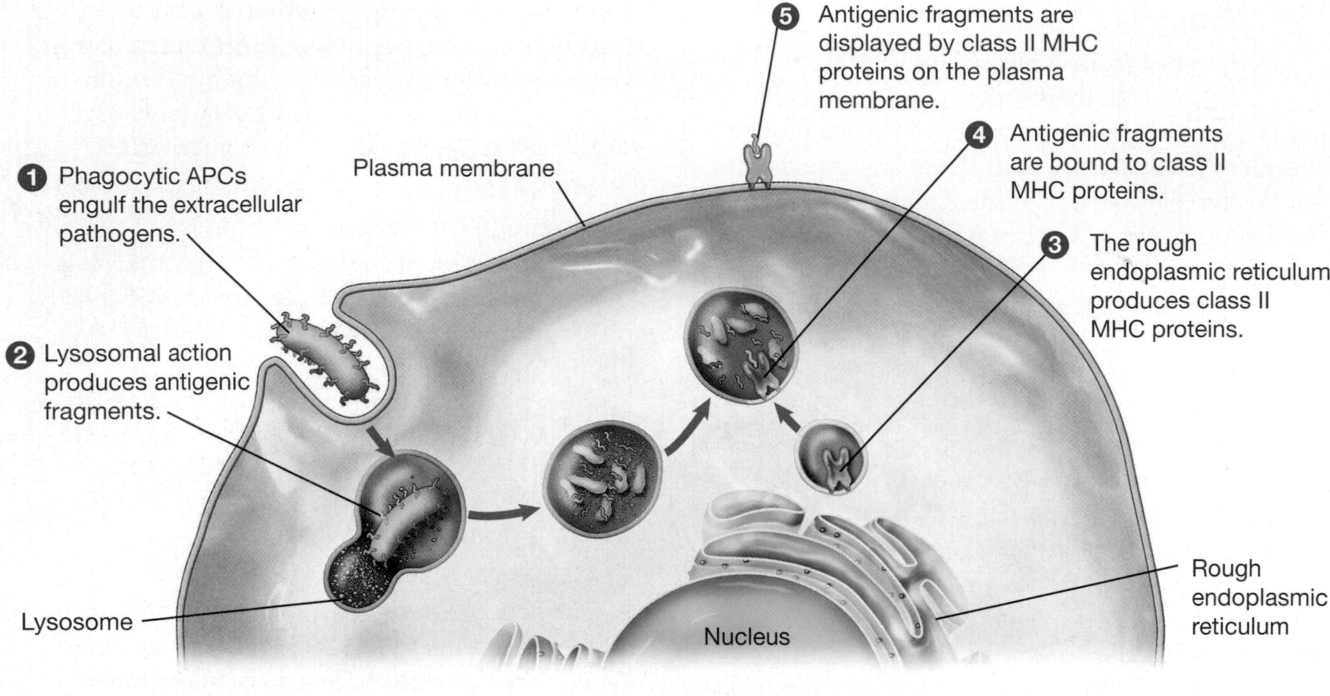

5 Antigenic fragments are displayed by class II MHC proteins on the plasma membrane.
4 Antigenic fragments are bound to class II MHC proteins.
1 Phagocytic APCs engulf the extracellular pathogens.
Plasma membrane
3 The rough endoplasmic reticulum produces class II MHC proteins.
2 Lysosomal action produces antigenic fragments.
Rough endoplasmic reticulum
Lysosome
Nucleus
Phagocytic Cell
© Body Scientific International

Figure 12.13 Diagram of antigen presentation by an antigen-presenting cell. Antigen-presenting cells (APCs) use class II MHC proteins to display fragments of foreign molecules (antigens) on their surface. (1) The process begins when the APC phagocytizes the foreign object, such as a bacterium. (2) A lysosome, which contains digestive enzymes, fuses with the engulfed object and breaks it down into many pieces. (3) Meanwhile, the cell is also producing class II MHC proteins packaged in vesicles. (4) A vesicle containing class II MHC proteins fuses with the vesicle containing digested antigenic fragments. (5) These digested fragments bind to the class II MHC proteins, which are then displayed on the cell membrane.

Humoral Immunity

Humoral immunity, also called *antibody-mediated immunity*, is effective against pathogens located outside of cells—such as extracellular viruses, bacteria, and bacterial toxins. Humoral immunity begins when a B cell encounters the antigen that binds to its antigen receptors. During this encounter, the B cell undergoes clonal selection, as described previously. The B cell divides repeatedly, making many copies of itself.

B cell reproduction is most strongly activated when the B cell, with an antigen bound to it, presents the antigen to a helper T cell that also has a receptor for that antigen. When the helper T cell detects presentation of an antigen by a B cell, it releases **interleukins** (IN-ter-loo-kinz), chemicals that stimulate an immune response. The interleukins fully activate the B cell by binding to it.

Plasma Cells

Some of the daughter cells produced by clonal selection become memory helper B cells, but most become plasma cells. The plasma cells have a cytoplasm full of rough endoplasmic reticulum (RER), a membranous network that is involved in protein synthesis.

In plasma cells, large quantities of antibodies are made in the RER and are secreted into the interstitial fluid. The antibodies made by the plasma cell "recognize" and bind to the same antigen that stimulated the original B cell. Thus, the clonal selection process for B cells produces an army of B cells, all of which make antibodies specifically directed at the invading antigen.

Antibodies

Antibodies are proteins that recognize particular antigens with great specificity. Antibodies are also called **immunoglobulins** (im-yoo-noh-GLAHB-yoo-linz) because they are involved with immune function and originally were thought of as globular in shape.

An antibody is a Y-shaped protein made up of four polypeptide chains (**Figure 12.14**). The tips of the Y are the parts that can bind to an antigen. The antigen-binding portions have a variable amino acid sequence that determines the antigen's specific target. The variable regions on the two arms of the Y match each other, so that each arm binds to the same antigen. The stem and lower parts of the arms of the Y do not vary; they are the same for all antibodies of a given class.

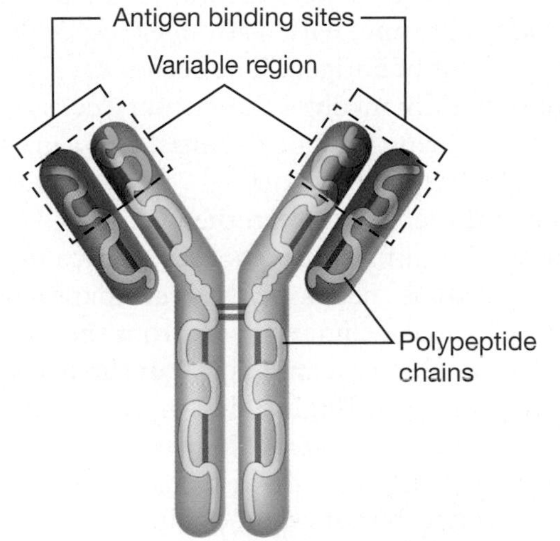

Figure 12.14 An antibody is a Y-shaped protein composed of four polypeptide chains. The tips of the arms of the Y have a variable amino acid sequence and are the sites at which antigens bind.

There are five classes of antibodies, which are described in **Figure 12.15**. Antibodies do not directly destroy antigens. Instead, they interfere with antigen function and mark the antigens for destruction. The formation of an *antigen-antibody complex* can eliminate the threat of an antigen through multiple mechanisms:

- An antibody can neutralize a virus or bacterial toxin (a toxic chemical secreted by a bacterium) by occupying the binding site that the virus or toxin would use to attach to a target cell.
- **Precipitation** causes small, soluble (dissolvable) antigen molecules, rather than whole cells, to clump together. The resulting antigen complexes are too big to remain dissolved in the bloodstream.

IgG	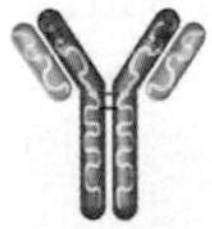	Immunoglobulin G (IgG), the most common type of circulating antibody, provides resistance against many infectious agents.
IgD	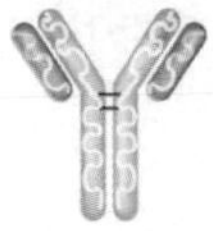	IgD is found in the membranes of B cells, where it forms the antigen receptors on the cell surface.
IgE	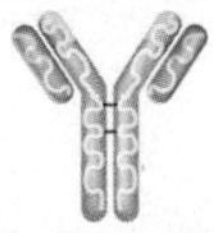	The stem of IgE binds to mast cells and basophils and causes them to release histamine and other chemicals that play roles in inflammation and allergy.
IgA	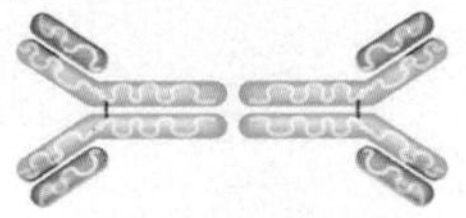	IgA is a dimer (made of two antibody subunits). It is found in secretions such as mucus, saliva, tears, and semen. It binds to antigens when they are still on the "outside" of the body and prevents them from crossing the epithelium and entering the body tissue.
IgM	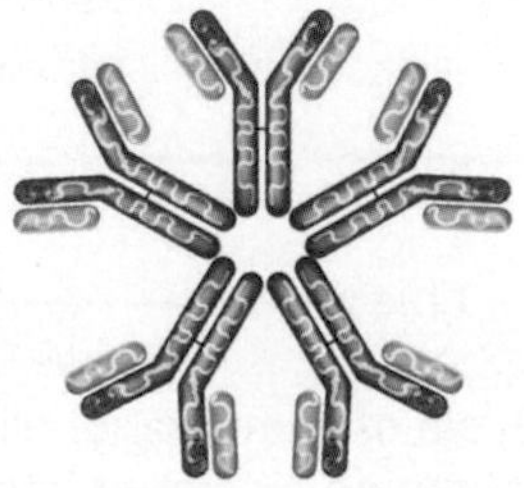	IgM is a pentamer (made of five antibody subunits). It is the first class of antibody secreted by activated B cells. It activates the complement system. Because it has ten binding sites, it is good at causing agglutination, or clumping up, of antigens.

Figure 12.15 Different classes of antibodies.

- Agglutination (a-gloo-ti-NAY-shun) is similar to precipitation, except that the antigens lie on the surface of a cell or virus; thus, the clumping process involves cells, viruses, or bacteria rather than small molecules. See Chapter 10 for more information about agglutination.
- Binding of an antibody to its target causes a slight change in shape along the stem of the Y. Binding sites on the antigen are exposed, activating the complement system. Antibodies and complement proteins on a pathogen make it more appealing to phagocytes.
- Antibody-antigen complexes stimulate inflammation by causing mast cells and basophils (a type of white blood cell) to release histamine and other chemicals.

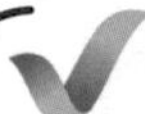

Check Your Understanding

1. What is another name for humoral immunity?
2. What is the functional difference between precipitation and agglutination?

Primary and Secondary Immune Responses

When an antigen enters the body for the first time, the immune system response is neither fast nor widespread. Because memory cells for the new antigen do not yet exist in the body, detection of the threat may take a while. When the threat is detected, the immune system response is limited. However, if the antigen returns, the immune system response will be faster and much stronger.

The **primary immune response** occurs when the body is first exposed to a foreign invader, such as a virus or bacterium. The **secondary immune response** occurs when the virus or bacterium enters the body for a second or subsequent time, with a stronger response to a lesser amount of antigen. The secondary immune response mainly involves the memory cells that developed during the body's initial exposure to the potentially harmful invader.

The difference between the primary and secondary immune responses, shown in **Figure 12.16**, is the reason that vaccination works. The word *vaccine* comes in part from the Latin word *vacca*, which means "cow." In the late 1700s Edward Jenner, an English doctor, noticed that milkmaids were much less likely than other people to contract smallpox, a disease characterized by rash and raised blisters on the skin. At the time it was known that the disease cowpox, which could infect people as well as cows, was similar to smallpox but less severe.

Jenner believed that the exposure of milkmaids to cowpox made them resistant to smallpox. He tested his idea by injecting pus from the blisters of people infected with cowpox into healthy individuals. He then tried to give those healthy individuals smallpox by injecting them with pus from patients infected with smallpox. (Such experiments would be prohibited, with good reason, by the human subjects protection board

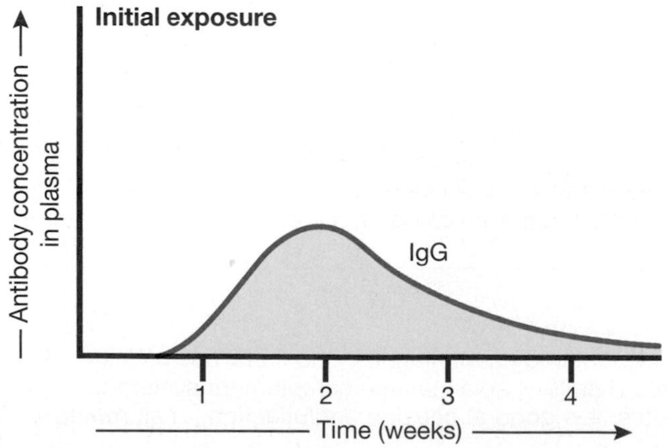

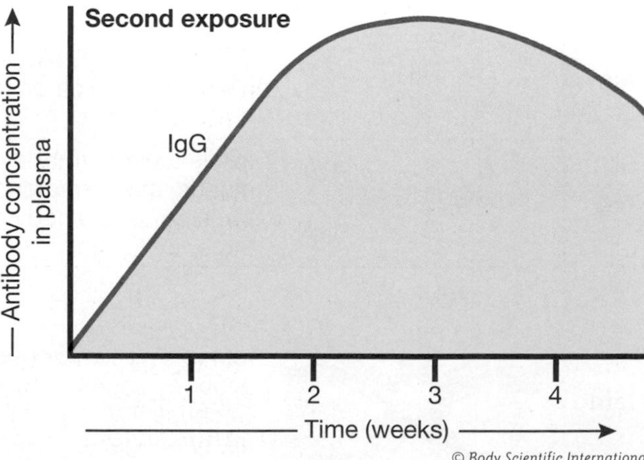

Figure 12.16 Primary and secondary immune responses. These graphs show the levels of immunoglobulin G (the most common antibody) in the blood plasma during an initial infection (left) and during a second infection (right). The response to the second exposure is larger and faster than the response to the first exposure.

of a modern hospital.) Jenner's series of careful experiments showed that a substance in the cowpox pus gave people a long-lasting immunity to smallpox.

The antibody-mediated immunity described earlier is also called **active immunity** because the antibodies are actively produced by the blood plasma cells of the body. **Passive immunity**, by contrast, is antibody-mediated immunity that comes from antibodies received from an outside source. In the case of infants, for example, the outside source of antibodies can be from breast milk, which is rich in antibodies. Another outside source is an injection of antibodies purified from the plasma of a blood donor.

Check Your Understanding

1. Why is a secondary immune response faster than the primary response?
2. What is the difference between active and passive antibody-mediated immunity?

Cellular Immunity

Cellular immunity, or *cell-mediated immunity*, is mediated by (that is, facilitated, or assisted, by) T cells. Cell-mediated immunity is not only mediated by cells; it is also directed at cells. When body cells are infected by a bacterium or virus, or when they become cancerous or precancerous, they display abnormal proteins on their surface. Cells of transplanted tissue also display foreign antigens. If the tissue is not well matched from donor to recipient, it will provoke a cell-mediated immune response.

Figure 12.17 illustrates how the cellular immune response is activated and how a specific T cell is selected for clonal reproduction. The cellular immune response begins when an antigen-presenting cell presents an antigen on its surface with a class II major histocompatibility (MHC) protein (**Figure 12.17A**). The APC encounters a T cell whose receptor matches the antigen. A glycoprotein known as CD4, which is found on the surface of helper T cells, "recognizes" and binds to part of the class II MHC protein on the APC (**Figure 12.17B**). This simultaneous binding of an antigen receptor to an antigen, and of a CD4 protein to a class II MHC protein, is a "double handshake" that activates the helper T cell. The helper T cell then divides rapidly, making many genetically identical copies (clones) of itself.

During the clonal selection process, the rapid cellular division of the helper T cell generates *active helper T cells* and some long-lived *memory helper T cells* (**Figure 12.17C**). An active helper T cell now helps activate another type of T cell: *cytotoxic T cells*, sometimes called *killer T cells*. Cytotoxic T cells have a CD8 glycoprotein that recognizes class I MHC molecules. (Recall that all nucleated cells use class I MHC proteins to display antigens.) When a cytotoxic T cell detects an antigen bound to its antigen receptors, *and* it detects with its CD8 molecule that the antigen is presented by a class I MHC protein, then the cytotoxic T cell is partially activated for clonal selection.

Complete activation of the cytotoxic T cell requires assistance from an activated helper T cell. Once the cytotoxic T cell is fully activated, it divides repeatedly, producing three types of cells: active cytotoxic T cells, memory cytotoxic T cells, and suppressor T cells. Active cytotoxic T cells seek out and destroy antigen-displaying cells that initiated the immune response. Both memory cytotoxic T cells and suppressor T cells prevent the cellular response from being too strong or too long-lasting.

An activated cytotoxic T cell binds to a cell displaying the foreign antigen recognized by that T cell. One way in which the activated cytotoxic T cell kills the target cell is by stimulating intracellular pathways that lead to apoptosis (programmed cell destruction). Another way in which the activated cytotoxic T cell kills the target cell is by releasing perforin molecules. Natural killer (NK) cells also use perforins to kill their targets (refer to Lesson 12.2). Perforin molecules insert themselves into the target cell membrane and assemble to form a relatively large opening, or perforation, in the cell. This large hole is lethal to the target cell.

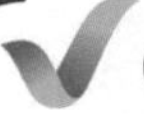

Check Your Understanding

1. What three types of T cells are involved in cell-mediated immunity?
2. What events must occur to activate a T cell for clonal selection?

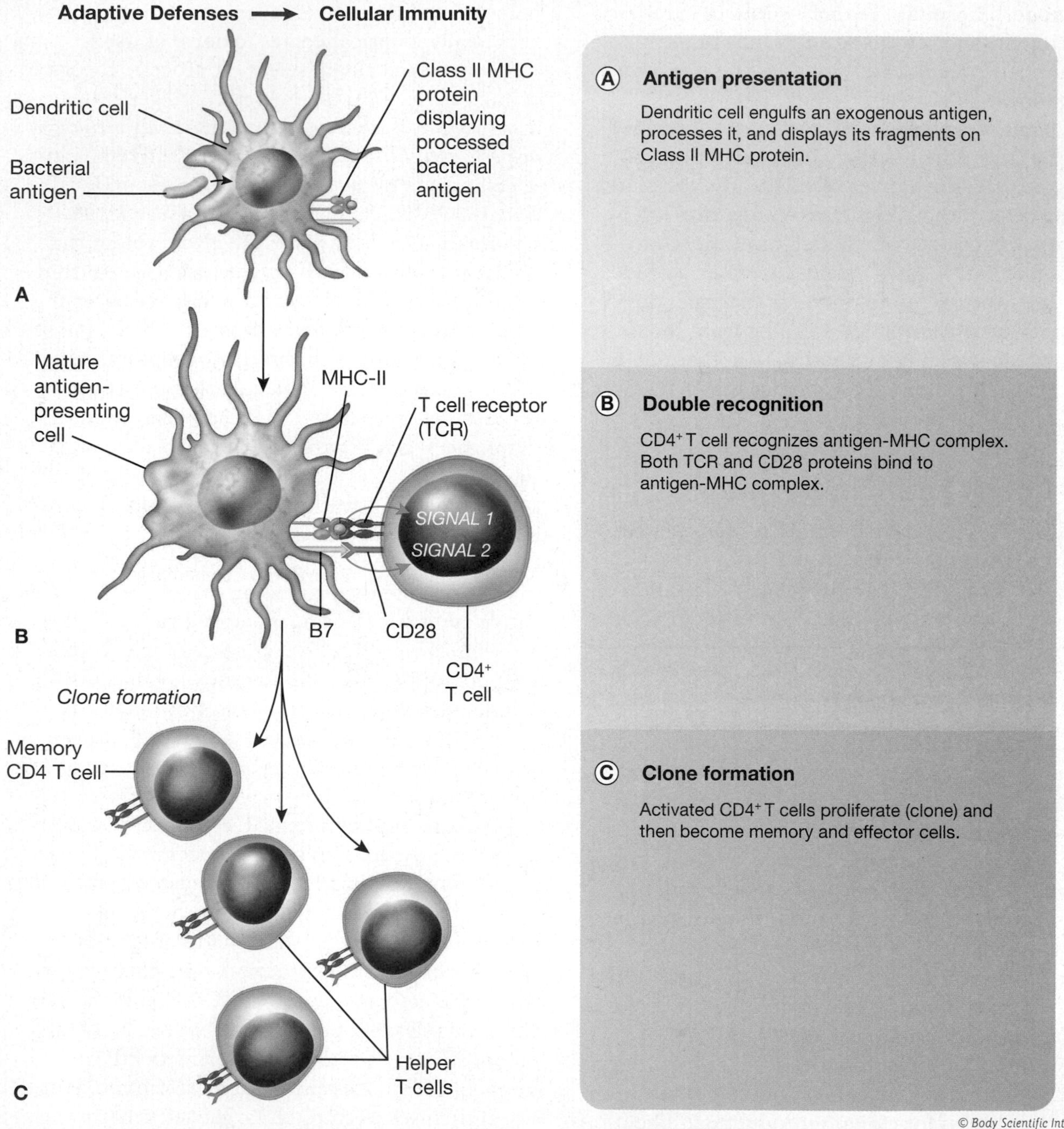

Figure 12.17 Activation and clonal selection of T cells. A—Antigen presentation. B—Double recognition. C—Clone formation.

LESSON 12.3 Review and Assessment

Mini Glossary

Make sure that you know the meaning of each key term.

active immunity immunity in which the blood plasma cells in the body make antibodies as a result of previous exposure to a disease or a vaccine

antigenic determinants the multiple foreign parts on the surface of an antigen molecule that may cause an immune response

antigen-presenting cells (APCs) cells that process protein antigens and present them on their surface in a form that can be recognized by lymphocytes (white blood cells)

apoptosis a programmed process of cellular self-destruction (cell suicide)

cellular immunity immunity that arises from the activation of T lymphocytes (T cells) by antigen-presenting cells; cell-mediated immunity

clonal selection repeated division of a lymphocyte that produces many exact genetic copies (clones) of itself

humoral immunity immunity associated with free antibodies that circulate in the blood; antibody-mediated immunity

immune system the cells and chemicals that contribute to the body's specific defenses against disease

immunoglobulins antibodies; proteins that recognize particular antigens with great specificity

interleukins chemicals released by helper T cells and other cells that stimulate an immune response

major histocompatibility complex glycoproteins (MHCs) family of proteins found on the surfaces of lymphocytes and other cells; help the immune system recognize foreign antigens and ignore "self" tissues

memory cells B lymphocytes and T lymphocytes in lymphatic tissues that can respond if a previously encountered antigen invades the body again

passive immunity immunity that comes from antibodies received from an outside source, such as breast milk

precipitation the formation of an insoluble complex, such as a clump of antigen molecules joined together by antibodies

primary immune response the initial immune system response to a foreign invader such as a virus or bacterium

secondary immune response immune system response to an infectious agent that it has encountered before

severe combined immune deficiency (SCID) a genetic disorder, present at birth, in which both B cell and T cell responses are significantly below normal

Know and Understand

1. Describe the genetic immune system deficiency that is more commonly known as "bubble boy disease."
2. Identify the types of cells that can act as antigen-presenting cells.
3. What is apoptosis?
4. Describe the structure of an antibody.
5. What type of immunity results when purified antibodies are injected from the plasma of a blood donor?

Analyze and Apply

6. Explain why only a fraction of lymphocytes will ever "meet" the antigen that binds to their specific antigen receptor.
7. What is the difference between an antigen and an antibody?
8. Describe the sequence of events that occurs when a lymphocyte meets an antigen.
9. Using the knowledge that you have learned about humoral immunity, list the steps that occur when a B cell undergoes clonal selection.
10. The neuromuscular system develops from head to toe during infancy. If a child is born with a neuromuscular disease, such as cerebral palsy, what symptoms do you think you would see?
11. If a cancer patient were experiencing a cell-mediated immune response, what symptoms would you expect to see?
12. Explain how vaccinations provide immunity.

IN THE LAB

13. After reading Lessons 12.2 and 12.3, you should have a good understanding of the difference between the nonspecific and specific defense systems of the body. Create a model, draw a picture with labels, or write an essay or a story in which you describe something that is protected or defended by both nonspecific and specific defenses. A garden, for example, might have a fence around it to keep out many different kinds of "invaders," yet the gardener might sprinkle snail bait in the garden for the specific purpose of preventing snails from eating his vegetables. Identify as many nonspecific and specific defenses as possible. In your model, picture, or written composition, compare your different defense mechanisms to the corresponding immune defenses studied in Lessons 12.2 and 12.3.
14. Using the internet and your knowledge of the lymphatic system, write a 250-word essay about David Vetter, the "bubble boy." Describe in detail the genetic disease with which he was affected.
15. Many parents are fearful of giving their children vaccines. Because of these fears, the government had to create new laws regarding childhood vaccines in order for children to enter school. Research these laws and create a poster or brochure that would explain the importance of childhood vaccines and the laws regarding them.

LESSON 12.4

Disorders and Diseases of the Immune System

Before You Read

Try to answer the following questions before you read this lesson.

- What causes an allergy?
- What is the difference between the human immunodeficiency virus (HIV) and acquired immunodeficiency syndrome (AIDS)?

Lesson Objectives

- Explain what cancer is and what happens during metastasis.
- Define the term *allergy* and explain the role of an antigen-presenting cell in an allergic response.
- Explain what an autoimmune disorder is and give one example.
- Describe how HIV is related to AIDS.

Key Terms

acquired immunodeficiency syndrome (AIDS)
allergen
allergen immunotherapy
allergy
anaphylaxis
autoimmune disorder
human immunodeficiency virus (HIV)
lymphedema
metastasis
opportunistic infection
tolerance

From allergies to AIDS, many health problems can be linked to a compromised immune system. This section explores some common disorders and diseases of the body's defense systems, along with their mechanisms. The table in **Figure 12.18** summarizes the etiology, prevention, pathology, diagnosis, and treatment of immune system disorders.

Cancer and Lymph Nodes

Cancer is a disease in which the normal control of cell division (mitosis) fails, and a cell starts to divide too fast and without limit. As a solid tumor grows, cancerous cells sometimes

CLINICAL CASE STUDY

Denzel, age 19, is a college freshman. It is February and he is not feeling well. Many of his classmates, including one of his lab partners, have been out sick in recent weeks. He thought about going to the Student Health Clinic for a flu shot before Christmas vacation, but he never got around to it. Now he wonders if he has the flu, and whether a shot could still help. He emails his professors to say he will not make it to classes, and he stays in bed. At noon he decides to go to the Student Health Clinic.

Ms. Tracey, nurse practitioner, sees Denzel. She checks his vital signs: blood pressure 122/78, pulse 96 beats per minute, respiratory rate 20 breaths per minute, temperature 101.3°F (38.5°C). His height and weight are within normal limits. He says he has a pretty bad headache, and his sinuses and his throat hurt. His entire body aches and he feels very tired, even though he has not done much in the last 24 hours. His symptoms started a little less than a day ago. Ms. Tracey listens to his heart and lungs. His heart sounds are normal and he has some wheezing in his lungs. His skin is warm and sweaty. His throat appears mildly inflamed. She collects some mucus from the back of his throat with a swab, for a rapid strep test. A few minutes later, the test comes back negative.

Ms. Tracey does not prescribe any medicine. Denzel lives in a dormitory at school, but his family home is only 40 minutes away. Ms. Tracey recommends that he go home to rest and recover. She recommends plenty of fluids. He can take ibuprofen or acetaminophen for relief of fever and for aches and pains.

Denzel goes home. After three days, he starts to feel better, and he returns to college on the fifth day. He stays healthy for the rest of the school year. As you read this section, try to determine the answers to the following questions.

1. Did Denzel have the flu?
2. Should Denzel get the flu vaccine to help him get better faster?
3. Why did Ms. Tracey *not* prescribe antibiotics or antiviral medication?
4. What was happening in Denzel's body, and in particular with his immune system, as he experienced and recovered from the infection?
5. Why do people need a new flu shot every year?

Diseases and Disorders of the Lymphatic and Immune Systems					
	Etiology	**Prevention**	**Pathology**	**Diagnosis**	**Treatment**
Lymphoma	cancer of lymphoid cells and tissues	none	swollen lymph nodes, fatigue, fever, night sweats, weight loss	physical exam; lymph node biopsy; bone marrow biopsy; blood tests; imaging	watch and wait in early stages; chemotherapy, immunotherapy, radiation therapy; bone marrow transplant
Lymphedema	swelling in one or both arms and/or legs, typically after damage to or removal of lymph nodes	if lymph nodes surgically removed, protect arms and legs from scrapes, heat, cold, injury, tight clothing	aching, tightness, heaviness, swelling of leg or arm; restricted motion; infections	physical exam; imaging tests	no cure, but symptoms treated with light exercise, massage, compression garments
Myalgic encephalomyelitis/ chronic fatigue syndrome (ME/CFS)	extreme physical and mental fatigue	none	extreme, long-lasting fatigue, sore throat, loss of concentration, headache, muscle aches, enlarged lymph nodes	physical exam; biomarker blood test in early development phase	treat symptoms: antidepressants, cognitive therapy, alternative medicine therapies
Measles (rubeola)	viral infection that can be serious or fatal for young children	vaccination	fever, dry cough, runny nose, sore throat, conjunctivitis, skin rash	physical exam; lab tests	post-exposure vaccination, immune serum globulin, medication to reduce fever, vitamin A
Mumps	viral infection that affects salivary glands	vaccination	swollen glands, fever, headache, muscle aches, weakness, fatigue	physical exam; blood tests	none, but recovery is generally spontaneous within 2 weeks
Rubella (German measles)	viral infection that causes a red rash but is not as infectious as rubeola (measles)	vaccination	mild fever, headache, inflamed eyes, enlarged lymph nodes, rash, aching joints	lab tests	bedrest, OTC pain relievers, isolation is advised
Tonsillitis	inflammation of the tonsils	wash hands thoroughly and often; do not share food, drink, dishes, utensils	sore throat, trouble swallowing, swollen tonsil(s)	physical exam; throat swab; blood tests (CBC)	home treatment: rest, fluids, throat lozenges, humidified air, antibiotics, surgical removal of tonsils

Figure 12.18

Goodheart-Willcox Publisher

break free from the tumor and migrate to other areas of the body. The process of cancer spreading from its initial location to another part of the body is called **metastasis** (meh-TAS-ta-sis). A cancer that has spread is said to be *metastatic*.

Metastatic cells can spread by entering a lymphatic vessel and traveling in the lymph to the nearest lymph node. When the cells reach the lymph node, they may get caught in the reticular tissue within the lymph node and continue growing. When some types of cancer have been diagnosed, it is standard for an oncologist (a doctor who specializes in cancer treatment) to get a sample of nearby lymph node tissue to determine whether the cancer has spread. The sample may be obtained by surgically removing one or more lymph nodes or by performing a needle biopsy using a syringe.

If cancer has metastasized to lymph nodes, then more lymph nodes may be removed to reduce the chance of further metastasis. Lymph node removal has risks. The biggest risk is that it disrupts the lymphatic drainage in the affected area of the body. As a result, fluid that leaks out of blood capillaries builds up in the interstitial space, causing tissue swelling and damage. This buildup of extracellular fluid is called **lymphedema** (limf-eh-DEE-ma).

Breast cancer often metastasizes to axillary (underarm) lymph nodes. Removal of axillary lymph nodes increases the risk of lymphedema of the arm—the most common type of lymphedema. Treatment options include a compression sleeve, physical therapy, and carefully designed, light exercise.

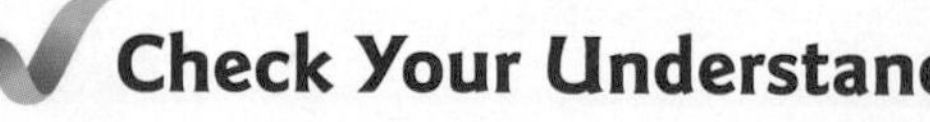

Check Your Understanding

1. How is cancer spread?
2. What is the cause of lymphedema?

Allergies

Do you sneeze, cough, or suffer from itchy, watery eyes when you are exposed to dust, pollen, or animal dander? If so, you are not alone. Some 55% of Americans have an allergy to one or more substances in the environment.

An **allergy** is an inappropriately strong response of the immune system to an environmental antigen, such as dust mites, pet dander, pollen, or certain foods (**Figure 12.19**). In such cases, the antigen is

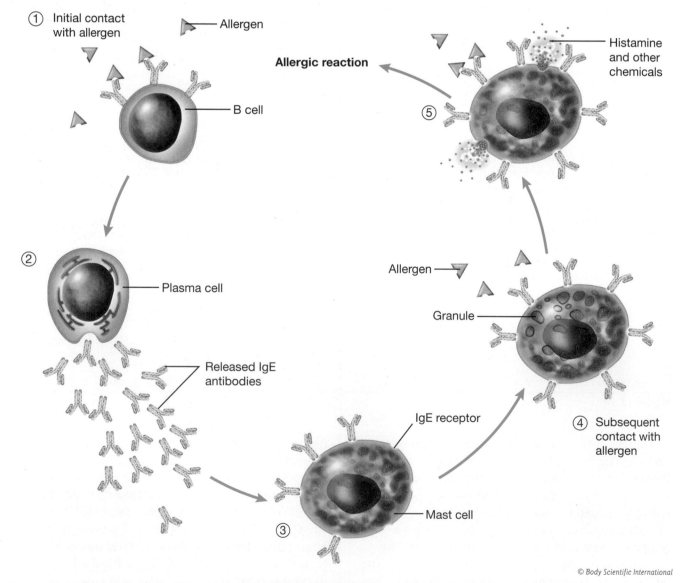

① Initial contact with allergen
Allergen
B cell
② Plasma cell
Released IgE antibodies
③ IgE receptor
Mast cell
④ Subsequent contact with allergen
Allergen
Granule
⑤ Histamine and other chemicals
Allergic reaction

Figure 12.19 Diagram of an allergic reaction. *Why do you think some people have allergies and others do not?*

not really a threat; the problem is an overreactive immune system.

Allergies arise when an antigen-presenting cell presents the antigen—an **allergen**—to a helper T cell in a person susceptible to allergies. This allergen presentation activates the helper T cell, which in turn activates B cells, causing them to produce a class of antibodies called *IgE antibodies*. The IgE antibodies interact with mast cells and basophils, which become sensitive to the allergen. The next time the allergen is encountered, basophils and mast cells respond by secreting large amounts of histamine.

Histamine causes an inflammatory response, and can also lead to symptoms such as a runny nose and watery, itchy eyes. In severe cases, such as with bee-sting allergies and certain nut allergies, exposure to the antigen causes large quantities of histamine to be released throughout the body. Excessive histamine in the body can lead to life-threatening symptoms. These include pulmonary obstruction due to inflammation and swelling of the airways and low blood pressure due to leakage of blood plasma into the interstitial space, through excessively leaky capillaries. Such a severe allergic reaction is called **anaphylaxis** (an-a-fi-LAK-sis).

Anaphylaxis can be treated with an injection of epinephrine (ehp-i-NEHF-rin), a hormone that opens up the airways and constricts (narrows) the blood vessels. **Figure 12.21** shows a woman administering epinephrine using an emergency auto-injector to treat an anaphylactic reaction. Antihistamine drugs, which block the effects of histamine, can be used to treat anaphylaxis as well as less severe allergic reactions.

What Research Tells Us

...about Antibody-Based Drugs

Many drugs have side effects that limit their usefulness because the drugs affect processes other than the specific disease mechanisms for which they are intended. Because antibodies bind very specifically, it has long been thought that they could make good drugs.

In the past 15 years, a growing number of antibody-based drugs have made it to market. They are made by fusing a B lymphocyte with a cultured cell derived from a cancerous lymph cell (**Figure 12.20**). The fused cell can divide without limit because it is derived from a cancer cell, and it makes one specific antibody because it is also derived from a B lymphocyte. The cell is allowed to divide, grow, and secrete its antibody product, which is harvested from the fluid bathing the cells. The antibody product is then packaged as a drug. Because the cells are genetic copies of the original fused cell, they are called *clones*; the antibodies they make are called *monoclonal antibodies* because they come from a single clone. You can recognize many drugs that are monoclonal antibodies because they usually have the word segment *-mab* (for "monoclonal antibody") in their generic name.

Infliximab (sold as Remicade®) is an antibody to tumor necrosis factor, a protein that plays an important role in rheumatoid arthritis, the disease for which it is most often prescribed. Trastuzamab (sold as Herceptin®) is an antibody to the human epidermal growth factor receptor 2 (HER2), which is found on the surface of some kinds of breast cancer cells. It is given as a chemotherapeutic agent to patients with HER2-positive breast cancer. Many more monoclonal antibody drugs exist, and the list continues to grow with advances in research.

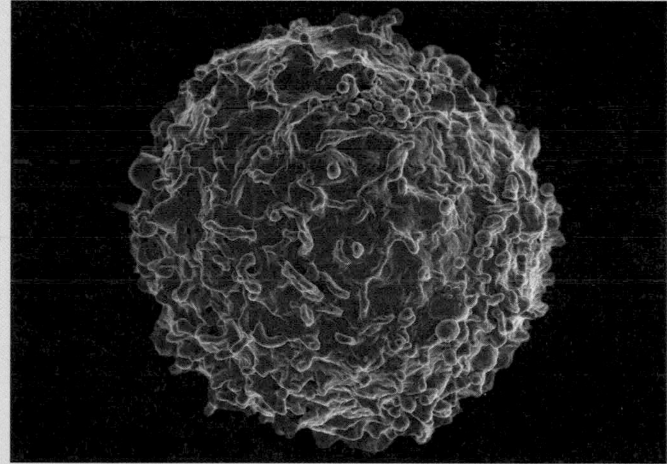

NIAID/Science Source

Figure 12.20 Micrograph of a lymphocyte.

Taking It Further

Working with another student or in a group, research monoclonal antibody drugs for cancer treatment. How do these drugs work? Why are they typically used? How are they given to patients? What are common side effects of these drugs? Prepare a report and share your findings with the class.

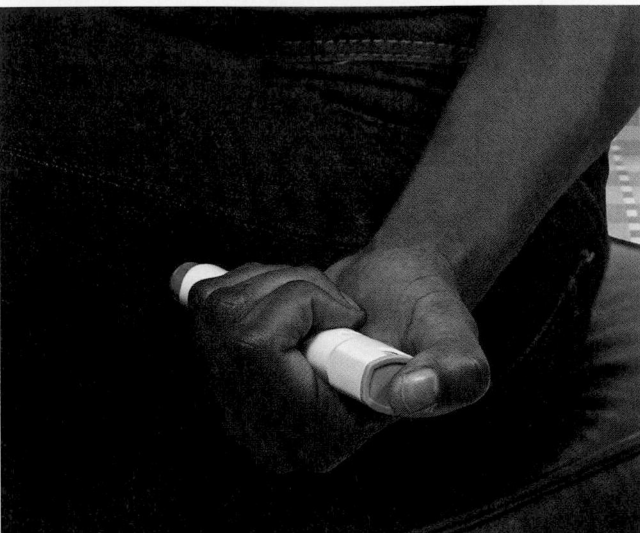

Rob Byron/Shutterstock.com

Figure 12.21 People with severe allergies that may result in an anaphylactic reaction may carry emergency "pens" like this one to inject a life-saving dose of epinephrine if they accidentally encounter the allergen.

Allergy shots, or **allergen immunotherapy**, are a longer-term treatment, aimed at preventing allergic reactions before they occur. In allergy-shot treatment, a specific allergen is injected underneath the skin, starting with tiny amounts and gradually building up to larger amounts. This gradual approach often leads to the development of immune system **tolerance** of the antigen. As a result, the allergic response may be reduced or eliminated.

In many cases, the person may not know what substance actually triggers an allergic reaction. Allergists often perform skin prick tests, also called scratch tests, in an attempt to determine what causes the person's allergies. These tests expose the patient to very low doses of various common allergens (**Figure 12.22**), and the size of the allergic response is measured in millimeters. After the allergen is identified, the patient is better able to avoid it, and if necessary, allergen immunotherapy can begin.

Check Your Understanding

1. What causes itchy, water eyes from exposure to dust, pollen, or animal dander?
2. What can excessive amounts of histamine do to the body?
3. Name two treatments for anaphylaxis.

Autoimmune Disorders

An **autoimmune disorder**, such as an allergy, is a condition in which the immune system overreacts to an antigen that, in and of itself, does not pose an actual threat. In an allergy, the antigen is a substance outside the body (that is, in the environment). In an autoimmune disorder, the antigen is part of the body's own tissue.

When the immune system perceives the body's own tissue as foreign, it attacks that tissue as it would attack an invading organism. The cause of autoimmune disorders is often unclear. An autoimmune disorder sometimes develops when a genetically susceptible person is exposed to an environmental antigen that resembles one of the body's own molecules. The immune response to the outside antigen produces collateral damage (unintended harm) to the body's own cells.

More than 80 different types of autoimmune disorders have been identified. Examples include:

- rheumatoid (ROO-ma-toyd) arthritis, in which the immune system attacks the synovial membrane that lines joint cavities
- multiple sclerosis, in which the immune system attacks the myelin sheath that surrounds nerve cells
- type 1 diabetes mellitus

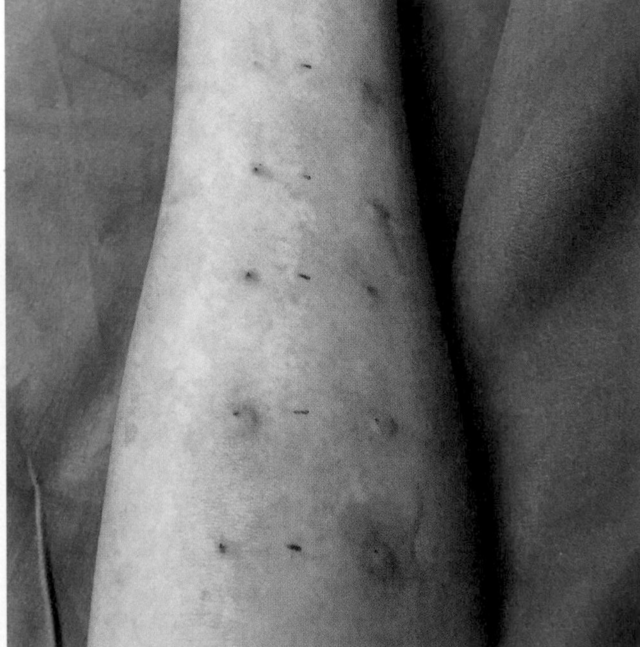

Hunna/Shutterstock.com

Figure 12.22 Allergy testing determines the level of a person's allergic response to several suspected allergens.

Multiple sclerosis is discussed in more detail in Chapter 6; rheumatoid arthritis, in Chapter 4; and type I diabetes mellitus, in Chapter 8.

In type 1 diabetes, cytotoxic T cells attack the cells in the pancreas that manufacture insulin, a hormone that regulates metabolism of carbohydrates and fats and regulates glucose levels in the blood. Unfortunately, the cytotoxic T cell attacks are usually very effective: they destroy all or most of the insulin-producing cells. Once the insulin-producing cells are gone, they do not grow back. Type 1 diabetes is also called *insulin-dependent diabetes* because individuals with this autoimmune disease require regular insulin injections from an outside source.

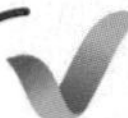

Check Your Understanding

1. Name three common autoimmune disorders.
2. Why is the attack of cytotoxic T cells in type 1 diabetes so harmful?

HIV and AIDS

As its name indicates, **human immunodeficiency virus (HIV)** is a virus that causes immune deficiency in humans. HIV is the virus that can lead to **acquired immunodeficiency syndrome (AIDS)**. HIV is commonly transmitted sexually, through sharing of needles during illegal drug use, or from mother to child during pregnancy, birth, or breastfeeding. Less common modes of transmission include blood transfusions or being accidentally "stuck" with a contaminated needle. The latter is a risk for healthcare workers.

Within a few weeks of infection, a person with HIV may develop flu-like symptoms that last one or two weeks. Others may not experience any symptoms at all. Although individuals infected with HIV may feel perfectly healthy, the virus is at work inside their bodies. Because HIV damages the immune system, it compromises the body's ability to fight disease-causing organisms.

As shown in **Figure 12.23**, the HIV virus infects lymphocytes that have the CD4 protein on their surface ($CD4^+$ cells). Most $CD4^+$ cells are helper T cells, and most helper T cells are $CD4^+$. After the virus uses the intracellular machinery to make copies of itself, it breaks open the cell, killing the cell and releasing new, infectious virus particles.

Of all the immune cells, the helper T cells are probably the cells that the body can least afford to lose. The helper T cells are essential for strong activation of both the humoral and cellular immune responses. When the concentration level of helper T cells drops below 200/mm^3, the immune system is seriously weakened, and the patient is said to have AIDS.

AIDS patients are highly susceptible to developing rare forms of cancer and **opportunistic infections**—unusual infections that are almost never seen in people with healthy immune systems. Multi-drug treatments for HIV are effective at suppressing viral reproduction for many years. However, these drugs can have serious side effects, such as nausea, vomiting, weight loss, and fatigue. Also, AIDS antiviral drugs are expensive and must be taken for life. Therefore, the scientific community continues its effort to create an HIV vaccine.

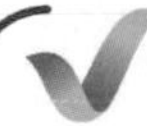

Check Your Understanding

1. List common modes of transmission for HIV.
2. What is an opportunistic infection?

LESSON 12.4 Review and Assessment

Mini Glossary

Make sure that you know the meaning of each key term.

acquired immunodeficiency syndrome (AIDS) a disease in which the immune system is greatly weakened due to infection with HIV, making a person more susceptible to rare cancers and opportunistic infections

allergen antigen that causes an inappropriately strong immune system response

allergen immunotherapy a long-term, preventive treatment for allergies; "allergy shots"

allergy an inappropriately strong response of the immune system to an environmental antigen, such as dust mites, pet dander, pollen, or certain foods

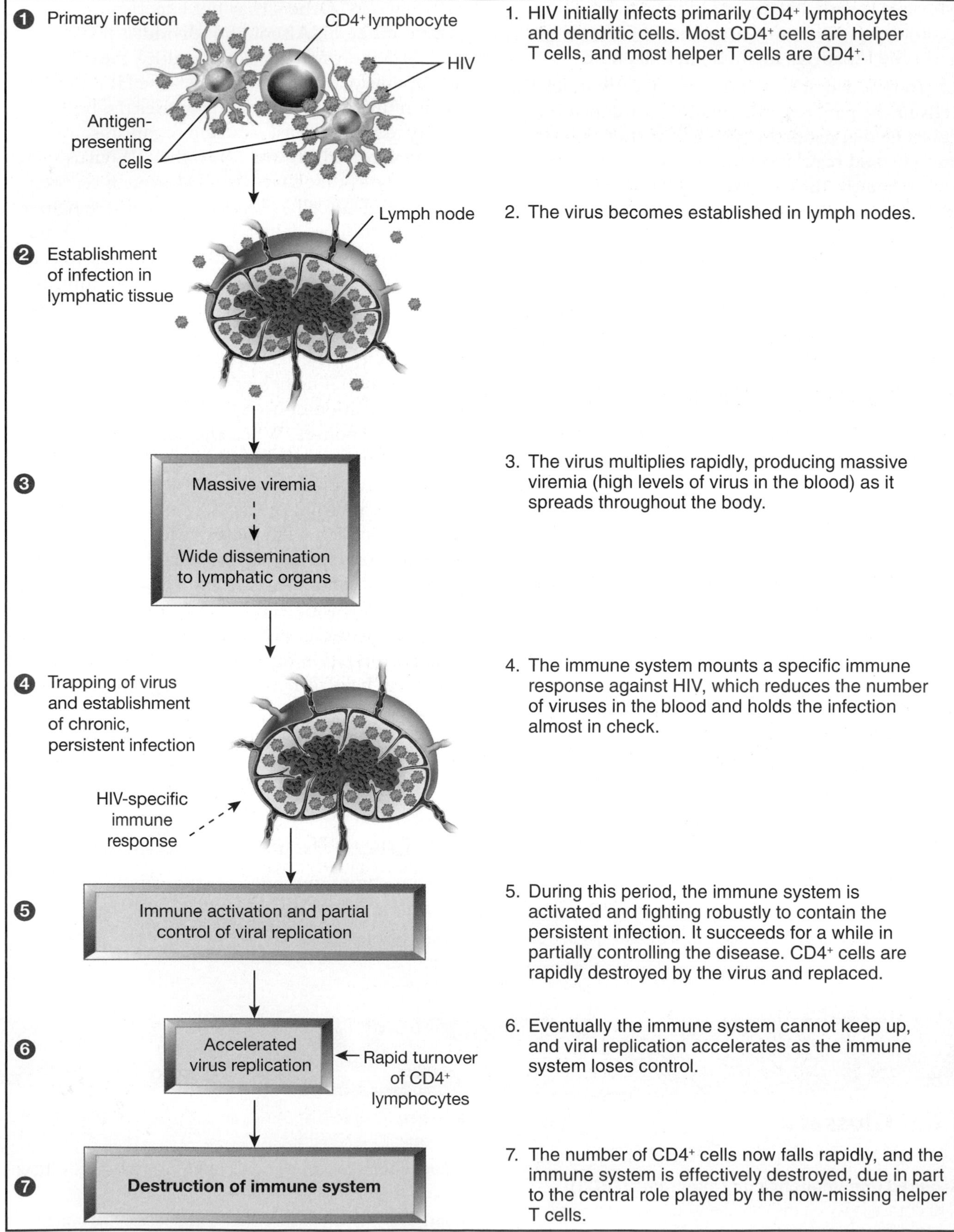

1 Primary infection
CD4+ lymphocyte
HIV
Antigen-presenting cells
1. HIV initially infects primarily CD4+ lymphocytes and dendritic cells. Most CD4+ cells are helper T cells, and most helper T cells are CD4+.
Lymph node
2 Establishment of infection in lymphatic tissue
2. The virus becomes established in lymph nodes.
3
Massive viremia
Wide dissemination to lymphatic organs
3. The virus multiplies rapidly, producing massive viremia (high levels of virus in the blood) as it spreads throughout the body.
4 Trapping of virus and establishment of chronic, persistent infection
HIV-specific immune response
4. The immune system mounts a specific immune response against HIV, which reduces the number of viruses in the blood and holds the infection almost in check.
5
Immune activation and partial control of viral replication
5. During this period, the immune system is activated and fighting robustly to contain the persistent infection. It succeeds for a while in partially controlling the disease. CD4+ cells are rapidly destroyed by the virus and replaced.
6
Accelerated virus replication
Rapid turnover of CD4+ lymphocytes
6. Eventually the immune system cannot keep up, and viral replication accelerates as the immune system loses control.
7
Destruction of immune system
7. The number of CD4+ cells now falls rapidly, and the immune system is effectively destroyed, due in part to the central role played by the now-missing helper T cells.

Figure 12.23 HIV infection and the development of AIDS.

anaphylaxis a severe and potentially life-threatening allergic reaction that may include airway obstruction and very low blood pressure

autoimmune disorder a condition in which the immune system attacks the body's own tissue

human immunodeficiency virus (HIV) the virus that causes AIDS

lymphedema a buildup of extracellular fluid in the body because of disruption in lymphatic drainage

metastasis the spreading of cancerous cells from their original location to another part of the body

opportunistic infection an infection that rarely or never occurs in people with a healthy immune system but that may occur in a person with a damaged immune system, such as from AIDS

tolerance reduction or elimination of the allergic response, which may occur after immunotherapy

Know and Understand

1. Describe the surgical procedure that is used to determine whether cancer has spread from its initial location to another part of the body.
2. List the potential risks associated with having a lymph node removed.
3. State the treatment options for a patient with lymphedema of the arm as a result of having an axillary lymph node removed.
4. Define IgE antibodies and describe how they are produced.
5. Identify the two types of cells responsible for secreting large amounts of histamine in response to an allergen.
6. Summarize the purpose of allergen immunotherapy.
7. What is an autoimmune disorder?
8. Explain the difference between HIV and AIDS.
9. Describe the process by which an antibody-based drug is made.

Analyze and Apply

10. Breast cancer can metastasize, or spread. Identify the area of the body where breast cancer often metastasizes, and label it on a diagram of the human body.
11. Based on what you have learned about severe allergies, describe two ways in which histamine could cause life-threatening symptoms.
12. One of the most important aspects of HIV/AIDS is prevention. There are several ways to prevent the spread of this disease, including a regimen called PrEP. Research this approach, how it works, and the medications involved. Write a one-page summary and cite your sources.
13. Choose an autoimmune disease to research. Write an essay about the disease process. Include information on treatments and support groups. As always, cite your sources.

IN THE LAB

14. You are a doctor who has just seen the following patients. What is your diagnosis for each patient? Use information that you learned in this lesson, as well as information from previous chapters.

    Patient A: tests show very high cell counts in certain lymph nodes; the patient is not currently experiencing any pain or fatigue

    Patient B: severe pain in the hands and feet; severe inflammation and swelling in the hands; fatigue

    Patient C: excessive sneezing, coughing, and watery eyes; symptoms began during a recent hiking trip

    Patient D: has two different infections; standard tests have failed to identify the cause of either infection; patient reports that she has been very healthy for the past two years
15. Using the Centers for Disease Control (CDC) website as a source, research anaphylaxis. Then create a poster illustrating the proper steps to follow when using an epinephrine injection pen for anaphylactic shock.
16. Create flashcards for all of the terms in this chapter. Use words and pictures to help you commit the terms to memory. Then use your cards to test a classmate. How many was your classmate able to get right? Did he or she find your pictures helpful? Switch places and answer the same questions for your classmate's set of cards.
17. Choose a disease or disorder that is prevalent in today's society, such as autism, VRSI, listeria, mumps, measles, or seasonal flu. Conduct an internet search to find out more about current research on this disease or disorder. Write a report of your findings. Be sure to list your sources.

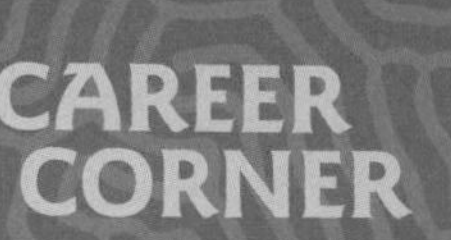

Anatomy & Physiology at Work

Careers in immunology and oncology involve extensive study of and work with the immune system. These careers in bioscience (that is, the scientific study of the body) require a high level of motivation, a great deal of education, and a lot of hard work. However, they can be highly challenging, rewarding, and profitable.

Immunologist

An immunologist may be a doctor, researcher, and/or college professor. Strong skills in mathematics, biology, and chemistry, along with a deep interest in scientific inquiry or human well-being, are important for success in the field of immunology.

Research immunologists typically work in a lab, performing scientific research in an effort to better understand the anatomy, physiology, and pathological conditions of the human immune system (**Figure 12.24**). Research immunologists study cells and genes in the body and conduct tests to determine how different chemicals interact with these cells and genes.

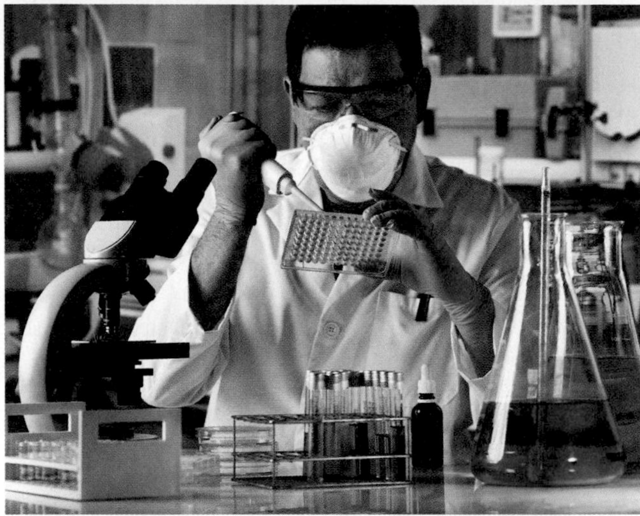

angellodeco/Shutterstock.com

Figure 12.24 Research immunologists study immune systems and associated diseases, often with the goal of finding vaccines and drugs to cure or lessen the damage done by certain diseases.

A career as a research immunologist requires a PhD from a university with an accredited program in immunology. The PhD degree, which may take five or more years to complete, involves extensive coursework and study in the areas of molecular and cellular biology, biochemistry, bacteriology, virology, and biostatistics, as well as ethical issues in scientific research.

Some medical doctors specialize in caring for patients with diseases of the immune system. Allergists and rheumatologists are two examples of this kind of medical specialist. Allergists treat patients with allergies. Rheumatologists treat patients with connective tissue diseases, many of which are autoimmune diseases. Both allergists and rheumatologists are medical doctors who, after completing four years of college and four years of medical school, have also completed a residency in pediatrics or internal medicine (three years) plus a fellowship in allergy or rheumatology (usually another two years).

Some immunologists forge a career in academia. These individuals continue to participate in research while teaching students enrolled in medical school or in an advanced immunology degree program at a college or university. To serve as a faculty member or administrator in higher education, an immunologist must have either a PhD or medical doctor (MD) degree.

Oncologist

An oncologist has an extraordinarily difficult job: diagnosing cancer and treating patients throughout the course of their disease, from diagnosis to recovery or death. While medical and surgical oncologists have similar responsibilities, surgical oncologists are qualified to perform operations on patients.

Typical job duties for both the medical oncologist and the surgical oncologist include making cancer diagnoses, preparing case histories, keeping records of physical examinations and test results, writing prescriptions, and monitoring treatment plans (**Figure 12.25**). Usually, the oncologist coordinates a cancer treatment team, which may include nurses, physician assistants, radiologists, rehabilitation therapists, dieticians, and social workers. Oncologists explain cancer development stages to patients, help educate them about their disease, discuss treatment options, and assist in pain management.

A career as an oncologist requires a degree from an accredited medical school, followed by an internal medicine residency and an oncology fellowship. In addition, oncologists may obtain board certification from an appropriate organization to demonstrate professional competence in their field.

Planning for a Health-Related Career

Do some research on the career of an immunologist or oncologist, or select a profession from the list of related career options. Using the internet or resources at your local library, find answers to the following questions:

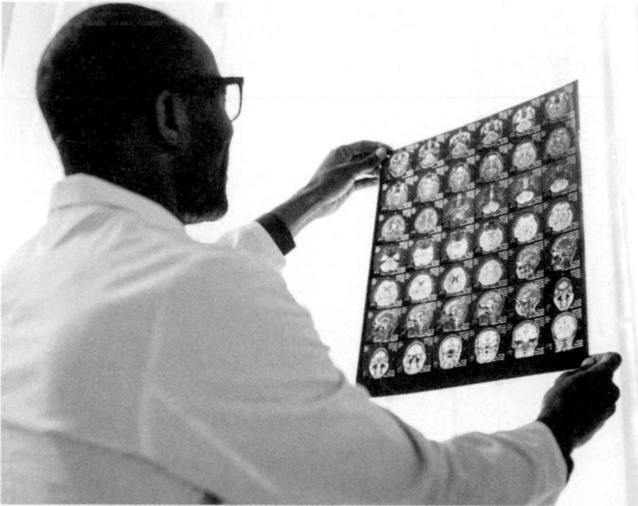

Auremar/Shutterstock.com

Figure 12.25 An important aspect of an oncologist's work is making a diagnosis.

1. What are the main responsibilities of the career that you have chosen to research?
2. What is the outlook for this career? Are workers in demand, or are jobs dwindling? For complete information, consult the current edition of the *Occupational Outlook Handbook*.
3. What special skills or talents are required? For example, do you need to be good at subjects such as biology, chemistry, and anatomy and physiology? Do you need to enjoy interacting with other people?
4. What personality traits do you think are needed to be successful in this job? For example, some characteristics of an effective oncologist are compassion, excellent analytical and problem-solving skills, and the ability to make sound clinical judgments under emotional pressure.
5. Does this career involve a great deal of routine, or is there variety among the day-to-day responsibilities?
6. Does the work require long hours, or is it a standard, "9-to-5" job?
7. What is the salary range for this job?
8. What do you think you would like about this career? Is there anything about it that you might dislike?

Related Career Options

- Biochemist
- Biologist
- Epidemiologist
- Geneticist
- Hematologist
- Histologist
- Medical physicist
- Medical scientist
- Microbiologist
- Oncology nurse
- Palliative care specialist
- Pathologist
- Pediatric immunologist
- Pediatric oncologist
- Radiation therapist
- Radiologist
- Toxicologist
- Virologist

CHAPTER

12 Review

›LESSON 12.1

The Lymphatic System

Key Points

- The lymphatic system includes lymphocytes, lymphatic vessels, lymphatic fluid, and lymphatic organs—lymph nodes, the spleen, and the thymus.
- Physical, cellular, and chemical mechanisms within the lymphatic and immune systems provide both specific and nonspecific defenses against microbial challenges to the body.

Key Terms

B lymphocytes (B cells)
cisterna chyli
endothelial cells
interstitial fluid
lingual tonsils
lymph
lymph nodes
lymphatic nodules
lymphatic trunks
lymphatic valves
lymphatic vessels
lymphocytes
macrophages
mucosa-associated lymphatic tissue (MALT)
natural killer (NK) cells
palatine tonsils
pathogens
pharyngeal tonsil
spleen
T lymphocytes (T cells)

›LESSON 12.2

Nonspecific Defenses

Key Points

- Challenges to human health come in many forms, including bacteria, fungi, viruses, and nonmicrobial organisms, such as helminthic parasites.
- The skin functions as a physical barrier against infectious agents, so when the integrity of your skin is breached, you are at a much greater risk for infection.
- Phagocytes, natural killer cells, the complement system, and interferons comprise the body's cellular and chemical defenses against disease.
- Injured tissues initiate an inflammatory response that, although uncomfortable, promotes repair of the injured tissue.
- Fever maintenance of body temperature at a higher-than-normal level.

Key Terms

alternative pathway
chain of infection
classical pathway
complement proteins
complement system
exocytosis
fever
germ theory of disease
inflammatory response
interferons
mast cells
monocytes
neutrophils
opsonins
phagocytes
phagocytosis
prostaglandins
pyrogens

➤ LESSON 12.3

Specific Defenses

Key Points

- Antigens enable the body to distinguish between "self" and "nonself" cells.
- Immune system cells include lymphocytes and antigen-presenting cells such as macrophages, dendritic cells, and B cells.
- Antibody-mediated immunity is called *humoral immunity*.
- A primary immune response occurs when the body is first exposed to a foreign invader. A secondary response occurs when the invader enters a second or subsequent time.
- Cellular immunity is mediated by T cells.

Key Terms

active immunity
antigenic determinants
antigen-presenting cells (APCs)
apoptosis
cellular immunity
clonal selection
humoral immunity
immune system
immunoglobulins
interleukins
major histocompatibility complex (MCH) glycoproteins
memory cells
passive immunity
precipitation
primary immune response
secondary immune response
severe combined immune deficiency (SCID)

➤ LESSON 12.4

Disorders and Diseases of the Immune System

Key Points

- The process by which cancer spreads from its initial location to another part of the body via the lymphatic system is called *metastasis*.
- Allergies are caused by an inappropriately strong immune response.
- Common autoimmune disorders include rheumatoid arthritis, multiple sclerosis, and type 1 diabetes.
- Human immunodeficiency virus (HIV) damages the immune system and compromises the body's ability to fight disease-causing organisms.

Key Terms

acquired immunodeficiency syndrome (AIDS)
allergen
allergen immunotherapy
allergy
anaphylaxis
autoimmune disorder
human immunodeficiency virus (HIV)
lymphedema
metastasis
opportunistic infection
tolerance

Assessment

›LESSON 12.1

The Lymphatic System

Learning Key Terms and Concepts

1. What two vital functions does the lymphatic system perform in the human body?
   A. returning fluid to the cardiovascular system and protecting the body from disease
   B. protecting the body from disease and transporting nutrients to body cells
   C. preventing plasma from leaving the cardiovascular system and maintaining the body's oxygen supply
   D. protecting the body from disease and maintaining a constant level of oxygenation
2. *True or False?* The normal leakage rate of blood plasma across the entire body is 2 to 3 mL per minute.
3. *True or False?* Lymph formation begins with fluid that leaks out of blood vessel capillaries.
4. *True or False?* The human body has a pump similar to the heart that helps propel lymph through the network of lymph vessels.
5. Lymph from the thoracic duct drains into the _____ vein.
6. *True or False?* During the process of lymph drainage, lymphatic fluid never rejoins the blood to once again become blood plasma.
7. B lymphocytes mature in the _____.
   A. spleen
   B. thymus
   C. bone marrow
   D. lymph nodes
8. When a monocyte migrates out of lymphatic circulation into the surrounding tissue, it develops into a _____.
   A. macrophage
   B. natural killer cell
   C. T lymphocyte
   D. B lymphocyte

Thinking Critically

9. Assume you are a doctor talking to the parents of a high school football player with a ruptured spleen. Evaluate the causes of this trauma and explain the diagnosis in a way that the parents and the athlete will understand.
10. Explain the process that causes your lymph nodes to become swollen in response to exposure to an infection.
11. Prepare an age-appropriate written explanation of the physiology of the lymphatic system for a junior high/middle school student.
12. Create a flowchart that demonstrates the flow of lymphatic drainage.

›LESSON 12.2

Nonspecific Defenses

Learning Key Terms and Concepts

13. The theory that microscopic organisms can cause disease in humans is known as the _____ theory of disease.
14. *True or False?* Most prokaryotes are too small to be seen under a light microscope.
15. *True or False?* Antibiotics can increase the risk of a fungal infection.
16. *True or False?* When skin has been cut or punctured, you are at a much greater risk for infection.
17. The process by which cells engulf and destroy foreign matter and cellular debris is called _____.
    A. exocytosis
    B. phagocytosis
    C. inflammation
    D. opsonization
18. _____ develop into macrophages when they leave the bloodstream and enter tissues.

19. The process by which cell membranes fuse together and then push debris from the cell vesicles to the outside of the cell is called _____.
20. The _____ system is a set of more than 30 proteins that circulate in the blood plasma and work together to destroy bacteria.
21. The process by which complement proteins make cells more attractive to phagocytes is called _____.
    A. opsonization
    B. activation
    C. phagocytosis
    D. precipitation

Thinking Critically

22. The complement system can be activated in two primary ways. Identify the two pathways and describe how each one is initiated.
23. Create a graph that shows the process of phagocytosis.
24. List five examples of barrier defenses, and explain how each barrier repels pathogens.

➤ LESSON 12.3

Specific Defenses

Learning Key Terms and Concepts

25. A(n) _____ is a large molecule on the surface of a cell that helps the body distinguish between "self" and "nonself" cells.
26. Which of the following *cannot* act as an antigen-presenting cell?
    A. macrophages
    B. histamines
    C. dendritic cells
    D. B cells
27. T lymphocytes travel to the _____ to complete their maturation.
28. A programmed process of cellular self-destruction is called _____.
    A. differentiation
    B. clonal selection
    C. apoptosis
    D. metastasis
29. *True or False*? Antibodies, also known as *immunoglobulins*, are Y-shaped.
30. How many classes of antibodies exist?

Thinking Critically

31. Explain how the immune system uses a vaccine to build a defense through the primary and secondary immune response.
32. Explain how clonal selection, or cloning of lymphocytes, works and what becomes of the clones.
33. The immune system is a complex system that is constantly finding, targeting, and eliminating bacteria, viruses, and other pathogens. How does the immune system identify the items for elimination?

➤ LESSON 12.4

Disorders and Diseases of the Immune System

Learning Key Terms and Concepts

34. A cancer that has spread is said to be _____.
35. About what percentage of Americans have an allergy to one or more substances in the environment?
    A. 14%
    B. 28%
    C. 35%
    D. 46%
36. A severe allergic reaction that may include pulmonary obstruction and low blood pressure is called _____.
    A. anaphylaxis
    B. encephalomyelitis
    C. lymphoma
    D. lymphedema
37. _____ is a hormone that opens up the airways and constricts the blood vessels.
    A. Antihistamine
    B. Anaphylaxis
    C. Immunoglobulin
    D. Epinephrine
38. Development of an immune system _____ of an antigen may reduce or eliminate an allergic response.
39. A condition such as an allergy, in which the immune system overreacts to an antigen that, in and of itself, does not pose an actual threat is called a(n) _____.

40. Which virus can lead to the development of AIDS?
    A. rubeola
    B. HIV
    C. rubella
    D. staphylococcus

Thinking Critically

41. Describe the process by which a patient transitions from HIV-positive status to a diagnosis of AIDS.
42. Considering that the immune system protects the body against illness and infection, why do you think cancer is able to thrive?
43. Write a paragraph describing what your life would be like and what adjustments you would make if you suddenly became allergic to your favorite food.
44. Find a current news article on a cancer of the immune system and summarize it. Be sure to specify the article and its source.
45. AIDS patients are highly susceptible to developing rare forms of cancer and opportunistic infections. Give one example of a cancer and one example of an infection commonly seen in AIDS patients.

Building Skills and Connecting Concepts

Analyzing and Evaluating Data

Instructions: The chart in **Figure 12.26** gives the percentages of the population (between 15 and 49 years of age) infected with HIV in 15 countries. Use the chart and your knowledge of geography (do some research if necessary) to answer the following questions.

Percentages of Age 15 to 49 Population with HIV in Select Countries

Country	%	Country	%
Argentina	0.5	Japan	0.1
Canada	0.2	Mexico	0.3
Chile	0.4	Mozambique	11.5
China	0.1	Nigeria	3.6
Colombia	0.5	South Africa	17.8
France	0.4	United Kingdom	0.2
Germany	0.1	United States	0.6
India	0.3		

Figure 12.26 — Goodheart-Willcox Publisher

46. What percentage of people between 15 and 49 years of age in the United States have contracted HIV? (Round your answer to the nearest whole number.)
47. List, in descending order, the six countries in the western hemisphere with the highest incidence of HIV, based on percentage of HIV infections.
48. Of the countries listed in the chart, is the average incidence of HIV greater in Asia or Europe?
49. What is the ratio of people in South Africa who have HIV compared to those in Japan, Germany, or China who have HIV?
    A. 64 to 1
    B. 18 to 1
    C. 180 to 1
    D. 22 to 1
50. According to this chart, what percent of the total populations of these 15 countries combined has HIV? Show your work.

Communicating about Anatomy & Physiology

51. **Speaking** Debate the topic of vaccines for children. Divide into two groups. Each group should gather information in support of either the "pro" argument (children should be vaccinated) or the "con" argument (children should not be vaccinated). Use definitions and descriptions from this chapter to support your side of the debate and to clarify word meanings as necessary. You will want to do further research to find expert opinions, costs associated with vaccines, and other relevant information.
52. **Listening** As classmates deliver their presentations, listen carefully to their arguments. Take notes on important points and write down any questions that occur to you. Later, ask questions to obtain additional information or clarification from your classmates as necessary.
53. **Writing** Review the list of careers in the Career Corner feature in this chapter. Write a persuasive essay encouraging someone to choose one of these careers. Include the benefits of the career, the schooling needed, what schools offer the training, and the expected pay. Your essay must be in APA format and must be a minimum of two pages. Pay close attention to correct spelling, grammar, and formatting. Be sure to list your sources.

Lab Investigations

54. Using the information in your textbook and from websites approved by your instructor, create a tool for the parent or guardian of a newborn child that offers a recommended vaccination schedule and allows the parent or guardian to keep track of vaccinations. Be sure to add a calendar or other tracking method that could be helpful. Print out the tool and give a copy to each student in the class.
55. In addition to creating the tracking tool described above, prepare an information sheet that lists and describes each vaccine, the disease that the vaccine prevents, the potential side effects of the disease, and the potential side effects of the vaccine. Be sure to cite the research sources that you used to prepare your information sheet. Print out copies and share them with your classmates.
56. Handwashing for at least 20 seconds, using soap, is the best way to break the chain of infection. Unfortunately, most people do not wash their hands properly, and some do not wash their hands at all. Working with a partner, perform a handwashing investigation as follows.

    Materials: blindfold, soap, running water, water-soluble paint, watch with a second hand

    Procedure: Team member A places paint in the palm of the hand, rubs it in, and allows it to dry. Team member B then blindfolds team member A and watches and times as team member A washes and dries his or her hands and records the time. Remove the blindfold and examine team member A's hands. Has all of the paint been removed? Then switch places, so that team member A watches and records while team member B performs the handwashing blindfolded. Finally, create a graph showing how long each participant washed his or her hands and the percentage of paint removed. Is there a correlation?

Building Your Portfolio

57. Take digital photographs of the models and projects you created as you worked through this chapter. Create a document or folder called "The Lymphatic and Immune Systems" and insert the photographs, along with written descriptions of what the models show and your reasons for creating them using the materials and forms you chose. Add the reports from your laboratory experiments and add this document or folder to your personal portfolio.

CHAPTER

13 The Digestive System and Nutrition

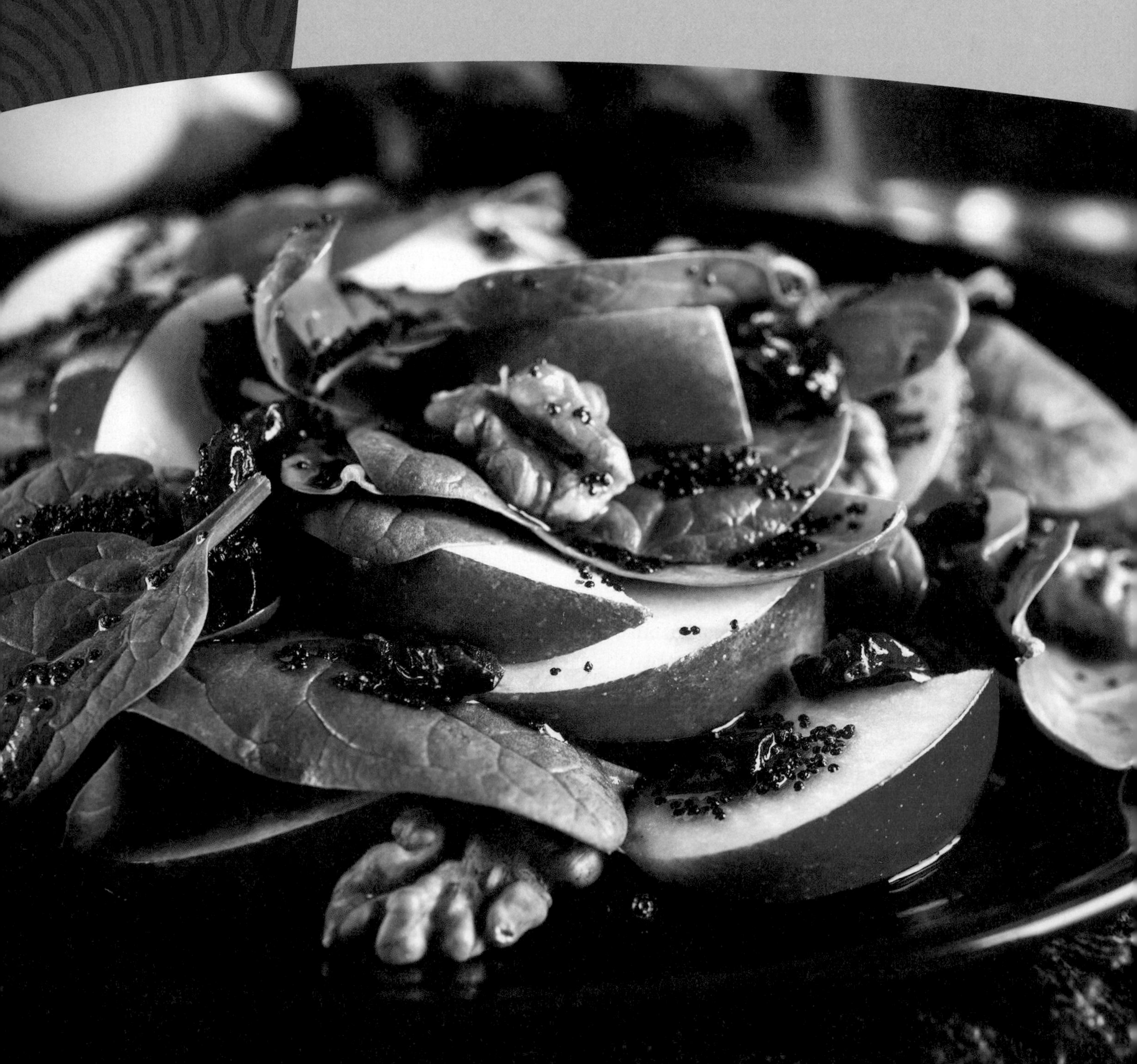

How do you get energy and nutrients for life from your food?

The human body needs energy to function. The ultimate source of that energy—the sun—is about 93 million miles away. The energy from sunlight is converted into chemicals by plants. The chemicals, including sugars such as glucose, fructose, and sucrose, store the energy. When people eat plants and animals (that also eat plants), the body obtains the fuel it needs.

However, people need more than just energy to survive and thrive. They also need certain molecular building blocks that enable the body to grow and maintain itself. This is where the digestive system comes in. The digestive system brings in all the molecules (except oxygen) that the body needs—including energy molecules.

Eating is the first step of the digestive process. Many more steps are involved in breaking down bite-sized fragments of food into microscopic pieces. These microscopic pieces are eventually absorbed into the blood. The digestive system also disposes of the parts of food that cannot be absorbed by the body. This chapter describes how the structures and functions of the digestive system work together to process and store the energy and nutrients needed for a healthy body.

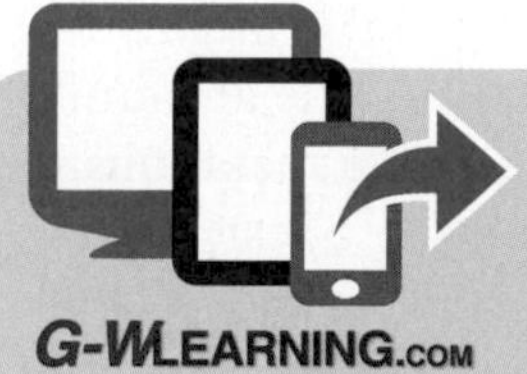

Click on the activity icon or visit www.g-wlearning.com/healthsciences/0202 to access online vocabulary activities using key terms from the chapter.

Chapter 13 Outline

◂ Elenadesign/Shutterstock.com

LESSON 13.1 Nutrition

Before You Read

Try to answer the following questions before you read this lesson.

- Which nutrients does the human body need in relatively large amounts?
- Which nutrients are needed in only small amounts?

Lesson Objectives

- Identify ways in which energy use by the body is measured.
- Describe the major categories of nutrients.

Key Terms

basal metabolic rate (BMR)	minerals
Calorie	monounsaturated fats
coenzymes	nutrients
energy	polyunsaturated fats
lipids	trans-unsaturated fats
macronutrients	vitamin deficiency
micronutrients	vitamins

The digestive system exists to provide nutrients to the body. This chapter discusses the nutrients found in the foods people eat, before examining the digestive system itself.

Energy

As you read this paragraph, your body is growing, moving, breathing, pumping blood, and staying warm. To perform these activities (and many others), your body needs **energy**, which is the ability of a physical system to do work.

Energy takes many forms. Heat is a form of energy, for example. Chemical energy, which is released during a chemical reaction, is the energy stored in the bonds of atoms and molecules. Kinetic energy is the energy of motion present in a moving object. Potential energy is stored energy, such as the energy stored in a stretched spring.

Measuring the Body's Energy Use

Just as there are many forms of energy, there are many ways to measure energy. The standard unit for measuring energy in the metric system is the joule. Electric companies use a unit of measure called the *kilowatt hour* (*kWh*) to calculate energy usage by their customers.

Food scientists are interested in the potential energy found in foods. Food energy is often measured in kilocalories. One kilocalorie is equal to the amount of heat energy required to raise the temperature of 1 kilogram of water by 1°C. Food scientists and nutritionists often use the term **Calorie**, with a capital C, to refer to one kilocalorie. The "Calories" on a food nutrition label are kilocalories. The uppercase *C* in Calorie is often reduced to a lowercase *c* in nonscientific writing. This is potentially confusing, but you will get used to it, with experience. For example, you might read that "a teaspoon of sugar has 16 calories". In fact, a teaspoon of sugar has 16 Calories, which equals 16 kilocalories.

Basal Metabolic Rate

Metabolic activities are the chemical and physical reactions that occur in an organism and that serve to keep it alive. Examples of metabolic activity include the beating of the heart and inspiration and expiration in the lungs. The sum of these activities is referred to as *metabolism* (meh-TAB-oh-lizm).

To perform metabolic activities, your body needs energy. The amount of energy it needs varies. Not surprisingly, your body requires more energy when you are physically active than when you are asleep, reading, or working online (**Figure 13.1**).

Scientists use a measure called the **basal metabolic rate (BMR)** to identify the amount of energy required to sustain a person's metabolism for one day if he or she is at complete rest.

BMR is expressed as Calories per day. For example, an average adult who weighs 150 pounds (68 kg) and has a body fat percentage of 25% (the

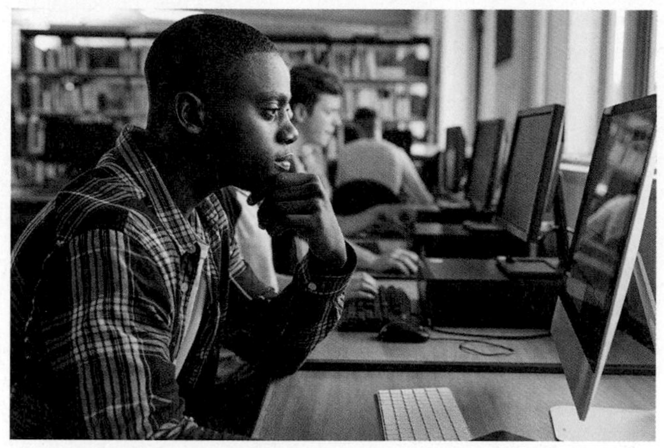
A

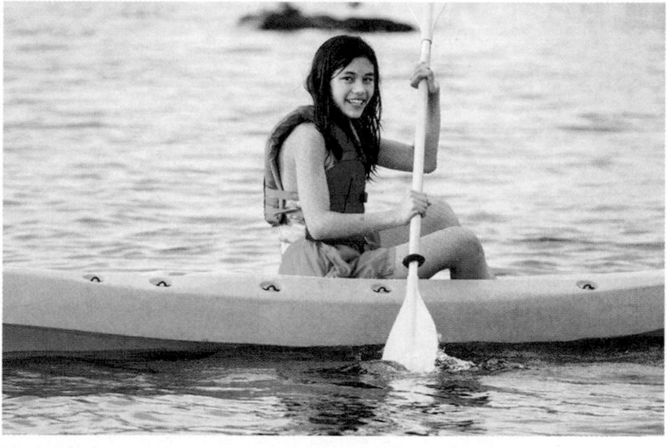
B

Monkey Business Images/Shutterstock.com, Jaren Jai Wicklund/Shutterstock.com

Figure 13.1 One of the factors in BMR is activity level. A—At rest, the body needs less energy, or fewer Calories. B—The body needs more energy as activity level increases.

fraction of body mass that is fat) has a BMR of just under 1,500 Calories per day. If this person is physically active during the day, a higher number of calories is required.

BMR can differ significantly from one individual to the next. Factors that influence BMR include a person's age, gender, height, body mass, and body fat percentage. Because few people are inactive all day, their bodies typically require 20% to 70% more Calories than indicated by the BMR. The more active you are, the more energy and Calories you need. If you walk a mile, for example, your body will use about 50 Calories above your BMR.

Moderately active boys between 14 and 18 years of age need between 2,400 and 2,800 Calories per day. Girls in this age range need about 2,000 Calories per day. However, teenagers who are physically active need more energy. Each day, active boys need up to 3,200 Calories, whereas active girls need about 2,400 Calories.

Check Your Understanding

1. How is kinetic energy different from potential energy?
2. What unit is used to count and measure energy in nutrition science?
3. How many Calories do moderately active teenage boys and girls need each day?

Macronutrients, Vitamins, and Minerals

Nutrients are substances that the body needs for energy, growth, and maintenance. Water is a nutrient. Nutrients include **macronutrients**—the carbohydrates, proteins, and lipids (fats) that you read about in Chapter 2.

Vitamins and minerals are also essential nutrients. Vitamins are organic compounds—carbon-based chemicals—that the body needs in small amounts to help regulate its processes. Minerals are elements, such as calcium and iron, that are required to maintain good health. Both vitamins and minerals are classified as **micronutrients**.

The *Dietary Guidelines for Americans* was created by the United States Department of Agriculture (USDA) and the US Department of Health and Human Services, with input from advisory panels of doctors and nutritionists. The guidelines state the levels of nutrients that you need to achieve a healthful diet. The *Dietary Guidelines* document is available online. Nutrition information can also be found by visiting the USDA's Food and Nutrition Information Center online, or by talking to the health and wellness teachers at your school.

Carbohydrates

Sugars and starches are foods, or ingredients in foods, that are classified as carbohydrates. Examples of sugar include fructose, which is found in fruits, and sucrose, more commonly known as table sugar. Some sources of starches include pasta, bread,

MEMORY TIP

A nutrient is classified as either a *macronutrient* or a *micronutrient*. *Macro-* means "large" and *micro-* means "small." However, in a discussion of nutrients, the terms *large* and *small* do not refer to size. Rather, these terms refer to the amounts of the nutrients the body needs.

Macronutrients are needed in quantities of tens or hundreds of grams each day. A gram is approximately one-thirtieth of an ounce. Micronutrients are needed in much smaller amounts. Except for a few minerals that are needed in quantities of one to five grams daily, the body requires only a fraction of a gram per day of most micronutrients. In most cases, people need less than 10 milligrams (mg) daily of the micronutrients, and in some cases less than 10 micrograms (mcg) daily. A milligram is one-thousandth of a gram, and a microgram is one-millionth of a gram.

and cereal (**Figure 13.2**). Once it has been fully digested, a gram of carbohydrate provides about 4 Calories of energy.

According to the USDA, about half of a person's energy (45% to 65%) should come from carbohydrates that are part of a healthful diet. No more than 10% of carbohydrate calories should come from sugars such as those found in soft drinks and other sweet foods. For example, if you consume a total of 2,000 Calories a day, about half of them should come from carbohydrates. This would equal about 250 grams (8 or 9 ounces) of carbohydrates per day. This does not mean that you should eat only 8 or 9 ounces of food. Remember that the 8 or 9 ounces is the weight of the carbohydrates alone. This measurement does not include, for example, the food's water weight, which is a significant part of the weight of most foods.

Proteins

Current dietary recommendations suggest that about a quarter (10% to 35%) of energy be derived from proteins. As explained in Chapter 2, proteins are made of amino acids. There are 20 common amino acids in the human body. Proteins contain varying amounts of the 20 amino acids. Nine of the amino acids are considered essential for adults, and twelve are considered essential for children. The body can produce nonessential amino acids if sufficient amounts of essential amino acids are present.

Meat, which is composed mostly of protein, provides a well-balanced mix of all 20 amino acids (**Figure 13.3**). You can also obtain sufficient protein, with all the essential amino acids, by eating a healthful vegetarian diet that includes legumes (beans, peas, or soy) and grains (rice, corn, or wheat).

Each gram of protein provides about 4 Calories of energy. In a diet of 2,000 Calories per day, this translates to 500 Calories, or 125 grams (about 4½ ounces) of protein per day.

Lipids

Fats, or **lipids**, include oils and solid fats. As described in Chapter 2, fats contain combinations of different types of fatty acids—saturated and unsaturated. Most saturated fatty acids come from

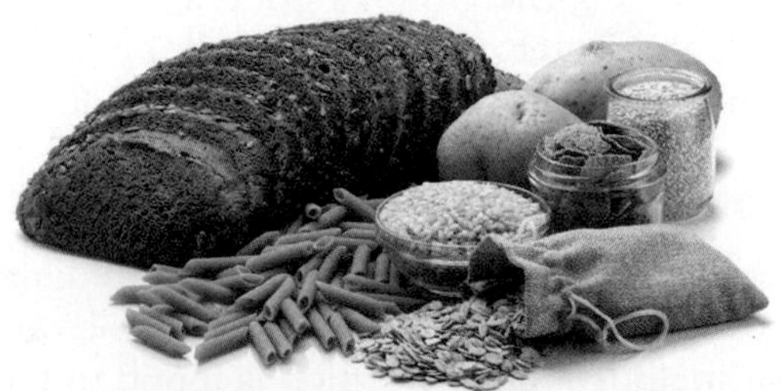

nehophoto/Shutterstock.com

Figure 13.2 Examples of carbohydrates. *In a well-balanced diet, what percentage of energy comes from carbohydrates?*

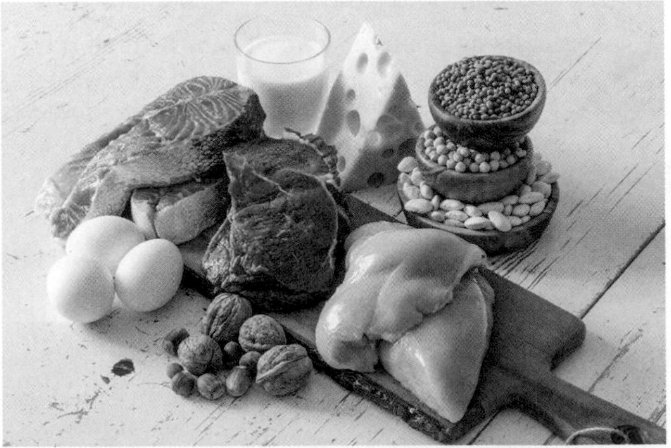

Oleksandra Naumenko/Shutterstock.com

Figure 13.3 Meat is one of the best dietary sources of protein and amino acids, but dairy and other foods also contain significant amounts of protein. *What are good sources of protein and amino acids for vegetarians?*

animal sources, such as meats and dairy products. Some oils that come from plants, such as coconut oil and palm oil, are also high in saturated fatty acids.

MEMORY TIP

Saturated fats are called *saturated* because their hydrocarbon chains are fully loaded, or *saturated*, with hydrogen atoms. Unsaturated fats are not fully loaded, or saturated, with hydrogen atoms.

Most unsaturated fatty acids come from plant sources. Unsaturated fatty acids are classified as **monounsaturated fats**, **polyunsaturated fats**, or **trans-unsaturated fats**. Corn and soybean oils are high in polyunsaturated fatty acids (**Figure 13.4**). Canola oil and olive oil are high in monounsaturated fatty acids. The majority of trans-unsaturated fats, or *trans fats*, are artificially produced.

Most fats that contain a high percentage of saturated and trans fats are solid at room temperature. Fats that contain a high percentage of monounsaturated and polyunsaturated fatty acids tend to be liquid at room temperature.

Many scientific studies have shown that diets high in saturated fatty acids and trans fats are unhealthful, especially for the cardiovascular system. Several studies have established the benefits of replacing saturated fats and trans fats in the diet with naturally unsaturated fats, especially monounsaturated fats.

Each gram of fat delivers about 9 Calories of energy—or about twice as much energy per gram as a gram of carbohydrate or protein. The *Dietary Guidelines for Americans* suggest that people between 4 and 18 years of age obtain 25% to 35% of their total calories in the form of fats. Therefore, if you consume 2,000 Calories a day, you should limit your intake of fats to 55 grams, or about 2 ounces. The guidelines also state that people who eat a healthful diet overall should keep their intake of saturated fats and trans fats to a minimum.

Vitamins

Vitamins are organic chemicals that are needed for your metabolism to function normally. The body needs only small amounts of vitamins to achieve good health. However, the body itself produces an insufficient amount of vitamins, so most vitamins must be obtained from food (**Figure 13.5**).

Vitamins are classified as either fat soluble or water soluble. A vitamin's solubility determines how the body absorbs, stores, and transports it. Fat-soluble vitamins enter the body with fats and can be stored in adipose tissue. Excess fat-soluble vitamins are not easily excreted from the body; they can be toxic, causing infection or disease. By contrast, fat does not play a role in the absorption of water-soluble vitamins. Water-soluble vitamins are generally not stored in the body. If you consume more water-soluble vitamins than you need, the excess is expelled from the body in urine.

Most water-soluble vitamins are **coenzymes** (koh-EHN-zighmz). A coenzyme is a molecule that combines with a protein to make a working enzyme. This coenzyme-protein combination can catalyze a chemical reaction.

The table in **Figure 13.6** lists and describes the functions of some of the vitamins that your body needs. Your recommended daily vitamin intake depends on your age, gender, and health status. Long-term lack of a particular vitamin is called a **vitamin deficiency**. Certain health problems

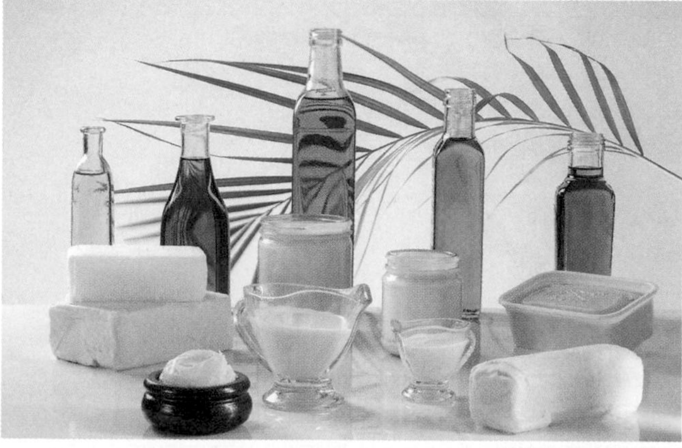

JPC-PROD/Shutterstock.com

Figure 13.4 Oils and fats are a necessary part of a healthy diet, but they should be used sparingly. *Which types of fats should be avoided to maintain a healthy diet?*

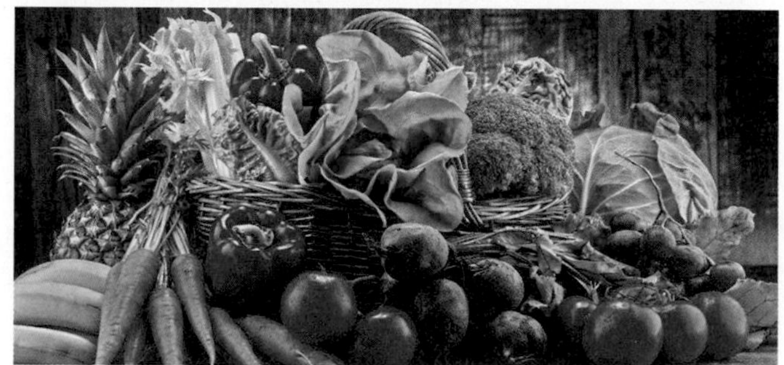

monticello/Shutterstock.com

Figure 13.5 Fruits and vegetables contain many of the vitamins and minerals that your body needs.

Micronutrients and Their Functions*	
Water-Soluble Vitamins	
Thiamine (B_1)	Coenzyme that works in multiple body systems; needed for many biochemical reactions; needed for the synthesis of acetylcholine, a chemical used by nerve cells
Riboflavin (B_2)	Coenzyme that works in multiple body systems; needed for cellular reactions in eyes, skin, intestinal epithelia, and blood cells
Niacin (B_3)	Coenzyme needed for breakdown of fats and for skin cell metabolism
Pantothenic acid (B_5)	Coenzyme that works in multiple body systems; used in the creation of several hormones; needed for biochemical processing of carbohydrates, lipids, and amino acids
B_6	Coenzyme that works in multiple body systems; needed for chemical reactions involving amino acids (the building blocks of proteins)
Biotin (B_7)	Coenzyme that plays a key role in metabolism of fatty acids, glucose, and amino acids.
Folate (Folic acid, B_9)	Needed for chemical reactions involving amino acids and nucleic acids
B_{12}	Plays a role in the formation of red blood cells and in chemical reactions involving nucleic acids (the building blocks of DNA and RNA)
Ascorbic acid (C)	Promotes protein synthesis, including collagen formation; an antioxidant that neutralizes free radicals, highly reactive chemicals that could otherwise cause damage
Fat-Soluble Vitamins	
A	Helps form light-sensitive chemical in the eyes; helps epithelial cells grow normally
D	Aids calcium and phosphorous absorption in the intestine, and prevents loss of those elements in the urine; needed for bone growth
E	Inhibits the breakdown of cell membranes; needed for red blood cell formation and for formation of DNA and RNA; an antioxidant that neutralizes free radicals
K	Plays a major role in blood clotting
Minerals	
Calcium (Ca)	Helps form and maintain healthy bones and teeth; decreases risk of developing some cancers; plays a role in regulation of blood pressure and immune system function
Fluoride (F)	Supports the deposition of calcium and phosphorus in bones and teeth; helps prevent cavities
Iodine (I)	A component of thyroid hormones that controls the regulation of body temperature, BMR, growth, and reproduction
Iron (Fe)	Part of hemoglobin and myoglobin, which transport oxygen in the body; component of many enzymes; essential for brain growth and function
Phosphorus (Ph)	An essential component of ATP; helps form and maintain healthy bones; helps activate and deactivate enzymes; a component of DNA and RNA
Potassium (K)	Plays a role in muscle contractions and the transmission of nerve impulses; helps regulate blood pressure
Sodium (Na)	Helps regulate water distribution and blood pressure; involved in nerve transmission and muscle function; aids in the absorption of some nutrients

*This is not a complete list of micronutrients or of their functions.

Goodheart-Willcox Publisher

Figure 13.6

are related to vitamin deficiency. For example, a vitamin D deficiency can cause osteoporosis, muscle weakness, or high blood pressure.

Minerals

Like vitamins, **minerals** are elements that the body needs in relatively small amounts; yet they are essential for the proper functioning of the body. The average daily recommended intake for different minerals varies. For example, about 4,700 mg of potassium is recommended each day. However, other minerals have daily recommended doses of only fractions of a milligram.

Minerals that are vital for good health include calcium and phosphorus, which are major components of bone. Iron helps red blood cells transport oxygen. Sodium is another required mineral, although the amount of sodium that the body needs is a subject of debate in the medical community.

Adults require about 1,000 mg of sodium per day. Government health organizations recommend that most people keep their sodium intake below 1,500 mg per day. However, most Americans consume an average of 3,400 mg of sodium each day because their diets are high in salt, or *sodium chloride*. Many Americans frequently eat high-salt foods, such as processed foods and meals from fast-food restaurants.

Strong evidence links a high-sodium diet to high blood pressure. People with high blood pressure have an increased risk of developing cardiovascular disease. The American Heart Association recommends that people strive to reduce their sodium intake.

Check Your Understanding

1. Which nutrients are classified as macronutrients?
2. Identify a food or ingredient that is a carbohydrate.
3. What are the building blocks of proteins?
4. What are sources of saturated fatty acids?

LESSON 13.1 Review and Assessment

Mini Glossary

Make sure that you know the meaning of each key term.

basal metabolic rate (BMR) the amount of energy required to sustain a person's metabolism for one day if he or she is at complete rest

Calorie the unit that food scientists use to measure the potential energy in foods; the amount of heat required to raise the temperature of 1 kilogram of water by 1°C; also called *kilocalorie*

coenzymes molecules that are necessary for the action of enzymes

energy the capacity of a physical system to do work

lipids substances found in oils and solid fats; can be classified either as saturated or unsaturated; also called *fats*

macronutrients substances such as carbohydrates, proteins, and lipids that the body requires in relatively large quantities

micronutrients vitamins and minerals that are essential to the body in small amounts

minerals elements that the body needs in relatively small amounts

monounsaturated fats one category of unsaturated fatty acids; sources include canola oil and olive oil

nutrients chemicals that the body needs for energy, growth, and maintenance

polyunsaturated fats one category of unsaturated fatty acids; sources include corn oil and soybean oil

trans-unsaturated fats one category of unsaturated fatty acids that are artificially produced; also called *trans fats*

vitamin deficiency the long-term lack of a particular vitamin in a person's diet; may result in health problems

vitamins organic chemicals needed by the body for normal functioning and good health

Know and Understand

1. List four different forms of energy.
2. List some of the factors that affect a person's basal metabolic rate (BMR).
3. Explain why some nutrients are called *micronutrients*.
4. According to current dietary recommendations, how much of a person's energy should be obtained from protein?
5. Why should people limit their intake of sodium?

Analyze and Apply

6. Explain why people need more energy each day than indicated by their BMR.
7. Compare and contrast saturated and unsaturated fats.
8. Explain why a person requires only small amounts of vitamins in his or her diet.
9. Compare micronutrients and macronutrients.
10. Give examples of four different sugars and list two sources for each.

IN THE LAB

11. Suppose that you are a dietitian and one of your patients recently suffered a heart attack. Tests show that your patient, who eats a high-fat diet, has significant plaque buildup in his arteries. Research low-fat diets and create a diet plan for your patient. Include healthful options for each meal (breakfast, lunch, and dinner), as well as for snacks.
12. Create a display to educate people about sugar content of common foods. Collect at least seven empty food wrappers and drink containers. Line them up from the least amount of sugar to the most. Place one sugar cube in front of each food for each tablespoon of sugar in the product. Share your display with the class.

LESSON 13.2

Anatomy and Physiology of the Digestive System

Before You Read

Try to answer the following questions before you read this lesson.

- Can you live without a gallbladder?
- What role does the liver play in digestion?

Lesson Objectives

- Describe how food is digested and absorbed.
- Identify the layers of the alimentary canal.
- Describe the function of each organ in the digestive system.

Key Terms

absorption	gingiva
bile	ingestion
chemical breakdown	mechanical breakdown
chyme	mucosa
defecation	muscularis externa
emulsification	peristalsis
esophagus	propulsion
gallbladder	serosa
gastrointestinal tract (GI tract)	submucosa

The digestive system consists of a tube running through the body with organs alongside it. Most of these organs secrete substances into the tube. Food goes in one end, is broken down, and is partly absorbed. The portions that are not absorbed exit through the other end of the tube.

This may be a very simple view of the digestive system, but it is a starting point. By the time you finish this lesson, you will be able to describe the structure and function of the digestive system in much greater detail.

The tube that runs through the body is called the **gastrointestinal** (gas-troh-in-TEHS-tin-ahl) **tract (GI tract)**, also known as the *alimentary* (al-i-MEHN-ter-ee) *canal*. The GI tract begins with the mouth and ends with the anus. The primary organs of the digestive system located between the mouth and anus include the pharynx, esophagus, stomach, small intestine, and large intestine.

Besides these primary organs, the digestive system includes accessory organs of digestion, such as the salivary glands, pancreas, liver, and gallbladder. These accessory organs are connected to the GI tract by ducts. The accessory organs secrete substances through the ducts that aid in chemical breakdown and absorption of food. **Figure 13.7** shows an overview of the GI tract and accessory organs of digestion. In total, the GI tract is approximately 9 meters (30 feet) long.

Activities of Digestion

There are different ways of understanding how the digestive system processes food. To help you understand how the system works, this section divides the digestion process into six different activities. **Figure 13.8** depicts these activities.

The first activity in the process of digestion is **ingestion**—getting the food into the body. Ingestion involves the mouth, including the teeth, lips, and tongue.

Propulsion begins after ingestion and continues all the way along the GI tract. Propulsion is initiated by swallowing at the pharynx and includes **peristalsis** (PER-i-STAHL-sis), the symmetrical contraction of muscles that moves food along the remainder of the GI tract.

MEMORY TIP

When used in an anatomical sense, the word *lumen* means "the open space inside a hollow tubular structure," such as the intestine or a blood vessel. At the hardware store, you will see the word *lumens* listed on a lightbulb package. In this context, the number of lumens indicates the brightness of the bulb. *Lumen* is Latin for "light." If the alimentary canal is a tunnel, then you could say there is light at the end of the tunnel—the lumens at the end of the lumen!

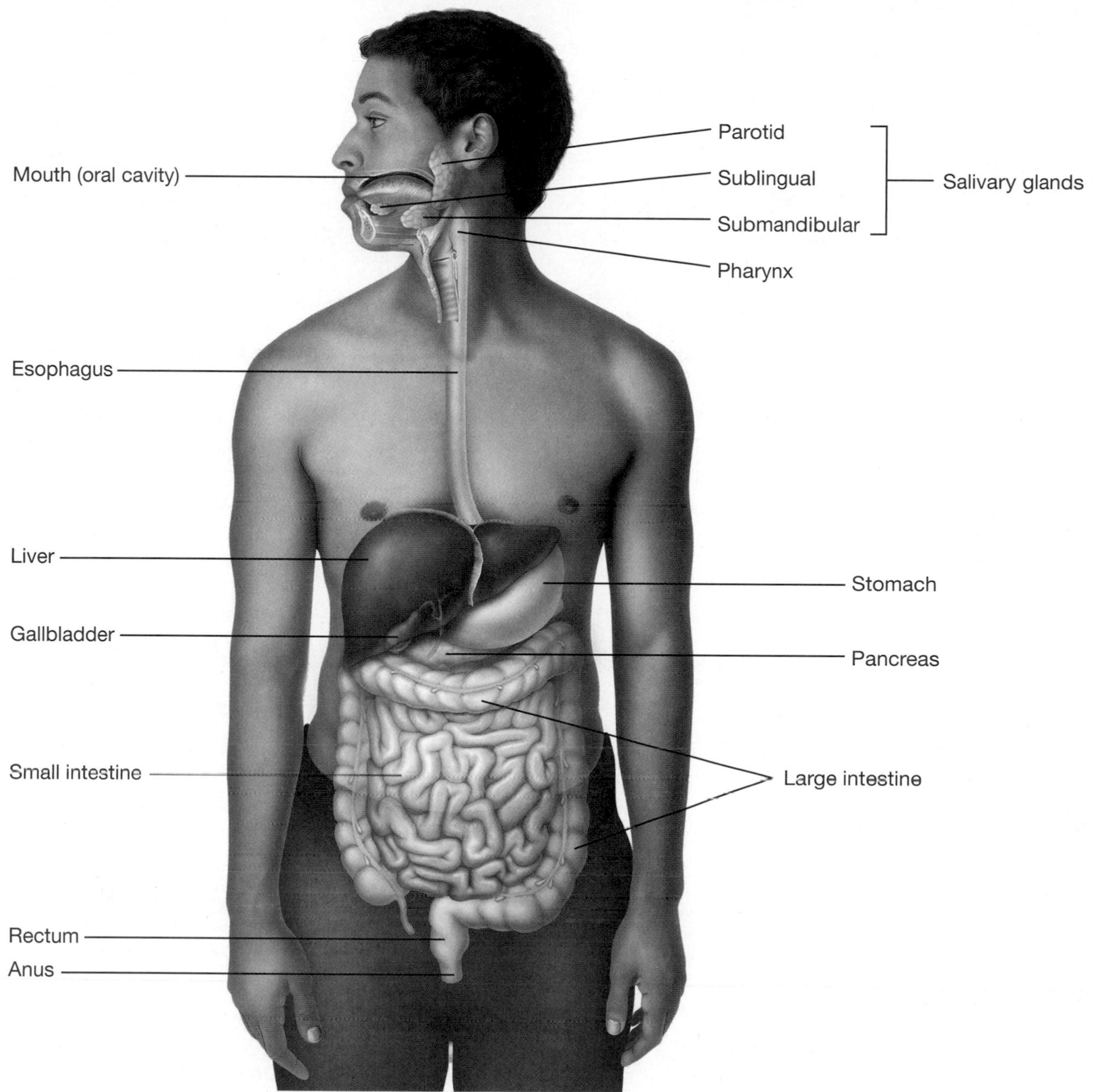

© Body Scientific International

Figure 13.7 The organs of the digestive system include those that are part of the GI tract as well as accessory, or helper, organs that aid in digestion and nutrient absorption. *Which organs shown here are considered accessory organs?*

The actual "digesting," or breaking down of the food particles, occurs in two ways: mechanical and chemical breakdown. **Mechanical breakdown** reduces food into smaller pieces and increases the surface area of the food. Chewing, churning in the stomach, and further churning by muscular contraction in the small intestine all contribute to the mechanical breakdown of food.

The **chemical breakdown** of food historically has been referred to as *digestion*. Enzymes in the lumen—the central opening of the GI tract into the stomach—and on the walls of the GI tract break large food molecules into smaller molecules.

Absorption, the fifth activity in digestion, involves the movement of small food molecules from the lumen of the small intestine into the blood. Once absorption has occurred, the blood carries the food to other parts of the body.

The final activity in the process of digestion is **defecation**—the expulsion of the food that was not absorbed. This waste matter, or feces, exits the body via the anus.

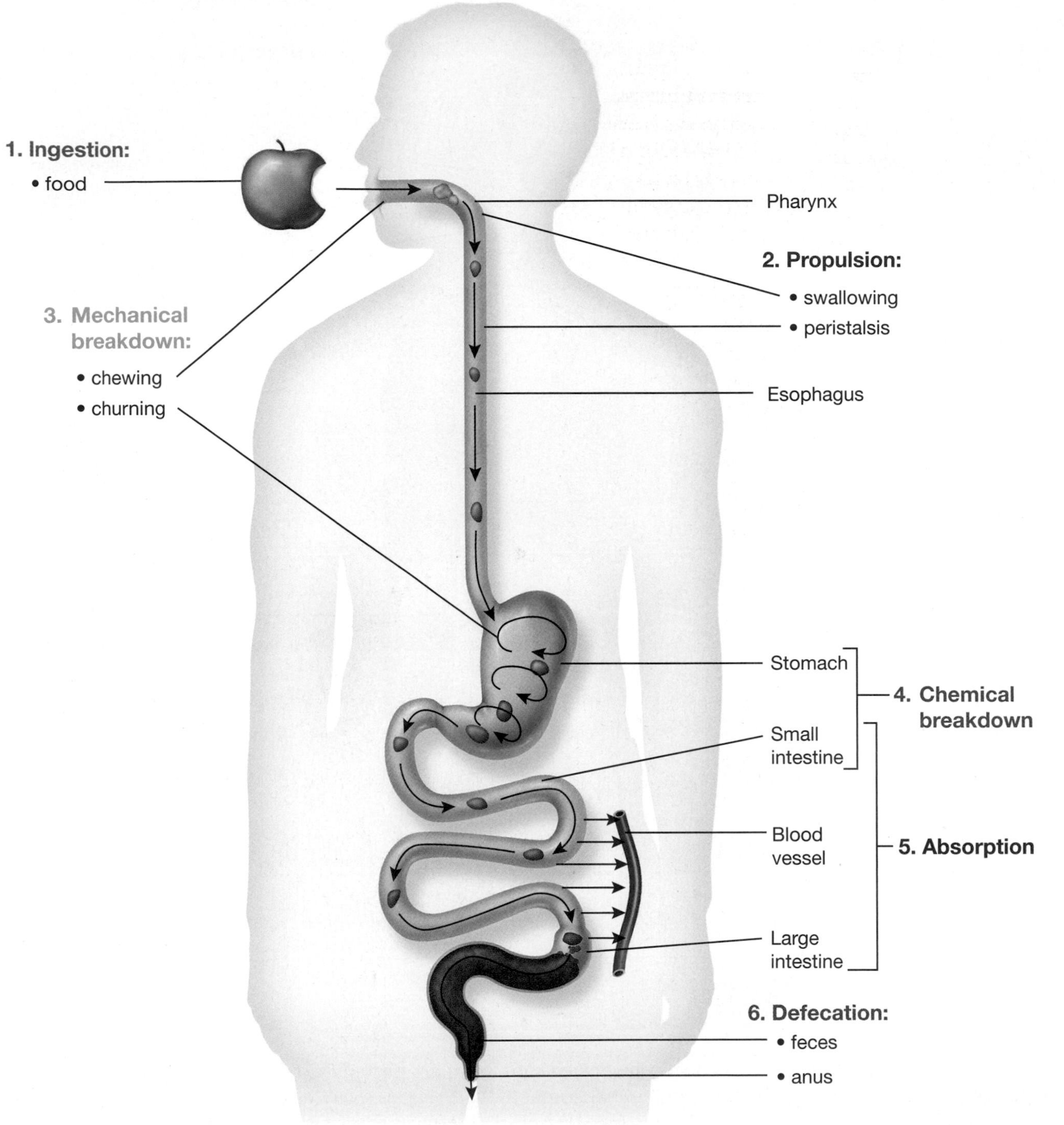

1. Ingestion:
• food
Pharynx
2. Propulsion:
• swallowing
• peristalsis
3. Mechanical breakdown:
• chewing
• churning
Esophagus
Stomach
Small intestine
4. Chemical breakdown
Blood vessel
5. Absorption
Large intestine
6. Defecation:
• feces
• anus

Figure 13.8 From ingestion to defecation, six activities are involved in digestion. *What process moves food into and through the GI tract during the propulsion stage?*

Check Your Understanding

1. List the structures of the GI tract, beginning with the mouth and ending with the anus.
2. Approximately how long is the entire GI tract?
3. List the accessory organs of digestion.

Layers of the GI Tract

The walls of the alimentary canal, or GI tract, have four basic layers. From the inside out, the layers are the mucosa, the submucosa (sub-myoo-KOH-sa), the muscularis externa, and the serosa (seh-ROH-sa) (**Figure 13.9**).

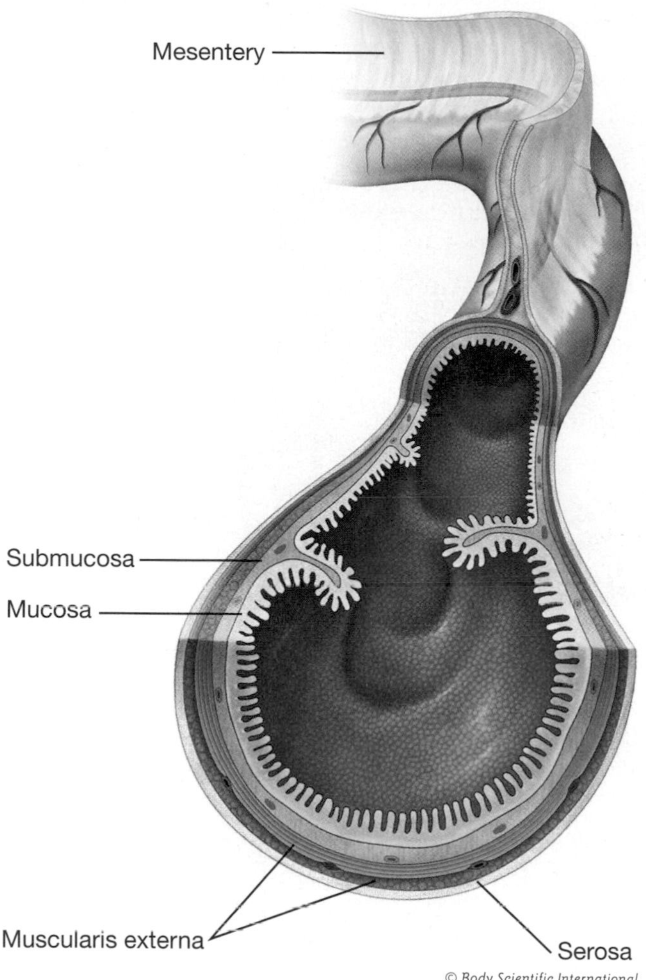

Figure 13.9 The layers of the walls of the GI tract, as seen in the small intestine. The mesentery helps ensure that the small intestines maintain their proper position as the body twists and moves.

Mucosa

The **mucosa**, or mucous membrane, is on the inside of the gastrointestinal tract, which means that it directly faces the outside world, because the lumen of the gut is connected to the outside world. Recall from Chapter 2 that epithelial tissue is found at the interface between the body and the outside world. It is therefore not surprising that the innermost layer of the mucosa is epithelial tissue, whose surface is covered by mucus secreted by cells or glands. The mucosa also has a slightly deeper sublayer of areolar connective tissue. This tissue contains blood vessels, lymphatic vessels, nerves, and, in some areas of the body, mucus-secreting glands.

Submucosa

Below the mucosa lies the **submucosa**, a layer of irregular dense connective tissue containing blood vessels, lymphatic vessels, and nerves. Lymphatic tissue and glands in some parts of the submucosa in the alimentary canal secrete substances that aid in digestion and absorption.

MEMORY TIP

When used to describe the layers of the GI tract walls, the word *deeper* means "farther away from" the lumen. The submucosa, whose name means "under the mucosa," is deeper than the mucosa. Thus, the submucosa is farther from the lumen than the mucosa.

A surgeon who has entered the abdominal cavity and is cutting into the GI tract will first slice into the serosa, then the muscularis externa, followed by the submucosa, and finally the mucosa. After cutting the mucosa, the surgeon will have reached the lumen.

Muscularis Externa

The **muscularis** (mus-kyoo-LAH-ris) **externa** surrounds the submucosal layer. In most of the GI tract, the muscularis externa has two layers of smooth muscle. The muscularis externa propels food through the GI tract by means of peristalsis. The muscularis externa also churns and breaks down the food mechanically.

The inner muscle layer has fibers that run in a circular manner around the lumen. The outer layer has fibers that run longitudinally, or lengthwise, along the canal. A layer of nerve fibers between the two layers regulates the activity of each layer.

Serosa

The outermost layer of the GI tract is the serosa. The **serosa** is so named because it is a serous membrane. Serous membranes are thin, slippery membranes that help minimize friction between organs and between organs and the body cavity wall (**Figure 13.10**).

In the abdominopelvic cavity, which contains most of the organs of digestion, the serous membrane is also known as the *peritoneum* (per-i-toh-NEE-um).

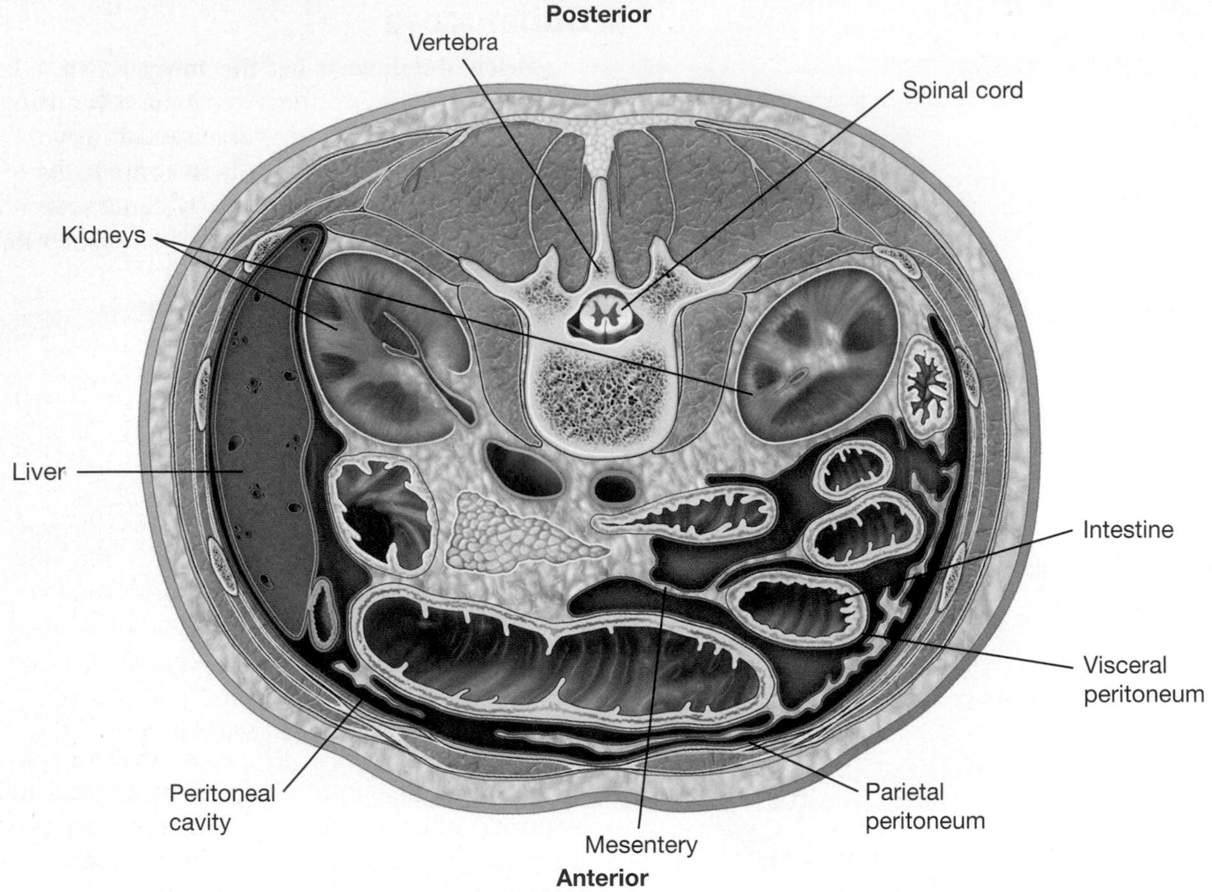

Figure 13.10 Transverse view of the abdominopelvic cavity. Some abdominal organs, such as the kidneys and pancreas, are retroperitoneal; that is, they lie behind the peritoneum.

The peritoneum is divided into two layers: the parietal and visceral. The parietal peritoneum lines the body wall. The visceral peritoneum wraps around the organs and forms the outer layer of those organs.

The parietal and visceral peritoneum are connected to each other by the *mesentery* (MEHS-ehn-ter-ee), a double layer of peritoneum. Blood and lymphatic vessels and nerves travel in the mesentery between the dorsal body wall and the organs of digestion. The mesentery also helps hold the abdominopelvic organs, particularly the small intestine, in their proper place.

The "empty space" between the parietal and visceral peritoneum is called the *peritoneal* (per-i-toh-NEE-al) *cavity*. It normally contains a small amount of watery fluid that allows the organs to move with minimal friction. Some organs—the kidneys and pancreas, for example—lie against the dorsal wall of the abdominopelvic cavity. These organs are said to be *retroperitoneal*, as **Figure 13.10** shows.

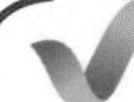

Check Your Understanding

1. List the layers of the walls of the alimentary canal, starting with the innermost layer.
2. What are the two layers of the peritoneum?

Digestive Organs and Their Functions

The digestive process involves several organs throughout the body. Some organs play a major role, while others aid in the process of digesting and absorbing nutrients.

The Oral Cavity

The mouth is also called the *oral cavity* (**Figure 13.11**). The mouth helps accomplish four of the six key activities of digestion: ingestion, mechanical breakdown, chemical breakdown, and propulsion.

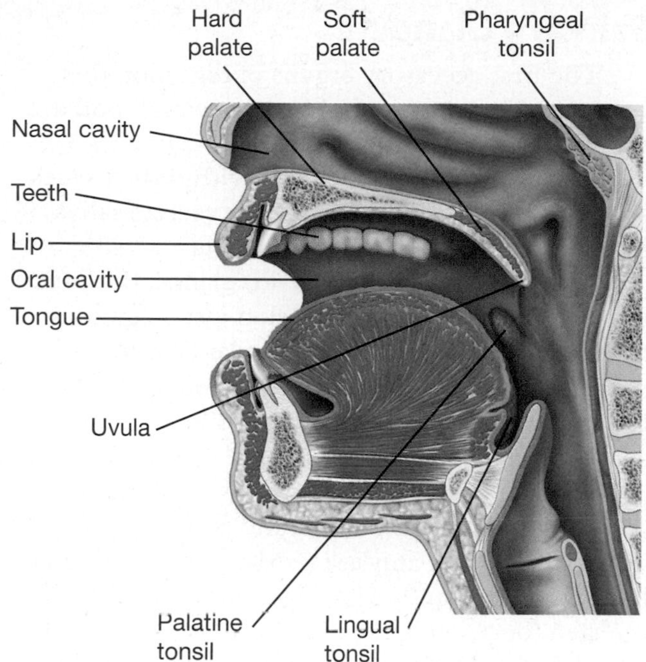

Figure 13.11 The oral cavity houses many digestive "tools" that begin the chemical and mechanical breakdown of food.

The epithelial lining of the mouth is the mucosa, which you learned about earlier in this lesson. The lips assist with ingestion by grabbing food and pulling it into the mouth. The lips also keep food and liquids from leaking out of the mouth. The lips contain the *orbicularis* (or-bik-yoo-LAH-ris) *oris* muscle. Like all skeletal muscles, this muscle is under voluntary control.

Anyone who has ever lost function in the lips understands the importance of this seemingly small body part. Loss of lip function can happen to a patient who has had a stroke. Strokes sometimes affect the nerves that control the lip muscles.

The tongue, like the lips, contains skeletal muscles. It has bumps, or papillae, on its surface. Some papillae house taste buds, whereas others simply help the tongue grip food better. Besides helping to provide the sense of taste, the tongue aids digestion by manipulating food in the mouth and moving chewed food to the back of the mouth for swallowing, or *deglutition*.

The cheeks form the lateral borders of the oral cavity, and the palate is the roof of the cavity. The front part of the palate, which is formed from parts of the maxillae and palatine bones, is called the *hard palate*. The posterior portion of the palate is called the *soft palate*. The soft palate is formed from a fold of mucous membrane.

The Nasal Cavity

The nasal cavity, the passageway for air entering and leaving via the nose, is located above the palate. When you look in your mouth, you can see the uvula (YOO-vyoo-la) hanging from the soft palate in the back. The uvula helps prevent food from entering the nasal cavity when you swallow.

Teeth and Gums

Teeth begin the mechanical breakdown of food by grinding or crushing the food after it enters the mouth. This process is known as *mastication*. When food is broken into smaller pieces, its surface area is increased. The enlarged surface area helps digestive enzymes chemically break down the food. The gum, or **gingiva** (JIN-ji-vuh), is a soft tissue that covers the necks of the teeth and the maxilla and mandible.

Types of Teeth

Children have 20 deciduous (temporary) teeth, which start to appear at around six months of age and are usually all visible by approximately two years of age. Starting around six years of age, 32 permanent teeth begin to form in the jawbones—16 in the mandible and 16 in the maxilla. As permanent teeth grow, they push out the deciduous teeth. The last permanent teeth, the wisdom teeth, usually do not appear until the late teens or early twenties.

The front four teeth on the top and bottom of the mouth are called *incisors*. Just lateral and posterior to the incisors, on each side of the mouth, are the canine teeth. Two molars follow each canine and complete a child's deciduous set of teeth, or *dentition*. The permanent dentition adds two premolars, or *bicuspids*, between the canines and the molars. A third molar, commonly known as a *wisdom tooth*, is also added to each side of the mouth (**Figure 13.12**).

The incisors are shaped to be good at cutting. The molars are good at crushing and grinding. The canines and premolars are intermediate, with the canines more adapted for cutting and the premolars more adapted for grinding and crushing.

Anatomy of the Tooth

The part of the tooth that projects out of the jawbone is called the *crown*. The part embedded in the jawbone is the *root*. The middle part, located between the crown and the root, is the *neck* (**Figure 13.13**).

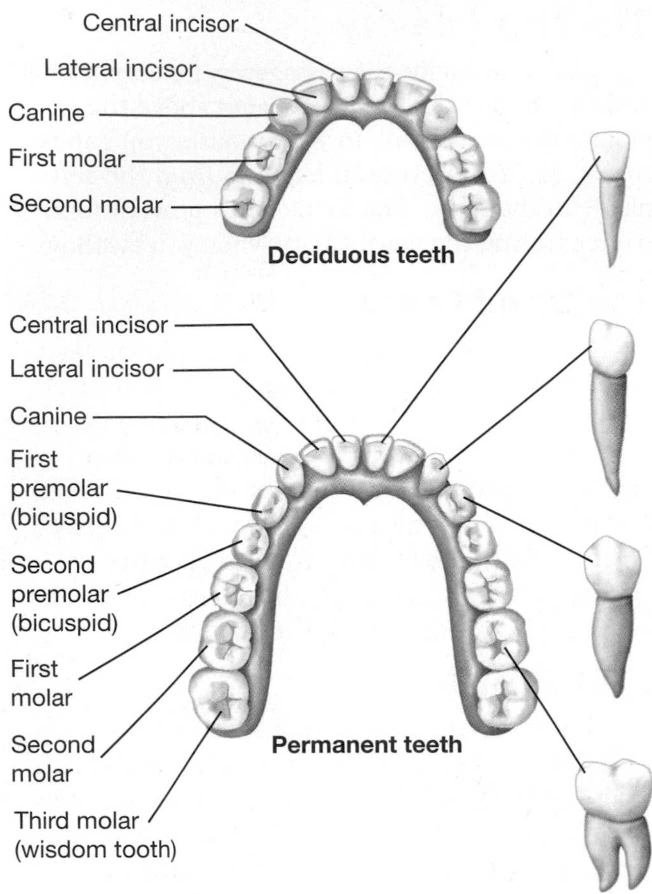

Figure 13.12 Deciduous teeth are eventually replaced by permanent teeth. The same permanent teeth appear on both the maxilla and mandible. *At what age do the permanent teeth begin to appear?*

The crown of each tooth has a coating of enamel. Enamel is the hardest material in the body, considerably harder than bone. The body of the tooth is made of *dentin*, a material that is similar to but harder and denser than bone. The *pulp cavity* is a hollow central region containing soft tissue, nerves, and blood vessels. The hollow *root canal* provides a passageway for nerves and blood vessels to reach the pulp cavity from the mandible or maxilla. The nerves that occupy the pulp cavity alert you to oral pain or sensitivity by sending signals via the nervous system.

Each tooth is securely anchored in its bony socket by the *periodontal* (per-ee-oh-DAHN-tal) *ligament*, a mesh of collagen fibers surrounding each root. Each incisor and canine has a single root; each premolar has one or two roots; and each molar has two or three roots.

Salivary Glands

The first accessory organs of digestion that contribute to the chemical breakdown of food are the three pairs of salivary glands (**Figure 13.7**). The salivary glands are located within the tissues surrounding the oral cavity. They secrete saliva into the mouth via connecting ducts.

The parotid (pah-RAHT-id) glands, the largest salivary glands, lie under the skin just below and in front of the ears. The submandibular (sub-man-DIB-yoo-lar) salivary glands lie on the medial side of the lower back part of the mandible. The sublingual salivary glands are under each side of the tongue.

Saliva is composed mostly of water. It also contains mucus, antibodies, and several enzymes, including salivary amylase (AM-il-ays) and lingual lipase (LIGH-pays). The water and mucus help moisten food, while the antibodies protect the mouth against bacterial infection. Salivary amylase breaks down complex carbohydrates (starches) into shorter chains of sugar subunits. Lingual lipase initiates the chemical breakdown of lipids.

MEMORY TIP

Many structures in and around the mouth contain the root word *gloss/o* or *–lingu/o*, both of which refer to the tongue.

- The hypoglossal (high-poh-GLAHS-al) and glossopharyngeal (glahs-oh-fah-RIN-jee-al) nerves go to the tongue region.
- The genioglossus (gee-nee-oh-GLAHS-us) and hyoglossus (high-oh-GLAHS-us) muscles form part of the tongue.
- The lingual frenulum (LING-gwahl FREHN-yoo-lum) is the thin band of tissue under the tongue that helps anchor it in the oral cavity.
- The lingual tonsil is at the back of the base of the tongue.

Pharynx

The pharynx (FAIR-ingks) is the region that connects the mouth and the nasal cavity to the trachea and the esophagus (**Figure 13.14**). As explained in Chapter 9, the pharynx plays an important role in respiration as well as digestion. From top to bottom, the pharynx is composed of three main parts:

- The nasopharynx (NAY-zoh-fair-ingks) connects the nasal cavity to the oropharynx. Only air passes through the nasopharynx.

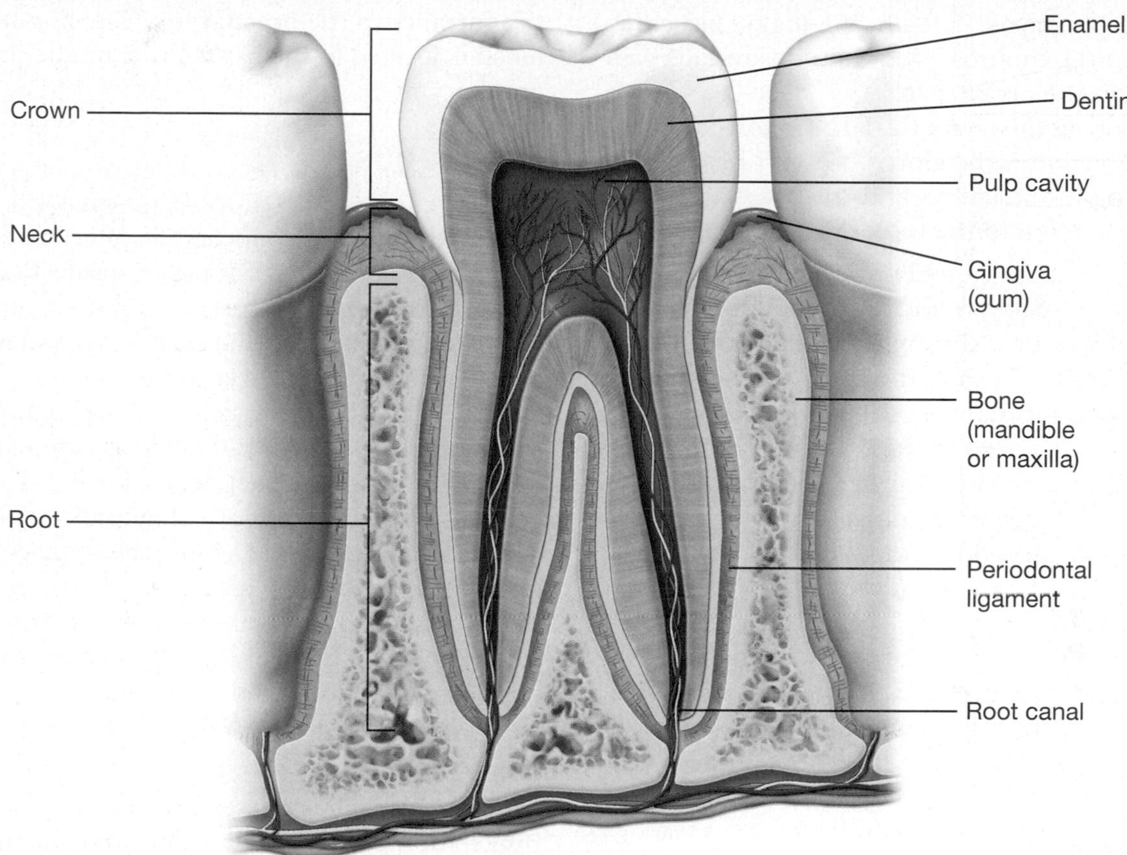

Figure 13.13 The structure of a tooth. *What material is harder than bone and protects the crown of a tooth?*

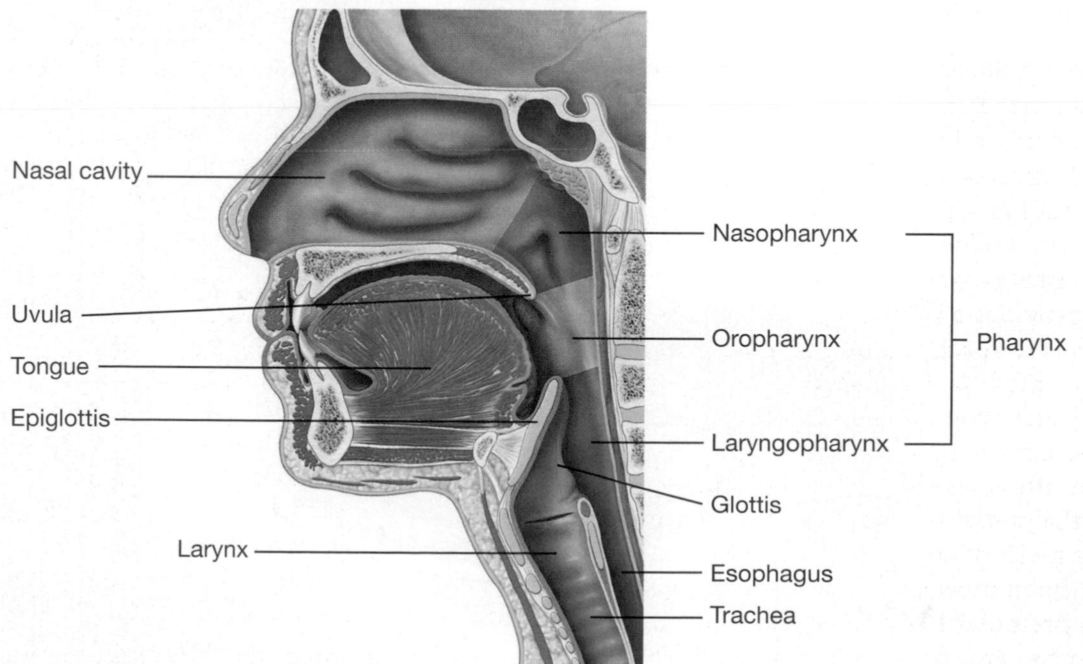

Figure 13.14 The pharynx is divided into three sections—the nasopharynx, oropharynx, and laryngopharynx. *The pharynx connects the mouth and nasal cavity to which structures?*

- The oropharynx (OR-oh-fair-ingks) lies at the back of the mouth. Food, liquids, and air pass through the oropharynx.
- The laryngopharynx (la-RING-goh-fair-ingks) includes the glottis (GLAHT-is)—the opening to the larynx and trachea—and extends down to the top of the esophagus.

The epiglottis is a fold of tissue on the front side of the oropharynx and laryngopharynx. Food, liquids, and air pass through the oropharynx and laryngopharynx. During the act of swallowing, coordinated contractions of the longitudinal and circular muscle layers in the walls of the pharynx push food through the pharynx and on to the esophagus. As food or liquid is swallowed, the epiglottis contracts downward to cover the glottis so that neither the food nor the liquid enters the trachea.

Figure 13.11 shows the tonsils, which are small bundles of lymphatic tissue. Like fortresses full of guards, the tonsils are full of lymphocytes that protect the body from infection. The pharyngeal tonsil, located on the posterior wall of the nasopharynx, is often referred to as the *adenoid*. A palatine tonsil lies on each side of the entrance to the oropharynx. The lingual tonsil is located at the base of the tongue, in the oropharynx.

Esophagus

The **esophagus** (eh-SAHF-a-gus) is a muscular tube that connects the pharynx to the stomach (**Figure 13.7**). It lies posterior to the trachea and heart and passes through an opening in the diaphragm, the muscle that separates the thoracic and abdominal cavities.

Just below the diaphragm, the esophagus reaches the stomach. When food enters the top of the esophagus during the act of swallowing, a wave of peristalsis begins. This wave of muscular contraction pushes food downward and into the stomach. At the junction of the esophagus and stomach, the *cardiac sphincter* allows food to move from the esophagus to the stomach, but closes to prevent the food from moving back into the esophagus.

Stomach

The stomach is a reservoir in which food is broken down both mechanically and chemically before it enters the small intestine (**Figure 13.15**).

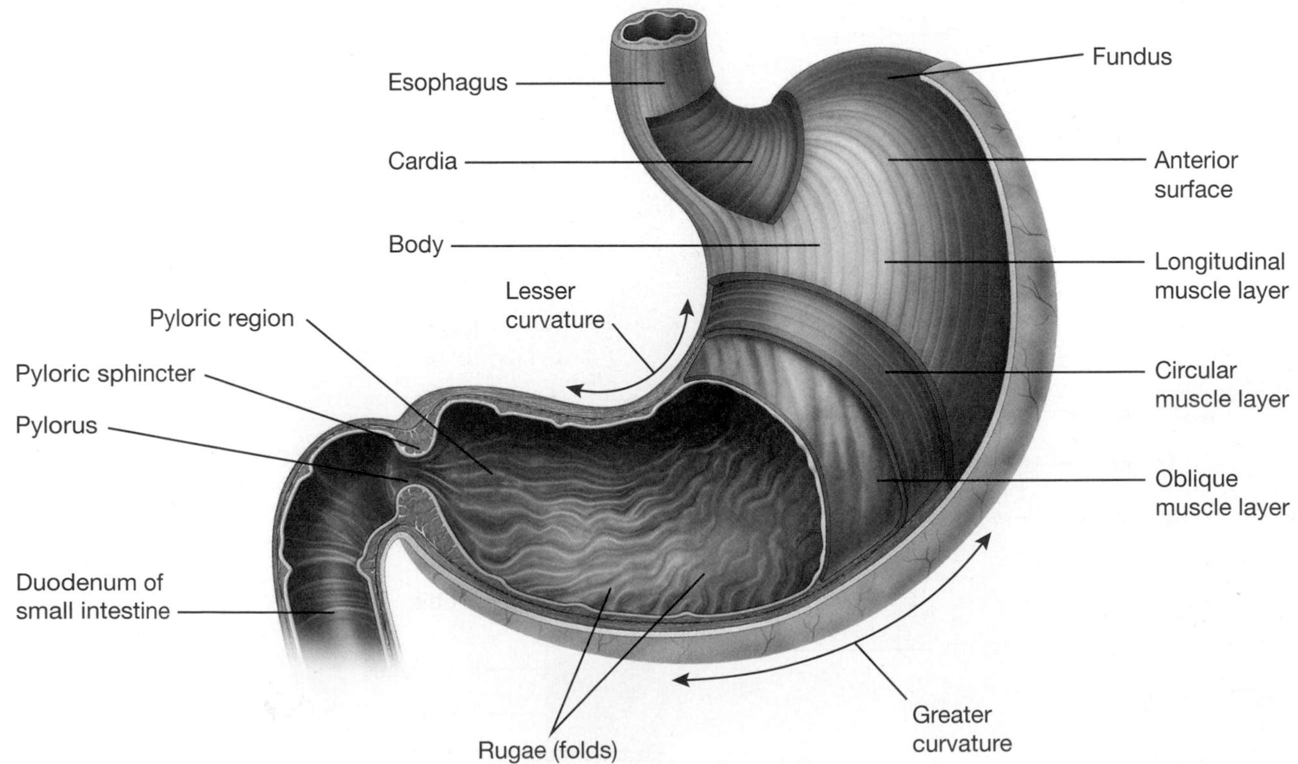

Figure 13.15 The stomach contains three layers of muscle, unlike most of the GI tract, which only has two layers. *What is the purpose of the oblique muscle layer in the wall of the stomach?*

Major regions of the stomach include the cardia, the fundus, the body, and the pyloric region.

The cardia (a term meaning "near the heart") is the region closest to the opening of the esophagus. The fundus is the upper end of the stomach, the body is the middle part, and the pyloric region is at the lower end.

The empty stomach has an internal volume of about 50 mL. However, the folds of the inside wall, called *rugae* (ROO-gee), are able to flatten. As the stomach stretches, the rugae flatten, increasing the stomach's volume. When full, the stomach can hold two liters or more, and the rugae flatten until they almost disappear.

The wall of the stomach contains three layers of muscle, unlike most of the GI tract, which has only longitudinal and circular muscle. The extra layer, called the *oblique* (ob-LEEK) muscle layer because its fibers run diagonally, sits beneath the circular and longitudinal muscle layers. The oblique muscle layer helps the stomach churn food and remains strong even when stretched.

The pylorus (pi-LOR-us) is the opening from the stomach into the small intestine. The wall of the pylorus contains the pyloric sphincter, a ring of circular smooth muscle that must relax to allow food to pass into the small intestine.

Lining of the Stomach

The lining of the stomach is a simple columnar epithelium made of mucus-secreting *goblet cells*. (For a review of columnar epithelial tissue, see Chapter 2.) A microscopic view of the stomach lining reveals millions of tiny openings called *gastric pits* (**Figure 13.16**). Each opening leads to a tubular gastric gland that secretes gastric juice. Gastric juice is also secreted as part of a parasympathetic nervous system response—seeing, smelling, and tasting food alerts the nervous system that digestion is about to begin.

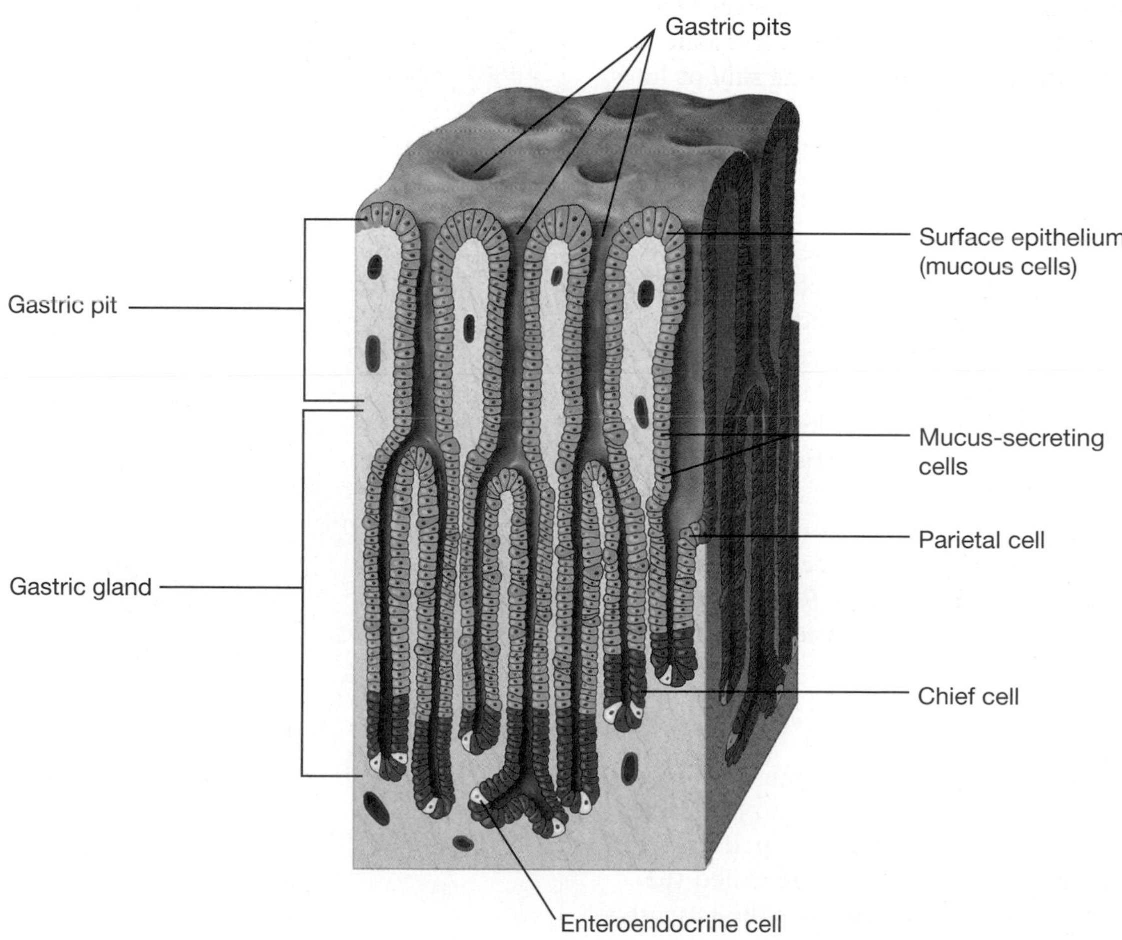

Figure 13.16 The lining of the stomach contains gastric pits and gastric glands. A gastric pit is a tubular opening in the stomach lining that connects to a deeper, tubular gastric gland.

The cells lining the gastric pits secrete mucus. The cells lining the gastric gland include mucus-secreting cells, parietal cells, chief cells, and enteroendocrine cells. The parietal cells secrete hydrochloric acid (HCl) and a glycoprotein called *intrinsic factor* that helps the body absorb vitamin B_{12}. The chief cells secrete the protein pepsinogen (pehp-SIN-oh-jehn). Enteroendocrine cells produce the hormone gastrin (GAS-trin), which stimulates the secretion of more gastric juice.

Hydrochloric acid secreted by the parietal cells makes the stomach contents very acidic, with a typical pH of 1.5 to 2.5. This acidic environment helps kill bacteria and aids in the conversion of inactive pepsinogen to active pepsin, a protein-digesting enzyme.

Chemical Reactions in the GI Tract and Stomach

The secretion of protein-digesting enzymes in the GI tract creates a potentially dangerous situation: the enzymes could start digesting, or breaking down, the body's own tissues. The body can avoid this dangerous situation as long as adequate mucus is produced. The mucus lines the stomach wall and protects it from the eroding effects of hydrochloric acid and protein-digesting enzymes such as pepsin.

In a process called *maceration* , food that enters the stomach mixes with the acidic gastric juice to form **chyme** (kighm). Active contractions of the muscular wall keep the mixture well stirred. Pepsin breaks down proteins in the food into shorter amino acid chains. Intrinsic factor binds to any vitamin B_{12} molecules present, enabling the vitamin to be absorbed when it later reaches the small intestine. The hormone gastrin and nerve impulses on the vagus nerve both stimulate secretion of gastric juice and churning activity of the stomach muscles. Relaxation of the pyloric sphincter allows chyme to enter the small intestine.

Small Intestine

The small intestine gets its name from its diameter, which is much smaller than that of the large intestine. If intestines were named for their length, the small intestine would be called the *long* intestine. The small intestine is the longest segment of the GI tract, with a length of about 7 or 8 yards (6 or 7 meters) when relaxed. Most chemical breakdown of food occurs in the small intestine, as well as some mechanical breakdown. In the mechanical process of *segmentation*, the circular muscles surrounding the small and large intestines rhythmically contract to help digest chyme. The small intestine is also the site of all food absorption and most water absorption.

Segments of the Small Intestine

The small intestine has three segments: the *duodenum* (doo-AH-deh-num), the *jejunum* (jeh-JOO-num), and the *ileum* (IL-ee-um), all shown in **Figure 13.17**. The duodenum is the first and shortest segment. It begins at the pyloric sphincter and continues for about 10 inches (about 25 centimeters).

The secretions of the liver, gallbladder, and pancreas enter the duodenum via the duodenal ampulla (doo-AH-deh-nal am-POOL-la), a small chamber in the wall of the duodenum. The duodenal papilla, a small cone of tissue on the wall of the duodenum, contains the opening of the duodenal ampulla.

The jejunum follows the duodenum and is about 8 feet (2.5 meters) long. The ileum is the last and longest segment of the small intestine, measuring between 12 and 13 feet (3.5 and 4 meters) long. Chemical digestion, absorption, and propulsion by peristalsis occur in all three segments of the small intestine.

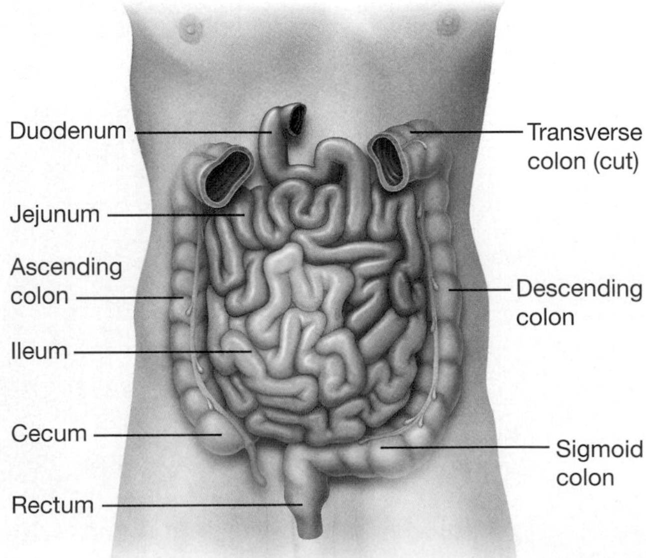

Figure 13.17 The small intestine is divided into three segments: the duodenum, jejunum, and ileum. *Which of the three segments of the small intestine is the shortest?*

The Lining of the Small Intestine

The surface area of the small intestine's lining is greatly increased by several structural features. The inner surface of the small intestine has circular folds that are large enough to see with the naked eye (**Figure 13.18A**). The surface of each fold is covered with finger-like projections called *villi*, and with tubular indentations called *intestinal crypts*, which are similar to gastric pits in the stomach (**Figure 13.18B**).

Each villus (the singular form of *villi*) contains a lymphatic capillary called a *lacteal* (LAK-tee-al), as well as blood capillaries. The epithelial cells of the villi have tiny, finger-like projections on the exposed surfaces of the cells, which face the lumen of the intestine. These microscopic projections are called *microvilli* (**Figure 13.18C**). The microvilli are collectively called the *brush border* because, when viewed with a microscope, they resemble a fuzzy edge on one side of the cell.

MEMORY TIP

Recall that a villus is made up of many cells and has lacteal and blood capillaries in its core. A microvillus, on the other hand, is much smaller than a single cell. It contains little more than cytoplasm and a few protein filaments for stiffening. The basic cellular information in Chapter 2 may also help you remember the difference between villi and microvilli.

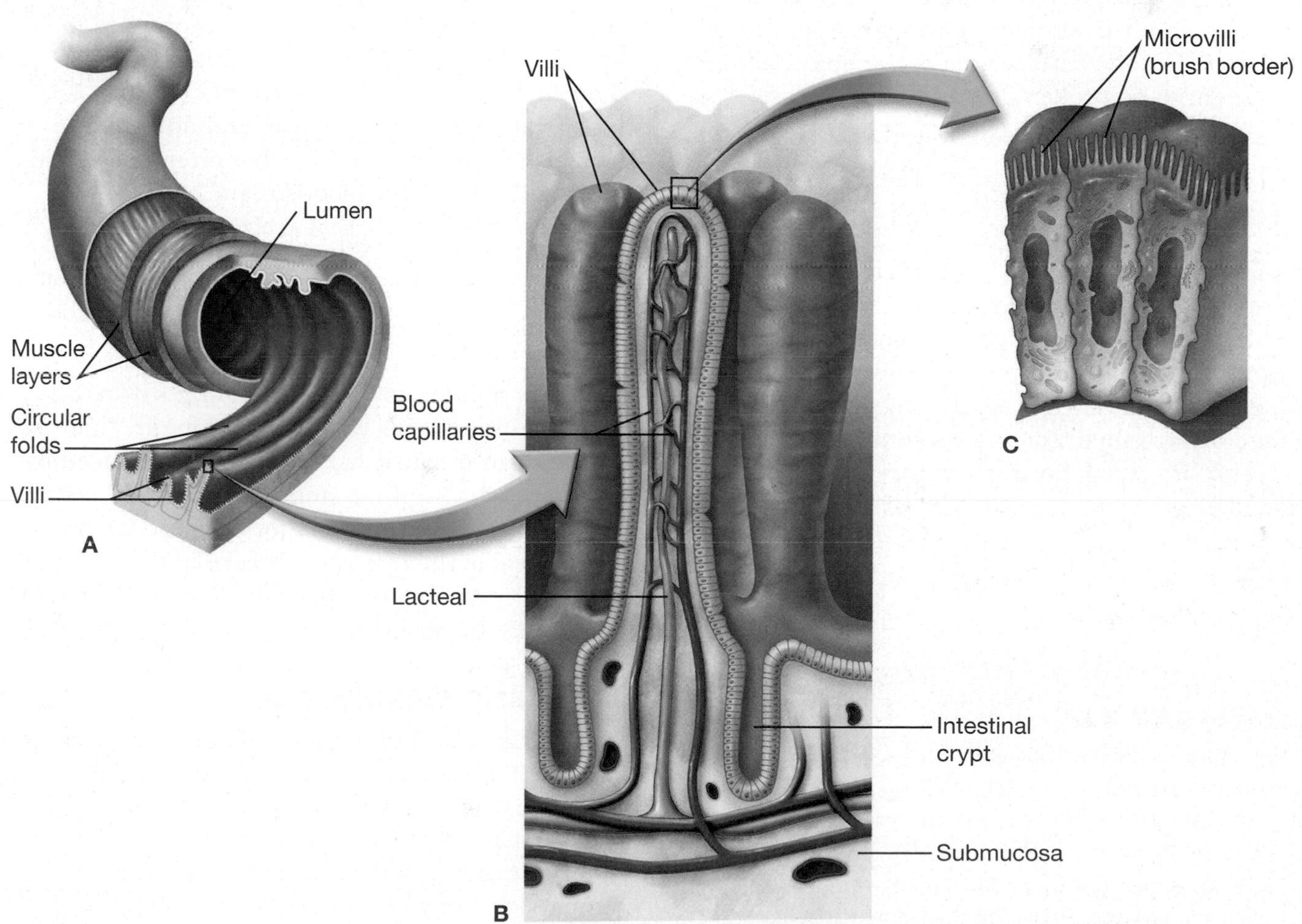

Figure 13.18 The wall of the small intestine. A—The lining of the small intestine contains circular folds. B—The surfaces of the folds are covered with villi and intestinal crypts. C—The epithelial cells covering the villi have microvilli on the part of the cell membrane that faces the lumen of the intestine.

Chemical Breakdown in the Small Intestine

Chyme enters the duodenum from the stomach, where it mixes with bile and pancreatic juice. Bile plays an important role in **emulsification**, the breakdown of large fat particles into smaller, more evenly distributed particles.

Pancreatic juice contains several chemicals, such as bicarbonate, pancreatic amylase, pancreatic lipase, and inactive pancreatic proteases. These chemicals break down the chyme and food particles in the duodenum.

- Bicarbonate is an alkaline molecule that neutralizes acidic chyme.
- Pancreatic amylase breaks down starches into chains that are as short as two sugar molecules (disaccharides).
- Pancreatic lipase breaks down lipids into their constituent fatty acids and monoglycerides. The emulsification of lipids by bile salts greatly increases the surface area of the lipids, allowing them to be broken down faster by lipase.

When inactive pancreatic proteases reach the duodenum, they are converted to their active forms. This happens because the pancreas, like the stomach, must avoid being digested by its own proteases. The pancreas protects itself by secreting proteases in an inactive form.

By the time carbohydrates and proteins approach the end of the small intestine, their chemical breakdown is nearly complete. The final stage of carbohydrate and protein breakdown occurs with brush border enzymes attached to the surfaces of the microvilli. Sucrase, for example, is a brush border enzyme that breaks sucrose (table sugar) into the single sugar molecules glucose and fructose.

MEMORY TIP

Many enzymes have names that end with the suffix *-ase*. These enzymes usually break down a molecule into smaller parts. *Proteases* break down proteins (long chains of amino acids) into short amino acid chains. *Lipases* break down lipids into free fatty acids and glycerol. *Amylases* break down starches into progressively shorter chains, ultimately producing chains that are two or three subunits long.

Absorption from the Small Intestine into the Blood

Absorption of food molecules into the blood occurs in all three segments of the small intestine. This process is enhanced by the large surface area created by the intestinal folds, villi, and microvilli.

Monosaccharides, such as glucose, and most amino acids are actively transported into the epithelial cells of the small intestine. The monosaccharides move from the epithelial cells into the blood capillaries within each villus. The blood in these capillaries, now rich in nutrients, is collected by the portal vein, which delivers the blood to the liver. In addition to serving as a transport system for oxygen and carbon dioxide, the blood helps the body absorb nutrients.

Free fatty acids and monoglycerides also enter the epithelial cells. The epithelial cells repackage these lipid subunits with proteins to form chylomicrons (KIGH-loh-migh-krahnz). The chylomicrons are too large to enter the blood capillaries, but they can and do enter the lacteals (**Figure 13.18**). The lymph in the lacteals eventually enters the bloodstream.

Most of the water that is absorbed into the blood is also absorbed in the small intestine. Water-soluble vitamins (vitamin C and most B vitamins) enter with the water.

Vitamin B_{12} is too large and electrically charged, though, to be absorbed on its own. So how does it make its way into the blood? Vitamin B_{12} binds to intrinsic factor, which is produced by the parietal cells of the stomach. Epithelial cells in the ileum have receptors for intrinsic factor, which enable them to actively take in the intrinsic factor-B_{12} combination. Fat-soluble vitamins (A, D, E, and K) are absorbed with lipids.

Liver and Gallbladder

The liver and the gallbladder are accessory organs of digestion. The **gallbladder** is the digestive organ that stores bile and delivers it to the duodenum when needed.

You can live without a gallbladder (many people do), but you cannot live without a liver. The digestive function of the liver and gallbladder is to make bile, store it, and deliver it in a timely manner to the duodenum. The duodenum uses bile to aid in the chemical breakdown of lipids.

Figure 13.19 shows the shape and position of both the liver and the gallbladder. The liver is the largest organ, by weight, in the abdominopelvic or thoracic cavity. It lies just under the diaphragm, primarily on the right side of the body.

Functions of the Liver

The liver has many functions. Most of its functions are metabolic, which means that they are related to the synthesis and processing of various chemicals. These functions help maintain a stable, healthy internal body environment—in other words, they maintain homeostasis. The specific metabolic functions of the liver include:

- maintenance of normal blood concentrations of glucose, lipids, and amino acids
- conversion of one nutrient type to another—for example, conversion of carbohydrates to lipids or, if necessary, amino acids to glucose
- synthesis and storage of glycogen and secretion of cholesterol, plasma proteins, and clotting factors
- storage of iron, lipids, and fat-soluble vitamins
- absorption and inactivation of toxins, hormones, immunoglobulins, and drugs

The Liver's Blood Supply

As explained in Chapter 11, the liver has an unusual blood supply. The liver receives oxygenated blood from the hepatic artery, which branches off the aorta. The blood leaves the liver via the hepatic vein, which drains into the inferior vena cava. So far, these circulatory processes are not unusual.

What is unusual is that the liver also receives deoxygenated, nutrient-rich blood from the stomach and intestines via the hepatic portal vein. This blood makes its way through the capillaries of the stomach, the small intestine, or the large intestine. In these organs, the blood loses its oxygen and absorbs whatever nutrients are present. Then it travels to the liver via the hepatic portal vein, and on through the liver capillaries.

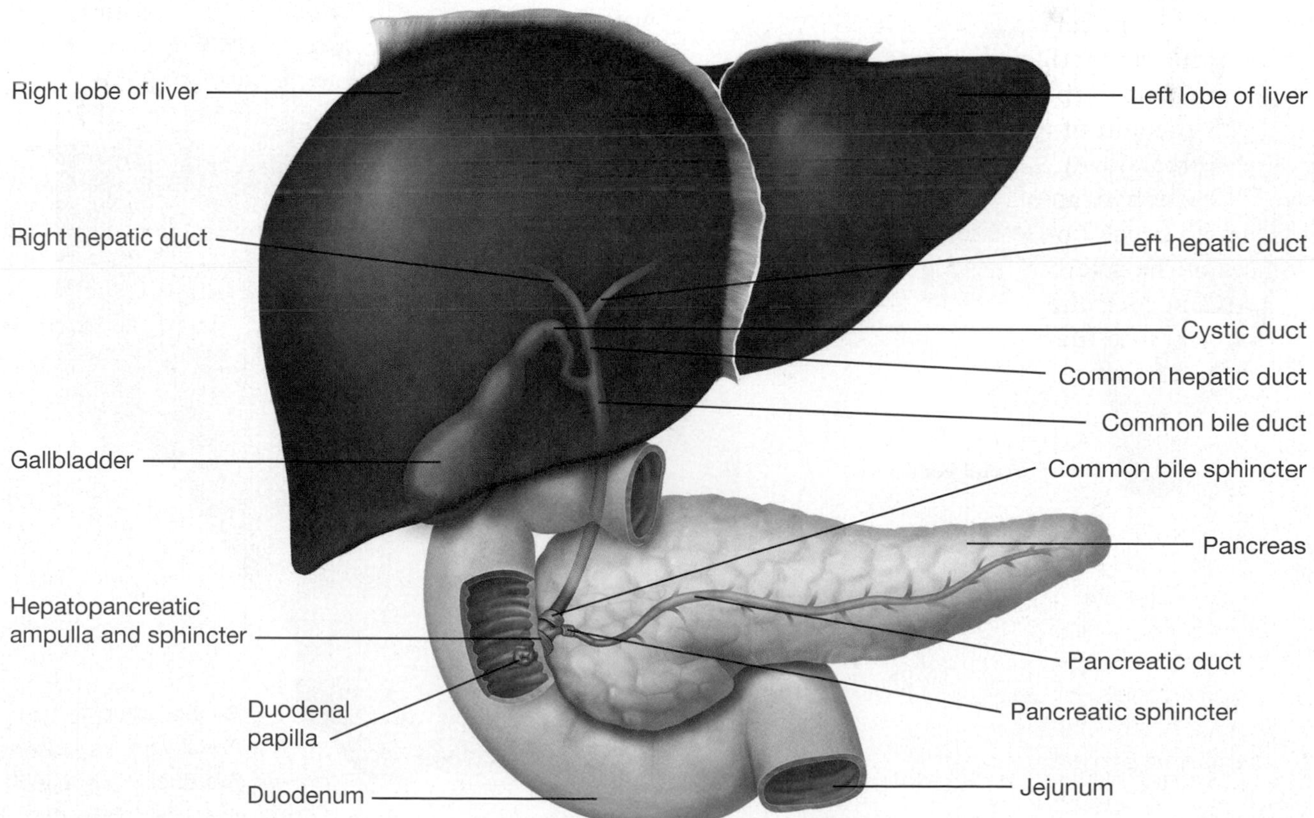

Figure 13.19 Anterior view of the liver, gallbladder, pancreas, and duodenum. *What are the digestive functions of the liver and gallbladder?*

Usually, blood goes through only one set of capillaries on its way from the arterial to the venous side of the circulatory system. In this case, however, it goes through two sets of capillaries.

The liver capillaries, called *sinusoids* (SIGH-nyoo-soyds), are "leakier" than most capillaries (**Figure 13.20**). Sinusoids contain fenestrations, or holes, in their walls, and lack a surrounding basement membrane, which is present in most capillaries. This leakiness makes it easy for nutrients to diffuse (spread out) from the capillaries to the hepatocytes (HEHP-a-toh-sights), or liver cells, and for proteins secreted by the hepatocytes to enter the capillaries.

Hepatic portal circulation serves an important function—delivering concentrated nutrients to the liver. Without this system, the nutrients from the stomach and intestines would be diluted, mixing with blood from the rest of the body. This would make the liver's job of processing and storing nutrients much harder.

MEMORY TIP

The combining form *hepat/o* means "liver." *Hepatocytes* are liver cells. *Hepatitis* is an inflammation of the liver. *Hepatic* blood vessels go to and from the liver.

Portare is a Latin word meaning "to carry." *Portal* veins *carry* blood from one capillary bed to another. The hepatic portal system is by far the largest portal system in the body. There is also a tiny, but important, portal circulation system between the hypothalamus and the pituitary gland in the brain.

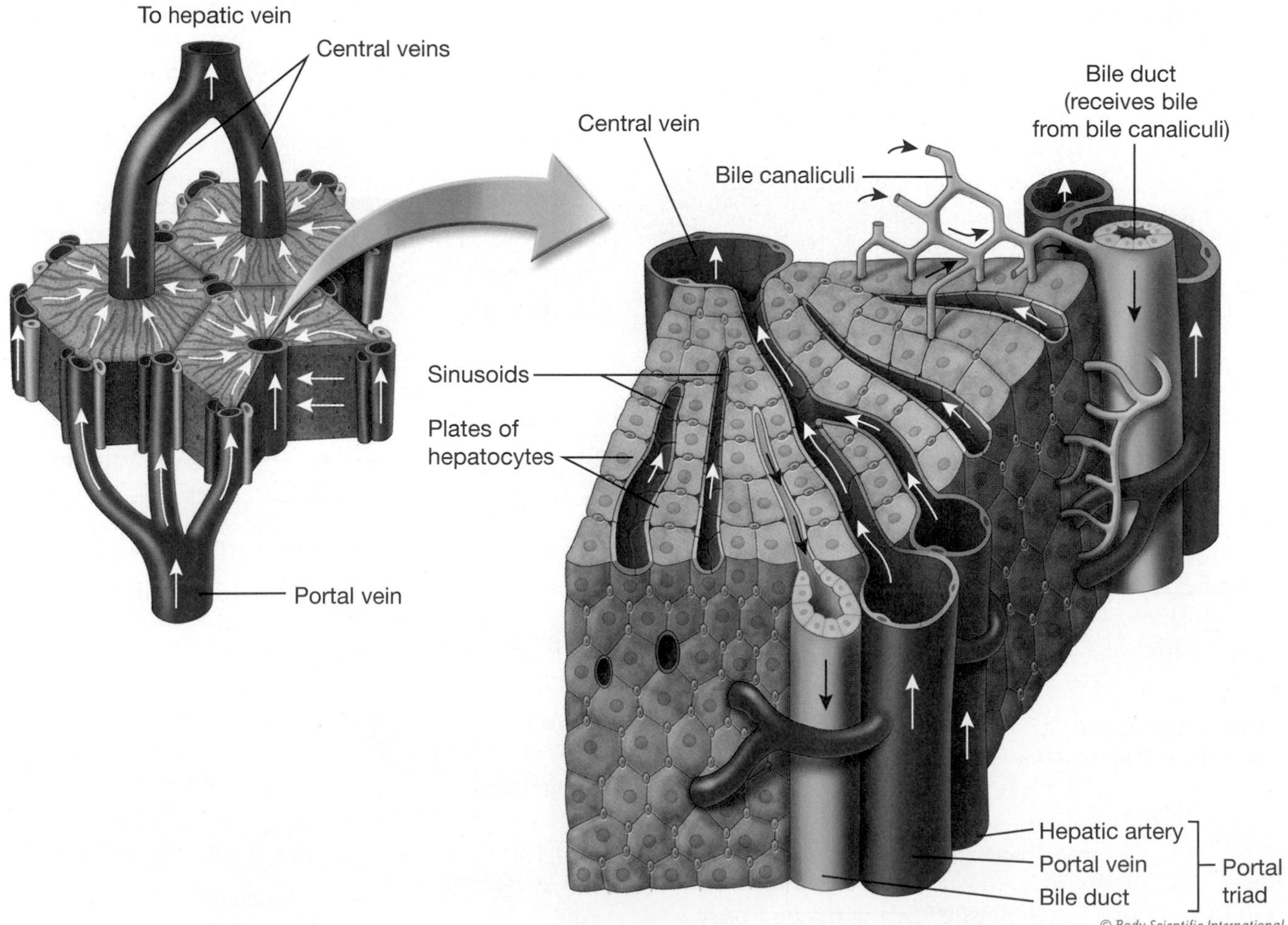

Figure 13.20 Detailed anatomy of a liver lobule. Blood flows from the triads "in" toward the central vein, through sinusoids (leaky capillaries), as indicated by the solid white arrows. Bile produced by hepatocytes is collected in bile canaliculi and flows "out" to the bile duct branches at the triads.

Liver Lobules

At a microscopic level, the liver is made up of a million or so functional units called *liver lobules* (**Figure 13.20**). A lobule is about one millimeter (a fraction of an inch) across. Each lobule includes hepatocytes, blood vessels, and *bile canaliculi* (kan-a-LIK-yoo-ligh)—"little canals"—and ducts that collect bile.

At each corner of each liver lobule is a portal triad that consists of a bile duct, a small hepatic artery, and a small portal vein. Blood enters the lobule through the portal vein and the hepatic artery. The blood flows through the sinusoids, exchanging nutrients, oxygen, and other substances with the hepatocytes. The blood is collected in the central vein, and from there it flows to the hepatic vein. The hepatic vein carries the blood from the liver to the vena cava.

Bile

While blood is flowing rapidly from the portal triads to the central vein, bile is moving slowly in the opposite direction. **Bile** is a watery solution containing *bile salts*, which are derived from cholesterol. When bile salts combine with fat droplets in chyme, the bile salts emulsify, or break apart, the fats. Bile salts are detergents, or emulsifying agents. Emulsification greatly increases the total surface area of fats, thus aiding their breakdown by lipases.

Bile is made and secreted by hepatocytes. It moves into the bile canaliculi, which carry it to the bile ducts at the triads. Small bile ducts join together to form the right and left hepatic ducts, which travel from the right and left lobes of the liver. These two ducts merge to form the common hepatic duct (**Figure 13.19**). The hepatic duct then joins with the cystic duct, coming from the gallbladder, to form the common bile duct. The common bile duct and the pancreatic duct meet at the wall of the duodenum to form a small chamber, the duodenal ampulla, which opens into the duodenum at the duodenal papilla (pa-PIL-a).

Bile Storage

The liver makes bile at a fairly steady rate of about one liter per day. However, the body does not need the bile at a steady rate. Bile is needed only after a meal, when there is chyme in the duodenum.

This mismatch between the liver's steady supply of bile and the body's intermittent demand for it is why people have gallbladders. The gallbladder releases bile after a meal that contains fat. Several sphincters work together to control bile outflow. These include the common bile sphincter, pancreatic sphincter, and the hepatopancreatic sphincter, which encircles the duodenal papilla.

When the body's demand for bile is low, bile coming down the hepatic duct travels up the cystic duct to be stored in the hollow gallbladder (**Figure 13.19**). Bile stored in the gallbladder becomes somewhat more concentrated because some of its water has been absorbed. When chyme—especially chyme containing a lot of fat—enters the duodenum, the muscular wall of the gallbladder contracts, squeezing out stored bile. At the same time, the common bile duct and hepatopancreatic sphincter relax, so that the bile can flow into the duodenum to emulsify the fat.

People with gallstones may have their gallbladder removed surgically. A person without a gallbladder still produces and secretes bile at a modest rate, but does not get the surge of bile that is needed to help digest a particularly fatty meal. Therefore, a person without a gallbladder should avoid large, fatty meals to prevent *steatorrhea*, the presence of excess fat in feces, which can cause fecal incontinence.

Pancreas

Like the liver and the gallbladder, the pancreas is an accessory organ of digestion. As **Figure 13.7** shows, the pancreas is nestled behind and underneath the stomach.

The pancreas is also part of the endocrine system and functions as both an endocrine and an exocrine gland. It secretes products into the blood (endocrine function) and into the lumen of the small intestine (exocrine function).

Like the liver, the pancreas has both digestive and metabolic functions. Its digestive function is to make and secrete pancreatic juice into the duodenum. Its metabolic function is to make the hormones insulin and glucagon and secrete them into the bloodstream.

Pancreatic Juices

Acinar cells in the pancreas produce and transport digestive enzymes that break down all the major classes of nutrients: proteases, amylases, and lipases. Pancreatic proteases are produced and secreted in an inactive form, to prevent self-digestion of the pancreas and its ducts. These inactive proteases are converted in the duodenum into the active proteases trypsin, chymotrypsin, and carboxypeptidase.

Pancreatic juice also contains pancreatic amylases that break down starches and pancreatic lipases that break down lipids. Pancreatic juice is alkaline due to the presence of bicarbonate. The bicarbonate in pancreatic juice neutralizes the hydrochloric acid in the chyme that comes from the stomach.

Glucose Regulation

The metabolic function of the pancreas is to secrete hormones that regulate the concentration of glucose in the blood. This is a classic example of hormonal regulation of the internal environment, for the purpose of maintaining homeostasis.

A high concentration of glucose in the blood causes beta cells in the pancreas to produce insulin and secrete it into the blood. The blood transports insulin, which binds to receptors on cells throughout the body. In the liver, insulin causes hepatocytes to extract more glucose from the blood and store it by converting it to glycogen. The binding of insulin to adipocytes (AD-i-poh-sights) causes greater glucose uptake and conversion of glucose to fat for storage. These actions cause the concentration of glucose in the blood to fall.

Glucagon is a hormone that is made and secreted by alpha cells in the pancreas when blood glucose levels are low. Like insulin, glucagon binds to receptors on cells throughout the body. However, its effects are opposite to those of insulin. Glucagon promotes conversion of glycogen to glucose in liver cells. Its actions have the overall effect of causing the concentration of glucose in blood to rise.

MEMORY TIP

To help you distinguish *glucagon* from terms such as *glucose* and *glycogen*, remember that "glucagon is secreted when glucose is gone."

Large Intestine

The large intestine has a larger diameter than the small intestine, but a shorter length; it measures about 5 feet (1.5 meters) when relaxed (**Figure 13.7**). The major segments of the large intestine are the cecum (SEE-kum), colon, rectum, and anal canal. The colon is the longest section of the large intestine. The anal canal terminates at the anus. The main functions of the large intestine are propulsion and elimination of waste. Absorption of water, electrolytes, and some vitamins are additional, but limited, functions.

A distinctive feature of the large intestine is the presence of large colonies of bacteria. These bacteria perform some helpful tasks, including synthesis of some B vitamins and vitamin K. The bacteria are usually not harmful, although the smelly gas they produce, which is occasionally expelled through the anus, is annoying.

The Cecum

The *cecum* is the first part of the large intestine to receive food from the small intestine. The end of the ileum connects to the cecum at the ileocecal (il-ee-oh-SEE-kal) valve. This valve is usually closed, but it opens in response to gastrin released by the stomach. It is also partially controlled by the nervous system. When the ileocecal valve opens, digested remnants of food travel from the ileum into the cecum.

The appendix hangs off the lowest part of the cecum. The appendix contains lymphocytes that help protect the body from infectious organisms in digested food. Unfortunately, these lymphocytes sometimes fail to protect the appendix itself from blockage, inflammation, and infection—appendicitis. The treatment for appendicitis is surgical removal of the appendix.

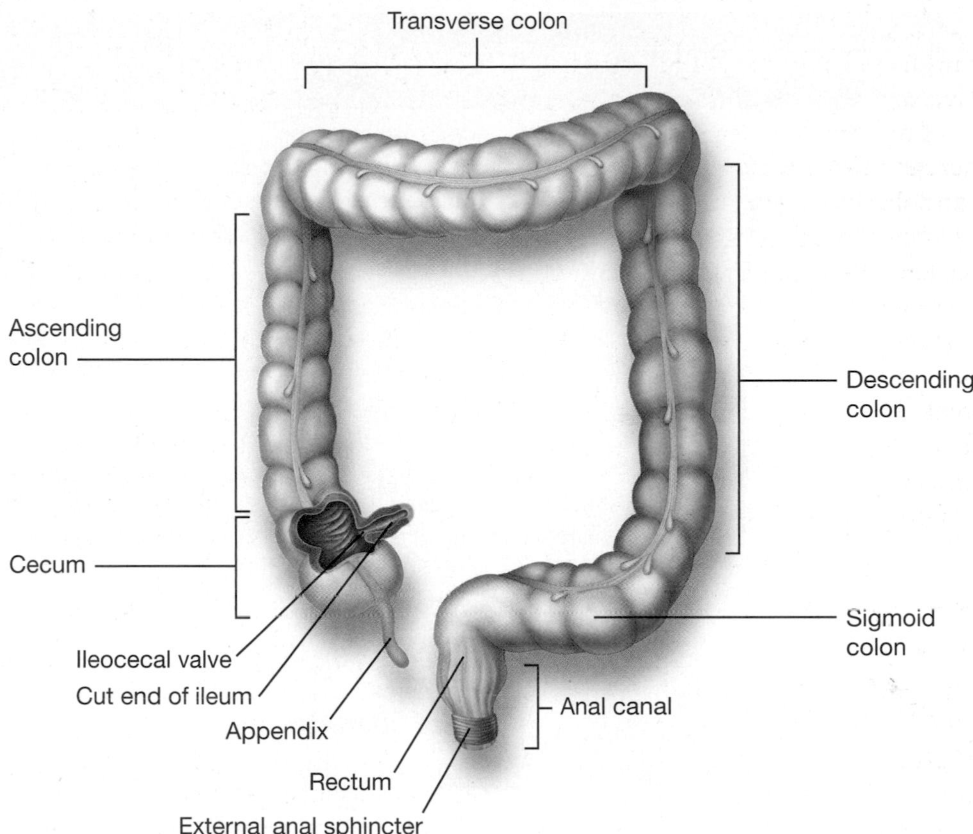

Figure 13.21 Anterior view of the large intestine. The small intestine has been removed.

The Colon

The colon has four major segments: the ascending, transverse, descending, and sigmoid colon. The ascending colon extends upward from the cecum to the right kidney, where it takes a 90-degree turn. Here the transverse colon begins. It crosses from right to left, and when it reaches the left edge of the abdominopelvic cavity, it turns down and becomes the descending colon. The descending colon leads to the sigmoid (SIG-moyd) colon, which twists around and ends at the rectum (**Figure 13.21**).

MEMORY TIP

Sigma is the name for the Greek letter *S*. The sigmoid colon is shaped like an *S*.

When what remains of food reaches the large intestine, almost all of its extractable nutrients have been harvested. During the 12 to 24 hours that the residue spends in the colon, additional water, some electrolytes (sodium and chloride), and water-soluble vitamins are absorbed. The colon absorbs less of these substances than the small intestine does. A process called *haustral churning*, which consists of slow contractions that help reabsorb water, compact the remains into feces, and prepare them for exit from the body.

Rectum, Anal Canal, and Anus

The final parts of the alimentary canal are the rectum, anal canal, and anus. The sigmoid colon empties into the rectum, a short segment whose lower end comprises the anal canal. The anus, which is the opening to the outside world, is usually closed due to constriction of the internal and external anal sphincters. The internal anal sphincter is made of smooth muscle. The external anal sphincter is composed of skeletal muscle.

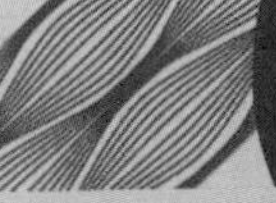

LIFE SPAN DEVELOPMENT: *The Digestive System*

By the beginning of the second trimester of intrauterine life, the fetal circulation is well-established. The fetus pumps blood through the placenta, where it receives nutrients from the mother's blood. The nutrient-rich blood then returns to the fetus. This process provides the fetus with the nutrients needed until birth. The newborn baby has no teeth and cannot chew. For this reason, it relies on a liquid diet. Breast milk is the ideal source of nutrition for an infant.

By the end of the first day after birth, bacteria are beginning to colonize in the infant gut. Over the first several months of life, the stomach develops the ability to make acid and secrete pepsin. The small intestine has a unique ability to absorb antibodies and growth factors that are present in breast milk. These substances promote infant growth and help protect the infant from infection. All twenty primary teeth are usually present by age three, allowing the child to chew food well. By this age, the child's gastrointestinal tract and accessory organs are well-developed and fully functional.

Inflammatory bowel diseases, including Crohn's disease and ulcerative colitis, often appear in early adulthood or even in late adolescence. Gallstones and stomach ulcers typically affect people in middle age. The typical age of onset of gallstones was middle age and elderly, but more young adults now seem to be developing gallstones. This trend is likely related to the increase in obesity rates, which is seen across all age groups.

The digestive system, like other organ systems, performs less well in old age. Gastrointestinal motility and secretory activity decrease as people age. Dental problems become more common and severe. Arthritis and dementia may make feeding difficult. For these and other reasons, elderly people are at greater risk for malnutrition than young and middle-age adults. Cancers of the digestive system are also more common in the elderly.

Life Span Review

1. What is the ideal source of nutrition for a newborn infant?
2. By what age is a child's gastrointestinal system fully functional?

Defecation, the elimination of solid waste, begins when waste reaches the rectum. The waste stretches the rectal wall, initiating reflex contractions of muscles in the sigmoid colon and rectum. These reflex contractions push the waste toward the anus, causing the internal anal sphincter to relax. As a skeletal muscle, the external anal sphincter is under voluntary control. It relaxes when the time is appropriate, allowing defecation to occur.

Check Your Understanding

1. How do the lips assist with ingestion?
2. How many permanent teeth are found in a healthy adult mouth?
3. What are *rugae*?
4. Name the three segments of the small intestine.
5. Describe the digestive functions of the liver and the gallbladder.
6. List the metabolic functions of the liver.

LESSON 13.2 Review and Assessment

Mini Glossary

Make sure that you know the meaning of each key term.

absorption the movement of food molecules from the small intestine into the blood

bile a watery substance produced by the liver that contains bile salts, which help emulsify fats

chemical breakdown the breakdown of large food molecules into smaller molecules by enzymes; historically referred to as *digestion*

chyme the mixture of food and digestive juice in the stomach and duodenum

defecation the discharge of feces from the anus

emulsification the breakdown of large fat particles into much smaller particles, aided by bile

esophagus the muscular tube that connects the pharynx and stomach

gallbladder the digestive organ that stores bile and delivers it to the duodenum when needed

gastrointestinal tract (GI tract) the stomach, small intestine, and large intestine; alimentary canal

gingiva soft tissue that covers the necks of the teeth, the mandible, and the maxilla; also called the *gum*

ingestion the intake of food and liquids via the mouth

mechanical breakdown the breakdown of food into smaller pieces, thus increasing its surface area

mucosa innermost layer of the GI tract, which directly faces the outside world

muscularis externa layer of the GI tract that surrounds the submucosal layer; propels food through the GI tract by peristalsis

peristalsis the symmetrical contraction of muscles that moves food along the GI tract

propulsion the movement of food through the gastrointestinal tract that is stimulated by swallowing at the pharynx and peristalsis, muscular contractions that move food through the rest of the GI tract

serosa the outermost layer of the GI tract

submucosa layer of the GI tract just deep to the mucosal layer; composed of irregular dense connective tissue containing blood vessels, lymphatic vessels, and nerves

Know and Understand

1. List the six activities of digestion.
2. Which layer of the GI tract directly faces the outside world?
3. The oral cavity helps to accomplish which four activities of digestion?
4. What is the purpose of the root canal in a tooth?
5. What substances combine to form saliva?
6. Where in the GI tract is the pyloric sphincter located?
7. List the chemicals found in pancreatic juice.
8. What does the combining form *hepat/o* mean?
9. What are the main functions of the large intestine?

Analyze and Apply

10. Evaluate the ways in which the structures and functions of the digestive system contribute to the processing and storage of energy in the body.
11. Explain the functions of the water, mucus, antibodies, and enzymes found in saliva.
12. Describe the purpose of the acidic environment in the stomach.
13. Explain why a person cannot live without a liver.
14. Describe how the pancreas regulates the concentration of glucose in the blood.

IN THE LAB

15. Using different colors of clay, create all the organs of the alimentary canal, as well as the accessory organs of digestion. On a piece of poster board or other heavy paper, assemble your digestive system by placing the organs that you created in the proper anatomical positions. Beside each organ, write its name and function (digestive and/or metabolic).
16. Conduct research to discover more about infant formula. Write an essay comparing breast milk to formula. Include examples of when each might be the best alternative for a newborn.
17. Perform an experiment to determine the effect of saliva on carbohydrates. Cut a slice of whole-wheat bread in half. Chew one-half of the bread for 3 minutes and swallow it. Pay attention to the changes in how the bread tastes over the 3 minutes, and record your findings. Now chew the other half of the bread, but only for 10 seconds. Then remove it from your mouth and place it in a baggie or other safe location for 5 minutes. Then chew the same piece of bread again for 2 minutes and record your observations. Explain what chemical actions have taken place.

LESSON 13.3

Disorders and Diseases of the Digestive System

Before You Read

Try to answer the following questions before you read this lesson.

- What is the source of the discomfort commonly known as heartburn?
- What is an ulcer?

Lesson Objectives

- Describe some of the common disorders and diseases of the gastrointestinal tract.
- Explain the effects of common diseases and disorders of the accessory organs.
- Identify cancers of the digestive system.

Key Terms

cholecystectomy
constipation
Crohn's disease
diarrhea
diverticulitis
diverticulosis
gallstones
gastroenteritis
gastroesophageal reflux
gastroesophageal reflux disease (GERD)
healthcare-associated infections (HAIs)
hepatitis
inflammatory bowel disease
pancreatitis
peptic ulcer
periodontal disease
plaque
ulcerative colitis

CLINICAL CASE STUDY

Roxana, age 76, has been driven by her son to her primary care provider, Dr. Maturin, without an appointment, because her belly hurts and she feels bloated and nauseated. Dr. Maturin sees her promptly. Roxana's vitals are: BP 132/78 mmHg, HR 78 bpm, respirations 18/minute, temperature 100.9°F (38.3°C). She is 5'1" tall and weighs 165 pounds. She says the pain has developed over the last two days. She reports that she has not vomited and that her most recent bowel movement did not appear bloody. Roxana experiences significant pain when the left lower quadrant of her abdomen is gently palpated. The other areas of her abdomen are much less sensitive and may be pressed and released quickly without causing major pain. Dr. Maturin does not feel any unusual masses. A blood sample shows normal hematocrit and hemoglobin levels and a slightly elevated white blood cell count. As you read this section, try to determine which of the following conditions Roxana most likely has, and hypothesize about the probable treatment plan and preventive measures for the future.

A. Appendicitis
B. Diverticulitis
C. Cholecystitis
D. Pancreatitis

Digestive ailments are some of the most common reasons people of all ages seek medical attention. Each time you eat, you ingest nonsterile foreign material, some of which contains potential pathogens. The digestive environment itself is harsh, with strong acids and enzymes that can be very damaging. Considering the state of the digestive environment, you might expect digestive illnesses to be even more common than they are.

Diseases of the GI Tract

Diseases of the digestive system are not limited to stomachaches. Both the alimentary canal and the accessory organs are subject to various diseases and disorders. The etiology, strategies for prevention, pathology, diagnosis, and treatments for common digestive diseases and disorders are summarized in **Figure 13.22**.

Diseases and Disorders of the GI Tract					
	Etiology	**Prevention**	**Pathology**	**Diagnosis**	**Treatment**
Gingivitis	inflammation caused by tartar buildup	brushing and flossing regularly; professional cleaning	redness, swelling, gum infection, eventual tooth loss	physical exam	improved oral hygiene, medicated rinse; antibiotics for infection
Gastroesophageal reflux disease (GERD)	movement of chyme from the stomach into the esophagus	maintain normal weight, do not smoke	painful burning sensation in the lower esophagus (heartburn)	physical exam, X-ray, endoscopy	lifestyle changes; medications to neutralize or reduce acid; surgery
Celiac disease (sprue) (gluten-sensitive enteropathy)	inflammatory immune reaction to gluten protein in rye, barley, and wheat, causing damage to the GI tract, especially the small intestine	none	constipation or diarrhea, nausea or vomiting, abdominal pain, fatigue, headache, joint pain, mouth ulcers	serology and genetic blood tests	permanent gluten-free diet
Peptic ulcer	break in the lining of the stomach, duodenum, or lower esophagus	none	burning pain, bloating, fatty food intolerance, heartburn, nausea	physical exam, lab tests for *H. pylori*, endoscopy, upper GI series of X-rays	depends on cause: antibiotics, medications to block acid production, antacids
Inflammatory bowel disease	chronic inflammation of the small or large intestine; includes ulcerative colitis and Crohn's disease	none	alternating pain and remission; diarrhea, malabsorption resulting in weight loss	physical exam; lab tests; various endoscopic and imaging procedures	steroids, lifestyle/ diet changes, medication, surgery
Irritable Bowel Syndrome (IBS)	chronic disorder of the large intestine involving cramping, abdominal pain, bloating, gas, diarrhea and/or constipation	none	abdominal pain and bloating, excess gas, diarrhea or constipation, mucus in the stool	physical exam, stool tests, colonoscopy, X-ray or CT scan	diet restrictions, regular exercise, get enough sleep, medications to help control symptoms
Diverticulosis and diverticulitis	outward-bulging pouches of mucosal and submucosal layers of intestine through the muscular layer; inflammation (diverticulitis)	maintain a healthy weight, exercise regularly, do not smoke	abdominal pain, nausea and vomiting, fever, diarrhea, sometimes constipation	physical exam, abdominal imaging by X-ray, CT scan, or colonoscopy; genetic testing	antibiotics, liquid or low-fiber diet; surgery for severe diverticulitis
Hemorrhoids	swollen veins in anus	hydrate; high-fiber foods, fiber supplements; regular exercise; avoid straining	pain, swelling, itching or lump near anus; blood in bowel movement	physical exam; digital rectal exam or colonoscopy	home treatments: high-fiber food, warm baths, cold packs, ointments; surgery if severe

Figure 13.22

Goodheart-Willcox Publisher

Gingivitis and Periodontal Disease

The health of the oral cavity, which is part of the GI tract, can affect the entire body. Gingivitis is an inflammation of the gingiva, or gum tissue (**Figure 13.23**). Gingivitis is the most common form of **periodontal disease**—disease that affects the supporting structure of the teeth.

Gingivitis is caused by long-term plaque accumulation on the teeth. **Plaque** is a sticky mixture of bacteria, food particles, and mucus that hardens to form *tartar* if it is not regularly removed by brushing and flossing. Buildup of plaque and bacteria activates an inflammatory response from the immune system. If not treated, gingivitis can cause damage to the jawbone around the tooth and weakening of the periodontal ligament that holds the tooth in its socket. Untreated gingivitis can eventually lead to tooth loss.

People with gingivitis are at an increased risk of developing cardiovascular disease. The inflammation of oral tissue is thought to shift the entire body into a pro-inflammatory state, increasing the likelihood of atherosclerosis, or hardening of the arteries.

Gastroesophageal Reflux Disease

Gastroesophageal (gas-troh-eh-sahf-oh-JEE-al) **reflux** is the movement of chyme from the stomach into the lower esophagus. The stomach wall is protected from the harmful effects of the acids in chyme by a thick layer of mucus, but the esophagus is unprotected. As a result, gastroesophageal reflux can cause a painful burning sensation commonly known as *heartburn*, due to its location in the esophagus near the heart.

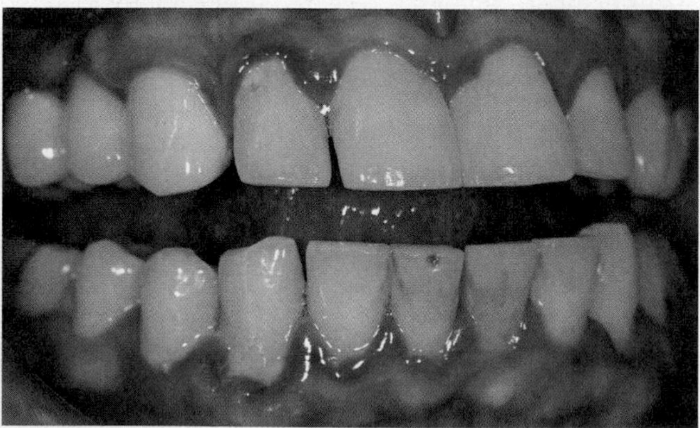

Dirk Saeger/Shutterstock.com

Figure 13.23 Gingivitis is an inflammation of the gum tissues, caused by plaque buildup on the teeth.

If gastroesophageal reflux occurs often, the lower esophagus can become chronically inflamed. This condition is called **gastroesophageal reflux disease (GERD)**. Pregnancy can cause GERD because the growing uterus pushes other abdominal organs up and out of their usual positions. GERD can also be caused by a hiatal (high-AY-tal) hernia, in which part of the stomach protrudes through the hiatus, or opening, in the diaphragm that normally accommodates the esophagus. Obesity and smoking also increase the risk of developing GERD.

Peptic Ulcers

A **peptic ulcer** is a break in the protective lining of the stomach, duodenum, or lower esophagus. Ulcers can be extremely painful because the break in the lining causes the deeper structures of the body to be exposed to, and damaged by, the acidic chyme and protein-digesting enzymes.

Most cases of peptic ulcer are caused by infection from the bacterium *Helicobacter pylori* (HEHL-i-koh-bak-ter pigh-LOR-igh), or *H. pylori*. The name of this bacterium reflects its helical shape and its discovery in tissue samples from the pyloric region of the stomach.

The long-held belief that stress or spicy food can cause ulcers is not supported by scientific evidence. Some evidence does suggest, however, that stress or spicy food can make an existing ulcer worse. Ulcer treatment includes antibiotics to kill the infectious bacteria. Drugs that slow down the release of acid in the stomach are often prescribed to reduce the painful symptoms.

Gastroenteritis

Gastroenteritis (gas-troh-ehn-ter-IGH-tis) is an inflammation of the stomach or intestine that produces nausea, vomiting, diarrhea, and/or abdominal pain. Gastroenteritis is often contagious and is sometimes called "stomach flu," although it is unrelated to influenza. The most common cause of gastroenteritis in children is infection with rotavirus. The goal of treatment is to reduce symptoms through restoration of lost fluid and electrolytes, preferably through oral rehydration therapy.

Inflammatory Bowel Disease

Inflammatory bowel disease is a disease in which the walls of either the small or large intestine become chronically inflamed. Inflammatory bowel disease often results in diarrhea and pain. The cause of this condition is not clear.

Ulcerative colitis (koh-LIGH-tis) is a form of inflammatory bowel disease that usually affects only the colon and the mucosal layer of the intestinal wall. **Crohn's disease** can affect all four layers of the digestive tract wall. Inflammation from Crohn's disease usually affects the small intestine or colon.

Patients with Crohn's disease and ulcerative colitis also suffer from malabsorption. This can result in weight loss when the illness flares up, requiring high-calorie supplements.

Each of these inflammatory diseases is characterized by alternating periods of pain and remission during which symptoms are mild. Treatment may include steroids to reduce inflammation during flare-ups. Lifestyle changes such as reduction of fiber in the diet also help.

Diverticulosis and Diverticulitis

Diverticulosis is the development of small outward-bulging pouches, or diverticula (singular: diverticulum), in the walls of the intestine. These bulges occur where the mucosal and submucosal layers of the wall push through weak spots in the muscular layer, which lies outside the mucosa and submucosa. **Diverticulitis**, also known as *diverticular disease*, is the development of inflammation in these diverticula. Diverticulitis causes abdominal pain, nausea and vomiting, fever, diarrhea, and sometimes constipation. Diverticulosis and diverticulitis are much more common in the large intestine than in the small intestine, and they usually appear in the descending or sigmoid colon. Most patients with diverticulosis do not develop diverticulitis.

Constipation and Diarrhea

Constipation and diarrhea are digestive ailments that are often symptoms of other diseases. **Constipation**, or difficulty with defecation, usually occurs when waste spends too much time in the colon. So much water is absorbed from the waste that the remaining waste becomes nearly solid, and therefore, more difficult to pass. Causes of constipation include weakness of the bowel muscle, lack of fiber, lack of exercise, and some prescription drugs.

Diarrhea is characterized and diagnosed by abnormally frequent, watery bowel movements. It occurs when waste does not spend enough time in the colon, where excess water would be absorbed. As a result, the waste contains more water than usual. Diarrhea also occurs when unusually large amounts of water are left in the waste despite normal travel time through the intestine.

Causes of diarrhea include dysentery (an infection of the intestines or stomach by a bacterium, virus, or parasites), food poisoning, inflammatory bowel disease, or milk consumption by a person with lactase deficiency. Lactase deficiency is the inability to break down lactose, or milk sugar. This condition is common in people who are not of European descent. Lactase deficiency causes no problems if milk and other dairy products are avoided.

Treatment for diarrhea and constipation depends on the cause. In cases of diarrhea, lost water and electrolytes may be replaced orally or by intravenous infusion. Diarrhea can be prevented in many cases by addressing the underlying causes: providing clean drinking water and food in parts of the world where it is lacking, practicing good hygiene to prevent fecal-oral transmission of pathogenic bacteria, and using antibiotics carefully.

Healthcare-Associated Infections

Healthcare-associated infections (HAIs) are infections that patients get in the course of receiving care at a healthcare facility such as a hospital, clinic, skilled care facility, or other healthcare setting. Some HAIs affect the GI tract predominantly and spread via GI-related pathways, including bacteria in feces of infected patients. Some patients may become carriers of disease while in a healthcare setting, and then spread the disease when they return to their home and community. HAIs are a significant cause of morbidity (sickness) and mortality (death), especially among older patients.

Examples of HAIs include infections associated with catheters in the veins and in the urinary tract, infections associated with artificial ventilators (ventilator-acquired pneumonia), surgical site infections, methicillin-resistant *Staphylococcus aureus* (MRSA, pronounced "mersah"), and *Clostridium difficile* (*C. difficile* or *C. diff.*, pronounced "see diff").

C. difficile infections are among the most common HAIs. They usually occur in hospitalized patients and residents of skilled care facilities who are on antibiotics. In some patients, the antibiotics can kill a significant fraction of the normal "good" bacteria in the colon. This allows *C. difficile* to multiply, producing toxins that cause inflammation of, and damage to, the mucosal layer of the colon. The symptoms of *C. difficile* infection often include watery diarrhea, abdominal cramping, loss of appetite, and malaise (feeling sick). Treatment may include removal of antibiotics that preceded the illness, the use of different antibiotics, and other measures that depend on the severity of the case and other factors.

Healthcare facilities must carefully follow procedures to reduce the incidence of HAIs. For example, antibiotics should be used carefully and conservatively. Excellent hand hygiene must be practiced by every person who enters and leaves patients' rooms. *Contact precautions* may be implemented. This means everyone entering the patient's room must wash their hands carefully and don a gown and gloves before entering, and they must wash their hands and discard the gown and gloves before leaving the room. All healthcare personnel must be educated about infection control practices. Use of devices such as catheters and ventilators must be kept to the minimum duration necessary.

Check Your Understanding

1. What is gingivitis?
2. Which bacterium causes most peptic ulcers?
3. What effect does malabsorption have on patients with Crohn's disease?
4. What is the usual cause of constipation?
5. Name two types of bacteria that commonly cause HAIs.

Diseases and Disorders of the Accessory Organs

Some gastrointestinal disorders are specific to the accessory organs. Examples include hepatitis, pancreatitis, and gallstones. **Figure 13.24** describes the etiology, prevention, pathology, diagnosis, and treatment of these disorders.

Hepatitis

Hepatitis is a group of diseases characterized by inflammation of and damage to the liver. Hepatitis has many possible causes, treatments, and prognoses (likely outcomes). Liver damage is the common feature among all types of hepatitis.

Causes of hepatitis include viral infection, excessive use of alcohol or drugs (prescription or illegal), and poisoning (such as from certain mushrooms). Acute hepatitis, which lasts for less than six months, may result in healing of the liver and a return to normal liver function. Unfortunately, acute hepatitis may also lead to progressive liver damage and death. Chronic hepatitis lasts longer than six months, and its symptoms are usually less severe.

Because the liver is the site of many biological and chemical processes, damage to this vital organ can cause a wide variety of symptoms. One common symptom of hepatitis is jaundice, or yellowed skin and whites of the eyes. A damaged liver is unable to discharge bilirubin, a product of red blood cell destruction, into the bile. As a result, people with hepatitis sometimes develop jaundice as bilirubin accumulates in the body.

Diseases and Disorders of the GI Accessory Organs					
	Etiology	**Prevention**	**Pathology**	**Diagnosis**	**Treatment**
Cirrhosis	scarring and fibrosis of the liver	maintain healthy weight; avoid alcohol; avoid needle sharing and unprotected intercourse	nausea, fatigue, jaundice, weight loss, bruising, swelling in legs or abdomen	blood tests, imaging, liver biopsy	treat alcohol dependence, lose weight; medication to control causes or symptoms; liver transplant
Hepatitis	inflammation of and damage to the liver	maintain good hygiene; vaccine for hepatitis A and B	abdominal pain, jaundice, dark urine, fever, joint pain, weakness, fatigue	physical exam for jaundice; lab tests for blood clotting and liver enzymes, tests for hepatitis viruses	depends on type and cause of hepatitis; medication is now available to cure hepatitis C
Pancreatitis	inflammation of and damage to the pancreas	reduce or avoid consumption of alcohol	upper abdominal pain that feels worse after eating; fever, nausea, vomiting	blood tests for elevated pancreatic enzymes; stool tests for fat levels; imaging	fasting for a few days; pain medications; rehydration
Gallstones	solid crystals that form from substances in bile	maintain healthy weight, exercise regularly, eat a high-fiber, low-fat, low-cholesterol diet	pain, inability to digest fat	abdominal ultrasound, CT scan, MRI, endoscopic retrograde cholangiopan-creatography (ERCP); blood tests	medications to dissolve the gallstone, or cholecystectomy

Figure 13.24

Goodheart-Willcox Publisher

Another symptom of hepatitis is the inability of blood to clot normally. The liver produces the clotting proteins that circulate in the blood, but a damaged liver does not produce enough of these proteins. One sign of hepatitis visible during laboratory analysis of blood samples is the presence of liver enzymes in the blood. These enzymes are released from dying liver cells.

At least five viruses are known to cause acute hepatitis; these are labeled *A* through *E*. Hepatitis viruses vary in severity and ease of spread. Proper hygiene is key for preventing the spread of viral hepatitis. Vaccines are available that provide immunity to hepatitis A and B.

Pancreatitis

Pancreatitis (pan-kree-uh-TIGH-tis) is an inflammation of the pancreas. It occurs when the pancreatic enzymes, especially proteases, become active while they are still in the pancreas. When this occurs, the pancreas starts to break down its own tissues, resulting in severe abdominal pain.

In the United States, most cases of pancreatitis are linked to alcoholism. There is no cure for pancreatitis; however, medication to reduce pain is often prescribed, and lost fluids are replenished.

Occasionally, pancreatitis is caused by a gallstone that lodges in the common outflow tract of the pancreas and gallbladder. This blockage prevents the release of pancreatic juice. Eventually, the enzymes in the juice become active and start damaging the tissue.

Gallstones

Gallstones are solid crystals that form from substances in bile (**Figure 13.25**). Gallstones are usually formed in the gallbladder and then

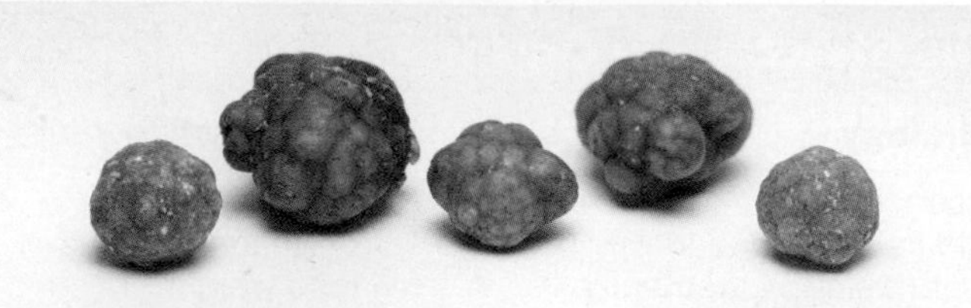

hamchoke punya/Shutterstock.com

Figure 13.25 Gallstones affect the ability of the gallbladder to secrete bile.

get stuck in the cystic duct or common bile duct. This blockage prevents further secretion of bile, resulting in pain and inability to digest fat.

Special drugs may be used to dissolve the gallstones, but usually the gallbladder is removed in a procedure called a **cholecystectomy** (koh-leh-sis-TEHK-toh-mee). This surgical procedure is often done laparoscopically (through a few small openings). After the gallbladder has been removed, a person should compensate for smaller amounts of bile by eating smaller, more frequent, and less fatty meals.

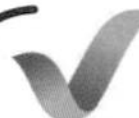

Check Your Understanding

1. List three common causes of hepatitis.
2. What causes pancreatitis?
3. What procedure is performed to remove gallstones?

Cancer

Cancers of the digestive system are among the most common forms of cancer. They can also be among the deadliest. In the United States, for example, colon cancer is the third most common cancer in men and women and the second leading cause of cancer-related deaths. Only lung cancer causes more deaths than cancers of the digestive system.

Typically, cancers of the digestive system grow slowly. In some cases, they are not detected until they have entered nearby body tissues. These cancers usually originate in the epithelial cells of the GI tract or the accessory organs of digestion. Primary tumors (tumors that are new and did not spread from another site) can arise anywhere in the GI system. Besides colon cancer, cancers of the rectum, the mouth, and the tissues surrounding the mouth are the most common. Cancers of the esophagus, stomach, pancreas, and liver are less common, but they result in high mortality rates.

Cancers of the digestive system can be serious, but screening and early detection play a big role in improving treatment outcomes. Currently, the intestines are the only organ in the digestive system that can be screened for cancer or precancerous growths (polyps). Colonoscopy, for example, is a common screening test for cancers of the colon and rectum. During a colonoscopy, a doctor looks at the entire length of the large intestine and rectum with a long, flexible scope called a *colonoscope*. A small video camera attached to the colonoscope enables the doctor to take pictures or video of the colon. Special instruments can be passed through the colonoscope to biopsy tissue samples, if necessary. Colonoscopies are typically done in a hospital outpatient department, clinic, or in a physician's office.

Check Your Understanding

1. What can be done to reduce the risk of cancers of the digestive system?
2. Which screening test is used to test for cancers of the colon and rectum?

LESSON 13.3 Review and Assessment

Mini Glossary

Make sure that you know the meaning of each key term.

cholecystectomy surgical removal of the gallbladder

constipation condition characterized by difficulty in defecating

Crohn's disease a chronic inflammatory bowel disease that usually affects the small intestine or colon

diarrhea the occurrence of frequent, watery bowel movements

diverticulitis development of inflammation in the diverticula

diverticulosis development of small outward-bulging pouches, or diverticula, in the walls of the intestine

gallstones solid crystals that form from substances in the bile of the gallbladder

gastroenteritis an inflammation of the stomach or intestine that produces nausea, vomiting, diarrhea, and/or abdominal pain

gastroesophageal reflux the movement of chyme from the stomach into the lower esophagus

gastroesophageal reflux disease (GERD) chronic inflammation of the esophagus caused by the upward flow of gastric juice

healthcare-associated infections (HAIs) infection that patients get in the course of receiving care in a healthcare facility

hepatitis a group of diseases characterized by inflammation of and damage to the liver

inflammatory bowel disease a condition in which the wall of the small and/or large intestine becomes chronically inflamed

pancreatitis inflammation of the pancreas

peptic ulcer a break in the lining of the stomach, duodenum, or lower esophagus

periodontal disease a disease that affects the supporting structure of the teeth and the gums

plaque a sticky mixture of bacteria, food particles, and mucus that hardens to form tartar if it is not regularly removed by brushing and flossing

ulcerative colitis an inflammatory bowel disease that usually affects the colon and the mucosal layer of the intestinal wall

Know and Understand

1. What causes gingivitis?
2. What is a hiatal hernia?
3. Why are ulcers painful?
4. Which digestive disorder is often called "stomach flu"?
5. What is an HAI?
6. Why is pancreatitis so painful?
7. Why do people with gallstones have a difficult time digesting fat?
8. Where do most cancers of the digestive system originate?

Analyze and Apply

9. What is the difference between diverticulosis and diverticulitis?
10. Explain why the buildup of plaque on the teeth and gums can be dangerous, potentially leading to heart disease.
11. Explain why GERD is common during pregnancy.
12. Why are peptic ulcers commonly treated with antibiotics?
13. Explain why patients with Crohn's disease and ulcerative colitis both suffer from malabsorption.
14. Explain the relationship between constipation and water absorption in the large intestine.

IN THE LAB

15. Create an informational pamphlet on the digestive system disorder of your choice. Include the following topics in your pamphlet: definition of the disorder, symptoms, causes, age groups affected, methods of diagnosis, treatments, and prognosis. Present your pamphlet to the class.
16. Assume that you are the infection control nurse at a healthcare facility. HAIs have increased in the digestive unit, and it is your job to decrease the number of infections. Develop a campaign you could use to educate physicians, nurses, housekeeping, staff members, and visitors to the facility. Create at least one poster and a plan of work to document your plan.

CAREER CORNER

Anatomy & Physiology at Work

The digestive system brings into your body the molecules that you need from nutrients in food. By eating a healthful and well-balanced diet, your body gets the molecules it needs the most. Many people have found challenging and fulfilling careers in promoting good nutrition and oral health, and in diagnosing and treating diseases of the digestive system.

Nutritionist or Dietitian

Nutritionists and dietitians are experts in food and nutrition. They advise people about the foods that they can eat to stay healthy, get healthy, or cope with disease. They work in many settings, including schools, cafeterias, skilled care facilities, hospitals, and companies that make prepared food.

One of the responsibilities of a nutritionist or dietitian is to educate people about proper nutrition and healthful lifestyles. Nutrition and lifestyle information and advice may be delivered in a one-on-one setting with individual patients, or it may be presented to small or large groups of people (**Figure 13.26**).

Some dietitians work with a variety of patients; others focus on helping people with a specific disease or disorder. For example, people with renal failure, or kidney disease, may be better able to manage their disease by adopting a particular diet. A dietitian specializing in patients with kidney disease would create a diet plan to meet the specific nutritional needs of these patients.

Most nutritionists and dietitians attend four years of college to obtain their bachelor's degree in nutrition, dietetics, or a related field. Many students are required to complete supervised, hands-on training during a postgraduate internship. Most states require that nutritionists and dietitians be licensed and state certified. These qualifications can be obtained by passing an exam.

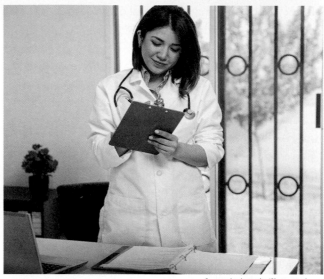

Supavadee butradee/Shutterstock.com

Figure 13.26 This dietitian is responsible for managing the nutritional needs of the people who live in this skilled care facility.

Dental Hygienist

Dental hygienists clean teeth, examine teeth and gums, and provide preventive dental care. During a typical cleaning, a dental hygienist focuses on removing plaque and tartar from the patient's teeth to help prevent cavities and gum diseases such as gingivitis (**Figure 13.27**). Dental hygienists may also take X-rays of the teeth.

One of the most important responsibilities of a dental hygienist is to educate patients on how to care for their teeth and gums. A dental hygienist might demonstrate the most effective way to brush teeth or the proper method of flossing, skills that are both necessary for achieving good oral health.

Dental hygienists work under the supervision of dentists. To become a dental hygienist, you must complete a two-year associate's degree program. High school coursework in biology,

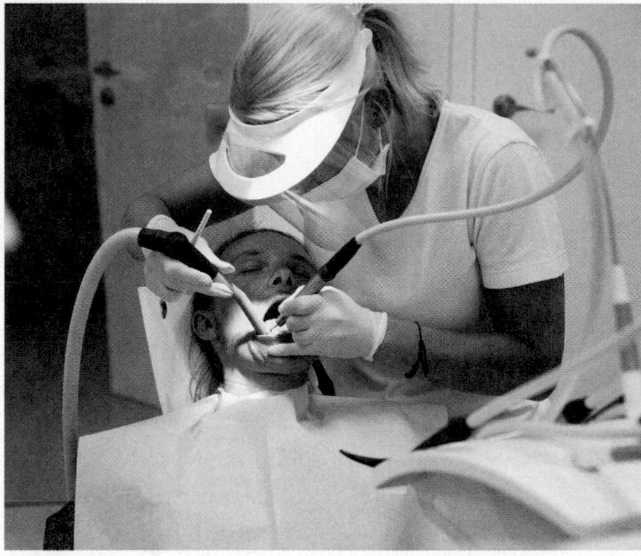

zlikovec/Shutterstock.com

Figure 13.27 This dental hygienist is performing a routine cleaning for a patient.

anatomy and physiology, and nutrition provides a good base of knowledge for future dental hygienists. In the United States, dental hygienists must pass a certification exam after they have earned their degree. The certification exam may include both written and practical portions.

Planning for a Health-Related Career

Do some research on the career of a dietitian, nutritionist, or a dental hygienist. You may choose instead to research a profession from the list of related career options. Using the internet or resources at your local library, find answers to the following questions:

1. What are the main tasks and responsibilities of a person employed in the career that you chose to research?
2. What is the outlook for this career? Are workers in demand, or are jobs dwindling? For complete information, consult the current edition of the *Occupational Outlook Handbook*, published by the US Department of Labor. This handbook is available online or at your local library.
3. What special skills or talents are required? For example, do you enjoy research? Do you need to be good at biology and anatomy and physiology? Do you need to enjoy communicating with other people?
4. What personality traits do you think are necessary for success in the career you have chosen to research? For example, a dental hygienist works closely with patients. Would you mind touching another person's face and mouth?
5. Does the work involve a great deal of routine, or are the day-to-day responsibilities varied?
6. Does the career require long hours, or is it a standard, "9-to-5" job?
7. What is the salary range for this job?
8. What do you think you would like about this career? Is there anything about it that you might dislike?

Related Career Options

- Chemical technician
- Dental assistant
- Dental laboratory technician
- Dentist
- Food science technician
- Food scientist
- Gastroenterologist
- Health educator
- Orthodontist
- Periodontist

CHAPTER

13 Review

LESSON 13.1

Nutrition

Key Points

- The body needs energy to perform metabolic activities; basal metabolic rate is a measure of the amount of energy needed to sustain a person for one day at complete rest.
- Nutrients include water, macronutrients (carbohydrates, proteins, and fats), vitamins, and minerals.

Key Terms

basal metabolic rate (BMR)
Calorie
coenzymes
energy
lipids
macronutrients
micronutrients
minerals
monounsaturated fats
nutrients
polyunsaturated fats
trans-unsaturated fats
vitamin deficiency
vitamins

LESSON 13.2

Anatomy and Physiology of the Digestive System

Key Points

- The activities of digestion include ingestion, propulsion, mechanical breakdown, chemical breakdown, absorption, and defecation.
- The GI tract, or alimentary canal, has four layers: the mucosa, submucosa, muscularis externa, and serosa.
- The digestive system includes the oral and nasal cavities, teeth and gums, salivary glands, pharynx, esophagus, stomach, small intestine, liver, gallbladder, pancreas, large intestine, rectum, anal canal, and anus.

Key Terms

absorption
bile
chemical breakdown
chyme
defecation
emulsification
esophagus
gallbladder
gastrointestinal tract (GI tract)
gingiva
ingestion
mechanical breakdown
mucosa
muscularis externa
peristalsis
propulsion
serosa
submucosa

LESSON 13.3

Disorders and Diseases of the Digestive System

Key Points

- Diseases and disorders of the GI tract include gingivitis and other periodontal disease, GERD, peptic ulcers, gastroenteritis, inflammatory bowel disease, diverticulosis, diverticulitis, constipation, diarrhea, and healthcare-associated infections.
- Diseases and disorders of the accessory organs include hepatitis, pancreatitis, and gallstones.
- Cancer of the digestive system organs usually originates in the epithelial cells of the GI tract or accessory digestive organs.

Key Terms

cholecystectomy
constipation
Crohn's disease
diarrhea
diverticulitis
diverticulosis
gallstones
gastroenteritis
gastroesophageal reflux
gastroesophageal reflux disease (GERD)
healthcare-associated infections (HAIs)
hepatitis
inflammatory bowel disease
pancreatitis
peptic ulcer
periodontal disease
plaque
ulcerative colitis

Assessment

➤ LESSON 13.1

Nutrition

Learning Key Terms and Concepts

1. Growing, moving, and breathing are activities that require the body to use _____.
2. Food scientists use the kilocalorie, or _____, to measure the potential energy in food.
3. The sum of all the chemical and physical reactions that occur in the body is called _____.
4. Active teenage girls typically need to consume about how many Calories per day?
   A. 2,000
   B. 2,400
   C. 2,800
   D. 3,200
5. Which of the following is *not* a nutrient?
   A. proteins
   B. vitamins
   C. bacteria
   D. water
6. Which of the following foods is classified as a carbohydrate?
   A. chicken breast
   B. rice
   C. olive oil
   D. butter
7. Proteins are made up of varying amounts of 20 different _____.
   A. vitamins
   B. lipids
   C. chromosomes
   D. amino acids
8. *True or False?* Protein delivers about twice as much energy as carbohydrates and fats.
9. _____ fatty acids are derived mainly from animal sources.
10. Unsaturated fatty acids may be either polyunsaturated, trans-unsaturated, or _____.
11. *True or False?* Fat-soluble vitamins can be stored in the body.
12. *True or False?* Water-soluble vitamins are usually stored in the body.

Thinking Critically

13. Why is basal metabolic rate (BMR) an insufficient method of calculating the required daily intake of an active teenager?
14. Using what you have learned about the different kinds of fats, explain which are healthful and which are unhealthful.
15. Too much of a good thing can be detrimental to the body. What might happen if you consume too much of minerals that are needed by the body in small amounts?
16. Using information from this chapter and previous chapters, explain what the building blocks of proteins are.

➤ LESSON 13.2

Anatomy and Physiology of the Digestive System

Learning Key Terms and Concepts

17. The gastrointestinal (GI) tract is also called the _____.
18. The _____ breakdown of food reduces food into smaller pieces through chewing and stomach churning.
19. The process of muscles contracting for the purpose of moving food particles along the GI tract is called _____.
    A. absorption
    B. peristalsis
    C. ingestion
    D. churning
20. The order of layers in the wall of the GI tract, starting from the innermost layer, is _____.
    A. submucosa, mucosa, serosa, and muscularis externa
    B. mucosa, submucosa, muscularis externa, and serosa
    C. serosa, submucosa, mucosa, and muscularis externa
    D. mucosa, serosa, submucosa, and muscularis externa
21. The mouth is also called the _____.

22. The three pairs of salivary glands in the mouth are the submandibular, parotid, and _____ salivary glands.
    A. periodontal
    B. submaxillary
    C. buccal
    D. sublingual
23. The muscular tube that connects the pharynx to the stomach is the _____.
    A. trachea
    B. small intestine
    C. esophagus
    D. colon
24. *True or False*? The folds in the wall of the stomach are called *rugae*.
25. The three segments of the small intestine, beginning with the segment closest to the stomach, are the _____.
    A. ileum, jejunum, and cecum
    B. duodenum, jejunum, and ileum
    C. cecum, colon, and ileum
    D. jejunum, ileum, and duodenum
26. The purpose of bile is to break apart, or _____, fats.
27. Bile is made by cells in the liver called _____ and stored in the gallbladder.
28. The pancreas produces two hormones, insulin and _____, and secretes them into the bloodstream.
29. The four major segments of the large intestine, starting with the segment closest to the small intestine, are the _____.
    A. cecum, rectum, colon, and anal canal
    B. cecum, anal canal, rectum, and colon
    C. anal canal, rectum, colon, and cecum
    D. cecum, colon, rectum, and anal canal

Thinking Critically

30. Using what you have learned about propulsion and peristalsis in the GI tract, explain what reverse peristalsis is and what might cause it.
31. Why is it important for a surgeon to know and understand the layers of the GI tract, particularly their order?
32. If a patient is diagnosed with colon cancer and has surgery to remove part of the colon, how does the process of elimination occur after the surgery?
33. What are the components of feces in a healthy person?

LESSON 13.3

Disorders and Diseases of the Digestive System

Learning Key Terms and Concepts

34. Gingivitis is an inflammation of the _____, or gum tissue.
35. Gingivitis results from long-term buildup of _____ on the teeth.
36. Because of its location, gastroesophageal reflux is commonly called _____.
37. Which bacterium causes most peptic ulcers?
38. Gastroenteritis in children is commonly caused by infection with _____.
    A. rotavirus
    B. hepatitis
    C. salmonella
    D. staphylococcus
39. _____ is a gastrointestinal disease that affects all four layers of the digestive tract wall.
    A. Diverticulosis
    B. GERD
    C. Crohn's disease
    D. Ulcerative colitis
40. _____ can be caused by waste spending too much time in the colon.
41. _____ occurs when waste does not spend enough time in the colon.
42. *True or False*? HAIs are infections that people get while they are in a healthcare facility.
43. _____ are solid crystals that form from bile and can block the secretion of bile into the small intestine.
44. Cancer of the digestive system organs usually originates in _____ cells of the GI tract.
    A. squamous
    B. blood
    C. nerve
    D. epithelial

Thinking Critically

45. Evaluate the cause and effect of periodontal disease on the structure and function of the cardiovascular system.
46. Why might chyme harm the esophagus but not the stomach?
47. In recent years, several alternatives to having a screening colonoscopy have been developed. What are they, and in your opinion, why have they been developed?

Building Skills and Connecting Concepts

Analyzing and Evaluating Data

Instructions: The bar graph in **Figure 13.28** shows the incidence of all cancer deaths in the United States in 2015. Use the graph to answer the following questions.

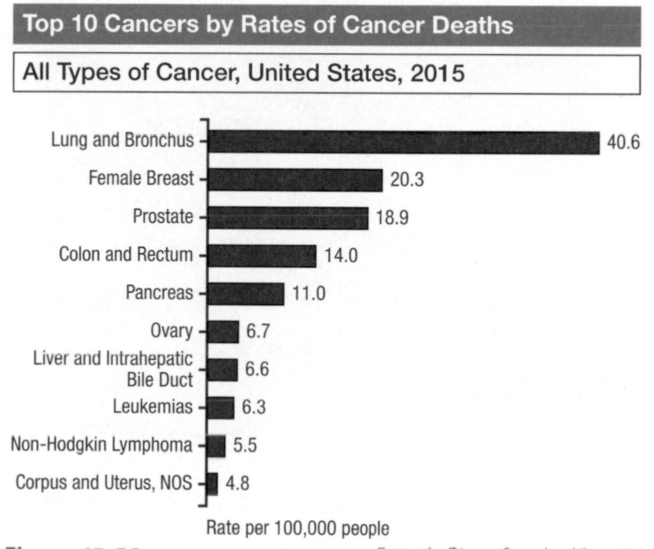

Figure 13.28

48. What is the percentage of people who died of cancers to the colon and rectum?
49. For every 100,000 people, how many died of cancers to the colon and rectum?
50. In 2015, how many people, per 100,000 people, died of *any* cancer related to the digestive system?
51. What percentage of the people who died of *any* cancer related to the digestive system died of pancreatic cancer? Round your answer to the nearest tenth of a percent.
52. How many more people, per 100,000, died of colon and rectum cancer than died of liver and bile duct cancer?

Communicating about Anatomy & Physiology

53. **Speaking** Working in groups of three students, create flash cards for the key terms in this chapter. On the front of the card, write the term. On the back of the card, write the pronunciation and a brief definition. Take turns quizzing one another on the pronunciations and definitions.
54. **Writing** Write a research essay on one of the diseases or disorders presented in this chapter. Your essay must include in-text citations and a resource page. The essay must be a minimum of three pages long and must be presented in APA format. Pay close attention to correct spelling, grammar, and format.

Lab Investigations

55. Analyze nutrient data on food labels of various snack foods.

    Materials: Snack food labels from potato and tortilla chips, cookies, candy, granola bars, fruit snacks, and doughnuts

    Check online to find the latest recommendations for healthy snacks.

    Create a spreadsheet that lists nutritional information for each snack food. Include the total amount of fat, saturated fat, trans fat, sugar, sodium, and any artificial sweeteners in your spreadsheet. Then create a report identifying the snacks that you evaluated to be the "healthiest" based on the data.
56. Using a model, label the anatomical structures of the digestive system. Explain the pathway of food from the mouth to the anus, identifying major landmarks. Remove the labels and repeat. Create a video of yourself pointing to and explaining the function of each anatomical part and explaining the pathway of food from the mouth to the anus. Ask your classmates to view your video and comment on how helpful your video was for their learning process.

Building Your Portfolio

57. Make digital copies of the reports you created and the research studies you performed as you worked through this chapter. Create a document or folder called "The Digestive System" and insert the documents. Add this document or folder to your personal portfolio.

CHAPTER

14 The Urinary System

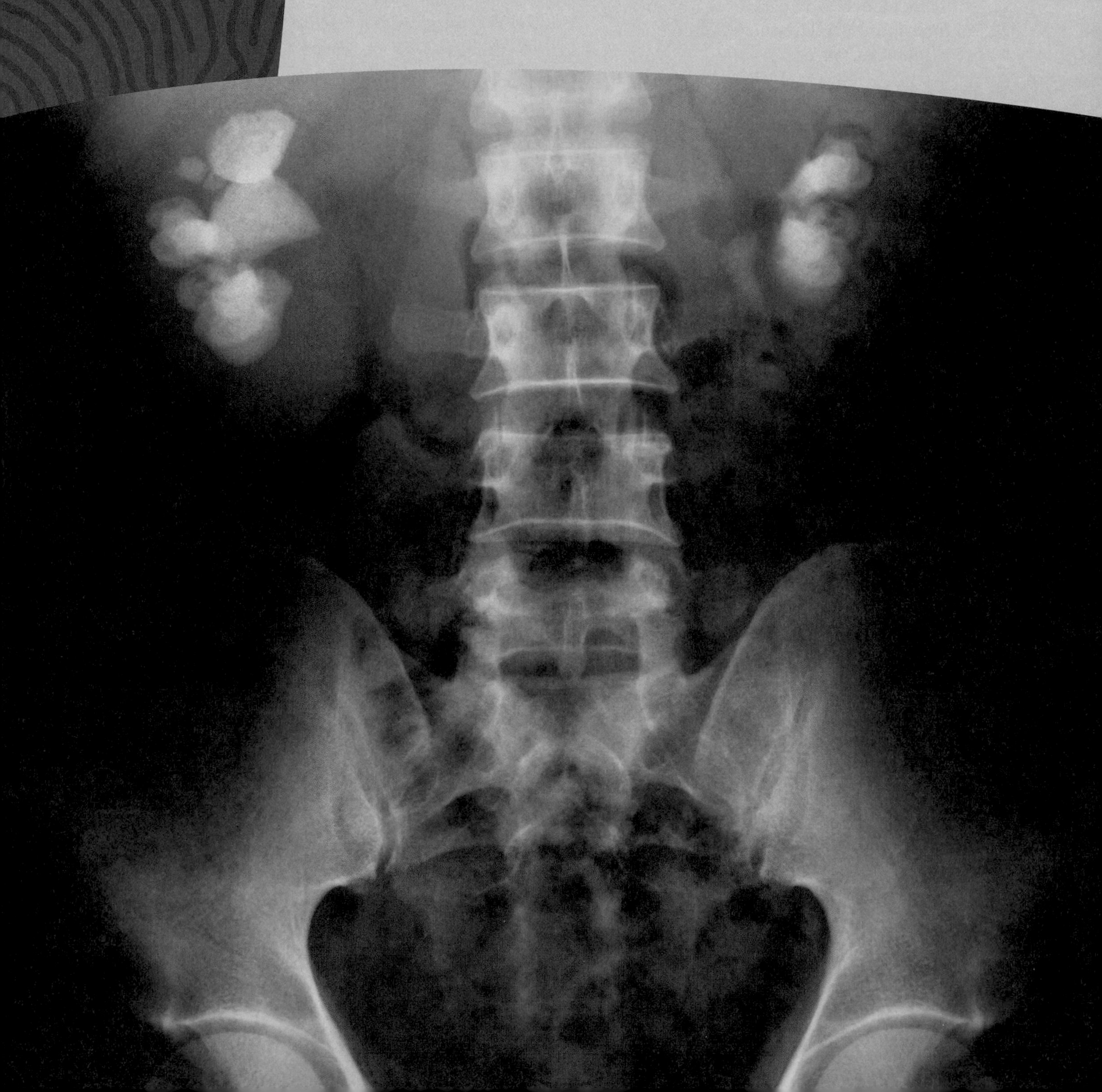

How are wastes filtered from the blood and flushed from the body?

A stable chemical environment inside the human body is essential for life and health. The biochemical reactions of life require watery surroundings and a stable level of electrolytes in the body fluids. Proteins will not fold properly—and enzymes will not work—if the fluid that surrounds them has an abnormal pH or osmolarity.

The urinary system adapts to changing conditions so that the body's internal environment stays constant. The key organs in the urinary system are the kidneys. These two organs are remarkable for the number of tasks they accomplish. The other organs of the urinary system—two ureters, the bladder, and the urethra—are also essential, but their functions are much simpler than those of the kidneys.

Lessons 14.1 and 14.2 of this chapter explore the anatomy and physiology of the kidneys. Lesson 14.2, which covers urine formation, storage, and excretion, discusses the ureters, bladder, and urethra. The last lesson describes tests of kidney function and diseases and disorders of the kidneys.

Chapter 14 Outline

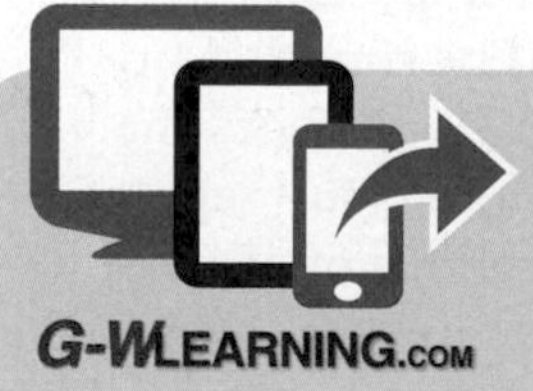

Click on the activity icon or visit www.g-wlearning.com/healthsciences/0202 to access online vocabulary activities using key terms from the chapter.

◂ Sutha Burawonk/Shutterstock.com

LESSON 14.1 The Kidney

Before You Read

Try to answer the following questions before you read this lesson.

- Where in the body are the kidneys located?
- Which blood vessels and nerves go to and from the kidneys?

Lesson Objectives

- Describe the location and size of the kidney.
- Know the basic anatomy of the kidney and its primary working unit, the nephron.
- Trace the flow of blood through the kidney.

Key Terms

collecting duct	renal corpuscle
distal convoluted tubule (DCT)	renal cortex
glomerulus	renal medulla
nephron	renal pelvis
nephron loop	renal tubule
proximal convoluted tubule (PCT)	vasa recta

The urinary system is composed of structures that excrete liquid waste in the form of urine, retain water and electrolytes, and maintain homeostasis. The kidneys are the main players in the urinary system. They purify many times their weight in fluid each day, eliminating waste from the blood while retaining valuable chemical compounds. The kidneys control the volume of water in the body, and in doing so they control blood volume and blood pressure.

The kidneys also regulate the pH and saltiness of blood. Physiologists and healthcare providers use the term *osmolality* (ahz-moh-LAL-i-tee) as a more precise term for saltiness. The osmolality of fluid is the number of dissolved molecules per unit volume of fluid. The kidneys control the concentration of various ions in the blood, including sodium, chloride, potassium, magnesium, and calcium. They make the hormones *erythropoietin* (eh-rith-roh-POY-eh-tin) and *renin*. They also convert vitamin D to its active form. In short, no human-engineered device comes close to doing what a kidney does, especially in such a small package.

Anatomy of the Kidney

The kidneys are located on either side of the spinal column, high in the lumbar (lower back) region (**Figure 14.1**). They are *retroperitoneal* (reht-roh-per-i-toh-NEE-al); that is, they lie behind the peritoneum, the membrane that lines the abdominopelvic cavity. (The prefix *retro-* means "back" or "located behind.") The two lowest ribs offer some protection to the kidneys against physical blows from behind.

Each kidney is about 4.3 inches (11 cm) long, 2.4 inches (6 cm) wide, and 1.2 inches (3 cm) thick—somewhat larger than a deck of cards. A kidney weighs about one-third of a pound (150 grams). The liver, located above the kidneys, pushes the right kidney to a slightly lower position than the left. Each kidney has a convex (outward-curving) lateral edge and a concave (inward-curving) medial surface. The indentation on the medial surface, where blood vessels and nerves enter the kidney, is called the *renal hilum* (REE-nal HIGH-lum). The kidney usually is cushioned by some fat. The small adrenal gland, an endocrine system organ, is located on top of the kidneys.

The frontal section through the kidney shown in **Figure 14.2** separates it into a "front half" and a "back half." The lighter-colored, outer part of the kidney is called the **renal cortex**, and is surrounded by the *renal capsule*. The darker, inner part, the **renal medulla**, is divided into *renal pyramids*. The base of each pyramid faces outward, toward the cortex. The rounded tip of the pyramid, the *papilla* (pa-PIL-a), faces the center of the kidney. The pyramids are separated by *renal columns*, inward extensions of cortex-like tissue. The **renal pelvis** is the deepest part of the kidney. Urine produced in the cortex and medulla seeps through *calyces* (singular: *calyx*) into the

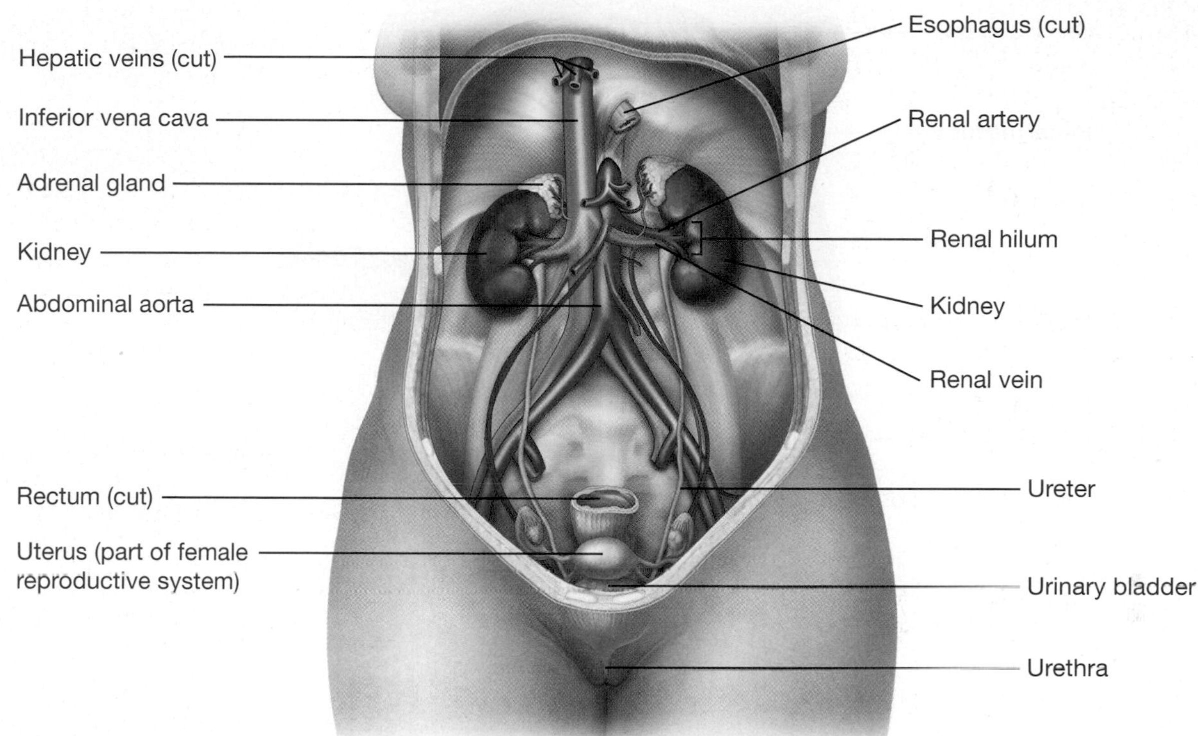

Figure 14.1 Urinary system anatomy. The kidneys lie against the posterior body wall, on either side of the spinal column. *Which vessel supplies blood to the kidneys? From which vessel does purified blood exit the kidneys?*

renal pelvis, which drains into the ureter (YOOR-eht-er), a tube that leads from the kidney to the urinary bladder (**Figure 14.1**).

Nerve and Blood Supply

The kidneys make up about 0.5% of total body weight, but they receive 20% to 25% of the blood pumped by the heart, under resting conditions. Therefore, the renal artery and renal vein, which connect each kidney to the nearby abdominal aorta, have a large diameter. The renal artery supplies blood to the kidneys. The renal vein drains purified blood from the kidneys.

The renal nerve fibers, which are mostly from the sympathetic division of the autonomic nervous system, discussed in Chapter 6, form an irregular mesh on the outside of the renal artery. The renal artery, vein, nerves, and ureter all connect to the kidney at the renal hilum.

The Nephron

The basic working unit of each kidney is the **nephron** (NEH-frahn), shown in **Figure 14.3**. Each kidney contains about one million nephrons. Each nephron has its own blood supply and creates urine, which passes through a collecting duct to the renal pelvis. Each nephron has two main parts: the **renal corpuscle** (KOR-puh-suhl), shown in **Figure 14.3A**, and the **renal tubule** (TOO-byool), shown in **Figure 14.3B**.

The renal corpuscle has a mass of capillaries called the **glomerulus** (glah-MER-yoo-lus) and a surrounding, cuplike *glomerular capsule*. Blood enters the glomerulus through an afferent arteriole, passes through the glomerulus, and exits via the efferent arteriole.

MEMORY TIP

Afferent comes from the Latin verb phrase *ad ferro*, which means "to carry toward." *Efferent* comes from the Latin *ex ferro*, which means "to carry away." The English word *ferry* has the same origin.

The glomerular capsule has an outer surface and an inner surface, and a hollow space in between called the *glomerular capsule space*. The inner surface of this space is formed by podocytes

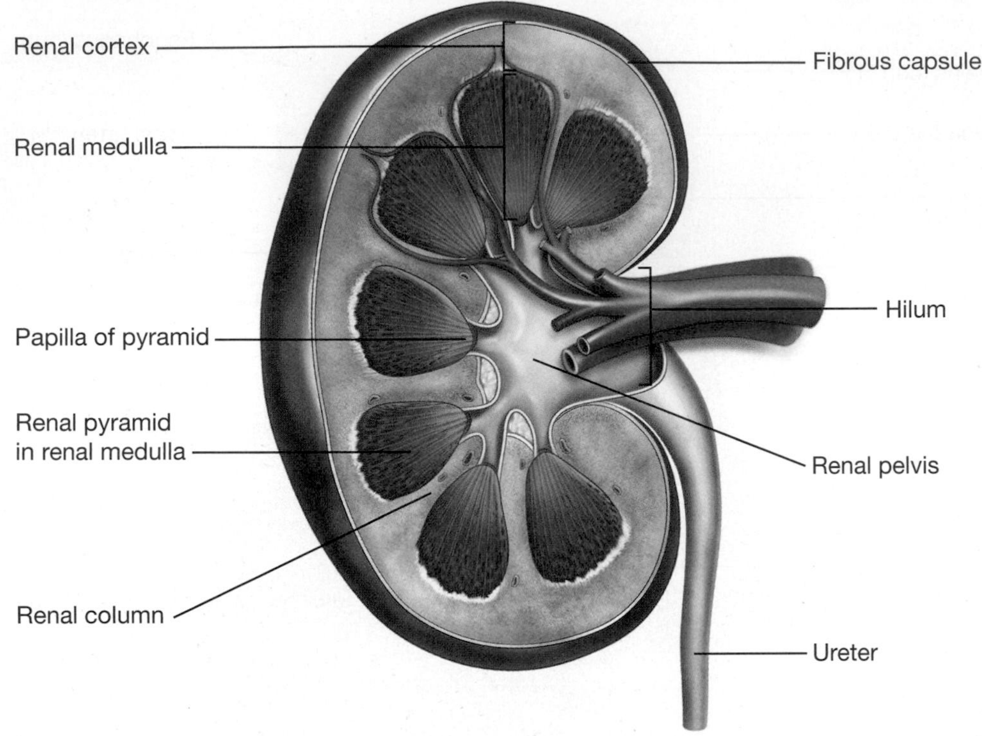

Figure 14.2 Frontal section through the kidney. The kidney has a light-colored cortex around the outside and a darker renal medulla inside. *Where are the "base" and the "tip" of a renal pyramid?*

(PAHD-oh-sights)—literally, "foot cells"—that wrap around the capillaries. The podocytes have finger-like processes that interlock with one another. Between the processes of the podocytes are tiny filtration slits.

To understand the relationship between the glomerulus and the glomerular capsule, imagine punching your fist into a big water balloon—softly enough that you do not pop the balloon. Your fist is like the ball of capillaries, and the balloon, now wrapped around your fist, is the capsule. The layer of the balloon against your fist is like the podocytes, and the space inside the balloon is like the glomerular capsule space.

As blood passes through the capillaries, a lot of the blood plasma leaks through the endothelial cells of the capillaries (which are much leakier than capillaries in most of the body), and through the filtration slits of the surrounding podocytes, into the glomerular capsule. After much processing, some of this fluid becomes urine.

The renal tubule and the capillaries that surround the tubule are shown in **Figure 14.3B**. The renal tubule has three main parts: the proximal convoluted tubule, the nephron loop, and the distal convoluted tubule.

The **proximal convoluted tubule (PCT)** begins at the glomerular capsule. The fluid in the glomerular capsule space passes into the PCT. The fluid then enters the **nephron loop** (also called the *loop of Henle*), first through the descending limb and then through the ascending limb. The descending limb and the lower part of the ascending limb have much thinner walls than the rest of the ascending limb and the proximal and distal convoluted tubules.

After the fluid reaches the end of the thick part of the ascending limb of the nephron loop, it enters the **distal convoluted tubule (DCT)**. The fluid that reaches the end of the distal convoluted tubule enters the **collecting duct**. Each collecting duct receives fluid from the distal convoluted tubules of several nephrons. The collecting ducts merge into larger ducts, which ultimately drain into the hollow renal pelvis.

The renal corpuscle and the proximal and distal convoluted tubules lie in the renal cortex. The nephron loops enter the renal medulla. The parallel nephron loops and surrounding capillaries give the renal cortex a striated (finely striped) appearance. Some nephrons, called *cortical nephrons*, have short nephron loops that penetrate only slightly into the medulla.

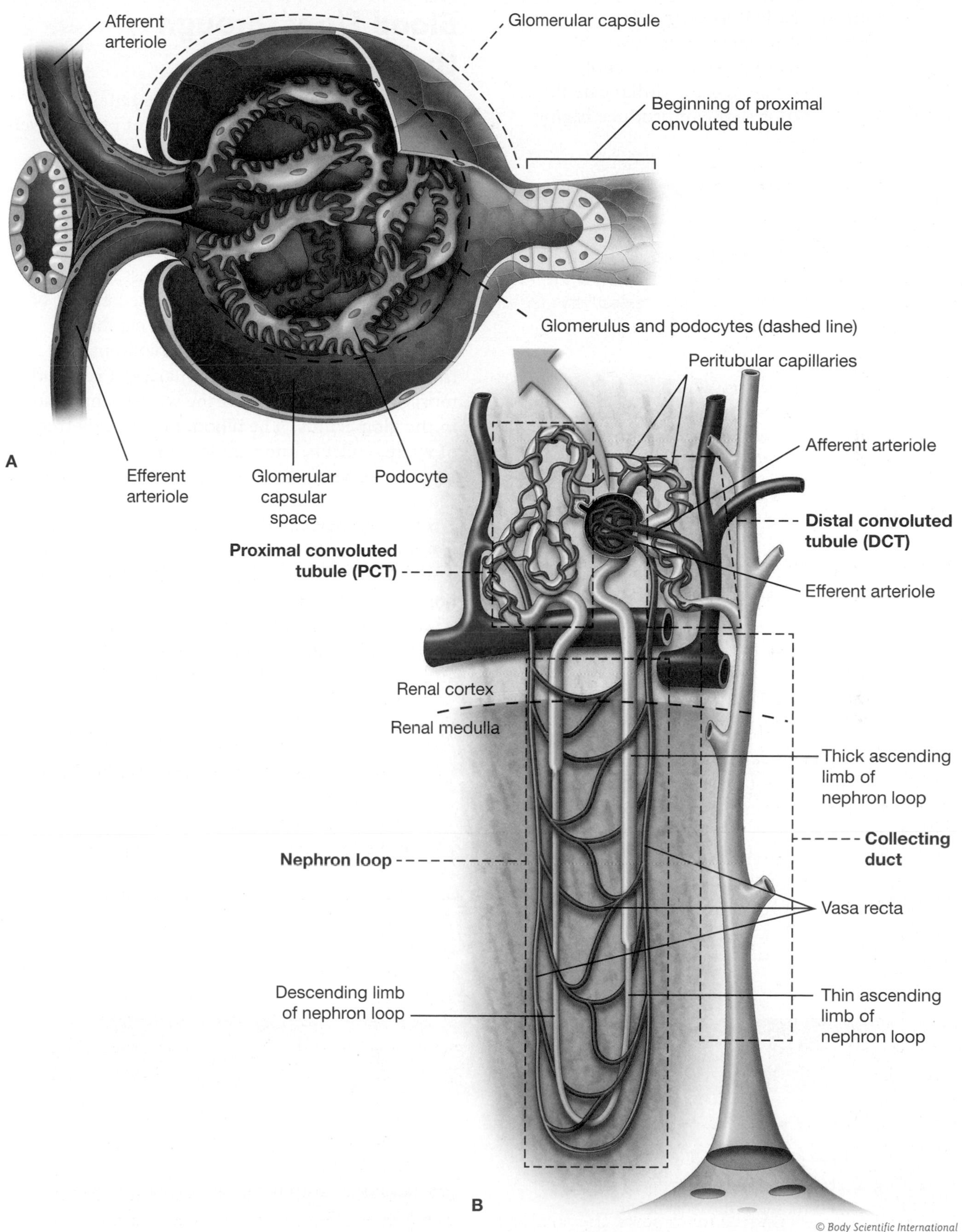

© Body Scientific International

Figure 14.3 Structure of a nephron. A—Renal corpuscle. B—Renal tubule and surrounding capillaries. The renal tubule includes the proximal convoluted tubule, the nephron loop, and the distal convoluted tubule. *Through which arteriole does blood enter the renal corpuscle? Through which arteriole does blood leave the corpuscle?*

Other nephrons, called *juxtamedullary* (juks-ta-MEHD-yoo-lair-ee) *nephrons*, have long nephron loops that penetrate deeply into the renal medulla. The juxtamedullary nephrons are the only nephrons that can produce highly concentrated urine.

MEMORY TIP

The word *juxtamedullary* is made up of the prefix *juxta-* (which means "next to" or "nearby") and the word *medullary*. The corpuscles of juxtamedullary nephrons lie *next to* the medulla.

The efferent arteriole, which carries blood out of the glomerulus, connects to a second set of capillaries called the *peritubular* (per-i-TOO-byuh-lar) *capillaries*. The peritubular capillaries surround the proximal and distal convoluted tubules. Many efferent arterioles from juxtamedullary nephrons give rise to capillaries that run parallel—first down and then up—with the long nephron loops. These capillaries are called **vasa recta** (Latin for "straight vessels").

Check Your Understanding

1. Where are the kidneys located in the abdominopelvic cavity?
2. What is the name of the outer part of the kidney, which is lighter in color than other parts?
3. What are the two main parts of a nephron?
4. Where are podocytes located?
5. What are the three main parts of the renal tubule?

Blood Flow through the Kidney

Blood enters the kidney via the renal artery and, after passing through a series of progressively smaller arteries, reaches the afferent arteriole at the entrance to the glomerulus. The blood then flows through the glomerular capillaries, and as it does, a significant fraction of the blood plasma enters the glomerular capsule space. The blood then exits the glomerulus, passes through the efferent arteriole, and enters a second set of capillaries—either the peritubular capillaries or the vasa recta. Finally, as the blood passes through the second set of capillaries, it reabsorbs most of the fluid—but not the waste—that it lost in the glomerulus. The blood, now largely free of waste, collects into venules, which merge to form larger veins, and exits the kidney via the renal vein.

In most parts of the body, blood passes from arteriole to capillary to venule, and then into larger veins. Kidney circulation is unusual because it does not follow this pattern. In the kidney, blood passes from afferent arteriole to capillaries to efferent arteriole to another set of capillaries, and only then to a venule and larger veins.

Check Your Understanding

1. Through what blood vessel does blood enter the kidney?
2. What is the purpose of the second set of capillaries through which blood passes in the kidneys?

LESSON 14.1 Review and Assessment

Mini Glossary

Make sure that you know the meaning of each key term.

collecting duct a tube that collects urine from several nephrons and carries it to the renal pelvis

distal convoluted tubule (DCT) the last part of a nephron through which urine flows before reaching the collecting duct

glomerulus a cluster of capillaries around the end of a renal corpuscle

nephron the fundamental excretory unit of each kidney

nephron loop the U-shaped part of the nephron that is between the proximal convoluted tubule and the distal convoluted tubule; has a descending limb and ascending limb; loop of Henle

proximal convoluted tubule (PCT) the part of the nephron between the glomerular capsule and the nephron loop; minerals, nutrients, and water are reabsorbed from the filtrate here

renal corpuscle the part of a nephron that consists of a glomerular capsule with its included glomerulus

renal cortex the lighter-colored, outer layer of the kidney that contains the glomeruli and convoluted tubules

renal medulla the darker, innermost part of the kidney

renal pelvis a funnel-shaped cavity in the center of the kidney where urine collects before it flows into the ureter

renal tubule the part of a nephron that leads away from a glomerulus and empties into a collecting tubule; consists of a proximal convoluted tubule, nephron loop, and distal convoluted tubule

vasa recta thin-walled blood vessels that begin and end near the boundary between the renal cortex and the renal medulla, and which extend deep into the renal medulla, running parallel to the nephron loops; play a role in the formation of concentrated urine

Know and Understand

1. The kidneys are retroperitoneal. What does that mean?
2. Where do the renal artery, renal vein, nerves, and ureter connect to the kidney?
3. What happens to urine that is produced in the renal cortex and the renal medulla?
4. What is the basic working unit of the kidney?
5. What are the names of the arteries that lead into and out of the glomerulus?
6. Which part of the renal tubule begins at the glomerular capsule?
7. Which type of nephron has long nephron loops that penetrate deeply into the renal medulla?
8. What happens to blood as it passes through the peritubular capillaries or the vasa recta?

Analyze and Apply

9. The kidneys, which make up about 0.5% of total body weight, receive 20% to 25% of the blood pumped by the heart (under resting conditions). What can you conclude about the kidneys based on this fact?
10. How does the flow of blood through the kidneys differ from the flow of blood through other parts of the body?

IN THE LAB

11. Build a three-dimensional kidney. You will need clay in several colors (brown, red, blue, yellow, orange, and white), pins, paper, tape, and textbook illustrations for reference. Include and label each of the following: fibrous capsule, renal hilum, renal cortex, renal medulla, renal pyramids, papilla, renal columns, renal pelvis, renal artery, renal vein, and ureter. Keep the following points in mind as you construct your 3-D model:
    A. Build your model so that it opens like a book, with the hilum serving as the "spine."
    B. Include arterioles and venules that branch off the renal artery and vein and go up between the renal pyramids into the renal cortex.
    C. Use brown clay for the majority of the kidney, red for the artery/arterioles, blue for the vein/venules, yellow for the ureter, white for the nerve, and orange for the adrenal gland.
12. According to the World Health Organization, "Organ transplant is often the only treatment for end state organ failure such as liver and heart failure. Kidney transplantation is generally accepted as the best treatment both for quality of life and cost effectiveness. Kidney transplantation is by far the most frequently carried out globally." Research the ethical dilemma in which disadvantaged individuals are exploited and encouraged to sell their organs and the efficacy of transplant tourism specifically in low-income countries. Site instances of exploitation, and suggest an alternative plan to protect disadvantaged individuals. Present your findings in an electronic presentation with a minimum of 10 slides.

LESSON 14.2

Urine Formation, Storage, and Excretion

Before You Read

Try to answer the following questions before you read this lesson.

- What are the three key steps involved in the formation of urine?
- How does the nervous system control the excretion of urine, and which muscles play a role?

Lesson Objectives

- Explain the process of urine formation.
- Understand how urine is stored in the body.
- List the steps in urine excretion.

Key Terms

aldosterone
angiotensin
antidiuretic hormone (ADH)
atrial natriuretic peptide (ANP)
detrusor
external urethral sphincter
glomerular filtration
glomerular filtration rate (GFR)
hydrostatic pressure
internal urethral sphincter
micturition
osmosis
osmotic pressure
reabsorption
renin
secretion
trigone
ureter
urethra
urinary bladder

To better understand how the body disposes of wastes, first consider two different ways that you could design a system for removing chemical wastes and toxins from fluid. Approach 1 would be to create a filter that allows wastes and toxins to pass through and does not allow anything "good" to pass through. Then you simply dispose of whatever substances pass across the filter.

Approach 2 would be to make a leaky filter with pores that allow water and other substances to pass through. Many good substances, as well as wastes, can pass through this nonselective filter. Therefore, you would need to pass the filtrate (fluid that has crossed the filter) through another stage of processing, in which the good substances, including most of the water, are pumped back into the body. After that stage, only wastes, toxins, and a little bit of water would remain on the filtered side. At that point, the remaining water and waste would be excreted.

Approach 1 sounds like it would be simpler and more efficient than Approach 2. However, the body uses Approach 2 for removing chemical wastes and toxins from fluid. Why?

It is impossible to predict all the different kinds of wastes and toxins an individual might need to excrete during his or her lifetime. Even if you did know exactly what you would need to excrete ahead of time, it probably would be impossible to make the hypothetical filter described in Approach 1 above. Why? In short, wastes and toxins sometimes are not very different from "good" molecules in size, electrical charge, and other properties.

Approach 2 presumably was favored by the human body because it works well even when the wastes and toxins are not known ahead of time. Approach 2 simply "throws out everything" and then selectively reclaims the good molecules, whose identity is known in advance.

Urine Formation

The first step in removing wastes and toxins from the body is the formation of urine. Three processes are involved in urine formation: filtration, reabsorption, and secretion. **Figure 14.4** shows a simplified view of where these processes occur in the nephron.

Filtration

Glomerular filtration, which occurs in the renal corpuscle, is the first step in urine formation. Glomerular filtration is the movement of water and solutes (dissolved substances) from the capillaries into the glomerular capsule space. The water that reaches the capsule is called the *glomerular filtrate*. To reach the glomerular capsule space, water and solutes must cross the capillary endothelial cells, the basement membrane (a layer of extracellular protein), and the podocytes of the glomerular capsule. These three structures are collectively known as the *filtration membrane*.

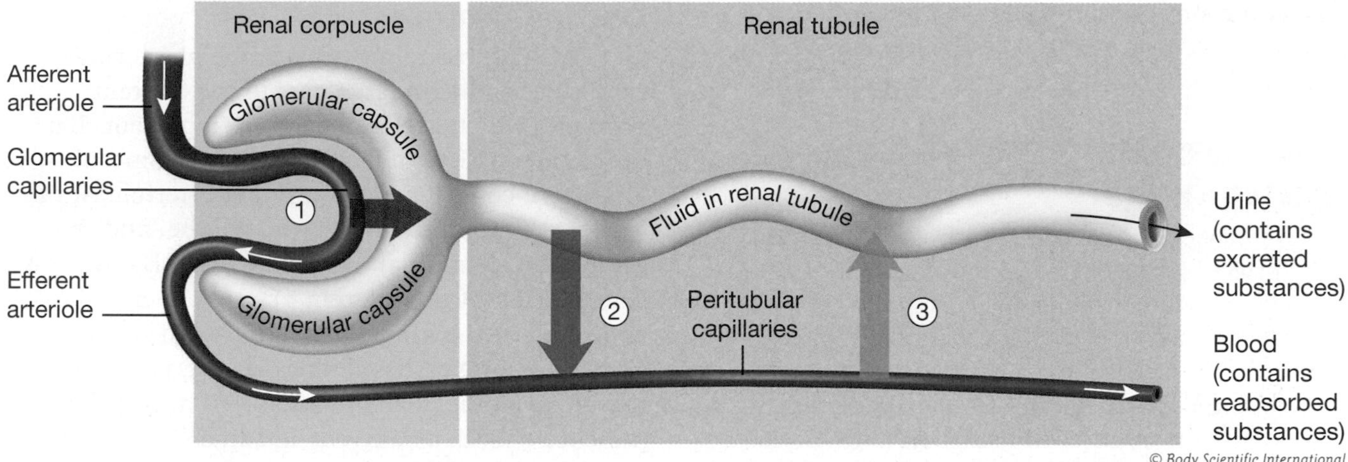

Figure 14.4 Formation of urine in the nephron—a functional view. 1. Filtration from the glomerular capillaries into the glomerular capsule (brown arrow) occurs in the renal corpuscle. 2. Reabsorption is the movement of water, ions, glucose, and other substances back into the capillaries (pink arrow). 3. Wastes and some ions, drugs, and toxins are secreted from the capillaries into the renal tubule (orange arrow).

Red and white blood cells are too large to cross the filtration membrane. Large and medium-sized proteins, such as albumin—the most common protein in blood plasma—are also prevented from crossing the filtration membrane. But water and small molecules and ions can cross this membrane. The list of substances that do cross the filtration membrane includes water, glucose, sodium, potassium, chloride, amino acids, urea (a waste product of metabolism), many kinds of prescription and over-the-counter drugs, and other molecules smaller than about 3 nanometers in diameter.

The total amount of water (in milliliters) filtered per minute is called the **glomerular filtration rate (GFR)**. A normal GFR value is about 125 mL per minute in males and 105 mL per minute in females. Laboratory tests are used to determine GFR, one of the most important benchmarks for assessing kidney health. If you multiply the normal GFR (the amount filtered per minute) by the number of minutes in a day, you get about 150 to 180 L of glomerular filtrate per day! Because human urine output is (fortunately) nowhere close to 180 L a day, you may guess that the majority of the filtrate eventually will be reclaimed by the body. The driving force for glomerular filtration is pressure: hydrostatic pressure and osmotic pressure.

Hydrostatic Pressure

You know **hydrostatic pressure** as "regular" pressure. It is the pressure of water in a balloon that makes the balloon swell. It is the pressure in pipes that makes water come out when you turn on the faucet. Water is pushed by hydrostatic pressure from where the pressure is high to where it is low.

In a glomerulus, the hydrostatic pressure in the capillaries is the blood pressure there—about 55 mmHg. This figure is considerably higher than the pressure of about 20 to 25 mmHg found in most capillaries. The pressure in the glomerular capsule space is only 15 mmHg, so there is a hydrostatic pressure difference of 40 mmHg pushing water from the capillaries into the capsule.

Osmotic Pressure

Unlike hydrostatic pressure, **osmotic** (ahs-MAHT-ik) **pressure** is a kind of pressure that people do not ordinarily notice. Osmotic pressure is created by the presence of dissolved substances in water. High osmotic pressure "pulls in" water from areas of low osmotic pressure. Hydrostatic pressure, by contrast, "pushes" water from areas of high to low pressure.

The more dissolved substances in a fluid, the higher its osmotic pressure. Therefore, water is drawn in to "salty" areas (ones that are full of dissolved substances) from areas that have fewer dissolved substances. The movement of water from an area of low osmotic pressure to an area of high osmotic pressure is called **osmosis** (ahz-MOH-sis).

In the renal corpuscle, the blood has a higher osmotic pressure than the filtrate because the proteins, which are too big to cross the filtration membrane, are present only on the "blood" side of the membrane. The molecules that are small enough to cross the membrane are present in equal concentrations on both sides, so they do not create an osmotic pressure difference. The osmotic pressure is about 30 mmHg higher in blood than in filtrate.

MEMORY TIP

Osmotic pressure is directly related to the amount of dissolved substances a fluid contains. When a cell or region contains the same amount of dissolved substances as the surrounding solution, the solution is considered *isotonic*. The prefix *iso-* means "same" or "equal"; the combining form *ton/o* means "tension." When the cell contains more dissolved substances (high osmotic pressure), it is *hypertonic*, and when it contains fewer dissolved substances (low osmotic pressure), it is *hypotonic*.

You can compare the size and direction of the pressure differences to determine the net amount and direction of pressure across the filtration membrane. Recall that the hydrostatic pressure is 40 mmHg higher in the capillary than in the glomerular capsular space, and the osmotic pressure is 30 mmHg higher in the capillary than in the capsular space. These pressures act in opposite directions: High hydrostatic pressure *pushes*, and high osmotic pressure *pulls*. Thus, there is a net filtration pressure of 10 mmHg pushing water from the capillary into the capsule (**Figure 14.5**).

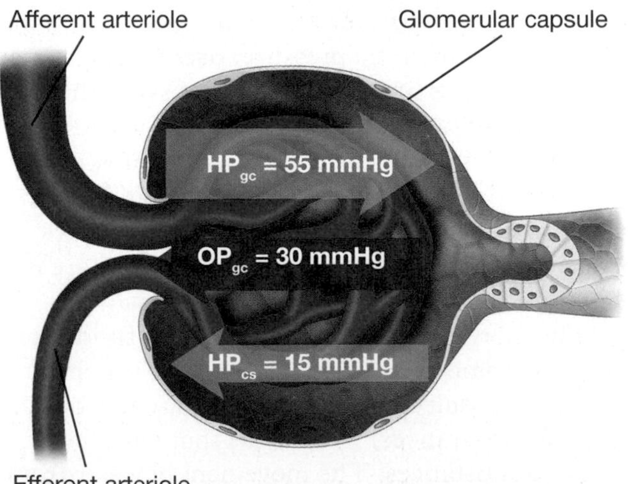

Figure 14.5 Pressures driving filtration. Hydrostatic pressure in the glomerular capillary (HP_{gc}) pushes water out of the capillary. Hydrostatic pressure in the capsular space (HP_{cs}) pushes back, from the capsule to the capillary. Osmotic pressure in the glomerular capillary (OP_{gc}) pulls water into the capillary. *What is the net filtration pressure of water being pushed out of the capillary?*

Pressure Controls

The high blood pressure in the glomerular capillaries is due in large part to the efferent arteriole, which acts as a constricting agent that limits the outflow of blood from the glomerulus. The more constricted the efferent arteriole is, the higher the glomerular pressure will be, and the greater the glomerular filtration will be. By contrast, constriction of the afferent arteriole, which lies upstream of the glomerulus, limits inflow to the glomerulus and causes glomerular pressure—and therefore glomerular filtration—to drop. The presence of both an afferent and an efferent arteriole provides the body with the ability to control glomerular pressure and glomerular filtration.

Hormones and sympathetic nerves to the kidney both have the ability to regulate the renal arterioles. The sympathetic nerves have a greater effect on the afferent arterioles than on the efferent arterioles. Sympathetic nerve activity rises during exercise and during stressful situations that evoke a fight-or-flight response.

When sympathetic nerve activity increases, the afferent arterioles constrict more than the efferent arterioles. This constriction causes a drop in glomerular capillary pressure and a decrease in glomerular filtration rate, for the reasons described above. The decrease in glomerular capillary pressure and GFR helps the body to reduce urine output and keeps blood volume high, which is useful during exercise. These physiological effects probably gave humans an advantage in surviving some fight-or-flight situations in the past.

Reabsorption

The filtrate from the glomerular capsule flows into the renal tubule. As it flows through the tubule and then into the collecting duct, most of the water and dissolved substances are reabsorbed into the blood in the capillaries surrounding the tubule. Most **reabsorption** occurs in the proximal convoluted tubule. The remainder occurs in the distal convoluted tubule and the collecting duct.

The epithelial cells that form the wall of the PCT have microvilli on their luminal (lumen-facing) side. These microvilli increase the surface area of the PCT, enhancing its reabsorptive ability. The major steps involved in reabsorption are shown in **Figure 14.6**.

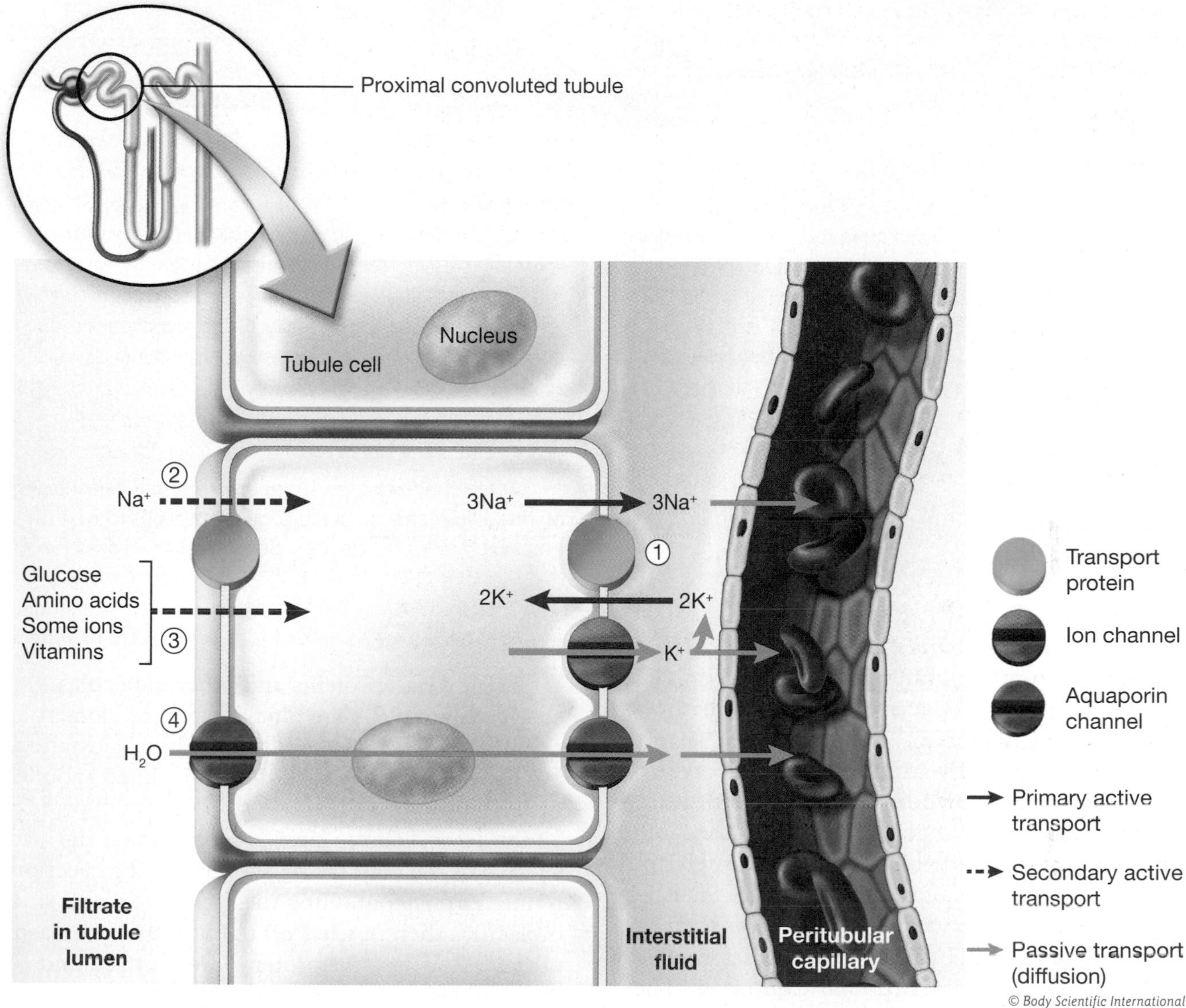

Figure 14.6 Reabsorption in the proximal convoluted tubule. The lumen of the tubule is at the far left, and the peritubular capillary is at the right. The cells lining the tubule have been enlarged to show details, and the microvilli on the luminal side of the cell have been omitted for clarity. 1. Sodium-potassium pumps (the green transport proteins shown above) actively pump sodium (Na^+) out of the tubule cell and potassium ions (K^+) into the cell. 2. Sodium flows down its energy gradient into the cell. 3. Glucose and amino acids are co-transported into the cell with sodium, by secondary active transport. 4. Water enters the cell from the tubule through aquaporin channels, and it leaves the cell on the capillary side through aquaporin channels.

Sodium

Sodium is the most abundant ion in the filtrate, and it is actively pumped out of the tubular epithelial cells by sodium-potassium pump proteins. These carrier proteins use ATP to move sodium from the cell into the interstitial space that surrounds the peritubular capillary.

The active excretion of sodium from the cell by the sodium-potassium pump leaves the cytoplasm of the cell with little sodium. Since there is a high concentration of sodium in the tubular fluid, sodium spreads into the cell from the tubule. The sodium that has been pumped out of the cells and into the space surrounding the capillaries then diffuses into the capillaries.

Secondary Active Transport

Cotransport proteins in the part of the cell membrane that faces the tubule bring sodium into the cell. Using the energy from this sodium entry,

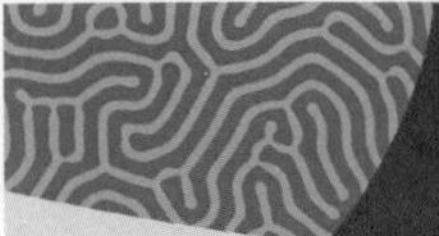

What Research Tells Us

...about Body Fluids

Water makes up 50% to 60% of the weight of a healthy young adult, with women being close to 50% and men closer to 60%. This amounts to about 40 liters (L) in a 70 kg male. Of this amount, about 25 L are intracellular fluid, and 15 L are extracellular. The intracellular fluid is located in the cytoplasm, nuclei, and organelles of the body cells. The extracellular fluid is the blood plasma (about 3 L) and the interstitial fluid (about 12 L). Interstitial fluid is between the cells but not in the circulation.

Water can move between the plasma and the interstitial fluid by crossing the walls of capillaries. This movement does not change the total amount of extracellular fluid, since the plasma and the interstitial fluid are both extracellular. Water can also move between the interstitial fluid and the intracellular space, by crossing cell membranes.

Capillaries and cell membranes are quite permeable to water. The water permeability of cell membranes is due in large part to the presence of aquaporin channels, which allow facilitated diffusion of water.

Taking It Further

Research the changes in the amounts and percentages of intracellular and extracellular fluids as people age. Write an essay explaining your findings. Be sure to cite your references.

the cotransport proteins pump various desirable substances from the lumen into the cell. This is an example of secondary active transport, which was discussed in Chapter 2.

In secondary active transport, the energy of one substance going "downhill" is used by a protein to pump another substance "uphill." Glucose, amino acids, some ions, and vitamins enter the cell from the tubule by means of secondary active transport with sodium. These valuable substances then move out of the cell by facilitated diffusion on side of the cell facing the peritubular capillaries. The substances then diffuse into the capillaries.

Osmotic Pressure

The positive charge on the sodium ions (Na^+) tends to draw negatively charged chloride (Cl^-) out of the tubule and into the peritubular capillaries. The active pumping of sodium into the interstitial space, and its diffusion into the peritubular capillaries, creates a relatively high osmotic pressure in the capillaries and in the interstitial space. The high osmotic pressure draws water by osmosis out of the tubule, through the cell, and into the interstitial space and the capillary. Aquaporin (ak-kwa-POR-in) channels in both sides of the cell allow facilitated diffusion of water into and out of the cell. Thus, the active pumping of sodium provides the driving force for reabsorption of glucose, amino acids, vitamins, chloride and some other ions, and water.

Endocytosis

Some small proteins and other molecules, such as vitamin B_{12}, are filtered from the glomerular capillary blood into the filtrate. These substances are recovered in the proximal convoluted tubule by *receptor-mediated endocytosis*. The small proteins and other molecules bind to receptors on the surface of the cells facing the tubule. The section of membrane containing these receptors and small molecules then pinches off to enter the cytoplasm of the cell, where the proteins are recycled and other molecules are processed as appropriate.

Secretion

At the same time that the "good" substances are being reabsorbed by the blood, wastes still in the blood are being actively secreted from the capillaries. Waste products, such as urea, that were not fully removed during filtration are actively pumped out of the capillaries and into the renal tubule by the cells that form the walls of the tubules. This active pumping of wastes from capillary blood into the tubules is called **secretion**. Unlike filtration, which is a passive process, secretion is active; that is, it uses chemical energy, often in the form of ATP, to move molecules.

Tubular epithelial cells—cells in the walls of the proximal and distal convoluted tubules and collecting duct—actively export certain molecules, such as urea and uric acid, into the lumen of the renal tubule. The lumen of the tubule contains the fluid that will eventually be eliminated from the body as urine. Exporting these molecules into the lumen of the renal tubule is the body's way of getting rid of them. This active export of molecules into the lumen is called *tubular secretion*.

The tubular epithelial cells can also secrete hydrogen ions (acid, H+) or bicarbonate ions (base, HCO_3^-) to maintain the pH of arterial blood at about 7.4. The renal tubule epithelial cells also secrete, or push out, some drugs, if they are present in the blood. Penicillin and aspirin are examples of drugs that are eliminated from the body by the kidneys in this manner.

The Renal Medulla

So far, this lesson has discussed mainly the reabsorption and secretion that take place in the proximal and distal convoluted tubules, both of which are located in the renal cortex. Now consider what happens to the wastes and the "good" substances as they travel down and then back up through the renal medulla (**Figure 14.7**).

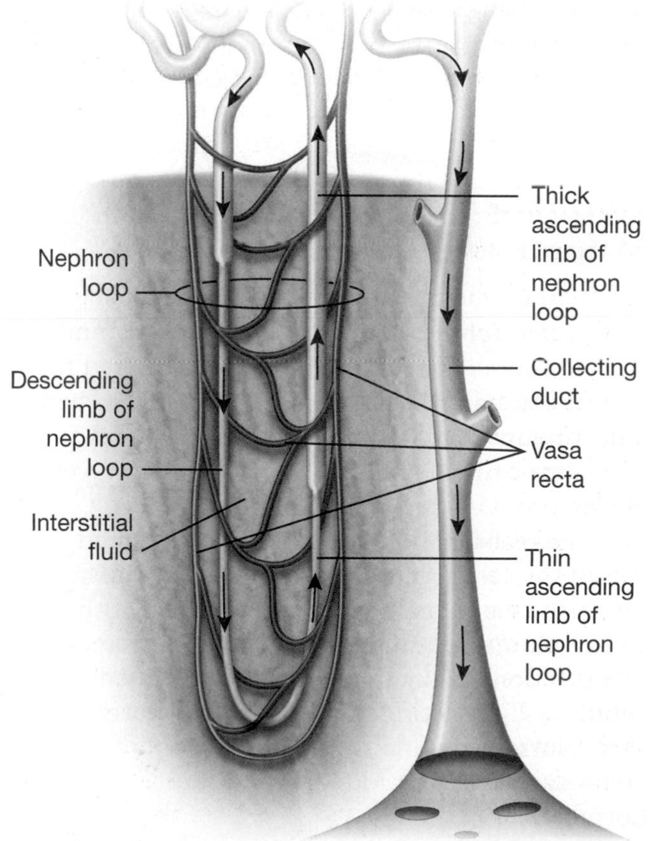

Figure 14.7 The renal medulla. Notice the change in thickness of the descending and ascending limbs. *Why are these changes significant?*

The thin descending limb of the nephron loop lacks the active pumping capability or intracellular machinery (such as mitochondria) of the PCT cells. Thus, no active reabsorption or secretion occurs in either the descending limb or the thin ascending limb of the nephron loop. Water can leave the filtrate in the descending limb but not in the ascending limb, whose cells lack aquaporin channels. The thick portion of the ascending limb, which *does* have pumping capability, actively reabsorbs sodium, but water cannot follow due to the lack of aquaporin channels in the ascending limb.

The reabsorption of sodium in the thick, ascending limb of the nephron loop, where water cannot be reabsorbed, and the permeability to water of the descending limb of the nephron loop, work together to create very salty interstitial fluid in the renal medulla.

Limited amounts of urea reenter the interstitial space as urine travels down the collecting duct. Reentry of urea within the interstitial space contributes to the high osmolality of the interstitial fluid in the renal medulla. The net result is that the deepest parts of the renal medulla can have an interstitial osmolality of about 1,200 milliosmoles (mOsm), about four times higher than normal interstitial fluid osmolality. Milliosmoles are a measurement of the number of ions, or particles, that contribute to the osmotic pressure of a solution. A milliosmole is equal to one-thousandth of an osmole per unit volume of fluid.

The Countercurrent Mechanism

The geometric arrangement of the nephron loop and the parallel vasa recta capillaries are key to renal medullary function, as shown in **Figure 14.8**. Capillary blood grows highly concentrated as it goes down the vasa recta into the renal medulla because osmosis draws water out of the capillary. As the blood ascends in the vasa recta, osmosis causes water to re-enter the capillaries. As a result, the blood leaving the vasa recta is no more and no less concentrated than it was when it entered, despite having passed through an area of very high interstitial fluid concentration. Thus, the deep parts of the renal medulla get the blood flow they need despite the high concentration of interstitial fluid, which is necessary for the production of highly concentrated urine.

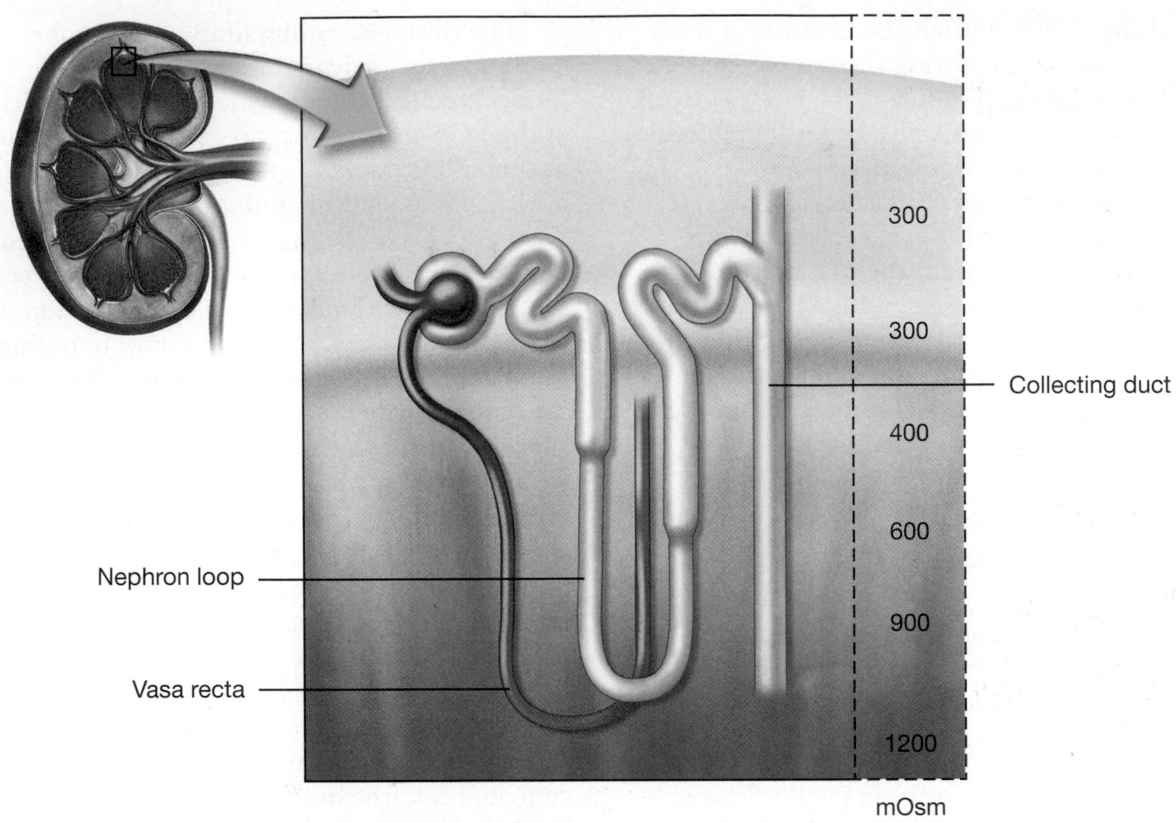

Figure 14.8 Water permeability of the descending limb of the nephron loop, and active sodium reabsorption from the ascending limb, establish the high osmolality of the deep renal medulla. The numbers on the right show the osmolality of the interstitial fluid, represented in milliosmoles (mOsm), in the renal medulla. *Does higher osmolality mean more or less "saltiness"?*

The geometric arrangement that makes this process possible is called a *countercurrent mechanism.* It is called *countercurrent* because the blood flows "down" the vasa recta, then back past itself in the opposite direction.

The flow of filtrate in the nephron loop is also a countercurrent arrangement because the filtrate flows down the descending limb, then up the ascending limb, adjacent to where it is going down. As with the vasa recta, the close proximity of these parallel pathways helps the kidney create and maintain high osmolality of the interstitial fluid in the deep parts of the renal medulla.

When urine travels down the collecting duct, through the deepest parts of the medulla, water can be reabsorbed from the collecting duct by osmosis into the highly concentrated interstitial fluid. When this occurs maximally, the urine can reach an osmolality of 1,200 milliosmoles because the water in the collecting duct reaches osmotic equilibrium with the interstitial space.

Hormonal Regulation of Urine Volume and Composition

By the time the filtrate reaches the distal convoluted tubule, about 80% of the water and 90% of the sodium and chloride that entered the glomerular capsular space have been reabsorbed. The amount of reabsorption in the proximal convoluted tubule and nephron loop is relatively constant.

The reabsorption in the distal convoluted tubule and collecting duct, however, is adjusted by hormones to maintain homeostasis. In other words, the "fine tuning" of urine volume and composition occurs in the distal convoluted tubule and collecting duct. Three key hormones that control this fine tuning are aldosterone, atrial natriuretic peptide, and antidiuretic hormone.

Aldosterone

A steroid hormone called **aldosterone** (al-DAHS-ter-ohn) is produced in the adrenal cortex. A drop in blood sodium concentration or a rise in blood potassium concentration directly stimulates the secretion of more aldosterone. A decrease in blood pressure also stimulates more aldosterone secretion, but by an indirect mechanism: decreased blood pressure causes greater secretion of the hormone **renin** (REE-nin), a protein, by the kidney.

Renin circulates in the blood and binds to the circulating protein angiotensinogen. Renin acts on angiotensinogen to produce **angiotensin** (an-jee-oh-TEHN-sin), a polypeptide hormone in the blood that constricts blood vessels and increases blood pressure. After binding to angiotensinogen, the renin cuts the angiotensinogen into two fragments, one of which is angiotensin I. An enzyme in the lungs, appropriately named *angiotensin-converting enzyme*, converts angiotensin I into angiotensin II by removing two amino acids. Angiotensin II stimulates adrenal cortical cells to secrete more aldosterone.

Aldosterone acts on the distal convoluted tubule cells and collecting duct to increase the amount of sodium reabsorption and potassium secretion. Because more sodium is reabsorbed than potassium is secreted, water follows the sodium and also is reabsorbed more when a greater amount of aldosterone is present. As a result, aldosterone causes a decrease in the volume and sodium content of urine, and an increase in its potassium content. The decreased urine volume means that more water is retained in the circulation, which causes blood pressure to rise. Thus, the decrease in blood pressure that led—via the renin-angiotensin mechanism—to more aldosterone secretion is corrected.

Atrial Natriuretic Peptide

A hormone made by the atria of the heart, **atrial natriuretic** (nay-tree-yoo-REHT-ik) **peptide (ANP)** is released in response to increased stretching of the atria, which occurs when blood volume is high. ANP inhibits sodium reabsorption in the collecting ducts, which causes decreased water reabsorption due to osmotic pressure effects. As a result, urine volume and sodium excretion increase, which tends to correct the high blood volume that stimulated ANP production.

Antidiuretic Hormone

A peptide hormone secreted by the pituitary gland, **antidiuretic** (an-tee-digh-yoo-REHT-ik) **hormone (ADH)**, is also known as *vasopressin*. ADH secretion increases when blood osmolality increases.

Blood osmolality increases when a person becomes dehydrated because water intake has not kept up with water loss. Antidiuretic hormone causes collecting duct cells to produce more aquaporin molecules and insert them in their own membranes. As a result, more reabsorption of water occurs in the collecting ducts, which produces more concentrated urine.

When a person is severely dehydrated and ADH levels are high, reabsorption of water in the collecting ducts is so effective that the urine leaving the collecting duct is extremely concentrated, with an osmolality of about 1,200 milliosmoles. In a well-hydrated person, ADH levels are low. As a result, little water is reabsorbed in the collecting duct, and urine osmolality can drop to between 50 and 100 milliosmoles.

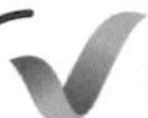

Check Your Understanding

1. Why is glomerular filtration rate important?
2. Do more dissolved substances in a fluid mean higher or lower osmotic pressure?
3. Where does most of the reabsorption of water and dissolved substances take place in the kidneys?
4. What substances are actively reabsorbed and secreted in the ascending and descending limbs of the nephron loop?
5. Describe the countercurrent mechanism in the vasa recta.
6. Does an increase in secretion of renin lead to higher or lower blood pressure?

Urine Storage

Urine is made continuously by the kidney. Unlike the respiratory system, which excretes waste (carbon dioxide) continuously, the urinary system excretes waste intermittently. Therefore, the body needs a place to store the urine until the time and place for elimination are appropriate. The body also needs plumbing—structures to take the urine from where it is made to where it is stored, and from where it is stored to the outside.

Ureters

Each kidney is connected by a **ureter** (YOOR-et-er) to the bladder (**Figure 14.1**). The renal pelvis connects to the hollow ureter, as shown in **Figure 14.2**. Each ureter is lined with epithelium and contains smooth muscle in its wall. The ureters connect to the bladder via the posterior wall of the bladder.

Urinary Bladder

The **urinary bladder** is a hollow, muscular organ that stores urine. It sits on the floor of the pelvic cavity, under the peritoneum, and its superior surface is directly covered by the peritoneum. In men, it is positioned directly in front of the rectum and above the prostate gland. In women, it is positioned in front of the vagina and uterus.

The bladder wall is made of smooth muscle, the **detrusor** (dee-TROO-zer), with a layer of epithelial cells on its interior. When the bladder is empty, it collapses, causing folds to develop in the walls and lining. A moderately full bladder may contain 500 mL of urine. An extremely full bladder can contain as much as 1,000 mL.

The bladder has three openings: one *ureteric orifice* for each of the two ureters, plus the opening of the urethra. The urethra connects to the bladder at the bladder neck. The imaginary triangle formed by the two ureteric orifices and the urethra is the **trigone** (TRIGH-gohn) of the bladder.

Urethra

The **urethra** (yoo-REE-thra) is a thin tube that connects the urinary bladder to the outside (**Figure 14.9**). It begins at the neck of the bladder,

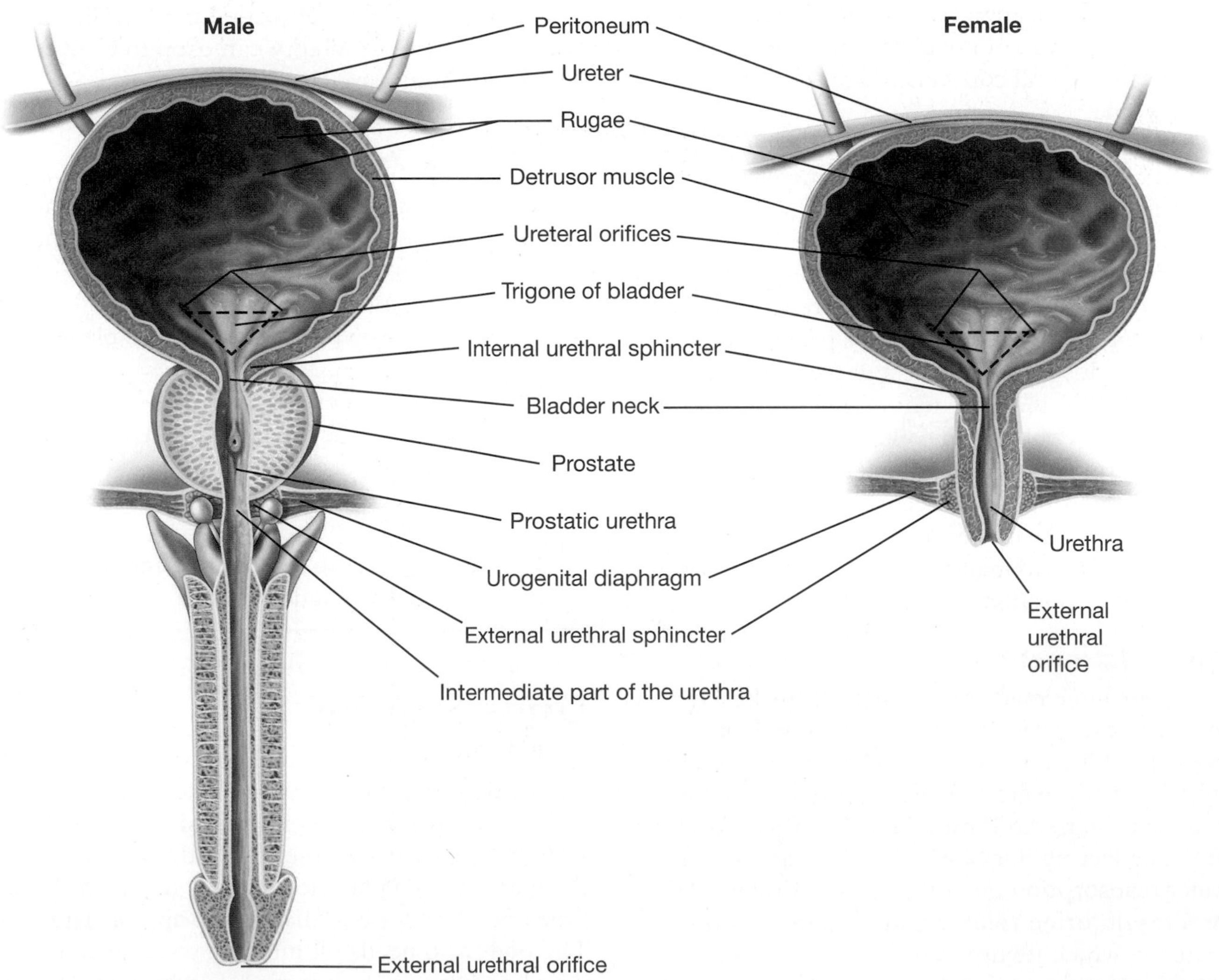

Figure 14.9 The male and female bladder and urethra. *Where is the bladder positioned in the male? Where is it positioned in the female? For both males and females, how many openings does the bladder have? (Note: The trigone is a clue.)*

in its midline. A layer of smooth muscle that encircles the urethra where it exits the bladder is called the **internal urethral sphincter**.

In men, the prostate gland lies directly below the bladder. The prostatic urethra is the portion of the urethra that passes through the prostate gland. The next part of the male urethra, the intermediate part, passes through the muscles of the pelvic floor, which make up the *urogenital* (yoor-oh-JEHN-i-tal) *diaphragm*. A ring of skeletal muscle, the **external urethral sphincter**, surrounds the intermediate part of the urethra where it passes through the urogenital diaphragm. The intermediate part continues to the base of the penis and becomes the *spongy urethra* as it passes down the length of the penis, finally opening to the outside at the external urethral orifice.

The total length of the male urethra is about 8 inches (20 cm). The intermediate part of the urethra and the spongy urethra also carry seminal fluid (see Chapter 15).

The female urethra is only about 1.5 inches (3 to 4 centimeters) long. Like the male urethra, it is surrounded by the external urethral sphincter as it passes through the urogenital diaphragm; its external opening is also called the *external urethral orifice*.

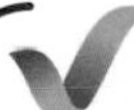

Check Your Understanding

1. Why would the bladder be unnecessary if the urinary system functioned more like the respiratory system?
2. Which structure in the urinary system leads to the outside of the body?

Urine Excretion

Thousands of collecting ducts in each kidney produce a steady trickle of urine into the renal pelvis. As fluid from the kidney enters the ureter, the ureter stretches. This stretching causes a wave of peristalsis to develop in the smooth muscle wall of the ureter. The wave of muscle contractions travels down the ureter, pushing the urine ahead of it.

The release of urine from the bladder is called *urination*, *voiding*, or **micturition** (mik-choo-RISH-un). Micturition requires contraction of the detrusor to force urine out of the bladder, and simultaneous relaxation of both the internal and external sphincters to open the pathway for release.

Because the internal sphincter is made of smooth muscle, it is controlled by the autonomic nervous system and is not consciously controlled. By contrast, the external urethral sphincter is made of skeletal muscle. This means that the external urethral sphincter is consciously controlled by somatic motor nerve fibers. (The autonomic and somatic branches of the nervous system are described in Chapter 6.) The autonomic reflexes of micturition occur in the spinal cord, and conscious control of the external urethral sphincter originates in the brain.

Figure 14.10 shows the pathways and actions involved in micturition. The numbers in the following description correspond to the numbers in the figure.

1. As the bladder fills, it stretches. Stretch receptors in the wall generate action potentials that excite sensory neurons in the bladder wall. These neurons send impulses to the sacral portion of the spinal cord.
2. Interneurons in the spinal cord signal motor neurons in the sacral cord that the bladder is stretched.
3. The sacral cord neurons send impulses back out to the bladder via parasympathetic nerve fibers.
4. The impulses sent to the bladder through the parasympathetic nerve fibers cause the detrusor to contract and the internal urethral sphincter to relax.
5. While the detrusor is contracting and the internal urethral sphincter is relaxing, the spinal cord sends an impulse to the brain, signaling that the bladder is stretched (from step 1).
6. The sensory message from the spinal cord activates the micturition reflex center in the brainstem, which sends impulses to the sacral cord.

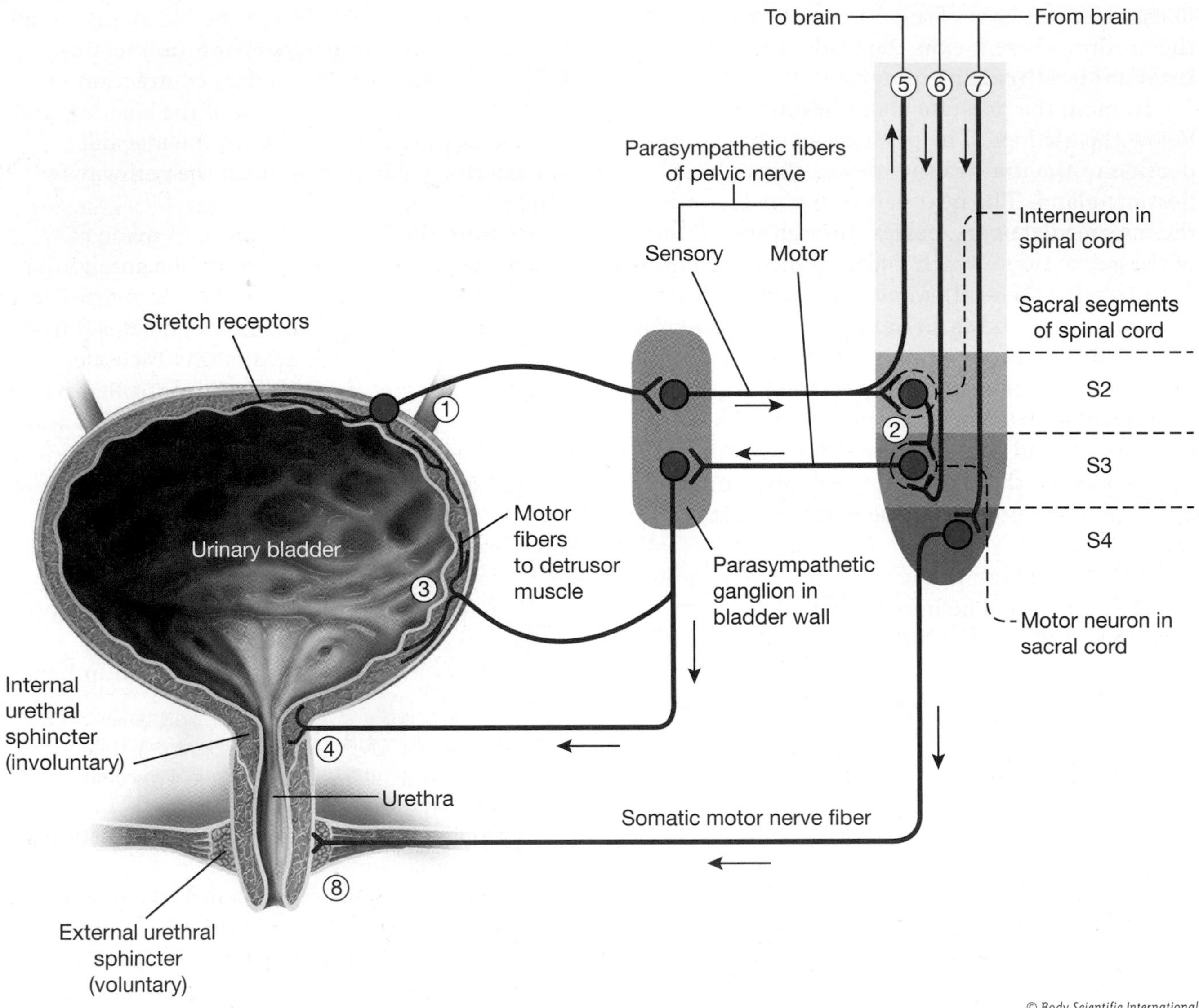

Figure 14.10 The pathways and actions involved in micturition. *Based on what you see in the drawing, how would you describe the brain's involvement in the micturition process?*

7. The detrusor contracts, and the internal urethral sphincter relaxes. At the same time, the person becomes consciously aware that the bladder is full. If the time is not right for urination, there is no change in the steady signal to the external urethral sphincter that causes it to stay contracted. If the time is right for urination, nerve impulses are sent from the brainstem to the sacral spinal cord.
8. From the sacral spinal cord, the nerve impulses travel to the external urethral sphincter, signaling it to relax. As a result, the pathway for micturition becomes fully open, the detrusor contracts, and the urine is expelled.

Early in childhood, people unconsciously learn that they can aid the expulsion of urine. They do this, without realizing it, by contracting the respiratory diaphragm and the skeletal muscles of the abdomen. This muscle contraction raises pressure in the abdominal cavity, which pushes down on the top of the bladder, thus helping to force urine out. This voluntary effort to raise intra-abdominal pressure is called the *Valsalva maneuver* and can also be useful in aiding defecation.

Check Your Understanding

1. What process moves urine through the ureters to the urinary bladder?
2. What is a Valsalva maneuver?

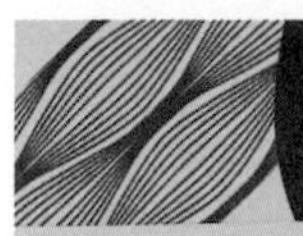

LIFE SPAN DEVELOPMENT: *The Urinary System*

The urinary and reproductive systems, also referred to during early development as the *urogenital system*, start to form in the fourth week of embryonic life. Two urogenital ridges form on either side of the midline in the mesoderm, or middle layer, of the embryo. Urogenital ridge cells in the future pelvic region of the embryo develop into the kidneys. As development continues and the embryo elongates, the kidneys move from the pelvis up into the abdomen, reaching their final position around the ninth week. The blood supply to the kidneys initially comes from the paired iliac arteries. As the kidneys move up, the renal arteries form, connecting the kidneys to the abdominal aorta, and the vascular connections to the iliac arteries degenerate. The bladder develops from the embryonic cloaca, which is the distal end of the early gut. A membrane develops in the cloaca, dividing into the bladder anteriorly and the rectum and anal canal posteriorly.

Sometimes one of the kidneys fails to develop. This usually does not cause problems, because a single healthy kidney is sufficient for normal renal function. Sometimes multiple renal arteries or veins form. This, too, does not cause difficulties in most cases. Occasionally the early kidneys in the pelvis are connected in the midline, forming a single U-shaped or "horseshoe" kidney. This kidney may not fully ascend into the abdomen. Patients with a horseshoe kidney are at increased risk for kidney stones and obstruction of the ureters.

Polycystic kidney disease (PKD) is a congenital abnormality in which fluid-filled cysts develop in the kidneys. It has varying severity. Most people with PKD do not develop symptoms, such as high blood pressure, pain, and kidney failure, until middle age. In more rare and severe cases, the kidneys fail very early in life.

Most metabolic wastes produced by the fetus are transferred into the mother's blood in the placenta and are excreted by the mother. Although the fetal kidneys are not the primary means of waste disposal during development, they do produce urine, and this urine makes up the majority of the amniotic fluid which bathes, surrounds, and protects the fetus. In rare cases, both kidneys fail to develop. This leads to insufficient amniotic fluid, which causes multiple developmental abnormalities. If a fetus with these abnormalities does survive to be born, it usually dies soon after birth.

A gradual decline in renal function is an inevitable consequence of aging. Glomerular filtration rate declines by about 1% per year after age 40. Chronic kidney disease, discussed in Lesson 14.3, affects 40% to 50% of adults age 70 and over in the United States.

Urinary incontinence, the leakage of urine from the body at unwanted times, and urinary retention, the inability to expel urine from the bladder when desired, both become more common with age. Urinary incontinence can be due to weakening of the pelvic floor muscles, which may be exacerbated by childbirth in women. In older men, hypertrophy, or excessive growth, of the prostate gland, can compress the urethra and is a cause of urinary retention.

Life Span Review

1. From what structure in the embryo does the bladder develop?
2. Name a common cause of urinary incontinence in older men and women.

LESSON 14.2 Review and Assessment

Mini Glossary

Make sure that you know the meaning of each key term.

aldosterone a steroid hormone produced in the adrenal cortex that regulates salt and water balance in the body by increasing the amount of sodium reabsorbed from urine

angiotensin a polypeptide hormone in the blood that constricts blood vessels and increases blood pressure

antidiuretic hormone (ADH) a peptide hormone secreted by the pituitary gland that constricts blood vessels, raises blood pressure, and reduces excretion of urine; vasopressin

atrial natriuretic peptide (ANP) a peptide hormone secreted by the atria of the heart that promotes excretion of sodium and water and lowers blood pressure

detrusor the smooth muscle that forms most of the bladder wall and aids in expelling urine

external urethral sphincter a ring of skeletal muscle that surrounds the intermediate part of the urethra where it passes through the urogenital diaphragm; this muscle is voluntarily controlled during release of urine from the body

glomerular filtration the movement of water and solutes (dissolved substances) from the capillaries into the glomerular capsular space; this is the first step in urine formation

glomerular filtration rate (GFR) the total amount of water filtered from the glomerular capillaries into the glomerular capsule per unit of time; usually measured in milliliters per minute

hydrostatic pressure the pressure exerted by a liquid as a result of its potential energy

internal urethral sphincter a layer of smooth muscle located at the inferior end of the bladder and the proximal end of the urethra; this muscle, which prohibits release of urine, is under involuntary control

micturition urination

osmosis the movement of water molecules from a region of low osmotic pressure to a region of high osmotic pressure

osmotic pressure a pressure created by the presence of dissolved substances in water

reabsorption the movement of water and dissolved substances from the filtrate (in a renal tubule) back into the blood

renin an enzyme made and secreted by the kidneys; aids in the production of angiotensin

secretion the active movement of substances from the blood into the filtrate, which will become urine

trigone the triangular region of the bladder formed by the two ureteric orifices and the internal urethral orifice

ureter a duct through which urine travels from the kidney to the bladder

urethra a thin tube that connects the urinary bladder to the outside environment

urinary bladder a hollow, muscular organ that stores urine

Know and Understand

1. What are the three major processes involved in urine formation?
2. During filtration in the glomerular capsule, water and solutes move from where to where? What is the water called after this movement?
3. What two types of pressure are involved in the filtration process that creates urine?
4. Name four substances that diffuse into the capillaries along with sodium as a result of secondary active transport.
5. List the three key hormones involved in "fine tuning" urine volume and composition.
6. How does the urinary system differ from the respiratory system in eliminating waste?
7. Which structure(s) contract and which structure(s) relax during micturition?

Analyze and Apply

8. Compare and contrast hydrostatic pressure and osmotic pressure.
9. Explain how and why the nervous system is involved in excreting urine from the body.
10. Explain the relationship between antidiuretic hormone and dehydration.
11. Glomerular filtration rate is often used as an indication of kidney function. Conduct research to determine a "normal" GFR. What factors affect the normal value?

IN THE LAB

12. Conduct an experiment to see how osmosis works. Place a few cherries in a bowl of water and put a lid on the bowl. Take the lid off the bowl the next day and examine the cherries. How have the cherries changed? How do you explain these changes? In your explanation, use terms that you learned in this lesson.
13. Measure and compare the amount of liquid ingested and urine produced for a 24-hour period. Specifically, measure the volumes of all liquids you consume for 24 hours, before each drink. Convert volumes measured in fluid ounces (if any) to milliliters, using the conversion factor of 1 fluid ounce equals 30 mL. During the same 24-hour period, measure your own urine output by urinating into a beaker with measuring lines on it. Maintain proper hygiene: Do not touch the beaker to your body; discard the urine into the toilet after each urination; wash your hands before and after each measurement. When the 24 hours are complete, compare the total volume you drank to the total urine volume voided. Are they equal? If not, which is greater? What could account or the difference, if any? (*Hints*: What are other ways that water enters the body or is produced in the body? What are other ways that water leaves the body?)

LESSON 14.3

Diseases and Disorders of the Urinary System

Before You Read

Try to answer the following questions before you read this lesson.

- What is renal dialysis, and who needs it?
- Why do women experience more urinary tract infections than men?

Lesson Objectives

- Explain how different tests of renal function work and what these tests tell us.
- Describe urinary system disorders, diseases, and treatment options.

Key Terms

chronic kidney disease	peritoneal dialysis
creatinine	proteinuria
cystitis	pyelonephritis
diabetic nephropathy	renal dialysis
hemodialysis	renal failure
kidney stone	urinalysis
lithotripsy	urinary tract infection (UTI)
osmotic diuresis	urine specific gravity

Many illnesses, of both renal and non-renal origin, cause changes in the urine. Therefore, the analysis of urine—**urinalysis**—is a standard part of a complete physical examination. This lesson discusses some non-renal medical conditions that create abnormalities in the urine and eventually lead to kidney damage. The lesson also identifies the causes and symptoms of several disorders and diseases of the urinary system, along with treatment options.

Assessing Renal Function

The amount, appearance, smell, and chemical content of urine can reveal clues to abnormalities in kidney function. Because the kidneys regulate the composition of blood, analysis of blood is also essential for evaluation of kidney function.

CLINICAL CASE STUDY

Louis is a 54-year-old man with a complicated medical history. He was diagnosed with type 1 diabetes mellitus when he was 17 years old. He has been monitoring his blood glucose and giving himself insulin injections to control his blood glucose ever since then. He knows that people with diabetes have a higher risk of chronic kidney disease and cardiovascular disease, so he has taken steps to reduce his risk: he does not smoke; he exercises regularly; he has maintained a normal body weight. He has regular medical care, and he takes medicine to control his blood pressure. He has stayed relatively healthy for several decades, but in the last year, he has started to feel more and more tired and unwell. His serum creatinine was 2.0 mg/dL two years ago, 2.5 last year, and 2.8 six months ago. These values correspond to glomerular filtration rates (GFRs) of 37, 28, and 24 mL/minute, two years, one year, and six months ago. Now his nephrologist says his creatinine is 3.2, his GFR is 21, and it is time to think seriously about renal replacement therapy. As you read this section, try to determine the answers to the following questions.

1. What condition, besides diabetes mellitus, does Louis have?
2. How is this condition diagnosed?
3. What does Louis's GFR indicate about his condition?
4. What options exist for Louis if his condition progresses to renal failure?

Physical Characteristics of Urine

Urine is normally clear and yellow (**Figure 14.11**). Cloudy urine may indicate a urinary tract infection. A color other than yellow may result from the presence of blood in the urine—which is never normal—or from certain vitamin supplements, drugs, or foods.

The pH of urine can vary from 4.5 to 8.0 under normal conditions. A urine pH of 6.0 is typical. The **urine specific gravity** is a measure of the urine's mass per unit volume, divided by the

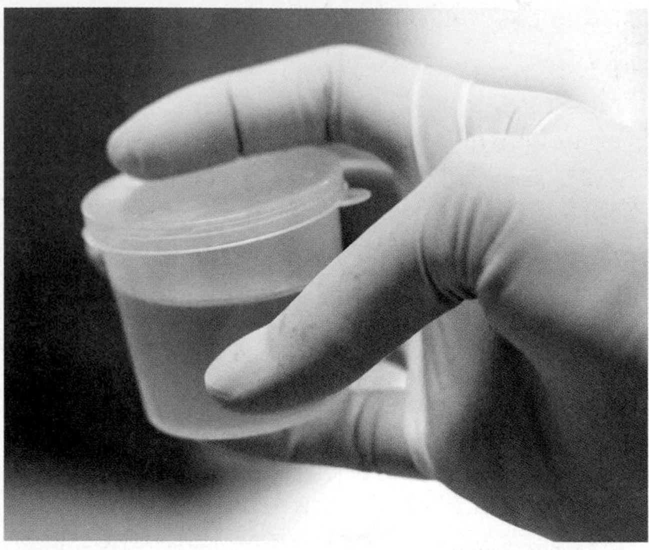

BENCHAMAT/Shutterstock.com

Figure 14.11 A sample of urine. Urine that is cloudy instead of clear indicates a possible urinary tract infection. *If the color of urine is not yellow, what are some possible causes?*

density of pure water. Normal urine has a specific gravity of 1.003 to 1.035, with higher numbers indicating more concentrated urine—that is, urine that contains more dissolved substances. A typical daily volume of urine is 1 pint to ½ gallon (0.5 to 2.0 L).

Chemical Composition of Urine

Urine is about 95% water. Urea is the most abundant solute in urine. It is a type of nitrogenous (nitrogen-containing) waste produced by the normal chemical breakdown of proteins. Potassium, chloride, sodium, and other ions are typically present in urine. The presence of red or white blood cells, protein, or glucose in urine is abnormal and usually leads to further testing to determine the cause.

Inexpensive test kits allow rapid measurement of many compounds in urine. The kits contain small plastic strips with chemicals that change color in response to the presence or concentration of various compounds in urine. A microscope is also essential for checking a urine sample for blood cells, bacteria, and other abnormalities.

Glomerular Filtration Rate

As explained in Lesson 14.2, the measurement of glomerular filtration rate (GFR) is a key part of assessing kidney function. One approach to measuring GFR is based on the idea that if a substance in blood plasma is easily filtered by the glomerulus, and is neither reabsorbed nor secreted by the renal tubules, then the rate at which that substance collects in the urine should be an indicator of GFR. If you can measure the concentration of this substance in blood and in urine, then you can use an equation to estimate GFR.

Inulin, a nontoxic polysaccharide derived from plants, meets these requirements and has been used by physiologists and clinicians to estimate GFR in research studies. Although inulin is considered an excellent way to measure GFR, it is not routinely used in humans because it requires an infusion of inulin into the patient's blood.

The most common way to estimate GFR is by measuring blood concentration of **creatinine** (kree-AT-in-in), a normal by-product of muscle metabolism that is produced at a steady rate. Creatinine is freely filtered by the glomerulus. (To a small extent, creatinine is also secreted by the tubule, which means it is not a perfect compound for measuring GFR.) If the GFR is high, creatinine is removed rapidly from the blood by glomerular filtration, and the creatinine blood concentration becomes low. If GFR is low, creatinine is not removed rapidly from the blood, and the creatinine blood concentration remains high.

Equations have been developed and tested that allow the estimation of GFR based on a patient's blood creatinine level. The most widely used equation includes correction factors to adjust for the age, gender, and race of the patient. All of these factors affect the normal values.

Check Your Understanding

1. Why is the analysis of urine a standard part of a complete physical examination?
2. What pH range is considered normal for urine?
3. When urine has a high specific gravity, what does this indicate?
4. What is the most common method of measuring glomerular filtration rate?

Urinary Diseases and Disorders

Diseases and disorders that affect the urinary system can have effects throughout the body, and in many different organ systems. This lesson describes a few of the major ones. **Figure 14.12** summarizes the etiology, prevention, pathology, diagnosis, and treatment of these disorders.

Diabetes

Diabetes, which means "passing through" in Greek, refers to conditions in which urine output is abnormally elevated—in other words, too much water is passing through the body. The two types of diabetes, as described in Chapter 8, are diabetes mellitus and diabetes insipidus. When the term *diabetes* is used alone, it refers to *diabetes mellitus*.

Diseases and Disorders of the Urinary System

	Etiology	Prevention	Pathology	Diagnosis	Treatment
Urinary incontinence	leaks of urine, loss of bladder control	avoid diuretic foods, drinks, medications; do not smoke; maintain healthy weight; pelvic floor exercises	small urine leaks with stress, overfull bladder; sudden urge to urinate	physical exam with urinalysis; diary of bladder intake and output; measure of residual urine	depends on underlying cause; may include behavior change, pelvic floor muscle training, medications, medical devices
Overactive bladder	frequent, sudden, and compelling need to pass urine	maintain healthy body weight; regular exercise; avoid "trigger" drinks	overly active detrusor muscle; may or may not include incontinence	review of symptoms and exclusion of other possible causes	behavioral therapy; drugs that affect autonomic nerves; surgery
Benign prostatic hyperplasia	enlargement of prostate	none	frequent and/or urgent need to urinate; dribbling at end/weak urination; blood in urine; UTI	physical exam including digital rectal exam; urine and blood tests	medication; minimally invasive therapies; surgery
Interstitial cystitis	chronic bladder pressure and pain; sometimes pelvic pain	none	persistent, frequent, urgent urination; pain during intercourse; bladder, pelvic, or perineum pain	physical exam including pelvic exam; bladder diary, urine test; cystoscopy	physical therapy; oral medications such as NSAIDs and tricyclic antidepressants; nerve stimulation
Glomerulonephritis	Inflammation of the glomeruli	control hypertension and blood sugar	Blood and/or protein in the urine; hypertension; fluid retention	urinalysis; blood tests; imaging (X-ray, CT scan, ultrasound); kidney biopsy	treat underlying cause when possible; dialysis for severe cases
Diabetes mellitus*	type 1: autoimmune disorder with little or no insulin production type 2: body cells do not take up glucose	type 1: maintain healthy weight; exercise regularly; eat a healthy diet type 2: awareness of family history	large amounts of urine; hyperglycemia	physical exam; measure of urine output; blood and urine glucose measurements	lifestyle modifications: lose weight, control blood pressure, exercise regularly; medications to control glucose levels
Diabetes insipidus*	hyposecretion of ADH, or inability of kidneys to use ADH	none	excessive thirst; frequent urination; dilute urine	blood tests for ADH, urinalysis	supplemental synthetic ADH

*Diabetes mellitus and diabetes insipidus are described in further detail in Chapter 8. Refer to Figure 8.19 for diabetes mellitus and Figure 8.12 for diabetes insipidus.

Goodheart-Willcox Publisher

Figure 14.12

Diabetes Mellitus

Diabetes mellitus is characterized by the production of large amounts of urine that contains glucose, a sweet, colorless sugar. (The Latin word *mellitus* means "sweet.") Diabetes mellitus develops in one of two ways: when the pancreas fails to produce the hormone insulin, or when the body's cells fail to respond to insulin.

Type 1 diabetes mellitus is an autoimmune disease in which the body's immune system attacks and destroys the insulin-producing cells of the pancreas. Type 2 diabetes mellitus is less well understood. Both types of diabetes involve an inability to metabolize glucose properly after carbohydrate digestion. As a result, blood glucose levels can soar.

MEMORY TIP

The word **diuresis** (digh-yoo-REE-sis) is made up of the prefix *dia-* meaning "through," the combining form *ur/o* meaning "urine," and the suffix *-sis*, which means "state of" or "condition." *Diuresis* literally means "state or condition of urine passing through"—in short, "urine production."

Antidiuretic hormone reduces diuresis. Diuretic drugs, which increase diuresis, are widely prescribed both to reduce blood pressure and to reduce the buildup of fluid in the body (edema) that occurs in patients with weak or failing hearts. "Loop diuretics" such as furosemide (trade name Lasix®) reduce sodium reabsorption in the ascending limb of the nephron loop. Other blood pressure-lowering agents work by inhibiting angiotensin-converting enzyme, by blocking the receptors for angiotensin, or by other mechanisms.

Figure 14.13 illustrates carbohydrate digestion and blood glucose regulation in a healthy person. Because a person with type 1 diabetes cannot make insulin, the blood glucose level soars after a carbohydrate-rich meal. This is because muscle cells and fat cells are not stimulated by insulin to take up and store glucose.

As discussed in Lesson 14.2, glucose normally is filtered by the glomerulus and fully reabsorbed in the renal tubule, due to cotransport with sodium in the tubule. In diabetes mellitus, so much glucose enters the filtrate from the glucose-rich plasma that the tubule cannot reabsorb it all—which is why the urine of patients with diabetes mellitus may have a sweet odor.

The excess glucose in the filtrate increases osmotic pressure, which interferes with normal water reabsorption in the tubule and collecting duct. The result is less water reabsorption and more urine production. This is an example of **osmotic diuresis**, an increase in urine production due to abnormally high osmolality of the filtrate.

There is no known way to prevent the autoimmune attack that causes type 1 diabetes. People can reduce the risk of developing type 2 diabetes mellitus by maintaining a healthy weight and diet, exercising regularly, reducing high blood pressure if it is elevated, and maintaining healthy blood cholesterol levels.

Type 1 diabetes mellitus is treated with lifelong injections or infusion of insulin. Patients must monitor their blood glucose levels by regular sampling. In recent years, continuous glucose monitors have replaced fingerstick sampling, and wearable insulin pumps have replaced self-administered injections for some patients. Medical technology is evolving rapidly in this area.

One of the most serious long-term consequences of poorly controlled diabetes mellitus is kidney damage, or **diabetic nephropathy** (neh-FRAHP-a-thee). Diabetes mellitus is the most common cause of chronic kidney disease and renal failure. **Proteinuria**, or excessive protein in the urine, is often the first sign of kidney damage, followed by a gradual decrease in glomerular filtration rate. Patients who control their blood glucose well have significantly lower risk of renal failure.

MEMORY TIP

The word *nephropathy* in the term *diabetic nephropathy* comes from the Greek words *nephros*, which means "kidney," and *pathos*, which means "disease" or "suffering."

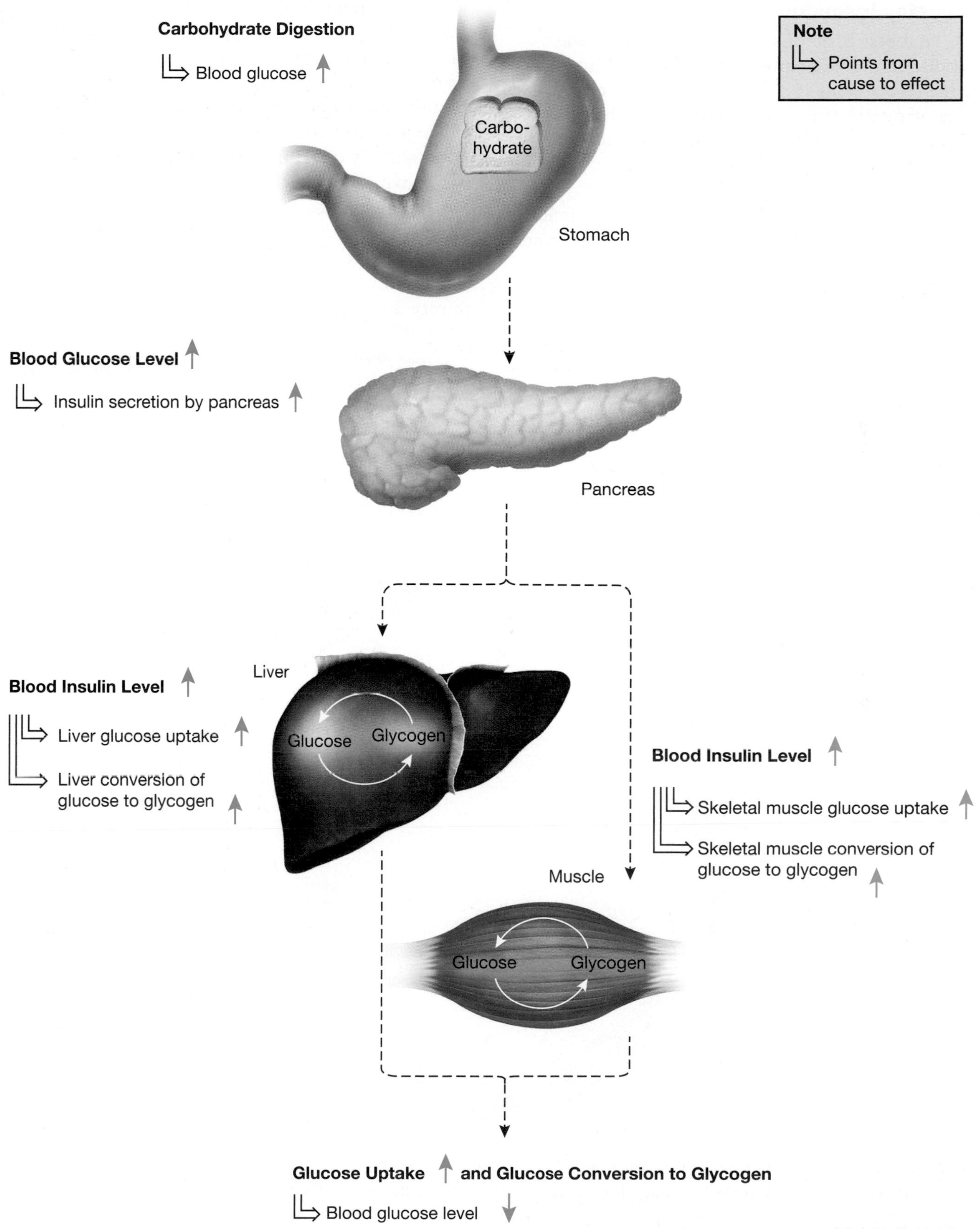

Figure 14.13 Effects of normal carbohydrate digestion on blood glucose and blood insulin levels. *How does diabetes mellitus cause a breakdown in the processes shown above?*

Diabetes Insipidus

Diabetes insipidus is characterized by the production of large amounts of highly diluted urine (more than 12 liters a day in severe cases). The urine specific gravity is less than the normal lower limit of 1.002, and the urine osmolality is also low, indicating that the urine is mostly water with very few substances dissolved in it.

Diabetes insipidus is usually caused by failure of the pituitary gland to produce normal amounts of antidiuretic hormone (ADH). This is called *central diabetes insipidus*, reflecting its origin in the central nervous system. It may result from trauma or surgery to the hypothalamic and pituitary region of the brain, or from a pituitary tumor. In a minority of cases, the disease is caused by unresponsiveness of the kidney to ADH: *nephrogenic diabetes insipidus*. This form of DI may be due to drugs that damage the kidney or to renal disease.

As explained in Lesson 14.2, ADH causes the collecting ducts to be permeable to water. The collecting ducts are the site for the final stage of water reabsorption. Therefore, collecting duct reabsorption is critical for the formation of concentrated urine. The regulation of blood osmolality by ADH in a healthy person is shown in **Figure 14.14**. In the absence of ADH, or if the kidney cannot respond to ADH, little or no water is reabsorbed as the urine flows down the collecting duct. As a result, urine output is much higher than normal, and the patient is always thirsty due to the constant loss of fluid.

MEMORY TIP

In the term *diabetes insipidus*, the Latin word *insipidus* means "weak." The urine of a person with diabetes insipidus could be considered to be weak because both its specific gravity and its urine osmolality are low.

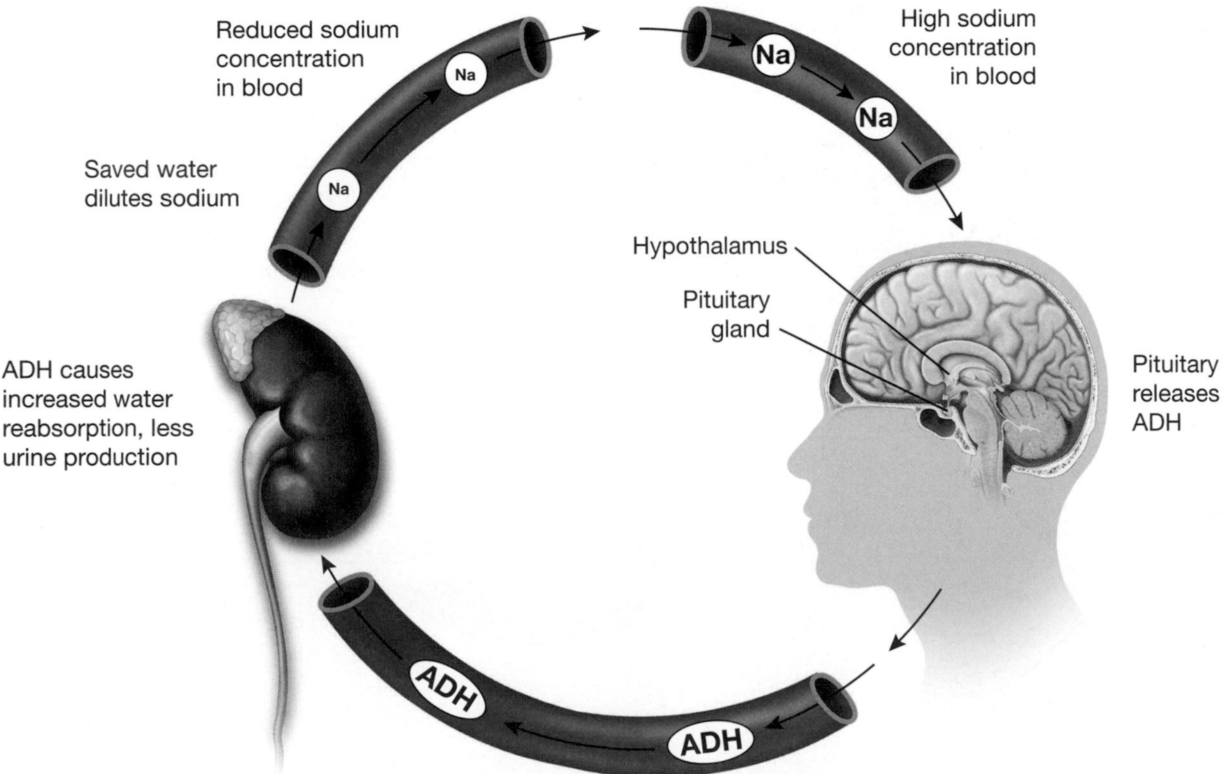

Figure 14.14 Regulation of blood osmolality by ADH. In a healthy person, regulation of blood sodium concentration and blood osmolality are roughly equivalent because sodium is the biggest contributor to blood osmolality. *What happens to urine output in a person with diabetes insipidus?*

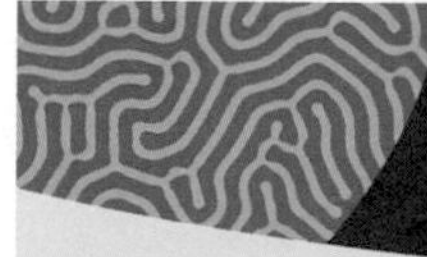

What Research Tells Us

...about Paired Kidney Transplants

The human kidney is one of the most commonly transplanted organs in the body. A kidney transplant is done when a person has chronic, or end-stage, renal failure. In the United States, the two leading causes of end-stage renal failure are diabetes and high blood pressure.

A transplanted kidney may come from a living donor or a recently deceased person. Research indicates that patients who get a kidney from a live donor have better health and life-expectancy outcomes than those who receive a cadaver kidney.

Unfortunately, there are far fewer kidneys available than there are patients who need them. Every person has two kidneys and can donate one of them, if health and compatibility requirements are met. Research shows that live donors do not have shorter or less healthful lives.

Live-donor transplants can be difficult to arrange. Often, a family member who is willing to donate a kidney is not immunologically compatible with the relative who needs a kidney. In other words, the kidney from the willing donor would be rejected by the recipient's body. To address this problem, doctors have sometimes performed "paired" kidney transplants.

For example, Bob is willing to donate a kidney to Mark, but Mark's blood type and body tissue are incompatible with Bob's. Meanwhile, Mallory is willing to donate a kidney to Pearl, but Pearl's blood type and body tissue are incompatible with Mallory's. Suppose that Bob is compatible with Pearl, and Mallory is compatible with Mark. If they all agree to make "crossed" donations, then both Mark and Pearl will get the kidneys they need (**Figure 14.15**).

Paired kidney transplants can work in even larger circles of donors and recipients. In 2011, a chain of 30 linked kidney transplants was completed—the largest paired-kidney transplant chain ever. This "pay-it-forward" chain took four months to complete and involved hospitals throughout the United States. Such a large chain of linked kidney transplants was possible due to significant advances in organ donor technology. For example, extremely precise and efficient methods were used to keep a kidney viable (healthy) while it was harvested at one hospital and then flown to a recipient in another location. Improved surgical techniques increased the odds of success for each operation. Also, computer technology played a key role in the linked-kidney transplant chain. Before the operations were arranged, a special software program was used to identify possible matches between the patients and willing donors who had joined a national registry.

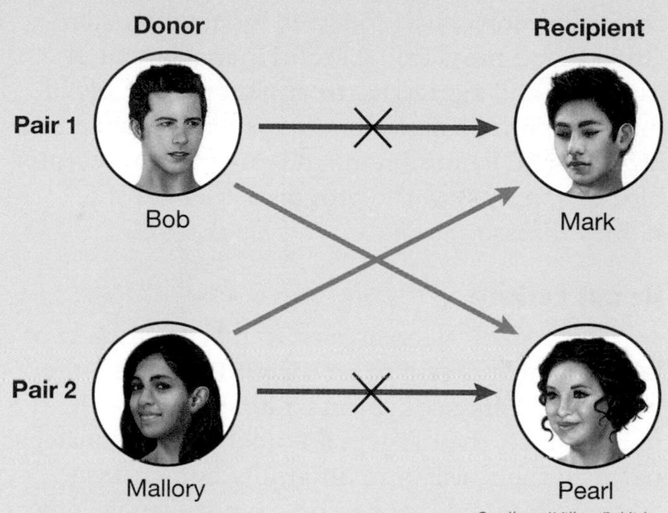

Figure 14.15 Paired kidney transplants with crossed kidney donation.

Taking It Further

1. Research the topic of kidney transplants in general or paired kidney transplants in particular. What is required of a donor? What are transplant risks for both the donor and the recipient? What does the procedure involve? What kind of medical care must the organ recipient continue to have after surgery? What happens when a person's body rejects a transplanted kidney?
2. Can you think of any ethical and legal issues that a paired kidney transplant might present for donors and recipients? Prepare an argument with supporting research, and present your case in an oral report to the class.

Chronic Kidney Disease

Chronic kidney disease is defined by evidence of kidney damage (usually proteinuria) or a glomerular filtration rate less than 60 mL per minute for at least 3 months. Chronic kidney disease develops slowly. Diabetes mellitus is the most common cause, followed by hypertension (high blood pressure). Careful management of diabetes, and aggressive treatment of high blood pressure with drugs such as angiotensin-converting enzyme (ACE) inhibitors and angiotensin receptor blockers, may slow the progression of chronic kidney disease.

Renal Failure

When GFR decreases to 15 mL per minute or less, a patient is said to have **renal failure**—the most severe stage of chronic kidney disease. In renal failure, the kidneys are unable to adequately perform their task of maintaining homeostasis. Without treatment, a person cannot survive long in this state. Waste products accumulate in the blood, and levels of pH and various ions are no longer well controlled. At this stage, the patient must receive renal dialysis, a medical procedure in which wastes are removed from the blood, or a kidney transplant.

Because the supply of donor kidneys is very limited, most patients with renal failure undergo dialysis. However, the process of dialysis compromises a patient's health and lowers life expectancy. Filtering the blood through a machine is not as good for one's health or life span as having a real kidney.

Renal Dialysis

Renal dialysis (digh-AL-i-sis) is the removal of wastes from the blood by artificial means. The two types of dialysis are hemodialysis and peritoneal dialysis. Both forms of dialysis remove water, urea, and some sodium from the body.

Hemodialysis

In **hemodialysis** (hee-moh-digh-AL-i-sis), blood is withdrawn from an artery, pumped through a dialyzer—a large machine positioned next to the patient—and then returned to the patient through a vein. The *dialyzer* (DIGH-a-ligh-zer) acts as an artificial kidney, although it does not perform all the functions of a real kidney (**Figure 14.16**).

In the dialyzer, the blood passes through thin tubes whose semipermeable walls make up the dialysis membrane. Dialysis fluid circulates around those tubes. Urea, other wastes, water, and some electrolytes diffuse out of the blood and into the dialysis fluid. The dialysis fluid is discarded, and the blood is returned to the body.

Peritoneal Dialysis

In **peritoneal dialysis**, dialysis fluid is added to the abdominopelvic cavity through a surgically implanted port in the abdomen. As the dialysis solution remains in the abdomen for an hour or more, it absorbs water and wastes from capillaries in the mesentery (the membrane that attaches the intestines to the wall of the abdomen) and elsewhere in the abdominopelvic cavity. The peritoneum itself serves as the dialysis membrane that separates the blood from the dialysis fluid.

Kidney Stones

A **kidney stone**, also called a *renal calculus*, is not really a stone. It is a solid crystalline mass that forms in the urine (**Figure 14.17**). Kidney stones are usually made of calcium-containing compounds, but they can also be composed of magnesium or uric acid.

Kidney stones usually form in the renal pelvis, but they may form in the ureter or bladder. Stones smaller than 0.2 inch (5 mm) in diameter may pass from the body in the urine without difficulty. If a larger stone develops in the kidney, it is carried by urine flow to the ureter, where it gets stuck. When a kidney stone becomes lodged in the ureter, intense pain usually occurs.

Lithotripsy (LITH-oh-trip-see) is the use of intense, ultrasonic sound waves to break up a kidney stone into pieces small enough to be passed from the body in the urine. The risk of additional kidney stone development can be reduced by drinking a lot of fluids. Greater fluid intake increases the volume and flow rate of urine, reducing the likelihood of crystallization.

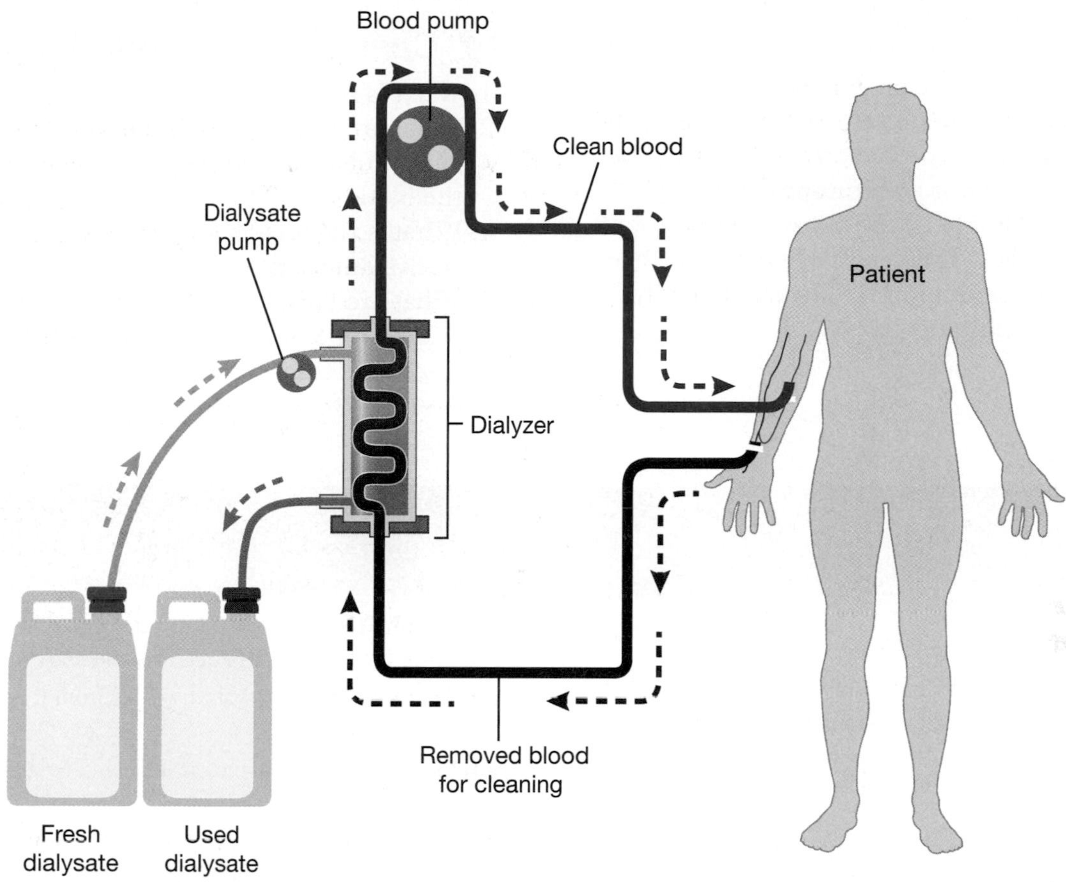

© Body Scientific International

Figure 14.16 Hemodialysis is the most common treatment for renal failure. Blood is withdrawn from an artery, usually in the forearm, and is pumped through a dialyzer. In the dialyzer, a semipermeable membrane separates the blood from dialysate. Dialysate is a fluid with a chemical composition similar to blood plasma. Wastes, including urea, cross from the blood into the dialysate. The "cleaned" blood returns to the body. The used dialysate is discarded.

Urinary Tract Infections

A **urinary tract infection (UTI)** is usually caused by bacteria that enter the urethra at its outside opening. If the bacteria reach the bladder, the resulting infection can lead to **cystitis** (sis-TIGH-tis), an inflammation of the urinary bladder epithelium. Urinary tract infections are more common in women than in men; women have a shorter urethra, so bacteria can more easily reach the bladder. Careful hygiene reduces the risk of developing UTIs; there is also evidence that increasing fluid intake may reduce risk.

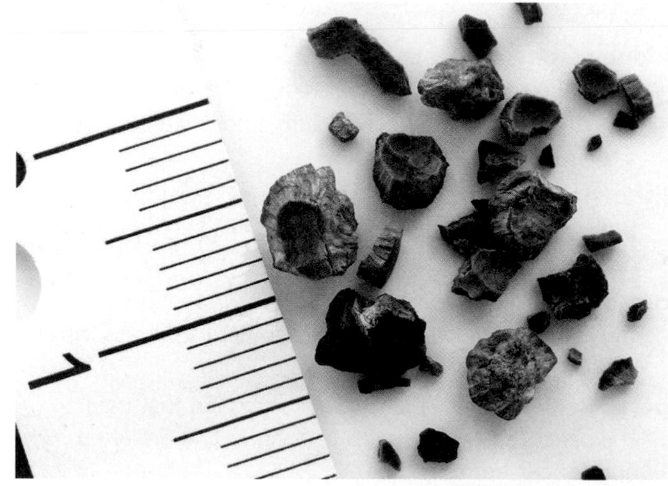

Piotr Malczyk/Shutterstock.com

Figure 14.17 Kidney stones. *At what size can kidney stones become lodged in the ureter?*

UTI symptoms include pain during urination, increased urinary frequency, fever, and sometimes cloudy or dark urine. If the bacteria travel up the ureters to the kidneys, the kidneys themselves can become infected. The resulting condition is **pyelonephritis** (pigh-eh-loh-neh-FRIGH-tis). Besides the symptoms already described, patients often experience back pain in the kidney region. UTIs are typically treated with antibiotics.

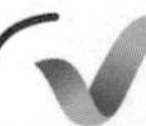

Check Your Understanding

1. What is renal failure?
2. What are two types of renal dialysis?
3. What substances does dialysis remove from the blood?
4. What is the ideal source of a kidney used for transplantation?
5. What are kidney stones composed of?
6. Which type of microorganism causes urinary tract infections?

LESSON 14.3 Review and Assessment

Mini Glossary

Make sure that you know the meaning of each key term.

chronic kidney disease a condition defined by evidence of kidney damage or a glomerular filtration rate of less than 60 milliliters per minute for at least three months

creatinine a normal by-product of muscle metabolism; it is produced by the body at a fairly steady rate and is freely filtered by the glomerulus

cystitis inflammation of the urinary bladder epithelium

diabetic nephropathy kidney disease

hemodialysis a procedure for removing metabolic waste products from the body; blood is withdrawn from an artery, pumped through a dialyzer, and then returned to the patient through a vein

kidney stone a solid crystalline mass that forms in the kidney and may become stuck in the renal pelvis or ureter; usually made of calcium, phosphate, uric acid, and protein

lithotripsy the use of intense, ultrasonic sound waves to break up a kidney stone into pieces small enough to be passed from the body in the urine

osmotic diuresis an increase in urine production caused by high osmotic pressure of the glomerular filtrate, which "pulls" more water into the filtrate

peritoneal dialysis a renal dialysis method that uses the patient's peritoneum to filter fluids and dissolved substances from the blood

proteinuria presence of excessive protein in the urine

pyelonephritis urinary tract infection in which one or both of the kidneys also become infected

renal dialysis the removal of wastes from the blood by artificial means

renal failure kidney failure, as indicated by a GFR of 15 mL/min. or less

urinalysis laboratory analysis of urine to test for the presence of infection or disease

urinary tract infection (UTI) an infection of the urethra, bladder, ureters, and/or kidney, usually caused by bacteria that enter the urethra at its outside opening

urine specific gravity the density (mass per unit volume) of urine, divided by the density of pure water

Know and Understand

1. Urine consists primarily of what substance? What is the most abundant solute in urine?
2. Why is blood creatinine concentration used to assess kidney function? Why is creatinine considered better than inulin for measuring GFR?
3. Why does the urine of many patients with diabetes mellitus have a sweet odor?
4. Why does the absence of antidiuretic hormone cause diabetes insipidus?
5. How is chronic kidney disease defined by glomerular filtration rate?
6. Which functions of the kidneys can be accomplished through renal dialysis? Which functions cannot be accomplished?

7. What are the two types of renal dialysis, and what is the difference between them?
8. How is lithotripsy used to treat kidney stones?
9. Why are urinary tract infections more common in women than in men?

Analyze and Apply

10. Compare and contrast the symptoms and the causes of diabetes mellitus and diabetes insipidus.
11. Suppose that you are a doctor or a nurse practitioner. One of your patients, a 24-year-old woman, complains of frequent, painful urination. She has a slight temperature. You request a urine sample from her. Her urine is dark and cloudy. What do you think may be causing her symptoms?
12. You have just completed your first half marathon and are drenched in perspiration. When you finally get the chance to urinate, you are surprised at the small amount of urine and its dark color. How would you explain the reason for your diminished urine output considering that you were careful to keep yourself hydrated during the run?
13. Urine is one of the body's waste products and is therefore in abundant supply. Using the internet, research the potential of using urine as part of the fertilization process in gardening. What benefits might this have for subsistence farmers in low-income countries? What are the disadvantages?
14. The presence of albumin and bilirubin in the urine is considered abnormal. Conduct research to find out what conditions may cause the presence of these substances in the urine.
15. In patients who have kidney disease, physicians often monitor intake and output of fluids. Common forms of fluid intake include oral (both liquids and in foods) and administration of intravenous fluids. Output includes micturition and vomit. However, other forms of fluid output also occur in healthy individuals on a daily basis. These include sweating, elimination of feces, and even exhaled water vapor. Conduct research to find out how much these additional forms of output add to a person's total fluid output. In your opinion, should they be included in an intake/output (I/O) analysis of kidney patients? Why or why not?

IN THE LAB

16. In this activity, you will measure pH and compare the pH of several substances to that of urine.

    Instructions: Using litmus paper, a liquid pH indicator, or a pH meter and probe, measure the pH of the following substances: distilled water, juice squeezed from a lemon, black coffee, household ammonia, bleach, vinegar, a carbonated beverage, milk of magnesia, and a solution of baking soda and water.

    Draw a pH "ruler" and mark it with the units 0 to 14. Recall that a neutral pH is 7. A solution with a pH below 7 is acidic, and a solution with a pH above 7 is alkaline. For each substance you test, determine whether the pH is neutral, acidic, or alkaline, and write its name in the corresponding area along the ruler.

    A urine pH of 6.0 is typical. Compare the pH of the tested substances with that of urine.
17. Diabetic ketoacidosis is a potentially fatal complication of type 1 diabetes. Find out more about ketoacidosis. What are the symptoms? What causes it? How is it related to high ketone levels in the urine? How can it be prevented, and if it occurs, what treatment is required? Create an instruction sheet for people who have diabetes; you may want to consider making it a card and laminating it so that it can be carried in a wallet or bag.

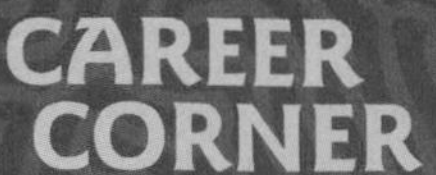

CAREER CORNER Anatomy & Physiology at Work

The urinary system performs the critical work of filtering waste products from the blood and maintaining a stable chemical environment inside the body. Many people have found fulfilling careers in the diagnosis and treatment of diseases and disorders of the urinary system. Two examples of these careers are nephrologist and renal dialysis technician.

Nephrologist

A nephrologist, or renal physician, is a medical doctor who specializes in the diagnosis and treatment of kidney diseases and disorders (**Figure 14.18**). Most nephrologists divide their time between seeing patients in office settings and in hospitals. Some work at kidney and dialysis centers. Renal patients usually see a nephrologist after being referred by their primary care physician.

Nephrologists diagnose kidney problems by ordering and interpreting tests, such as blood tests, urinalyses, ultrasound procedures, and biopsies, in which a small piece of tissue is removed from the kidney and examined for signs of disease. Nephrologists also manage the care of patients with chronic kidney disease, including patients on dialysis. Patients who need surgery—to remove kidney stones or to treat kidney cancer, for example—are referred to another type of doctor called a *urologist*.

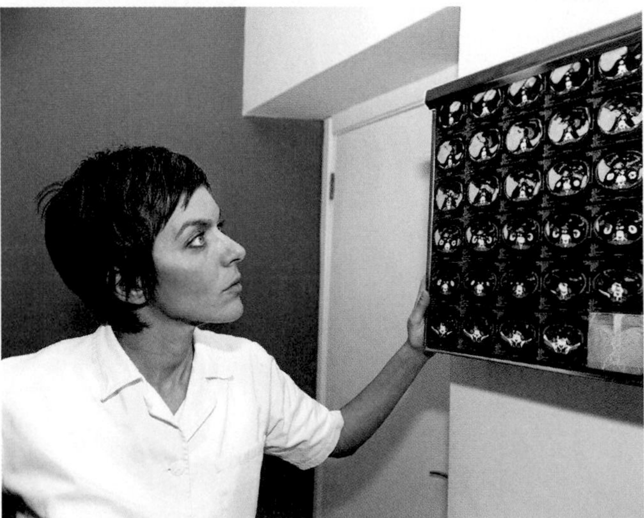

smart.art/Shutterstock.com

Figure 14.18 A nephrologist explains a patient's test results.

A nephrologist's patients have a variety of illnesses and disorders, several of which are covered in this lesson. They may have infections or kidney stones. They may have kidney problems brought on by pregnancy or by a genetic condition. However, many of the nephrologist's patients have chronic kidney disease caused by conditions such as hypertension or diabetes. After assessing the seriousness of the renal disease, nephrologists may prescribe medication to lower blood pressure, prescribe renal dialysis, or refer patients for kidney transplantation.

In the United States, a nephrologist has a bachelor of science degree and a medical doctor (MD) degree. Medical school is followed by three years of training in internal medicine and then by a nephrology fellowship lasting two or three years. A physician who has completed this training is eligible to take the examination to become a board-certified nephrologist.

Renal Dialysis Technician

Renal dialysis technicians perform and monitor the dialysis treatment of kidney patients. They work under the supervision of a registered nurse. Most renal dialysis technicians are employed in dialysis facilities, most of which are located in hospitals and outpatient facilities.

Following a prescription written by a doctor, renal dialysis technicians prepare the dialysate, the solution that is used in the dialysis treatment. They test and prepare the dialysis equipment. They also prepare patients for dialysis, which involves inserting needles for access to an artery and a vein (**Figure 14.19**).

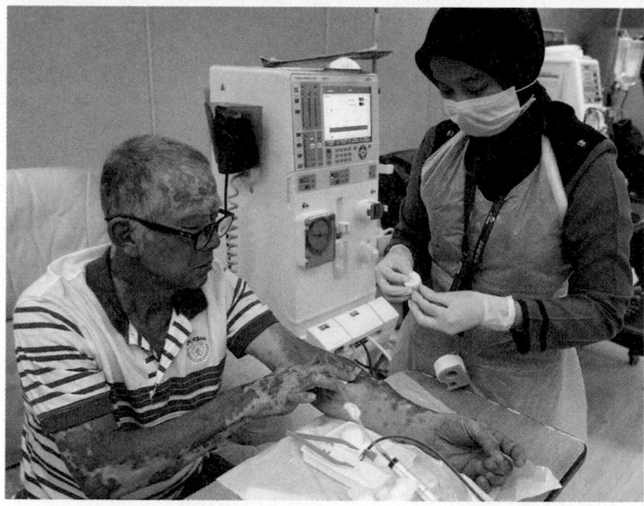
Djohan Shahrin/Shutterstock.com

Figure 14.19 A renal dialysis technician prepares a patient for dialysis.

While patients are undergoing treatment, renal dialysis technicians monitor and adjust the dialysis machinery. They monitor patients and measure blood-flow rates and fluid removal rates. They must be prepared for dialysis-related emergencies. Renal dialysis technicians are responsible for maintaining dialysis machines in proper working order. Because they work directly with patients, renal dialysis technicians must have good communication skills and be able to respond to their patients' emotional needs.

To become a renal dialysis technician, you must have a high school diploma and certification. Certification requirements vary by state, but usually involve passing an examination and successfully completing up to 18 months of on-the-job training.

Planning for a Health-Related Career

Do some research on the career of a nephrologist or a renal dialysis technician. Alternatively, select a profession from the list of related career options. Using the internet or resources at your local library, find answers to the following questions:

1. What are the main tasks and responsibilities of a person employed in the career that you chose to research?
2. What is the outlook for this career? Are workers in demand, or are jobs dwindling? For complete information, consult the current edition of the *Occupational Outlook Handbook*, published by the US Department of Labor. This handbook is available online or at your local library.
3. What special skills or talents are required? For example, do you need to be good at biology and anatomy and physiology? Would you be able to master the operation of complex machinery used to treat patients?
4. What personality traits do you think are necessary for success in the career that you chose to research? For example, renal dialysis technicians must have excellent interpersonal, communication, and problem-solving skills.
5. Does the work involve a great deal of routine, or are the day-to-day responsibilities varied?
6. Does the career require long hours, or is it a standard, "9-to-5" job?
7. What is the salary range for this job?
8. What do you think you would like about this career? Is there anything about it that you might dislike?

Related Career Options

- Diabetes educator
- Home health and personal care aide
- Renal dietitian
- Renal nurse
- Renal social worker
- Transplant surgeon
- Urologist

CHAPTER 14 Review

> LESSON 14.1

The Kidney

Key Points

- The main functions of the kidney are to eliminate waste from the blood while retaining valuable chemical compounds and to control blood volume and blood pressure.
- Blood enters the kidney through the renal artery, passes from an afferent arteriole to capillaries to an efferent arteriole to another set of capillaries, and only then to a venule and larger veins before leaving the kidney through the renal vein.

Key Terms

collecting duct
distal convoluted tubule (DCT)
glomerulus
nephron
nephron loop
proximal convoluted tubule (PCT)
renal corpuscle
renal cortex
renal medulla
renal pelvis
renal tubule
vasa recta

> LESSON 14.2

Urine Formation, Storage, and Excretion

Key Points

- Three steps are involved in urine formation: filtration, reabsorption, and secretion. Three hormones—aldosterone, atrial natriuretic peptide, and antidiuretic hormone—are key to "fine tuning" urine volume and composition.
- Urine is stored in the bladder, which stretches as it fills. The stretching generates actions in the nervous system that eventually signal the detrusor to contract and the internal urethral sphincter to relax.
- When the "time is right," the brain sends signals that cause the external urethral sphincter to relax, and the urine is expelled.

Key Terms

aldosterone
angiotensin
antidiuretic hormone (ADH)
atrial natriuretic peptide (ANP)
detrusor
external urethral sphincter
glomerular filtration
glomerular filtration rate (GFR)
hydrostatic pressure
internal urethral sphincter
micturition
osmosis
osmotic pressure
reabsorption
renin
secretion
trigone
ureter
urethra
urinary bladder

> LESSON 14.3

Diseases and Disorders of the Urinary System

Key Points

- The amount, color, pH, and specific gravity of urine are characteristics that can indicate abnormalities in kidney function.
- Diabetes mellitus and hypertension are the two main causes of chronic kidney disease, which can progress to renal failure. Other common disorders and diseases include kidney stones and urinary tract infections.

Key Terms

chronic kidney disease
creatinine
cystitis
diabetic nephropathy
hemodialysis
kidney stone
lithotripsy
osmotic diuresis
peritoneal dialysis
proteinuria
pyelonephritis
renal dialysis
renal failure
urinalysis
urinary tract infection (UTI)
urine specific gravity

Assessment

› LESSON 14.1
The Kidney

Learning Key Terms and Concepts

1. A(n) _____ gland is located on top of each kidney.
2. The lighter-colored, outer part of the kidney is the renal _____.
3. Approximately how many nephrons does each kidney contain?
   A. 1,000
   B. 100,000
   C. 1 million
   D. 10 million
4. The three main parts of the renal tubule are the proximal convoluted tubule, the distal convoluted tubule, and the _____.
5. *True or False*? Cortical nephrons are the only nephrons that produce highly concentrated urine.
6. Where are the peritubular capillaries located?
7. The blood vessel that carries blood into the kidney is the _____.

Thinking Critically

8. Compare and contrast the cortical nephrons and the juxtamedullary nephrons.
9. Why do you think the descending limb and the lower part of the ascending limb have thinner walls than the rest of the ascending limb and the proximal and distal convoluted tubules?
10. Compare and contrast blood flow through the kidneys with blood flow through the heart. Explain the uniqueness of each in relation to arteries, veins, and capillaries.

› LESSON 14.2
Urine Formation, Storage, and Excretion

Learning Key Terms and Concepts

11. The formation of urine comprises three processes: filtration, _____, and secretion.
12. The endothelial cells, basement membrane, and podocytes combine to form the _____.
13. Which of the following is an important benchmark in assessing kidney health?
   A. PCT
   B. ADP
   C. ADH
   D. GFR
14. *True or False*? Hydrostatic pressure is influenced by the amount of dissolved substances in water.
15. *True or False*? In the renal corpuscle, the blood has a higher osmotic pressure than the filtrate.
16. The _____ on the wall of the proximal convoluted tubule increase the surface area of the proximal convoluted tubule, enhancing its reabsorptive ability.
17. The _____ channels allow water to easily enter and exit cells during reabsorption.
18. Which of the following is *not* an accurate description of the interstitial fluid in the renal medulla?
   A. watery
   B. salty
   C. concentrated
   D. higher than normal osmolality
19. A decrease in blood sodium or an increase in potassium results in secretion of _____ by the adrenal cortex.
20. The tube that leads from the kidney to the bladder is the _____.
21. *True or False*? The detrusor muscle must relax for urine to be excreted.
22. *True or False*? The brain plays a role in excretion of urine.

Thinking Critically

23. The external and internal sphincter muscles are controlled in different ways. Explain.
24. Explain why a GFR of 125 mL/minute indicates that the body is reabsorbing most of the glomerular filtrate.
25. Compare and contrast the functions of the three key hormones involved in urine volume and composition.

> LESSON 14.3

Diseases and Disorders of the Urinary System

Learning Key Terms and Concepts

26. Approximately what percentage of urine is water?
27. Which of the following is normally present in normal urine?
    A. urea
    B. white blood cells
    C. glucose
    D. protein
28. *True or False?* Creatinine is a normal by-product of muscle metabolism.
29. When GFR is high, creatinine concentration is _____; when GFR is low, creatinine concentration is _____.
30. *True or False?* In diabetes, too much water is passing through the body.
31. A deficiency in which hormone is linked to the development of diabetes mellitus?
32. *True or False?* Type 1 diabetes mellitus is a kidney disease.
33. An increase in urine production due to abnormally high osmolality of the filtrate is called _____.
34. The first sign of kidney damage is often an excessive amount of protein in the urine, a condition known as _____.
35. What are the two main causes of chronic kidney disease?
36. The purpose of dialysis is to remove _____ from the blood.

Thinking Critically

37. What are the two types of renal dialysis, and how do they work?
38. What are kidney stones? How can they be treated and prevented?
39. A urinary tract infection may affect which organs of the urinary system?
40. Carbohydrate digestion is impaired in a person who has diabetes mellitus. What can you conclude about the ideal diet of a person with this disease? Which types of foods should be avoided?
41. Suppose that you are a patient with renal failure. Compare and contrast a kidney transplant with renal dialysis in terms of benefits and costs.

Building Skills and Connecting Concepts

Analyzing and Evaluating Data

Instructions: Figure 14.20 shows selected urine measurements over a period of time for a 30-year-old adult male. Answer the questions using the data and what you have learned in this chapter.

Selected Urine Measurements				
Test	**1**	**2**	**3**	**4**
Specific gravity	1.023	1.031	1.027	1.046
Daily volume	1.25 L	1.20 L	1.15 L	1.0 L
GFR	125 mL/m	95 mL/m	80 mL/m	75 mL/m

Figure 14.20 Goodheart-Willcox Publisher

42. Is the specific gravity of the patient's urine trending higher or lower?
43. Would the patient's urine be "saltier" in test 2 or test 4?
44. By what percentage did the patient's daily volume of urine production drop between test 1 and test 4?
    A. 80%
    B. 2%
    C. 8%
    D. 20%
45. How would you assess this patient's kidney health? Give specific reasons for your assessment.

Communicating about Anatomy & Physiology

46. **Writing and Speaking** Create a picture book for preschool-aged children that describes the journey of grape juice through the urinary system. Use simple explanations about the urinary system. Include drawings with the text. Test your book by sharing it with a preschool-aged child after getting a parent's permission.
47. **Speaking** With a partner, role-play the following situation: A doctor must explain to a patient with renal failure why he or she must start renal dialysis. One student plays the role of the doctor; the other acts as the patient. Use your own words to explain how renal dialysis works. As the doctor explains the dialysis process, the patient should ask questions if the explanation is unclear. Switch roles and repeat the activity.

Lab Investigations

48. Perform this experiment to mimic the inner workings of the human kidneys. Materials: Two clear glass jars, one regular coffee filter, large rubber band, chalk, water, red food coloring.

    Mix one-half spoonful of crushed chalk with one-half cup of water in a clear glass jar. Add a few drops of food coloring. (The water represents blood; the chalk represents toxins in the blood.) Place the coffee filter over the top of the second glass jar and secure it with the rubber band. (The coffee filter represents the kidneys filtering toxins from the blood.) Pour the chalk-and-water mixture through the coffee filter into the second jar.

    Observe what happens to the chalk (toxins) as the colored water (blood) drips into the jar. Develop a brief, written summary that explains how the results of this experiment help illustrate the glomerular filtration process in the kidneys.

49. James Staffer is three hours post-op after abdominal surgery. He has a nasogastric tube in place connected to suction. In addition, he has an intravenous (IV) drip infusing via a cannula in his left arm. Using the information provided below, determine his total input and output for 10 hours. Record your notes in a chart similar to the one in **Figure 14.21**. Use military time and metric quantities.

    Notes: 1 glass = 8 oz.; 1 soup bowl = 16 oz.; 1 cup = 8 oz.; 1 oz. = 30 mL

    0600 Drank 2 glasses of water
    Voided 300 mL of urine
    0800 Ate breakfast: 1 glass of apple juice, 1 cup of coffee, 1 bowl of cereal with 30 mL of milk
    0900 Voided 200 mL of urine
    Drank half a glass of apple juice
    1000 Nasogastric tube irrigated with 40 mL of normal saline and replaced to suction with a return of 15 mL
    1200 Ate lunch: 1 8-oz. glass of apple juice, 1 soup bowl of broth, 1/2 cup of tea
    1300 Absorbed 300 mL of IV solution
    1400 Voided 200 mL of urine
    1500 Vomited 150 mL of coffee ground emesis
    1600 Drank 1 glass of ginger ale
    1800 Voided 300 mL of urine
    Nasogastric drainage emptied and measured 200 mL of light brown clear drainage

Building Your Portfolio

50. Take digital photographs of the models and projects you created as you worked through this chapter. Create a document called "The Urinary System" and insert the photographs, along with written descriptions of what the models show and your reasons for creating them using the materials and forms you chose. Also gather your lab reports and summaries. Add these documents to your personal portfolio.

	Intake			Output		
Time	**Oral**	**IV**	**NG tube**	**Urine**	**NG tube**	**Emesis**
0600						
0700						
0800						

Figure 14.21

Goodheart-Willcox Publisher

CHAPTER

15 The Male and Female Reproductive Systems

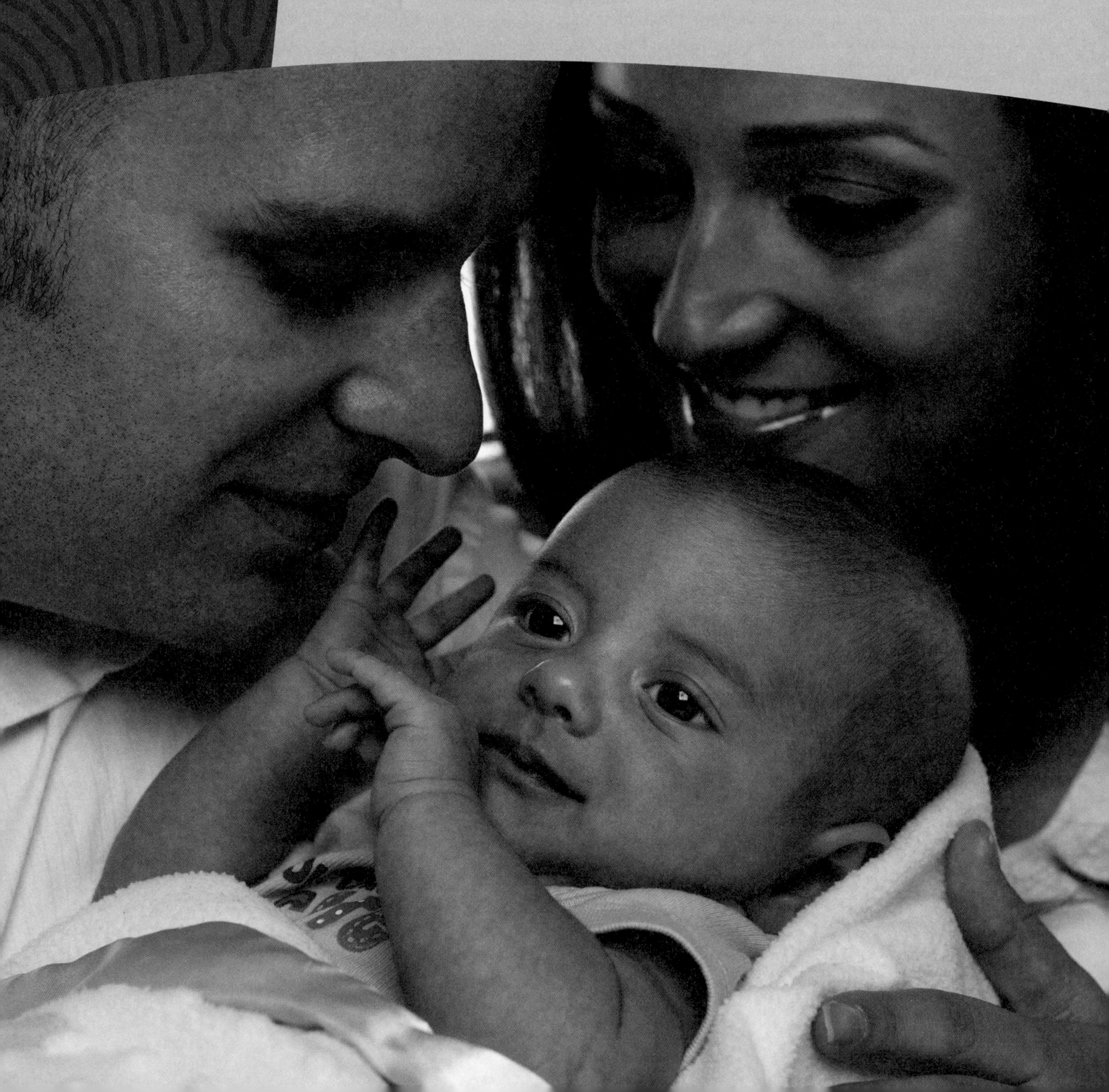

How did genetic material from your biological parents become the blueprint for who you are?

Reproduction, pregnancy, and childbirth are among the most significant, if not *the* most significant, of life's events. It is not unreasonable to say that all the other physiological systems in the body function in part to help ensure that people live long enough to reproduce and care for their young until they can take care of themselves.

In the human reproductive system, major structural and functional differences exist between the sexes, unlike with most other anatomical systems. The male system has two principal functions, and the female reproductive system has five.

This chapter begins by reviewing the differences between meiosis and mitosis—important information to have in mind during the later discussion of the generation of sperm and eggs. The chapter then explores the anatomy and physiology of the male reproductive system, followed by the anatomy and physiology of the more complicated and multi-functional female reproductive system. Pregnancy, childbirth, and lactation (the production and secretion of breast milk) are also discussed. Finally, the chapter reviews some of the more common disorders and diseases of the male and female reproductive systems.

Click on the activity icon or visit www.g-wlearning.com/healthsciences/0202 to access online vocabulary activities using key terms from the chapter.

Chapter 15 Outline

◂ Andy Dean Photography/Shutterstock.com

LESSON 15.1

Reproduction and Development of the Human Reproductive Systems

Before You Read

Try to answer the following questions before you read this lesson.

- What is sexual reproduction?
- How is genetic diversity created during human reproduction?

Lesson Objectives

- Describe the main difference between sexual reproduction and asexual reproduction.
- Differentiate between mitosis and meiosis.
- Describe the development of the reproductive systems during the embryonic and fetal stages and during puberty.

Key Terms

centromere	genotype
chromatids	haploid
chromosomes	meiosis
crossovers	menarche
diploid	phenotype
epigenetics	puberty
fertilization	zygote
gametes	

This lesson examines both sexual and asexual reproduction. It then compares the two different processes—mitosis and meiosis—involved in cell reproduction. Finally, it describes the development of the male and female reproductive systems.

Reproduction

When most animals, including humans, reproduce, their offspring receive genetic material from both parents. Each parent contributes half of the genetic material for each offspring. This type of reproduction is called *sexual reproduction*.

Another way of reproducing involves only one parent. In this case, the offspring are clones, or genetic copies, of the parent. This method is called *asexual reproduction*.

Asexual reproduction is not uncommon in the plant kingdom. It occurs more rarely in a few animal species, including flatworms. Asexual reproduction is simple because only one parent is required and no "sorting" of genetic material is needed. Genetic diversity still occurs because of mutations that arise every now and then.

Sexual reproduction, which involves two parents, offers the advantage of producing individuals who are genetically different from their parents. Sexual reproduction is more complicated than asexual reproduction, and the additional steps required mean more opportunities for things to "go wrong."

Sexual reproduction requires that each parent produce **gametes** (GAM-eets), cells for reproduction that contain half as many **chromosomes** as a normal cell. Such cells are called **haploid** (HAP-loyd) cells. Chromosomes are structures in the nuclei of body cells that contain a person's individual DNA and genes. **Fertilization** is the formation of a single cell containing the genetic material from two gametes—one gamete from each parent. The fertilized cell produced by the combining of gametes is called a **zygote** (ZIGH-goht). The zygote is the single cell from which a new individual will develop.

The **phenotype**, or observable features, of the new individual depend in part on its **genotype**, or genetic makeup, which is established at fertilization. Other factors that influence phenotype are the environment and epigenetics. **Epigenetics** refers to processes, molecules, and molecular modifications, other than changes in DNA sequence, that can affect gene expression and can be passed on from one generation to the next. Epigenetics is a very active area of research.

Check Your Understanding

1. Is genetic diversity possible in asexual reproduction? Explain.
2. At what point is a person's genetic makeup determined?

Mitosis versus Meiosis

Chapter 2 introduced mitosis. This section describes a similar-sounding cell division process—**meiosis**. Mitosis occurs in all of the body's tissues, throughout life, as the body grows and renews itself. Meiosis, on the other hand, occurs only in the sex organs, and produces a special kind of cell. Looking at these processes side by side will help you understand them both better.

Mitosis

The development of a zygote into an adult requires that one cell give rise to trillions of cells. Mitosis is the process of cell division by which this growth occurs. In mitosis, one cell divides to make two "daughter" cells. The two daughter cells are genetically identical to the mother cell, except for the occasional mutation. The process of mitosis is shown in the left panel of **Figure 15.1**.

Before mitosis begins, the parent cell has 23 pairs of chromosomes—22 similar pairs, plus

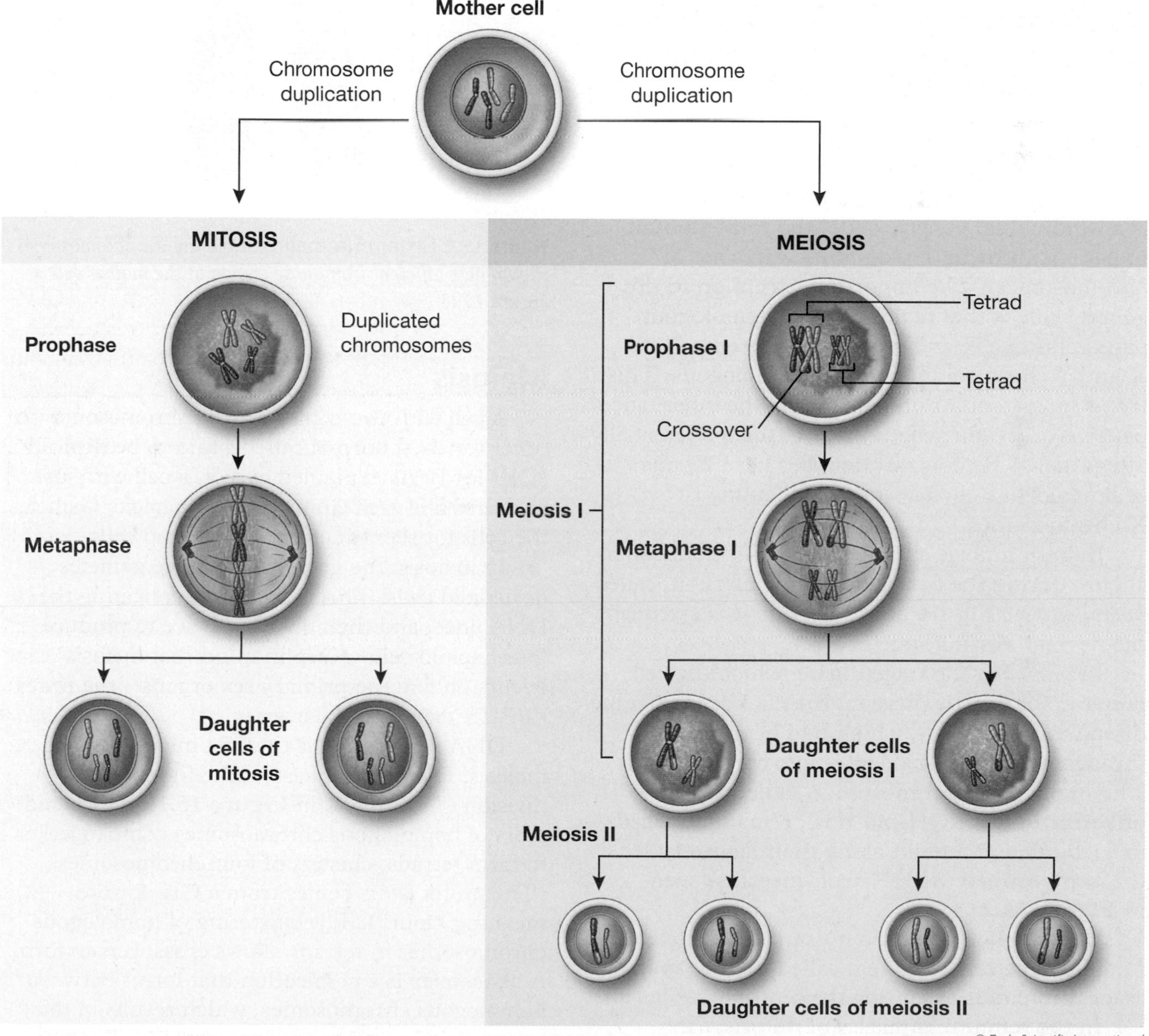

Figure 15.1 Comparison of mitosis with meiosis. An abbreviated look at mitosis is provided here. For a more complete look at the process, see **Figures 2.20** and **2.21** in Chapter 2. Also note that to more clearly illustrate the process, only 2 of the 23 pairs of chromosomes are shown. *How many pairs of homologous chromosomes are in the genome of a male? A female? During which stage in mitotic division does DNA condense into chromosomes?*

two X chromosomes if female, or an X and a Y chromosome if male. The two members of a chromosomal pair are called *homologous* (hoh-MAHL-uh-gus) *chromosomes*. For the purpose of explanation, only 2 of the 23 pairs are shown in the figure.

Homologous chromosomes are very similar, but they are not quite identical. The parent cell inherited one of each of 23 chromosomes from each parent. Therefore, you can think of the purple chromosomes shown in the parent cell in **Figure 15.1** as chromosomes from the mother, and you can think of the green chromosomes as being from the father—or vice versa. A complete diagram would depict 23 purple chromosomes and 23 green chromosomes.

Because humans have two homologous versions of each chromosome, they have two versions of each gene in their genome—one gene from each parent. (Recall from Chapter 2 that a genome is an individual genetic code, the total amount of genetic information contained in a set of chromosomes.) The important exception to this general rule is that males have 22 homologous pairs, plus one X and one Y chromosome. The X and Y chromosomes are not homologous. This fact is important for understanding the inheritance patterns of certain genetic diseases that preferentially affect males. By contrast, females have 23 pairs of homologous chromosomes, including two X chromosomes.

In both mitosis and meiosis, DNA duplication occurs during the first stage of cell division, called *interphase* (see **Figure 2.20**). Interphase is essentially the normal, resting state of a cell.

In *prophase*, the stage during which the cell prepares for mitotic division, the nuclear membrane dissolves. The DNA, which had been spread throughout the cell, condenses into chromosomes. The duplicated chromosomes, called sister **chromatids** (KROH-ma-tids), remain attached to each other at a point along their length called the **centromere** (SEHN-troh-meer), as seen in **Figure 15.2**.

In *metaphase*, the chromosomes line up in the middle of the cell. A protein called *separase* splits the sister chromatids by cutting the centromeres in half.

In the remaining phases of mitosis, each chromosome is pulled to one side of the cell or the other, and the cytoplasm divides (**Figure 2.21**). The result is two cells, each with 46 chromosomes that are identical to the 46 chromosomes in the mother cell.

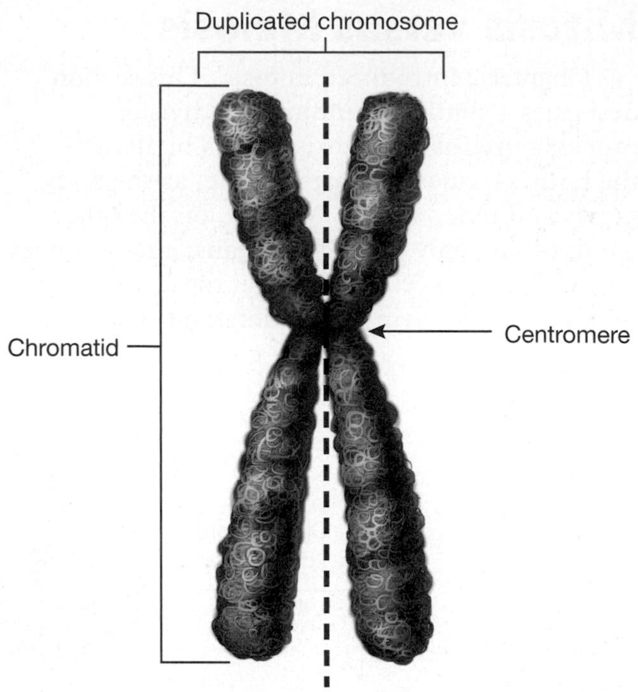

© Body Scientific International

Figure 15.2 Sister chromatids. *How are the chromosomes shown here different from those shown in the mother cell in Figure 15.1?*

Meiosis

A cell with two copies of each chromosome—in other words, a normal cell—is said to be **diploid** (DIP-loyd). As explained earlier, a cell with just one version of each chromosome is haploid. Gametes, the cells for reproduction, are haploid cells.

In meiosis, the goal is to produce gametes, or haploid cells. This is done by duplicating the DNA once, and then dividing twice to produce four haploid cells. Keep in mind that meiosis occurs only in the primary sex organs—the testes (TEHS-teez) and the ovaries.

DNA duplication is the first major task of meiosis. During prophase of the first meiotic division ("Meiosis I" in **Figure 15.1**), duplicated pairs of homologous chromosomes come together to form tetrads, clusters of four chromosomes. (The prefix *tetra-* comes from a Greek word meaning "four"). The clustering of homologous chromosomes in tetrads allows crossovers to form. A **crossover** is a connection that forms between homologous chromosomes, which results in the swapping of portions of chromosomes. Tetrads and crossovers form in meiosis but not in mitosis. Crossovers generate additional genetic diversity in the gametes.

When chromosomes separate in the first meiotic division, the sister chromatids are not separated as they are in mitosis. The daughter cells of the first meiotic division contain 23 *duplicated* chromosomes. Due to crossing over, these duplicates are not exactly identical. By contrast, the daughter cells of mitosis contain 23 pairs of *homologous* chromosomes—in other words, 46 *different* chromosomes. Remember that homologous chromosomes consist of "one from dad and one from mom," whereas duplicated chromosomes are two copies of the same chromosome (from *either* mom or dad).

In the first meiotic division, the segregation of chromosomes to one or the other daughter cell is random. The other chromosome always goes to the other daughter cell. This process continues for all 23 pairs of chromosomes.

When one flips a coin 23 times, more than 8 million possible outcomes can occur. Similarly, each mother cell that undergoes meiosis can produce 8 million different possible daughter cells in the first meiotic division, and that does not even take into account the additional genetic diversity generated by crossovers.

In the second meiotic division ("Meiosis II" in **Figure 15.1**), the two daughter cells of Meiosis I divide without chromosome duplication. Sister chromatids are cut apart, and the four resulting cells contain 23 chromosomes each. These haploid cells are the final product of meiosis.

Check Your Understanding

1. What is the end result of mitosis?
2. How is a gamete different from normal cells in the human body?
3. What is the end result of the second meiotic division?

Development and Puberty

The male and female reproductive systems, unlike the other organ systems, do not become functional until later in life. The development and adult functioning of the reproductive system is closely regulated by the endocrine system, discussed in Chapter 8. This section includes references to parts of the reproductive system that will be described more fully in Lessons 15.2 and 15.3.

The Y chromosome contains a gene called *SRY*, which stands for "sex-determining region Y." The gene encodes a protein called a *transcription factor*, which controls when other genes are *transcribed*—in other words, when they are switched on or off. By regulating other genes, the SRY gene acts as a molecular switch that triggers a cascade of events leading to the development of male sex organs. A zygote *with* a normal Y chromosome therefore becomes a male. A zygote *without* a Y chromosome develops into a female.

Embryonic and Fetal Development

During the first six to seven weeks of development, male and female embryos are visually indistinguishable. Reproductive organs begin to develop in the fifth week, and for the next two weeks they develop in the same way in both males and females.

In the seventh week of development, the SRY gene starts to take effect in embryos that have a Y chromosome. Male sex organs begin to develop, starting with the testes. The cells in the developing testes secrete testosterone, which causes the penis, scrotum, and male accessory organs to develop.

Embryos that do not have an SRY gene start to develop ovaries in the eighth week. In the absence of testosterone, female accessory organs and external genitals develop. In the final two months of gestation, the testes descend from the pelvic cavity into the scrotum in males. In females, the ovaries descend somewhat, but they remain within the pelvic cavity.

The body's default is to develop female reproductive anatomy. The presence of a Y chromosome and the resulting production of testosterone cause male anatomical structures to develop. Therefore, the great majority of individuals who are XY develop male reproductive organs and anatomy. *Intersex individuals* are those whose reproductive system anatomy and physiology are not purely male or purely female. This can occur for a variety of reasons, including lack of enzymes that make and activate testosterone, or lack of cell surface receptors that can respond to testosterone, or translocation of the SRY gene to an X chromosome. Intersex individuals may have external genitals that are neither fully male nor fully female, or they may have external genitals that appear normal but which do not match their genetic sex.

At the time of childbirth, the blood levels of follicle-stimulating hormone (FSH) and luteinizing hormone (LH) in the newborn are high. However, these levels decline rapidly and remain low for 8 to 14 years, until the onset of puberty. Because FSH and LH are low, the testes do not produce testosterone, and the ovaries do not produce estrogen or progesterone. Thus, the reproductive organs remain nonfunctional for the first 8 to 14 years of life.

Puberty

The typical human life span includes a series of stages—from birth to death—that are collectively referred to as the human growth and development cycle. Certain physical, cognitive, and socioemotional milestones characterize each stage. The stages are: infancy (birth to age 1), toddlerhood (ages 1 to 3), early childhood (ages 3 to 5), middle childhood (ages 6 to 10), adolescence (ages 11 to 19), early adulthood (ages 20 to 39), middle adulthood (ages 40 to 65), and older adulthood (ages 66 and up).

Puberty is the final maturation of the reproductive system. Lasting several years, it marks the time when sexual reproduction becomes possible. Puberty normally starts between 8 and 13 years of age in females and between 9 and 14 years of age in males. Adolescence begins with the appearance of secondary sex characteristics (described below) and ends when adult height has been reached.

The initial stimulus for puberty is elevated secretion of gonadotropin-releasing hormone, or GnRH. This hormone is secreted by the hypothalamus in the brain. GnRH causes the pituitary to produce more FSH and LH. In turn, FSH and LH stimulate production of gonadal hormones—testosterone in males and estrogen and progesterone in females. The rising levels of gonadal hormones stimulate maturation of the reproductive organs and cause the appearance of secondary sex characteristics (**Figure 15.3**).

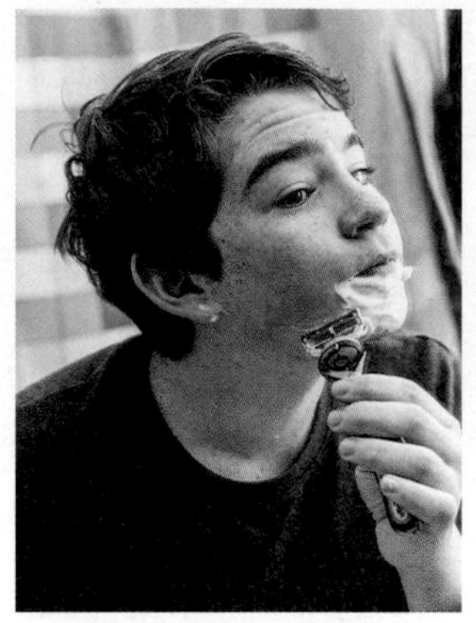

A

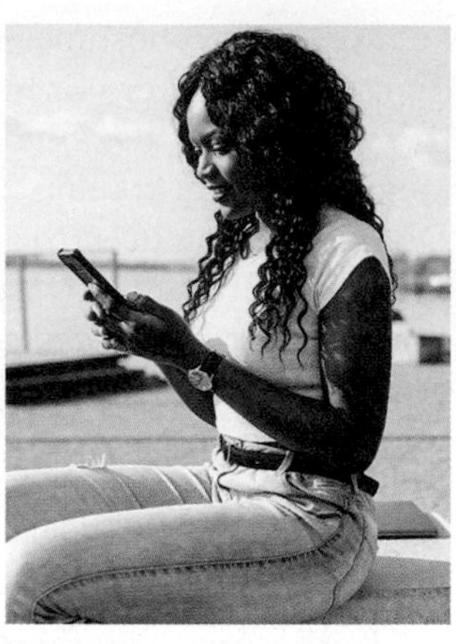

B

Arina P Habich/Shutterstock.com, Standret/Shutterstock.com

Figure 15.3 Secondary sex characteristics appear at puberty. Both males and females develop underarm and pubic hair. A—Males develop facial hair. B—Females develop breasts and a wider pelvis that eventually aids in childbirth. *What additional secondary sex characteristics appear at puberty for males? What additional characteristics appear for females?*

Female development

In females, the first phase of puberty is marked by breast growth, followed by the development of secondary sex characteristics: growth of axillary (underarm) and pubic hair, and gradual changes in the width of the pelvis and the size of the pelvic outlet to facilitate pregnancy and childbirth. In addition, skeletal growth accelerates.

About two years after the beginning of puberty, **menarche** (MEHN-ar-kee)—the first menstrual bleeding—occurs. Ovulation cycles typically are irregular for the first one or two years. They become more regular as puberty reaches its conclusion. At this time, the epiphyseal plates in the long bones close, causing height growth to stop.

Male development

In males, the first visible phase of puberty is marked by growth of the scrotum and testes. As in females, secondary sex characteristics appear, with a key difference: besides pubic and axillary hair growth, an increase in the size of the larynx and the length of the vocal folds causes the voice to deepen. The penis grows larger in proportion to body size.

During the early years of puberty, males typically experience erections at unexpected times, as well as occasional emission of semen during sleep. (The discharge of semen during sleep is called a *nocturnal emission*.) By the end of puberty, mature sperm are present in semen. As in females, the epiphyseal plates close, and the long bones in the body stop growing.

Check Your Understanding

1. What is the function of the SRY gene?
2. Which hormone initiates puberty when its level is elevated?
3. Name at least one secondary sex characteristic shared by males and females.

LESSON 15.1 Review and Assessment

Mini Glossary

Make sure that you know the meaning of each key term.

centromere the point or region on a chromosome that divides the chromosome into two arms and functions as the point of attachment for the sister chromatids; provides movement during cell division

chromatids paired strands of a duplicated chromosome that become visible during cell division and that are joined by a centromere

chromosomes rod-shaped structures in the nuclei of body cells that contain individual DNA and genes

crossovers connections that form between homologous chromosomes during meiosis, resulting in the swapping of portions of chromosomes

diploid a cell having two sets of chromosomes: one set from the mother and one set from the father

epigenetics processes, molecules, and molecular modifications, other than changes in DNA sequence that can affect gene expression and can be passed on from one generation to the next

fertilization the formation of a single cell that contains the genetic material from two gametes, one from each parent

gametes mature haploid male or female cells that unite with cells of the opposite sex to form a zygote; eggs and sperm

genotype genetic makeup

haploid having a single set of unpaired chromosomes

meiosis a type of cell division that produces eggs (in females) or sperm (in males), daughter cells with half the chromosome number of the parent cell

menarche the first menstrual bleeding

phenotype the observable features of an individual, which are established at fertilization

puberty the final maturation of the reproductive system

zygote a diploid cell produced by the fusion of a sperm with an egg; a fertilized egg

Know and Understand

1. What are the offspring of asexual reproduction called?
2. How many pairs of chromosomes are in a normal human cell?
3. How many pairs of homologous chromosomes do males have? How many do females have?
4. What is the difference between haploid and diploid cells?
5. What is the first major event of meiosis?
6. What role do crossovers play in genetic diversity?
7. What are the age ranges for the onset of puberty in males and in females?

Analyze and Apply

8. Compare and contrast asexual and sexual reproduction, identifying and explaining as many differences as possible.
9. Compare and contrast mitosis and meiosis, explaining as many similarities and differences as possible.
10. Explain the differences between the embryonic and fetal development of the male sex organs as compared to the female sex organs.
11. Explain the role of a chromosome.

IN THE LAB

12. In this activity, you will demonstrate how meiotic cell division creates a gamete with half the chromosomes of other cells, and how random assignment of chromosomes creates gametes with many different combinations of chromosomes. You will start with 46 chromosomes (23 from the mother and 23 from the father).

    Materials: small bowl, 23 pennies (chromosomes from the mother), 23 nickels (chromosomes from the father), 1 quarter, 2 sets of coin-sized labels numbered 1–23.

    Procedure: Place the pennies in a row across the desk, evenly spaced. Place a nickel next to each penny. Place a numbered label beside each penny-nickel pair. For example, the first penny and nickel should be labeled "1," the next penny and nickel should be labeled "2," and so forth, through the 23 pairs. Flip the quarter. If it lands heads up, place the penny from the first penny-nickel pair into the bowl. If it lands tails up, place the nickel from the first penny-nickel pair into the bowl. Continue flipping the quarter for each penny-nickel pair until you have 23 coins in the bowl. Record the numbers of the pennies and nickels in the bowl. Repeat 5 times. How many times did you get the exact same combination of coins? According to the lesson, how many combinations may occur if you repeated this forever? Plot the outcomes in a spreadsheet, and share your findings with the class.
13. Using a high-powered microscope and prepared slides, view both the female and male gametes. Draw what you see on a sheet of paper. Trade drawings with another student and ask the student to label the parts of the gametes.

LESSON 15.2 Male Reproductive System

Before You Read

Try to answer the following questions before you read this lesson.

- What are the primary and accessory male reproductive organs?
- Where are sperm cells created?

Lesson Objectives

- Describe the anatomy of the male reproductive system.
- Explain the functions of the male reproductive system.

Key Terms

bulbourethral glands	prostate gland
ductus deferens	semen
ejaculation	seminal glands
epididymis	seminiferous tubules
erection	sperm
gonads	spermatogenesis
penis	

The male reproductive system differs from the female reproductive system because, although the final goal of both is to produce offspring, males and females have different roles to play in the process. This lesson explains male reproductive anatomy and its functions in the production of offspring.

Male Reproductive Anatomy

For both males and females, the primary reproductive organs are the **gonads** (GOH-nads), the sites in which gametes are made. In males, the gonads are the testes, also called the *testicles*; the gametes are called *sperm*. **Sperm** are the male haploid cells that can fertilize an egg to make a zygote.

The *accessory reproductive organs* in the male reproductive system are the other structures needed for sperm maturation and delivery of sperm to the female. These include the external genitals—the penis and scrotum—and the internal structures, including five accessory glands. These glands are the prostate, the two seminal glands, and the two bulbourethral (bul-boh-yoo-REE-thral) glands.

Scrotum and Testes

The scrotum is a pouch of skin that hangs outside the body below the pelvic cavity, in the midline and anterior to the anus (**Figure 15.4**). The scrotum contains the two testes and associated ducts.

The external location of the scrotum causes the temperature of the testes to be about 93.2°F (34°C), which is cooler than the core body temperature of 98.6°F (37°C). Sperm formation is most vigorous at this cooler temperature. Two muscles—the cremaster and the dartos—work together to maintain optimum temperature of the scrotum. When the scrotum is cold, the cremaster and dartos muscles contract to pull the organ closer to the body. When the scrotum is warm, the cremaster and dartos relax to allow the scrotum more freedom and greater surface area.

The testes (singular *testis*) inside the scrotum are the two primary male reproductive organs. **Figure 15.4** shows one testis and the **epididymis** (ehp-i-DID-i-mis), a structure that holds the testes in place. The testis contains a dense network of small tubes in which sperm forms. These are called **seminiferous tubules**.

The seminiferous tubules connect to the tubules of the epididymis, which lies on the posterior side of the testis. The tubules in the upper part of the epididymis converge to form the duct of the epididymis. This duct travels down, behind and to the side of the testis, to the bottom of the testis, where it bends back upward. As the duct runs upward, it is known as the **ductus deferens** (DEHF-eh-rehnz), or the *vas deferens*. The ductus deferens and the arteries and veins that supply and drain the testis and epididymis ascend in the spermatic cord and then enter the pelvic cavity (**Figure 15.5**).

Penis

The **penis** is designed to deliver sperm to the female reproductive tract. The shaft of the penis leads to the *glans penis*, the enlarged end. The *prepuce* (PREE-pyoos), or foreskin, is a loose fold of skin that covers much of the glans penis.

Circumcision is the surgical removal of the prepuce. This practice may be done for religious, cultural, or hygienic reasons. Circumcision has been shown to reduce the risk of certain sexually

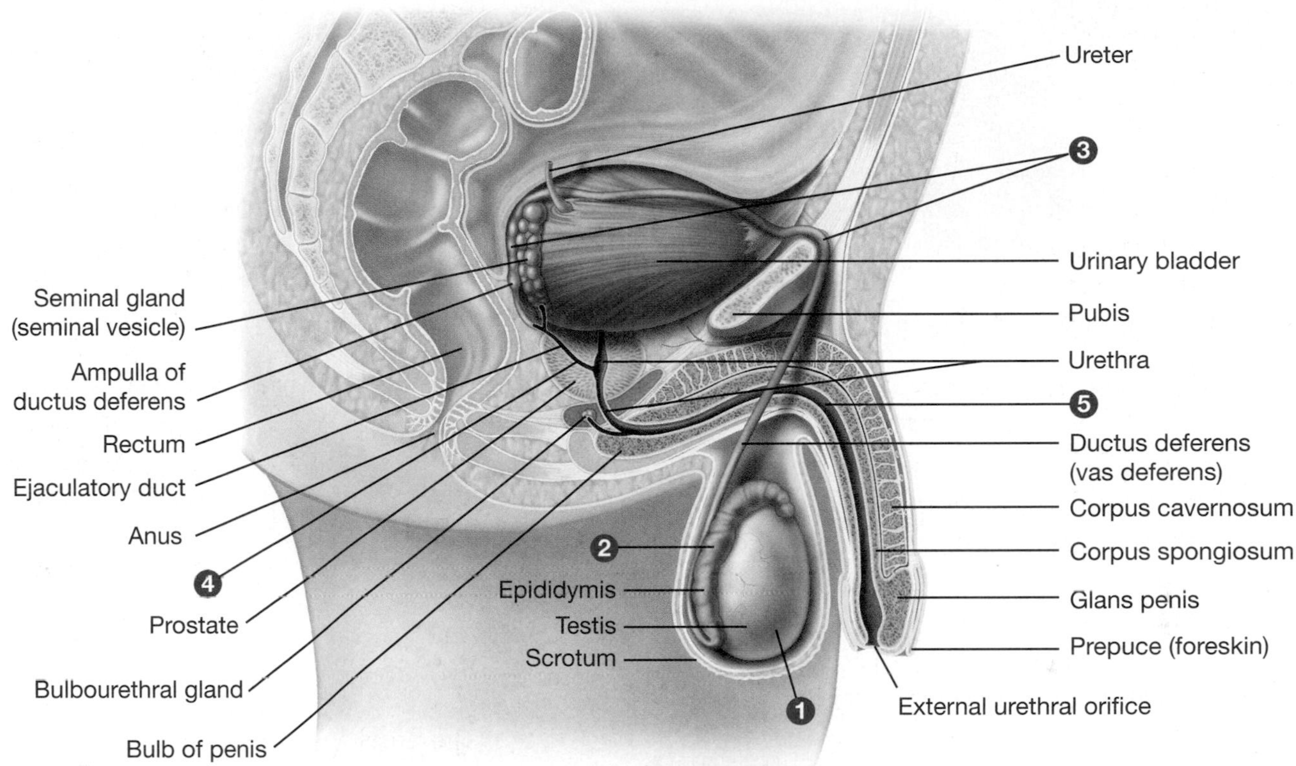

Figure 15.4 Sagittal view of the male reproductive organs. 1—Sperm form in the testes (one testis shown here). 2—Sperm spend 10 to 14 days in the epididymis before they reach full maturation. 3—Smooth muscle in the ductus deferens propels sperm toward the urethra. 4—Sperm from the ductus deferens and fluid from the seminal gland pass through the ejaculatory duct into the urethra. The prostate gland also secretes fluid into the urethra. 5—During ejaculation, semen moves through the urethra and out of the body. *How does the anatomy of the scrotum enhance the production of sperm?*

transmitted diseases. However, some cultures oppose infant circumcision as an unnecessary medical procedure.

The shaft of the penis contains erectile tissue and the urethra. Recall from Chapter 14 that the opening at the outer end of the urethra is the external urethral orifice. The erectile tissue in the shaft is separated into two *corpora cavernosa*, which lie parallel to each other and extend the length of the shaft, and one *corpus spongiosum* (spun-jee-OH-sum). These tissues contain spaces in which blood can pool. During sexual arousal, the erectile tissues become enlarged and rigid due to engorgement with blood.

Ducts of the Male Reproductive System

The male duct system (shown in **Figure 15.4** and **Figure 15.5**) transports sperm from the testes, where it is formed, to the external urethral orifice at the tip of the penis. Sperm from the seminiferous tubules of each testis enter the epididymis. The duct of the epididymis carries sperm to the ductus deferens. The two ductus deferens carry sperm from the scrotum into the pelvic cavity, inside the body.

Each ductus deferens proceeds from front to back along the upper lateral border of the bladder. At the posterior side of the bladder, the ductus deferens turns downward and widens slightly to form a chamber called the *ampulla* (am-POO-la) of the ductus deferens. The outlet of the ampulla and the duct from the seminal gland merge to form the *ejaculatory duct*, which is much shorter than the ductus deferens. The ejaculatory duct from each side enters the prostate and, in the center of the prostate, joins the urethra. The urethra carries urine out of the body during micturition, and it conveys sperm out of the body during sexual intercourse.

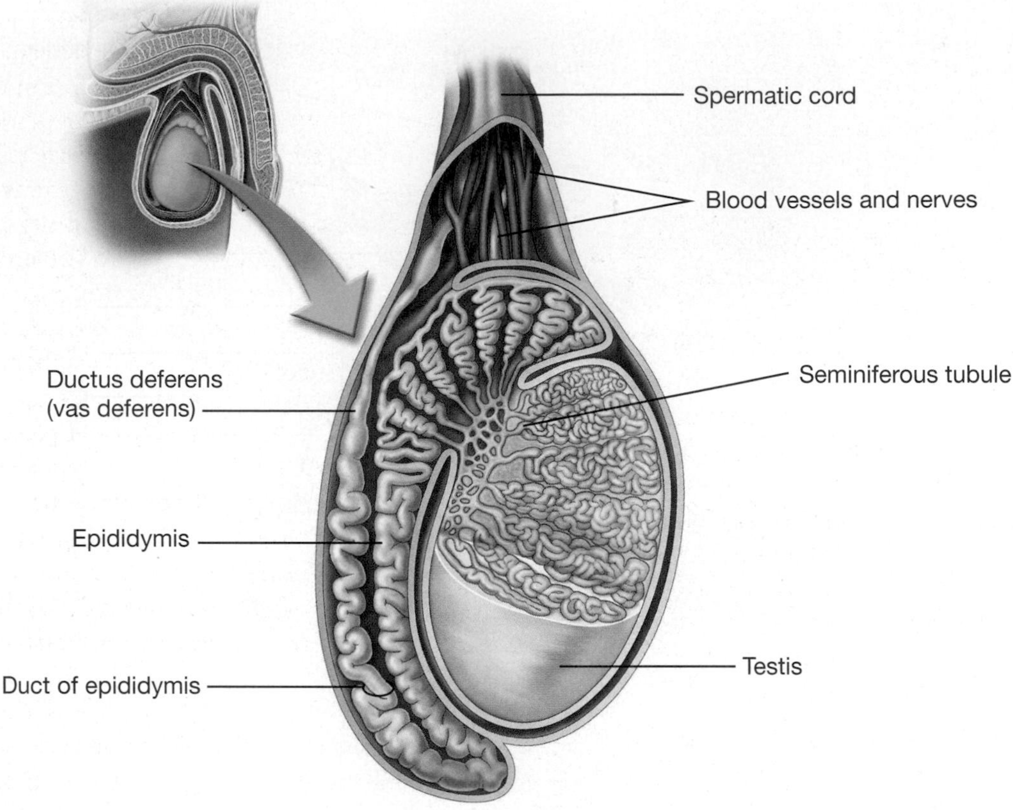

© Body Scientific International

Figure 15.5 A testis and epididymis. *Do sperm form in the epididymis or the seminiferous tubules?*

Accessory Glands and Semen

Semen is the fluid that contains sperm, which is delivered to the female during intercourse. Sperm cells make up only about 10% of the volume of semen. Most seminal volume comes from the accessory glands of the male reproductive system.

The two **seminal glands**, or *seminal vesicles*, produce up to 70% of the volume of semen. The **prostate gland** sits directly under the bladder. The urethra passes through the middle of the prostate gland as it descends from the bladder. The glandular tissue of the prostate secretes fluid that makes up one-quarter to one-third of seminal volume. Several ducts from the prostate join the urethra as it passes through the prostate. The two small **bulbourethral glands** lie below the prostate. Their ducts join the urethra and contribute a small amount of fluid to semen.

During ejaculation, the total volume of semen ejected typically is 2 to 5 mL. Semen contains 20 million to 150 million sperm cells per milliliter (**Figure 15.6**).

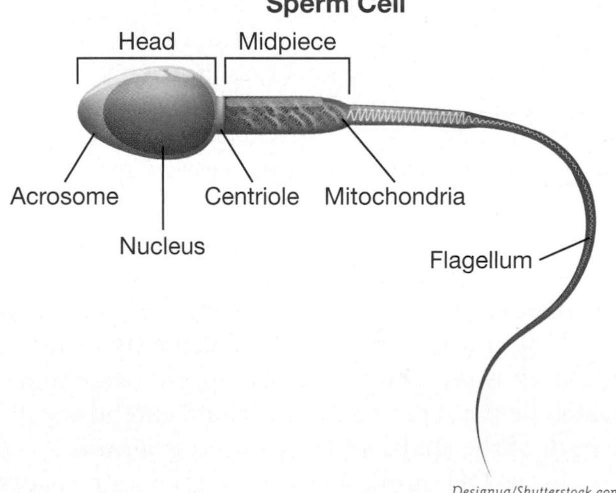

Designua/Shutterstock.com

Figure 15.6 A sperm cell. *What is the name of the fluid that contains sperm? Name the three glands that contribute to the development of this fluid.*

Check Your Understanding

1. In what part of the testes do sperm form?
2. Sperm make up what percentage of the total volume of semen?

Male Reproductive Physiology

The male reproductive system has two principal functions. Its functions are to create sperm and to deliver those sperm to the site of fertilization.

Sperm Formation

Sperm formation, or **spermatogenesis** (sper-mat-oh-JEHN-i-sis), occurs in the walls of the seminiferous tubules of the testes. Stem cells called *spermatogonia* (sper-mat-oh-GOH-nee-a) undergo mitosis. One of the two daughter cells remains as a stem cell for future division, and the other daughter cell becomes a *primary spermatocyte* (sper-MAT-oh-sight).

The primary spermatocyte is diploid—it has 46 chromosomes. The first meiotic division yields two secondary spermatocytes, and the second meiotic division produces four *spermatids* (SPER-mat-ids). The spermatids are gametes: they are haploid, with 23 chromosomes each.

Each immature spermatid develops a *flagellum* (fla-JEHL-um), or tail, which it will use to move up the female reproductive tract. Once the spermatid has a flagellum, it is released into the lumen of the seminiferous tubule. At this stage it is referred to as a *sperm*, although it is not yet mature. From the development of a primary spermatocyte to the release of sperm into the seminiferous tubule, the process takes 9 to 10 weeks. Immature sperm move from the seminiferous tubules of the testes to the epididymis where they spend about three weeks achieving maturation.

Sexual Response

The male sexual response has two complementary components: erection and ejaculation. **Erection** permits the penis to gain entry to the female reproductive tract. During erection, the penis enlarges and stiffens in response to sexual stimulation. Neural impulses travel along parasympathetic nerve fibers to the erectile tissues of the penis, triggering the production and release of nitric oxide (NO). The nitric oxide causes the arterioles in the penis to relax; as a result, more blood fills the tissue, and the penis becomes erect.

Ejaculation is the ejection of semen from the body. When sexual stimulation is sufficient, a burst of activity occurs on sympathetic nerves leading to the male reproductive tract. These nerve impulses cause peristaltic contractions of smooth muscle in the male duct system, and of smooth muscle in the male accessory glands. The nerve impulses also cause contraction of the urethral sphincter at the base of the bladder, which prevents mixing of urine with semen. The burst of nerve activity, ejaculation of semen, and the pleasurable sensation are called an *orgasm*.

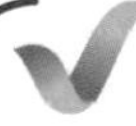

Check Your Understanding

1. What is spermatogenesis?
2. What is the purpose of the flagellum on a sperm?

LIFE SPAN DEVELOPMENT: *Adult Male Reproductive System*

Male reproductive function declines gradually with age, but it does not cease completely, as it does in women. The concentration of testosterone in the blood decreases in aging men. The reduced level of testosterone is associated with a decrease in exercise capability, an increase in body fat, and a decrease in libido (sexual drive). Decreased bone strength and cognitive decline are also associated with lower testosterone levels. Erectile dysfunction, the inability to have or maintain an erection, becomes more common with aging. The motility and viability of the sperm cells in semen also decreases with aging.

Benign prostatic hyperplasia, the enlargement of the prostate gland, usually begins by age 45 and continues until death. This growth of the prostate compresses the urethra and makes urination difficult, as discussed in Chapter 14.

Life Span Review

1. What happens to the level of testosterone in males as they age?
2. Name five consequences of the change in testosterone levels in older men.

LESSON 15.2 Review and Assessment

Mini Glossary

Make sure that you know the meaning of each key term.

bulbourethral glands two small glands at the base of the penis that secrete mucus into the urethra

ductus deferens the secretory duct of the testis, which extends from the epididymis and joins with the excretory duct of the seminal gland; vas deferens

ejaculation the discharge of sperm from the ejaculatory duct during the male sexual response

epididymis a system of small ducts in the testis in which sperm mature

erection the condition of erectile tissue when filled with blood, which permits the penis to gain entry to the female reproductive tract

gonads the organs that produce gametes (oocytes and sperm): the ovaries in females and the testes in males

penis the reproductive organ that delivers sperm to the female reproductive tract

prostate gland the gland that sits directly under the bladder and surrounds the beginning of the urethra in the male; produces about one-third of the fluid volume of semen

semen the fluid that contains sperm, which is delivered to the female during intercourse; penile ejaculate

seminal glands glands that produce up to 70% of the volume of semen; seminal vesicles

seminiferous tubules small tubes in the testes in which sperm form

sperm (singular or plural) the male gamete; a haploid cell that can fertilize an egg to make a zygote

spermatogenesis sperm formation

Know and Understand

1. Where are gametes made?
2. Where within the testes do sperm form?
3. From a reproductive standpoint, what is the penis designed to accomplish?
4. Trace the path of sperm from the testes to the external urethral orifice, naming each duct and organ through which the sperm travel.
5. What is the name of the fluid that contains sperm as they travel through the male reproductive system?
6. What is the name of the stem cells in which the production of sperm cells begins?
7. What is the purpose of a flagellum?
8. What is the role of sympathetic nerves in stimulating ejaculation?

Analyze and Apply

9. Compare the structures and functions of spermatogonia, spermatocytes, and spermatids.
10. Explain how the anatomy of the male reproductive system makes erection possible.
11. Consider the information in Lessons 15.1 and 15.2. Then compare and contrast the male and female gametes.
12. Mr. Erikson is a 67-year-old male who explains to his physician that he is having increasing difficulty with urination, and that he just has not been very interested in sexual intercourse lately. Other than these symptoms, he has no complaints, but his wife is concerned that he may have a urinary tract infection or even prostate cancer, so he agreed to have the physician "check it out." The physical exam was normal, and blood tests revealed no abnormalities except for a decrease in testosterone level. What do you think is wrong with Mr. Erikson? Should the physician take action? Explain.

IN THE LAB

13. Using 3×5 cards, create flash cards for terminology pertaining to the male reproductive system. Use all of the key terms, as well as any other unfamiliar terms in this lesson. Write the term on one side and the definition on the other side. You may wish to draw pictures on the definition side to help you remember the term. Use the flash cards to quiz yourself; then quiz your lab partner.
14. When the temperature of the scrotum rises above the optimal level, the cremaster and dartos muscles relax. This causes the surface area of the scrotum to increase, which lowers its temperature. Demonstrate how surface area affects the transfer of heat and temperature.

    Materials: 2 disposable vinyl gloves, 2 large bottles, 2 large beakers (1,000 mL), string or rubber bands, warm water, ice, thermometer.

    Procedure: Fill a large bottle with water and ice. Fill the other bottle with warm water. Pour the ice water into the two beakers. Tie off the five fingers of one glove, decreasing its surface area, and pour 7 fluid ounces of the warm water into it. Immediately immerse the glove into a beaker, holding the open end out of the water. After 3 minutes, measure and record the temperature of the water inside the glove. Repeat the procedure with the other glove, but do not tie off the fingers. How do the water temperatures inside the gloves compare? What can you conclude about the relationship between surface area and heat transfer?

LESSON 15.3 Female Reproductive System

Before You Read

Try to answer the following questions before you read this lesson.

- What are the primary and accessory female reproductive organs?
- What happens during the ovarian and the uterine cycles?

Lesson Objectives

- Describe the internal and external anatomy of the female reproductive system.
- List the steps in oogenesis.
- Identify the monthly changes in the ovaries and the uterus, and the major hormones involved in the reproductive process. Explain how these changes prepare the body for fertilization and pregnancy.

Key Terms

cervix	oocyte
clitoris	oogenesis
corpus luteum	ovarian cycle
labia majora	ovaries
labia minora	ovulation
lactiferous duct	uterine cycle
mammary glands	uterine tubes
menopause	uterus
menstrual cycle	vagina

Female Reproductive Anatomy

In females, the gonads are the **ovaries** and the gametes are called *ova*, or eggs. The ovaries are the primary female reproductive organs—the organs in which gametes are made (**Figure 15.7**). Accessory organs include the uterine tubes, uterus, vagina, and vulva.

The Ovaries

Just as the testes produce sperm and secrete the hormone testosterone, the ovaries produce oocytes and secrete the hormones estrogen and progesterone. The two oval-shaped ovaries, which are about 1.2 inches (3.0 cm) long and 0.6 inch (1.5 cm) wide, are positioned against the posterior wall of the pelvic cavity. The ovaries, like the testes, have a fibrous outer covering, as the right ovary in **Figure 15.7** shows. Unlike the testes, however, the ovaries do not contain ducts. Instead, they contain many ovarian follicles.

Each follicle inside the ovaries contains a single **oocyte** (OH-oh-sight), or egg cell, and multiple surrounding cells. At any given time, the ovaries contain follicles in various stages of maturation. *Primordial* (prigh-MORD-ee-al) *follicles* are the most plentiful and least mature. They contain a single layer of cells surrounding the oocyte.

A *primary follicle* is slightly larger than a primordial follicle, but still has only a single layer of cells surrounding the oocyte. Secondary and vesicular follicles are larger and have more cells surrounding the oocyte. Each month one follicle reaches maturity, and the oocyte that it contains is released from the ovary during **ovulation**.

Ducts of the Female Reproductive System

There are a couple of significant differences between the female and male reproductive duct systems. One major difference is the open-ended design of the female system. In males, sperm are formed in the seminiferous tubules of the testes, which connect directly to the duct system that carries the sperm out of the body. In females, the duct system is open at the ovarian end (**Figure 15.7**).

Another significant difference is that the female urethra is completely separate from the reproductive tract. In males, by contrast, the urethra serves a dual purpose: it is both the outlet for the urinary system and the terminal portion of the reproductive tract.

Uterine Tubes

Each of the two **uterine** (YOOT-er-in) **tubes** (also called *fallopian tubes*) begins at the lateral end of its ovary and curves up and around the ovary to terminate at the top lateral portion of the uterus. The hollow tube is open at the ovary. It has fringe-like projections called *fimbriae* (FIM-bree-igh),

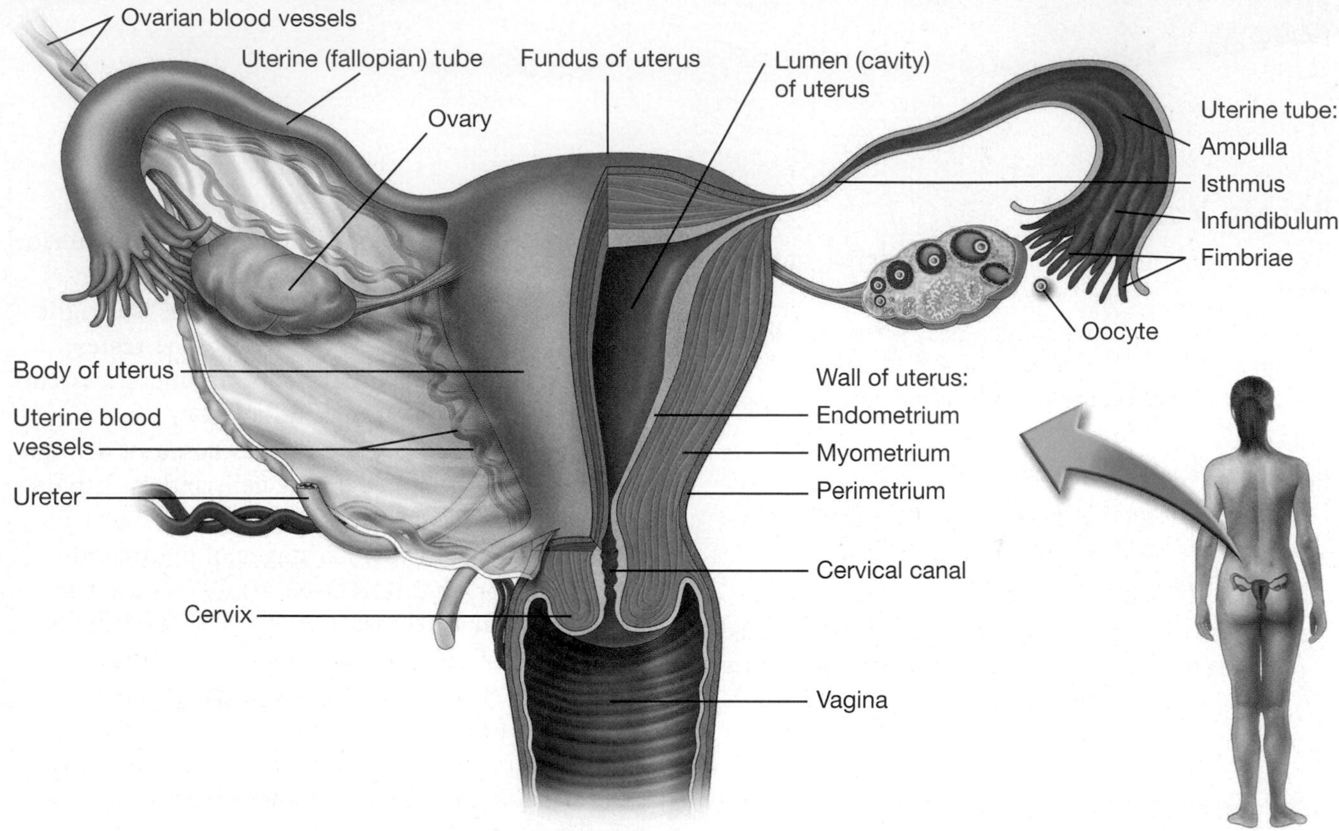

Figure 15.7 The female reproductive organs, posterior view. A cutaway view of one ovary shows development of an oocyte. *How are the ovaries similar to and different from the testes in the male?*

which wrap part of the way around the ovary. The cells lining the uterine tube, including the fimbriae, have vibrating cilia, which are short, microscopic, hair-like structures.

At the time of ovulation, the cilia of the fimbriae sweep fluid and, usually, the ovulated oocyte into the uterine tube. Cilia in the tube, and peristaltic contractions of the smooth muscle in the wall of the tube, move the oocyte toward the uterus. The uterine tube passes through the wall of the uterus and opens into the lumen, or cavity, of the uterus.

The open-ended design of the female duct system has one great benefit and several drawbacks. The benefit is that it provides an ovulated oocyte with a means of entry into the reproductive tract. Once in the reproductive tract, the oocyte can be fertilized, and it can develop into an embryo and then a fetus. The fetus evolves into a newborn human being, which emerges from the mother's body during childbirth.

On the other hand, because the female duct system is open at the ovaries, the oocyte released each month is not always captured by the fimbriae. The oocyte usually dies soon thereafter, but on rare occasions a sperm reaches the oocyte and fertilizes it while it sits in the pelvic cavity. If this happens, the fertilized egg may implant on the wall of the pelvic cavity. A fertilized egg that implants in the pelvic cavity, or in the uterine tube rather than in the uterus, is called an *ectopic pregnancy*.

An ectopic pregnancy cannot survive because the embryo is in an environment that is not designed to support development. Inevitably, a spontaneous abortion (naturally occurring premature termination of pregnancy) will end an ectopic pregnancy. This type of spontaneous abortion is a medical emergency that can involve significant internal bleeding.

The Uterus

The **uterus** (YOOT-er-us), also known as the *womb*, is a hollow, muscular organ located in front of the rectum and behind the bladder. It usually lies with its upper end, or *fundus*, tipped forward over the bladder (**Figure 15.8**). Its purpose is to receive and nourish a fertilized egg and to expel the fetus by forceful, muscular contractions during childbirth about nine months later.

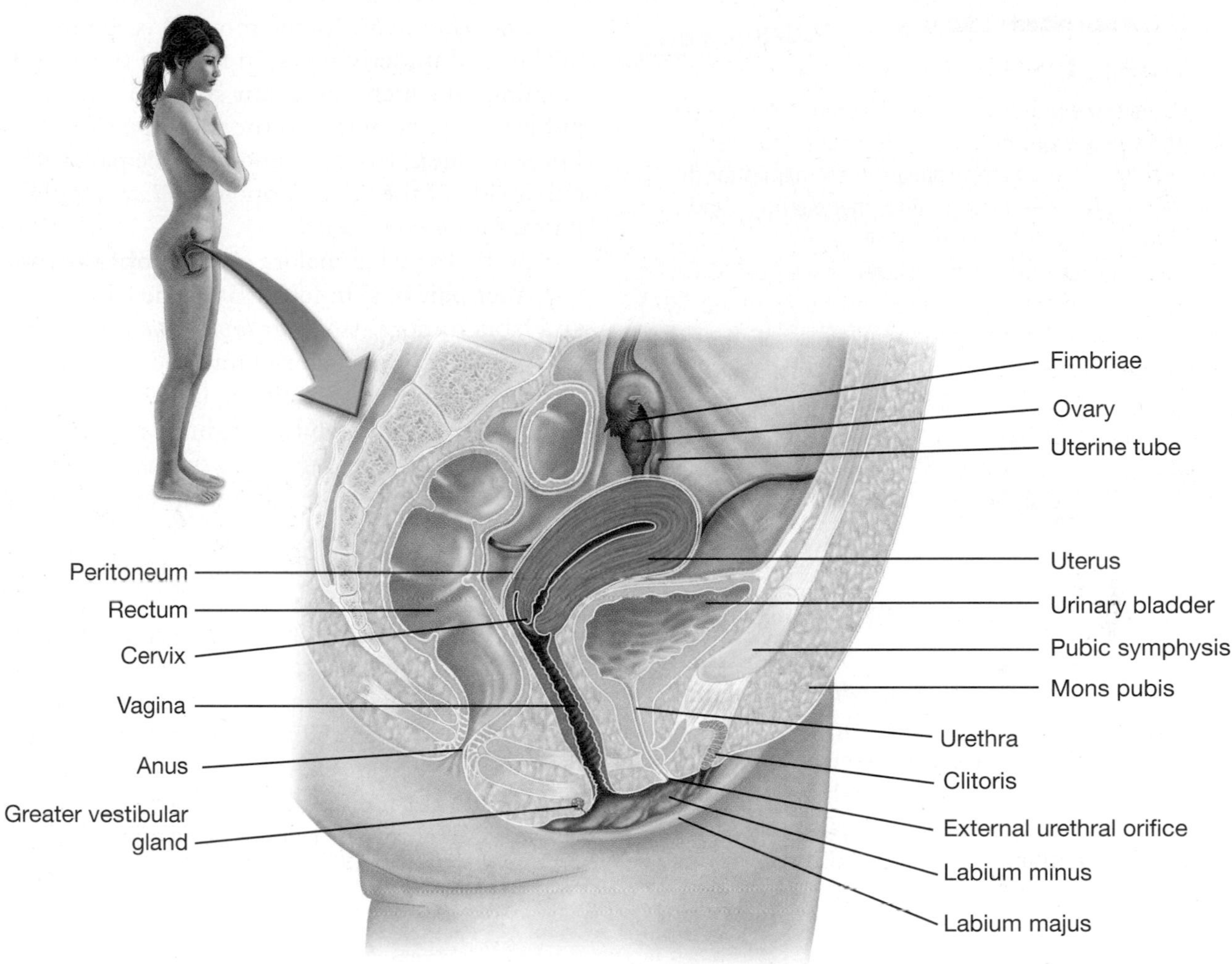

Figure 15.8 The female reproductive organs, midsagittal section. *What is the purpose of the uterus?*

The wall of the uterus has three layers, which are visible in **Figure 15.7**. The *perimetrium* (per-i-MEE-tree-um) is the thin, membranous outer layer. The *myometrium* (migh-oh-MEE-tree-um), which comprises the bulk of the uterine wall, is made of smooth muscle. The *endometrium* (ehn-doh-MEE-tree-um) is the mucosal tissue that forms the innermost layer of the uterus.

The endometrium is perhaps the most fascinating layer of the uterus for a couple of reasons. First, it undergoes significant changes on a four-week cycle. Second, it is the layer that receives, envelops, and nourishes a fertilized egg.

The layer of the endometrium that is closer to the lumen is called the *functional layer*, or *stratum functionalis*. The functional layer grows thicker under the influence of hormones and is shed during menstruation (discussed later in this section). The basal layer, or *stratum basalis*, is the deeper layer of the endometrium. The basal layer is not shed during menstruation.

The narrow lower end of the uterus is called the **cervix** (SER-viks). The cervix, or cervical canal, is the narrow passageway that connects the lumen of the uterus to the lumen of the vagina.

The Vagina

The **vagina** is a thin-walled tubular structure below the uterus. It is sometimes called the *birth canal* because the infant passes through the vagina during birth. During intercourse, sperm are delivered to the lumen of the vagina. In normal, healthy adult women, the pH of the vagina is rather acidic, which helps prevent bacterial infection. Apart from childbirth or intercourse, the walls of the vagina usually touch each other. This means that the lumen is a *potentially* open space rather than an actual open space.

MEMORY TIP

The Greek word *metra* means "womb." *Metra* comes from the Greek word *meter*, which means "mother." The combining form *metr/o* appears in the names for the walls of the uterus—*endometrium*, *myometrium*, and *perimetrium*.

The combining form *end/o* means "inside" or "within." Thus, the *endometrium* is the innermost layer of the uterine wall. The combining form *my/o* means "muscle." The *myometrium*, the middle layer of the uterine wall, is composed of muscle. Finally, the combining form *pe/r-* means "surrounding" or "enclosing." The *perimetrium* is the outer layer of the uterine wall—the layer that surrounds the myometrium and the endometrium.

The External Genitalia

The reproductive structures on the outside of the body are the *external genitalia*. The female external genitalia are shown in **Figure 15.9**. The *vulva* is another name for the external genitalia in females. The vulva includes the labia, mons pubis, clitoris, and vestibule, and the area between the mons pubis and the anus is generally referred to as the *perineum* (peh-rih-NEE-um).

The *mons pubis* (pubic mound) is the region of skin and underlying fat in front of the vaginal opening on which pubic hair starts to grow during puberty. Just posterior to the mons pubis are the **labia majora**, two skin folds that lie parallel on either side of the vaginal opening. *Labia majora* is plural for *labium majus*.

Inside the labia majora are the **labia minora**, a smaller pair of skin folds. Both the labia majora and labia minora (singular *labium minus*) limit entry of infectious material into the reproductive tract. Within the labia minora is the *vestibule*, the recessed area in which the vaginal and urethral openings lie. The two *greater vestibular glands* secrete lubricating mucus onto the epithelium of the vestibule.

The **clitoris** (KLIT-or-is), a small structure at the anterior end of the vestibule, is composed of erectile tissue. The clitoris is derived from the same embryologic precursor as the erectile tissue of the penis. The clitoris is covered anteriorly by a skinfold called the *prepuce*, and the exposed tip is called the *glans*. (As you can see, these terms echo the names of similar structures in the penis.) The clitoris is richly endowed with sensory nerve endings.

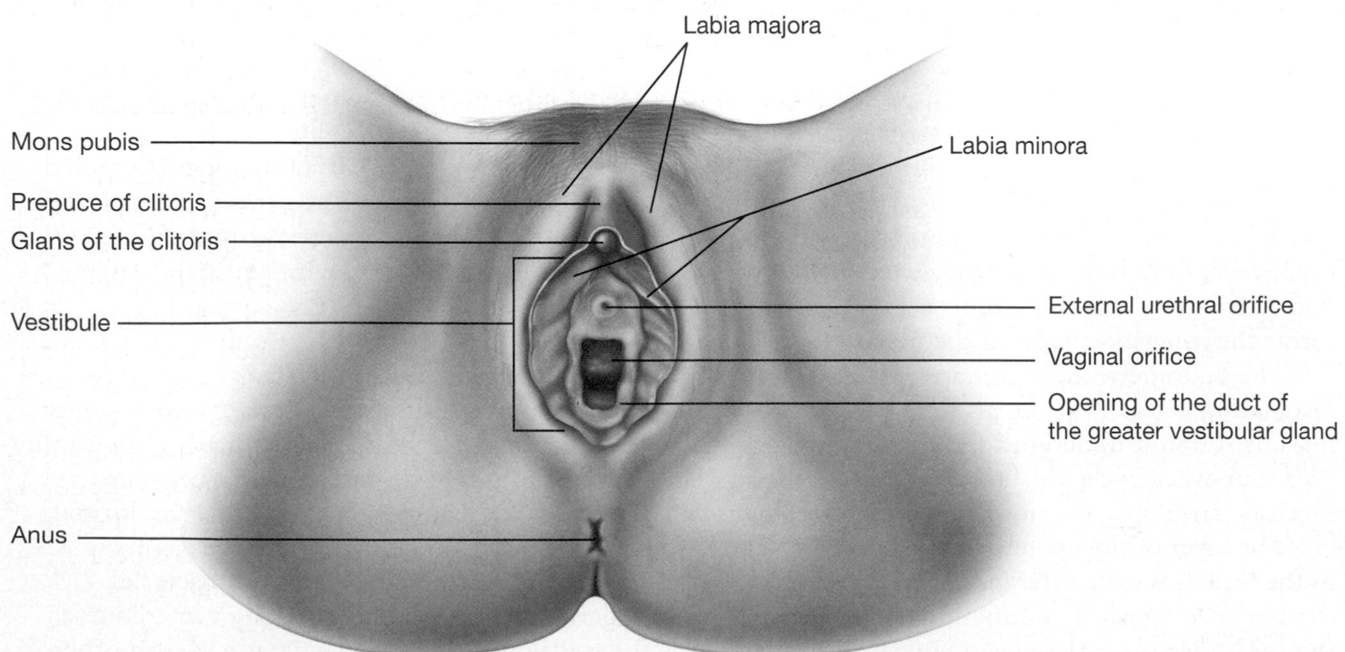

Figure 15.9 The female external genitalia. *Which part of the female external genitalia is derived from the same embryologic precursor as the erectile tissue of the penis?*

The Mammary Glands

The female **mammary glands** produce milk for the newborn baby. Increased estrogen in females during puberty stimulates maturation of the mammary glands. The mature mammary gland is capable of lactation, or milk production, but does not produce milk unless stimulated to do so by the hormone prolactin, which is released after childbirth. **Figure 15.10** shows the structure of a lactating mammary gland.

The mammary glands are modified sweat glands. Like sweat glands, they are part of the skin. Each mammary gland lies on top of the *pectoralis major*, the most superficial muscle of the anterior chest wall. On the surface of the breast is the protruding nipple, which is surrounded by a ring of pigmented skin called the *areola* (uh-REE-oh-la).

The mammary gland contains 15 to 20 lobes internally, each of which has many smaller lobules capable of producing milk. Each lobe secretes its milk into a **lactiferous** (lak-TIF-er-us) **duct** that opens at the nipple. When the breast is not lactating, the glandular tissue remains undeveloped and occupies very little space. The size of the nonlactating breast is determined by the amount of adipose (fat) tissue and interspersed glandular tissue.

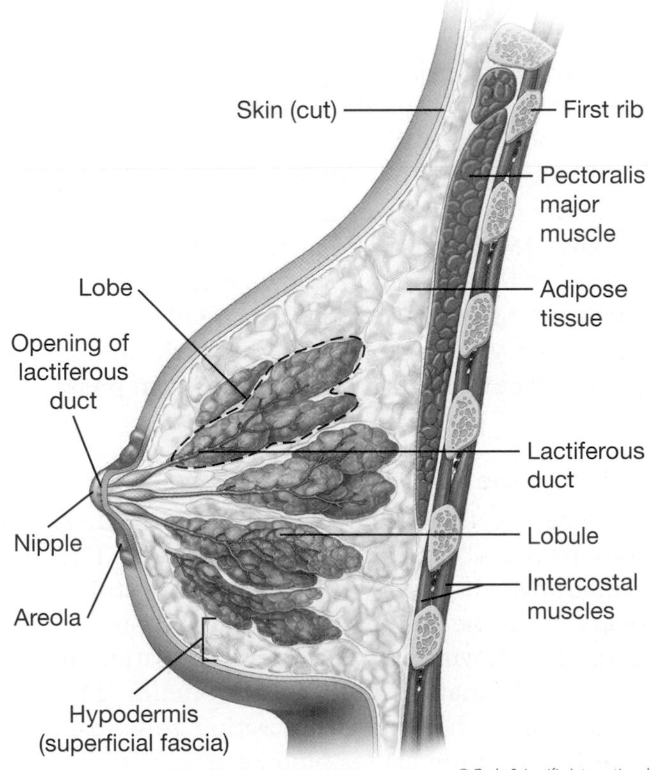

Figure 15.10 A lactating mammary gland.

Check Your Understanding

1. Which reproductive organs in the female are the counterpart to the testes in the male?
2. What are the two major differences between the duct systems of the male and female reproductive systems?
3. What three layers make up the wall of the uterus?
4. What is the name of the narrow passageway that connects the lumen of the uterus to the lumen of the vagina?
5. Which gland of the female reproductive system is a modified sweat gland?

Female Reproductive Physiology

The female reproductive system has five functions. These are to generate eggs, to deliver the eggs for fertilization, to nourish the developing embryo and fetus, to give birth, and to provide nourishment after birth.

Oogenesis

Oogenesis (oh-oh-JEHN-eh-sis) is the process by which oocytes, or egg cells, are generated. Because gametes must be haploid, the oogenetic process involves meiosis. Oogenesis is similar to spermatogenesis, but also differs from it.

Oogenesis begins in the ovaries of the female fetus before birth. *Oogonia*, diploid stem cells that correspond to spermatogonia in males, undergo mitosis and produce primary oocytes, which correspond to primary spermatocytes. Each primary oocyte is surrounded by a single layer of follicle cells, thus forming a *primordial follicle*.

The oocyte in the primordial follicle starts the process of meiosis before the female fetus is born; however, meiosis stops partway through the first meiotic division. About one to two million oocytes are present as primordial follicles at birth. About one-quarter to one-half million of these oocytes survive to puberty. This number is more than enough because only one oocyte is released per month for a period of 30 to 40 years, for a total of fewer than 500 oocytes over a lifetime.

At puberty, the increased level of follicle-stimulating hormone triggers a small number of follicles to develop further each month. One of these follicles becomes the dominant follicle and its oocyte completes the first meiotic division, producing two unequal daughter cells. The *secondary oocyte* gets half the chromosomes and almost all the cytoplasm and organelles. The other cell—a polar body (nonfunctional cell)—gets half the chromosomes and practically nothing more.

The secondary oocyte begins to undergo the second meiotic division, but again meiosis stops partway through. The oocyte is released from the ovary—that is, ovulation occurs. If the oocyte is fertilized, the second meiotic division of the oocyte resumes and is completed.

The second meiotic division follows the same unequal pattern as the first, yielding a tiny polar body and a large haploid oocyte. Meanwhile, the first polar body may or may not complete the second meiotic division. The end result of the process is one haploid oocyte and two or three polar bodies.

The Menstrual Cycle

The **menstrual cycle** is the "monthly" cycle of the female reproductive system. It spans 28 days on average, but the actual duration of the cycle varies from about 21 to 40 days. During this cycle, the ovaries and the uterus undergo changes, as do several key hormones (**Figure 15.11**). These changes are referred to as the *ovarian cycle* and the *uterine cycle,* but keep in mind that all of these changes are occurring at the same time, as part of one monthly cycle.

The Ovarian Cycle

The **ovarian cycle** is the sequence of events associated with maturation and release of an oocyte. The cycle has two main phases: the *follicular phase*, which lasts from day 1 to day 14, and the *luteal phase*. Ovulation, the release of the oocyte, marks the end of the follicular phase and the beginning of the luteal phase. These changes in the ovary are also illustrated in **Figure 15.12**.

Follicular Phase

Each month, several primordial follicles from each of the two ovaries develop into primary follicles. Gradually, one of the primary follicles becomes dominant. This means that only one follicle, from one ovary, develops fully and is released (ovulated) each month.

The maturation of the primordial follicles into one dominant *primary follicle* marks the initial stage of follicular development. The cells of the primary follicle surrounding the oocyte then divide. When these cells become more than one layer thick, they are called *granulosa* (gran-yoo-LOH-sa) *cells*; at this stage, the follicle is called a *secondary follicle*.

The secondary follicle grows and the oocyte develops a clear, extracellular glycoprotein coat called the *zona pellucida* (peh-LOO-si-da). Spaces filled with clear liquid begin to appear in the follicle, around the oocyte. The follicle is now called a *late secondary follicle*.

When the fluid-filled spaces in the follicle merge into a single, large, fluid-filled *antrum* (cavity), the follicle is called a *vesicular follicle*. As the follicle develops first into a late secondary follicle, and then into a vesicular follicle, the growing number of granulosa cells, triggered by FSH, secrete greater amounts of estrogen.

Figure 15.11C shows the steady rise of estrogen from day 5 to day 14. The rising estrogen level inhibits release of FSH from the hypothalamus during this time, which is why the FSH level decreases slightly from about day 6 to day 12. The large vesicular follicle now bulges against the ovarian wall (**Figure 15.12**, step 4).

At about this time, the pituitary gland starts to secrete more FSH and LH. The high level of LH causes the primary oocyte to complete its first meiotic division, and the secondary oocyte begins its second meiotic division.

The surge in LH then causes the bulging vesicular follicle to rupture the ovarian wall (**Figure 15.12**, step 5). The result is ovulation—the release of the secondary oocyte and a layer of surrounding cells, called the *corona radiata*, into the pelvic cavity. This release concludes the follicular phase of the ovarian cycle, and the luteal phase begins.

Luteal Phase

The oocyte normally is swept into the uterine tube by the vibrating cilia of the fimbriae. The remaining cells of the follicle, which are still in the ovary, form the **corpus luteum** (Latin for "yellow body"). LH, which surged during ovulation, helps stimulate formation of the corpus luteum. The disruption of the estrogen-secreting granulosa cells by ovulation causes blood estrogen levels to plummet after ovulation.

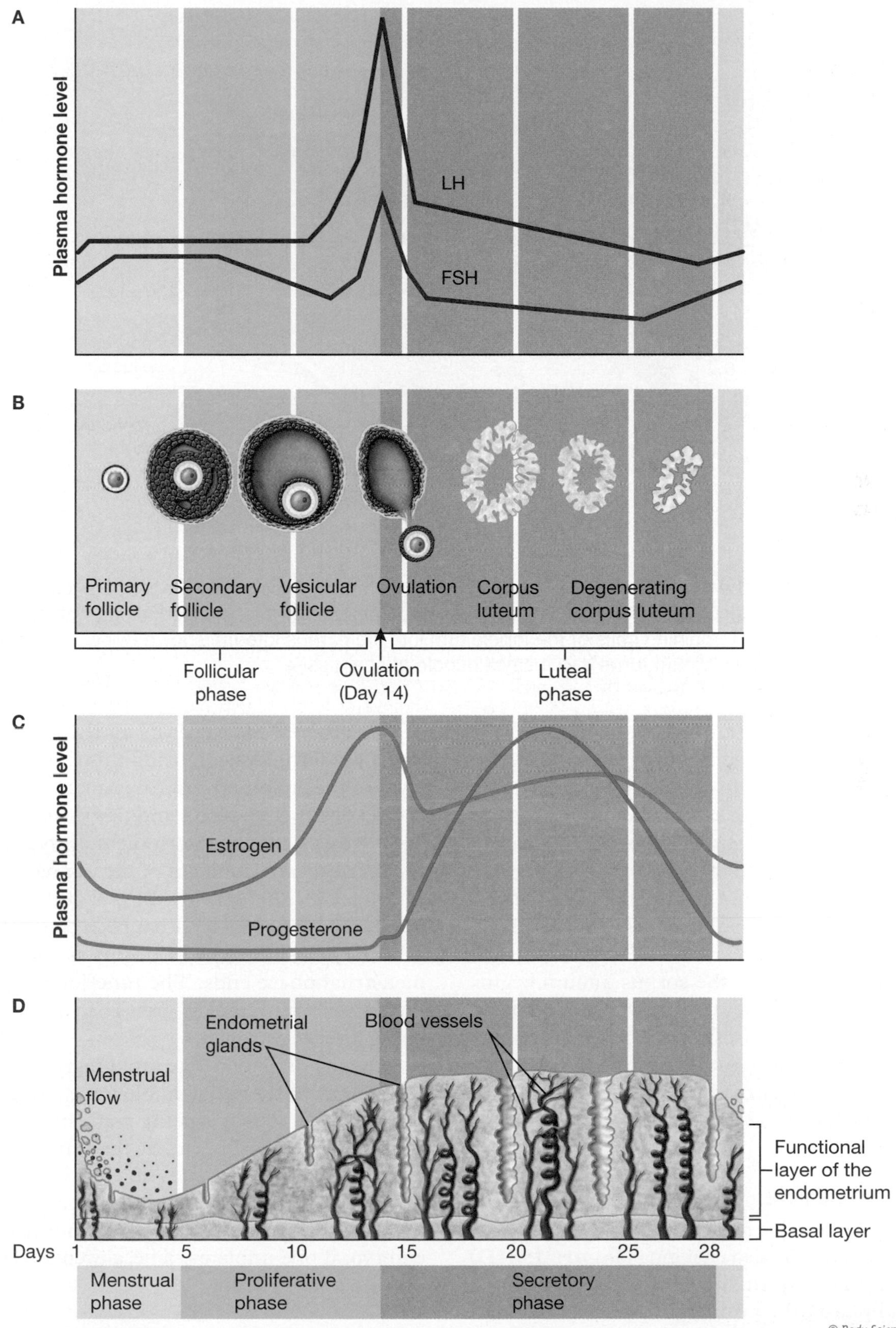

© Body Scientific International

Figure 15.11 Hormonal and structural changes during the female sexual cycle. The events of one complete female cycle, lasting about 28 days, are shown. The time scale, shown horizontally at the bottom, applies to all four panels of the figure. In these drawings, the ovulated oocyte is *not* fertilized. If it *were* fertilized, then the events of the second half of the cycle would be quite different for all four panels.

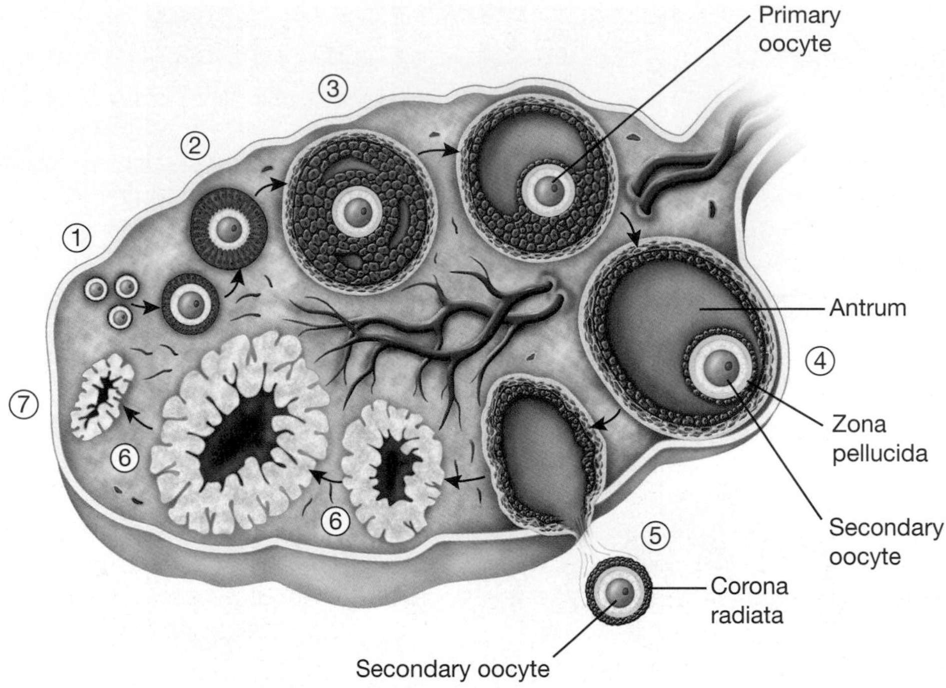

Figure 15.12 Changes in the ovary during the ovarian cycle. 1—Primary follicles. 2—Secondary follicle. 3—Late secondary follicle. 4—Vesicular follicle. 5—Ovulation. The secondary oocyte is released, along with surrounding corona radiata cells. 6—Remaining cells of the follicle turn into the corpus luteum (shown twice). 7—If fertilization does not occur, the corpus luteum turns into a small bundle of scar tissue.

The cells of the corpus luteum begin to secrete progesterone, and the progesterone level in the blood rises steadily during the early part of the luteal phase as the corpus luteum grows. The corpus luteum secretes modest amounts of estrogen, leading to a slight rebound of estrogen levels in the early part of the luteal phase. These changes in progesterone and estrogen levels are shown in **Figure 15.11C**.

After about 10 days, the corpus luteum begins to disintegrate if the oocyte has not been fertilized. This disintegration causes the progesterone and estrogen levels to drop in the late luteal phase. The corpus luteum turns into a small bundle of scar tissue called the *corpus albicans* (Latin for "white body").

The Uterine Cycle

While the ovaries are undergoing their changes, the uterus is also changing (**Figure 15.11D**). The three phases of the **uterine cycle** are the menstrual phase, the proliferative phase, and the secretory phase.

The *menstrual phase* lasts for the first four to five days of the cycle. During this time, the outer layer of the endometrium (the functional layer) breaks down. The blood and tissue that are lost during this stage pass from the uterus, through the cervical canal, and out of the vagina, producing the *menstrual discharge*. By the end of the menstrual phase, the functional layer has been completely shed.

The *proliferative phase* begins as soon as the menstrual phase ends. The functional layer of the endometrium rapidly grows back, aided by the rising level of estrogen.

During ovulation, the rapid regrowth of the endometrium slows down. Now the rising level of progesterone, which is being made by the corpus luteum in the ovaries, causes the functional layer of the endometrium to develop a dense network of blood vessels. The endometrium also develops nutrient-secreting glands that will nourish an embryo, if one implants. These events take place in the *secretory phase*.

LIFE SPAN DEVELOPMENT: *Female Reproductive System*

Menopause is the termination of the monthly female reproductive cycle, and with it comes the end of female reproductive capability. Menopause is a part of normal development. The age at menopause in the United States varies from the late 40s to the mid-50s. Smokers experience menopause approximately two years earlier than non-smokers.

The transition from regular monthly cycles to menopause occurs over two to eight years and is called *perimenopause.* During this time, the cycle duration and amount of monthly menstrual flow become more variable. The number of follicles in the ovaries, which is about 200,000 to 400,000 at puberty, decreases to about 25,000 by the late 30s, and to zero by the time of menopause, due to follicular degeneration. Many women experience hot flashes during perimenopause: an increase in skin temperature, local flushing, sweating, and increased heart rate for one to five minutes per episode. During peri- and post-menopause, glandular (milk-producing) tissue in the breast decreases in volume and is partly replaced with adipose and connective tissue.

The levels of estrogen and progesterone are very low after menopause. The decrease in circulating estrogen is associated with a loss of bone mass, increased risk for osteoporosis, a rise in LDL ("bad cholesterol"), a decrease in HDL ("good cholesterol"), and an increase in the risk of cardiovascular disease. Estrogen-replacement therapy, also known as *hormone replacement therapy,* can reduce the symptoms of menopause and the risk of osteoporosis, but it increases the risk of breast cancer and heart disease.

Life Span Review

1. At what approximate age do females in the United States undergo menopause?
2. What effect does menopause have on the female hormones estrogen and progesterone?

If fertilization does not occur, the corpus luteum begins to disintegrate, and the progesterone level in the blood falls. As a result, the blood vessels in the functional layer deteriorate, leading to tissue breakdown and bleeding. Thus, a new cycle begins.

Female Sexual Response

As with males, sexual excitement in females activates neural reflexes from the sympathetic and parasympathetic divisions of the autonomic nervous system. Sexual stimulation, which can involve psychological and tactile (touch) stimuli, activates parasympathetic nerves to the erectile tissue of the clitoris, which becomes engorged with blood. In addition, autonomic nerves activate smooth muscle fibers in the nipple, causing it to become erect. Increases in both vestibular gland and vaginal wall secretions stimulate production of lubricating fluid that facilitates intercourse.

Orgasm is marked by intense pleasure and rhythmic contraction of smooth muscle in the reproductive tract that may help move sperm toward the oocyte. In females, orgasm is not required for conception. In males, however, orgasm and associated ejaculation are required for successful delivery of sperm and fertilization.

Check Your Understanding

1. What is oogenesis?
2. What event triggers completion of the second meiotic division of the oocyte?
3. What are the two main phases of the ovarian cycle?
4. Why does FSH level decrease from day 6 to day 12 of the ovarian cycle?
5. What happens to the corpus luteum if the oocyte has not been fertilized within 10 days of ovulation?

LESSON 15.3 Review and Assessment

Mini Glossary

Make sure that you know the meaning of each key term.

cervix the narrow, lower end of the uterus that has the opening through which a baby passes during childbirth

clitoris a cylindrical body of erectile tissue that lies at the anterior end of the vulva

corpus luteum the remaining cells of the follicle, which are still in the ovary after an oocyte is released into the pelvic cavity during ovulation

labia majora two skin folds posterior to the mons pubis that lie parallel on either side of the vaginal opening

labia minora a smaller set of skin folds inside the labia majora

lactiferous duct a duct through which milk is secreted and which opens at the nipple

mammary glands the milk-producing glands in the female

menopause the termination of the monthly female reproductive cycle

menstrual cycle a hormone-driven cycle of changes to the ovaries and uterus that lasts roughly 28 days and includes both the ovarian cycle and the uterine cycle

oocyte egg cell

oogenesis the process by which oocytes, or female gametes, are generated

ovarian cycle the sequence of events associated with maturation and release of an oocyte

ovaries the primary female reproductive organs, in which gametes are made

ovulation the release of an oocyte, or egg, from the ovarian follicle

uterine cycle the monthly cycle of changes that the uterus undergoes; includes the menstrual, proliferative, and secretory phases

uterine tubes tubes in which the oocyte is fertilized; begin at the lateral end of the ovary and go up and around the ovary to terminate at the top lateral portion of the uterus

uterus a hollow, muscular organ located in front of the rectum and behind the bladder; the womb

vagina a thin-walled, tubular structure below the uterus; birth canal

Know and Understand

1. Explain how the female reproductive system is organized, including subdivisions of each component.
2. What does each follicle in an ovary contain?
3. Where does the uterine tube begin and end?
4. What is an ectopic pregnancy, and why is it a medical emergency?
5. What is the narrow lower end of the uterus called?
6. Describe the anatomy of the vulva.
7. What is the function of the female mammary glands?
8. What sequence of events occurs during the ovarian cycle?
9. List the names of the uterine cycle phases, and describe what occurs during each phase.

Analyze and Apply

10. Analyze the similarities and differences between the ovarian and uterine cycles.
11. Compare and contrast the three phases of the uterine cycle.
12. Menopause is a natural occurrence for every female, but it can also occur due to factors other than age. Conduct research on this topic if necessary, and then describe factors other than aging that can result in menopause.
13. What triggers the female menstrual cycle?
14. Compare the functions of the female reproductive system with those of the male reproductive system.

IN THE LAB

15. Since the female duct system is open at the ovary, what moves the oocyte from the ovary to the uterus where it implants? Using four different colors of clay, create models of these four structures: uterus, uterine tube (with fimbriae), ovary, and oocyte. Arrange your models as they appear in **Figure 15.7**. Demonstrate how an oocyte is swept into the uterine tube and into the uterus. Explain what can happen to the oocyte when it is not captured by the fimbriae.
16. Compare and discuss mammary glands and their functions in humans and animals. Choose three animals to use in your comparison. Form a hypothesis about the breast milk from each. Next, analyze the composition of human breast milk and that of the animals you have chosen. Look for differences and similarities, and think about why they may exist. Publish your results in a research documentation format. Pay close attention to correct spelling, grammar, and format.

LESSON 15.4

Fertilization, Pregnancy, and Birth

Before You Read

Try to answer the following questions before you read this lesson.

- What is the placenta, and how does it help the embryo and fetus develop?
- What are the stages of labor?

Lesson Objectives

- Describe the events that lead to fertilization of an oocyte.
- Describe the physiological changes that occur in the mother and developing child during pregnancy.
- Explain the sequence of events involved in childbirth.
- Explain how breast milk is produced and secreted.

Key Terms

amniotic fluid	human chorionic gonadotropin (hCG)
blastocyst	implantation
capacitation	lactation
dilation	let-down reflex
embryo	parturition
expulsion	placenta
fetus	umbilical cord
gestation	
gestational age	

As explained earlier in this chapter, the process of bringing a new child into the world begins when a male gamete unites with a female gamete. This lesson describes the events that occur from fertilization through childbirth.

Fertilization of the Oocyte

Fertilization occurs when the chromosomes of the oocyte and the sperm unite to produce a zygote, the first cell of a new individual. As explained in Lesson 15.1, each gamete—the oocyte and the sperm—has 23 chromosomes. Thus, fusion of the gametes produces a zygote with a full set of 46 chromosomes.

An ovulated oocyte can live for, at most, about 24 hours before it is fertilized. If the ovulated oocyte is not fertilized within this time frame, it dies. By contrast, sperm can live for up to 5 days in the female reproductive tract. This means that for fertilization to be successful, intercourse must occur no more than 5 days before ovulation and no more than 24 hours after ovulation.

The Journey of the Sperm

During a single act of intercourse, as many as several hundred million sperm are deposited in the vagina. If a sperm had a mind, there would be only one thing on it: find the egg and fertilize it.

Each sperm's flagellum wiggles back and forth, propelling the sperm through the female reproductive tract. The oocyte, if present, will be in the distal third of the uterine tube, which is as far as it will have advanced during its one day of viability. Thus, the sperm must travel from the vagina to the cervical canal, through the cervical canal to the uterus, through the uterus to the uterine tube, and then along the uterine tube to the oocyte.

Many sperm are lost at each stage of the journey. Some sperm leak out of the vagina, and many others do not encounter the cervical opening. Of those that do enter the uterus, most do not make it to the uterine tube that contains an oocyte at the other end. Eventually, a few thousand sperm may reach the oocyte. Although sperm can make this journey of 4 to 6 inches (10 to 15 cm) within 5 to 10 minutes, they require as much as 10 hours in the female reproductive tract for capacitation.

Capacitation (ka-pas-i-TAY-shun) is the process by which sperm becomes able to penetrate and fertilize an oocyte. Each sperm contains at the tip of its head a bundle of *acrosomal* (ak-roh-SOHM-al) *enzymes* that allow it to digest the protective glycoproteins surrounding the oocyte. When sperm first arrive in the vagina, this package of enzymes is well shielded from accidental release by a cell membrane thickened with extra cholesterol. The sperm are unable to fertilize the oocyte until the protective cap is worn away by contact with the fluids of the female, a process that takes up to 10 hours.

Sperm Penetration

When a sperm reaches the oocyte, contact with the oocyte's zona pellucida induces release of the acrosomal enzymes, which start to bore a hole toward the oocyte membrane (**Figure 15.13**). The acrosomal enzymes of hundreds of sperm are required to drill holes all the way through the zona pellucida. Eventually, a late-arriving sperm moves through the holes in the zona pellucida and binds to specific receptors on the oocyte membrane. This binding causes the membranes of the two cells to join together, and the nucleus of the sperm, which contains the sperm's chromosomes, enters the cytoplasm of the oocyte.

Protection against Polyspermy

If more than one sperm succeeds in penetrating the oocyte—an outcome called *polyspermy* ("many sperm")—the oocyte will have too many chromosomes and will not survive. The body has a system to protect against this possibility by figuratively "closing the door" as soon as one sperm merges with it.

Sperm entry causes sodium channels in the cell membrane to open, which results in the entry of sodium into the oocyte and the release of stored calcium ions from the oocyte. The rise in calcium in the cell reactivates meiosis, which was arrested partway through the second meiotic division. The rise in calcium also triggers the release of chemicals into the space just outside the oocyte. These chemicals react with water to form a protective shield around the oocyte. The net effect of the sodium entry, the calcium release, and the chemical reaction is to prevent additional sperm from fertilizing the oocyte.

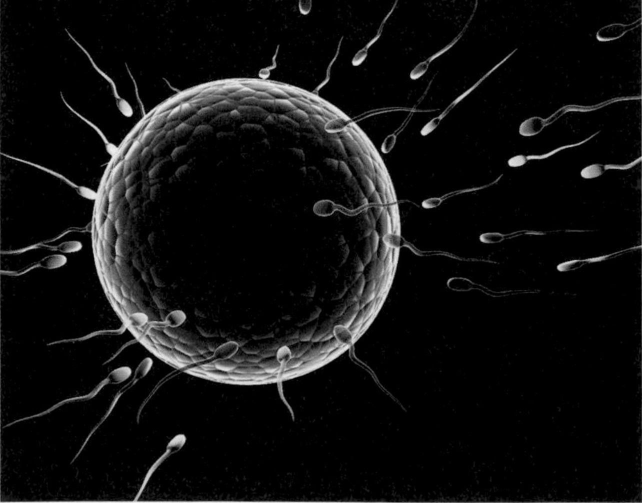

Nejron Photo/Shutterstock.com

Figure 15.13 Sperm attempting to penetrate an oocyte. *What enables sperm to penetrate the cell membrane of an egg?*

Completion of Meiosis and Fertilization

Completion of the second meiotic division of the oocyte generates two haploid daughter cells: a tiny, nonviable (nonfunctional) polar body, and the rest of the oocyte. The nuclear membranes of the sperm and the oocyte then dissolve, and their chromosomes intermingle. Fertilization is now complete. The oocyte and the sperm have become a zygote.

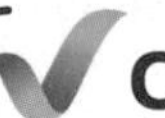

Check Your Understanding

1. What is the first cell of a new individual called?
2. When must intercourse occur for fertilization to be successful?
3. How is sperm propelled through the female reproductive tract?
4. How long can an ovulated, but unfertilized, oocyte live?
5. How far, in inches, does sperm travel to reach an oocyte?

Pregnancy

Pregnancy, or **gestation**, is the period from fertilization to birth. It lasts approximately 265 days. It is conventional to measure pregnancy duration from the first day of the last menstrual period because that is a date that the woman is likely to know. When measured this way, the typical duration of pregnancy is about 280 days, or 40 weeks, or 9 months plus 1 week.

From Fertilization to Implantation

After the zygote has been formed (**Figure 15.14B**), it continues its slow movement toward the uterus. During its 4- to 5-day trip in the uterine tube, the zygote divides without changing its overall size. Thus, it develops a larger number of smaller cells.

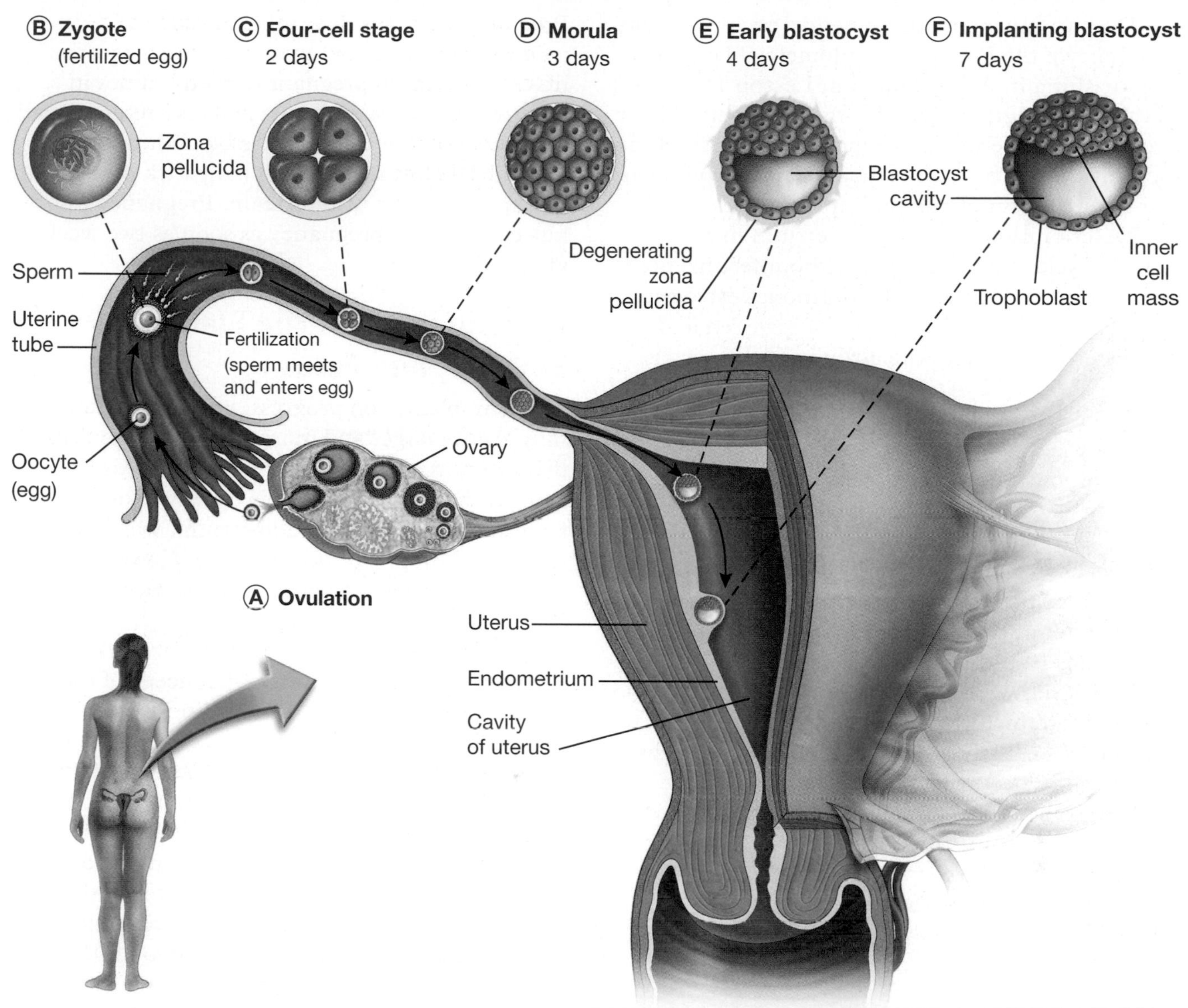

© Body Scientific International

Figure 15.14 Ovulation to fertilization to implantation. A—An oocyte is released from the ovary. B—The egg is fertilized by a sperm. The zygote divides by mitosis. C—The embryo reaches the four-cell stage. D—The embryo becomes a morula, a solid ball of cells. E—A fluid-filled cavity develops in the embryo, now called a *blastocyst*. F—The blastocyst implants on the endometrium.

As **Figure 15.14D** shows, 3 days after fertilization the zygote is a solid ball of 16 cells called a *morula*. By day 4, a **blastocyst** (BLAS-toh-sist), or fluid-filled cavity, develops inside the ball of cells. The blastocyst enters the uterine cavity and sheds the zona pellucida. Cell division continues, and by day 7 the blastocyst develops an inner cell mass and a thin layer of surrounding *trophoblast* (TROH-foh-blast) *cells*. At this point, the endometrium is at the peak of its development: it has grown thick and full of blood vessels to nourish an embryo and fetus.

As **Figure 15.11D** shows, peak development of the endometrium occurs around day 15 of the uterine cycle. **Implantation**, the binding of the blastocyst to the endometrium, begins around this time. The blastocyst gradually burrows into the endometrium, and the nearby endometrial cells proliferate, or grow quickly in number. In 5 days (now 12 days after fertilization), the blastocyst is fully embedded in the endometrium. Implantation is complete, and the blastocyst becomes known as an **embryo**.

Despite implantation, a potential problem awaits the embryo: the loss of the endometrial layer that is nourishing it. As explained in Lesson 15.3—and as shown in **Figure 15.11D**—the endometrial layer begins to degenerate at around day 27 or 28 of the monthly cycle. This is 13 or 14 days after fertilization, just after the completion of implantation.

Deterioration of the endometrium in a normal cycle (that is, a cycle without fertilization) results from a decline in the hormones estrogen and progesterone. The decline of estrogen and progesterone is due to the atrophy of the corpus luteum at the end of the month.

If the endometrial layer were to be shed, as it usually is during this phase of the cycle, then the embryo would be lost. This does not happen, however, because the trophoblast cells secrete a hormone called **human chorionic gonadotropin** (kor-ee-ON-ik goh-na-doh-TROH-pin) **(hCG)**, which prevents atrophy of the corpus luteum. The corpus luteum continues to secrete progesterone and estrogen so that the endometrium is not shed.

The levels of hCG, estrogen, and progesterone in the blood during pregnancy are shown in **Figure 15.15**. The rise in estrogen and progesterone after week 12 occurs because the placenta (discussed in the next section) develops and starts to secrete these hormones. At the same time, hCG secretion diminishes and the corpus luteum, which has completed its mission, atrophies.

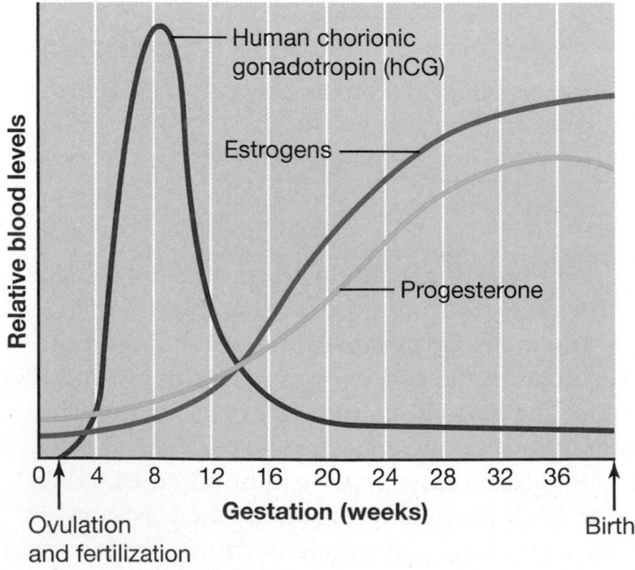

Figure 15.15 Hormone levels in the mother's blood during pregnancy. *How do pregnancy test kits work?*

Pregnancy test kits determine whether hCG is present in the urine. Such tests work because hCG is present in pregnant women but not in nonpregnant women. When hCG is present, small amounts "spill over" from the blood into the urine. Most kits require that a dipstick or test strip be exposed to the urine stream. Pregnancy test kits can detect a pregnancy as soon as two weeks after conception.

Development of the Placenta, Embryo, and Fetus

As implantation progresses, the inner cell mass grows larger and more complex as its cells divide and rearrange. When the embryo is tiny, it can get the nutrients it needs by simple diffusion from the tissue of the endometrium, which has a rich blood supply for this purpose. However, as the embryo grows, it needs more nutrients than the endometrium can supply.

The **placenta** is the organ that grows in the uterus to meet the nutritional needs of the embryo, which is called a **fetus** after 8 weeks of development. The placenta of a 13-week-old fetus, shown in **Figure 15.16**, contains cells of the fetus and cells of the mother. The placenta spreads out like a pancake on the wall of the uterus.

The placenta contains intertwining blood vessels from the cardiovascular systems of the fetus and the mother. The cardiovascular system is the first organ system of the embryo to function in a meaningful way. Just three and one-half weeks after fertilization, when the embryo is only one-quarter inch (6 mm) long, the immature heart begins to pump newly formed blood cells through newly formed blood vessels. Neither the embryo nor the fetus can receive oxygen (O_2) or expel carbon dioxide (CO_2) by breathing, and neither can obtain nourishment by eating. The placenta takes care of these needs.

Fetal vessels carry blood, pumped by the fetal heart, through the **umbilical cord** to and from the placenta. In the placenta, fetal capillaries are surrounded by cavities filled with maternal blood. The maternal and fetal blood do not actually mix; however, the thin layer of cells that separates them allows easy diffusion of nutrients from maternal blood to fetal blood, and diffusion of wastes in the reverse direction. Unfortunately, alcohol or drugs, if present in the mother's blood, also reach the fetus by this pathway and affect its development.

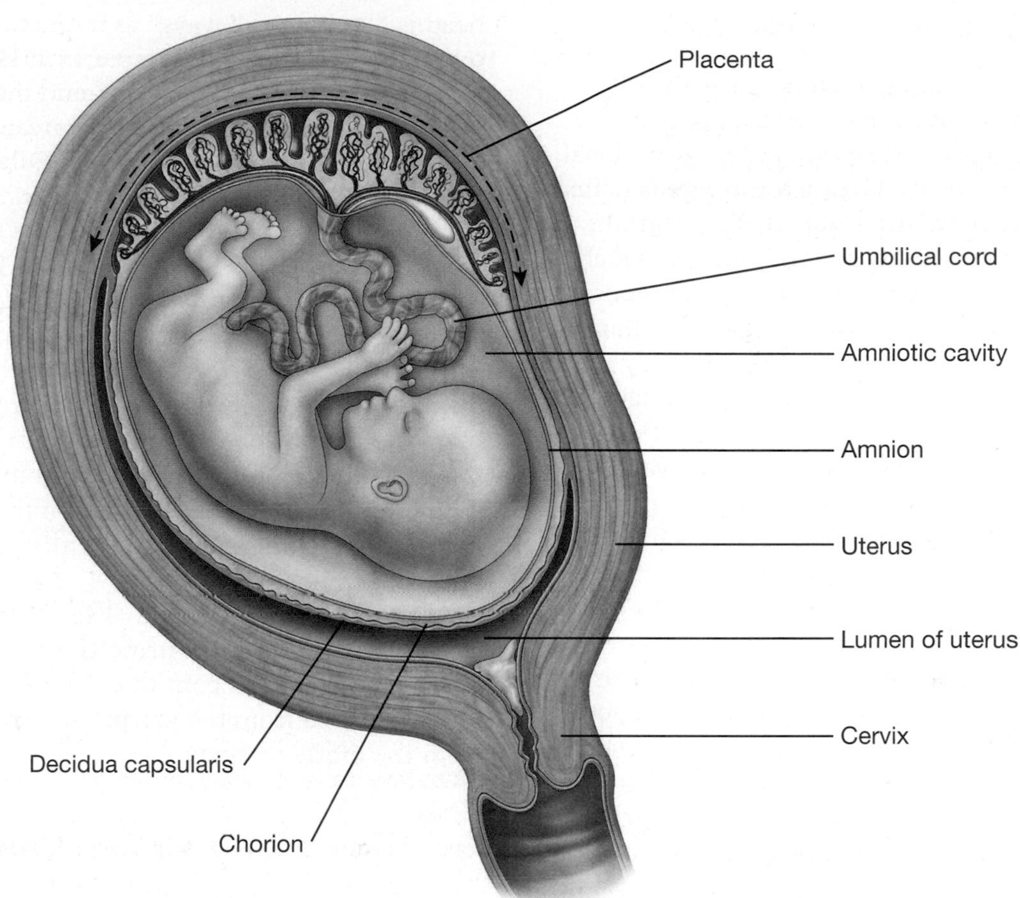

Figure 15.16 A 13-week-old fetus (end of first trimester). The fetus is about 10 centimeters long (crown to rump). The placenta is attached to the wall of the uterus. The fetus is bathed in amniotic fluid contained in a sac whose layers are (from inner to outer) the amnion, the chorion, and the decidua capsularis. *The placenta takes over for what structure in providing nourishment to the embryo?*

As **Figure 15.16** shows, the fetus fills up the uterine cavity by week 13. It is surrounded by a set of membranes and bathed in clear **amniotic** (am-nee-AHT-ik) **fluid**. The inner membrane of its sac is called the *amnion*. Outside the amnion is the *chorion*, which, like the amnion, is derived from the fetal tissue. The outermost membrane is called the *decidua capsularis* (Latin for "capsule that falls off, or sheds"); this membrane is derived from the mother's tissue. The umbilical cord, which contains two arteries and one vein, connects the fetus to the placenta.

Obstetrical ultrasound is widely used to monitor fetal development and to diagnose abnormalities in pregnancy and development. Ultrasound in the first trimester, or 13 weeks of gestational age, is important for confirming that a normal pregnancy is occurring in the uterus and for ruling out possible problems, such as ectopic pregnancy. The measurement of crown-rump length in the first trimester can be used to estimate fetal age, with an accuracy of about 5 days. In the second trimester, fetal age and expected due date are best estimated with ultrasound by measuring the femur length, head circumference, biparietal (transverse head) diameter, and abdominal diameter.

Check Your Understanding

1. How long is gestation when measured from the first day of the last menstrual period?
2. What is the term for the process by which the blastocyst binds to the endometrium?
3. At what point in its development does the embryo become a fetus?
4. Which organ system is the first to function in a meaningful way in an embryo?

Childbirth

Childbirth, or **parturition** (part-uh-RISH-un), normally occurs when the fetus is 36 to 40 weeks old. This corresponds to a "gestational age" of 38 to 42 weeks. **Gestational age** is defined as the time since the first day of the pregnant woman's last menstrual period. This is a widely used clinical measure of the duration of pregnancy. Gestational age is about two weeks more than actual fetal age, because conception typically occurs about two weeks after the first day of the last menstrual period.

Toward the end of gestation, high levels of estrogen and progesterone cause the uterine muscle cells to become more sensitive to oxytocin (ahk-see-TOH-sin), a hormone that plays a key role in labor. Oxytocin is released by the pituitary glands of both the fetus and the mother.

Fetal oxytocin causes the placenta to release the hormone *relaxin* and *prostaglandins*, lipid compounds that trigger uterine muscle contractions. Once the uterine muscle has started to contract, the baby's head is pushed into the cervical opening, causing mechanical receptors to be stretched there. These receptors send messages to the brain that stimulate maternal oxytocin release, causing even more vigorous contractions of the uterine muscle and even greater stretching of the cervical receptors. This is an example of physiological *positive feedback*: an action triggers a response that, in turn, causes the original action to occur with greater strength and frequency.

Stages of Labor

The stages of labor are dilation, expulsion, and delivery of the placenta. When the time for birth arrives, most fetuses are in the head-down position, called the *vertex presentation*. The vertex presentation, which causes the baby's head to exit the mother's body first, is shown in **Figure 15.17**. A rump-first position, or *breech presentation*, makes delivery much more difficult.

The **dilation** stage begins with uterine contractions and ends with a full widening of the cervical canal. In early dilation (**Figure 15.17A**), the cervix is several centimeters dilated, and the baby's head is "looking sideways" as it enters the pelvic outlet. In late dilation (**Figure 15.17B**), the cervix is fully dilated (10 centimeters), and the baby's head starts to rotate to a "looking-to-the-rear" orientation as it moves deeper into the pelvis. Dilation, which can last from 6 to 12 hours or longer, is usually the longest part of labor.

The **expulsion** stage (**Figure 15.17C**), the period from full dilation to delivery of the baby, lasts less than an hour in most cases. Strong contractions of the uterus, each lasting a minute or longer, occur at two- to three-minute intervals, forcing the baby's head out. Once the head has emerged, the rest of the body usually follows quickly. The baby is still connected to the mother by the umbilical cord, which is clamped and cut.

Delivery of the placenta (**Figure 15.17D**) is the last stage of birth. During this stage, strong uterine contractions continue, causing detachment of the placenta from the uterine wall and expulsion from the mother's body.

Check Your Understanding

1. What are the stages of labor?
2. Describe the difference between vertex presentation and breech presentation during the delivery of a baby.

Lactation

Lactation is the production of milk by the mother. Breast milk is an important source of nutrition for the developing infant. It contains amino acids, fats, carbohydrates, and vitamins that are well absorbed by the infant's digestive system. Breast milk also contains antibodies from the mother that help protect the infant from infection while its own immune system is immature. Successful lactation requires activation of the normally inactive milk-producing cells of the mammary gland, as well as delivery of the milk through ducts to the baby. The two processes are regulated by two different hormones.

Umbilical cord
Placenta
Uterus
Vagina
Cervix
A

Pubic symphysis
Sacrum
B

C

Uterus
Placenta (detaching)
Umbilical cord
D

© Body Scientific International

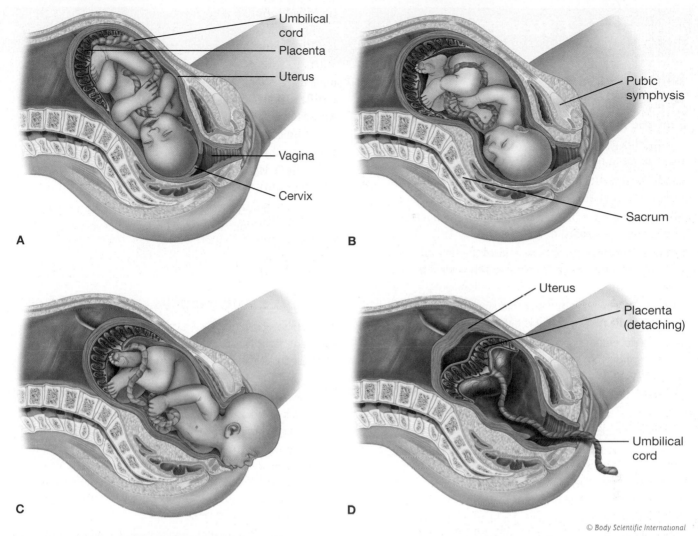

Figure 15.17 The stages of labor. A—Early dilation. B—Late dilation. C—Expulsion. D—Delivery of the placenta. *About how wide is the typical cervix when it is fully dilated?*

Late in pregnancy, high levels of estrogen and progesterone stimulate the hypothalamus in the brain to produce *prolactin-releasing factor*, a hormone that triggers the release of the hormone prolactin from the pituitary gland. Prolactin stimulates the secretory cells of the mammary glands to produce milk.

Following birth, the infant suckling at the nipple activates receptors that trigger the release of the hormone oxytocin from the mother's pituitary. Oxytocin, which was also important for labor and delivery, causes the **let-down reflex**—the contraction of smooth muscle cells in the mammary glands, which allows milk to be squeezed toward and out of the nipple.

Check Your Understanding

1. What is the term for the production of milk by the mother?
2. Briefly explain the mechanism that triggers milk production.

LESSON 15.4 Review and Assessment

Mini Glossary

Make sure that you know the meaning of each key term.

amniotic fluid a clear fluid in which the embryo, and then the fetus, is suspended

blastocyst a fluid-filled cavity

capacitation the process by which sperm becomes able to penetrate and fertilize an oocyte

dilation the stage of labor during which the opening of the cervix dilates, or widens

embryo the developing human from the time of implantation to the end of the eighth week after conception

expulsion the stage of labor that starts at full dilation and ends when the baby is delivered

fetus a developing human from eight weeks after conception to birth

gestation the period of human development between fertilization and birth

gestational age time since the first day of a woman's last menstrual period before pregnancy

human chorionic gonadotropin (hCG) a hormone secreted by the trophoblast cells of the embryo that prevents deterioration of the corpus luteum and stimulates progesterone production in the placenta

implantation the binding of the blastocyst to the endometrium

lactation secretion of milk by the mammary glands

let-down reflex contraction of smooth muscle cells in the mammary glands that allows milk to be squeezed toward and out of the nipple

parturition childbirth

placenta the organ that grows in the uterus to meet the nutritional needs of the embryo and fetus

umbilical cord the cord that connects the fetus to the placenta

Know and Understand

1. Describe what occurs during capacitation.
2. How is sperm able to penetrate the zona pellucida of the oocyte?
3. What is polyspermy, and how is it prevented?
4. What is human chorionic gonadotropin hormone, and what is its purpose?
5. Which hormones are secreted by the placenta?
6. How do the embryo and, later, the fetus receive oxygen and nutrients, and how do they expel carbon dioxide and waste?
7. What does breast milk contain that makes it an important source of nutrition for the developing infant?
8. What is the let-down reflex?

Analyze and Apply

9. How is childbirth—in particular, the roles of fetal and maternal oxytocin—an example of a positive feedback system?
10. Events in hospitals, including childbirth, are documented using a 24-hour notation, often called *military time*. This differs from the time notation people usually use, which is based on a 12-hour clock. For example, in the 12-hour system, there is a 1:00 AM and a 1:00 PM. In 24-hour notation, these same times are noted as 0100 and 1300. Conduct research to find out more about military time, and write a report explaining why this system is used in healthcare.
11. You are a doctor with a patient who is reluctant to breast-feed her newborn infant. What would you say to convince her of the benefits of breast feeding?
12. Assume that you are a childbirth educator and you must explain childbirth to your class of newly pregnant women. What would you say? Would you use any props? If so, what?
13. Do you think the infant experiences any pain or distress when the umbilical cord is clamped and cut after birth? Explain.
14. Obstetrical ultrasound is widely used to monitor fetal development and to diagnose abnormalities in pregnancy and development. Conduct research to determine which parts of the fetal anatomy can be seen and checked using this method.

IN THE LAB

15. Diffusion is movement of material from a place where it is concentrated to a place where it is less concentrated. This occurs in the placenta when nutrients pass from maternal blood, through a layer of cells, and into fetal blood. Using the membrane that separates an eggshell from the egg white, demonstrate the process of diffusion through a membrane.

    Materials: 2 raw eggs, 1 to 2 L of white vinegar, 3 beakers (one 1,000 mL and two 250 mL), 100 mL of corn syrup, 100 mL of distilled water, a food scale, measuring tape, and plastic wrap.

    Procedure: Place the uncracked eggs in the 1,000 mL beaker and cover with vinegar. Set aside. After four days, very gently rinse the eggs with cool water until the shells dissolve. Measure and record the weight, length, and circumference of each egg. Then place each egg in a 250 mL beaker. Cover one with distilled water and the other with corn syrup. Set aside. After one day, rinse off the eggs and measure them again. Describe your observations about the change in the size of each egg before and after soaking. In which direction is diffusion occurring in each instance?

16. Develop a better appreciation for embryonic and fetal growth by making life-size models of the embryo and fetus at different ages.

    Materials: About 2.5 pounds (at least 1.1 kg) of modeling clay or Play-Doh® or home-made playdough (search online for "homemade playdough recipe"), ruler, scale or balance that can measure with 1-gram accuracy.

    Procedure: The table in **Figure 15.18** shows the length and weight of the embryo and fetus at different gestational ages. Make models of the embryo and fetus at each age that have the correct length, weight, and shape. (For shape, find images online.) Work collaboratively with other students to make models for every other week, through 22 weeks of gestational age.

    Modeling clay has a density of about 2 grams per cubic centimeter (g/cc). Play-Doh has a density of about 1.2–1.3 g/cc. Embryonic and fetal density is about 1 g/cc. Therefore, the models will have somewhat smaller volumes than a fetus of the same weight. In other words, the models will be a bit on the skinny side, although the weights are correct. To make models with the right volume, increase the weight of the model, at each age, by a factor of 2 or 1.3, for modeling clay or Play-Doh respectively.

Embryo/Fetus Statistics

Gestational age (weeks)	8	10	12	14	16	18	20	22
Weight (grams)	1	4	15	45	100	190	300	430
Length* (mm)	15	30	55	90	120	140	260	280

* The crown-to-rump length is shown for weeks 6 through 18 because the legs are underdeveloped and curled up under the body in early life. At weeks 20 and 22, the crown-to-heel length is shown.

Figure 15.18 *Goodheart-Willcox Publisher*

LESSON 15.5

Disorders and Diseases of the Reproductive Systems

Before You Read

Try to answer the following questions before you read this lesson.

- Why are some people, either male and female, infertile?
- What types of cancer affect the reproductive system?

Lesson Objectives

- Describe common causes of male and female infertility.
- Identify common sexually transmitted diseases, and describe their symptoms and treatments.
- Identify cancers that affect the reproductive system.

Key Terms

amenorrhea
chlamydia
endometriosis
genital herpes
gonorrhea
human papillomavirus (HPV)
impotence
infertility
pelvic inflammatory disease (PID)
sexually transmitted infection (STI)
uterine fibroids

CLINICAL CASE STUDY

Jenna, age 28, goes to her primary care provider because she cannot get pregnant. She and her husband have been trying for almost a year. She reports that her menstrual periods are irregular and infrequent. Her body mass index is 31 kg/m^2. When asked by the PCP, Jenna says she had laser hair removal for her upper lip and chin a few years ago. A blood sample is obtained. The blood chemistry analysis shows an above-normal level of LH and a normal level of FSH. Her testosterone level is above normal for a female, and her progesterone level is normal. Her fasting levels of insulin and glucose are above normal. All other hormone levels are normal. A pregnancy test confirms that she is not pregnant.

The PCP refers Jenna to a medical imaging center to get an ultrasound of her ovaries. As you read this section, try to determine the answers to the following questions.

1. What condition does Jenna probably have?
2. What other aspects of Jenna's presentation are notable?
3. Why was Jenna referred to an imaging center for ultrasound of her ovaries?
4. What treatment options are available for Jenna?

Disorders of the human reproductive system impair the ability to reproduce. Infertility is one common reproductive disorder. Also, because the male and female reproductive systems are open to the outside environment, they are vulnerable to infection and disease. Reproductive system diseases, including those that are sexually transmitted, require immediate medical attention because they can easily be spread to healthy individuals. Cancers of the reproductive system are among the most prevalent of all cancers. This lesson describes common disorders and diseases of the male and female reproductive systems, their signs and symptoms, and their treatments. Additional disorders are described in the table in **Figure 5.19**.

Infertility

Infertility is the inability to get pregnant. It is defined clinically as the inability of a couple to conceive after at least one year of unprotected intercourse. Infertility may be due to either male or female causes (**Figure 15.20**).

Male Infertility

Two common causes of male infertility are insufficient healthy-sperm count and the inability to release sperm. An insufficient quantity of healthy sperm, often called *low sperm count*, has numerous possible causes, many of which are treatable. These causes include abnormal levels of the hormones that regulate sperm production

Diseases and Disorders of the Reproductive Systems

	Etiology	Prevention	Pathology	Diagnosis	Treatment
Endometriosis	growth of endometrial tissue outside of the uterus	none	painful intercourse, menstrual periods, and/or bowel movements; heavy menstrual bleeding; fatigue; nausea	physical exam; laparoscopy and biopsy; MRI; ultrasound	pain medication; hormone therapy; surgery, if needed
Dysmenorrhea (painful menstruation)	abdominal cramps may be due to elevated prostaglandin levels or sensitivity	stop smoking; regular exercise	cramps before and during period; nausea; headaches; dizziness	history and physical exam; ultrasound; imaging; laparoscopy	pain relievers (NSAIDs); oral birth control; surgery; alternative therapies
Vaginal yeast infection (Candidiasis)	fungal infection of vulva and/or vagina	wear loose cotton underwear and no tight pants at the crotch; minimize antibiotics; keep area dry and unscented	vaginal rash; pain; discharge; itching; burning; swelling	pelvic exam and test of secretions	antifungal medication
Trichomoniasis	parasitic STI	practice safe sexual intercourse; use condoms correctly	foul-smelling vaginal or penile discharge; genital itching; painful urination	microscopic examination of vaginal fluid (females) or urine (males); rapid antigen tests; nucleic acid amplification tests	medication (metronidazole or Tindamax)
Syphilis	bacterial STI; can be passed from mother to child at childbirth	practice safe sexual intercourse; avoid recreational drugs	primary: painless sore on genitals, rectum, or mouth; secondary: rash, muscle aches, fever, swollen lymph nodes; latent: no symptoms; tertiary: damage to brain, nerves, eyes, heart, and other organs, and death	blood tests; lumbar puncture to test CSF	penicillin
Erectile dysfunction	frequent inability to attain or maintain an erection for sexual intercourse	exercise; stop smoking; reduce or eliminate alcohol intake; reduce stress	lack of sexual desire; inability to attain or maintain an erection	history and physical exam, including psychological; blood test; urine test; ultrasound	medication; penis pumps/surgery; exercise; counseling; alternative therapies

Figure 15.19

Goodheart-Willcox Publisher

(LH and FSH); chronic, warm temperature of the testes, which need to be somewhat below normal body temperature for optimum sperm production; smoking; heavy use of alcohol, cocaine, or marijuana; use of anabolic steroids (body-building drugs); exposure to environmental toxins; and older age. If infertility is related to low sperm count—as is frequently the case—further investigation often can help determine a cause, and, if applicable, appropriate treatment can be given.

The inability to release sperm can be caused by impotence or damage to the ducts that convey sperm and other components of semen. **Impotence**, or the inability to maintain an erection, is also called *erectile dysfunction (ED)*. Causes of ED include damage to the nerves or blood vessels of erectile tissues, side effects of some medications, prostate surgery, older age, stress, and psychological factors. The male duct system can be damaged by injury or by scarring from disease.

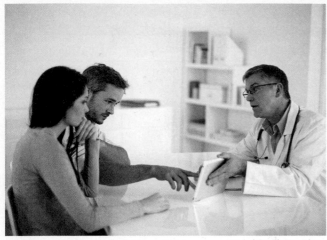

Jack Frog/Shutterstock.com

Figure 15.20 Doctors may recommend that couples make lifestyle changes to increase their chances of pregnancy. *What recommendations might they make?*

Female Infertility

Causes of female infertility include failure to ovulate, inability of the egg to reach the uterine tube and travel to the uterus, and inability of the blastocyst to implant successfully on the endometrium.

Failure to ovulate is usually accompanied by abnormal menstrual periods—either a complete absence of menstrual periods, called **amenorrhea** (a-mehn-oh-REE-a), or cycles of unusual or unpredictable length. Failure to ovulate is often associated with abnormal levels of FSH or LH, or both. Causes include polycystic ovarian syndrome (PCOS) and abnormalities of the pituitary gland, which secretes FSH and LH or the hypothalamus, which secretes GnRH. Other causes of failure to ovulate include scarring of the ovaries, failure of the mature follicle to rupture, and premature menopause.

Inability of the oocyte to enter and make it through the uterine tube usually results from scarring and damage to the tube. Uterine tube damage can be caused by diseases of the reproductive tract (usually sexually transmitted diseases); abdominal cavity infection (appendicitis, for example); previous surgery, which can cause scarring or *adhesions* (areas where tissues stick together inappropriately); ectopic pregnancy; or congenital abnormalities.

Failure of the blastocyst to implant on the endometrium can have multiple causes. These causes include scars or adhesions on the endometrium from previous infections or surgery; **endometriosis** (ehn-doh-mee-tree-OH-sis), the growth of endometrial cells outside the uterus (usually in the abdominal cavity), which produces inflammation and alters the balance between progesterone and estrogen; **uterine fibroids**, benign tumors of the muscular layer of the uterus; and abnormalities of the blastocyst itself.

Treatment for Infertility

A variety of treatments are available for male and female infertility, and they depend on the identified cause. Treatments include:

- lifestyle changes (less alcohol, drug, or tobacco use in males can help stabilize or increase sperm count, and reduced stress can be helpful for both sexes)
- drugs to induce ovulation
- surgery to correct anatomical issues

When these treatments fail, a variety of assisted reproductive technologies is available. The most common is *in vitro fertilization (IVF). In vitro fertilization* literally means "fertilization in glass"). IVF requires harvesting one or more oocytes from the mother and combining them in a petri dish with sperm collected from the father. Fertilization occurs in the dish; then the embryo is transferred into the uterus for implantation.

Check Your Understanding

1. What is the clinical definition of infertility?
2. What are the two most common causes of male infertility?
3. What are the three most common causes of female infertility?
4. How can male and female infertility be treated?

Sexually Transmitted Infections

A **sexually transmitted infection (STI)** is an infection that can be passed from one person to another by sexual intercourse or genital contact. This lesson discusses the most common sexually transmitted infections: AIDS, gonorrhea, chlamydia, genital herpes, human papillomavirus, and pelvic inflammatory disease.

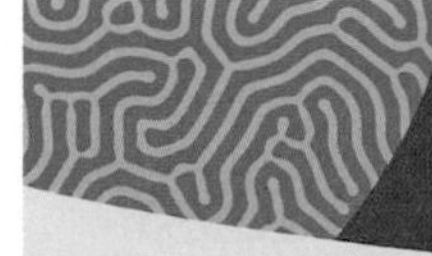

What Research Tells Us

...about Egg Freezing as a Solution for Infertility

More women than ever are waiting until their 30s or 40s to have children. As a result, age-related infertility concerns have grown more common.

Aging can cause infertility for several reasons. A woman in her 30s or 40s has a smaller number of eggs in her ovaries, and the ovaries do not release eggs as often as they did when the woman was younger. Also, the eggs tend to be less healthy. To complicate matters, only about 25% of all fertilized eggs implant in the uterus. Miscarriage, in which the fetus is spontaneously expelled from the body, is more common in women as they age.

New technologies are available to help women who, for medical, economic, or other reasons, are postponing childbirth until later in life. One of these technologies is *oocyte cryopreservation*, more commonly known as *egg freezing*. It is less controversial than embryo cryopreservation because the oocyte is not fertilized, and so is not, by itself, a potential person.

The road to egg freezing begins when a fertility specialist—a medical doctor—prescribes drugs that stimulate a woman's ovaries to produce multiple eggs. The doctor then uses a needle and ultrasound imaging for guidance to harvest eggs from the ovaries. The eggs and some surrounding fluid from the pelvic cavity are extracted and placed in a flat dish. A laboratory technician identifies individual eggs through a microscope and withdraws them from the dish for freezing.

If isolated eggs were simply placed in a freezer, ice crystals would form inside them, causing irreversible damage. For this reason, various strategies have been devised to limit ice crystal formation and preserve the viability of the eggs. The two broad strategies used are *dehydration* followed by slow freezing, and *vitrification*.

In dehydration followed by slow freezing, chemicals are used to draw as much water as possible out of the eggs before they are slowly cooled. When the eggs reach approximately –20°F to –40°F (–30°C to –40°C), they are plunged into liquid nitrogen for long-term storage. Liquid nitrogen is simply nitrogen gas (the main component of air) that has been refrigerated to –321°F (–196°C) or cooler. At –321°F, nitrogen gas liquefies. In vitrification, the eggs are placed in a very small volume of chemical preservative solution for less than a minute, after which they are quickly cooled by direct exposure to liquid nitrogen.

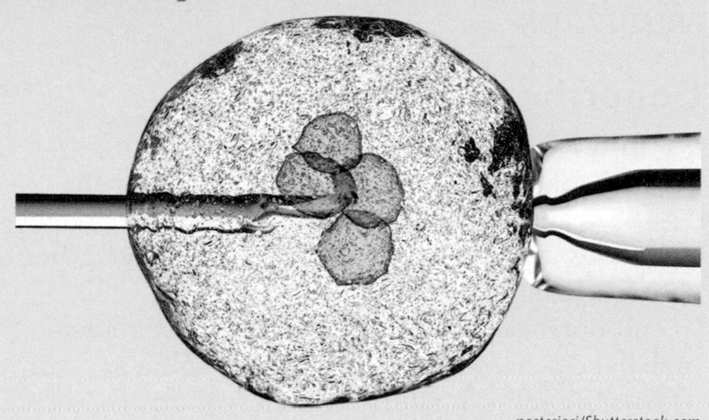

posteriori/Shutterstock.com

Figure 15.21 A human oocyte about to be injected with sperm. This procedure, called *intracytoplasmic sperm injection*, is one type of *in vitro* fertilization.

When a woman is ready to have children, the eggs are removed from the liquid nitrogen storage tank and thawed. In a procedure called *intracytoplasmic sperm injection (ICSI)*, each egg is fertilized by injection with a single sperm (**Figure 15.21**). When an egg has developed into an embryo, it is implanted into the uterus through a catheter, a flexible tube that is easily inserted into small openings in the body.

In October 2012, the American Society of Reproductive Medicine (ASRM) reclassified oocyte cryopreservation as a proven treatment for infertility. Previously, the process was considered experimental. The ASRM based its decision on analyses of many scientific studies. The studies showed that rates of fertilization and birth, and the health outcomes of the resulting children, were just as good with eggs that had been frozen as they were with *in vitro* fertilization (IVF) of fresh eggs that had never been frozen.

Taking It Further

Desiree is a 36-year-old, single female undergoing chemotherapy treatment for breast cancer. She has always wanted to have a child. When Desiree's oncologist informs her that the chemotherapy drugs may cause sterility, Desiree decides to have her eggs frozen, which will allow her to postpone pregnancy until she is cancer free. Do research on the health and financial risks, as well as ethical considerations, associated with egg freezing. Develop a "pro" argument in favor of Desiree's decision or a "con" argument against it. Support your argument with facts from expert sources. Present your case to the class.

HIV and AIDS

Acquired immune deficiency syndrome (AIDS) is the most lethal sexually transmitted infection. It is caused by the human immunodeficiency virus (HIV), which is shown in **Figure 15.22**. See Chapter 12 for a more detailed discussion of HIV/AIDS.

Gonorrhea

In the United States, **gonorrhea** (gahn-oh-REE-a) infection rates have been falling for the past 35 years. Gonorrhea still is, however, a common infectious disease, especially among teenagers and young adults.

Gonorrhea may cause pain during urination, unusual discharge of fluid from the vagina or penis, or no symptoms at all. In women, gonorrhea can damage the endometrium and uterine tubes and can lead to infertility, even if the infection produces no symptoms. Because gonorrhea is caused by a bacterium, it can be successfully treated with antibiotics.

Chlamydia

Chlamydia (klah-MID-ee-a) is the most commonly reported STI in the United States. Its incidence has been rising.

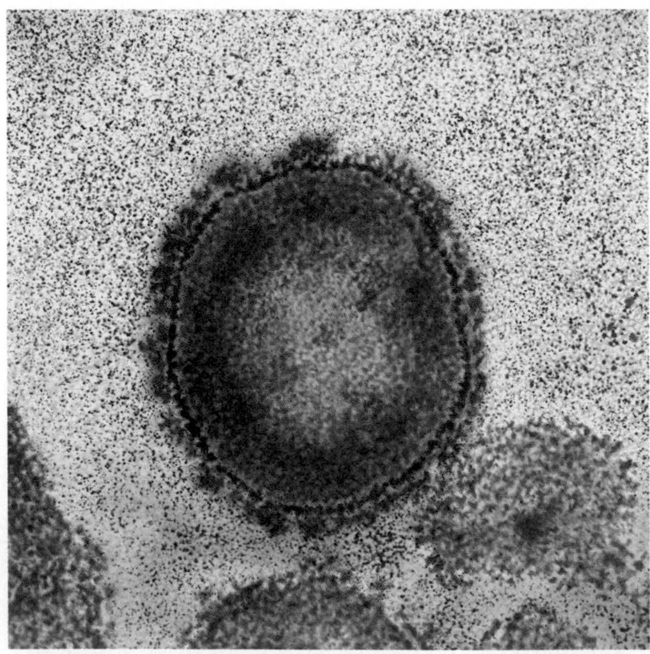

NIBSC/Science Source

Figure 15.22 A micrograph of an HIV virus cell. *What is the name of the virus that causes AIDS?*

Chlamydia often causes no symptoms, but it can damage the female reproductive tract, leading to infertility and increased risk of ectopic pregnancy. Chlamydia can be easily and successfully treated with antibiotics. The CDC recommends that all sexually active young women get an annual screening test for chlamydia.

Genital Herpes

Genital herpes is caused by *herpes simplex virus type 1 (HSV-1)* or *herpes simplex virus type 2 (HSV-2)*. It is a common STI: genital HSV-2 infects about one out of six Americans between 14 and 49 years of age.

Genital herpes may cause blisters or sores in the genital or anal area or near the mouth, or it may cause no symptoms. In fact, most people with genital herpes are unaware that they have it. Pregnant women who have—or have been exposed to—genital herpes need to discuss this fact with their healthcare provider. This consultation is recommended because this STI can spread from a pregnant mother to her unborn child, with serious or fatal results. There is no cure for genital herpes, but the condition is manageable with antiviral drugs.

Human Papillomavirus

Human papillomavirus (HPV) causes genital warts and cervical cancer. The most common STI in the United States, human papillomavirus infects both men and women. Some 6 million new infections emerge each year, and one-half of all sexually active adults will be infected with HPV at some point in their lives.

HPV may produce no symptoms. In most people, the immune system eliminates HPV, but it takes about two years to do so. A vaccine is now available to prevent HPV.

Pelvic Inflammatory Disease

Pelvic inflammatory disease (PID) is an inflammation of the uterus, uterine tubes, ovaries, and/or other organs of the peritoneal (abdominopelvic) cavity. PID is caused by a bacterial infection. It is a potentially serious complication of chlamydia and gonorrhea in females.

The symptoms of pelvic inflammatory disease may include mild to severe pelvic pain, fever, and painful urination. When the symptoms are mild, PID often goes unrecognized. PID can be effectively treated with antibiotics. Prompt treatment is important to prevent permanent damage to the reproductive organs, including scarring of the uterine tubes. Such damage can cause infertility and increase the risk of ectopic pregnancy.

Detection and Prevention

Sexually transmitted infections can infect any sexually active person. A person with symptoms—such as a discharge of unusual fluid from the genitals, burning during urination, or unusual sores, growths, or a rash—should stop having sex and see a healthcare provider immediately. The use of a condom during sex helps prevent the spread of most STIs. However, abstinence from sexual activity is the only foolproof method of preventing STIs.

Check Your Understanding

1. How do sexually transmitted diseases spread from one person to another?
2. Why is genital herpes a concern for pregnant women?
3. Which STI can cause infected women to develop cervical cancer?

Cancers of the Reproductive Systems

Cancers of the reproductive systems in males and females are among the most common and among the deadliest cancers. When detected early, however, these cancers often can be successfully treated. Millions of people in the United States are cancer survivors. In discussions of cancer, you will often see the words *incidence* and *mortality*. *Incidence* refers to the number of people who get the disease; *mortality* refers to the number of people who die from it.

Prostate Cancer

After skin cancer, the cancer with the highest incidence among men in the United States is prostate cancer. After lung cancer, prostate cancer is the second most frequent cause of cancer mortality among men. Older men and men with a family history of prostate cancer are among those with an increased risk of developing prostate cancer.

Most prostate cancers, which are slow-growing, originate in the gland cells that produce the fluid added to semen. Screening tests are available for prostate cancer, the most common of which is the *prostate-specific antigen (PSA) test*. The PSA test is valuable in the early detection and treatment of prostate cancer, and it saves lives. However, the test sometimes produces false-positive results, prompting a series of follow-up tests and treatments that have risks of their own. Furthermore, the PSA test may not distinguish between rapidly growing, malignant tumors and slow-growing tumors that might safely be left alone.

Treatment of prostate cancer includes surgery to remove cancer cells, radiation therapy, and chemotherapy. Radiation therapy is the use of X-rays to kill cancerous cells. Radiation therapy for prostate cancer is sometimes delivered to the tumor by surgically implanting radioactive "seeds"—each about the size and shape of a grain of rice—into the prostate gland. This method, known as *brachytherapy*, may have fewer unwanted side effects than other treatment options.

Testicular Cancer

Testicular cancer is the most common solid malignant cancer in young (ages 20–35) men in the United States. However, it is relatively uncommon, making up about 0.5% of new annual cancer cases in the United States. Men who have a close relative (especially a father or brother) who has had testicular cancer are at six to 10 times greater risk than other men of developing testicular cancer. The standard treatment for testicular cancer is surgical removal of the cancerous testis, and radiation therapy or chemotherapy or both, if the disease has spread beyond the testis. Testicular cancer is curable. About two-thirds of new cases have not spread beyond the testis at the time of diagnosis, and those patients have a 5-year survival rate exceeding 99%. The 5-year survival is about 95% among those whose cancer has spread to nearby lymph nodes, and 75% among those whose cancer has metastasized to distant body areas.

Cancers of the Female Reproductive Tract

The three most commonly diagnosed cancers of the female reproductive tract—and the deadliest (not including breast cancer)—are uterine, ovarian, and cervical cancers. These cancers affect about 70,000 American women annually and cause more than 20,000 deaths each year.

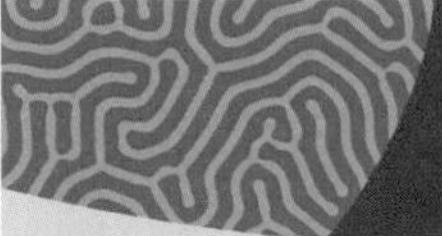

What Research Tells Us

...about Radioactivity in Healthcare

Radioactive compounds are chemicals containing atoms that spontaneously change from one element to another. When this change occurs, energy is released. This energy-releasing process is called *radioactivity*, and the energy emitted is called *ionizing radiation*, because it has the ability to knock electrons off of molecules, thus creating ions. Ionizing radiation can also break the chemical bonds that hold molecules together.

Isotopes and Radioactivity

An atom is radioactive if the combination of protons and neutrons in its nucleus is unstable. A carbon atom with six protons and six neutrons (carbon-12) is stable, and therefore not radioactive. But a carbon atom with six protons and eight neutrons (carbon-14) is not stable. It is a carbon *isotope* (containing the same number of protons but a different number of neutrons) that has a very small chance, each minute, of undergoing radioactive decay. If that happens, one of the neutrons in the nucleus turns into a positively charged proton plus an electron. The electron has a great deal of energy and flies away from the atom. It is the ionizing radiation in this reaction. The proton stays in the nucleus, so the nucleus now consists of seven protons and seven neutrons. This is a nitrogen-14 atom. Thus a carbon atom has become a nitrogen atom. It takes about 5,400 years for half the atoms in a sample of pure carbon-14 to turn into nitrogen atoms.

Soon after the discovery of radioactivity, scientists learned that radioactive chemicals could be both useful and harmful in medicine. Ionizing radiation from radioactive chemicals, called *radioisotopes*, could kill cancer cells, but it could also cause burns and increase the risk of getting cancer later.

Radiopharmaceuticals

The medical use of radioactive chemicals (*radiopharmaceuticals*) is called *nuclear medicine* and involves both diagnosis and treatment of disease. The most common use of radiopharmaceuticals is to diagnose cancer that is impossible to see with other imaging modalities. Cancer cells are more metabolically active than normal cells, so they take up glucose more than most cells. Fluorodeoxyglucose (FDG) is a radioactive glucose-like molecule that accumulates in metabolically active cells, including cancer cells. The radiation emitted by the radioactive fluorine atoms is detected, and its location inside the body is calculated. An image made this way is called a positron emission tomography (PET) scan, because the ionizing radiation is emitted in the form of positron particles. PET scans are used to identify cancers and to see if cancer has spread. Similar chemicals and techniques can be used to identify areas of damaged cardiac muscle and to identify areas of abnormal brain tissue.

Radiopharmaceuticals are also used to treat disease, particularly cancer, by delivering ionizing radiation to cells. The radiation kills the cells by damaging their DNA. For example, a patient with thyroid cancer can take a pill containing radioactive iodine. Thyroid cells take up iodine strongly, because iodine is a key component of thyroid hormone, as explained in Chapter 8. The radioactive iodine kills the cancerous thyroid gland cells. Another approach, called *brachytherapy*, is to implant pellets (often called *seeds*) containing radioactive material into a solid tumor. Because the pellets are inside the tumor, the cancer cells receive an intense dose of damaging radiation, and healthy tissues outside the tumor receive less radiation. Brachytherapy is used to treat tumors of the prostate, breast, and other organs.

Taking It Further

Conduct research to find out more about the use of radioisotopes in healthcare and in healthcare research. Include fluorine-18, rubidium-82, and iodine-123 in your research. For what healthcare purposes are these radioisotopes used?

Uterine Cancer

Cancer of the uterus is the most frequently diagnosed cancer of the female reproductive tract. Uterine cancer almost always develops in cells of the endometrium, the inner lining of the uterus. For this reason, *endometrial cancer* is another term for uterine cancer. Abnormal uterine bleeding often reveals the presence of uterine cancer before it spreads within the body. Surgical removal of the entire uterus (known as *hysterectomy*), uterine tubes, and ovaries is the standard initial treatment. More than 80% of uterine cancer patients survive for at least five years after diagnosis.

Ovarian Cancer

Cancer of the ovary is the fifth most common cause of cancer-related death among women in the United States. Ovarian cancer causes more deaths than any other cancer of the female reproductive tract. Unlike uterine cancer, ovarian cancer usually does not cause any symptoms until the disease has spread beyond its initial site. For this reason, the average five-year survival rate of ovarian cancer patients is about 40%. The standard initial treatment is surgical removal of the uterus, uterine tubes, and ovaries. In most cases, surgery is followed by chemotherapy. Currently, there are no effective screening tests for ovarian cancer.

Cervical Cancer

Although the cervix is part of the uterus anatomically, cervical cancer is considered a different type of cancer from uterine cancer. Among cancers of the female reproductive tract, cervical cancer is the third most commonly diagnosed, and it ranks third as a cause of death among US women, after uterine and ovarian cancers. The *Papanicolaou test*, or *Pap smear*, is a screening test that has significantly reduced cervical cancer mortality over the last 35 years. It is used not only to detect cervical cancer but also to detect precancerous conditions in the cervix. Cervical cancer develops slowly, and the Pap smear allows early detection and surgical treatment.

Most cervical cancers are caused by high-risk forms of human papillomavirus. HPV also causes most anal cancers and about half of all vaginal, vulvar, and penile cancers. Health professionals expect that over the next few years, the incidence and mortality rates of cervical cancer, and perhaps those of other reproductive system cancers, will drop because of widespread use of vaccines that protect against HPV infection.

Breast Cancer

Breast cancer is a type of cancer that forms in the tissues of the breast—usually in the ducts and lobules. Males can develop breast cancer, but females typically are affected. After skin cancer, breast cancer is the most commonly diagnosed cancer among women in the United States. More women die from breast cancer than from any other cancer, with the exception of lung cancer. However, the breast cancer death rate has been declining due to early detection and more effective treatment therapies.

Factors that raise a woman's risk of developing breast cancer include advanced age, a family history of breast cancer, menarche at an early age, late onset of menopause, being overweight, and never having given birth.

Early detection of breast cancer improves the odds of successful treatment. For this reason, regular clinical breast examinations and mammography are recommended. Mammography involves the production of an X-ray image (mammogram) of the breast to detect a tumor while it is still small. A yearly mammogram is recommended for women 40 years of age and older. In addition, many women regularly examine their own breasts for lumps and other unusual changes. This is called a *breast self-exam*. If a woman discovers an abnormality during a breast self-exam, she should contact a doctor.

Breast cancer is treated with surgery to remove cancer cells and with radiation therapy and/or chemotherapy to kill cancer cells. Treatment options, such as what kind of surgery to have or which drugs to use, depend on the specific clinical details of each case. Surgery options range from a "lumpectomy," in which only a small region of cancer tissue is removed, to a radical mastectomy, in which all the breast tissue and surrounding lymph nodes are removed.

Check Your Understanding

1. What is brachytherapy?
2. Name three common cancers of the female reproductive tract.

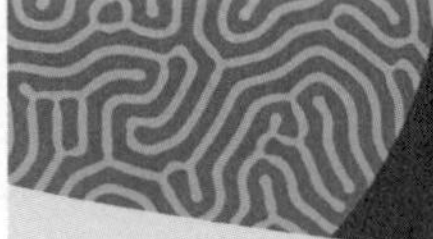

What Research Tells Us

...about Genetic Research and Cancer Treatment Breakthroughs

Cancers of the reproductive tract, like cancers of other organs and tissues, are diseases in which cells grow "out of control," as seen in **Figure 15.23**. As explained in Chapter 2, cancer cells have mutations in their DNA. Often, these mutations result from damage to the genes that regulate cell division. Cells become cancerous because the mechanisms that regulate cell division—which act as "brakes" on cell division—no longer work.

Advances in technology are making it possible for scientists to decipher more information about the genetic makeup of cancer cells. Likewise, this technology is enabling scientists to identify people who, because of their genetic constitution, are more likely to develop cancer. These advances are leading to earlier detection of cancer as well as potentially significant changes in cancer care.

Genes Associated with Cancer

Researchers have found that a person's genetic makeup can make him or her more likely to develop cancer. This information can be used to detect cancer at its earliest stage, when it can be successfully treated. For example, women who inherit a mutant form of the BRCA1 or BRCA2 gene have a significantly elevated risk of developing breast or ovarian cancer. These genes, named for their association with breast cancer, provide the genetic codes for proteins that repair damaged DNA. When the BRCA1 and BRCA2 genes are damaged, cells are less able to repair the DNA damage that can occur as people grow and age. As a result, the risk of further gene mutation, and thus the risk of cancer, increases.

A woman can be tested for the mutant forms of the BRCA1 and BRCA2 genes. If she has the mutation, she can undergo periodic screenings to detect precancerous changes in cells.

Women with damage to the BRCA1 or BRCA2 genes account for only about 15% of breast cancer cases. The remainder of cases do not have a direct hereditary cause and may arise from gene mutation that occurs randomly throughout life.

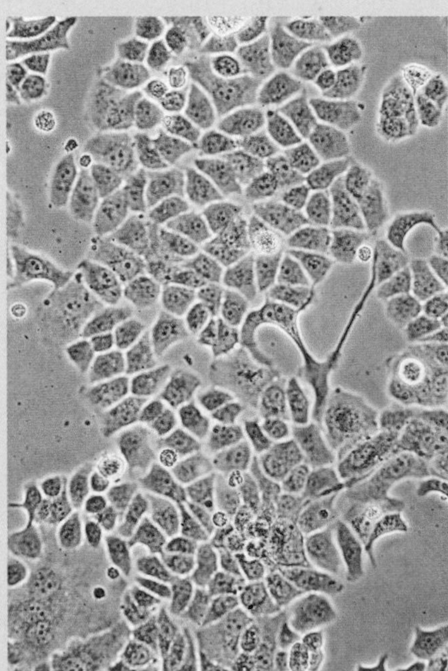

Paul Hakimata Photography/Shutterstock.com

Figure 15.23 Microscopic view of ductal breast cancer cells in a tissue culture.

New Cancer Treatments

Besides alerting women to a potential genetic vulnerability to cancer, advances in technology are reducing the time and cost required to determine the DNA sequence of cancer cells from individual patients. These technological benefits can lead to improved cancer care. For example, some tumors have a genetic mutation that makes them responsive to certain anti-cancer drugs. A doctor and patient with this knowledge could choose drug therapy accordingly.

Currently, more information is available on cancer cell mutations than there are drug therapies to effectively target and treat these mutations. Medical researchers continue their efforts to develop drugs tailored to the specific DNA mutations identified in different types of cancer cells.

Taking It Further

1. Why does damage to genes that regulate cell division often cause cancer?
2. How can doctors use a patient's genetic information to detect cancer at its earliest stage?
3. How can doctors use genetic information about cancer cells to treat cancer patients?

LESSON 15.5 Review and Assessment

Mini Glossary

Make sure that you know the meaning of each key term.

amenorrhea complete absence of menstrual periods

chlamydia a sexually transmitted disease that often causes no symptoms, but can damage the female reproductive tract and lead to infertility and increased risk of ectopic pregnancy

endometriosis the growth of endometrial cells outside the uterus, usually in the abdominal cavity

genital herpes a sexually transmitted disease that may cause blisters or sores in the genital or anal area or near the mouth; may have no symptoms

gonorrhea a sexually transmitted disease that may cause pain during urination, unusual discharge of fluid from the vagina or penis, or no symptoms at all; can lead to infertility

human papillomavirus (HPV) a sexually transmitted disease that causes genital warts and can cause cervical cancer

impotence the inability of a male to maintain an erection

infertility the inability of a couple to get pregnant

pelvic inflammatory disease (PID) an inflammation of the uterus, uterine tubes, ovaries and/or other organs of the peritoneal (abdominopelvic) cavity

sexually transmitted infection (STI) an infection transmitted through sexual contact

uterine fibroids benign tumors of the muscular layer of the uterus

Know and Understand

1. Clinically, what is meant by the phrase *low sperm count*?
2. What is another name for impotence?
3. Which hormones, when present at abnormal levels, can result in failure to ovulate?
4. What are some causes of uterine tube damage?
5. What are uterine fibroids?
6. What is the most lethal STI?
7. Which STI is the most common in the United States, affecting 50% of all sexually active adults at some point in their lives?
8. Which screening tests are used to detect cancers of the prostate, cervix, and breast respectively?

Analyze and Apply

9. Compare and contrast male and female infertility.
10. How can a sexually active lifestyle increase a person's risk of becoming infertile? What can people do to help ensure that their reproductive systems function normally when they want to have children?
11. Explain the meanings of the words *incidence* and *mortality* as they relate to discussions of cancer.
12. An older term for *sexually transmitted infections (STIs)* is *sexually transmitted diseases (STDs)*. What do you think is the reasoning behind this change in accepted terminology?
13. Do you think condoms can protect against STIs, pregnancy, and cancer? Explain your answer.

IN THE LAB

14. Working in a small group, pick one of the sexually transmitted infections discussed in this lesson that is of particular interest to you and the members of your group. Create an educational presentation using presentation software or online tools that represents the causes, symptoms, and treatments for that condition. Share your presentation with the class.
15. Collect slides of cells from various reproductive cancers, including breast, prostate, testicular, ovarian, and uterine cancer. Using a high-powered microscope, review each slide. In your lab book, describe what each type of cell looks like: size, color, and shape. One aberration that can be observed in cancer cells is the presence of multiple centrosomes during interphase. Explain why having multiple centrosomes is a problem for cells.

CAREER CORNER

Anatomy & Physiology at Work

The basic role of the male and female reproductive systems is to ensure that genes are passed on to a new generation through reproduction, pregnancy, and childbirth. Many people have found careers in the promotion of reproductive health and in the diagnosis and treatment of diseases and disorders of the reproductive system.

Diagnostic Medical Sonographer

A diagnostic medical sonographer uses ultrasonic imaging equipment to diagnose and monitor medical conditions. Ultrasonic imaging uses sound waves (ultrasound) to generate pictures of structures inside the body. The technique is called *ultrasound imaging* because it uses sound frequencies far beyond those that can be detected by the human ear. The pictures created by ultrasound imaging are called *sonograms*, and the procedure itself is sometimes called an *ultrasound*. An echocardiogram is one type of sonogram. These images are studied by diagnostic medical sonographers and doctors to diagnose health problems.

Diagnostic medical sonographers may specialize in one or more parts of the body. For example, obstetric sonographers perform ultrasound imaging of organs and tissues of the female reproductive system. Their patients are often pregnant women who have ultrasounds to monitor the health and growth of the fetus. A video display screen allows the obstetric sonographer to share ultrasound images with expectant mothers.

Diagnostic medical sonographers work in hospitals, doctors' offices, and medical laboratories (**Figure 15.24**). They must be able to use complex, computerized imaging equipment and assess the images they produce to ensure that they are sufficiently clear and detailed. They are also responsible for maintaining the equipment they use. Because they work with patients, diagnostic medical sonographers must possess good communication and interpersonal skills. They explain ultrasound test procedures, answer patients' questions, and provide comfort and reassurance to nervous or distraught patients.

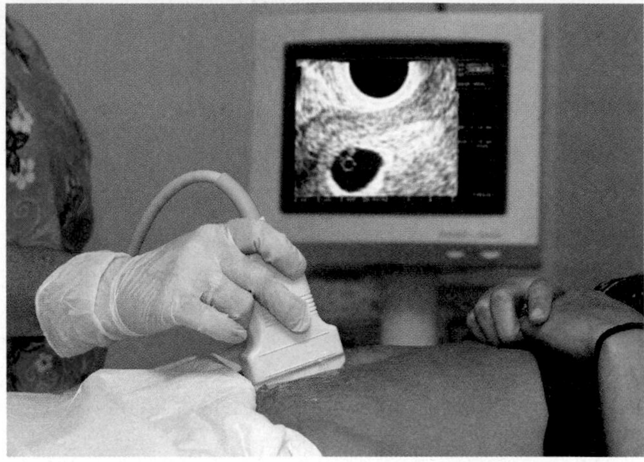

Steven Frame/Shutterstock.com

Figure 15.24 A diagnostic medical sonographer shows a patient ultrasound images of the fetus that she is carrying.

The minimum requirement to become a diagnostic medical sonographer is an associate's degree or a postsecondary certificate awarded by a community college. Many employers require that sonographers have professional certification. To be certified, they must earn a diagnostic medical sonography degree or complete a certificate program from an accredited college, or complete a health-related program and have appropriate clinical experience. They must also pass an examination. Certification examinations are given by the American Registry for Diagnostic Medical Sonography. Professional certification is also required in some states.

Job opportunities for diagnostic medical sonographers are plentiful. In fact, the demand for diagnostic medical sonographers is expected to grow faster than the average for many other professionals.

Obstetrician-Gynecologist

An obstetrician-gynecologist (ob-gyn) is a physician who specializes in the healthcare of women, including the diagnosis and treatment of disorders of the female reproductive system. The ob-gyn also provides routine physical care to teenage girls and women. According to the American College of Obstetricians and Gynecologists, a teenage girl should make her first visit to a gynecologist between the ages of 13 and 15.

Ob-gyns examine patients and take their medical histories. They order and conduct routine diagnostic tests—for example, breast exams, pelvic exams, and Pap tests—to check for infections or disease, such as sexually transmitted diseases or cancer. They prescribe medications and counsel women on reproductive health, birth control, fertility, menstrual irregularities, and sexual problems. They care for women before, during, and after childbirth, and they perform surgical procedures. Ob-gyns work in hospitals, clinics, and in their own medical offices (**Figure 15.25**).

Training to become an ob-gyn begins with four years of college, followed by four years of medical school. The ob-gyn candidate then completes three or four years of residency training in obstetrics and gynecology. During this time, the medical resident treats patients under the supervision of senior doctors. An ob-gyn often works long and irregular hours, including nights and weekends. Ob-gyns must be available when their patients are ready to give birth.

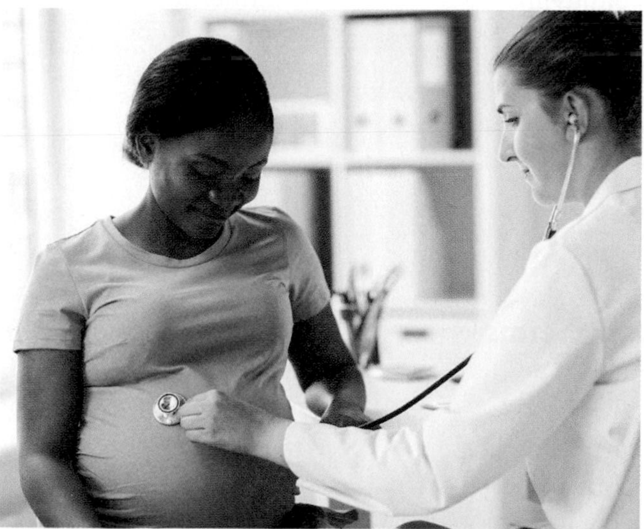

Syda Productions/Shutterstock.com

Figure 15.25 An obstetrician-gynecologist examines a pregnant patient during a routine visit.

Planning for a Health-Related Career

Do some research on the career of an obstetrician-gynecologist or a diagnostic medical sonographer. Otherwise, select a profession from the list of related career options. Find answers to the following questions:

1. What are the main tasks and responsibilities of a person employed in this career?
2. What is the outlook for this career? Are workers in demand, or are jobs dwindling?
3. What special skills or talents are required? For example, do you need to be good at science and comfortable with new and ever-changing technologies? Do you need to enjoy interacting with other people?
4. What personality traits do you think are necessary for success in the career that you have chosen to research?
5. Does the work involve a great deal of routine, or are the day-to-day responsibilities varied?
6. Does the career require long hours, or is it a standard, "9-to-5" job?
7. What is the salary range for this job?
8. What do you think you would like about this career? Is there anything about it that you might dislike?

Related Career Options

- Genetic counselor
- Marriage and family therapist
- Medical laboratory technician or technologist
- Neonatal nurse practitioner
- Nurse-midwife
- Reproductive endocrinologist
- Surgical technologist
- Urologist

CHAPTER 15

Review

> LESSON 15.1

Reproduction and Development of the Human Reproductive Systems

Key Points

- Of the two types of reproduction—asexual and sexual—sexual reproduction is more complicated.
- Mitosis is the cell division process that occurs in all of the body's tissues throughout life. Meiosis occurs only in the sex organs and produces gametes.
- Unlike other organ systems, the reproductive systems do not become fully functional until later in life, beginning at puberty.

Key Terms

centromere
chromatids
chromosomes
crossovers
diploid
epigenetics
fertilization
gametes
genotype
haploid
meiosis
menarche
phenotype
puberty
zygote

> LESSON 15.2

Male Reproductive System

Key Points

- The primary organs of the male reproductive system are the testes; accessory organs include the penis and scrotum and five accessory glands: the prostate, the two seminal glands, and the two bulbourethral glands.
- Sperm are produced in the testes and then delivered to the external urethral orifice through a series of ducts; semen is ejaculated as a result of nerve impulses that cause peristaltic contractions.

Key Terms

bulbourethral glands
ductus deferens
ejaculation
epididymis
erection
gonads
penis
prostate gland
semen
seminal glands
seminiferous tubules
sperm
spermatogenesis

> LESSON 15.3

Female Reproductive System

Key Points

- The primary organs in the female reproductive system are the ovaries; accessory organs include uterine tubes, uterus, vagina, and vulva.
- During the female's monthly cycle, the ovaries, uterus, and hormones undergo changes. Ovulation occurs when a follicle reaches maturity and the oocyte is released from the ovary.

Key Terms

cervix
clitoris
corpus luteum
labia majora
labia minora
lactiferous duct
mammary glands
menopause
menstrual cycle
oocyte
oogenesis
ovarian cycle
ovaries
ovulation
uterine cycle
uterine tubes
uterus
vagina

LESSON 15.4

Fertilization, Pregnancy, and Birth

Key Points

- Fertilization occurs when the chromosomes of the oocyte and the sperm unite to produce a zygote.
- After fertilization, the zygote travels through the uterine tube and into the uterus, where it implants and develops into a fetus. Fetal vessels carry blood through the umbilical cord to and from the placenta, which grows to meet the nutritional needs of the fetus.
- The stages of labor are dilation, expulsion, and delivery of the placenta.
- Lactation, the production of milk by the mother, is regulated by hormones.

Key Terms

amniotic fluid
blastocyst
capacitation
dilation
embryo
expulsion
fetus
gestation
gestational age
human chorionic gonadotropin (hCG)
implantation
lactation
let-down reflex
parturition
placenta
umbilical cord

LESSON 15.5

Disorders and Diseases of the Reproductive Systems

Key Points

- Infertility is the inability of a couple to conceive after at least one year of unprotected intercourse.
- A sexually transmitted infection is an infection that can be passed from one person to another by sexual intercourse or genital contact.
- Sexually transmitted infections include HIV/AIDS, gonorrhea, chlamydia, genital herpes, and HPV.
- Cancers of the reproductive system are some of the most common and deadliest types of cancer.

Key Terms

amenorrhea
chlamydia
endometriosis
genital herpes
gonorrhea
human papillomavirus (HPV)
impotence
infertility
pelvic inflammatory disease (PID)
sexually transmitted infection (STI)
uterine fibroids

Assessment

LESSON 15.1

Reproduction and Development of the Human Reproductive Systems

Learning Key Terms and Concepts

1. A person's _____ consists of his or her observable characteristics, which are determined at fertilization by genetic makeup.
2. *True or False*? Homologous chromosomes are the two identical chromosomes that make up one of the 23 pairs in a mother cell.
3. Which of the following most directly helps create genetic diversity?
   A. DNA
   B. mitosis
   C. crossovers
   D. SRY genes

4. Does the presence of a Y chromosome indicate development of a male or a female?
5. Adolescence officially begins with the appearance of _____ characteristics.
6. Which of the following hormones is *not* involved in stimulating puberty: follicle stimulating hormone, luteinizing hormone, oxytocin, or gonadotropin-releasing hormone?
7. *True or False*? By the end of puberty, mature sperm are present in semen.

Thinking Critically

8. Imagine that you have been asked to teach a lesson on the differences between mitosis and meiosis to an eighth-grade biology class. How would you explain the differences to the class?
9. How is genetic diversity created during human reproduction?
10. Genotype is one of three factors that determine phenotype. What are the other two?

➤ LESSON 15.2

Male Reproductive System

Learning Key Terms and Concepts

11. Testes are the organ in which the male gametes, called _____, are made.
12. At which temperature would you expect sperm production to be *most* vigorous?
    A. 98.6°F
    B. 101.1°F
    C. 93.2°F
    D. 97.4°F
13. The _____ glands make the greatest contribution to the volume of semen.
14. One of the functions of the male reproductive system is to deliver sperm to the site of _____.
15. How many chromosomes does a spermatid have?
16. *True or False?* When a spermatid develops a flagellum and is released into the seminiferous tubule, it is a mature sperm.

Thinking Critically

17. Compare sperm cells to other cells in the human body. How are they different? How are they similar?
18. If a male gets testicular cancer in one testis, will he still produce sperm in the other?
19. If a male has a vasectomy, what part of the anatomy is affected? Can it be reversed later?

➤ LESSON 15.3

Female Reproductive System

Learning Key Terms and Concepts

20. Each follicle in a woman's ovary contains a single _____, or egg cell.
21. How many ovarian follicles reach maturity each month?
22. The projections called _____ that project from the uterine tubes help sweep an ovulated oocyte into the uterine tube.
23. A fertilized egg that implants on the wall of the pelvic cavity causes a(n) _____ pregnancy.
24. The pH of the vagina is acidic in healthy adult women in order to help prevent _____ infection.
25. Which hormone stimulates milk production by the female mammary glands after childbirth?
26. Which of the following functions is not a primary function of the female reproductive system?
    A. giving birth
    B. protecting from STIs
    C. generating eggs
    D. nourishing a newborn child
27. After ovulation, what happens to the levels of estrogen and progesterone in the blood?
    A. estrogen level falls, progesterone level rises
    B. estrogen level rises, progesterone level falls
    C. both estrogen and progesterone levels rise
    D. both estrogen and progesterone levels fall

Thinking Critically

28. Describe the step-by-step process that occurs during ovulation.
29. Describe where the uterus is located. What is the purpose of the uterus in reproduction?
30. Compare and contrast the anatomy of the ovary and the testis.
31. Compare and contrast the functions of the male and female reproductive systems.
32. Compare the risks and benefits of hormone replacement therapy for women after menopause.
33. A woman is born with all the eggs she will ever have. Do those eggs change as the woman ages?

›LESSON 15.4

Fertilization, Pregnancy, and Birth

Learning Key Terms and Concepts

34. *True or False*? A gamete has 46 chromosomes.
35. *True or False*? After intercourse, a few thousand sperm may reach the oocyte.
36. The function of _____ enzymes in sperm is to digest the protective glycoproteins surrounding an oocyte.
37. Which structure connects the fetus to the placenta?
38. Which stage of labor usually lasts the longest?
39. Which hormone stimulates the let-down reflex?

Thinking Critically

40. Describe how pregnancy-test kits work.
41. Where is the placenta located, and what is its function?
42. Explain why it is important for pregnant women to avoid drinking alcohol and taking drugs that are illegal or not prescribed. How can these substances reach the developing fetus?
43. What procedure might be done if there is a complication during labor or delivery? What are the pros and cons of this procedure?
44. The purpose of lactation after childbirth is to provide nutrition for the newborn, but some women choose not to breast-feed their babies. Why do you think this is so? What are the pros and cons of breast-feeding?

›LESSON 15.5

Disorders and Diseases of the Reproductive Systems

Learning Key Terms and Concepts

45. The inability of a couple to conceive after a year of unprotected intercourse is known as _____.
46. Which of the following glands secretes GnRH?
    A. pituitary
    B. testis
    C. hypothalamus
    D. ovary
47. The clinical name for freezing eggs as a solution to infertility is _____.
48. *True or False*? Gonorrhea and chlamydia *cannot* be successfully treated with antibiotics.
49. *True or False*? Genital warts are caused by human papillomavirus.
50. The STI that is a possible complication of gonorrhea in females is _____.
51. A PSA test is performed to screen for _____ cancer.
52. *True or False*? The breast cancer death rate has been declining in recent years.

Thinking Critically

53. Why are the male and female reproductive systems vulnerable to infection and disease?
54. What is the difference between infertility and impotence?
55. What is in vitro fertilization (IVF)? Briefly describe how the procedure is performed.
56. What is the relationship between gene mutation and cancer development?
57. Evaluate the cause and effect of the human papillomavirus on the structure and function of the female reproductive system.
58. You are a doctor who treats infertile couples. A new patient complains that she is not pregnant although she and her husband have been trying for six months. What would you tell this patient? Write a "prescription" for lifestyle changes that could help increase their chances of conceiving.
59. Are there vaccines against any of the common STIs? If so, which ones?

Building Skills and Connecting Concepts

Analyzing and Evaluating Data

Instructions: Figure 15.26 shows the rate of HPV infection among surveyed females in the United States. Several factors are linked to the rate of infection among certain demographic groups. Use the chart to answer the questions.

HPV Infection Rates Among Surveyed US Females		
Factor	**Demographic Group**	**Rate of Infection**
Age	14–19	40%
	20–24	50%
	25–29	28%
	30–39	37%
	40–49	25%
	50–59	20%
Race/ Ethnicity	African-American	39%
	Caucasian	24%
	Hispanic	24%
Economic Status	Below the poverty line	38%
	At/above the poverty line	24%

Figure 15.26 *Goodheart-Willcox Publisher*

60. Which race/ethnicity is most likely to become infected with HPV?
61. What is the difference in HPV infection rate between those at or above the poverty line and those below the poverty line?
62. How much more likely is a woman between 14 and 19 years of age to become infected with HPV than a woman between 50 and 59 years of age?
63. Why do you think that females 20-24 years of age are more likely to become infected with HPV than other age groups?
64. Develop a scatter plot using the data provide on HPV infection rates.

Communicating about Anatomy & Physiology

65. **Speaking** Pick a figure in this chapter, such as Figure 15.4, 15.7, or 15.14. Working with a partner, tell and then retell the important information being conveyed by that figure.
66. **Reading and Speaking** Cancer screenings can detect cancer at an early stage, but the value of some of these tests for people who have no symptoms or no risk factors has recently come into question. Research the debate surrounding either prostate or breast cancer screenings. Choose a position (yes or no), and develop an argument in response to the following question: Do the benefits of cancer screenings outweigh the risks involved?
67. **Writing** Choose one STI presented in this chapter, and create a flyer directed at preteens to help prevent the spread of the disease. It must include statistics relative to their age group, must be colorful, and must be at their reading level. Include signs and symptoms and resources in your local area that you have verified.

Lab Investigations

68. Create a trifold board with another team member that will educate your peers about teen pregnancy. Develop a graph with statistics on teen pregnancy, including information on the dangers of smoking, drinking and poor nutrition. Research agencies in your area that can assist pregnant and parenting teens and include this information on your board. Present your board with all of your findings in class, at a health fair, or at an open house. Be prepared to answer questions from the public.

Building Your Portfolio

69. Take digital photographs of the models and projects you created as you worked through this chapter. Create a document or folder called "The Reproductive Systems" and insert the photographs, along with written descriptions of what the models show and your reasons for creating them using the materials and forms you chose. Add the reports from your laboratory experiments, and add this document or folder to your personal portfolio.

Appendix A **Metric-English Conversion Factors**

Quantity	When you know English units	Multiply by	To get metric units[1]
Length	inches	2.54	centimeters
	inches	0.0254	meters
	feet	30.5	centimeters
	feet	0.305	meters
Area	square inches	6.45	square centimeters
	square feet	0.929	square meters
Volume[2]	fluid ounces	29.4	milliliters
	pints	0.473	liters
	quarts	0.946	liters
Weight	ounces	28.3	grams
	ounces	0.283	kilograms
	pounds	0.454	kilograms
Pressure	pounds per square inch	51.7	millimeters of mercury
	pounds per square inch	6.89	kilopascals
Flow	gallons per minute	3.79	liters per minute
Mass	slug	0.0685	kilogram
Force	pound	0.225	newton
Torque	foot-pounds	0.738	newton-meters
Temperature[3]	Fahrenheit	5/9 × (F-32)	Celsius

[1] To convert from metric to English units, divide metric units by the number shown.
[2] For volume, note that 1 milliliter = 1 cubic centimeter.
[3] For temperature, use the formula F = (9/5 × C) + 32 to convert metric to US units.

Goodheart-Willcox Publisher

Appendix B **Basic Mathematical Operations**

As you study anatomy and physiology, you will encounter situations in which you need to use basic math skills. This appendix provides a brief review of some commonly used mathematical concepts and operations.

Negative Numbers

Negative numbers are indicated by a minus sign (–). The following rules apply to arithmetic operations involving negative numbers:

1. Addition of a negative number yields the same result as subtraction of a positive number of the same magnitude:

   $7 + (-3) = 4$ $\quad$ $25 + (-10) = 15$

   $7 - 3 = 4$ $\quad$ $25 - 10 = 15$

2. Subtraction of a negative number yields the same result as addition of a positive number of the same magnitude:

   $7 - (-3) = 10$ $\quad$ $25 - (-10) = 35$

   $7 + 3 = 10$ $\quad$ $25 + 10 = 35$

3. Multiplication or division of a positive number and a negative number yields a negative result:

   $3 \times (-7) = -21$ $\quad$ $81 \div (-9) = -9$

4. Multiplication or division of two negative numbers yields a positive result:

   $(-5) \times (-6) = 30$ $\quad$ $(-35) \div (-5) = 7$

Exponents

Exponents are superscripted numbers that immediately follow a *base number*, indicating the number of times that base number is to be self-multiplied to yield the result:

$2^3 = 2 \times 2 \times 2 = 8$

$6^2 = 6 \times 6 = 36$

$3^4 = 3 \times 3 \times 3 \times 3 = 81$

Square Roots

Taking the square root of a number is the opposite of squaring a number (multiplying a number by itself). The square root of a number is the number that yields the original number when the square root is multiplied by itself. For example, the square root of 81 is 9 and the square root of 25 is 5.

$9 \times 9 = 81$ $\quad$ $5 \times 5 = 25$

Using mathematical notation, these relationships are expressed as:

$\sqrt{81} = 9$ $\quad$ $\sqrt{25} = 5$

Averages

It is often useful to know the average value in a set of numbers, or data set. To calculate an average, add all the numbers together and divide that sum by the total number of values in the data set. Consider this set of numbers:

7 23 33 55 57 62 87 90

When you add all the numbers together, the sum is 414. There are 8 numbers in the data set. Dividing 414 by 8 yields 51.75, which is the average ($414 \div 8 = 51.75$).

Ratios

A ratio is a comparison of two values. The ratio comparing the numbers 3 and 1 can be expressed as 3 to 1, 3:1, or 3/1. A science experiment (or a cooking recipe) may call for a mixture of two substances in a 3:1 ratio. If a larger amount than the 3:1 measurement yield is needed, the 3:1 ratio can be multiplied. For example, if 3 cups of flour and 1 cup of sugar do not yield enough cookie dough, the 3:1 ratio can be multiplied by 2. To maintain the correct ratio of ingredients, both sides of the ratio must be multiplied by the same number:

To double the amounts:
$3:1 \times 2 = (3 \times 2):(1 \times 2) = 6:2$

To triple the amounts:
$3:1 \times 3 = (3 \times 3):(1 \times 3) = 9:3$

Fractions

A fraction is used to represent a part of a whole. One half, one third, and one fourth can be represented numerically with fractions as 1/2, 1/3, and 1/4. The top half of the fraction is called the *numerator* and the bottom half is the *denominator.*

Adding Fractions

To add two fractions with the same denominator, add the numerators and place the sum over the same denominator:

$$\frac{1}{5} + \frac{3}{5} = \frac{4}{5}$$

To add two fractions with different denominators, the fractions must first be expressed with the same denominator, known as the *least common denominator* (*LCD*). The fractions can then be added by adding the numerators over the LCD.

Example: To find the sum of 2/9 and 3/12, first find the LCD. To do that, note that the *greatest common factor* (*GCF*) of 9 and 12—the largest whole number that divides evenly into both numbers—is 3. Divide one of the denominators by the GCF and multiply the answer by the other denominator:

$9 \div 3 = 3$

$3 \times 12 = 36$, so the LCD is 36.

Express the fractions using the LCD:

$$\frac{2}{9} \times \frac{4}{4} = \frac{8}{36} \qquad \frac{3}{12} \times \frac{3}{3} = \frac{9}{36}$$

Now add the numerators:

$$\frac{8}{36} + \frac{9}{36} = \frac{17}{36}$$

Multiplying Fractions

To multiply two fractions, multiply the numerators, multiply the denominators, and place the product of the numerators over the product of the denominators:

$$\frac{2}{9} \times \frac{3}{12} = \frac{6}{108}$$

Multiply the numerators ($2 \times 3 = 6$)

Multiply the denominators ($9 \times 12 = 108$)

Place the product of the numerators over the product of the denominators (6/108)

Then simplify the fraction by dividing by the largest whole number that goes evenly into both the numerator and denominator; in this case, 6:

$$\frac{6 \div 6}{108 \div 6} = \frac{1}{18}$$

Dividing Fractions

To divide one fraction by another, invert the denominator fraction and multiply the inverted fraction by the numerator fraction. This involves multiplying the numerators together and the denominators together, then placing the product of the numerators over the product of the denominators. To divide 2/9 by 3/12:

$$\frac{\frac{2}{9}}{\frac{3}{12}} = \frac{2}{9} \times \frac{12}{3} = \frac{24}{27}$$

Invert 3/12 to 12/3.

Multiply 2/9 x 12/3

Multiply the numerators (2 x12 = 24)

Multiply the denominators (9 x 3 = 27)

Place the product of the numerators over the product of the denominators

Simplify the fraction:

$$\frac{24 \div 3}{27 \div 3} = \frac{8}{9}$$

Percentages

A *percentage* is a part of 100. Thus, 37% represents 37 parts of 100. To find the percentage when the number of parts does not equal 100, first change the percentage to a decimal by dividing it by 100. Then multiply the decimal by the total number of parts.

Example: Find 37% of 80

$$\frac{37}{100} = 0.37$$

$80 \times 0.37 = 29.6$

Therefore, 29.6 is 37% of 80.

To determine the percentage of the number 55 that equals 42, divide 42 by 55 and then multiply the product by 100%:

$$\frac{42}{55} \times 100 = 0.764 \times 100 = 76.4\%$$

Appendix C Anatomy and Physiology Word Elements

Many word parts that are routinely used in the study of anatomy and physiology come from Greek and Latin. The meanings of these word parts offer clues to the meanings of words used to describe structures, functions, and processes. For example, the word *physiology* is made up of physio- ("function") and -logy ("study of"). Thus, physiology is the study of how living things function or work.

The following combining forms, prefixes, and suffixes are used throughout the text. This list is not exhaustive; only commonly used forms are presented.

A

ab- away from, off (*abdominal aorta, abduction*)

abdomen/o abdomen (*abdominal, abdominopelvic cavity*)

acous/o, acoust/o hearing, sound (*external acoustic meatus*)

acr/o- extremity, highest or farthest point (*acromegaly, acromion*)

ad- to, toward, near (*adduction*)

adip/o- fat or fatty tissue (*adipocyte, adipose tissue*)

af- toward (*afferent nerves, afferent pathway*)

-agon to gather, assemble (*agonist, antagonist*)

alb/i, alb/o, albin/o white (*albinism*)

amni- fetal sac (*amnion, amniotic fluid*)

amph-, amphi/o on both sides, around (*amphiarthrosis*)

an- not, without (*anaerobic, anemia*)

ana- apart (*anatomy, anaphase*); up, build up (*anabolism*)

andr/o male (*androgen*)

angi/o blood vessel (*angioplasty, angiography, angiotensin*)

antero forward, from front to back (*anteroposterior*)

anti- against (*antibiotic, antidiuretic hormone*)

apo- above, away, off, separated from (*apocrine glands, aponeurosis*)

aque/o water (*aquaporins, aqueous humor*)

arteri/o artery (*arterial, arterioles*)

arthr/o joint (*synarthroses, diarthrodial*)

articul/o joint (*articular fibrocartilage, articulating bones*)

-ase enzyme (*amylase, polymerase*)

ather/o fat, plaque (*atherosclerosis*)

atri/o heart, entryway (*atrium, interatrial septum*)

audi/o, audit/o hearing (*auditory canal, audiologist*)

aur/i, aur/o, auricul/o ear, hearing (*auricle*)

aut/o self (*autoimmune disease, autonomic nervous system*)

axi/o axis, straight line (*axial skeleton, axon*)

B

bar/o pressure, weight (*baroreceptors, barometric*)

bi- two, twice, double (*bicarbonate, biceps*)

bi/o life (*biopsy, microbial*)

bil/i bile (*bilirubin*)

blast/o bud, germ, precursor (*blastocyst, osteoblast*)

brachi/o arm (*biceps brachii*)

bronch/i, bronch/o airway (*bronchus, bronchodilator*)

C

calc/o, calci/o calcium, stone (*hypercalcemia, calcitonin*)

calori- heat (*Calorie, caloric*)

carcin/o cancer (*carcinogen*)

cardi/o heart (*cardiovascular*)

carp/o wrist (*metacarpals, radiocarpal*)

centr/i, centr/o middle, center (*centromere, centriole*)

cephal/o head (*diencephalon, brachiocephalic artery*)

cerebr/o brain (*cerebrum*)

cervic/o neck, narrow part (*cervical*)

circ/um- around, about (*circumduction*)

-clast break (down), destroy (*osteoclasts*)

clavicul/o hammer, club, key (*clavicle, acromioclavicular joint*)

-cle little (*corpuscle*)

co- with, together (*cotransport*)

col-, col/o, col/ono- large intestine (*colonoscopy*)

com- with, together (*complement system, compression*)

contus/o bruise (*contusion*)

coron/o heart, crown (*coronary, corona radiata*)

corp/o, corpor/o body (*corpus luteum, corpora cavernosa*)

corti- covering (*cortical*)

cost/o rib (*intercostal nerves, sternocostal joints*)

cox/a, cox/o hip (*coxal bone*)

crani/o skull (*cranium*)

-crin/o secrete, separate (*endocrine, exocrine*)

cry/o cold (*cryotherapy, oocyte cryopreservation*)

-cule, -culus small (*molecule, canaliculus*)

cutane/o skin (*subcutaneous fascia, musculocutaneous*)

cyst/i, cyst/o bladder (*cystitis, cholecystectomy*)

-cyte, cyt/o cell (*lymphocyte, cytoplasm*)

D

de- down, away from, cessation (*dehydration, defibrillation*)

dendr/o tree, branch (*dendrites, oligodendrocytes*)

-derma, dermat/o, derm/o skin (*epidermal, dermatologist*)

-desis binding, tying together (*diapedesis*)

desm/o bond, ligament (*desmosomes, syndesmosis*)

di- two, apart, separate, through (*diuresis, antidiuretic hormone*)

dia- across, separate, through (*diaphragm, dialysis*)

dif- apart, separate (*differentiate, diffusion*)

digit- finger (*extensor digitorum*)

dilat/o widening, expanding, stretching (*dilation*)

dipl/o double (*diploid*)

dis- apart, separate (*dissect, dislocation*)

dist/o far, distant (*distal convoluted tubule*)

dors/i, dors/o back, back of body (*dorsal, latissimus dorsi*)

duc-, duct/o to lead, carry (*abduction, adduction*)

dynam/o strength, force, power, energy (*dynamic lung volume, dynamometer*)

dys- bad, abnormal, painful (*muscular dystrophy, dyspnea*)

E

e- out (*ejaculate, eversion*)

-eal pertaining to (*pineal, esophageal*)

ec-, ect/o out, outside, away (*ectopic*)

-ectomy incision, surgical removal (*cholecystectomy, mastectomy*)

-edema swelling (*lymphedema, myxedema*)

ef- out, out of (*efferent, effusion*)

-el, -elle small (*organelle, fontanel*)

electr/o electricity (*electrocardiogram, electrolytes*)

em- in, within (*embolism*)

-ema condition (*emphysema*)

-emia blood condition (*anemia, leukemia*)

en- in, into (*enzyme*)

encephal/o brain (*diencephalon*)

end/o in, inside, within (*endometrium*)

enter/o intestine (*gastroenterologist*)

epi- on, upon, above (*epidermis, epididymis*)

epitheli/o skin (*epithelium*)

erythr/o red (*erythrocyte*)

-esis action, condition, state of (*erythropoiesis, synthesis*)

estr/o female (*estrogen*)

ex-, exo- out, out of, away, away from (*exocytosis, exophthalmos*)

extra- outside (*extracellular*)

F

femor/o thigh bone (*femoral*)

fer-, -ferent to carry (*afferent, efferent*)

fibr/o fiber (*fibroblast*)

fil/a, fil/o, filament/o thread, thread-like (*microfilament, filtration*)

flex/o bend (*dorsiflexion*)

fore- before (*forearm*), in front (*forehead*)

-form, -iform having the shape or form of (*fusiform, deformed*)

G

gastr/o stomach (*gastric, gastroesophageal*)

-gen, -genic, -genesis producing, bringing about (*gluconeogenesis, oogenesis*)

germi- sprout, bud (*germinate, germinal*)

gest/o to carry (ingest); pregnancy (*gestation, progesterone*)

gingiv/o pertaining to the gums (*gingivitis*)

glauc/o having a blue or blue-gray color (*glaucoma*)

-glia glue (*neuroglia, microglia*)

globu- sphere, ball (*globulin, hemoglobin*)

gloss/o, glott/o tongue (*glossopharyngeal*)

gluc/o sugar, glucose (*glucose, glucocorticoid*)

glyc/o sugar, glucose (*glycogen, hypoglycemia, glycolysis*)

-gnosis knowledge (*diagnosis, prognosis*)

gon/o, gonad/o semen, seed, pertaining to reproduction (*spermatogonia, gonadotropic*)

gyn/o, gynec/o woman, female (*gynecology*)

H

hapl/o single, simple (*haploid*)

hema-, hemo-, hemat/o blood (*hematopoiesis, hematocrit*)

hemi- half (*hemisphere*)

-hemia blood condition (*polycythemia*)

hepat/o liver (*hepatitis*)

hist/o tissue (*histology*)

hom/o like, similar (*homologous*)

home/o unchanging, constant (*homeostasis*)

humer/o shoulder (*humerus*)

hydr/o water (*hydrophobic*)

hyper- above, above normal, excessive (*hypertrophy, hyperopia*)

hypo- under, below normal (*hypoxia, hyposecretion*)

I

-ia condition (*anemia, pneumonia*)

-iasis abnormal condition (*psoriasis*)

-iatr/o doctor, medicine (*pediatric*)

-ic, -ical pertaining to (*anatomical, biological*)

-icle, -icul small (*ossicle, canaliculus*)

-ics knowledge (*kinetics, genetics*)

-immun/o protection, safety (*autoimmune, immunotherapy*)

in- in, into, not (*inspiration*)

-in(e) protein, enzyme, chemical compound (*penicillin, creatinine*)

infra- below, beneath, inferior to (*infraspinous fossa*)

inter- between, among (*interstitial, intervertebral*)

intra- within, into (*intracellular*)

-ism process (*metabolism*); condition or disorder (*gigantism, astigmatism*)

is/o same, equal (*isometric*)

-ite little (*dendrite*)

-itis inflammation (*gingivitis*)

-ium structure, tissue (*cranium, endomysium*)

J

jaund/o yellow (*jaundice*)

jug- to join (*jugular*)

juxta- beside, next to (*juxtamedullary nephrons*)

K

kerat/o hard, horn-shaped tissue (*keratinocytes*)

kin/e, kin/o, kines/o, kinesi/o movement, motion (*kinetic, cytokinesis*)

L

lacrim/o tear (*lacrimal glands*)
lact/i, lact/o milk (*lactation*)
laryng/o voice box (*laryngeal*)
later/o side (*lateral rotation*)
-lepsy, -leptic seizure (*epilepsy, epileptic*)
-let small (*platelet*)
leuk/o white (*leukocytes, leukemia*)
lig/o to tie, bind (*ligament*)
lingu/a, lingu/o tongue (*lingual tonsil*)
lip/o fat (*lipocyte*)
lith/o stone (*lithotripsy*)
-(o)logy study of (*biology, physiology*)
-lucent, -lucid clear, light, shining (*zona pellucida, stratum lucidum*)
lumb/o lower back (*lumbar*)
lun- moon, crescent (*semilunar valves*)
lute/o yellow (*corpus luteum*)
-lymph, lymph/o lymph (*endolymph, lymphocytes*)
lys/o, lyt/o, -lyt/ic separate, break apart, break down, destroy (*lysosome, glycolysis*)

M

macro- large (*macrophage*)
mal/i bad (*malfunction, malignant*)
mamm/o breast (*mammogram*)
medi/o, mediastin/o middle (*medial, mediastinum*)
medull/o middle, deep part, marrow (*medullary canal, medulla oblongata*)
meg/a, megal/o, -megaly large, enlargement (*acromegaly, megakaryocytes*)
melan/o black color (*melanocyte, melanoma*)
men/o month, menses, menstruation (*amenorrhea, menarche*)
mening/o, meningi/o membrane (*meningitis*)
meta- after, beyond; change (*metaphase, metacarpal*)
-meter instrument or device used to measure (*spirometer, sphygmomanometer*)
metri- length, measure (*metric system*)
metri-, metr/o uterus, womb (*endometrium*)
micro- small; millionth (*microscope, microbiology*)
mon/o one, single (*monomer, monosaccharide*)
morph/o form, shape (*polymorphism*)
-mortem, mort/o death (*mortality, post-mortem*)
muc/o, mucos/o mucus (*mucosal*)
multi- many (*multicellular*)
muscul/o muscle (*musculoskeletal*)
muta- change (*mutation*)
mysi-, my/o, myos/o muscle (*myositis, epimysium*)
myel/o bone marrow (*myeloid*); spinal cord (*myelin*)

N

nas/o nose (*nasolacrimal, nasopharynx*)
natr/i, natr/o sodium (*hyponatremia, natriuretic*)
neo- new (*gluconeogenesis, neonatal*)
nephr/o kidney (*nephron*)
neur/o nerve (*neuromuscular, neuroscience*)
neutr/o neutral, neither (*neutrophil, neutralization*)
nucle/o nucleus (*nuclear membrane, deoxyribonucleic acid*)
nutri/o, nutrit/o nourish (*nutrient, nutrition*)

O

obstetr/o pregnancy; birth (*obstetrician*)
ocul/o eye (*oculomotor, orbicularis oculi*)
odont/o tooth (*periodontal disease*)
-ole little, small (*arteriole, nucleolus*)
-oma tumor, mass (*carcinoma, hematoma*)
onc/o tumor (*oncologist*)
-opia vision condition (*myopia, hyperopia*)
ophthalm/o eye (*ophthalmologist, exophthalmos*)
-opsy view of (*biopsy*)
optic/o eye, vision (*optic chiasma*)
or/o mouth (*oropharynx*)
orbi- circle (*orbicularis*)
-orexia appetite (*anorexia*)
orth/o straight (*orthopedic, orthodontist*)
-ose sugar (*glucose, fructose*)
-osis process (*mitosis, apoptosis*); disease, abnormal condition (*tuberculosis, cirrhosis*)
osseo- bony (*osseous tissue, interosseous membrane*)
ossi- bone (*ossification*)
ost/e, oste/o bone (*osteoporosis*)
ov/o, ovul/o egg (*ovum, ovulation*)
ox/o oxygen (*hypoxic, oxyhemoglobin*)

P

para- near, next to, beside (*parathyroid, parasites*)
-partum birth; labor (*parturition, postpartum*)
path/o disease (*pathology*); feeling, emotion (*sympathetic*)
pector/o chest (*pectoral girdle, pectoralis major*)
ped/o child (*pediatrician*); foot (*tinea pedis*)
pelv/i, pelv/o hip (*pelvic*)
pend/o to hang (*appendix, appendicular*)
-penia deficiency (*osteopenia*)
penna- thread (*unipennate*)
penta- five, fifth (*pentapeptide, pentamer*)
peri- around (*periosteum, peritoneum*)
-phage, phag/o eat, swallow (*esophagus, phagocytosis*)
phalang/o fingers, toes (*phalanges*)
pharyng/o throat (*pharyngeal*)
phil/o loving, attracted to (*hydrophilic*)
phleb/o vein (*phlebotomist*)
-phob/o, -phobia fear (*hydrophobic*)
phon/o, -phonia voice, sound (*phonetic*)
phot/o light (*phototherapy*)
physi/o, physic/o nature, function (*physiology, physician*)
-physis growth (*diaphysis, epiphysis*)
-plasm shaped, molded (*cytoplasm, endoplasmic*)
-plasty surgical repair (*rhinoplasty*)
-plegia, -plegic paralysis (*paraplegia*)
pleur/o lung (*pleurisy*)
plex/o network of nerves (*brachial plexus*)
-pnea breath, breathing (*dyspnea*)
pneum/o, pneumon/o lung, air (*pneumonia*)
pod/o foot (*podocyte*)
-poiesis formation (*hematopoiesis, erythropoiesis*)
-poietin substance that forms (*erythropoietin, thrombopoietin*)

poly- many, much (*polymer, polysaccharide*)

-porosis condition of holes, spaces (*osteoporosis*)

post- after, behind (*postmenopausal*)

poster/o back of (the body), behind (*posterior*)

pre- before, in front of (*precursor, preganglionic*)

presby/o old age (*presbyopia*)

pro- before, in front of (*prostate*); promote (*progesterone*)

prot/o first (*protoplasm*)

proxim/o near (*proximal*)

pseudo false (*pseudopod*)

psych/o mind (*psychological*)

pulmon/o lung (*pulmonary*)

puls/o, pulsat/o to beat, vibrate, push against (*pulsation, propulsion*)

pyr/o, pyret/o, pyrex/o fire; fever (*pyrogen*)

Q

quadri- four (*quadriceps*)

quater- fourth (*quaternary structure*)

R

radiat- radiating (*corona radiata*)

radi/o X-ray; radioactive; (*radiography*)

re- back, again, backward (*reabsorption, remodeling*)

-receptor, -ceptor receiver (*chemoreceptor*)

ren/o kidney (*renal cortex*)

respir/o breathe (*respiratory*)

reticul/o network (*reticular connective tissue*)

retr/o back, backward, behind (*retroperitoneal*)

rhin/o nose (*rhinoplasty*)

-rrhage, -rrhagia bursting forth of blood (*hemorrhagic stroke*)

-rrhea flow, discharge (*diarrhea, amenorrhea*)

S

sacchar/o sugar (*polysaccharide*)

sacr/o posterior section of pelvic bone (*sacroiliac joint*)

scapul/o shoulder blade (*scapulothoracic joint, subscapular*)

-scope, scop/o, -scopy see (*microscope, colonoscope*)

sect/o to cut (*dissection*)

semi- half (*semicircular canals, semilunar valves*)

semin/i semen, seed (*seminal glands, seminiferous tubules*)

-sis state of, condition (*stenosis*); process (*mitosis, glycolysis*)

son/o sound (*sonogram*)

-spasm sudden contraction of muscles (*bronchospasm*)

sperm/o, spermat/o sperm cells (*spermatid, spermatocyte*)

-sphyxia pulse (*asphyxiation*)

spir/o to breathe (*respiration, spirometer*)

stas/i, stat/i stop, remain, stay the same (*homeostasis*)

-static pertaining to stopping or controlling (*homeostatic, hydrostatic*)

sten/o narrow, constricted (*valvular stenosis*)

stern/o chest, breast (*sternum*)

steth/o chest (*stethoscope*)

strept/o twisted chains (*streptococcus*)

stri/a striped (*striated*)

sub- under, below (*subcutaneous*)

super- above, beyond (*superior, superficial*)

sym- together, with (*symphysis, symmetrical*)

syn- together, with (*synthesis, synarthroses*)

synaps/o, synapt/o to join, make contact (*synaptic*)

systol/o contraction (*systolic*)

T

tars/i, tars/o ankle, hindfoot (*metatarsal*)

tendin/o, ten/o tendon (*tendinitis*)

tens/o stretched, strained (*tensile*)

tetra- four (*tetramer, tetrad*)

therm/o heat (*hyperthermia, thermometer*)

thorac/o, -thorax chest, pleural cavity (*cardiothoracic*)

thromb/o blood clot (*thrombosis, thrombocytes*)

tom/o to cut (*splenectomy, cholecystectomy*)

tox/o, toxic/o poison (*cytotoxic*)

trans- across, through (*neurotransmitter, transverse plane*)

tri- three (*adenosine triphosphate, triglycerides*)

-tropin to act upon, stimulate (*adrenocorticotropin, gonadotropin*)

U

-ul, -ule little, small (*trabecula, glomerulus*)

ultra- beyond, excessive (*ultraviolet, ultrasonic*)

-um structure, tissue, substance (*cerebrum, sodium*)

uni- one (*unipennate, unipolar*)

-uresis urination (*diuresis*)

ur/i, ur/o, -uria, urin/o urine, urination (*polyuria, urinalysis*)

-us structure, thing (*fetus, hypothalamus*)

uter/o womb (*uterus, uterine*)

V

valv/o, valvu/o valve (*valvular stenosis*)

vas/o, vascul/o vessel (*vasa recta, vascular, vas deferens*)

ven/i, ven/o vein (*venous, venule, intravenous*)

ventil/o to oxygenate (*ventilation, hyperventilation*)

ventr/o, ventricul/o belly side of body, lower part (*ventral, ventricle*)

vers/o, -verse, -version turning (*eversion, inversion*)

vertebr/o spine; backbone (*intervertebral*)

vir/o virus (*viral, virology*)

viscer/o internal organs (*visceral pleura, visceral pericardium*)

vit/a, vit/o life (*vitamin, vital signs*)

vitr/e, vitr/o glass (*vitreous humor, in vitro*)

X

xanth/o yellow (*xanthosis*)

xiph/o sword-shaped (*xiphoid process*)

Y

-y condition, process (*thermoplasty*)

Z

zo/o life (*zoology*)

zyg/o union, junction, pair (*zygote*)

Appendix D Common Medical Abbreviations

A

ACTH adrenocorticotropin hormone
AD Alzheimer's disease
ADH antidiuretic hormone
ADP adenosine diphosphate
AED automatic external defibrillator
AIDS acquired immunodeficiency syndrome
ALL acute lymphocytic leukemia
ALS amyotrophic lateral sclerosis
AML acute myeloid leukemia
ANP atrial natriuretic peptide
ANS autonomic nervous system
APC antigen-presenting cell
ATP adenosine triphosphate
AV atrioventricular (node; valves)

B

BMI body mass index
BMR basal metabolic rate
BPM beats per minute

C

CLL chronic lymphocytic leukemia
CML chronic myeloid leukemia
CNS central nervous system
CO_2 carbon dioxide
COPD cardiopulmonary disease
CP cerebral palsy
CPR cardiopulmonary resuscitation
CT computed tomography

D

DNA deoxyribonucleic acid
DO doctor of osteopathic medicine
DOMS delayed-onset muscle soreness
DPT doctor of physical therapy

E

ECG electrocardiogram
ED erectile dysfunction
EIB exercise-induced bronchospasms
EKG electrocardiogram (*variant of* ECG)
EMD electromechanical delay
EMT emergency medical technician
EPO erythropoietin
ERV expiratory reserve volume

F

FEV_1 forced expiratory volume in one second
FEV_1/FVC forced expiratory volume in one second/forced vital capacity
fMRI functional magnetic resonance imaging
FRC functional residual capacity
FSH follicle-stimulating hormone
FT fibers fast-twitch fibers

G

GERD gastroesophageal reflux disease
GFR glomerular filtration rate
GH growth hormone
GI gastrointestinal
GnRH gonadotropin-releasing hormone

H

H_2O water
HbA1c glycosylated hemoglobin (test)
hCG human chorionic gonadotropin
HDL high-density lipoprotein
HIV human immunodeficiency virus
HPV human papillomavirus
HR heart rate
HSV-1 herpes simplex virus type 1
HSV-2 herpes simplex virus type 2

I

IRV inspiratory reserve volume
IV intravenous
IVF in vitro fertilization

L

L/min liters per minute
LBP low back pain
LDL low-density lipoprotein
LH luteinizing hormone

M

MAC membrane attack complex
MALT mucosa-associated lymphatic tissue
MAP mean arterial pressure
MD medical doctor; muscular dystrophy
mg/DL milligrams per deciliter
MHC major histocompatibility complex glycoproteins
mL/beat milliliters per beat
mmHG millimeters of mercury
MRA magnetic resonance angiography
MRI magnetic resonance imaging
mRNA messenger RNA (ribonucleic acid)
MS multiple sclerosis

N

NCV nerve conduction velocity
NK cells natural killer cells

O

O_2 oxygen
OD optometry degree

P

PA physician assistant
PACs premature atrial contractions
PCOS polycystic ovarian syndrome
PCT proximal convoluted tubule
PD Parkinson's disease
PET positron emission tomography
pH acid-base balance
PID pelvic inflammatory disease
PNS peripheral nervous system
PRO prolactin
PSA test prostate-specific antigen test
PTH parathyroid hormone
PVCs premature ventricular contractions
PVD peripheral vascular disease

Q

Q cardiac output

R

RBC red blood cell
RNA ribonucleic acid
rRNA ribosomal RNA (ribonucleic acid)
RT respiratory therapist
RV pulmonary ventilation residual volume

S

SA sinoatrial (node)
SCID severe combined immune deficiency
SNS sympathetic nervous system
ST fibers slow-twitch fibers
STD sexually transmitted disease
SV stroke volume

T

T_3 triiodothyronine
T_4 thyroxine
TB tuberculosis
TBI traumatic brain injury
TIA transient ischemic attack
TLC total lung capacity
tRNA transfer RNA (ribonucleic acid)
TSH thyroid-stimulating hormone
TV tidal volume

U

UTI urinary tract infection
UVB ultraviolet B

V

VC vital capacity

W

WBC white blood cell

Glossary

A

ABCD rule The American Cancer Society's rule for determining the presence of melanoma. (3)

abdominal cavity space bounded by the abdominal walls, the diaphragm, and the pelvis (1)

abdominopelvic cavity continuous internal opening that includes the abdominal and pelvic cavities (1)

abduction movement of a body segment away from the body in the frontal plane (5)

absorption the movement of food molecules from the small intestine into the blood (13)

acceleration the change in velocity of an object to which the force is applied (1)

acetylcholine a neurotransmitter chemical that stimulates muscle (5)

acquired immunodeficiency syndrome (AIDS) a disease in which the immune system is greatly weakened due to infection with HIV, making a person more susceptible to rare cancers and opportunistic infections (12)

acromegaly a rare condition in which the anterior pituitary hypersecretes growth hormone, causing an increase in overall body size; gigantism (8)

action potential the electric charge produced in nerve or muscle fiber by stimulation (5); nerve impulse caused by a wave of depolarization along the length of a neuron (6)

active immunity immunity in which the blood plasma cells in the body make antibodies as a result of previous exposure to a disease or a vaccine (12)

active transport a process that requires energy to move against a concentration gradient, from an area of lower concentration to one of higher concentration (2)

acute bronchitis a temporary inflammation of the mucous membranes that line the trachea and bronchial passageways; causes a cough that may produce mucus (9)

acute flaccid myelitis (AFM) a rare, but serious neurologic condition that occurs primarily in children; attacks the gray matter in the spinal cord, affecting the muscles and reflexes (6)

acute lymphocytic leukemia (ALL) the most common form of leukemia in adults over 70 years of age; characterized by overproduction of lymphocytes (10)

acute myeloid leukemia (AML) the most common form of leukemia in adults; develops when the bone marrow produces too many myeloblasts (10)

Addison disease a condition caused by hyposecretion of adrenal corticoid hormones that causes muscle atrophy, a bronze skin tone, low blood pressure, kidney damage, hypoglycemia, severe loss of fluids and electrolytes, and a general feeling of weakness (8)

adduction movement of a body segment closer to the body in the frontal plane (5)

adenosine triphosphate (ATP) a nucleotide composed of an adenine base, a sugar, and three phosphate groups (2)

adipose tissue tissue that consists almost entirely of adipocytes, or fat cells, with little extracellular matrix (2)

adrenal cortex outer layer of the adrenal glands, which itself has three layers that secrete steroid hormones (8)

adrenal medulla the part of the adrenal glands that functions as a part of the nervous system; it secretes the hormones epinephrine and norepinephrine (catecholamines) during the fight-or-flight response (8)

adrenocorticotropin (ACTH) tropic hormone secreted by the anterior pituitary that acts on the adrenal cortex to stimulate release of steroid hormones (8)

afferent nerves sensory transmitters that send impulses from receptors in the skin, muscles, and joints to the central nervous system (6)

agglutination the process by which red blood cells clump together, usually in response to an antibody; can block small blood vessels and cause hemolysis (10)

agonist role played by a skeletal muscle to cause a movement (5)

aldosterone the principal mineralocorticoid hormone produced by the adrenal cortex; stimulates the kidneys to reabsorb sodium and water from urine and to eliminate potassium (8); a steroid hormone produced in the adrenal cortex that regulates salt and water balance in the body by increasing the amount of sodium reabsorbed from urine (14)

allergen antigen that causes an inappropriately strong immune system response (12)

allergen immunotherapy a long-term, preventive treatment for allergies; "allergy shots" (12)

allergy an inappropriately strong response of the immune system to an environmental antigen, such as dust mites, pet dander, pollen, or certain foods (12)

all-or-none law the rule stating that the fibers in a given motor unit always develop maximum tension when stimulated (5)

alternative pathway one of the two primary ways in which the complement system can be activated; this pathway is triggered when the C3b complement protein binds to foreign material (12)

alveolar capillary membrane gas-exchange structure that contains the alveoli and the capillaries surrounding the alveoli (9)

alveoli air sacs in the lungs from which gas is exchanged with the capillaries (9)

Alzheimer's disease (AD) condition of dementia involving a progressive loss of brain function with major consequences for memory, thinking, and behavior (6)

Note: The number in parentheses following each definition indicates the chapter in which the term can be found.

amenorrhea absence of a menstrual period in women of reproductive age (4, 15)
amino acids the building blocks of proteins (2)
amniotic fluid a clear fluid in which the embryo, and then the fetus, is suspended (15)
amphiarthrosis joint type that permits only slight motions (4)
anaphylaxis a severe and potentially life-threatening allergic reaction that may include airway obstruction and very low blood pressure (12)
anatomical position erect standing position with arms at the sides and palms facing forward (1)
anatomy the study of the form or structure of living things, including plants, animals, and humans (1)
androgens male sex hormones (8)
anemia a condition characterized by a decrease in the number of red blood cells or an insufficient amount of hemoglobin in the red blood cells (10)
aneurysm abnormal ballooning of a blood vessel, usually an artery, due to a weakness in the wall of the vessel (11)
angina pectoris condition characterized by severe, constricting pain or sensation of pressure in the chest, often radiating to the left arm; caused by an insufficient supply of blood to the heart (11)
angiotensin a polypeptide hormone in the blood that constricts blood vessels and increases blood pressure (14)
anorexia nervosa condition characterized by body weight 15% or more below the minimal normal weight range, extreme fear of gaining weight, an unrealistic body image, and amenorrhea (4)
antagonist role played by a skeletal muscle acting to slow or stop a movement (5)
anterior (ventral) body cavity continuous internal opening that includes the thoracic and abdominopelvic cavities (1)
antibody a cell that circulates in plasma and attacks red blood cells with foreign antigens, or antigens that are different from those of the host (10)
antidiuretic hormone (ADH) hormone produced in the hypothalamus and stored in the posterior pituitary; decreases urine output by stimulating the kidneys to increase water reabsorption (8); a peptide hormone secreted by the pituitary gland that constricts blood vessels, raises blood pressure, and reduces excretion of urine; vasopressin (14)
antigen a protein on the surface of RBCs that is used to identify blood type; a molecule on the surface of cells that identifies cells as either "self" or "nonself" (foreign) cells (10)
antigenic determinants the multiple foreign parts on the surface of an antigen molecule that may cause an immune response (12)
antigen-presenting cells (APCs) cells that process protein antigens and present them on their surface in a form that can be recognized by lymphocytes (white blood cells) (12)
antihistamines medications that work to curb the activity of histamines (7)
aorta a large arterial trunk that arises from the base of the left ventricle and channels blood from the heart into other arteries throughout the body (11)
aortic arch the curved portion of the aorta between the ascending and descending parts of the aorta (11)
aortic valve the semilunar valve between the left ventricle and the aorta that prevents blood from flowing back into the left ventricle (11)
aplastic anemia a rare but serious condition in which the bone marrow is incapable of making new red blood cells (10)
apocrine glands sweat glands located in the genital and armpit areas that secrete a milky fluid consisting of sweat, fatty acids, and proteins (3)
aponeurosis a flat, sheetlike fibrous tissue that connects muscle or bone to other tissues (5)
apophysis site at which a tendon attaches to bone (4)
apoptosis a programmed process of cellular self-destruction (cell suicide) (12)
appendicular skeleton the bones of the body's appendages; the arms and legs (4)
aqueous humor the clear, watery fluid that fills the anterior chamber of the eye; provides nutrients for the lens and cornea and helps maintain intraocular pressure (7)
areolar connective tissue connective tissue that has a gel-like extracellular matrix that holds water well and serves as a support for overlying epithelia (2)
arteries vessels that carry blood away from the heart (11)
arterioles microscopic arteries that connect with capillaries (11)
arthritis family of more than 100 common pathologies associated with aging, characterized by joint inflammation accompanied by pain, stiffness, and sometimes swelling (4)
articular cartilage dense, white, connective tissue that covers the articulating surfaces of bones at joints (4)
articular fibrocartilage tissue shaped like a disc or partial disc called a meniscus that provides cushioning at a joint (4)
asthma disease of the lungs characterized by recurring episodes of airway inflammation causing bronchospasms and increased mucus production (9)
astrocytes glial cells that link neurons to capillaries and control the chemical environment to protect the neurons from any harmful substances in the blood (6)
atherosclerosis hardening of the arteries (11)
atlas the first cervical vertebra; specialized to provide the connection between the occipital bone of the skull and the spinal column (4)
atoms tiny particles of matter (1)
atrial fibrillation condition in which the atria contract in an uncoordinated, rapid manner (rate above 350 bpm), causing the ventricles to contract irregularly (11)
atrial natriuretic peptide (ANP) a peptide hormone secreted by the atria of the heart that promotes excretion of sodium and water and lowers blood pressure (14)
atrioventricular (AV) node a small mass of tissue that transmits impulses received from the sinoatrial node to the ventricles via the bundle of His (11)
atrioventricular (AV) valves the two valves (tricuspid and mitral) situated between the atria and the ventricles (11)
auditory canal a short, tubelike structure that connects the outer ear to the eardrum (7)

auricle the irregularly shaped outer portion of the ear (7)
autoimmune disorder a condition in which the immune system attacks the body's own tissue (12)
autonomic nervous system branch of the nervous system that controls involuntary body functions (6)
autonomic reflexes involuntary stimuli transmitted to cardiac and smooth muscle (6)
avulsion a fracture caused when a tendon or ligament pulls away from its attachment to a bone, taking a small chip of bone with it (4)
axial skeleton central, stable portion of the skeletal system, consisting of the skull, spinal column, and thoracic cage (4)
axis the second cervical vertebra; specialized with an upward projection called the odontoid process, on which the atlas rotates (4)
axon a long, thin fiber connected to the motor neuron cell body (5)
axon terminals offshoots of the axon that branch out to connect with individual muscle fibers (5)

B

ball-and-socket joint synovial joint formed between one bone end shaped roughly like a ball and the receiving bone reciprocally shaped like a socket (4)
baroreceptors pressure-sensitive nerve endings in the atrium, aortic arch, and carotid arteries (11)
basal cell carcinoma the most common form of skin cancer and the least malignant type (3)
basal metabolic rate (BMR) the amount of energy required to sustain a person's metabolism for one day if he or she is at complete rest (13)
base pairs pairs of complementary nucleic acid bases; that is, A and T or C and G (2)
bending a loading pattern created by a combination of off-center forces (1)
bile a watery substance produced by the liver that contains bile salts, which help emulsify fats (13)
blastocyst a fluid-filled cavity (15)
B lymphocytes (B cells) lymphocytes that mature in the bone marrow before moving out to the blood and the rest of the body; also called B cells (12)
bone marrow material with a rich blood supply found within the marrow cavity of long bones; yellow marrow stores fat, and red marrow is active in producing blood cells (4)
bony labyrinth winding tunnels located in the inner ear (7)
brachial artery the artery located at the fold of the elbow where the brachial pulse is detected (11)
bradycardia a normal heart rhythm but with a rate below 60 bpm; a condition common among athletes (11)
bronchioles the thin-walled branches of the bronchi; the smallest air-conducting passageways of the bronchi. The terminal bronchioles conduct a small amount of gas exchange in the respiratory zone. (9)
bronchospasms spasmodic contractions of the bronchial muscles that constrict the airways in the lungs during an asthma attack (9)
buffy coat a thin layer of white blood cells and platelets that lies between the red blood cells and plasma in a blood sample that has gone through a centrifuge (10)
bulbourethral glands two small glands at the base of the penis that secrete mucus into the urethra (15)
bulimia nervosa disordered eating that involves a minimum of two eating binges a week for at least three months; an associated feeling of lack of control; use of self-induced vomiting, laxatives, diuretics, strict dieting, or exercise to prevent weight gain; and an obsession with body image (4)
bundle of His a slender bundle of modified cardiac muscle that conducts electrical impulses from the AV node to the left and right bundle branches to Purkinje fibers in the ventricle (11)
bursae small capsules lined with synovial membranes and filled with synovial fluid; they cushion the structures they separate (4)
bursitis inflammation of one or more bursae (4)

C

calcitonin hormone produced and released by the parafollicular cells of the thyroid gland that helps maintain calcium homeostasis (8)
Calorie the unit that food scientists use to measure the potential energy in foods; the amount of heat required to raise the temperature of 1 kilogram of water by 1 °C; also called kilocalorie (13)
capacitation the process by which sperm becomes able to penetrate and fertilize an oocyte (15)
capillaries small, thin-walled vessels where oxygen and carbon dioxide gas exchange occurs (11)
capillary beds network of intertwined vessels formed by multiple capillaries (11)
carbaminohemoglobin hemoglobin molecule with carbon dioxide molecules attached; transports carbon dioxide to the lungs where it can be expelled from the body (10)
cardiac circulation blood circulation through the coronary arteries, providing the heart with nutrients and removing wastes (11)
cardiac cycle the events that occur during a single heartbeat (11)
cardiac output (CO) the amount of blood pumped from the heart per minute (11)
cardiomyopathy heart failure caused by infection and weakening of the myocardium, or heart muscle (11)
carotid artery the artery located on the side of the neck, where the carotid pulse is felt (11)
carpal bones bones of the wrist (4)
cartilage a connective tissue that provides support and flexibility to parts of the skeleton (2)
catecholamines hormones released into the blood during times of physical or emotional stress (8)
cells the smallest living building blocks of all organisms (1)

cellular immunity immunity that arises from the activation of T lymphocytes (T cells) by antigen-presenting cells; cell-mediated immunity (12)

cellulitis a bacterial infection characterized by an inflamed area of skin that is red, swollen, and painful (3)

central chemoreceptors chemical receptor cells that monitor changes in the pH of the cerebrospinal fluid in an effort to regulate carbon dioxide levels and respiration (9)

central nervous system (CNS) the brain and spinal cord (6)

centrioles short cylinders made of nine triplets of parallel microtubules (2)

centromere the point or region on a chromosome that divides the chromosome into two arms and functions as the point of attachment for the sister chromatids; provides movement during cell division (15)

cerebellum section of the brain that coordinates body movements, including balance (6)

cerebral palsy (CP) a group of nervous system disorders resulting from brain damage before or during birth, or in early infancy (6)

cerebrospinal fluid (CSF) fluid in the subarachnoid space that cushions the brain and spinal cord (6)

cerebrovascular accident a sudden blockage of blood flow, or rupture of an artery in the brain, that causes brain cells to die from lack of oxygen (11)

cerebrum the largest part of the brain, consisting of the left and right hemispheres (6)

ceruminous glands secretors of cerumen, or earwax; located in the auditory canal (7)

cervical region the first 7 vertebrae, comprising the neck (4)

cervix the narrow, lower end of the uterus that has the opening through which a baby passes during childbirth (15)

chain of infection the disease process for infections, starting with the causative pathogen and ending with the actual infection (12)

channel proteins molecules with a hollow central pore that allows water or small, charged particles of certain substances to pass into or out of the cells (2)

chelation therapy a procedure in which excess metals, such as iron, are removed from the blood (10)

chemical breakdown the breakdown of large food molecules into smaller molecules by enzymes; historically referred to as digestion (13)

chlamydia a sexually transmitted disease that often causes no symptoms, but can damage the female reproductive tract and lead to infertility and increased risk of ectopic pregnancy (15)

cholecystectomy surgical removal of the gallbladder (13)

chondroblasts cells that secrete the extracellular matrix of cartilage (2)

choroid the middle layer of the wall of the eye (7)

chromatids paired strands of a duplicated chromosome that become visible during cell division and that are joined by a centromere (15)

chromosome one DNA molecule and the proteins around which it coils (2); rod-shaped structure in the nucleus of body cells that contains individual DNA and genes (15)

chronic bronchitis a long-lasting respiratory condition in which the airways of the lungs become obstructed due to inflammation of the bronchi and excessive mucus production (9)

chronic kidney disease a condition defined by evidence of kidney damage or a glomerular filtration rate less than 60 milliliters per minute for at least three months (14)

chronic lymphocytic leukemia (CLL) a form of leukemia characterized by extremely high levels of lymphocytes; most often found in middle-age adults (10)

chronic myeloid leukemia (CML) a form of leukemia characterized by overproduction of granulocytes (10)

chronic obstructive pulmonary disease (COPD) any lung disorder characterized by a long-term airway obstruction, making it difficult to breathe (9)

chyme the mixture of food and digestive juice in the stomach and duodenum (13)

cilia hair-like projections that actively flex back and forth to move fluid or mucus across the outside of a cell (2)

ciliary body the structure between the choroid and the iris that anchors the lens in place (7)

ciliary glands modified sweat glands located between the eyelashes (7)

circumduction rotational movement of a body segment such that the end of the segment traces a circle (5)

cisterna chyli an enlarged lymphatic vessel located just in front of the vertebral column, at the diaphragm level, at which the two lumbar trunks and the intestinal trunk converge (12)

citric acid cycle a chain of reactions, catalyzed by enzymes in the mitochondrial matrix, in which pyruvate is broken down into individual carbon atoms, which combine with oxygen molecules to make CO_2 (2)

classical pathway a mode of complement system activation in which a circulating complement protein recognizes an antibody bound to foreign material (12)

clavicle doubly curved long bone that forms part of the shoulder girdle; the collarbone (4)

clitoris a cylindrical body of erectile tissue that lies at the anterior end of the vulva (15)

clonal selection repeated division of a lymphocyte that produces many exact genetic copies (clones) of itself (12)

coagulation the process by which the enzyme thrombin and the protein fibrinogen combine to form fibrin, a fiber that weaves around the platelet plug to form a blood clot; takes between 2 and 15 minutes to complete (10)

coccyx 4 fused vertebrae at the base of the spine forming the tailbone (4)

cochlea a snail-shaped structure in the inner ear that enables hearing (7)

cochlear duct the portion of the membranous labyrinth inside the cochlea (7)

codon a set of three bases in DNA or RNA that codes for one amino acid (2)

coenzymes molecules that are necessary for the action of enzymes (13)

collecting duct a tube that collects urine from several nephrons and carries it to the renal pelvis (14)

combined loading the simultaneous action of two or more types of forces (1)
complement proteins proteins in the blood that work with immune system cells and antibodies to defend the body against infection (12)
complement system a system of more than 30 proteins that circulate in the blood plasma through the body and work together to destroy foreign substances; complements, or balances out, the specific and nonspecific defense systems of the body (12)
compression a squeezing force that creates compression in the structure to which it is applied (1)
compressive strength the ability of a material to withstand compression (inward-pressing force) without buckling (2)
concentric a type of contraction that results in shortening of a muscle (5)
conductivity the ability of a neuron to transmit a nerve impulse (6)
condyloid joint type of diarthrosis in which one articulating bone surface is an oval, convex shape, and the other is a reciprocally shaped concave surface (4)
cones sensory cells in the retina that are sensitive to bright light and provide color vision (7)
conjunctiva a delicate external membrane that covers the exposed eyeball and lines the eyelid (7)
connective tissue supporting tissue, which consists mainly of an extracellular matrix (2)
constipation condition characterized by difficulty in defecating (13)
contractility the ability to contract or shorten (5)
control center system that receives and analyzes information from sensory receptors, then sends a command stimulus to an effector to maintain homeostasis (1)
contusion the bruises or bleeding within a muscle that result from an impact (5)
conversion factor a number that can be used to multiply the units of one measurement system into units in another measurement system (1)
cornea a transparent tissue over the anterior center of the eye (7)
coronary artery disease a narrowing of one or more of the coronary arteries due to a buildup of plaque; coronary heart disease (11)
coronary sinus large venous channel between the left atrium and left ventricle on the posterior side of the heart that empties into the right atrium at the junction of the four chambers (11)
corpus callosum a large, myelinated tract connecting the left and right hemispheres of the brain; contains more than 200 million axons (6)
corpus luteum the remaining cells of the follicle, which are still in the ovary after an oocyte is released into the pelvic cavity during ovulation (15)
cortical bone dense, solid bone that covers the outer surface of all bones and is the main form of bone tissue in the long bones (4)
cortisol a glucocorticoid hormone produced by the adrenal cortex that works with cortisone to maintain blood glucose levels via gluconeogenesis (8)
cortisone a glucocorticoid hormone produced by the adrenal cortex that works with cortisol to maintain blood glucose levels via gluconeogenesis (8)
cranial cavity opening inside the skull that holds the brain (1)
cranial nerves 12 pairs of nerves that originate in the brain and relay impulses to and from the PNS (6)
craniosacral branch the parasympathetic branch of the autonomic nervous system, in which nerves originate in the brainstem or sacral region of the spinal cord (6)
cranium fused, flat bones surrounding the back of the head (4)
creatinine a normal by-product of muscle metabolism; it is produced by the body at a fairly steady rate and is freely filtered by the glomerulus (14)
Crohn's disease a chronic inflammatory bowel disease that usually affects the small intestine or colon (13)
cross bridges connections between the heads of myosin filaments and receptor sites on the actin filaments (5)
crossovers connections that form between homologous chromosomes during meiosis, resulting in the swapping of portions of chromosomes (15)
Cushing syndrome a disorder of the adrenal cortex caused by hypersecretion of cortisol; symptoms include weight gain, high blood glucose levels, hypertension, and osteoporosis (8)
cutaneous membrane another name for skin (3)
cystitis inflammation of the urinary bladder epithelium (14)
cytokinesis division of the cytoplasm during cell division (2)
cytoplasm the part of the cell that contains all of the organelles inside the cell membrane except the nucleus (2)
cytoskeleton a network of proteins that defines the shape of a cell and gives it mechanical strength (2)

D

data set systematically collected and recorded observations (1)
decubitus ulcers ulcers caused by an area of localized pressure that restricts blood flow to one or more areas of the body (3)
defecation the discharge of feces from the anus (13)
deformation change in shape (1)
delayed-onset muscle soreness (DOMS) muscle pain that follows participation in a particularly long or strenuous activity; begins 24–73 hours later, and involves multiple, microscopic tears in the muscle tissue that cause inflammation, pain, swelling, and stiffness (5)
dementia an organic brain disease involving loss of function in two or more areas of cognition (6)
dendrites branches of a neuron that collect stimuli and transport them to the cell body (6)
deoxyribonucleic acid (DNA) a polymer of nucleotides with the bases adenosine, guanine, cytosine, and thymine (2)
depolarize to contract; the atria and ventricles depolarize as the heart beats (11)
depolarized a condition in which the inside of a cell membrane is more positively charged than the outside (6)

dermis layer of skin between the epidermis and hypodermis; includes nerve endings, glands, and hair follicles (3)
detrusor the smooth muscle that forms most of the bladder wall and aids in expelling urine (14)
diabetes insipidus a disorder resulting from hyposecretion of antidiuretic hormone (ADH) by the posterior pituitary (8)
diabetes mellitus (DM) a disease that results from the body's inability to produce sufficient amounts of insulin to regulate blood glucose levels (8)
diabetic nephropathy kidney disease (14)
diapedesis the passage of blood, or any of its formed elements, through the blood vessel walls into body tissues (10)
diaphysis the shaft of a long bone (4)
diarrhea the occurrence of frequent, watery bowel movements (13)
diarthrosis freely movable joint; also known as synovial joint (4)
diastole the period of relaxation in the heart when the chambers are filling with blood (11)
diencephalon area of the brain that includes the epithalamus, thalamus, and hypothalamus; also known as the interbrain (6)
diffusion the movement of material from a place where it is concentrated to a place where it is less concentrated (2)
dilation the stage of labor during which the opening of the cervix dilates, or widens (15)
diploid a cell having two sets of chromosomes: one set from the mother and one set from the father (15)
dislocation injury that involves displacement of a bone from its joint socket (4)
distal convoluted tubule the last part of a nephron through which urine flows before reaching the collecting duct (14)
diverticulitis development of inflammation in the diverticula (13)
diverticulosis development of small outward-bulging pouches, or diverticula, in the walls of the intestine (13)
dorsal ramus posterior spinal nerves that transmit motor impulses to the posterior trunk muscles and relay sensory impulses from the skin of the back (6)
dorsiflexion movement of the top of the foot toward the lower leg (5)
downregulated decreased (8)
ductus arteriosus a short, broad vessel in the fetus that connects the left pulmonary artery with the descending aorta, allowing most of the blood to bypass the infant's lungs (11)
ductus deferens the secretory duct of the testis, which extends from the epididymis and joins with the excretory duct of the seminal gland; vas deferens (15)
dwarfism a condition in which the pituitary gland hyposecretes growth hormone, resulting in an adult height of less than four feet (8)
dysrhythmia an irregular heartbeat or rhythm (11)

E

eccentric contraction accompanied by lengthening of a muscle (5)
eccrine glands sweat glands located over the majority of the body that produce a clear, acidic fluid that consists of approximately 99% water, but it also contains waste products such as urea, uric acid, salts, and vitamin C (3)
effector unit that receives a command stimulus from the control center and causes an action to help maintain homeostasis (1)
efferent nerves motor transmitters that carry impulses from the central nervous system out to the muscles and glands (6)
ejaculation the discharge of sperm from the ejaculatory duct during the male sexual response (15)
elastic a response that occurs when force is removed and the structure returns to its original size and shape (1)
elasticity the ability of a material to spring back to its original shape after being stretched (2, 5)
electrolyte a substance that dissolves in water into particles with positive and negative charges (2)
embryo the developing human from the time of implantation to the end of the eighth week after conception (15)
emphysema chronic inflammation of the lungs characterized by an abnormal increase in the air spaces near the bronchioles; causes an accumulation of carbon dioxide in the lungs (9)
emulsification the breakdown of large fat particles into much smaller particles, aided by bile (13)
endocarditis inflammation of the innermost lining of the heart, including the inner surface of the chambers and the valves (11)
endocardium the innermost layer of the heart, which lines the interior of the heart chambers and covers the valves of the heart (11)
endocrine gland a gland that secretes its product into the interstitial space (2)
endocytosis process in which a region of a cell membrane forms a pocket into the cell and then pinches off to form membrane-bound sac, or vesicle, inside the cytoplasm (2)
endolymph a thick fluid inside the membranous labyrinth (7)
endometriosis the growth of endometrial cells outside the uterus, usually in the abdominal cavity (15)
endomysium a fine, protective sheath of connective tissue around a skeletal muscle fiber (5)
endoneurium a delicate, connective tissue that surrounds each nerve fiber (6)
endoplasmic reticulum (ER) a network of membranes in the cytoplasm (2)
endosteum membrane lining the medullary cavity (4)
endothelial cells cells that form the walls of lymphatic capillaries; their overlapping structure helps fluid enter the lymphatic capillaries and makes it hard for the fluid to leave (12)
energy the capacity of a physical system to do work (13)
enzymes proteins that speed up specific biological reactions (2)

ependymal cells glial cells that form a protective covering around the spinal cord and central cavities within the brain (6)
epicardium the outermost layer of the heart and the innermost layer of the pericardial sac (11)
epidermal dendritic cells skin cells that initiate an immune system response to the presence of foreign bacteria or viruses (3)
epidermis the outer layer of skin (3)
epididymis a system of small ducts in the testis, in which sperm mature (15)
epigenetics processes, molecules, and molecular modifications, other than changes in DNA sequence, that can affect gene expression and can be passed on from one generation to the next (15)
epiglottis a flap of cartilaginous tissue that covers the opening to the trachea; diverts food and liquids to the esophagus during swallowing (9)
epilepsy a group of brain disorders characterized by repeated seizures over time (6)
epimysium the outermost sheath of connective tissue that surrounds a skeletal muscle (5)
epinephrine the chief neurohormone of the adrenal medulla that is used as a heart stimulant, a vasoconstrictor (which narrows the blood vessels), and a bronchodilator (which relaxes the bronchial tubes in the lungs) (8)
epineurium the tough outer covering of a nerve (6)
epiphyseal plate growth plate near the ends of long bones where osteoblast activity increases bone length (4)
epiphysis the bulbous end of a long bone (4)
epithalamus the uppermost portion of the diencephalon; includes the pineal gland and regulates sleep-cycle hormones (6)
epithelial membranes thin sheets of tissue lining the internal and external surfaces of the body (3)
epithelial tissue a class of tissue that includes epithelia and glands (2)
erection the condition of erectile tissue when filled with blood, which permits the penis to gain entry to the female reproductive tract (15)
erythroblastosis fetalis a severe hemolytic disease of a fetus or newborn caused by the production of maternal antibodies against the fetal red blood cell antigens, usually involving Rh incompatibility between the mother and fetus (10)
erythrocytes red blood cells; contain hemoglobin, a protein responsible for oxygen and carbon dioxide exchange (10)
erythropoiesis the process by which red blood cells are produced (10)
erythropoietin a hormone secreted by the kidneys that stimulates the production of red blood cells (10)
esophagus the muscular tube that connects the pharynx and stomach (13)
estrogens female sex hormones (8)
Eustachian tube a channel that connects the middle ear to the pharynx and serves to equalize pressure on either side of the tympanic membrane (7)
eversion movement in which the sole of the foot is rolled outward (5)
exocrine gland a gland that secretes its product to the outside world (2)
exocytosis process in which a small, membrane-bound vesicle in the cytoplasm fuses with the cell's membrane to export molecules that were inside the vesicle to the outside (2); the process in which cell membranes fuse together and then push debris from the cell vesicles to the outside of the cell (12)
exophthalmos condition in which the eyes bulge outward (8)
expiration the process by which air is expelled from the lungs; exhalation (9)
expiratory reserve volume (ERV) the additional amount of air that can be exhaled, or forced from the lungs, immediately after a normal exhalation (9)
expulsion the stage of labor that starts at full dilation and ends when the baby is delivered (15)
extensibility the ability to be stretched (5)
extension movement that returns a body segment to anatomical position in the sagittal plane (5)
external respiration the process by which gas exchange occurs between the alveoli in the lungs and the pulmonary blood (9)
external urethral sphincter a ring of skeletal muscle that surrounds the intermediate part of the urethra where it passes through the urogenital diaphragm; this muscle is voluntarily controlled during release of urine from the body (14)
extracellular fluid the liquid—consisting mostly of water—that surrounds a typical cell (2)
extracellular matrix the solid or gel-like substance that surrounds a typical cell (2)
extrinsic muscles muscles attached to the outer surface of the eye that are responsible for changing the direction of viewing (7)

F

facial bones bones of the face (4)
fascicle a bundle of muscle fibers (5)
fast-twitch type of muscle that contracts quickly (5)
fatty acid a hydrocarbon chain with a carboxylic acid group at one end (2)
female athlete triad a combination of disordered eating, amenorrhea, and osteoporosis (4)
femur thigh bone (4)
fertilization the formation of a single cell that contains the genetic material from two gametes, one from each parent (15)
fetal circulation the process by which an unborn infant receives oxygen and nutrients and disposes of waste products (11)
fetus a developing human from eight weeks after conception to birth (15)
fever the maintenance of body temperature at a higher-than-normal level (12)

fibrin a long, thread-like fiber created by the combination of thrombin and fibrinogen; weaves around the platelet plug to form a blood clot (10)

fibula bone of the lower leg; does not bear weight (4)

first-degree burns burns that affect only the epidermal layer of skin (3)

fissures the uniformly positioned, deep grooves in the brain (6)

flexion forward movement of a body segment away from anatomical position in the sagittal plane (5)

follicle-stimulating hormone (FSH) tropic hormone secreted by the anterior pituitary that stimulates production of estrogen and eggs in women and production of sperm in men (8)

fontanel openings in the infant skull through which a baby's pulse can be felt; these openings enable compression of the skull during birth and brain growth during late pregnancy and early infancy (4)

foramen ovale opening in the septal wall between the atria; normally present only in the fetus (11)

force push or pull acting on a structure (1)

forced expiratory volume in one second (FEV_1) the amount of air that a person can expire in one second (9)

forced expiratory volume in one second/forced vital capacity (FEV_1/FVC) the overall expiratory power of the lungs (9)

formed elements the solid components of blood; red blood cells, white blood cells, and platelets (10)

fourth-degree burns full-thickness burns that destroy both the skin and underlying tissues including muscles, tendons, ligaments, and bone (3)

fracture any break or disruption of continuity in a bone (4)

Frank-Starling law an increase in blood volume in the ventricles of the heart causes an increase in stroke volume (11)

frontal lobes sections of the brain located behind the forehead (6)

frontal plane an invisible, vertical flat surface that divides the body into front and back halves (1)

functional residual capacity (FRC) the amount of air that remains in the lungs after a normal expiration; ERV + RV (9)

G

gallbladder the digestive organ that stores bile and delivers it to the duodenum when needed (13)

gallstones solid crystals that form from substances in the bile of the gallbladder (13)

gametes mature haploid male or female cells that unite with cells of the opposite sex to form a zygote; eggs and sperm (15)

ganglion a mass of nervous tissue composed mostly of nerve cell bodies (6)

gastroenteritis an inflammation of the stomach or intestine that produces nausea, vomiting, diarrhea, and/or abdominal pain (13)

gastroesophageal reflux the movement of chyme from the stomach into the lower esophagus (13)

gastroesophageal reflux disease (GERD) chronic inflammation of the esophagus caused by the upward flow of gastric juice (13)

gastrointestinal tract (GI tract) the stomach, small intestine, and large intestine; alimentary canal (13)

gene a segment of DNA containing all the codons to make one polypeptide chain (2)

gene therapy the intentional alteration of a person's DNA in order to cure disease (2)

genital herpes a sexually transmitted disease that may cause blisters or sores in the genital or anal area or near the mouth; may cause no symptoms (15)

genotype genetic makeup (15)

germ theory of disease the theory, now proven, that microscopic organisms, or "germs," can cause disease in humans (12)

gestation the period of human development between fertilization and birth (15)

gestational age time since the first day of a woman's last menstrual period before pregnancy (15)

gingiva soft tissue that covers the necks of the teeth, the mandible, and the maxilla; also called the gum (13)

glands epithelial cells that are organized to produce and secrete substances (2)

gliding joint type of diarthrosis that allows only sliding motion of the articulating bones (4)

glomerular filtration the movement of water and solutes (dissolved substances) from the capillaries into the glomerular capsular space; this is the first step in urine formation (14)

glomerular filtration rate (GFR) the total amount of water filtered from the glomerular capillaries into the glomerular capsule per unit of time; usually measured in milliliters per minute (14)

glomerulus a cluster of capillaries around the end of a renal corpuscle (14)

glucagon hormone secreted by alpha cells in the islets of Langerhans of the pancreas; increases blood glucose levels by causing the breakdown of glycogen stored in the liver (8)

glucose the main form of sugar that circulates in the blood (2)

glycogen a polymer of glucose found in animals; stored form of glucose (2)

glycolysis the breakdown of a glucose molecule into two pyruvate molecules (2)

glycoproteins proteins with carbohydrate groups attached (2)

goiter an enlarged thyroid gland caused by insufficient amounts of iodine or a thyroid disorder (8)

Golgi apparatus a set of membranous discs in the cytoplasm (2)

gonads the organs that produce gametes (oocytes and sperm): the ovaries in females and the testes in males (15)

gonorrhea a sexually transmitted disease that may cause pain during urination, unusual discharge of fluid from the vagina or penis, or no symptoms at all; can lead to infertility (15)

Graves disease an autoimmune disorder that causes an overactive thyroid gland and outward bulging of the eyes (8)

growth hormone (GH) nontropic hormone produced by the anterior pituitary that is responsible for growth and development of the muscles, cartilage, and long bones of the body (8)
gustatory sense the sense of taste (7)

H

haploid having a single set of unpaired chromosomes (15)
Haversian canals major passageways running in the direction of the length of long bones, providing paths for blood vessels (4)
Haversian system a single Haversian canal along with its multiple canaliculi, which branch out to join with lacunae, forming a comprehensive transportation matrix for supply of nutrients and removal of waste products; also called an osteon. (4)
healthcare-associated infections (HAIs) infection that patients get in the course of receiving care in a healthcare facility (13)
heart block a condition in which the impulses traveling from the SA node to the ventricles are delayed, intermittently blocked, or completely blocked by the AV node (11)
heart murmurs extra or unusual sounds heard by a stethoscope during a heartbeat; may be harmless or indicative of a problem with one of the heart valves (11)
hematocrit the percentage of total blood volume that is composed of red blood cells (10)
hematopoiesis process of red blood cell formation and development (4, 10)
hemodialysis a procedure for removing metabolic waste products from the body; blood is withdrawn from an artery, pumped through a dialyzer, and then returned to the patient through a vein (14)
hemoglobin an essential molecule of the red blood cell that serves as the binding site for oxygen and carbon dioxide; composed of two molecules: globin and heme (10)
hemolysis the rupture of red blood cells as a result of disease or old age (10)
hemophilia a condition in which blood does not clot properly due to the absence of a clotting factor (10)
hemostasis the sequence of events that causes a blood clot to form and bleeding to stop (10)
hepatic portal circulation blood circulation through the liver, helping to regulate the levels of nutrients (carbohydrates, proteins, and fats) in the blood (11)
hepatitis a group of diseases characterized by inflammation of and damage to the liver (13)
Hering-Breuer reflex an involuntary impulse triggered by stretch receptors in the bronchioles and alveoli that halts inspiration and initiates exhalation (9)
hernia a balloon-like section of the lining of the abdominal cavity that protrudes through a hole or weakened section of the muscles (5)
herpes simplex virus type 1 the form of herpes that generates cold sores or fever blisters around the mouth (3)
herpes simplex virus type 2 the genital form of herpes (3)
herpes varicella (chickenpox) a highly contagious, common childhood disease that is characterized by extremely itchy, fluid-filled blisters (3)
herpes zoster (shingles) a disease that involves a painful, blistering rash accompanied by headache, fever, and a general feeling of unwellness (3)
hinge joint type of diarthrosis that allows only hingelike movements in forward and backward directions (4)
histamines molecules that trigger a reaction to irritation of the nasal membranes, which produces nasal congestion and drainage (7)
histology the study of tissues (2)
homeostasis a state of regulated physiological balance (1)
homeostatic imbalance a state in which there is a diminished ability for the organ systems to keep the body's internal environment within normal ranges (1)
homeostatic mechanisms the processes that maintain homeostasis (1)
hormonal control type of endocrine control in which endocrine organs are stimulated by hormones from other endocrine organs, starting with the hypothalamus (8)
hormones chemical messengers secreted by the endocrine glands (8)
human chorionic gonadotropin (hCG) a hormone secreted by the trophoblast cells of the embryo that prevents deterioration of the corpus luteum and stimulates progesterone production in the placenta (15)
human genome the DNA sequence of a human (2)
human immunodeficiency virus (HIV) the virus that causes AIDS (12)
human papillomavirus (HPV) a group of approximately 150 viruses that cause warts (3); a sexually transmitted disease that causes genital warts and that can cause cervical cancer (15)
humerus major bone of the upper arm (4)
humoral control type of endocrine control in which levels of various substances in body fluids are monitored for homeostatic imbalance (8)
humoral immunity immunity associated with free antibodies that circulate in the blood; antibody-mediated immunity (12)
hydrostatic pressure the pressure exerted by a liquid as a result of its potential energy (14)
hypercalcemia a condition caused by the hypersecretion of parathyroid hormone (PTH), leading to increased blood calcium levels and increased calcium absorption by the kidneys (8)
hyperextension backward movement of a body segment past anatomical position in the sagittal plane (5)
hyperglycemia a condition in which blood glucose levels become elevated (8)
hypertension condition that occurs when the force of blood against the arterial wall remains elevated for an extended period of time; high blood pressure (11)

hyperthyroidism a condition characterized by a visibly enlarged thyroid gland in the neck; overactive thyroid gland (8)
hyperventilation excessive ventilation that leads to abnormal expulsion of carbon dioxide (9)
hypodermis the layer of tissue beneath the dermis, which serves as a storage repository for fat (3)
hypothalamic nonreleasing hormones hormones produced in the hypothalamus and carried by a vein to the anterior pituitary, where they stop certain hormones from being released; hypothalamic inhibiting hormones (8)
hypothalamic releasing hormones hormones produced in the hypothalamus and carried by a vein to the anterior pituitary, where they stimulate the release of hormones from the anterior pituitary (8)
hypothalamus a portion of the diencephalon that regulates functions such as metabolism, heart rate, and blood pressure (6)
hypothesis an educated guess about what the outcome of a study will be (1)
hypothyroidism a condition caused by an underactive thyroid gland (8)
hypoxia condition of not having enough oxygen (9)

I

immune system the cells and chemicals that contribute to the body's specific defenses against disease (12)
immunoglobulins antibodies; proteins that recognize particular antigens with great specificity (12)
impetigo a bacterial infection common in elementary school children that is characterized by pink, blister-like bumps, usually on the face (3)
implantation the binding of the blastocyst to the endometrium (15)
impotence inability of a male to maintain an erection (15)
incus one of the three ossicles; tiny bone in the middle ear that attaches to the malleus and transmits sound from the malleus to the stapes (7)
inferior vena cava largest vein in the human body that returns deoxygenated blood to the right atrium of the heart from body regions below the diaphragm (11)
infertility the inability of a couple to get pregnant (15)
inflammatory bowel disease a condition in which the wall of the small and/or large intestine becomes chronically inflamed (13)
inflammatory response physiological response to tissue injury or infection, also called inflammation; the four signs of inflammation are heat, redness, swelling, and pain (12)
influenza a viral infection that affects the respiratory system; the flu (9)
ingestion the intake of food and liquids via the mouth (13)
insertion muscle attachment to a bone that tends to move when the muscle contracts (5)
inspiration the process by which air flows into the lungs; inhalation (9)
inspiratory reserve volume (IRV) the amount of air that can be inhaled immediately after a normal inhalation (9)
insulin a hormone that promotes glucose uptake in body tissues (8); hormone secreted by beta cells in the pancreas that lowers blood glucose levels (8)
insulin resistance a condition common in type 2 diabetes in which the pancreas secretes insulin, but the body's insulin receptors are downregulated, causing elevated blood glucose levels (8)
integumentary system enveloping organ of the body that includes the epidermis, dermis, sudoriferous and sebaceous glands, and nails and hair (3)
interatrial septum the wall that separates the right and left atria in the heart (11)
interferons proteins released by cells that have been infected with viruses; interfere with virus reproduction (12)
interleukins chemicals released by helper T cells and other cells that stimulate an immune response (12)
internal respiration the process of gas exchange between the tissues and arterial blood (9)
internal urethral sphincter a layer of smooth muscle located at the inferior end of the bladder and the proximal end of the urethra; this muscle, which prohibits release of urine, is under involuntary control (14)
interneurons neurons that form bridges to transmit nerve impulses between afferent and efferent neurons (6)
interstitial fluid fluid in the spaces between cells (12)
interventricular septum thick wall that divides the two ventricles in the heart (11)
intervertebral discs fibrocartilaginous cushions between vertebral bodies that allow bending of the spine and help to create the normal spinal curves (4)
inversion movement in which the sole of the foot is rolled inward (5)
iris the anterior portion of the choroid, which gives the eye its color (7)
iron-deficient anemia the most common anemia; caused by an insufficient dietary intake of iron, loss of iron from intestinal bleeding, or iron-level depletion during pregnancy (10)
irritability the ability to respond to a stimulus (5)
ischemia a lack of blood flow, usually due to the narrowing of a blood vessel (11)
isometric a type of contraction that involves no change in muscle length (5)

J

jaundice a blood disorder characterized by yellow-colored skin and whites of the eyes (10)

K

keratin a tough protein found in the skin, hair, and nails (3)
keratinocytes cells within the epidermis that produce keratin (3)

ketoacidosis condition in which the pH of the blood is decreased, making the blood dangerously acidic; results from using fats for fuel, which produces ketone bodies in the blood (8)

kidney stone a solid crystalline mass that forms in the kidney and that may become stuck in the renal pelvis or ureter; usually made of calcium, phosphate, uric acid, and protein (14)

kinetics the analysis of the actions of forces (1)

L

labia majora two skin folds posterior to the mons pubis that lie parallel on either side of the vaginal opening (15)

labia minora a smaller set of skin folds inside the labia majora (15)

lacrimal glands tear secretors; located above the lateral end of each eye (7)

lactation secretion of milk by the mammary glands (15)

lactiferous duct a duct through which milk is secreted and which opens at the nipple (15)

lacunae tiny cavities laid out in concentric circles around the Haversian canals (4)

laryngitis inflammation of the larynx, or voice box (9)

larynx a triangular-shaped space inferior to the pharynx that is responsible for voice production; the voice box (9)

lateral rotation outward (lateral) movement of a body segment in the transverse plane (5)

left bundle branch the left branch arising from the bundle of His, through which electrical impulses are transmitted through the left ventricle (11)

lens a transparent, flexible structure that is curved outward on both sides (7)

let-down reflex contraction of smooth muscle cells in the mammary glands that allows milk to be squeezed toward and out of the nipple (15)

leukemia a cancer caused by the production of an extremely high number of immature white blood cells in the bone marrow (10)

leukocytes white blood cells; fight infection and protect the body through various mechanisms (10)

ligaments bands composed of collagen and elastic fibers that connect bones to other bones (4)

limbic system the part of the brain that is responsible for emotions (7)

lingual tonsils two masses of lymphatic tissue that lie on either side of the base of the tongue (12)

lipids fatty molecules that dissolve poorly in water but dissolve well in a nonpolar solvent; fats and oils (2); substances found in oils and solid fats; can be classified either as saturated or unsaturated (13)

lipocytes fat cells (3)

lithotripsy the use of intense, ultrasonic sound waves to break up a kidney stone into pieces small enough to be passed from the body in the urine (14)

lobes the four regions of the brain—frontal, parietal, occipital, and temporal (6)

lower extremity bones of the hips, legs, and feet (4)

lumbar region low back region of the spine composed of 5 vertebrae (4)

lumen the hollow inside portion of a body cavity or tube (2)

luteinizing hormone (LH) tropic hormone secreted by the anterior pituitary that stimulates the ovaries to produce progesterone and estrogen and the release of eggs in women; in men, it stimulates the interstitial cells of the testes to produce testosterone (8)

lymph clear, transparent, sometimes faintly yellow fluid that is collected from tissues throughout the body and flows in the lymphatic vessels (12)

lymphatic nodules small, localized clusters of dense tissue formed by lymphocytes and macrophages (12)

lymphatic trunks large lymphatic vessels that drain lymph from different parts of the body (12)

lymphatic valves tissue flaps that act as one-way valves inside the lymphatic vessels (12)

lymphatic vessels vessels that carry lymph (12)

lymphedema a buildup of extracellular fluid in the body because of disruption in lymphatic drainage (12)

lymph nodes small, bean-shaped structures found along the lymphatic vessels throughout the body (12)

lymphocytes white blood cells that are abundant in lymphatic tissue (12)

M

macronutrients substances such as carbohydrates, proteins, and lipids that the body requires in relatively large quantities (13)

macrophages cells that phagocytize (surround and destroy) foreign cells, such as bacteria and viruses (12)

major histocompatibility complex glycoproteins (MHCs) family of proteins found on the surfaces of lymphocytes and other cells; help the immune system recognize foreign antigens and ignore "self" tissues (12)

malignant melanoma cancer of the melanocytes; the most serious form of skin cancer (3)

malleus one of the three ossicles; tiny bone in the middle ear that transmits sound from the tympanic membrane to the incus (7)

mammary glands the milk-producing glands in the female (15)

mandible jaw bone (4)

mass the quantity of matter contained in an object (1)

mast cells connective tissue cell with granules (particles) that contain histamine, a compound which, when eleased into surrounding fluid, activates an inflammatory response (12)

maxillary bones two fused bones that form the upper jaw, house the upper teeth, and connect to all other bones of the face, with the exception of the mandible (4)

mean arterial pressure (MAP) measure of the overall pressure within the cardiovascular system, which determines blood flow to various organs (11)

mechanical breakdown the breakdown of food into smaller pieces, thus increasing its surface area (13)

mechanoreceptors chemical receptor cells that detect muscle contraction and force generation during exercise; they quickly increase respiration rates when exercise begins (9)
medial rotation inward (medial) movement of a body segment in the transverse plane (5)
mediastinum the area of the thoracic cavity between the lungs; houses the heart, great blood vessels, trachea, esophagus, thoracic duct, thymus gland, and other structures (9)
medulla oblongata the lower portion of the brainstem; regulates heart rate, blood pressure, and breathing, and controls several reflexes (6)
medullary cavity central hollow in the long bones (4)
meiosis a type of cell division that produces eggs (in females) or sperm (in males); daughter cells with half the chromosome number of the parent cell (15)
melanin a pigment that protects the body against the harmful effects of ultraviolet ray damage from the sun (3)
melanocytes specialized cells in the skin that produce melanin (3)
melatonin hormone produced by the pineal gland that causes sleepiness (8)
membranes thin sheets or layers of pliable tissue (3)
membranous labyrinth membrane-covered tubes inside the bony labyrinth (7)
memory cells B lymphocytes and T lymphocytes in lymphatic tissues that can respond if a previously encountered antigen invades the body again (12)
menarche the first menstrual bleeding (15)
meninges three protective membranes that surround the brain and spinal cord (6)
meningitis an infection-induced inflammation of the meninges surrounding the brain and spinal cord (6)
menopause the termination of the monthly female reproductive cycle (15)
menstrual cycle a hormone-driven cycle of changes to the ovaries and uterus that lasts roughly 28 days and includes both the ovarian cycle and the uterine cycle (15)
Merkel cells touch receptors in the skin (3)
messenger RNA (mRNA) single-strand RNA molecule whose base sequence carries the information needed by a ribosome to make a protein (2)
metabolic rate the speed at which the body consumes energy (1)
metabolism all chemical reactions that occur within an organism to maintain life (1)
metacarpal bones the five interior bones of the hand, connecting the carpals in the wrist to the phalanges in the fingers (4)
metastasis the spreading of cancerous cells from their original location to another part of the body (12)
metatarsal bones small bones of the ankle (4)
metric system international system of measurement that is used in all fields of science (1)
microglia glial cells that absorb and dispose of dead cells and bacteria (6)
micronutrients vitamins and minerals that are essential to the body in small amounts (13)
microvilli finger-like extensions that increase the surface area of a cell (2)
micturition urination (14)
midbrain relay station for sensory and motor impulses; located on the superior end of the brainstem (6)
middle ear cavities openings in the skull that serve as chambers for transmitting and amplifying sound (1)
minerals elements that the body needs in relatively small amounts (13)
mitochondria organelles in the cytoplasm that make ATP (2)
mitosis the division of a cell nucleus and chromosomes into two nuclei, each with its own set of identical chromosomes (2)
mitral valve the valve that closes the orifice between the left atrium and left ventricle of the heart; bicuspid valve (11)
mitral valve prolapse an incomplete closing of the mitral valve, causing blood to flow backward into the left atrium when the left ventricle contracts (11)
molecules combinations of two or more atoms (1)
monocytes leukocytes that develop into phagocytizing macrophages when they migrate out of lymphatic circulation into surrounding tissue (12)
monounsaturated fats one category of unsaturated fatty acids; sources include canola oil and olive oil (13)
motor neuron a nerve that stimulates skeletal muscle tissue (5)
motor unit a single motor neuron and all of the muscle fibers that it stimulates (5)
mucosa innermost layer of the GI tract, which directly faces the outside world (13)
mucosa-associated lymphatic tissue (MALT) lymphatic tissue found in mucous membranes that line passageways open to the outside world; these include the respiratory, gastrointestinal, urinary, and reproductive tracts (12)
mucous membranes thin sheets of tissue lining the body cavities that open to the outside world (3)
mucus a slippery solution that protects the mucous membranes and aids in transporting substances (3)
multiple myeloma a cancer of the plasma cells in bone marrow (10)
multiple sclerosis a chronic, slowly progressive disease of the central nervous system that destroys the myelin sheath of nerve cell axons (6)
muscle cramps moderate to severe muscle spasms that cause pain (5)
muscle fiber an individual skeletal muscle cell (5)
muscle strain an injury that occurs when a muscle is stretched beyond the limits to which it is accustomed (5)
muscular dystrophy (MD) a group of similar, inherited disorders characterized by progressively worsening muscle weakness and loss of muscle tissue (5)
muscularis externa layer of the GI tract that surrounds the submucosal layer; propels food through the GI tract by peristalsis (13)
myelin sheath the fatty bands of insulation surrounding axon fibers (6)

myocardial infarction tissue death that occurs in a segment of heart muscle from blockage of a coronary artery; heart attack (11)
myocarditis inflammation of the myocardium, the middle layer of the heart (also known as the heart muscle) (11)
myocardium the middle layer of the heart, which makes up about 2/3 of the heart muscle (11)
myocytes mature muscle cells (5)
myositis ossificans a condition in which a calcium mass forms within a muscle three to four weeks after a muscle injury (5)
myxedema a condition in adults with hyperthyroidism that causes weight gain; a swollen, puffy face; low body temperature; dry skin; and decreased mental acuity (8)

N

nares the two openings in the nose through which air enters; nostrils (9)
nasal cavity opening within the nose (1)
nasal conchae three uneven, scroll-like nasal bones that extend down through the nasal cavity (9)
nasopharyngitis inflammation of the nasal passages and pharynx; the common cold (9)
natural killer (NK) cells lymphocytes that play an important role in the nonspecific defense system of the body by killing virus-infected cells and cancer cells (12)
negative feedback mechanism that reverses a condition that has exceeded the normal homeostatic range to restore homeostasis (1)
neonatal hypothyroidism hypothyroidism that occurs in infants and children; may develop congenitally or following birth (8)
nephron the fundamental excretory unit of each kidney (14)
nephron loop the U-shaped part of the nephron that is between the proximal convoluted tubule and the distal convoluted tubule; has a descending limb and ascending limb; loop of Henle (14)
net force the single force resulting from the summation of all forces acting on a structure at a given time (1)
neural control type of endocrine control in which nerve fibers stimulate the endocrine organs to release hormones (8)
neuroglia non-neural tissue that forms the interstitial or supporting elements of the CNS; also known as glial cells (6)
neuromuscular junction the link between an axon terminal and a muscle fiber (5)
neurotransmitters chemicals that act as messengers between an axon of one neuron and a dendrite on another, or between an axon and a muscle fiber (6)
neutrophils the most common type of white blood cell; can slip out of capillaries and into surrounding tissue, where they destroy bacteria and cellular debris (12)
non-steroid hormones hormones composed of protein, or peptide hormones and amino acid-derived hormones (8)
norepinephrine a neurotransmitter released by postganglionic neurons in the sympathetic nervous system (6)
nucleic acids key information-carrying molecules in cells (2)
nucleotides subunits that make up nucleic acids (2)
nucleus a rounded or oval mass of protoplasm within the cytoplasm of a cell that contains the cell's DNA and is bounded by a membrane (2)
nutrients chemicals that the body needs for energy, growth, and maintenance (13)

O

occipital lobes sections of the brain located behind the parietal lobes; integrate sensory information from the skin, internal organs, muscles, and joints (6)
olfactory bulb the thickened end of the olfactory nerve that sends sensory impulses to the olfactory region of the brain (7)
olfactory hairs threads that extend from the olfactory receptor cells into the nasal cavity (7)
olfactory nerve a cranial nerve that sends impulses to the olfactory cortex of the brain (7)
olfactory region a dime-sized area at the top of each nasal cavity that houses sensors responsible for smell (7)
olfactory sense the sense of smell (7)
oligodendrocytes glial cells that wrap around nerve fibers and produce a fatty insulating material called myelin to insulate some neurons (6)
oocyte egg cell (15)
oogenesis the process by which oocytes, or female gametes, are generated (15)
opportunistic infection an infection that rarely or never occurs in people with a healthy immune system but that may occur in a person with a damaged immune system, such as from AIDS (12)
opposition touching any of your four fingers to your thumb; this movement enables grasping of objects (5)
opsonins proteins that make cells more attractive to phagocytes (12)
optic chiasma the point at which the optic nerves cross (7)
optic nerve transmitter of visual sensory signals to the occipital lobe of the brain (7)
optic tracts the continuation of the optic nerve fibers beyond the optic chiasma (7)
oral cavity opening within the mouth (1)
orbital cavities openings that hold the eyes (1)
organ body part organized to perform a specific function (1)
organ of Corti a spiral-shaped ridge of epithelium in the cochlear duct lined with hair cells that serve as hearing receptors (7)
organ system two or more organs working together to perform specific functions (1)
origin muscle attachment to a relatively fixed structure (5)
osmosis the movement of water molecules from a region of low osmotic pressure to a region of high osmotic pressure (14)
osmotic diuresis an increase in urine production caused by high osmotic pressure of the glomerular filtrate, which "pulls" more water into the filtrate (14)

osmotic pressure a pressure created by the presence of dissolved substances in water (14)
ossicles the body's three smallest bones—the malleus, incus, and stapes; found in the middle ear (7)
ossification process of bone formation (4)
osteoarthritis degenerative disease of articular cartilage, characterized by pain, swelling, range-of-motion restriction, and stiffness (4)
osteoblasts specialized bone cells that build new bone tissue (4)
osteoclasts specialized bone cells that resorb bone tissue (4)
osteocytes mature bone cells (4)
osteon a Haversian system (4)
osteopenia reduced bone mass without the presence of a fracture (4)
osteoporosis condition in which bone mineralization and strength are so abnormally low that regular, daily activities can result in painful fractures (4)
oval window a membrane-covered opening that connects the middle ear to the inner ear (7)
ovarian cycle the sequence of events associated with maturation and release of an oocyte (15)
ovaries the primary female reproductive organs, in which gametes are made (15)
ovulation the release of an oocyte, or egg, from the ovarian follicle (15)
oxyhemoglobin hemoglobin molecule with attached oxygen molecules; transports oxygen from the lungs to the body tissues (10)
oxytocin hormone produced in the hypothalamus and stored in the posterior pituitary; facilitates childbirth and causes the mammary glands to secrete breast milk (8)

P

palate the structure consisting of hard and soft components that separates the oral and nasal cavities; the roof of the mouth (9)
palatine tonsils two masses of lymphatic tissue that lie in the back of the mouth, on the left and right sides; the largest and most commonly infected tonsils (12)
palpitations sensation of rapid heartbeat (11)
pancreatitis inflammation of the pancreas (13)
papillae tiny bumps on the tongue that house taste buds (7)
papillary layer the outer layer of the dermis (3)
papillary muscles small, muscular bundles attached at one end to the chordae tendineae and at the other to the innermost or endocardial wall of the ventricles; maintain tension on the chordae tendineae as the ventricles contract (11)
parallel a type of muscle fiber arrangement in which fibers run largely parallel to each other along the length of the muscle (5)
paraplegia disorder characterized by loss of function in the lower trunk and legs (6)
parathyroid hormone (PTH) hormone produced by the parathyroid glands that works with calcitonin to maintain calcium homeostasis (8)
paravertebral ganglia mass of nerve cell bodies close to the spinal cord (6)
parietal lobes sections of the brain located behind the frontal lobes; integrate sensory information from the skin, internal organs, muscles, and joints (6)
Parkinson's disease (PD) a chronic nervous system disease characterized by a slowly spreading tremor, muscular weakness, and rigidity (6)
parturition childbirth (15)
passive immunity immunity that comes from antibodies received from an outside source, such as breast milk (12)
passive transport a method of transport that does not require any energy (2)
patella kneecap (4)
pathogens disease-causing agents (12)
pectoral girdle bones surrounding the shoulder, including the clavicle and scapula (4)
pelvic cavity internal opening that holds the reproductive and excretory organs (1)
pelvic inflammatory disease (PID) an inflammation of the uterus, uterine tubes, ovaries and/or other organs of the peritoneal (abdominopelvic) cavity (15)
pelvis bones of the pelvic girdle and the coccyx at the base of the spine (4)
penis the reproductive organ that delivers sperm to the female reproductive tract (15)
pennate a type of muscle fiber arrangement in which each fiber attaches obliquely to a central tendon (5)
peptic ulcer a break in the lining of the stomach, duodenum, or lower esophagus (13)
peptide bond the chemical bond that links two amino acids by connecting the amino group of one amino acid to the acid group of another (2)
perforating (Volkmann's) canals large canals that connect the Haversian canals; oriented across bones and perpendicular to Haversian canals (4)
pericarditis inflammation of the pericardial sac that surrounds the heart (11)
perilymph a clear fluid that fills the bony labyrinth (7)
perimysium a connective tissue sheath that envelops each primary bundle of muscle fibers (5)
perineurium a protective sheath that surrounds a bundle of nerve fibers (6)
periodontal disease a disease that affects the supporting structure of the teeth and the gums (13)
periosteum fibrous connective tissue membrane that surrounds and protects the shaft (diaphysis) of long bones (4)
peripheral chemoreceptors sensory receptor cells located in the aortic arch and carotid arteries that are sensitive to changes in blood oxygen level (9)
peripheral nervous system (PNS) all parts of the nervous system external to the brain and spinal cord (6)

peripheral neuropathy a disease or degenerative state of the peripheral nerves often associated with diabetes mellitus; marked by muscle weakness and atrophy, pain, and numbness (8)
peripheral vascular disease (PVD) condition caused by a narrowing of the arteries in the legs (11)
peristalsis a wave of symmetrical squeezing of the digestive tract walls that occurs during digestion to move food along the GI tract (5, 13)
peritoneal dialysis a renal dialysis method that uses the patient's peritoneum to filter fluids and dissolved substances from the blood (14)
peritonitis inflammation of the peritoneum, the membrane lining the inner wall of the abdomen and covering the abdominal organs (3)
pernicious anemia a severe anemia caused by the inability of the intestines to absorb vitamin B_{12}, which is essential for the formation of red blood cells; usually develops in older adults (10)
pH a measure of the acidity or alkalinity of a solution (2)
phagocytes cells that engulf and consume bacteria, foreign material, and debris (12)
phagocytosis the process by which a cell engulfs and destroys foreign matter and cellular debris (12)
phalanges bones of the fingers (4)
pharyngeal tonsil lymphatic tissue that lies at the back of the nasopharynx, the part of the throat above the palate, and opens into the nasal cavity; commonly called the adenoid (12)
pharyngitis inflammation of the pharynx, or throat (9)
pharynx the muscular passageway that extends from the nasal cavity to the mouth and connects to the esophagus; the throat (9)
phenotype the observable features of an individual, which are established at fertilization (15)
phlebotomy the drawing of blood; a standard treatment for polycythemia (10)
phospholipids a lipid-containing phosphate group (2)
physiology the study of how living things function or work (1)
pivot joint type of diarthrosis that permits rotation around only one axis (4)
placenta the organ that grows in the uterus to meet the nutritional needs of the embryo and fetus (15)
plantar flexion downward motion of the foot away from the lower leg (5)
plantar warts warts that develop on the soles of the foot, grow inward, and can become painful (3)
plaque a sticky mixture of bacteria, food particles, and mucus that hardens to form tartar if it is not regularly removed by brushing and flossing (13)
plasma the liquid component of blood (10)
plasma membrane the membrane that defines the outer shell of a cell (2)
plastic permanent deformation of an object that occurs when a force causes a deformation that exceeds the object's elastic limit (1)
platelet plug gathering of platelets that forms a small mass at the site of an injury (10)
platelets part of the formed elements of the blood; play a vital role in blood clotting (10)
pleural sac the thin, double-walled serous membrane that surrounds the lungs (9)
pleurisy inflammation of the pleura, the membrane that encases the lungs (3)
plexuses complex interconnections of nerves (6)
pneumonia an infection of the lungs that causes inflammation; caused by a virus, bacterium, fungus, or—in rare cases—parasites (9)
polarized a condition that occurs when the inside of a cell membrane is more negatively charged than the outside (6)
polycythemia a condition in which the bone marrow manufactures too many red blood cells; caused by prolonged altitude exposure and a genetic mutation (10)
polymer a molecule made of many similar subunits (2)
polypeptide a long chain of amino acids (2)
polyunsaturated fats one category of unsaturated fatty acids; sources include corn oil and soybean oil (13)
pons the section of the brain that plays a role in regulating breathing (6)
pores of Kohn small openings in the alveolar walls that allow gases and macrophages to travel between the alveoli (9)
positive feedback mechanism that further increases a condition that has exceeded the normal homeostatic range (1)
posterior (dorsal) body cavity continuous internal opening located near the back of the body that includes the cranial and spinal cavities (1)
postganglionic neuron the second neuron in a series that transmits impulses from the CNS (6)
precapillary sphincter a band of smooth muscle fibers that encircles the capillaries at the arteriole-capillary junctions and controls blood flow to the tissues (11)
precipitation the formation of an insoluble complex, such as a clump of antigen molecules joined together by antibodies (12)
preganglionic neuron the first neuron in a series that transmits impulses from the CNS (6)
premature atrial contractions (PACs) condition in which an irritable piece of atrial heart tissue fires before the SA node, causing the atria to contract too soon (11)
premature ventricular contractions (PVCs) condition in which Purkinje fibers fire before the SA node, causing the ventricles to contract prematurely (11)
pressure force distributed over a given area (1)
primary bronchi the two passageways that branch off the trachea and lead to the right and left lungs (9)
primary immune response the initial immune system response to a foreign invader such as a virus or bacterium (12)
primary motor cortex outer region of the brain in the frontal lobes that sends neural impulses to the skeletal muscles (6)
primary somatic sensory cortex outer region of the brain in the parietal lobes that interprets sensory impulses received from the skin, internal organs, muscles, and joints (6)

process an outgrowth or projection on a bone or other body tissue (4)

prolactin hormone secreted by the anterior pituitary that stimulates the growth of mammary glands and milk production in women; it is also present in men, but its purpose is unknown (8)

pronation medial rotation of the forearm (palm down) (5)

propulsion the movement of food through the gastrointestinal tract that is stimulated by swallowing at the pharynx and peristalsis; muscular contractions that move food through the rest of the GI tract (13)

prostaglandins fatty acids involved in the control of inflammation and body temperature (12)

prostate gland the gland that sits directly under the bladder and surrounds the beginning of the urethra in the male; produces about one-third of the fluid volume of semen (15)

proteinuria presence of excessive protein in the urine (14)

proteome all of the proteins that are expressed by (made by) a particular cell or organism (2)

proximal convoluted tubule (PCT) the part of the nephron between the glomerular capsule and the nephron loop; minerals, nutrients, and water are reabsorbed from the filtrate here (14)

psoriasis a common skin disorder that involves redness, irritation, and scales (flaky, silver-white patches) that itch, burn, crack, and sometimes bleed (3)

puberty the final maturation of the reproductive system (15)

pulmonary circulation circulation of oxygen-poor blood from the right ventricle, through the lungs, and returning to the left atrium with oxygen-rich blood (11)

pulmonary valve semilunar valve located between the right ventricle and the pulmonary artery (11)

pulmonary ventilation the process of continuously moving air in and out of the lungs (9)

pupil the opening through which light rays enter the eye (7)

Purkinje fibers part of the impulse-conducting network of the heart that rapidly transmits impulses throughout the ventricles, causing ventricular contraction (11)

pyelonephritis urinary tract infection in which one or both of the kidneys also become infected (14)

pyrogens chemicals that tend to cause fever by raising the set-point temperature of the neurons in the hypothalamus (12)

Q

quadrant four divisions of a whole; for example, the human abdomen is often divided into four quadrants for descriptive purposes. (1)

quadriplegia disorder characterized by loss of function below the neck (6)

R

radial artery the artery located on the thumb side of the wrist, where the radial pulse is detected (11)

radial deviation rotation of the hand toward the thumb (5)

radius smaller of the two bones in the forearm; rotates around the ulna (4)

reabsorption the movement of water and dissolved substances from the filtrate (in a renal tubule) back into the blood (14)

receptor transmitter that senses environmental changes (1)

reflexes simple, rapid, involuntary, programmed responses to stimuli (6)

refractory period the time between the completion of the action potential and repolarization (6)

remodeling process through which adult bone can change in density, strength, and sometimes shape (4)

renal corpuscle the part of a nephron that consists of a glomerular capsule with its included glomerulus (14)

renal cortex the lighter-colored, outer layer of the kidney that contains the glomeruli and convoluted tubules (14)

renal dialysis the removal of wastes from the blood by artificial means (14)

renal failure kidney failure, as indicated by a GFR of 15 mL/min. or less (14)

renal medulla the darker, innermost part of the kidney (14)

renal pelvis a funnel-shaped cavity in the center of the kidney where urine collects before it flows into the ureter (14)

renal tubule the part of a nephron that leads away from a glomerulus and empties into a collecting tubule; consists of a proximal convoluted tubule, nephron loop, and distal convoluted tubule (14)

renin an enzyme made and secreted by the kidneys; aids in the production of angiotensin (14)

repolarization the reestablishment of a polarized state in a cell after depolarization (6)

repolarize to relax; the atria and ventricles repolarize as the heart beats (11)

research question a question to be answered or a problem to be solved in a research study (1)

residual volume (RV) the volume of air that never leaves the lungs, even after the most forceful expiration (9)

respiration the process by which the lungs provide oxygen to body tissues and dispose of carbon dioxide; breathing (9)

respiratory gas transport the process by which oxygen and carbon dioxide are transported to and from the lungs and tissues (9)

reticular connective tissue a type of tissue that contains reticular fibers and is found in lymph nodes, bone marrow, and the spleen (2)

reticular layer the layer of skin superficial to the papillary layer (3)

retina the innermost layer of the eye, containing light-sensitive nerve endings that send impulses through the optic nerves to the brain (7)

Rh factor the antigen of the Rh blood group that is found on the surface of red blood cells; people with the Rh factor are Rh+ and those lacking it are Rh– (10)

rheumatoid arthritis autoimmune disorder in which the body's own immune system attacks healthy joint tissues; the most debilitating and painful form of arthritis (4)

RhoGAM an immune serum that prevents a mother's blood from becoming sensitized to foreign antibodies from her fetus (10)

ribonucleic acid (RNA) one of two kinds of information-carrying nucleic acids found in cells; ribonucleic acid (2)

ribosomes very large enzymes that make polypeptides (2)

right bundle branch the right branch arising from the bundle of His, through which electrical impulses are transmitted through the right ventricle (11)

rods sensory cells in the retina that are activated in dim light (7)

rule of nines a method used in calculating body surface area affected by burns (3)

S

sacrum five fused vertebrae that form the posterior of the pelvic girdle (4)

saddle joint type of diarthrosis in which the articulating bone surfaces are both shaped like the seat of a riding saddle (4)

sagittal plane an invisible, vertical flat surface that divides the body into right and left halves (1)

saltatory conduction the rapid skipping of an action potential from node to node on myelinated neurons (6)

sarcolemma the delicate membrane surrounding each striated muscle fiber (5)

sarcomeres units composed of actin and myosin that contract inside the muscle fiber (5)

satellite cells glial cells that serve as cushioning support cells within the PNS (6)

scapula shoulder blade (4)

Schwann cells glial cells that wrap around the axons of some neurons in the PNS, providing them with a myelin sheath that speeds up their rate of transmission (6)

science a systematic process that creates new knowledge and organizes it into a form of testable explanations and predictions about an aspect of the universe (1)

scientific method a systematic process that can be used to answer questions or find solutions to problems (1)

scientific theory an explanation of some aspect of the natural world that is based on rigorously tested, repeatedly confirmed research (1)

sclera the tough, fibrous outer layer of the eye (7)

sebaceous glands glands located all over the body that produce sebum (3)

sebum an oily substance that helps to keep the skin and hair soft (3)

secondary immune response immune system response to an infectious agent that it has encountered before (12)

second-degree burns burns that involve damage to both the epidermis and the upper portion of the underlying dermis; characterized by blisters (3)

secretion the active movement of substances from the blood into the filtrate, which will become urine (14)

semen the fluid that contains sperm, which is delivered to the female during intercourse; penile ejaculate (15)

semicircular canals inner ear channels containing receptor hair cells that play an important role in balance (7)

semilunar valves valves situated at the opening between the heart and the aorta and at the opening between the heart and the pulmonary artery; they prevent backflow of blood into the ventricles (11)

seminal glands glands that produce up to 70% of the volume of semen; seminal vesicles

seminiferous tubules small tubes in the testes in which sperm form (15)

septum the structure made of cartilage that divides the left and right air passages in the nose (7)

serosa the outermost layer of the GI tract (13)

serous fluid a thin, clear liquid that serves as a lubricant between parietal and visceral membranes (3)

serous membranes thin sheets of tissues that line body cavities closed to the outside world (3)

severe combined immune deficiency (SCID) a genetic disorder, present at birth, in which both B cell and T cell responses are significantly below normal (12)

sexually transmitted infection an infection transmitted through sexual contact (15)

shear a force that acts along a surface and perpendicular to the length of a structure (1)

shin splint the name for pain localized to the anterior lower leg (5)

sickle cell anemia a disease in which the red blood cells are shaped like a sickle, or crescent, rather than a disk; caused by irregularly shaped hemoglobin molecules in the red blood cells (10)

simple epithelia epithelia that have a single layer of cells (2)

sinoatrial (SA) node a small mass of specialized tissue located in the right atrium that normally acts as the pacemaker of the heart, causing it to beat at a rate between 60 and 100 bpm (11)

sinuses the air-filled cavities that surround the nose (9)

sinusitis inflammation of the sinuses (9)

skull the part of the skeleton composed of all of the bones of the head (4)

slow-twitch type of muscle that contracts slowly and is fatigue resistant (5)

sodium-potassium pump a pumping mechanism powered by ATP molecules that actively transports potassium and sodium ions into and out of the cell, respectively, against their gradients in order to accomplish repolarization of the cell (6)

somatic nervous system branch of the nervous system that stimulates the skeletal muscles (6)

somatic reflexes involuntary stimuli transmitted to skeletal muscles from neural arcs in the spinal cord (6)

sperm (singular or plural) the male gamete; a haploid cell that can fertilize an egg to make a zygote (15)

spermatogenesis sperm formation (15)

spinal cavity the internal opening that houses the spinal cord (1)

spinal cord a column of nerve tissue that extends from the brainstem to the beginning of the lumbar region of the spine (6)
spinal nerves neural transmitters that branch from the left and right sides of the spinal cord (6)
spleen the largest lymphatic organ in the body, located in the abdomen below the diaphragm; filters blood and activates an immune response if necessary (12)
sprain injury caused by abnormal motion of the articulating bones that results in overstretching or tearing of ligaments, tendons, or other connective tissues crossing a joint (4)
squamous cell carcinoma a type of rapidly growing cancer that appears as a scaly, reddened patch of skin (3)
stapes one of the three ossicles; tiny bone in the middle ear that attaches to the incus on one side and the oval window on the other (7)
statistical inference the practice of generalizing the findings of a research study to a large population (1)
statistical significance an interpretation of statistical data indicating that the results of a study can legitimately be generalized to the population represented in the study sample (1)
sternum breastbone (4)
steroid hormones lipid (fat-based) hormones (8)
steroids a class of lipids with a structure that is different from other lipids; cholesterol, testosterone, and estrogen are three well-known steroids (2)
stratified epithelia epithelia that have multiple layers of cells (2)
stratum basale the deepest layer of the epidermis (3)
stratum corneum the outer layer of the epidermis (3)
stratum granulosum a layer of somewhat flattened cells lying just superficial to the stratum spinosum and inferior to the stratum lucidum (3)
stratum lucidum the clear layer of thick skin found only on the palms of the hands, fingers, soles of the feet, and toes (3)
stratum spinosum the layer of cells in the epidermis superior to the stratum basale and inferior to the stratum granulosum (3)
stress force distribution inside a structure (1)
stress fracture tiny, painful crack in bone that results from overuse (4)
stroke volume the volume of blood pumped from the heart per beat (11)
subcutaneous fascia the tissue that connects the skin to underlying structures; the hypodermis (3)
submucosa layer of the GI tract just deep to the mucosal layer; composed of irregular dense connective tissue containing blood vessels, lymphatic vessels, and nerves (13)
sudoriferous glands sweat glands that are distributed in the dermis over the entire body (3)
superior vena cava second largest vein in the body that returns deoxygenated blood to the right atrium of the heart from the upper half of the body (11)
supination lateral rotation of the forearm (palm up) (5)
surfactant a phospholipid that reduces the surface tension in the alveoli and prevents them from collapsing (9)
suspensory ligaments tiny structures that attach the lens of the eye to the ciliary body (7)
sutures joints in which irregularly grooved, articulating bone sheets join closely and are tightly connected by fibrous tissues (4)
symphysis type of amphiarthrosis joint in which a thin plate of hyaline cartilage separates a disc of fibrocartilage from the bones (4)
synapse the intersection between a neuron and another neuron, a muscle, a gland, or a sensory receptor (6)
synaptic cleft the tiny gap that separates the axon terminal and muscle fiber (5)
synarthrosis fibrous joint that can absorb shock, but permits little or no movement of the articulating bones (4)
synchondrosis type of amphiarthrosis joint in which the articulating bones are held together by a thin layer of hyaline cartilage (4)
syndesmosis joint at which dense, fibrous tissue binds the bones together, permitting extremely limited movement (4)
synovial fluid a clear liquid secreted by synovial membranes that provides cushioning for and reduces friction in synovial joints (3)
synovial joint a diarthrodial joint (4)
synovial membrane the lining of the synovial joint cavity that produces synovial fluid (3)
systemic circulation circulation of oxygenated blood through the arteries, capillaries, and veins of the circulatory system, from the left ventricle to the right atrium (11)
systole a period of contraction when the chambers are pumping blood out of the heart (11)

T

tachycardia a normal heart rhythm but with a rate above 100 bpm (11)
tarsal bones bones of the ankle (4)
tarsal glands secretors of an oily substance; located in the eyelids (7)
tastants compounds that stimulate the gustatory hairs to send nerve impulses to the brain (7)
taste buds sensory receptors for taste (7)
taste pores very small openings in the top of the taste buds through which gustatory hairs project (7)
temporal lobes the most inferior portions of the brain; responsible for speech, hearing, vision, memory, and emotion (6)
tendinitis inflammation of a tendon, usually accompanied by pain and swelling (5)
tendinosis degeneration of a tendon believed to be caused by microtears in the tendon connective tissue (5)
tendon tissue band composed of collagen and elastic fibers that connects a muscle to a bone (4)

tendon sheaths double-layered synovial structures surrounding tendons subject to friction given their position close to bones; secrete synovial fluid to promote free motion of the tendons during joint movement (4)
tensile strength the ability to withstand tension (outward pulling force) without tearing or breaking (2)
tension a pulling force that creates tension in the structure to which it is applied (1)
tetany a condition of sustained muscular contraction (8)
thalamus the largest portion of the diencephalon; communicates sensory and motor information between the body and the cerebral cortex (6)
thalassemia a condition that affects the body's ability to produce fully developed hemoglobin and red blood cells; Cooley's anemia (10)
third-degree burns burns that destroy the entire thickness of the skin (3)
thoracic cage bony structure surrounding the heart and lungs in the thoracic cavity; composed of the ribs, sternum, and thoracic vertebrae (4)
thoracic cavity the internal opening that houses the heart and lungs (1)
thoracic region the 12 vertebrae in the middle of the back (4)
thoracolumbar branch the sympathetic nerves that lie near the thoracic and lumbar regions of the spine (6)
thymosin hormone produced by the thymus that is essential for the development of white blood cells called T lymphocytes, or T cells (8)
thyroid cartilage the largest cartilaginous plate in the larynx; the Adam's apple (9)
thyroiditis inflammation of the thyroid gland (8)
thyroid-stimulating hormone (TSH) tropic hormone secreted by the anterior pituitary that acts on the thyroid gland to stimulate release of two thyroid hormones, thyroxine (T_4) and triiodothyronine (T_3) (8)
thyroxine (T_4) hormone secreted by the thyroid gland that works with T_3 to control the rate of energy metabolism and heat production in the body; called T_4 because it contains four iodine atoms (8)
tibia major weight-bearing bone of the lower leg (4)
tidal volume (TV) the amount of air inhaled in a normal breath (9)
tinea a fungal infection that tends to occur in areas of the body that are moist (3)
tissues organized groups of similar cells (1)
T lymphocytes (T cells) lymphocytes that complete their maturation in the thymus before they move out to the blood and the rest of the body; also called T cells (12)
tolerance reduction or elimination of the allergic response, which may occur after immunotherapy (12)
tonsillitis inflammation of the tonsils (9)
tonsils clusters of lymphatic tissue in the pharynx that function as the first line of defense against infection (9)
torque the rotary effect of a force (1)
torsion a loading pattern that can cause a structure to twist about its length (1)
total lung capacity (TLC) a combination of the vital capacity plus the residual volume; IRV + TV + ERV + RV (9)
trabecular bone interior, spongy bone with a porous, honeycomb structure (4)
trachea the air tube that extends from the larynx into the thorax, where it splits into the right and left bronchi; the windpipe (9)
transcription the production of RNA from DNA (2)
transfer RNA (tRNA) a molecule that binds to the mRNA-ribosome complex and helps assemble amino acids into polypeptides (2)
transient ischemic attack (TIA) a temporary lack of blood flow to the brain (11)
trans-unsaturated fats one category of unsaturated fatty acids that are artificially produced; also called trans fats (13)
transverse plane an invisible, horizontal flat surface that divides the body into top and bottom halves (1)
traumatic brain injury (TBI) mild or severe trauma that can result from a violent impact to the head (6)
tricuspid valve the valve that closes the orifice between the right atrium and right ventricle of the heart; composed of three cusps (11)
triglycerides compounds composed of a glycerol molecule with three fatty acids attached (2)
trigone the triangular region of the bladder formed by the two ureteric orifices and the internal urethral orifice (14)
triiodothyronine (T_3) hormone secreted by the thyroid gland that works with T_4 to control the rate of energy metabolism and heat production in the body; called T_3 because it contains three iodine atoms (8)
tropic hormones pituitary hormones that act on other endocrine glands; tropins (8)
tuberculosis (TB) a highly contagious bacterial infection caused by Mycobacterium tuberculosis (9)
unica externa the outermost layer of a blood vessel, composed mostly of fibrous connective tissue that supports and protects the vessel (11)
tunica intima the innermost layer of a blood vessel, composed of a single layer of squamous epithelial cells over a sheet of connective tissue; its smooth, frictionless surface allows blood to flow smoothly through the vessel (11)
tunica media the thicker middle layer of a blood vessel that contains smooth muscle cells, elastic fibers, and collagen; its muscle cells are directed by the sympathetic nervous system to increase or decrease blood flow to tissues as needed (11)
tympanic cavity the middle ear (7)
tympanic membrane a sheet of tissue at the end of the auditory canal; also known as the eardrum (7)

U

ulcerative colitis an inflammatory bowel disease that usually affects the colon and the mucosal layer of the intestinal wall (13)
ulna larger bone of the lower arm (4)

ulnar deviation rotation of the hand toward the little finger (5)

umbilical cord the cord that connects the fetus to the placenta (15)

universal donor a person with type O blood; type O blood has no antigens that can be attacked by the host's blood, so it can be donated to anyone (10)

universal recipient a person with type AB blood; type AB blood has neither A nor B antibodies, so a universal recipient can safely receive a transfusion of any blood type (10)

upper extremity bones of the shoulders, arms, and hands (4)

upregulated increased (8)

ureter a duct through which urine travels from the kidney to the bladder (14)

urethra a thin tube that connects the urinary bladder to the outside environment (14)

urinalysis laboratory analysis of urine to test for the presence of infection or disease (14)

urinary bladder a hollow, muscular organ that stores urine (14)

urinary tract infection (UTI) an infection of the urethra, bladder, ureters, and/or kidney, usually caused by bacteria that enter the urethra at its outside opening (14)

urine specific gravity the density (mass per unit volume) of urine, divided by the density of pure water (14)

uterine cycle the monthly cycle of changes that the uterus undergoes; includes the menstrual, proliferative, and secretory phases (15)

uterine fibroids benign tumors of the muscular layer of the uterus (15)

uterine tubes tubes in which the oocyte is fertilized; begin at the lateral end of the ovary and go up and around the ovary to terminate at the top lateral portion of the uterus (15)

uterus a hollow, muscular organ located in front of the rectum and behind the bladder; the womb (15)

V

vagina a thin-walled, tubular structure below the uterus; birth canal (15)

valvular stenosis a narrowing of the heart valve due to stiff or fused valve cusps (11)

vasa recta thin-walled blood vessels that begin and end near the boundary between the renal cortex and the renal medulla, and which extend deep into the renal medulla, running parallel to the nephron loops; play a role in the formation of concentrated urine (14)

vasoconstriction narrowing of the blood vessels, which decreases blood flow (11)

vasodilation widening of the blood vessels, which increases blood flow (11)

veins vessels that carry blood to the heart (11)

ventral ramus anterior spinal nerves that communicate with the muscle and skin of the anterior and lateral trunk (6)

ventricular fibrillation a life-threatening condition in which the heart ventricles quiver at a rate greater than 350 bpm (11)

ventricular tachycardia a life-threatening arrhythmia in which the ventricles, rather than the SA node, initiate the heartbeat; the heart rate is between 150 and 250 bpm, requiring swift medical attention (11)

venules the smallest veins; connect the capillaries with the larger systemic veins (11)

vertebrae the bones making up the spinal column (4)

vestibule a chamber in the inner ear that contains the three semicircular canals (7)

vestibulocochlear nerve a cranial nerve that rises from the cochlear and vestibular nerves (7)

vital capacity (VC) the total amount of air that can be forcibly expired from the lungs after a maximum inspiration (9)

vital signs measurements of pulse and blood pressure (11)

vitamin deficiency the long-term lack of a particular vitamin in a person's diet; may result in health problems (13)

vitamins organic chemicals needed by the body for normal functioning and good health (13)

vitreous humor gel-like substance that fills the posterior chamber of the eye; contributes to intraocular pressure (7)

vomer a plow-shaped bone that comprises most of the bony nasal septum (4)

W

weight force equal to the gravitational acceleration exerted on the mass of an object (1)

Z

zygote a diploid cell produced by the fusion of a sperm with an egg; a fertilized egg (15)

Index

A

B

C

D

E

F

G

H

I

J

K

N

O

P

Q

R

S

T

U

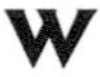